Oxford Textbook of

Heart Failure

Oxford Textbook of
Heart Failure

Edited by
Theresa A. McDonagh
Roy S. Gardner
Andrew L. Clark
Henry J. Dargie

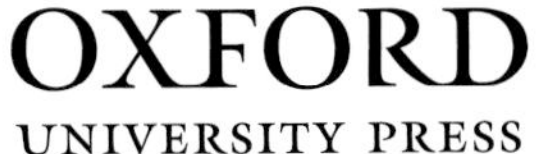

OXFORD
UNIVERSITY PRESS

Great Clarendon Street, Oxford OX2 6DP

Oxford University Press is a department of the University of Oxford.
It furthers the University's objective of excellence in research, scholarship,
and education by publishing worldwide in

Oxford New York

Auckland Cape Town Dar es Salaam Hong Kong Karachi
Kuala Lumpur Madrid Melbourne Mexico City Nairobi
New Delhi Shanghai Taipei Toronto

With offices in

Argentina Austria Brazil Chile Czech Republic France Greece
Guatemala Hungary Italy Japan Poland Portugal Singapore
South Korea Switzerland Thailand Turkey Ukraine Vietnam

Oxford is a registered trade mark of Oxford University Press
in the UK and in certain other countries

Published in the United States
by Oxford University Press Inc., New York

British Library Cataloguing in Publication Data
Data available

Library of Congress Cataloging in Publication Data
Data available

Typeset by Glyph International, Bangalore, India
Printed in China
on acid-free paper through
Asia Pacific Offset

ISBN 978-0-19-957772-9

10 9 8 7 6 5 4 3 2 1

Preface

Medical students in the 1980s and earlier were taught that heart failure was characterised by a miserable prognosis and that there was very little that could be done for patients beyond giving diuretics and preparing for an unavoidably short prognosis. Trainees contemplating a career as an academic cardiologist were warned to avoid the field of heart failure as recently as 1990, as everything was known and the prognosis was still bleak: surely the field of interventional cardiology was a better one to pursue?

We all know now how things have progressed: perhaps more than any other field in cardiology (and, indeed, medicine), the management of patients with heart failure has dramatically changed, fuelled by the quality of evidence-based medicine provided by large randomised controlled treatment trials. Although little perhaps has advanced in acute heart failure, chronic heart failure has become just that: a chronic condition rather than an inevitable death sentence. Those of us who manage patients with chronic heart failure practise with the certainty of a large evidence-base informing much of what we do, from arriving at the original diagnosis, through medical and device therapy, to general strategies of care. We know that what we do approximately doubles life-expectancy for patients.

Heart failure is a condition touching the lives of many, from basic scientists, to physicians in emergency rooms, to nurses running home care services. The requirements for a good heart failure service range from the relatively inexpensive use of pharmacological agents through well-structured diagnostic, treatment, and monitoring programmes, to expensive interventions such as implantable cardioverter-defibrillators, left ventricular assist devices, and even transplantation.

We hope that this book will have something to offer all those managing the range of patients with heart failure. A particular concern has been to offer chapters on the comorbidities patients suffer: most patients in clinical trials are a decade or so younger and have far fewer comorbidites than patients with heart failure in the typical clinic. We have tried to cover the whole spectrum of management through the whole clinical course of heart failure, and hope in so doing that this is a book that many will find useful as a reference point, but also as a practical guide in how to manage our patients.

Acknowledgements

Most importantly, we would like to thank all those colleagues who have taken on the responsibility of writing chapters for the book. We know it has been an added burden in already very full lives, and are grateful for their efforts in making the book a success. We have also been greatly supported by the staff at Oxford University Press, to whom we are indebted.

Contents

PART VI
The diagnosis of heart failure

PART VII
Noninvasive investigation

PART VIII
Invasive investigation

PART IX
Prognostication

PART X
Comorbidities: the patients with heart failure and . . .

PART XI
Medical therapy for chronic heart failure

PART XII
Medical therapy for acute heart failure

PART XIII
Nonpharmacological management

PART XIV
Device therapy for heart failure

PART XV
Surgical therapy for heart failure

PART XVI
Ventilatory strategies in heart failure

PART XVII
Disease management

PART XVIII
Future therapies

List of contributors

Stamatis Adamopoulos Second Department of Cardiology, Onassis Cardiac Surgery Centre, Athens, Greece

Nicholas R. Banner Consultant in Cardiology, Transplant Medicine and Circulatory Support, Harefield Hospital, Middlesex, UK; and National Heart and Lung Institute, Imperial College London, UK

Jeroen J. Bax Leiden University Medical Center, Leiden, The Netherlands

Pushan Bharadwaj Consultant in Nuclear Medicine, Raigmore Hospital,Inverness, UK

Emma J. Birks Professor of Medicine, Medical Director of Heart Failure, Transplantation and Mechanical Support, University of Louisville, Kentucky, USA

Lynda Blue British Heart Foundation, Healthcare Professionals Project Manager, London, UK

Margaret M. Burke Consultant Histopathologist, The Royal Brompton and Harefield NHS Foundation Trust, Harefield Hospital, Middlesex, UK

Badrinathan Chandrasekaran Clinical Fellow, Wessex Cardiothoracic Centre, Southampton General Hospital, Southampton UK

Raj K. Chelliah Department of Cardiology, Hull & York Medical School, University of Hull, UK

Andrew L. Clark Professor and Honorary Consultant Cardiologist, Academic Department of Cardiology, Hull &York Medical School, University of Hull, UK

John G.F. Cleland Professor of Cardiology, Academic Department of Cardiology, Hull & York Medical School, University of Hull, UK

Andrew J.S. Coats Deputy Vice-Chancellor, Faculty of Medicine, The University of Sydney, Australia

Alison P. Coletta Castle Hill Hospital, Castle Road, Cottingham, UK

Derek T. Connelly Consultant Cardiologist, Glasgow Royal Infirmary, UK

Tamera J. Corte Royal Brompton Hospital, National Heart and Lung Institute, London, UK

Peter J. Cowburn Consultant Cardiologist, Wessex Cardiothoracic Centre, Southampton General Hospital, Southampton, UK

Martin R. Cowie Professor of Cardiology, Imperial College London; and Honorary Consultant Cardiologist, Royal Brompton Hospital, London

Henry J. Dargie Consultant Cardiologist, Golden Jubilee National Hospital, Glasgow, UK

Martin Denvir Senior Lecturer and Honorary Consultant Cardiologist, Centre for Cardiovascular Science, University of Edinburgh and Royal Infirmary of Edinburgh, UK

Gregory Ducroq Service de Cardiologie, Groupe Hospitalier Bichat, Paris, France

Alison Duncan Department of Echocardiography, The Royal Brompton Hospital, London, UK

Perry M. Elliott The Heart Hospital, London, UK

Desmond Fitzgerald UCD Conway Institute, Dublin, Ireland

Stephen J. Fuller Research Fellow, Institute for Cardiovascular and Metabolic Research, School of Biological Sciences, University of Reading, UK

Roy S. Gardner Consultant Cardiologist, Scottish Advanced Heart Failure Service, Golden Jubilee National Hospital, Glasgow, UK

Panagiota Georgiadou Second Department of Cardiology, Onassis Cardiac Surgery Centre, Athens, Greece

Darren Green Clinical Research Fellow, University of Manchester, Salford Royal Hospital, UK

Mike Greenstone Hull & York Medical School, University of Hull, UK

Kaushik Guha Imperial College London, UK

Sian Harding, Professor of Cardiac Pharmacology, Imperial College London, UK

Suzanna Hardman Consultant Cardiologist with an Interest in Community Cardiology, Clinical & Academic Department of Cardiovascular Medicine, Whittington Hospital, London, UK and Honorary Senior Lecturer University College London

Simon P. Hart Hull & York Medical School, University of Hull, UK

Nathaniel M. Hawkins Liverpool Heart and Chest Hospital, Liverpool, UK

Bernard Iung Service de Cardiologie, Groupe Hospitalier Bichat, Paris, France

Colette E. Jackson BHF Cardiovascular Research Centre, University of Glasgow, UK

Andrew Jamieson Honorary Senior Clincal Lecturer, University of Glasgow, UK

Miriam Johnson Hull & York Medical School, University of Hull; St Catherine's Hospice, Scarborough, UK

Philip A. Kalra Consultant and Honorary Professor in Nephrology, Salford Royal Hospital and University of Manchester, UK

Andre Keren The Heart Institute, Hadassah University Hospital, Jerusalem, Israel

Stanley H. Korman Department of Genetics and Metabolic Diseases, Hadassah - Hebrew University Medical Center, Jerusalem, Israel

Giuseppe Limongelli Department of Cardiology, Monaldi Hospital, Second University of Naples, Naples, Italy

Alexander Lyon Walport Clinical Lecturer in Cardiology, Imperial College London, UK

Theresa A. McDonagh Consultant Cardiologist, King's College Hospital, London, UK

Anne McEntegart Consultant Rheumatologist, Stobhill Hospital, Glasgow, UK

John J.V. McMurray Western Infirmary, Glasgow and University of Glasgow, UK

Alexandre Mebazaa University Paris 7, Hopital Lariboisiere, Paris, France

Mhamed Mebazaa Emergency Room, Hôpital Monji Slim, La Marsa, Tunisia

Yvonne Millerick Lead Nurse/Senior Lecturer, Caring Together Heart Failure Palliative Care Programme, Glasgow Caledonian University, Glasgow, UK

Andrew Murday Consultant Cardiac Surgeon, West of Scotland Heart and Lung Centre, Golden Jubilee National Hospital, Glasgow, UK

Rachel C. Myles Clinical Lecturer in Cardiology, University of Glasgow, UK

Ashley M. Nisbet Specialist Registrar in Cardiology, NHS Greater Glasgow & Clyde, UK

C. Parsai Cardiovascular Magnetic Resonance Unit, Royal Brompton and Harefield NHS Trust, London, UK

John R. Pepper Consultant Cardiothoracic Surgeon, The Royal Brompton Hospital, London, UK

Susanna Price Consultant Cardiologist and Intensivist, The Royal Brompton Hospital, London, UK

Massimo F. Piepoli Consultant Cardiologist, Heart Failure Unit, Cardiology Department, G. da Saliceto Hospital, Piacenza, Italy

S.K. Prasad Consultant Cardiologist, The Royal Brompton Hospital, London, UK

Sushma Rekhraj Cardiovascular Clinical Research Fellow, Ninewells Hospital and Medical School, Dundee, UK

Jillian P. Riley Head of Postgraduate Education (Nursing and Allied Professions), Royal Brompton & Harefield NHS Foundation Trust; Course Director, MSc Cardio-respiratory Nursing, Imperial College, London

Joanne D. Schuijf Department of Cardiology, Leiden University Medical Center, Leiden, The Netherlands

Andre R. Simon Consultant Cardiac Surgeon and Director of Transplantation, The Royal Brompton and Harefield NHS Foundation Trust, Harefield Hospital, Middlesex, UK; and National Heart and Lung Institute, Imperial College, Dovehouse Street, London, UK

Anita K. Simonds Consultant in Respiratory Medicine, The Royal Brompton Hospital. London, UK

Mark S. Slaughter Professor and Chief, Division Cardiothoracic Surgery and Surgical Director Heart Failure, Transplantation and Mechanical Support, University of Louisville, USA

Godfrey L. Smith Professor of Cardiovascular Physiology, Integrative & Systems Biology, University of Glasgow, UK

Iain Squire Professor of Cardiovascular Medicine, Department of Cardiovascular Sciences, University of Leicester, UK

Allan Struthers Department of Clinical Pharmacology and Therapeutics, Ninewells Hospital and Medical School, Dundee, UK

Peter H. Sugden Professor in Biomedical Sciences, Institute for Cardiovascular and Metabolic Research, School of Biological Sciences, University of Reading, Reading, UK

Lorna Swan Consultant Cardiologist, The Royal Brompton Hospital, London, UK

Benjamin R. Szwejkowski Cardiovascular Clinical Research Fellow, Ninewells Hospital and Medical School, Dundee, UK

Laurens F. Tops Department of Cardiology, Leiden University Medical Center, Leiden, The Netherlands

Azam Torabi Department of Cardiology, Hull & York Medical School, University of Hull, UK

Shahana Uddin Consultant Intensivist, Kings's College Hospital, London, UK

S. Richard Underwood Professor of Cardiac Imaging, The Royal Brompton Hospital, London, UK

Alec Vahanian Groupe Hospitalier Bichat, Rue Henri-Huchard, Paris, France

Peter van der Meer Department of Cardiology, University Medical Center Groningen, The Netherlands

Dirk J. van Veldhuisen Department of Cardiology, University Medical Center Groningen, Groningen, The Netherlands

Ali Vazir Specialist Training Registrar, Clinical & Academic Department of Cardiovascular Medicine, Whittington Hospital, London UK

Vassilios Voudris Second Department of Cardiology, Onassis Cardiac Surgery Centre, Athens, Greece

Nicola L. Walker Consultant Cardiologist, Golden Jubilee National Hospital, Glasgow, UK

Klaus K. Witte Senior Lecturer and Honorary Consultant Cardiologist, University of Leeds and Leeds General Infirmary, UK

S.J. Wort National Heart and Lung Institute, Imperial College London, UK

Jufen Zhang Department of Cardiology, Hull & York Medical School, University of Hull, UK

List of abbreviations

AA	aldosterone antagonist
ACE	angiotensin converting enzyme
ACEi	angiotensin converting enzyme inhibitor
ACHD	adult congenital heart disease
ACR	acute cellular rejection
ACS	acute coronary syndrome
ACTH	adrenocorticotrophic hormone
ACTIV	acute and chronic therapeutic impact of a vasopressin antagonist
ADH	anti-diuretic hormone
AF	atrial fibrillation
AHA	American Heart Association
AHeFT	American Heart Failure Trial
AHF	acute heart failure
AIF	apoptosis inducing factor
AIV	anterior interventricular vein
AKI	acute kidney injury
ALS	advanced life support
AMI	acute myocardial infarction
AMPK	AMP-activated protein kinase
AMR	antibody-mediated rejection
ANP	atrial natriuretic peptide
AP	action potential
APD	action potential duration
APT	amiodarone pulmonary toxicity
AR	aortic regurgitation
ARB	angiotensin receptor blocker
ARVC	arrhythmogenic right ventricular cardiomyopathy
ARVD	atherosclerotic renovascular disease
AS	aortic stenosis
ASD	atrial septal defects
ASTRAL	Angioplasty and Stenting for Renal Artery Lesions
AT	anaerobic threshold
ATLAS	Assessment of Treatment with Lisinopril and Survival
AUC	area under the curve
AV	aortic valve; atrioventricular
AVID	Antiarrhythmics Versus Implantable Defibrillator
AVP	arginine vasopressin
BB	β-blocker
BiPAP	bilevel positive airway pressure
BIPS	Bezafibrate Infarction Prevention Study
BMI	body mass index
BNP	B-type natriuretic peptide
BSA	body surface area
CABG	coronary artery bypass grafting
CACT	carnitine/acylcarnitine translocase
CAD	coronary artery disease
CAM	cell adhesion molecules
CASH	Cardiac Arrest Study of Hamburg
CAV	cardiac allograft vasculopathy
CCTGA	congenitally corrected transposition of the great arteries
CDG	congenital disorders of glycosylation
CHD	coronary heart disease
CHF	chronic heart failure
CHO	Chinese hamster ovary
CHS	Cardiovascular Health Study
CI	cardiac index
CIDS	Canadian Implantable Defibrillator Study
CK	creatine kinase
CKD	chronic kidney disease
CMR	cardiac magnetic resonance
CNP	C-type natriuretic peptide
CNS	central nervous system
CO	cardiac output
COMET	Carvedilol Or Metoprolol European Trial
CONSENSUS	Cooperative North Scandinavian Enalapril Survival Study
COPD	chronic obstructive pulmonary disease
CPAP	continuous positive airway pressure
CPET	cardiopulmonary metabolic exercise testing
CPG	Committee for Practice Guideline
CPR	cardiopulmonary resuscitation
CR	cardiac rehabilitation
CRP	C-reactive protein
CRT	cardiac resynchronization therapy
CS	coronary sinus
CSA	central sleep apnoea
CSD	cardiac support device
CVC	central venous cannulation
CVP	central venous pressure
DCCT	Diabetes Control and Complications Trial
DCM	dilated cardiomyopathy
DCT	distal convoluted tubule
DEFINITE	Defibrillators in Non-Ischemic Cardiomyopathy Treatment Evaluation
DFT	diastolic filling time
DIABHYCAR	Type 2 DIABetes, Hypertension, Cardiovascular, Events and Ramipril study
DINAMIT	Defibrillator in Acute Myocardial Infarction Trial
DM	diabetes mellitus
DMARD	disease-modifying antirheumatic drugs
DVT	deep venous thrombosis
EARTH	Endothelin A Receptor Antagonist Trial in Heart

EBCT	electron beam CT
ECHOES	Echocardiographic Heart of England Screening Study
EDV	end-diastolic volume
EF	ejection fraction
ELISA	enzyme-linked immunosorbent assay
ELITE	Evaluation of Losartan in The Elderly
EPC	endothelial progenitor cells
EPHESUS	Eplerenone Post-acute MI Heart failure Efficacy and Survival Study
ER	endoplasmic reticulum
ERO	effective regurgitant orifice
ERS	European Respiratory Society
ERT	enzyme replacement therapy
ESA	erythropoiesis-stimulating agents
ESC	European Society of Cardiology
ESICM	European Society of Intensive Care Medicine
ESR	erythrocyte sedimentation rate
ESS	Epworth sleepiness score
ESV	end-systolic volume
ETF	electron transfer flavoprotein
ETF	electron transfer flavoprotein
EVEREST	efficacy of vasopressin antagonism in decompensated heart failure
FADD	Fas-associated death domain
FAOD	fatty acid oxidation disorders
FBC	full blood count
FDA	Food and Drug Administration
FDG	fluoro-D-glucose
FGF	fibroblast growth factor
FMR	functional mitral regurgitation
FRC	functional residual capacity
FVC	forced vital capacity
GCV	great cardiac vein
GFR	glomerular filtration rate
GJ	gap junctions
GPRD	General Practice Research Database
GSD	glycogen storage disorders
GSF	Gold Standards Framework
HAART	highly active antiretroviral therapy
HASTE	half-Fourier acquisition single-shot turbo spin-echo
HBI	home-based intervention
HEAAL	Heart failure Endpoint evaluation of Angiotensin II Antagonist Losartan
HeFNEF	heart failure with normal (preserved) ejection fraction
HELLP	haemolysis, elevated liver enzymes, low platelets
HF	heart failure
HFNS	heart failure nurse specialists
HFSA	Heart Failure Society of America
HFSS	Heart Failure Survival Score
HH	hereditary haemochromatosis
HLA	human leucocyte antigen
HLS	hypoplastic left heart syndrome
HMR	heart to mediastinal ratio
HOT	Hypertension Optimal Treatment Study
HRQL	health-related quality of life
HSCT	haematopoietic stem cell transplantation
IABP	intra-aortic balloon pump
ICD	implantable cardioverter defibrillator
ICU	intensive care unit
IDCM	idiopathic dilated cardiomyopathy
IE	infective endocarditis
IHD	ischaemic heart disease
INR	international normalized ratio
IPF	idiopathic pulmonary fibrosis
IRIS	Immediate Risk Stratification Improves Survival
ISHLT	International Society of Heart and Lung Transplantation
IVC	inferior vena cava
JVP	jugular venous pressure
KCCQ	Kansas City Cardiomyopathy Questionnaire
LBBB	left bundle branch block
LCFA	long-chain fatty acids
LCHAD	long-chain hydratase and hydroxyacyl-CoA dehydrogenase
LGE	late gadolinium enhancement
LHON	Leber hereditary optic neuropathy
LTOT	long-term oxygen therapy
LV	left ventricle/left ventricular
LVAD	left ventricular assist device
LVD	left ventricular dysfunction
LVDD	left ventricular diastolic dysfunction
LVEDP	left ventricular end-diastolic pressure
LVEF	left ventricular ejection fraction
LVESV	left ventricular end-systolic volumes
LVESVI	left ventricular end-systolic volume index
LVH	left ventricular hypertrophy
LVMI	left ventricular mass index
LVSD	left ventricular systolic dysfunction
MAD	multiple acyl-CoA dehydrogenases
MADIT	Multicenter Automatic Defibrillator Trial
MDC	Metoprolol in Dilated Cardiomyopathy
MDCT	multidetector row CT
MDRD	Modification of Diet in Renal Disease
MELAS	mitochondrial encephalomyopathy with lactic acidosis and stroke-like episodes
METEOR	Multicentre Evaluation of Tolvaptan Effect on Remodelling
MI	myocardial infarction
MIBI	methoxyisobutylisonitrile
MLHFQ	Minnesota Living with Heart Failure Questionnaire
MLP	muscle LIM protein
MPS	myocardial perfusion scintigraphy
MS	mitral stenosis
MSNA	muscle sympathetic nerve activity
MTP	mitochondrial trifunctional protein
MUGA	multiple gated acquisition
MUSTT	Multicenter UnSustained Tachycardia Trial
MVV	maximum voluntary ventilation
NAD	nicotinamide adenine dinucleotide
NFAT	nuclear factor of activated T-cells
NHLBI	National Heart, Lung and Blood Institute
NHYA	New York Heart Association
NNH	number needed to harm
NP	natriuretic peptides
NPR	natriuretic peptide receptor
NPV	negative predictive value
NRF	nuclear respiratory factors
NSAID	nonsteroidal anti-inflammatory drug
NYHA	New York Heart Association
OMT	optimal medical therapy
OSA	obstructive sleep apnoea
PAC	pulmonary artery catheter
PAFC	pulmonary artery flotation catheter
PAH	pulmonary arterial hypertension
PCI	percutaneous coronary intervention
PCR	polymerase chain reaction
PCWP	pulmonary capillary wedge pressure
PD	peritoneal dialysis
PDGF	platelet-derived growth factor
PEA	pulseless electrical activity
PEEP	positive end-expiratory pressure
PEF	peak expiratory flow
PET	positron emission tomography
PH	pulmonary hypertension
PIV	posterior interventricular vein
PLE	protein-losing enteropathy
PMC	percutaneous mitral commissurotomy

PND	paroxysmal nocturnal dyspnoea
PPAR	peroxisomal proliferator-activated receptor
PSA	prostate specific antigen
PSIR	phase-sensitive inversion recovery
PTLD	post-transplant lymphoproliferative disease
PVAD	paracorporeal ventricular assist device
PVI	pulmonary vein isolation
PVLV	posterior vein of the left ventricle
PVR	pulmonary vascular resistance
PWV	pulse wave velocity
QALY	quality-adjusted life year
QoL	quality of life
RA	rheumatoid arthritis; right atrium/atrial
RAAS	renin–angiotensin–aldosterone system
RALES	Randomized Aldactone Evaluation Study
RANKL	RANK ligand
RANTES	regulated upon activation, normal T cell expressed and secreted
RAS	renal artery stenosis
RBBB	right bundle branch block
RCT	randomized controlled trial
RDI	respiratory disturbance index
RDW	red cell distribution width
REM	rapid eye movement
RESOLVD	Randomized Evaluation of Strategies for Left Ventricular Dysfunction
RHC	right heart catheterization
RNVG	radionuclide ventriculography
ROC	receiver operating curve
ROS	reactive oxygen species
RQ	respiratory quotient
RR	relative risk
RRR	relative risk reduction
RRT	renal replacement therapy
RV	right ventricle/ventricular
RVEDP	right ventricular end diastolic pressure
RWMA	regional wall motion abnormalities
RXR	retinoid X receptors
SAVE	Survival and Ventricular Enlargement
SCD	sudden cardiac death
SCDHeFT	Sudden Cardiac Death in Heart Failure Trial
SDB	sleep-disordered breathing
SHF	systolic heart failure
SHFM	Seattle Heart Failure Model
SICM	scanning ion-conductance microscopy
SIGN	Scottish Intercollegiate Guidelines Network
SLE	systemic lupus erythematosus
SOLVD	Studies of Left Ventricular Dysfunction
SoV	sinus of Valsalva
SPECT	single photon emission CT
SPICE	Study of Patients Intolerant of Converting Enzyme
SR	sarcoplasmic reticulum; sinus rhythm
SSFP	steady-state free precession
STICH	Surgical Treatment for Ischemic Heart
STIR	short-tau inversion recovery
SU	sulphonylurea drug
SVC	superior vena cava
SVR	systemic vascular resistance
TAPSE	tricuspid annular plane systolic excursion
TARA	Trial of Atorvastatin in Rheumatoid Arthritis
TAT	transverse-axial tubular
TAVI	transcatheter aortic valve implantation
TCA	tricarboxylic acid
TDI	tissue Doppler imaging
TGF	transforming growth factor
TLC	total lung capacity
TLR	Toll-like receptors
TMS	tandem mass spectrometry
TNF	tumour necrosis factor
TOE	transoesophageal echocardiogram
TOR	target of rapamycin
TR	tricuspid regurgitation
TREAT	Trial to Reduce Cardiovascular Events with Aranesp Therapy
TS	tricuspid stenosis
TSE	turbo-spin echo
TTC	triphenyltetrazolium chloride
TZD	thiazolidenedione drug (glitazone)
UA	unstable angina
UGDP	Universities Group Diabetes Project
UKPDS	United Kingdom Prospective Diabetes Survey
UPR	unfolded protein response
VAD	ventricular assist device
VC	vital capacity
VE	minute ventilation
VEGF	vascular endothelial growth factor
VF	ventricular fibrillation
VHD	valvular heart disease
VHeFT	Vasodilator Heart Failure Trial
VPB	ventricular premature beats
VRS	ventricular restoration surgery
VSD	ventricular septal defect; ventricular systolic dysfunction
VT	ventricular tachyarrhythmia; ventricular tachycardia
VTI	velocity time integral
WASH	Warfarin-Aspirin Study in Heart
WCC	white cell count
WRF	worsening renal function

PART I

What is heart failure?

1

What is heart failure?

Andrew L. Clark

It is a commonplace in writings about heart failure (HF) that it has become an 'epidemic' in Western societies in particular. In truth, the incidence of HF is not rising, but the prevalence is. HF is thus not a true epidemic, which properly is a rise in the age-specific incidence. The major causes for its increasing prevalence are threefold: although the incidence of acute myocardial infarction may be falling, more patients survive acute coronary disease and go on to develop chronic HF; treatment of chronic HF has dramatically improved, and so many more patients survive for much longer; and the population generally is ageing—and HF is a disease of older people.

Although HF is a modern blight, it has been known for thousands of years. There is some suggestion from the Ebers papyrus (dated around 1500 BCE) that the ancient Egyptians recognized it ('When there is inundation of the heart, the saliva is in excess, and therefore the body is weak'), and Hippocrates (460–370 BCE) gave a much quoted description of cardiac cachexia: 'The flesh is consumed and becomes water … the abdomen fills with water; the feet and legs swell; the shoulders, clavicles, chest, and thigh melt away.'[1]

It was not until after Harvey described the circulation of the blood that the HF syndrome truly began to be related to the heart, with Richard Lower perhaps giving the first textbook discussion of HF in 1669.[2] Treatment for HF with venesection, perhaps one of the few instances in which the procedure might be helpful, was formally described in 1696.[3] William Withering described the formal use of *Digitalis* extracts, giving birth to clinical pharmacology,[4] although cardiac glycosides had undoubtedly been used for hundreds, and perhaps thousands,[5] of years previously.

The modern era of HF treatment truly began with the discovery of mercurial,[6] and then thiazide and subsequently loop, diuretics in the late 1950s and early 1960s. Perhaps the most important single trial in HF therapy demonstrating the beneficial effects of angiotensin converting enzyme (ACE) inhibitors was published in 1987.[7]

Definition of heart failure

Neither the epidemiology of a condition not its treatment can properly be understood unless properly defined. The term 'heart failure' is usually used freely between clinicians to describe what is wrong with individual patients, yet despite the fact that HF is so very common, it is very difficult to define it satisfactorily (Box 1.1).[8] Some difficulties arise because of the effects of modern treatment: although it may be reasonable to define acute HF in terms of some haemodynamic variable, the situation becomes very different in chronic treated HF.

Older general definitions of HF centred on haemodynamic changes, and were phrased in terms of inadequacy of cardiac output in response to normal filling pressure of the heart, with the inadequacy of the output thought of in terms of being inadequate to meet the requirements of the metabolizing tissues.[9] These sorts of definition are of some value in thinking about the pathophysiology of patients being admitted acutely with salt and water retention or pulmonary oedema, but less so in thinking about patients with chronic HF.

Patients with chronic HF, particularly when adequately treated, have normal resting cardiac output and normal left ventricular filling pressure. Their metabolizing tissues are well enough perfused that they are usually asymptomatic at rest: chronic treated HF is a condition of exercise limitation. Even so, for many patients, cardiac output and oxygen consumption go up as normal during modest exercise, only falling below normal towards peak exercise.

Ultimately, HF is a clinical syndrome characterized by a constellation of symptoms and signs, and not a discrete diagnosis. Much epidemiological work has defined HF in terms of those symptoms and signs, but simply defining the syndrome by its symptoms and signs may mistakenly include many patients without cardiac pathology.[10,11] The situation is even worse if simply considering *treatment* for HF as being adequate to define the presence of HF in epidemiological studies: such an approach may lead to gross overdiagnosis.[12]

The key combination is to recognize that HF is accompanied by a recognizable constellation of symptoms and signs, coupled with objective evidence that there is an abnormality of the heart consistent with the diagnosis. This is the line now taken by the European Society of Cardiology,[13] with the added clause that in doubtful cases, a response to treatment directed at HF sustains the diagnosis.

Box 1.1 Some definitions of heart failure

A condition in which the heart fails to discharge its contents adequately.

Thomas Lewis, 1933

A state in which the heart fails to maintain an adequate circulation for the needs of the body despite a satisfactory filling pressure.

Paul Wood, 1950

A pathophysiological state in which an abnormality of cardiac function is responsible for the failure of the heart to pump blood at a rate commensurate with the requirements of the metabolising tissues.

Eugene Braunwald, 1980

The state of any heart disease in which, despite adequate ventricular filling, the heart's output is decreased or in which the heart is unable to pump blood at a rate adequate for satisfying the requirements of the tissues with function parameters remaining within normal limits.

H. Denolin *et al.*, 1983

A clinical syndrome caused by an abnormality of the heart and recognised by a characteristic pattern of haemodynamic, renal, neural and hormonal responses.

Philip Poole-Wilson, 1985

... syndrome ... which arises when the heart is chronically unable to maintain an appropriate blood pressure without support.

Peter Harris, 1987

A syndrome in which cardiac dysfunction is associated with reduced exercise tolerance, a high incidence of ventricular arrhythmias and a shortened life expectancy.

Jay Cohn, 1988

... a complex clinical syndrome that can result from any structural or functional cardiac disorder that impairs the ability of the ventricle to fill with or eject blood.

ACC and AHA Task Force on Practice Guidelines. 2009 Focused Update Incorporated into the ACC/AHA 2005 Guidelines for the Diagnosis and Management of Heart Failure in Adults. *Circulation* 2009;**119:**e391–e479

A syndrome in which the patients should have the following features: symptoms of HF, typically shortness of breath at rest or during exertion, and/or fatigue; signs of fluid retention such as pulmonary congestion or ankle swelling, and objective evidence of an abnormality of the structure or function of the heart at rest.

The Task Force for the Diagnosis and Treatment of Acute and Chronic Heart Failure 2008 of the European Society of Cardiology. (*European Heart Journal* 2008;**29:**2388–2442)

Adapted from Poole-Wilson PA. History, definition and classification of heart failure. In Poole-Wilson, Colucci WS, Massie BM, Chatterjee K, Coast AJS (eds) *Heart failure*. Churchill Livingstone, New York, 1997, p. 270.

Such an approach is pragmatic, at least, and is rooted in clinical life. Some problems do arise in borderline cases. In an elderly patient, for example, breathlessness is a very common symptom, and peripheral oedema is a very common physical sign: if an echocardiogram shows left ventricular hypertrophy, can the patient truly be defined as having HF? The missing part of the equation is some objective test, independent of cardiac imaging, which allows the clinician to be sure that the cardiac abnormality is the cause of the patient's symptoms.

The natriuretic peptides may offer at least a partial solution in this regard. These hormones and their derivatives, released from the heart in response to cardiac stretch, should be raised in patients with HF. The next step in defining HF is likely to include natriuretic peptide level. In an untreated patient, if the natriuretic peptide level is normal, then there will be an alternative cause for the patient's symptoms.

Heart failure as an evolutionary disease

Why does HF present clinically as it does? This seems an odd question, as clinicians are so familiar with the clinical syndrome, but it is not immediately obvious why a patient whose heart function declines should start to retain fluid and develop neurohormonal activation. Harris emphasized the importance of blood pressure in the evolution of terrestrial animals.[14] In order to perfuse a large body unsupported by water; in order to allow rapid movement of that body; and in order to excrete the high level of waste products incurred by having a large, rapidly moving body, high blood pressure is fundamental—certainly compared with the blood pressure needed to service a fish.

An array of very powerful defensive mechanisms has evolved to maintain that high blood pressure at more-or-less all costs. The responses of the body to a fall in blood pressure induced by, say, haemorrhage, are very similar to those induced by HF. Vasoconstriction, salt and water retention and neurohormonal activation are the responses to both conditions. The clinical pattern of HF can thus be viewed as a consequence of mammalian evolution and the vital importance of maintaining high blood pressure.

Descriptions of heart failure

Older textbooks of cardiology abound in paired descriptions of HF: forward versus backward; right versus left; high versus low output; systolic versus diastolic; acute versus chronic. Some of the terms are now largely redundant but are worth considering in brief.

Forward HF refers to the notion that there is primarily failure of forward pump function leading to inadequate perfusion of peripheral tissues, particularly skeletal muscle, causing fatigue and exercise intolerance. Conversely, backward failure is thought to arise from the need to maintain cardiac output via increased left ventricular filling pressure, which results in left atrial hypertension and thus lung congestion and breathlessness.

Right HF suggest that the HF is predominantly due to failure of the right ventricle with consequent systemic venous congestion and 'backward' failure, whereas left HF leads to pulmonary venous hypertension and pulmonary oedema together with the consequences of reduced pump function. Such a classification is not very helpful: the commonest cause of right HF is left HF, and the two rarely occur as separate entities.

High-output cardiac failure is a rarity caused by excessive vasodilation together with salt and water retention; it should not be thought of as being primarily a cardiac condition. It is more correctly thought of as circulatory failure. Diastolic versus systolic HF remains a controversial distinction: some investigators report that up to half of patients with HF have impaired ventricular relaxation as their primary pathophysiological problem. In consequence, there is decreased stroke volume and the syndrome of HF. The implication is that had the heart been able to fill more completely, then there would be no HF.

The distinction between acute and chronic HF is clinically helpful, as long as the terms are understood correctly. The word 'acute' is often taken, wrongly, to mean 'severe', and should be used to mean 'presenting suddenly'. In very broad-brush terms, acute HF refers to patients presenting as emergencies to hospital, usually with either pulmonary oedema or with fluid retention. Such patients are often presenting for the first time, but may be patients having an exacerbation of their chronic, previously stable, HF. They have acutely abnormal haemodynamics.

In contrast, most patients with chronic HF have been treated medically and will usually have few if any symptoms or signs at rest. The term 'congestive' HF, often used to describe patients in this condition (particularly in North America), is inappropriate: patients with treated chronic HF should not be congested.[15]

Clinical course of heart failure

The prognosis of both acute and chronic HF is bleak, although improved dramatically by modern therapy, with an average life expectancy from diagnosis of around 3 years (depending on the population studied),[16] and a prognosis worse than for many kinds of cancer.[17] Such statistics disguise the fact that for the individual patient, the course of HF can be highly variable, and is much less predictable than the course of other malignant diseases (Fig. 1.1).

The initial presentation of HF is usually acute. The commonest cause of HF is coronary heart disease, and so an acute myocardial infarction is a common initial precipitant. With treatment, a number of outcomes is then possible: the patient might return to normal with impaired left ventricular function; the patient might reach a plateau of impaired function; or the patient might decline relentlessly toward death or transplantation.

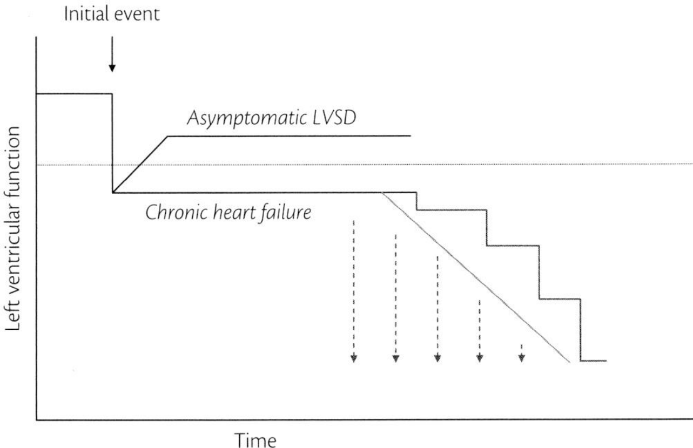

Fig. 1.1 Possible trajectories of heart failure. Following an initial heart failure event, a patient might recover to be left with asymptomatic left ventricular dysfunction, or settle into a state of chronic heart failure. As time passes, left ventricular function tends to decline further, either gradually, or in a stepwise manner. At any time, sudden death may occur.

Following an initial event and recovery or stabilization, a patient may continue unchanged for several years, or may have repeated episodes of decompensation of chronic HF. Each time, it is less likely that there will be complete recovery of the myocardium, and progressively left ventricular function worsens in a stuttering, stepwise course. As a general rule, such a trajectory often follows the pattern of a flat stone skimming across water: decompensation episodes become longer and the intervals between episodes shorten.

For some patients, the decline in left ventricular function is more gradual than punctuated: in this scenario, a patient may enter a 'vicious cycle' of decline (see below). An alarming feature of HF is that at any time in its clinical course, patients are at risk of sudden death.

A less common way for HF to present is with a less abrupt onset and gradually progressive symptoms of breathlessness, fatigue and peripheral oedema. The typical patient presenting this way may have had a remote myocardial infarct or have underlying valvular heart disease or dilated cardiomyopathy. Such a patient will usually present through primary care, and the diagnosis can be delayed in consequence—the range of causes of breathlessness is very broad.

Occasional patients appear completely to recover from an episode of HF. Such a recovery may happen in patients with a discrete episode of illness, such as acute myocarditis or postpartum cardiomyopathy. Some patients with dilated cardiomyopathy may apparently return to having normal left ventricular systolic function with medical therapy, and it can be difficult to judge in such circumstances whether medication should stop or continue indefinitely.[18]

Models of progression

Much of the thinking about the clinical course of HF has focused on potential vicious circles of decline (better thought of as spirals—the starting point is not regained). With all of the potential spirals, an abnormality induced by HF results in further deterioration in heart function, thereby worsening the HF. These models are helpful in thinking about the pathophysiology of HF, and in suggesting avenues for therapeutic development.

Haemodynamic model

The haemodynamic model of HF decline is the traditional way of looking at the pathophysiology of HF (Fig. 1.2). Initial damage to the heart is detected by body systems (particularly via a fall in blood pressure and in renal perfusion) and causes consequent haemodynamic changes to maintain tissue perfusion. Salt and water retention help to maintain output via the Frank–Starling relation by increasing preload; and vasoconstriction maintains blood pressure, but at a cost of increasing afterload. The increases in preload and afterload, however, exacerbate the heart's problems, leading to further decline.

Treatments based on the haemodynamic understanding of HF have not proved very successful: positive inotropic drugs have almost uniformly proved unsuccessful, and abrupt changes in haemodynamics (as with vasodilators or even heart transplantation) do not lead to immediate improvements in exercise function.

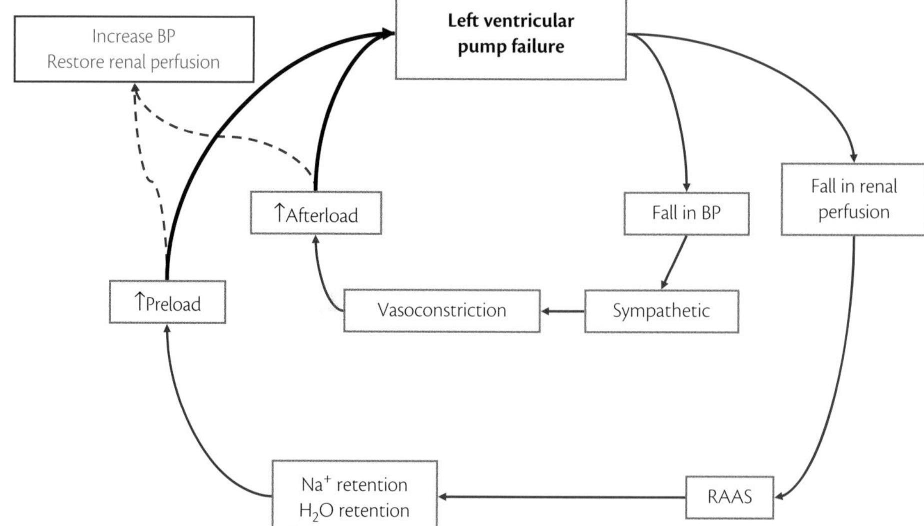

Fig. 1.2 The traditional haemodynamic model of heart failure. Initial ventricular damage leads to haemodynamic responses that tend to preserve blood pressure and renal function (blue arrows), but at a cost of increasing preload and afterload and thereby feeding back to cause further damage to the heart (black arrows).

Neurohormonal model

The neurohormonal model[19] has been particularly fruitful in guiding new treatments for HF. Note that the effectors in this model are the sympathetic nervous system and the renin–angiotensin system. These hormones have much more widespread effects than just their haemodynamic actions, causing direct harm to the heart, for example, by inducing programmed cell death and fibrosis. Thus neurohormonal activation leads to worsening HF.

As a guide to therapeutic advance, the neurohormonal model has been particularly helpful, underlying the development of modern therapy with ACE inhibitors, β-blockers, and aldosterone antagonists.

Peripheral model

The peripheral model (Fig. 1.3)[20] draws attention to the changes that happen in the periphery as a consequence of HF, particularly to skeletal muscle. Perhaps in part due to poor perfusion, perhaps due to lack of fitness, and perhaps due to neurohormonal and cytokine activation, a skeletal myopathy develops. The myopathy is a major cause of symptoms, particularly fatigue and breathlessness, but also causes sympathetic activation, leading to further damage to the heart. The peripheral model suggests that intervention to preserve skeletal muscle function or even reverse the myopathy may be helpful in managing HF.

A problem in thinking about the pathophysiology of decline in terms of vicious cycles or spirals is the implication that there is a continuing rapid downhill trajectory as HF inexorably declines. Untreated HF may behave in this way, but treated HF is typically much more stable—a punctuated equilibrium—presumably as a consequence of treatment.

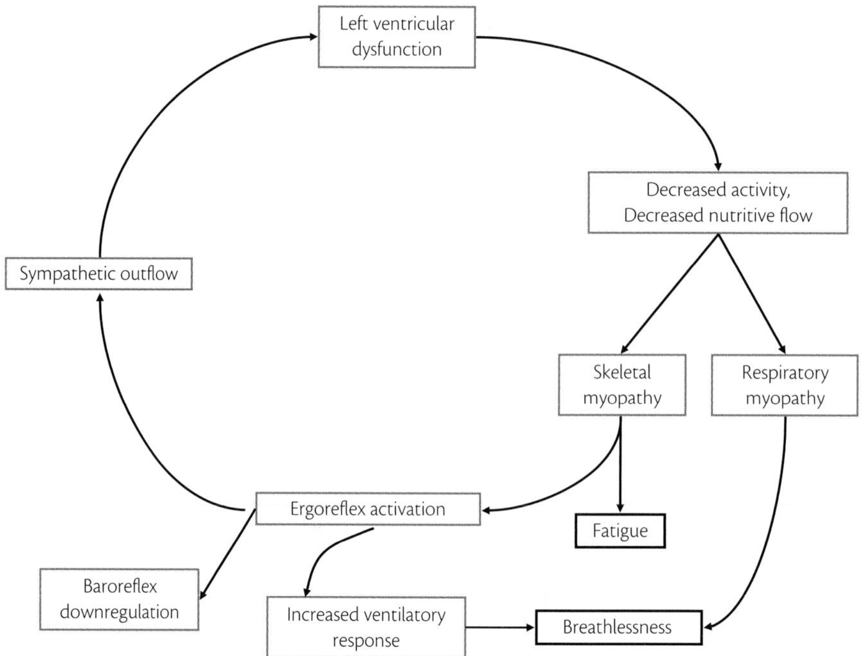

Fig. 1.3 A peripheral model of heart failure. Heart failure leads to a skeletal myopathy which is responsible for the symptoms of heart failure. The resulting activation of the ergoreflex causes sympathetic nervous system activation which feeds back to cause further damage to the heart.

References

1. Katz AM, Kat PB. Diseases of heart in works of Hippocrates. *Br Heart J* 1962;**24**:257–64.
2. Lower R. *Tractatus de corde, item de motu, et colore sanguinis et chyli in eum transitu,* 1st ed. J. Allestry, London, 1669.
3. Baglivi G. *De Praxi medica.* Roma, 1696.
4. Withering W. *An account of the foxglove and some of its medical uses—practical remarks on dropsy and other diseases,* 1st ed. M. Swinney, Birmingham, 1785.
5. Somberg J, Greenfield D, Tepper D. Digitalis: 200 years in perspective. *Am Heart J* 1986;**111**:615–20.
6. Pugh LG, Wyndham CL. The circulatory effects of mercurial diuretics in congestive heart failure. *Clin Sci (Lond)* 1949;**8**:11–19.
7. The CONSENSUS Trial Study Group. Effects of enalapril on mortality in severe congestive heart failure. Results of the Cooperative North Scandinavian Enalapril Survival Study (CONSENSUS). *N Engl J Med* 1987;**316**:1429–35.
8. Poole-Wilson PA. History, definition and classification of heart failure. In Poole-Wilson, Colucci WS, Massie BM, Chatterjee K, Coast AJS (eds) *Heart failure.* Churchill Livingstone, New York, 1997.
9. Denolin H, Kuhn H, Krayenbuehl HP, Loogen F, Reale A. The definition of heart failure. *Eur Heart J* 1983;**4**:445–8.
10. Remes J, Miettinen H, Reunanen A, Pyörälä K. Validity of clinical diagnosis of heart failure in primary health care. *Eur Heart J* 1991;**12**:315–21.
11. Marantz PR, Tobin JN, Wassertheil-Smoller S, *et al.* The relationship between left ventricular systolic function and congestive heart failure diagnosed by clinical criteria. *Circulation* 1988;**77**:607–12.
12. Clarke KW, Gray D, Hampton JR. Evidence of inadequate investigation and treatment of patients with heart failure. *Br Heart J* 1994;**71**:584–7.
13. Task Force for Diagnosis and Treatment of Acute and Chronic Heart Failure 2008 of European Society of Cardiology. ESC Guidelines for the diagnosis and treatment of acute and chronic heart failure 2008: the Task Force for the Diagnosis and Treatment of Acute and Chronic Heart Failure 2008 of the European Society of Cardiology. Developed in collaboration with the Heart Failure Association of the ESC (HFA) and endorsed by the European Society of Intensive Care Medicine (ESICM). *Eur Heart J* 2008;**29**:2388–442.
14. Harris P. Evolution and the cardiac patient. *Cardiovasc Res* 1983;**17**: 313–19; 373–8; 437–45.
15. Anand IS, Veall N, Kalra GS, *et al.* Treatment of heart failure with diuretics: body compartments, renal function and plasma hormones. *Eur Heart J* 1989;**10**:445–50.
16. Cowie MR, Wood DA, Coats AJ, *et al.* Survival of patients with a new diagnosis of heart failure: a population based study. *Heart* 2000;**83**:505–10.
17. Stewart S, MacIntyre K, Hole DJ, Capewell S, McMurray JJ. More 'malignant' than cancer? Five-year survival following a first admission for heart failure. *Eur J Heart Fail* 2001;**3**:315–22.
18. Anguita M, Arizón JM, Bueno G, Concha M, Vallés F. Spontaneous clinical and hemodynamic improvement in patients on waiting list for heart transplantation. *Chest* 1992;**102**:96–9.
19. Packer M. The neurohormonal hypothesis: a theory to explain the mechanism of disease progression in heart failure. *J Am Coll Cardiol* 1992;**20**:248–54.
20. Clark AL, Poole-Wilson PA, Coats AJS. Exercise limitation in chronic heart failure: the central role of the periphery. *J Am Coll Cardiol* 1996;**28**:1092–1102.

2

Heart failure syndromes

Andrew L. Clark

Heart failure (HF) is a protean condition, presenting acutely to hospital in most cases, but presenting with a more insidious course to primary care physicians in many cases.[1] Patients may only be diagnosed as having a primary cardiac problem after being seen by respiratory physicians or even, on occasion, after gastrointestinal workup for hepatomegaly (with or without jaundice) or weight loss. Nevertheless, there are common presenting clinical syndromes in patients with HF (Box 2.1) which should prompt different initial treatment strategies.

Acute heart failure

As a pragmatic definition, acute HF is HF necessitating emergency admission to hospital. Attempts have been made to classify acute HF into different types,[2] but the classification schemes often read as arbitrary, and resemble the Borges classification system for animals.[3] For the majority of patients, the problem of acute HF is that of 'fluid in the wrong place'; if that fluid is in the lungs, the patient has pulmonary oedema, but if predominantly in the tissues, the patient may present with anasarca (Greek ανα-, throughout; σαρχ, σαρκ-, flesh). Of course, patients will lie somewhere along a spectrum. Most patients will have some degree of pulmonary congestion even if the dominant problem is one of fluid retention; conversely, many patients with frank pulmonary oedema will have some evidence of ankle oedema.

Precipitants of acute heart failure

A large number of patients presenting with acute HF will have a background history of antecedent stable chronic HF. For patients presenting with pulmonary oedema, there will often be an obvious precipitant of the immediate crisis, and the trigger should be sought and treated (Box 2.2). Failure of compliance is the commonest identified trigger in several studies, with perhaps half of all admissions being potentially preventable if compliance had been better.[4,5]

Other common triggers include further ischaemic events in patients with ischaemic heart disease underlying their HF, and arrhythmia. Particularly in older patients, intercurrent illness, and especially chest infection, is a common precipitant (Fig. 2.1).[6]

The immediate precipitant does affect prognosis. Where uncontrolled hypertension is the culprit, the prognosis is good: however, patients admitted because of pneumonia, worsening renal function, or ischaemia have a worse prognosis.[6]

The fact that poor compliance is such a common trigger in all populations studied emphasizes the importance of patient education and follow-up to try to prevent recurrences. Although it is difficult to provide proof, increased numbers of admissions are certainly associated with a worse long-term prognosis.[7]

Pulmonary oedema

Pathophysiology

If the left ventricle fails acutely, cardiac output is maintained by the Frank–Starling mechanism: an increase in the left ventricular end-diastolic pressure, representing the preload of the left ventricle, leads to an increase in stroke work. However, the increase in pressure inevitably causes an increase in pulmonary venous, and then capillary, pressure.

The balance of forces keeping fluid within blood vessels is largely a balance between the hydrostatic pressure tending to force fluid out and the colloid osmotic pressure tending to keep fluid in. If the left ventricle fails, the rise in pulmonary capillary pressure required to maintain left ventricular output will exceed the combined resistance of the colloid osmotic pressure and the alveolar basement membrane and the capacity of the pulmonary lymphatics to drain tissue fluid.[8] At this point, fluid will start to accumulate in the pulmonary interstitium, then the alveoli, and ultimately the airways (see Fig. 2.2).

As fluid accumulates, so the lungs become stiffer and the work of breathing increases; bronchospasm (so-called 'cardiac asthma') can be a prominent feature; and at the same time, gas exchange is hampered by fluid filling the alveoli. The sympathetic response worsens the situation by causing tachycardia and peripheral vasoconstriction, thereby increasing the afterload against which the failing left ventricle is trying to eject blood.

Clinical syndrome

Pulmonary oedema is an acute medical emergency and an exceptionally alarming experience for the patient. The typical clinical

Box 2.1 Heart failure syndromes

- Acute heart failure
  - Pulmonary oedema
  - Anasarca
  - Cardiogenic shock
- Chronic heart failure
- Cardiac cachexia
- Sudden death

Box 2.2 Precipitants of acute heart failure

- Acute ischaemia
- Arrhythmia
  - Atrial fibrillation or flutter
  - Ventricular tachycardia
- Mechanical disaster
  - Papillary muscle rupture
- Intercurrent illness
  - Pneumonia
  - Influenza
- Noncompliance
- Pulmonary embolus
- Environment
  - Salt and or fluid load
  - Drugs

picture is well known. Symptoms tend to be of very abrupt onset, typically appearing over the course of less than an hour, but may be preceded by a day or so of worsening breathlessness and nocturnal dyspnoea. The patient rapidly becomes extremely breathless and distressed; speaking more than a few words at a time becomes impossible, and the need to breathe becomes overwhelming. The fearful sensation of impending death, *angor animi*, is very common. The patient needs to sit upright, often forwards, and might die if forced to lie flat. As the alveoli fill with fluid, the patient will cough, often violently, and will expectorate quantities of pink-tinged frothy fluid.

There is invariably a huge sympathetic nervous system response: the periphery becomes shut down due to vasoconstriction with associated pallor and coldness of the skin. Profuse sweating is commonly seen.

Common physical findings include sinus tachycardia, or arrhythmia, commonly atrial fibrillation or ventricular tachycardia. Hypertension is common, either as a precipitant or as a consequence of the sympathetic activity. The jugular venous pressure may be raised, but there are often no signs of peripheral oedema as the syndrome develops abruptly: there has been no time for the patient to become fluid overloaded. The problem is not one of excess fluid; rather, fluid in the wrong body compartment.

The cardiac findings depend upon the previous history, and may include a displaced and dyskinetic apex beat. A gallop rhythm is very common, with third, fourth, and summation sounds difficult to distinguish given the tachycardia. The chest may be silent *in extremis*, but is usually filled with a variety of fine and coarse crackles, and wheezes. In cases presenting early or with mild pulmonary oedema, the classical finding of fine late inspiratory crackles at the bases may be heard (see Fig. 2.3).

Natural history

Modern treatment of acute pulmonary oedema has changed the natural history of pulmonary oedema, and the outlook depends upon the severity of the syndrome as well as the underlying causes. Grading systems for recording severity are available, with the Killip class[9] and an assessment based on the combination of perfusion and congestion[10] commonly used (Table 2.1). The gradings are primarily designed for use in people with HF following acute myocardial infarction, but are helpful in assessing prognosis whatever the underlying cause of the pulmonary oedema.

Patients with acute pulmonary oedema typically present outside office hours, and it is striking that they either improve rapidly or die, so that within a few hours the immediate clinical outcome is obvious.

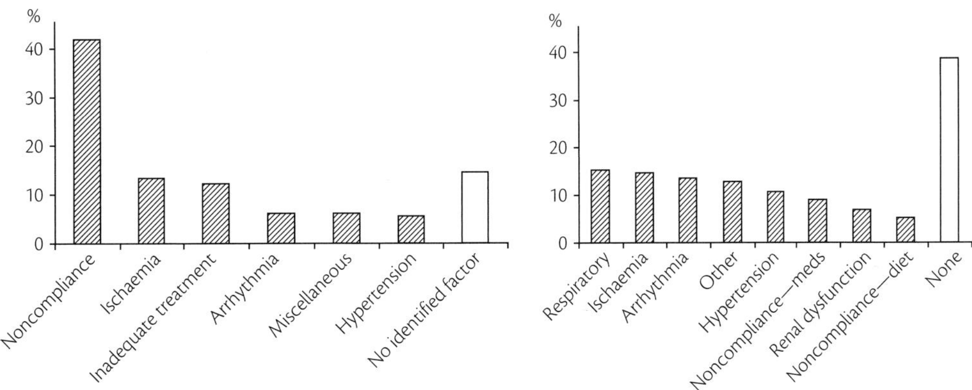

Fig. 2.1 Precipitants of admission to hospital with acute heart failure in two patient cohorts. Note that the totals may exceed 100% as an individual patient may have more than one precipitant.

Data from Michalsen A, *et al.* Preventable causative factors leading to hospital admission with decompensated heart failure. *Heart* 1998;**80**:437–41 (left) and Fonarow GC, *et al.* Factors identified as precipitating hospital admissions for heart failure and clinical outcomes: findings from OPTIMIZE-HF. *Arch Intern Med* 2008;**168**:847–54 (right).

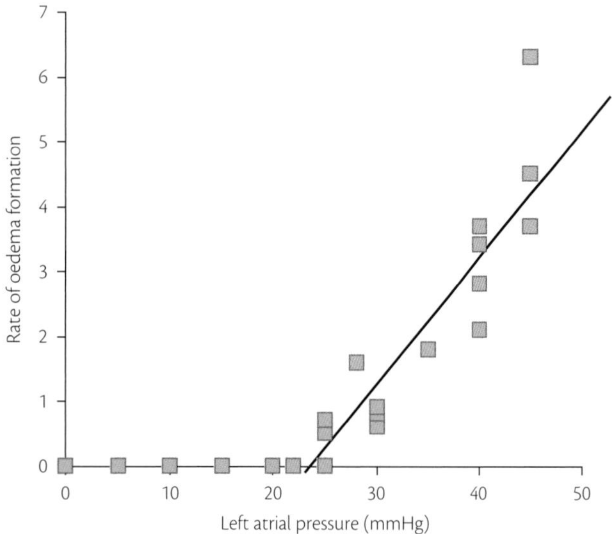

Fig. 2.2 The rate of pulmonary oedema formation is dependent on exceeding a critical left ventricular end-diastolic pressure.
Data from Guyton AC, Lindsey AW. Effect of elevated left atrial pressure and decreased plasma protein concentration on the development of pulmonary edema. *Circ Res* 1959;**7**:649–57.

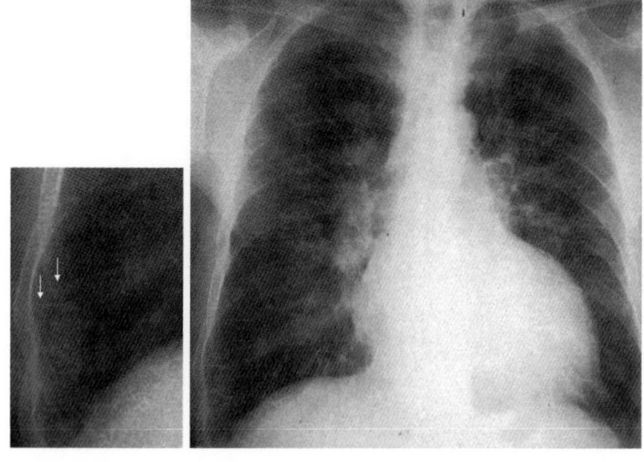

Fig. 2.3 Plain chest radiograph of a patient presenting with early pulmonary oedema. The heart is enlarged and the hila prominent. The enlarged section highlights interstitial lines (arrowed) of developing interstitial fluid (known as Kerley B lines). On examination, the patient had fine late inspiratory crackles at the bases.

Anasarca

Pathophysiology

At the other end of the spectrum of acute HF are patients presenting with fluid retention. This is a far more gradual process that that underlying acute pulmonary oedema. By the time patients present, they may have accumulated over 20 Lof excess fluid (and it requires approximately 5 L excess before ankle oedema appears).

The underlying pathophysiology is the neurohormonal response to poor renal perfusion and fall in arterial blood pressure. The kidneys 'try' to maintain normal perfusion by the release of renin, ultimately leading to aldosterone release and salt and water retention by the kidneys. In addition, antidiuretic hormone (ADH; arginine vasopressin) is released from the anterior pituitary gland. ADH is high relative to serum sodium, and causes water retention and the production of hypertonic urine, coupled with thirst, which results in increased fluid intake.[11]

The excess fluid increases the venous hydrostatic pressure which results in the Starling forces in the capillaries favouring fluid loss from the vessels and accumulation in the tissues.

Table 2.1 Grading systems for severe heart failure

Killip class	Clinical state	Hospital mortality (%)
1	No signs of heart failure	6
2	Third heart sound, basal crackles	17
3	Acute pulmonary oedema	38
4	Cardiogenic shock	81

From Killip T 3rd, Kimball JT. Treatment of myocardial infarction in a coronary care unit. A two year experience with 250 patients. *Am J Cardiol* 1967;**20:**457–464.

		Congestion			
		No		Yes	
Low perfusion	No	Warm and dry	1	Warm and wet	1.8
	Yes	Cool and dry		Cool and wet	2.5

The hazard ratio for the combined endpoint of death or transplantation is shown. There were too few patients in 'cool and dry' to give definitive statistical results.
From Nohria A, *et al.* Clinical assessment identifies hemodynamic profiles that predict outcomes in patients admitted with heart failure. *J Am Coll Cardiol* 2003;**41:**1797–1804.

Clinical syndrome

Where the excess fluid accumulates is a function of gravity. The ankles are usually first affected, commonly with swelling that increases during the day and may have gone by the next morning as a consequence of several hours' leg elevation. The oedema progressively rises up the legs, and then affects the abdominal wall. Pleural effusions and ascites are common at this stage, and pericardial effusions may become large.

The prominent physical finding is, of course, peripheral oedema, which is pitting. Sinus tachycardia or atrial fibrillation are usual findings together with low systemic blood pressure. The jugular venous pressure is invariably raised, and there may be evidence of tricuspid regurgitation in the jugular venous waveform. There is often a dilated heart with prominent third heart sound. The lung fields may be clear, or there may be some evidence of pulmonary oedema.

Natural history

There is some evidence that strict bed rest might result in a reduction in oedema,[12] but without therapy anasarca or 'dropsy' becomes a chronic state. Surprisingly large volumes of excess fluid are sometimes tolerated for many months before a patient finally presents (Fig. 2.4). Modern diuretic therapy means that the majority of patients progress at this stage to having chronic HF.

Chronic heart failure

The vast majority of patients with HF receive active treatment so that following a presentation with an acute episode of HF, congestion is removed. The chronic HF syndrome is what affects patients with heart failure once they are taking appropriate combination therapy with diuretics (as needed), angiotensin converting enzyme (ACE) inhibitors, β-blockers, and sometimes aldosterone antagonists. For these patients, the term 'congestive' HF is inappropriate—they should not be congested at all with suitable use of diuretics.

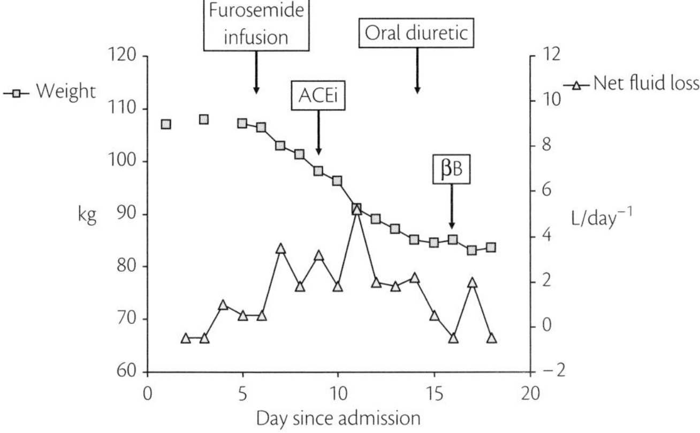

Fig. 2.4 Clinical course of a patient presenting with anasarca. The patient lost 25 kg during his admission, representing 25 L of excess fluid. ACEi, ACE inhibitor; βB, β-blocker.

The symptoms of chronic HF are most commonly breathlessness and fatigue on exertion, leading to exercise limitation and consequent decline in quality of life. The severity of symptoms is most commonly measured using the New York Heart Association (NYHA) scale (Table 2.2).[13] Unfortunately, the NYHA system is only weakly related to measures of exercise capacity, and bears no relation to left ventricular function at rest. It is often not clear from clinical studies whether the patients themselves are recording the score (which should surely be the case, as it is a subjective scoring system) or the physicians caring for the patients. When physicians score the patients, the NYHA system becomes a composite score of overall severity of HF rather than being a pure symptom score.[14]

Another limitation is that patients are forced into one of four categories, and in practice, most patients recruited to clinical trials are in either class II or class III (those in class I have no symptoms and might thus be thought not to have HF; those in class IV are bedbound). Further, there is a temptation to describe populations of patients by their 'average' NYHA class. This is inappropriate—no individual patient can have anything other than an integer score, and the scale is nonlinear.

Other scoring systems are better matched to the complexity of symptom assessment, and are better able to define subtle differences both between patients and in response to therapy. They are more cumbersome to administer in practice than the NYHA score. The Minnesota Living with Heart Failure self-assessment questionnaire is the most widely used, and is a series of 21 questions, each scored from zero to 5.[15,16] The Kansas City questionnaire[17] has the advantage of asking patients about how symptoms have changed and gives a better idea of the trajectory of an individual's clinical course.

Table 2.2 The New York Heart Association classification of symptoms in chronic heart failure

Class	Symptoms
I	No symptoms during ordinary activity
II	Mild symptoms during activity with some limitation
III	Marked limitation in exercise capacity with symptoms on mild exertion
IV	Symptoms at rest

A functional assessment is very helpful in trying to get an objective measure of a patient's symptoms. Incremental exercise tests with metabolic gas exchange measurements are often thought to be the best single assessment, but the equipment required is not universally available. Many patients are unable to manage an incremental exercise test. The six-minute walk test[18,19] is easy to administer, can be attempted by the great majority of patients, and is reproducible.

Pathophysiology

Central haemodynamics

Why chronic HF causes shortness of breath and fatigue has traditionally been attributed to abnormal central haemodynamics. It might be supposed that 'forward' failure leads to inability adequately to perfuse exercising skeletal muscle, thereby resulting in fatigue; and 'backward' failure leads to a rise in pulmonary venous pressure, stiff (or even oedematous) lungs, thereby resulting in breathlessness. However, against this hypothesis is the fact that there is no relation between exercise capacity and central haemodynamics (at least at rest); some patients with very severe left ventricular dysfunction have near normal exercise capacity;[20] acute correction of central haemodynamics (e.g. with positive inotropic drug therapy or even heart transplantation[21]) does not result in acute correction of exercise limitation. During early stages of exercise, the cardiac output responses are often normal in HF.

Some light is thrown on the issue by the observation that different kinds of exercise can lead to different symptoms in the same individual: rapidly incremental tests are more likely to cause limiting breathlessness,[22] whereas slower tests, although eliciting the same exercise performance, are more likely to cause fatigue. Cycle exercise is more often stopped by fatigue than breathlessness than is treadmill exercise, even when the same level of exercise is performed.[23, 24]

Some work has suggested that right ventricular function and pulmonary haemodynamics might be key determinants of exercise capacity, but some patients with the Fontan circulation (who thus have no right ventricle in the circulation) have near normal exercise capacity.[25]

Pulmonary physiology

The lungs are abnormal in many patients with chronic HF, in terms both of spirometric variables and of diffusion capacity.[26] In some studies, exercise capacity correlates closely with some spirometric variables.[27] However, about one-third of patients being assessed for transplantation will have normal spirometry and diffusion.[28]

One possibility is that pulmonary dead space might be increased. Dead space is that component of air in the respiratory tract not available for gas exchange. Anatomical dead space is the fixed dead space formed from the airways. It could plausibly be increased by an altered ventilatory pattern: the same minute ventilation achieved with double the respiratory rate and half the tidal volume will double anatomical dead space. Physiological dead space, on the other hand, is made up of alveoli that are ventilated but not perfused—'wasted' or inefficient ventilation.

However, there is no dead space receptor that might sense the increase and drive an excessive ventilatory response. In contrast to what might be expected, patients with chronic HF have better than normal arterial blood gases during exercise,[29] suggesting that the primary abnormality driving an excessive ventilatory response to exercise must lie elsewhere.

Skeletal muscle

Abnormalities of skeletal muscle in chronic HF range from ultrastructural,[30] through histological[31] and metabolic,[32] to changes in gross function (weakness and early fatigue[33]) and reduction in bulk.[34] The key feature distinguishing patients with abnormal exercise capacity is differences in skeletal muscle function: those with normal exercise capacity have normal (or near normal) skeletal muscle.[20] That these changes might cause the sensation of fatigue is easy to picture.

A unifying picture to explain the origin of symptoms comes from the ergoreflex (see Fig. 1.3). The ergoreflex is neurally mediated and arises from exercising muscle in proportion to work done. The strength of the signal is also proportional to the amount of muscle doing the work—the stimulus is greater when arm muscle is used to perform a given workload compared with leg muscle.[35]

Stimulation of the ergoreflex both increases ventilation and causes sympathetic nervous system activation. In patients with chronic HF, the ergoreflex is enhanced in proportion to the degree of exercise limitation and ventilatory abnormality.[36]

The ergoreflex model explains the two common chronic HF symptoms, and also helps explains other features of the syndrome. The origin of the sympathetic activation is not immediately obvious as the baroreflexes are down-regulated in HF.[37] Ergoreflex stimulation causes sympathetic activation. In addition, the chemoreflexes are enhanced in chronic HF, and they, too, are associated with baroreflex down-regulation.[38] Indeed, the peripheral model gives a new understanding of autonomic nervous system changes in chronic HF;[39] in the normal state, the main inputs into autonomic nervous system control from the cardiovascular system are the baroreceptors and cardiopulmonary receptors, with parasympathetic modulation being the major output; in HF, chemoreceptors and ergoreceptors are the most important inputs, and sympathetic activation results.

Natural history

There is, of course, nothing 'natural' about the outcome of patients with chronic HF. The marked improvements in prognosis that have come with modern medical therapy[40] (Fig. 2.5) are shown by the falling event rates among patients in the placebo groups of clinical trials. For very many patients, chronic HF can be stable for many years, but for some, it can be a progressive illness resulting in early death or transplantation.

Cardiac cachexia

That chronic heart disease can result in cachexia has been known for many hundreds of years. Quite how it comes about remains unknown, and anecdotally its frequency seems to be falling, perhaps as a consequence of widespread use of β-blockers. Part of the difficulty in discussing the syndrome is the lack of a universally recognized definition of cachexia. Clinicians know it when they see it, but defining it is a different matter. It is best thought of as a process of active weight loss rather than referring to a patient who is simply thin; but how much weight loss, and loss from which body compartment (fat, muscle, or bone) is not satisfactorily determined.

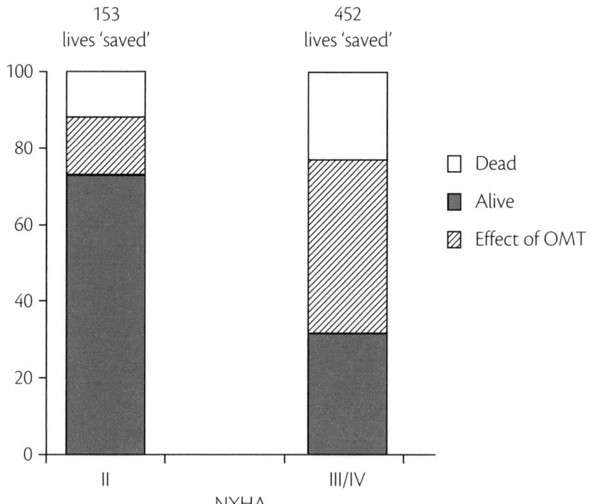

Fig. 2.5 The effect of modern medical therapy in chronic heart failure. The bars represent the 2-year outcome of 1000 patients with either mild (NYHA II/III) or severe (NYHA III/IV) heart failure. The red blocks represent the patients who would have survived and the white bars those who would have died without treatment. The shaded blocks represent the patients whose death would have been prevented by optimal medical therapy (OMT) with ACE inhibitor, β-blocker, and aldosterone antagonist.

Adapted from Cleland JG, Clark AL. Delivering the cumulative benefits of triple therapy to improve outcomes in heart failure: too many cooks will spoil the broth. *J Am Coll Cardiol* 2003;**42**:1234–7.

Partly as a result of the lack of an agreed definition, the epidemiology of cardiac cachexia is unclear. Data from clinical trial databases suggests that weight loss is common,[41] with over 40% of patients losing 5% or more of their body weight during 3 years of follow-up in the SOLVD trial (Fig. 2.6).

The weight loss in cachexia is from all body compartments, not simply lean muscle. Muscle loss is common from early in the

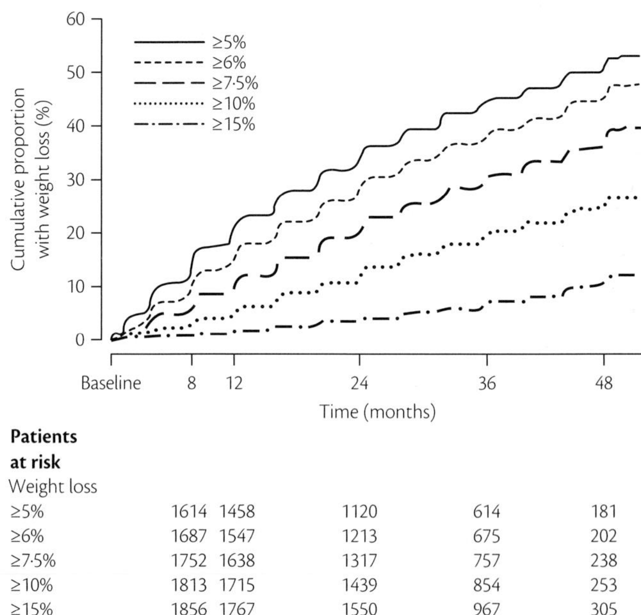

Fig. 2.6 Cumulative incidence of weight loss during follow-up in the SOLVD trial.
From Anker SD, *et al.* Prognostic importance of weight loss in chronic heart failure and the effect of treatment with angiotensin-converting-enzyme inhibitors: an observational study. *Lancet* 2003;**361**:1077–83, with permission.

course of chronic HF,[42] but loss of nonlean tissue is also seen[43] and patients are more prone to osteoporosis than normal individuals.[44] Patients with cachexia tend to have more advanced HF. The loss of bulk contributes to the general sense of fatigue and the activation of the ergoreflexes outlined above.

Origins of cachexia

Chronic HF seems to be an inherently catabolic state.[45,46] This is seen even at the level of increased hepatic fibrinogen synthesis.[47] Part of the explanation may be the continuous neurohormonal activation of HF. Sympathetic activation causes an increase in basal metabolic rate,[48,49] glycogenolysis, and lipolysis.[50] In animal models, high levels of angiotensin II are also associated with profound weight loss.[51,52] In normal individuals, infusions of catabolic hormones (hydrocortisone, glucagon, and adrenaline) induce hyperglycaemia, hyperinsulinaemia, insulin resistance, and negative nitrogen balance—precisely the changes seen in the cachexia syndrome.[53,54]

Other neurohormonal changes are commonly seen in chronic HF which are much more prevalent in patients with cachexia. In general, there seems to be a shift in the normal balance between catabolic and anabolic hormonal factors, so that patients develop resistance to the effects of both insulin[55] and growth hormone[56] and a decrease in the ratio of anabolic to catabolic steroid.[57] Additional procatabolic changes include the production of tumour necrosis factor (TNFα),[58] which is itself related to the changes in neurohormones.[59] These changes are strongly related to the alterations in body compartments,[60] suggesting that there is indeed an aetiological link between neurohormonal activation and weight loss.

One fascinating potential explanation which explains the otherwise slightly mysterious rise in TNFα is the possibility that bowel wall oedema, possibly caused by recurrent episodes of decompensation, allows the translocation of bacterial endotoxin across the bowel wall.[61] Bacterial endotoxin is the most potent natural stimulus for TNFα production. In support of this notion, circulating endotoxin is high during episodes of decompensation, and declines with treatment.[62] A further observation is that the endotoxin hypothesis may explain the apparent protective effects of cholesterol in patients with chronic HF:[63] endogenous lipoproteins act as a sump for endotoxin.[64]

Other potential contributors to cachexia are poor dietary intake, although there is only small-scale evidence for such a phenomenon.[65,66] There is some evidence that malabsorption (possibly as a consequence of gut oedema) may be a cause of impaired nutrition and fat malabsorption in particular.[67] Malaise, lethargy, nausea, lack of motivation, and poor mobility may contribute, particularly in elderly people.[68]

Treatment of cachexia

Hyperalimentation does not seem to offer any substantial benefit to stable patients with chronic HF,[69] but there is no large-scale intervention trial looking at its possible benefits in a cachectic population. There is some evidence that micronutrient supplementation may be helpful.[70] Other dietary approaches are being considered (reviewed[71] with many suggestions focusing on possible anti-inflammatory strategies), but none has so far proved to be effective.

Conventional HF therapy does affect cachexia. ACE inhibitors, or at least enalapril, reduce the risk of weight loss (Fig. 2.7).[72,73]

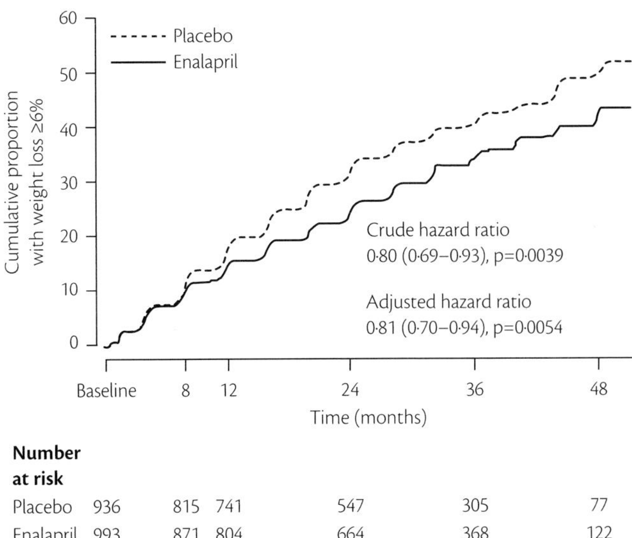

Fig. 2.7 Effect of the ACE inhibitor enalapril on the risk of developing ≥6% weight loss in the SOLVD trial.
From Anker SD, *et al.* Prognostic importance of weight loss in chronic heart failure and the effect of treatment with angiotensin-converting-enzyme inhibitors: an observational study. *Lancet* 2003;**361**:1077–83, with permission.

Similar effects have been reported with the angiotensin receptor antagonist candesartan.[74] β-Adrenoceptor antagonism causes a fall in basal metabolic rate,[75] an effect that may underlie the increase in weight seen in some patients on long-term β-blocker therapy.[76,77] There is some evidence that β-blockers may reduce the risk of cardiac cachexia developing,[78] and may reverse it once it has occurred.[79]

Natural history

The major clinical impact of cachexia is on outcome. Defined as unintentional weight loss of at least 7.5%, cachexia was associated with a mortality of 50% at 18 months.[80] In fact, decreasing body mass and not just an active process of cachexia is inversely related to survival.[81,82] Increasing body mass is strongly associated with survival following left ventricular assist device implantation.[83] The situation following cardiac transplantation is more complex. Weight at transplantation does not have a major impact on outcome,[84] but because thinner patients have a worse prognosis, there is more to be gained from transplantation for underweight patients.

Sudden death

It may seem odd to consider 'sudden death' to be a clinical syndrome, but one of the peculiarities of chronic HF is that patients are at risk of dying suddenly at any point in their clinical course. Approximately half the patients dying from HF die from progressive disease, but the others die suddenly. The mode of death in HF depends upon the severity of the HF syndrome (see Fig. 2.8). With worsening NYHA class of symptoms, so the likelihood of a death being sudden declines, with sudden death predominating as the mode of death in patients with milder symptoms. Note, however, that the likelihood of dying is much lower in patients with mild symptoms, so the absolute number of sudden deaths increases with worsening symptoms.

Patients with chronic HF are prone to tachyarrhythmias, both atrial and ventricular. The cause of sudden death has traditionally

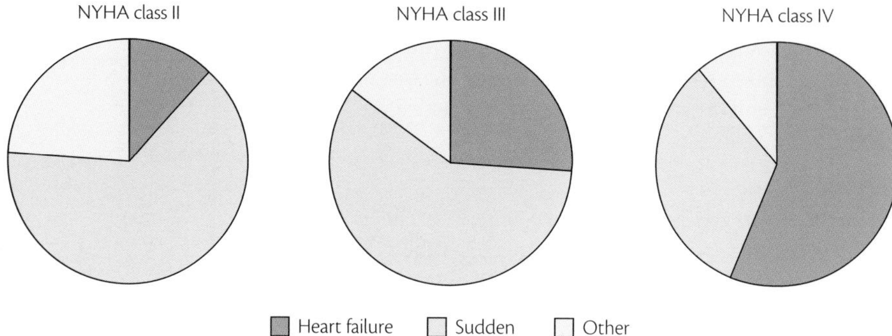

Fig. 2.8 The proportion of patients dying suddenly by NYHA class. Note, however, that the proportion of patients dying falls with increasing NYHA class, and so the likelihood of dying suddenly actually increases.

been considered to be a ventricular arrhythmia—either ventricular tachycardia or fibrillation (Fig. 2.9). However, it is important to remember that conduction system disease is very common in HF, and so patients are at risk of bradycardia as well.

A difficulty in understanding the pathophysiology of sudden death is the lack of an agreed definition of sudden death.[85] A further consideration is that most patients with chronic HF have underlying coronary heart disease, and so are potentially at risk from further ischaemic events. Although sudden deaths are commonly presumed to be due to arrhythmia, post-mortem studies of patients with HF dying suddenly show that very many are secondary to ischaemic events.[86,87] These ischaemic events are mostly not detected in life, leading to a false impression of how common arrhythmic death is. The importance lies in appreciating that therapies targeted specifically at sudden death (e.g. with implantable cardioverter-defibrillators) are not able to eradicate sudden death, which will still continue to happen.

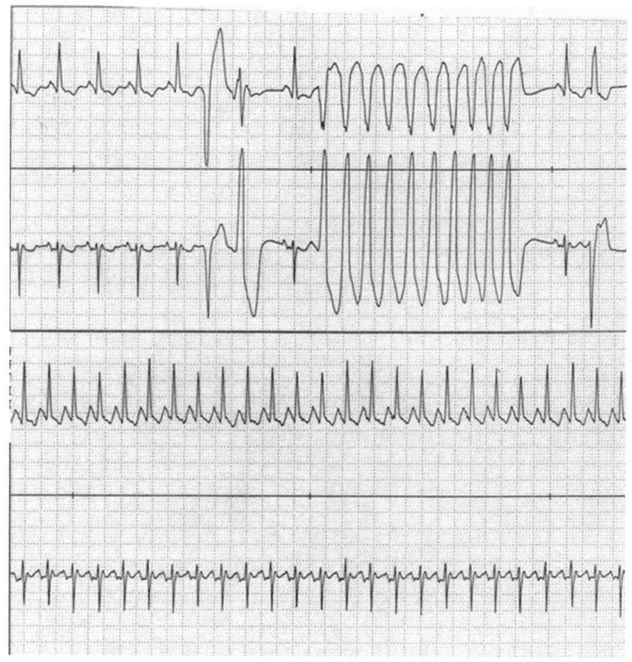

Fig. 2.9 An extract from a 24-h Holter recording of a patient with chronic heart failure showing both nonsustained ventricular tachycardia (top panel) and atrial flutter (bottom panel).

References

1. Cowie MR, Wood DA, Coats AJ, *et al.* Incidence and aetiology of heart failure; a population-based study. *Eur Heart J* 1999;**20**:421–8.
2. Nieminen MS, Böhm M, Cowie MR, *et al.* ESC Committee for Practice Guideline (CPG). Executive summary of the guidelines on the diagnosis and treatment of acute heart failure: the Task Force on Acute Heart Failure of the European Society of Cardiology. *Eur Heart J* 2005;**26**:384–416.
3. Borges JL. John Wilkins' analytical language. In Weinberger E *et al.* (ed. and trans.) *The total library: non-fiction 1922–86,* pp. 229–32. Penguin, London, 2001.
4. Ghali JK, Kadakia S, Cooper R, Ferlinz J. Precipitating factors leading to decompensation of heart failure. Traits among urban blacks. *Arch Intern Med* 1988;**148**:2013–16.
5. Michalsen A, König G, Thimme W. Preventable causative factors leading to hospital admission with decompensated heart failure. *Heart* 1998;**80**:437–41.
6. Fonarow GC, Abraham WT, Albert NM, *et al.*; OPTIMIZE-HF Investigators and Hospitals. Factors identified as precipitating hospital admissions for heart failure and clinical outcomes: findings from OPTIMIZE-HF. *Arch Intern Med* 2008;**168**:847–54.
7. Setoguchi S, Stevenson LW, Schneeweiss S. Repeated hospitalizations predict mortality in the community population with heart failure. *Am Heart J* 2007;**154**:260–6.
8. Guyton AC, Lindsey AW. Effect of elevated left atrial pressure and decreased plasma protein concentration on the development of pulmonary edema. *Circ Res* 1959;**7**:649–57.
9. Killip T 3rd, Kimball JT. Treatment of myocardial infarction in a coronary care unit. A two year experience with 250 patients. *Am J Cardiol* 1967;**20**:457–64.
10. Nohria A, Tsang SW, Fang JC, *et al.* Clinical assessment identifies hemodynamic profiles that predict outcomes in patients admitted with heart failure. *J Am Coll Cardiol* 2003;**41**:1797–804.
11. Anand IS, Ferrari R, Kalra GS, Wahi PL, Poole-Wilson PA, Harris PC. Edema of cardiac origin. Studies of body water and sodium, renal function, hemodynamic indexes, and plasma hormones in untreated congestive cardiac failure. *Circulation* 1989;**80**:299–305.
12. McDonald CD, Burch GE, Walsh JJ. Prolonged bed rest in the treatment of idiopathic cardiomyopathy. *Am J Med* 1972;**52**:41–50.
13. The Criteria Committee of the New York Heart Association. *Nomenclature and criteria for diagnosis, 9th edition.* Little, Brown. Boston, 1994.
14. Goode KM, Nabb S, Cleland JG, Clark AL. A comparison of patient and physician-rated New York Heart Association class in a community-based heart failure clinic. *J Card Fail* 2008;**14**:379–87.
15. Rector TS, Francis GS, Cohn JN. Patients' self-assessment of their congestive heart failure. Part 1. Patient perceived dysfunction and its poor correlation with exercise tests. *Heart Fail* 1987;**3**:192–6.
16. Rector TS, Francis GS, Cohn JN. Patients' self-assessment of their congestive heart failure. Part 2: content, reliability and validity of

a new measure, the Minnesota Living with Heart Failure questionnaire. *Heart Fail* 1987;**3**:196–209.

17. Green CP, Porter CB, Bresnahan DR, Spertus JA. Development and evaluation of the Kansas City Cardiomyopathy Questionnaire: a new health status measure for heart failure. *J Am Coll Cardiol* 2000; **35**:1245–55.
18. Olsson LG, Swedberg K, Clark AL, Witte KK, Cleland JG. Six minute corridor walk test as an outcome measure for the assessment of treatment in randomized, blinded intervention trials of chronic heart failure: a systematic review. *Eur Heart J* 2005;**26**:778–93.
19. Ingle L, Rigby AS, Carroll S, *et al.* Prognostic value of the 6min walk test and self-perceived symptom severity in older patients with chronic heart failure. *Eur Heart J* 2007;**28**:560–8.
20. Harrington D, Anker SD, Coats AJ. Preservation of exercise capacity and lack of peripheral changes in asymptomatic patients with severely impaired left ventricular function. *Eur Heart J* 2001;**22**:392–9.
21. Marzo KP, Wilson JR, Mancini DM. Effects of cardiac transplantation on ventilatory response to exercise. *Am J Cardiol* 1992;**69**:547–53.
22. Lipkin DP, Canepa-Anson R, Stephens MR, Poole-Wilson PA. Factors determining symptoms in heart failure: comparison of fast and slow exercise tests. *Br Heart J* 1986;**55**:439–45.
23. Fink LI, Wilson JR, Ferraro N. Exercise ventilation and pulmonary artery wedge pressure in chronic stable congestive heart failure. *Am J Cardiol* 1986;**57**:249–53.
24. Witte KKA, Clark AL. Cycle exercise causes a lower ventilatory response to exercise in chronic heart failure. *Heart* 2005;**91**:225–6.
25. Clark AL, Swan JW, Laney R, Connelly M, Somerville J, Coats AJS. The role of right and left ventricular function in the ventilatory response to exercise in chronic heart failure. *Circulation* 1994;**89**:2062–9.
26. Puri S, Baker BL, Dutka DP, Oakley CM, Hughes JMB, Cleland JGF. Reduced alveolar-capillary membrane diffusing capacity in chronic heart failure. *Circulation* 1995;**91**:2769–74.
27. Kraemer MD, Kubo SH, Rector TS, Brunsvold N, Bank AJ. Pulmonary and peripheral vascular factors are important determinants of peak exercise oxygen uptake in patients with heart failure. *J Am Coll Cardiol* 1993;**21**:641–8.
28. Wright RS, Levine MS, Bellamy PE, *et al.* Ventilatory and diffusion abnormalities in potential heart transplant recipients. *Chest* 1990;**98**:816–20.
29. Clark AL, Coats AJS. Usefulness of arterial blood gas estimations during exercise in patients with chronic heart failure. *Br Heart J* 1994;**71**: 528–30.
30. Sullivan MJ, Green HJ, Cobb FR. Skeletal muscle biochemistry and histology in ambulatory patients with long-term heart failure. *Circulation* 1990;**81**:518–27.
31. Lipkin DP, Jones DA, Round JM, Poole-Wilson PA. Abnormalities of skeletal muscle in patients with chronic heart failure. *Int J Cardiol* 1988;**18**:187–95.
32. Massie BM, Conway M, Yonge R, *et al.* Skeletal muscle metabolism in patients with congestive heart failure: relation to clinical severity and blood flow. *Circulation* 1987;**76**:1009–19.
33. Buller NP, Jones D, Poole-Wilson PA. Direct measurements of skeletal muscle fatigue in patients with chronic heart failure. *Br Heart J* 1991;**65**:20–4.
34. Volterrani M, Clark AL, Ludman PF, *et al.* Determinants of exercise capacity in chronic heart failure. *Eur Heart J* 1994;**15**:801–9.
35. Clark AL, Piepoli M, Coats AJS. Skeletal muscle and the control of ventilation on exercise; evidence for metabolic receptors. *Eur J Clin Invest* 1995;**25**:299–305.
36. Piepoli M, Clark AL, Volterrani M, Adamopoulos S, Sleight P, Coats AJS. Contribution of muscle afferents to the hemodynamic, autonomic, and ventilatory responses to exercise in patients with chronic heart failure: effects of physical training. *Circulation* 1996;**93**:940–52.
37. Ellenbogen KA, Mohanty PK, Szentpetery S, Thames MD. Arterial baroreflex abnormalities in heart failure: reversal after orthotopic cardiac transplantation. *Circulation* 1989;**79**:51–8.
38. Ponikowski P, Chua TP, Piepoli M, *et al.* Augmented peripheral chemosensitivity as a potential input to baroreflex impairment and autonomic imbalance in chronic heart failure. *Circulation* 1997;**96**:2586–94.
39. Clark AL, Cleland JGF. The control of adrenergic function in heart failure: therapeutic interventions. *Heart Failure Reviews* 2000;**5**:101–14.
40. Cleland JG, Clark AL. Delivering the cumulative benefits of triple therapy to improve outcomes in heart failure: too many cooks will spoil the broth. *J Am Coll Cardiol* 2003;**42**:1234–7.
41. Anker SD, Negassa A, Coats AJ, *et al.* Prognostic importance of weight loss in chronic heart failure and the effect of treatment with angiotensin-converting-enzyme inhibitors: an observational study. *Lancet* 2003;**361**:1077–83.
42. Mancini DM, Walter G, Reichnek N, *et al.* Contribution of skeletal muscle atrophy to exercise intolerance and altered muscle metabolism in heart failure. *Circulation* 1992;**85**:1364–73.
43. Anker SD, Clark AL, Teixeira MM, Hellewell PG, Coats AJS. Loss of bone mineral in patients with cachexia due to chronic heart failure. *Am J Cardiol* 1999:**83**:612–15.
44. Shane E, Mancini D, Aaronson K, *et al.* Bone mass, vitamin D deficiency, and hypoparathyroidism in congestive heart failure. *Am J Med* 1997;**103**:197–207.
45. Riley M, Elborn JS, McKane WR, Bell N, Stanford CF, Nicholls DP. Resting energy expenditure in chronic cardiac failure. *Clin Sci* 1991;**80**:633–9.
46. Poehlman ET, Scheffers J, Gottlieb SS, Fisher ML, Vaitekevicius P. Increased metabolic rate in patients with congestive heart failure. *Ann Intern Med* 1994;**121**:860–2.
47. Witte KK, Ford SJ, Preston T, Parker JD, Clark AL. Fibrinogen synthesis is increased in cachectic patients with chronic heart failure. *Int J Cardiol* 2008;**129**:363–7.
48. Staten MA, Matthews DE, Cryer PE, Bier DM. Physiological increments in epinephrine stimulate metabolic rate in humans. *Am J Physiol* 1987;**253**:E322–30.
49. Simonsen L, Bulow J, Madsen J, Christensen, NJ. Thermogenic response to epinephrine in the forearm and abdominal subcutaneous adipose tissue. *Am J Physiol* 1992;**263**:E850-E855.
50. Lafontan M, Berlan M. Fat cell adrenergic receptors and the control of white and brown fat cell function. *J Lipid Res* 1993;**34**:1057–91.
51. Brink M, Wellen J, Delafontaine P. Angiotensin II causes weight loss and decreases circulating insulin- like growth factor I in rats through a pressor-independent mechanism. *J Clin Invest* 1996;**97**:2509–16.
52. Brink M, Price SR, Chrast J, *et al.* Angiotensin II induces skeletal muscle wasting through enhanced protein degradation and down-regulates autocrine insulin-like growth factor I. *Endocrinology* 2001;**142**:1489–96.
53. Bessey PQ, Watters JM, Aoki TT, Wilmore DW. Combined hormonal infusion simulates the metabolic response to injury. *Ann Surg* 1984;**200**:264–81.
54. Watters JM, Bessey PQ, Dinarello CA, Wolff SM, Wilmore DW. Both inflammatory and endocrine mediators stimulate host responses to sepsis. *Arch Surg* 1986;**121**:179–90.
55. Swan JW, Anker SD, Walton C, *et al.* Insulin resistance in chronic heart failure: relation to severity and aetiology of heart failure. *J Am Coll Cardiol* 1997:**30**:527–32.
56. Niebauer J, Pflaum C-D, Clark AL, *et al.* Deficient insulin-like growth factor-I in chronic heart failure predicts altered body composition, anabolic deficiency, cytokine and neurohormonal activation. *J Am Coll Cardiol* 1998;**32**:393–7.
57. Anker SD, Chua TP, Ponikowski P, *et al.* Hormonal changes and catabolic/anabolic imbalance in chronic heart failure and their importance for cardiac cachexia. *Circulation* 1997;**96**:526–34.

58. McMurray J, Abdullah I, Dargie HJ, Shapiro D. Increased concentrations of tumour necrosis factor in 'cachectic' patients with severe chronic heart failure. *Br Heart J* 1991;**66**:356–8.
59. Anker SD, Clark AL, Kemp M, *et al.* Tumour necrosis factor and steroid metabolism in chronic heart failure: possible relation to muscle wasting. *J Am Coll Cardiol* 1997;**30**:997–1001.
60. Anker SD, Ponikowski PP, Clark Al, *et al.* Cytokines and neurohormones relating to body composition alterations in the wasting syndrome of chronic heart failure. *Eur Heart J* 1999;**20**:683–93.
61. Sandek A, Bauditz J, Swidsinski A, *et al.* Altered intestinal function in patients with chronic heart failure. *J Am Coll Cardiol* 2007;**50**:1561–9.
62. Niebauer J, Volk HD, Kemp M, *et al.* Endotoxin and immune activation in chronic heart failure: a prospective cohort study. *Lancet* 1999;**353**:1838–42.
63. Rauchhaus M, Clark AL, Doehner W, *et al.* The relationship between cholesterol and survival in patients with chronic heart failure. *J Am Coll Cardiol* 2003;**42**:1933–40.
64. Rauchhaus M, Coats AJ, Anker SD. The endotoxin-lipoprotein hypothesis. *Lancet* 2000;**356**:930–3.
65. Carr JG, Stevenson LW, Walden JA, Heber D. Prevalence and haemodynamic correlates of malnutrition in severe congestive heart failure secondary to ischaemic or idiopathic dilated cardiomyopathy. *Am J Cardiol* 1989;**63**:709–13.
66. Broqvist M, Arnqvist H, Dahlstrom U, *et al.* Nutritional assessment and muscle energy metabolism in severe chronic congestive heart failure-effects of long-term dietary supplementation. *Eur Heart J* 1994;**15**:1641–50.
67. King D, Smith ML, Chapman TJ, *et al.* Fat malabsorption in elderly patients with cardiac cachexia. *Age Ageing* 1996;**25**:144–9.
68. Bates CJ, Prentice A, Cole TJ, *et al.* Micronutrients: highlights and research challenges from the 1994–5 National Diet and Nutrition Survey of people aged 65 years and over. *Br J Nutr* 1999;**82**:7–15.
69. Broqvist M, Arnqvist H, Dahlström U, Larsson J, Nylander E, Permert J. Nutritional assessment and muscle energy metabolism in severe chronic congestive heart failure—effects of long-term dietary supplementation. *Eur Heart J* 1994;**15**:1641–50.
70. Witte KK, Nikitin NP, Parker AC, *et al.* The effect of micronutrient supplementation on quality-of-life and left ventricular function in elderly patients with chronic heart failure. *Eur Heart J* 2005;**26**:2238–44.
71. Kalantar-Zadeh K, Anker SD, Horwich TB, Fonarow GC. Nutritional and anti-inflammatory interventions in chronic heart failure. *Am J Cardiol* 2008;**101**(11A):89–103E.
72. Adigun AQ, Ajayi AA. The effects of enalapril-digoxin-diuretic combination therapy on nutritional and anthropometric indices in chronic congestive heart failure: preliminary findings in cardiac cachexia. *Eur J Heart Fail* 2001;**3**:359–63.
73. Anker SD, Negassa A, Coats AJ, *et al.* Prognostic importance of weight loss in chronic heart failure and the effect of treatment with angiotensin-converting-enzyme inhibitors: an observational study. *Lancet* 2003;**361**:1077–83.
74. Kenchaiah S, Pocock SJ, Wang D, *et al.*; CHARM Investigators. Body mass index and prognosis in patients with chronic heart failure: insights from the Candesartan in Heart failure: Assessment of Reduction in Mortality and morbidity (CHARM) program. *Circulation* 2007;**116**:627–36.
75. Monroe MB, Seals DR, Shapiro LF, Bell C, Johnson D, Parker Jones P. Direct evidence for tonic sympathetic support for resting metabolic rate in healthy adult humans. *Am J Physiol* 2001;**280**: E740–4.
76. Rossner S, Taylor CL, Byington RP, Furberg CD. Long term propranolol treatment and changes in body weight after myocardial infarction. *Br Med J* 1990;**300**:902–3.
77. Sharma AM, Pischon T, Hardt S, Kunz I, Luft FC. Hypothesis. Beta-adrenergic receptor blockers and weight gain: a systematic analysis. *Hypertension* 2001;**37**:250–4.
78. Anker SD, Coats AJS, Roecker EB, Scerlag A, Packer M. Does carvedilol prevent and reverse cardiac cachexia in patients with severe heart failure? Results of the COPERNICUS study. *Eur Heart J* 2002;**23**:394 (abstract).
79. Hryniewicz K, Androne AS, Hudaihed A, Katz SD. Partial reversal of cachexia by beta-adrenergic receptor blocker therapy in patients with chronic heart failure. *J Card Fail* 2003;**9**:464–8.
80. Anker SD, Ponikowski P, Varney S, *et al.* Wasting as independent risk factor for mortality in chronic heart failure. *Lancet* 1997;**349**:1050–3.
81. Davos CH, Doehner W, Rauchhaus M, *et al.* Body mass and survival in patients with chronic heart failure without cachexia: the importance of obesity. *J Card Fail* 2003;**9**:29–35.
82. Horwich TB, Fonarow GC, Hamilton MA, MacLellan WR, Woo MA, Tillisch JH. The relationship between obesity and mortality in patients with heart failure. *J Am Coll Cardiol* 2001;**38**:789–95.
83. Clark AL, Loebe M, Potapov EV, *et al.* Ventricular assist device in severe heart failure: effects on cytokines, complement and body weight. *Eur Heart J* 2001;**22**:2275–83.
84. Clark AL, Knosalla C, Birks E, *et al.* Heart transplantation in heart failure: The prognostic importance of body mass index at time of surgery and subsequent weight changes. *Eur J Heart Fail* 2007;**9**:839–844.
85. Narang R, Cleland JG, Erhardt L, *et al.* Mode of death in chronic heart failure. A request and proposition for more accurate classification. *Eur Heart J* 1996;**17**:1390–403.
86. Uretsky BF, Thygesen K, Armstrong PW, *et al.* Acute coronary findings at autopsy in heart failure patients with sudden death: results from the assessment of treatment with lisinopril and survival (ATLAS) trial. *Circulation* 2000;**102**:611–16.
87. Orn S, Cleland JG, Romo M, Kjekshus J, Dickstein K. Recurrent infarction causes the most deaths following myocardial infarction with left ventricular dysfunction. *Am J Med* 2005;**118**:752–8.

PART II

Epidemiology

3

The epidemiology of heart failure

Kaushik Guha and Theresa A. McDonagh

Introduction

Over the last 30 years we have gone from famine to feast in terms of the epidemiological data now published for heart failure (HF). The field started with the seminal publication on the natural history of HF from the Framingham study in 1971 showing a prevalence of HF of 0.8% in those aged between 50 and 59, rising to 9.1% in those over 80 years with incidence rates of 0.2% at age 54 and 0.4% at age 85 (Fig. 3.1).[1] This was followed by a large European study, 'The men born in 1913', which gave similar figures of a prevalence of 2.1% at age 50 and 13% at age 67 and incidence rates of 0.15% and 1% respectively at ages 50 and 67.[2]

These landmark studies relied on a clinical diagnosis of HF, based on symptoms, signs, and scoring systems to identify cases. More modern epidemiological studies have used definitions of HF which include objective measures of cardiac function in their definition, in keeping with current European and United States guidelines for the diagnosis of HF. Initial studies focused on systolic dysfunction because they reported at much the same time as the HF treatment trials which also enrolled patients with systolic HF. More recently attention has turned to describing the epidemiology of HF with preserved systolic function, in addition.

When describing the epidemiology of HF, it is worth bearing in mind that estimates of incidence and prevalence will vary according to the definition of HF used and the type of cohort being studied. This is especially important when assessing work which has objectively measured left ventricular systolic function. Variables such as left ventricular ejection fraction are normally distributed, so the cut point chosen is a critical determinant of the eventual results.

The present chapter aims to outline the contemporary epidemiology of HF by describing its prevalence, incidence, aetiology and mortality as well as describing the trends which are occurring in the area. It will discuss hospitalization rates, prognosis and economic burden in both Europe and the United States.

Prevalence studies (see Table 3.1)

Community-based studies

Many studies have been conducted in primary care or across geographical health care communities to estimate the prevalence of HF. One of the first was conducted in north-west London and reviewed 30 204 case records, yielding a crude prevalence of HF of 3.8/100 cases in the general population with a marked rise from those under 65 to those above 65 years of age, where the rate rose from 0.6 per 1000 to 28.0 per 1000.[3]

More recent data is available from the Scottish Continuous Morbidity scheme which covers 57 general practices in Scotland with access to GP Read codes for HF in 307 741 patients.[4] The calculated prevalence within the general population in Scotland was 7.1 per 1000, increasing in the population above 85 years old to 90.1 per 1000. The population identified by primary care was more elderly, and had more comorbidities than in population-based studies or clinical trial populations. The findings have been corroborated in a European study based in Utrecht, Netherlands. It found that patients with HF who were under the supervision of a cardiologist compared to a general practitioner were more likely to be male, younger (in their sixties), and to have an ischaemic aetiology.[5] When considering such data it must be remembered that the signs and symptoms of HF are neither sensitive nor specific. Studies evaluating referrals from primary care, when compared to expert cardiological assessment, have revealed only approximately 30% of patients may actually have HF.[6,7]

A recent study in Sweden reiterated this salient point. Random primary health care centres were picked from across the country. Medical records were interrogated and variables recorded. Approximately 30% of the participants had had an echocardiogram. The majority were labelled as having HF on the basis of signs and symptoms and basic investigations including chest radiographs and the electrocardiogram. There was also an underuse of evidence-based therapies.[8]

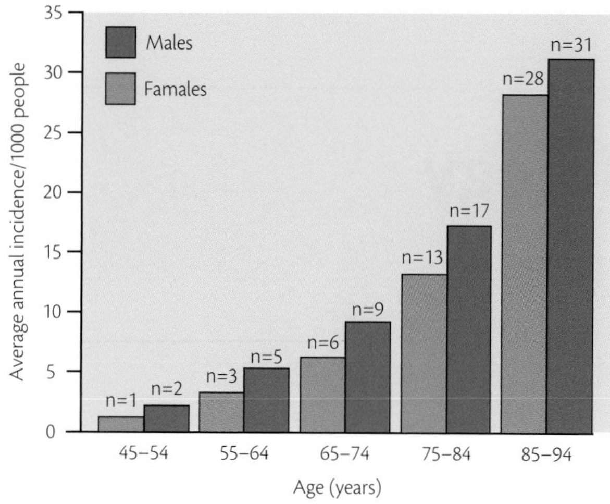

Fig. 3.1 Incidence of heart failure within the Framingham cohort.

Population-based studies using echocardiography

Systolic dysfunction

The North Glasgow MONICA Study was the first to report on the prevalence of left ventricular systolic dysfunction in a random sample of the general population of 2000 men and women aged 25–74 years.[9] In this cohort, 2.9% had significant left ventricular systolic dysfunction, of whom just over half had symptoms of breathlessness or were taking a loop diuretic. The estimated prevalence of HF was thus 1.5%, with 1.4% having the important precursor of HF, asymptomatic systolic dysfunction (ALVSD). The prevalence rose with age and was higher in men than women (Fig. 3.2).[9]

Many studies have reported subsequently both in Europe and in the United States. Data from these cohorts is fairly consistent for the general population. Prevalence rates for left ventricular systolic dysfunction (LVSD) were 1.8–3.5% in the ECHOES study from the English Midlands, with 50% of the LVSD being asymptomatic; in the US Olmsted county study 2.2% had HF validated using the Framingham criteria, and of these 56% had systolic dysfunction.[10,11]

When we look at population-based studies which have included much older subjects, the prevalence rates increase markedly. In the Helsinki Ageing Study of 501 subjects aged 75–86 years, clinical HF was found in 8.2% overall, 2.3% had systolic dysfunction, and 9% had ASLVD.[12] In the Rotterdam Study of 2267 men and women aged 55–95, 3.7% had fractional shortening of less than 25% (5.5% men and 2.2% women) and 2.2% had asymptomatic LVSD (see Fig. 3.3).[13] Similar findings were reported in a United Kingdom study of 817 subjects aged 70–84 years from Poole (on the south

Table 3.1 Prevalence of symptomatic and asymptomatic LVSD in populations with a calculated prevalence of manifest heart failure where applicable

Authors	Name of study	No. of patients (no. of cases of heart failure)	Location	Age range	Percentage symptomatic LVSD	Percentage ASLVD	Prevalence of HF <65 years of age	Prevalence of HF >65 years of age
Parameshwar *et al.*, 1992	Prevalence of heart failure in 3 GP practices	30 204 (117)	North-west London, UK	5–99	28% had echoes		0.6 per 1000	27.7 per 1000
Murphy *et al.*, 2004	National survey of heart failure	307,741 (2186)	Scotland, UK	0–>85	–		7.1 per 1000 (though not <65)	>85–90.1 per 1000
Rutten *et al.*, 2003	A questionnaire based survey of heart failure	(202)	Utrecht, Netherlands	40–95	53 % had echoes 97% LVSD			
McDonagh *et al.* 1997	MONICA	1640 (43)	North Glasgow, UK	25–74	2.9% LVSD	1.4% ALVSD	15 per 1000	
Davies *et al.*, 2001	ECHOES	3960 (72)	West Midlands, UK		1.8% LVSD 3.5% preserved EF	0.9% ALVSD	31 per 1000 (>45 years of age)	
Kupari *et al.*, 1997	Helsinki Ageing Study	501 (41)	Helsinki, Finland	75–86	4.1 % HEFPEF 3.9 % LVSD	9% ASLVD		(75–86) 82 per 1000
Mosterd *et al.*, 1999	Rotterdam Heart Study	2267 (88)	Rotterdam, Netherlands	55–94	3.7% LSVD	1.4% ASLVD	Men: 7 per 1000 (55–64) Women: 6 per 1000 (55–64)	Men: 37 per 1000 (65–74) 144 per 1000 (75–84) 59 per 1000 (85–94) Women: 16 per 1000 (65–74) 121 per 1000 (75–84) 140 per 1000 (85–94)
Morgan *et al.*, 1999	Poole Heart Study	817 (61)	Poole, Dorset, UK	70–84	7.5 % LVSD	3.9 % ASLVD		

ASLVD, asymptomatic left ventricular systolic dysfunction; LVSD, left ventricular systolic dysfunction.

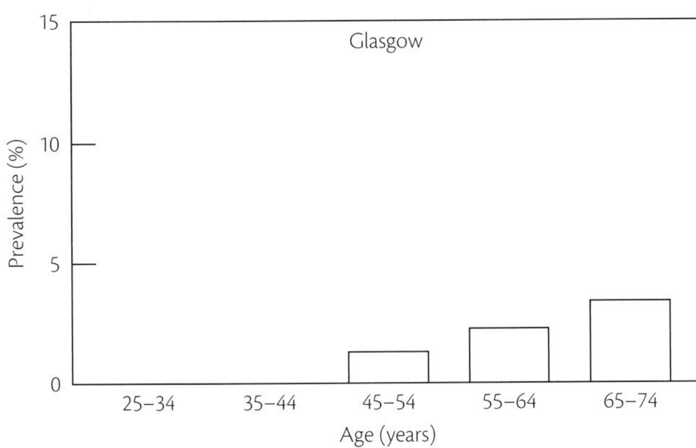

Fig. 3.2 Prevalence of left ventricular systolic dysfunction in the North Glasgow MONICA cohort.

coast of England) which demonstrated that 7.5% had LVSD (12.2% men and 2.9% women) and 52% of those with LVSD were previously undiagnosed.[14]

Heart failure with normal ejection fraction

Many of the population-based cohorts reviewed above concentrated on finding systolic dysfunction, as it is, to date, the only type of HF for which we have evidence-based treatment. Many of the cohorts have also by default or design been able to comment on the prevalence of HF with normal ejection fraction (HeFNEF). Hogg *et al.* reviewed the epidemiological data for HeFNEF. The prevalence ranged for 1.5% to 4.8% depending on the study. There was a definite increase in the proportion of HF due to HeFNEF in cohorts that contained more elderly individuals.[15] In the ECHOES study of the general population, 1.1% had definite HF and a LVEF greater than 50%,[10] whereas in the Helsinki Ageing Study, 72% of all the HF identified occurred with a normal LVEF.[11] In the United States, the Rochester Epidemiology Project found similar results in a random sample of 2042 subjects over 45 years, with 44% of subjects having HF with a LVEF greater than 50%.[11]

Even higher prevalence rates have been found in a recent large cross-sectional study from Portugal.[16] This showed the prevalence of HF was 16.1% in the population above 80 years old. The prevalence was roughly split equally between normal and reduced ejection fraction.

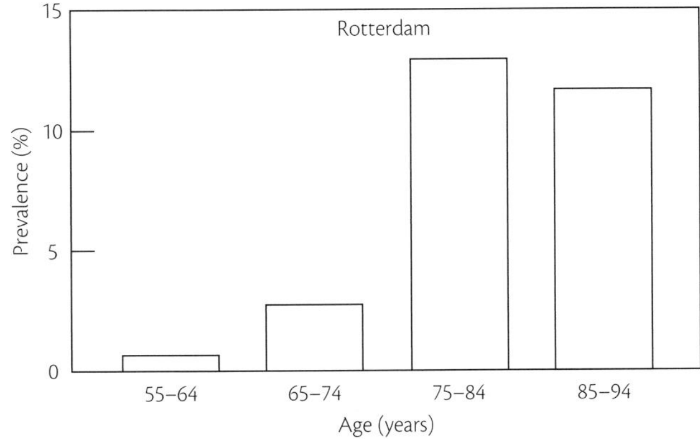

Fig. 3.3 Prevalence of left ventricular systolic dysfunction within the Rotterdam study.

The above studies all confirm one thing: a large prevalence of HF which increases exponentially with age. It is unsurprising, therefore, that the current burden of HF within the European Union member states is estimated to be approximately 15 million[17] and, according to the American Heart Association, more than 5 million Americans have HF.[18]

Incidence

Contemporary studies of incidence are far fewer than those for prevalence (Table 3.2).

The incidence of HF was ascertained in the west London district of Hillingdon. Here, all incident cases of HF were identified via either a specialist referral clinic or emergency admission.[19] The district contained 151 000 patients covered by 82 general practices. Using both portals of entry in the study, 220 new cases were identified. Participants had a full clinical assessment, standard investigations including a chest radiograph and ECG and 99% of the study population had an echocardiogram. The results were then shown to a panel of three cardiologists who made the gold standard diagnosis. The documented incidence rose from 0.02/1000 per year in the 25–34 age group to 11.6/1000 in those aged over 85 (Fig. 3.4).[19] There was a preponderance of impaired systolic function. The study confirmed that HF is predominantly a disease of elderly people, with a median age of first presentation of 76 years.

Incidence data for the United States are available from the Cardiovascular Health Study (CHS) showing an incidence rate of 19.3/1000 person-years in 5.5 years of follow-up.[20] Data are also available for incidence from general practice records. From the General Practice research database (GPRD) in the United Kingdom (administered by the Office of National Statistics), 696 884 potential patients aged above 45 years old were identified.[21] The records were interrogated and were categorized on the basis of records and medication prescription patterns. Using this approach, 6478 patients with definitive HF, 14 050 with possible HF, and 6076 with diuretics but a non-heart-failure diagnosis were identified. The overall incidence of definitive HF was 9.3/1000 per year, but if the possible HF group was included, the incidence increased to 20.2/1000 per year. The mean age of the definite HF population was 77 years. More recently, data from the Scottish Continuous Morbidity Recording data set showed an overall incidence of 2/1000 population per year: it was 25/1000 per year in men over the age of 85 years.[22]

The majority of epidemiological surveys have concentrated on white populations, with a bias towards relatively affluent areas of the Western world. However, data from more diverse populations are now emerging. Recent work from an elderly institutionalized population in Memphis and Pittsburgh showed some differences in incidence with race, at least in the United States. The annual incidence rate in African Americans was 1.63% and in white Americans 1.19%.[23] In addition, a recent study in a younger population of 5115 participants between 18 and 30 years old at baseline followed for 20 years from Oakland, California; Chicago, Illinois; Minneapolis, Minnesota; and Birmingham, Alabama showed a mean age of onset of HF of 39 years.[24] The cumulative incidence for black men and women respectively was 0.9% and 1.1%. There was also a high prevalence of asymptomatic echocardiographic LV systolic impairment. Rates of 9% in whites and 13% in African Americans were documented. This work highlights the need for more studies of incidence in ethnically diverse populations.

Table 3.2 Studies demonstrating incident rates of heart failure within different populations

Study	Name of study	Number of patients	Location	Age range	Mean/ median age of diagnosis (years)	Incidence of heart failure <65 years of age	Incidence of heart failure >65 years of age
McKee *et al.*, 1971	Framingham		Framingham, USA	45–94		2 per 1000 (45–54 years)	40 per 1000 (85–94 years)
Erikkson *et al.*, 1989	The men born in 1913	973	Gothenburg, Sweden	67			10 per 1000
Cowie *et al.*, 1999	Hillingdon Heart Study	151 000	Hillingdon, north-west London, UK	29–95	76	0.02 per 1000 (25–34 years) 0.2 per 1000 (35–44 years) 0.2 per 1000 (45–54 years) 1.2 per 1000 (55–64 years)	3 per 1000 (65–74 years) 7.4 per 1000 (75–84 years) 11.6 per 1000 (85–94 years)
Murphy *et al.*, 2004	GP database, Continuous Morbidity Recording scheme	307 741 (2186 cases)	Scotland, UK	45–85	–	1.3 per 1000 (45–64 years)	6.1 per 1000 (65–74) 16 per 1000 (75–84 years)
De Giuli *et al.*, 2005	GP Research Database	696 884 (6478 cases)	UK	45–101	77	3.4 per 1000 (55–64 years)	25.5 per 1000 (75–84 years)
Kalogeropoulos *et al.*, 2009	ABC Study	2934 (258)	Pittsburgh, and Memphis, Tennesee, USA	70–79	73.6		13.6 per 1000
Bibbins-Domingo *et al.*, 2009	CARDIA Study	5115(27)	Birmingham, Alabama, Chicago, Illinois, Minneapolis, Oakland, California, USA	18–30	39.1	African American male (cumulative incidence) 0.9% African American female (cumulative incidence) 1.1% White male (cumulative incidence) 0% White female (cumulative incidence) 0.08%	–

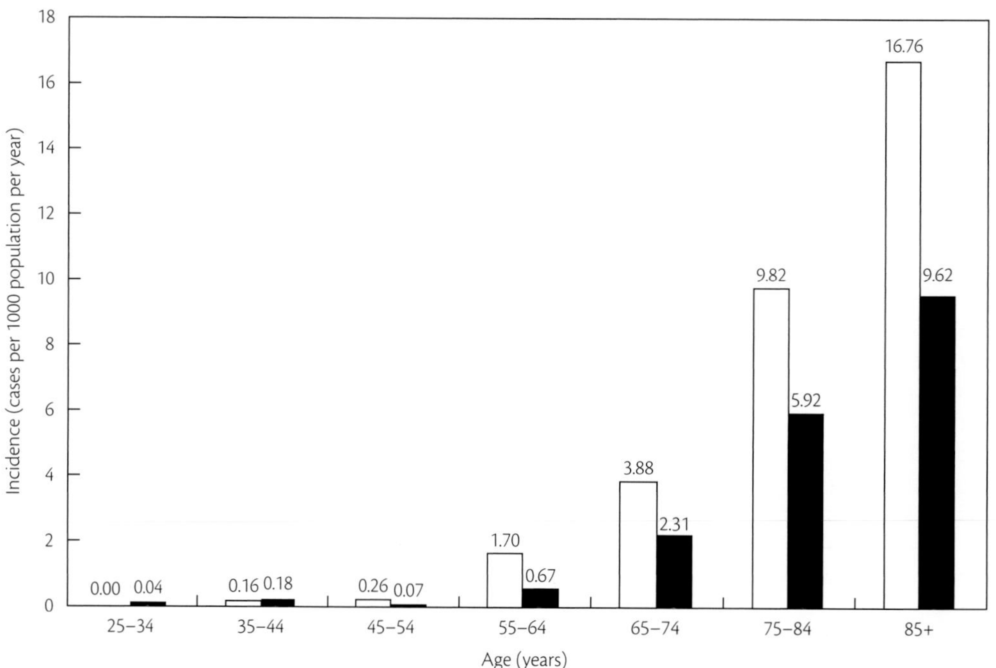

Fig. 3.4 Incidence of heart failure by sex and age group in Hillingdon Heart Failure Study.

Trends in incidence and prevalence

Data from the Framingham study has not shown any increase in incidence since the 1970s, dispelling the theory that we are experiencing an epidemic of HF. Similarly, data from Medicare records show a slight reduction in incidence from 57.5/1000 to 48.4/1000 person-years in the 80–84 year age group in the period 1994–2003. However, despite the slight reduction in incidence, the prevalence rate rose markedly from 90/1000 to 120/1000.[25] These trends will continue with the changing demography of most Western populations, with more elderly individuals and a greater number of survivors from cardiovascular disease earlier in life.

Aetiology

Determining the exact aetiology of HF in patients in epidemiological studies can be difficult. The commonest cause within the Western world currently is ischaemic heart disease (IHD), which represents a change in aetiology over time. When the Framingham study first reported, the predominant aetiological factor was hypertension. In this study, the influence of coronary heart disease has increased over time by 40% in men and 20% in women.

In the North Glasgow MONICA Study, over 95% of patients with symptomatic LV systolic dysfunction had some evidence of prior IHD, although hypertension was also common in this group, occurring in 68%. Other data from prevalence studies show similar results. In the ECHOES study, 53% of those with systolic dysfunction had evidence of IHD and 42% had hypertension; in the Helsinki Ageing Study it was 54% both for hypertension and for IHD. US data from the CHS confirm similar results with the population attributable risk for HF being 13.1%for coronary heart disease and 12.8% for hypertension. Both are clearly important aetiological factors.[20]

In the original Hillingdon study of incident HF, 41% of the HF cohort was due to coronary artery disease and much less, 6%, had hypertension.[26] A subsequent study carried out in Bromley (south London) looked into putative ischaemic aetiologies in more depth. All incident cases of HF were identified and referred to a specialist dedicated clinic or identified via tracking patients during their hospitalization. In this study 332 patients were identified and 99 of the 136 cases under the age of 75 years also underwent coronary angiography. An ischaemic aetiology was eventually attributed to 52% of the 136 cases.[27]

Hypertension as a cause of HF still seems to predominate in those with HF and normal ejection fraction, where IHD seems less prominent. Patients with HeFNEF tend to be older and are more likely to be female. Both ischaemia and hypertension are still common; a recent study by Zile showed a prevalence rate of hypertension of 82% and congestive heart disease (CHD) of 45% in patients with HeFNEF.[28]

The traditional risk factors that lead to myocardial disease have been extensively studied in predominately white populations. Increasing awareness that the same diseases may manifest and act differently in certain ethnic populations has led to some recent studies. Hypertension is a contributory factor in young African Americans below the age of 39 and results in a HF incidence 20 times the rate of whites.

South Asians seem to have a susceptibility to premature accelerated coronary artery disease.[29,30] A series of studies looking at South Asians hospitalized with HF in Leicestershire, United Kingdom and Toronto, Canada has shown that admission rates for HF were higher than in the white population, and there was more evidence of diabetes and hypertension. These findings may mean that the coronary artery disease leads to the development of HF at a younger age in a South Asian population.[31–33]

Traditionally, HF in the developing world has been viewed as a result of either infective or nutritional disease. Rheumatic heart disease is still endemic in sub-Saharan Africa.[34] However, the epidemiological data from traditional developing areas of the world is limited. Certain areas of the world which were previously viewed as 'developing' are now undergoing epidemiological transition to a more affluent, sedentary, urbanized population. This also means an epidemiological transition in terms of cardiovascular disease from infective and nutritionally based heart disease to that of atherosclerosis and progressive coronary artery disease.

Comorbidities

Because of its high prevalence within elderly populations, HF is commonly associated with numerous comorbidities, including renal impairment, anaemia, diabetes mellitus, obstructive sleep apnoea, and chronic obstructive pulmonary disease. These all have an adverse impact on survival when associated with HF.[35]

Anaemia was present in 51% of patients with HF in the Rochester Epidemiology Project. Severely impaired renal function was present in 10%. These rates are increased in patients presenting with acute HF syndromes; renal dysfunction occurred in 20% of those admitted with decompensated HF in the Euroheart Failure Survey II.[36]

Prognosis

The 32-year follow-up of the Framingham study signposted the awful mortality rate associated with HF. The probability of dying from HF was 62% for men and 42% for women at 5 years of follow-up from incident diagnosis. However, data from the Framingham study have shown consistent improvements in survival over time for both men and women.[37] In Europe, the mortality of incident HeFNEF also seems to be falling. In the initial Hillingdon study, 25% of patients were dead at 6 months, but in the more recent cohort of this study (from 2004–5), the figure had dropped to 14%.[38] The fall was independent of confounding variables and is linked to the increased usage of renin–angiotensin system inhibitors and β-blockers.

Although mortality is higher in studies of incident HF, it is also high in prevalent cases. In the ECHOES study, the 5-year survival rate was 53% for those with HF due to impaired systolic function (Fig. 3.5).[39] Survival for those with HeFNEF was a little better, at 62%. In contrast, the Mayo Clinic data showed that survival in the community with HF was similar for those with systolic and nonsystolic HeFNEF.[15] However, more recently the Mayo Clinic group reported on 4596 patients, of whom 47% had normal LVEF, between 1987 and 2001.[40] The survival rate was slightly better in the population with HeFNEF. However, the mortality rate declined in the population with systolic dysfunction during the study period, whereas patients with normal ventricular function had no change in mortality rates throughout the study period. More studies need to be done to clarify whether the mortality rates of these two types of HF do indeed differ.

The mortality rate for asymptomatic LV systolic dysfunction in the population is also high, with 21% of the population in the

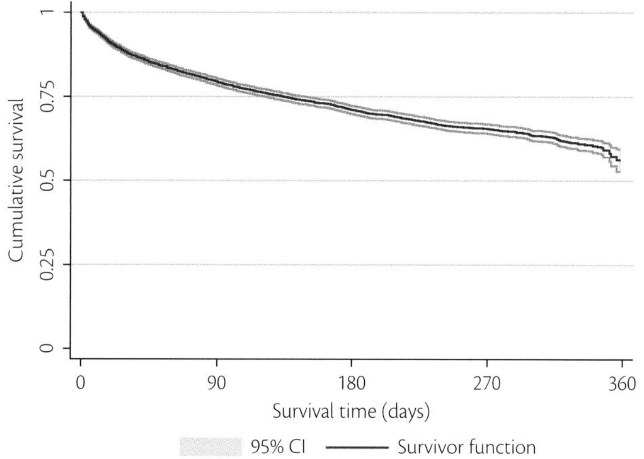

Fig. 3.5 Overall annual mortality from the ECHOES study.

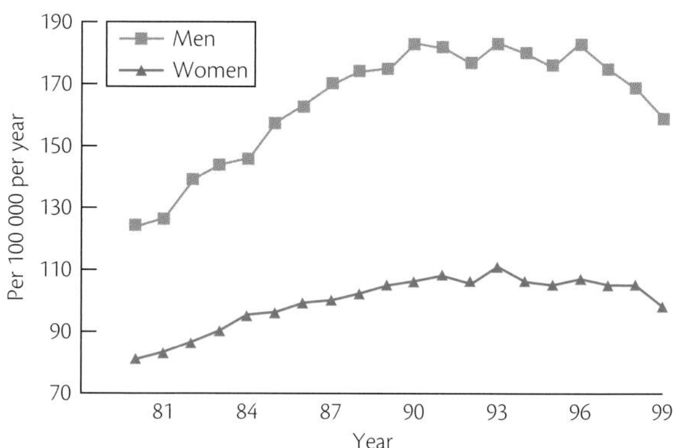

Fig. 3.7 Heart failure hospitalization rate in the Netherlands, 1980–1999.

North Glasgow MONICA cohort dead at 4 years, with no significant difference in survival between those with symptoms of HF and those with asymptomatic LV dysfunction. This finding emphasizes the need for early detection and treatment of the precursor phase of HF.

Data derived from hospitalized patients in Scotland also show a trend to towards improved survival. Between 1986 and 2003, median survival after a first admission to hospital with HF improved in men from 1.3 to 2.3 years and in women from 1.3 to 1.8 years (Fig. 3.6).[41] The poorer survival between those with acute HF syndromes requiring admission, compared to population-based surveys of prevalence is underscored by data from large European and US registries. In the EuroHeart Failure II survey, in-hospital mortality was 6.6%.[33] This varied with presentation but was nearly 40% in those presenting with cardiogenic shock. In a recent audit of acute hospital admissions within the United Kingdom results were poorer, with an in-hospital mortality of 15%.[42] In-hospital mortality in the United States is better, running at 4% in the OPTIMISE HF registry.[43]

In summary, mortality from HF remains high and the 5-year prognosis is worse than for either breast or bowel cancer.[44]

Morbidity and hospitalization

Part of the enormous morbidity incurred by HF patients relates to frequent hospitalizations. Advanced HF patients who have been hospitalized experience rehospitalization rates at 6 months of 36–45%.[45,46] In the 1990s, studies in the Netherlands, Scotland, the United States and Sweden documented increasing trends of admissions relating to HF.[47,48] The rise in hospital admissions was accompanied by increasing expenditure. In Scotland, 0.2% of the population were hospitalized per year and admissions relating to HF accounted for more than 5% of all adult general medical admissions.[49] Some evidence has now emerged that HF admissions may have peaked in certain European countries during the mid 1990s. Data from Scotland on 116 556 patients identified from hospital discharge records during the period 1986–2003 showed that rates of admission rose and peaked in the mid 1990s and subsequently fell by 2003;[38] there are similar findings from the Netherlands (Fig. 3.7).[50]

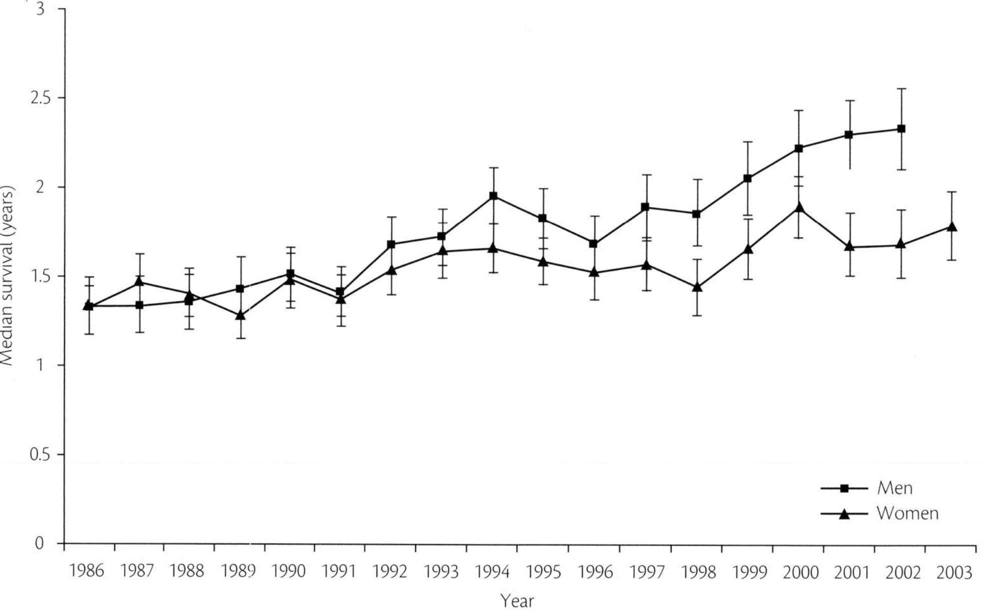

Fig. 3.6 Trends in median survival in Scotland, 1986–2003.

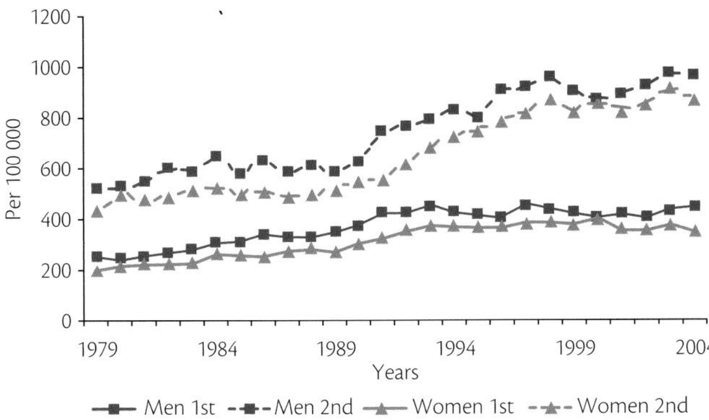

Fig. 3.8 Age-adjusted hospitalization rates for heart failure, National Discharge Survey 1979–2004.

The most recent American data, however, initially seem to contradict this finding. For the period between 1979–2004, HF admissions were recorded using the National Hospital Discharge Survey. The rate of admission tripled from 1 274 000 in 1979 to 3 860 000 in 2004 (Fig. 3.8).[51] However, lengths of stay and mortality have decreased in the United States according to data from the ADHERE registry.[42]

Health economics

Because of its high prevalence and hospitalization and rehospitalization rates, HF places a large economic burden on health care budgets. In the United States, the total expenditure on HF in 2007 was more than $33 billion (£21 billion, €24 billion).[52] The statistics are mirrored in European settings. In the United Kingdom, HF consumes 1–2% of the National Health Service budget which is approximately £1.2 billion (€1.3 billion, US$1.8 million).[53] It is the leading cause of hospitalization in the elderly population in the United Kingdom. Approximately 60% of the total expenditure within the United Kingdom on HF is spent on hospital admissions. In Europe, the situation is similar with HF consuming approximately 1% of health care budgets. The length of stay also contributes to the expense, with median hospital stay for HF in Europe being 9 days.[54] The estimates of cost are likely to be underestimates as true costs should include all primary care consultations, secondary care referrals, diagnostics, prescribing habits, further therapies including devices and care networks, and surgical intervention including transplantation.

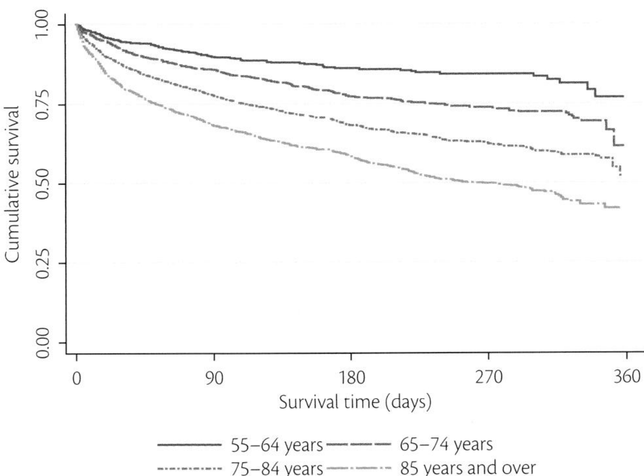

Fig. 3.9 Overall annual mortality stratified by age, from the ECHOES study.

Conclusions

Despite the advances that have been made in its treatment over the course of the last 20 years, which have seen mortality rates for those in clinical trials of HF therapies fall to less than 10% per year, epidemiological studies show that HF remains a common, lethal, disabling, and expensive condition. Its principal causes are IHD and hypertension, which often coexist. It also has a detectable asymptomatic precursor which is as prevalent as manifest HF itself. As the burden of HF increases with the ageing of our populations, we need to focus our efforts on better detection and prevention of the asymptomatic syndrome to improve its epidemiology in the future (Fig. 3.9).[39]

References

1. McKee PA, Castelli WP, McNamara PM, Kannel WB. The natural history of congestive heart failure. *N Engl J Med* 1971;**285**(26):1441–6.
2. Erikkson H, Svarsudd S, Larsson B, *et al.* Risk factors for the study of heart failure in the general population. The study of men born in 1913. *Eur Heart J* 1989;**10**:647–56.
3. Parameshwar J, Shackell MM, Richardson A, Poole-Wilson PA, Sutton GC. Prevalence of heart failure in three general practices in north-west London. *Br J Gen Prac* 1992;**42**:287.
4. Murphy NF, Simpson CR, Macalister FA, *et al.* National survey of the prevalence, incidence, primary care burden, and treatment of heart failure in Scotland. *Heart* 2004;**90**:1129–36.
5. Rutten FH, Grobee DE, Hoes AW. Diagnosis and management of heart failure: a questionnaire among general practitioners and cardiologists. *Eur J Heart Fail* 2003;**5**:345–8.
6. Remes J, Miettinen H, Reunanen A, Pyorala K. Validity of clinical diagnosis of heart failure in primary health care. *Eur Heart J* 1991;**12**:315–21.
7. Cowie MR, Struthers AD, Wood DA, *et al.* Value of natriuretic pepetides in assessment of patients with possible new heart failure in primary care. *Lancet* 1997;**350**:1349–53.
8. Dahlstrom U, Hakansson J, Swedberg K, Waldenstrom A. Adequacy of diagnosis and treatment of chronic heart failure in Sweden. *Eur J Heart Fail* 2009;**11**:92–8.
9. McDonagh TA, Morrison CE, Lawrence A, *et al.* Symptomatic and asymptomatic left ventricular systolic dysfunction in an urban population. *Lancet* 1997;**350**:829–33.
10. Davies M, Hobbs F, Davis R, *et al.* Prevalence of left-ventricular systolic dysfunction and heart failure in the Echocardiographic Heart of England Screening study: a population based study. *Lancet* 2001;**358**:439–44.
11. Senni M, Tribouilloy CM, Rodeheffer RJ, *et al.* Congestive heart failure in the community: a study of all incident cases in Olmsted County, Minnesota, in 1991. *Circulation* 1998;**98**(21):2282–9.
12. Kupari M, Lindroos M, Iivanainen AM, Heikkilä J, Tilvis R. Congestive heart failure in old age: prevalence, mechanisms, and 4 year prognosis in the Helsinki Ageing Study. *J Intern Med* 1997;**241**(5):387–94.
13. Mosterd A, Hoes AW, de Brunye DC, *et al.* Prevalence of heart failure and left ventricular dysfunction in the general population. *Eur Heart J* 1999;**20**:447–55.
14. Morgan S, Smith H, Simpson I, *et al.* Prevalence and clinical characteristics of left ventricular dysfunction among elderly patients in general practice setting: cross sectional survey. *BMJ* 1999;**318**:368–72.

15. Hogg K, Swedberg K, McMurray J. Heart failure with preserved left ventricular systolic function: epidemiology, clinical characteristics and prognosis. *J Am Coll Cardiol* 2004;**43**:317–27.
16. Ceia F, Fonseca C, Mota T, *et al.* Prevalence of chronic heart failure in Southwestern Europe. (EPICA Study). *Eur J Heart Fail* 2002;**4**:531–9.
17. Dickstein K, Cohen-Solal A, Fillipatos G, *et al.* ESC Guidelines for the diagnosis and treatment of acute and chronic heart failure. *Eur Heart J* 2008;**29**:2388–442.
18. Hunt SA, Abraham WT, Chin M, *et al.* ACC/AHA Guidelines for the diagnosis and management of chronic heart failure in the adult. *J Am Coll Cardiol* 2005;**46**:1116–43.
19. Cowie MR, Wood DA, Coats AJS, *et al.* Incidence and aetiology of heart failure: A population based study. *Eur Heart J* 1999;**20**:421–8.
20. Gottdiener JS, Arnold AM, Aurigemma GP, *et al.* Predictors of congestive heart failure in the elderly: the Cardiovascular Health Study. *J Am Coll Cardiol* 2000;**35**:1628–37.
21. De Giuli F, Khaw KT, Cowie MR, Sutton GC, Ferrari R, Poole-Wilson PA. Incidence and outcome of persons with a clinical diagnosis of heart failure in a general practice population of 696,884 in the United Kingdom. *Eur J Heart Fail* 2005;**7**:295–302.
22. Murphy NF, Simpson CR, McAlister FA, *et al.* National survey of the prevalence, incidence, primary care burden, and treatment of heart failure in Scotland. *Heart* 2004;**90**:1129–36.
23. Kalogeropoulos A, Georgiopoulou V, Kritchevsky SB, *et al.* Epidemiology of incident heart failure in a contemporary elderly population. The health, ageing & body composition study (Health ABC Study). *Arch Intern Med* 2009;**169**(7):708–15.
24. Bibbins-Domingo K, Pletcher MJ, Lin F, *et al.* Racial differences in incident heart failure in young adults. *N Engl J Med* 2009;**360**(12): 1179–90.
25. Curtis LH, Whellan DJ, Hammill BG, *et al.* Incidence and prevalence of heart failure in elderly persons, 1994–2003. *Arch Intern Med* 2008;**168**(4):418–24.
26. Parameshwar J, Poole-Wilson PA, Sutton GC. Heart failure in a district general hospital. *J Roy Coll Phys Lond* 1992;**26**(2):139–42.
27. Fox KM, Cowie MR, Wood DA, *et al.* Coronary artery disease as the cause of incident heart failure in the population. *Eur Heart J* 2001;**28**:228–36.
28. Zile MR, Baicu CF, Bonnema DD. Diastolic heart failure: definitions and terminology. *Prog Cardiovasc Dis* 2005;**47**(5):305–15.
29. Wild S, McKeigue P. Cross sectional analysis of mortality by country of birth in England and Wales, 1970–92. *BMJ* 1997;**314**:705–10.
30. Sheth T, Nair C, Nargundkar M, *et al.* Cardiovascular and cancer mortality among Canadians of European, south Asian and Chinese origin from 1979 to1993: an analysis of 1.2 million deaths. *CMAJ* 1999;**161**:132–8.
31. Blackledge HM, Newton J, Squire IB. Prognosis for South Asian and white patients newly admitted to hospital with heart failure in the United Kingdom:historical cohort study. *BMJ* 2003;**327**:526–31.
32. Newton JD, Blackledge HM, Squire IB. Ethnicity and variation in prognosis for patients newly hospitalised for heart failure: a matched historical cohort study. *Heart* 2005;**91**:1545–50.
33. Singh N, Gupta M. Clinical characteristics of South Asian patients hospitalized with heart failure. *Ethn Dis* 2005;**15**:615–19.
34. Brink AJ, Aalbers J. Strategies for heart disease in sub-Saharan Africa. *Heart* 2009;**95**(19):1559–60.
35. McMurray JJV, Pfeffer MA. Heart failure. *Lancet* 2005;**365**:1877–89.
36. Nieminen MS, Brutsaert D, Dickstein K, *et al.* EuroHeart Failure Survey II (EHFS II): a survey on hospitalized acute heart failure patients: description of population. *Eur Heart J* 2006;**27**(22):2725–36.
37. Ho KKL, Anderson KM, Kannel WB, Grossman W, Levy D. Survival after the onset of congestive heart failure in Framingham study subjects. *Circulation* 1993;**88**:107–15.
38. Mehta PA, Dubrey SW, McIntyre HF, *et al.* Improving survival in the 6 months after diagnosis of heart failure in the past decade: population based data from the UK. *Heart* 2009;**95**:1851–6.
39. Hobbs FD, Roalfe AK, Davis RC, *et al.* Prognosis of all-cause heart failure and borderline left ventricular systolic dysfunction: 5 year mortality follow-up of the Echocardiographic Heart of England Screening Study (ECHOES). *Eur Heart J* 2007;**28**(9):1128–34.
40. Owan TE, Hodge DO, Herges RM, *et al.* Trends in prevalence and outcome of heart failure with preserved ejection fraction. *N Engl J Med* 2006;**355**:251–9.
41. Jhund PS, Macintyre K, Simpson CR, *et al.* Long term trends in first hospitalization for heart failure and subsequent survival between 1986–2003. A population study of 5.1 million people. *Circulation* 2009;**119**:515–23.
42. Nicol ED, Fitall B, Roughton M, *et al.* NHS heart failure survey: a survey of heart failure admissions to England, Wales & Northern Ireland. Heart 2008;**94**:172–7.
43. Fonarow GC, Abraham WT, Albert NM, *et al.* Day of admission and clinical outcomes for patients hospitalized for heart failure: findings from the Organized Program to Initiate Lifesaving Treatment in Hospitalized Patients With Heart Failure (OPTIMIZE-HF). *Circ Heart Fail* 2008;**1**:50–7.
44. Stewart S, MacIntyre K, Hole DJ, Capewell S, McMurray JJV. More malignant than cancer? Five year survival after a first hospitalization with heart failure. *Eur J Heart Fail* 2001;**3**:315–22.
45. Fonarow GC, Heywood JT, Heidenreich PA, *et al.* Temporal trends in clinical characteristics, treatments, and outcomes for heart failure hospitalizations in 2002–2004.: findings from the ADHERE registry. *Am Heart J* 2007;**153**:1021–8.
46. O'Connor CM, Abraham WT, Albert NM, *et al.* Predictors of mortality after discharge in patients hospitalized with heart failure: an analysis from the Organized Program to Initiate Lifesaving Treatment in Hospitalized patients with heart failure. (OPTIMIZE-HF). *Am Heart J* 2008;**156**:662–73.
47. Reitsma JB, Mosterd A, de Craen AJ, *et al.* Increase in hospital admission rates for heart failure in The Netherlands, 1980–1993. *Heart* 1996;**76**:388–92.
48. Stewart S, MacIntyre K, MacLeod MM, *et al.* Trends in hospitalization for heart failure in Scotland, 1990–1996. An epidemic that has reached its peak? *Eur Heart J* 2001;**22**:209–17.
49. McMurray J, McDonagh T, Morrison CE, Dargie HJ. Trends in hospitalization in Scotland during 1980–1990. *Eur Heart J* 1993;**14**:1158–62.
50. Mosterd A, Hoes AW. Clinical epidemiology of heart failure. *Heart* 2007;**93**:1137–46.
51. Fang J, Mensah GA, Croft JB, Keenan NL. Heart failure related hospitalization in the US, 1979–2004. *J Am Coll Cardiol* 2008;**52**: 428–34.
52. Rosamond W, Flegal K, Friday G, *et al.* Heart disease and stroke statistics: 2007 update: a report from the American Heart Association Statistics Committee and Stroke Statistics Subcommittee. *Circulation* 2007;**115**:e69–171.
53. *National Heart Failure Audit 2008–2009*. NHS Information Centre, 2009.
54. Errikson H. Heart failure. A growing public health problem. *J Intern Med* 1995;**237**:135.

PART III

The aetiology of heart failure

4

The classical causes of heart failure

Roy S. Gardner and Colette E. Jackson

Introduction

Heart failure (HF) is the complex clinical syndrome that may result from a broad spectrum of structural or functional cardiac and non-cardiac diseases (see Table 4.1), often causing the classical triad of symptoms: breathlessness, fatigue, and fluid retention. It is not a single disease entity, but rather a process that may potentially complicate most forms of cardiac pathology, particularly in their final stages.

The aetiology of HF can be described in many ways. First, it can be categorized into a disorder of the myocardium, endocardium, pericardium, or great vessels. Myocardial disorders are the most common cause, and these are subdivided into those with reduced and those with normal left ventricular ejection fraction (LVEF). Reduced systolic function HF can also be classed as ischaemic or nonischaemic HF, the latter term only applied when an ischaemic cause has been excluded. Nonischaemic causes of left ventricular systolic dysfunction (LVSD) include hypertension, valvular heart disease, arrhythmias, alcohol, dilated cardiomyopathy, and peripartum cardiomyopathy.

The 'classical causes' are the common cardiovascular conditions that result in HF. These exhibit geographical variation and depend on the population being studied. In Western countries, coronary heart disease (CHD) and hypertension are the commonest causes of HF.[1] However, valvular heart disease (particularly degenerative), arrhythmias, and alcohol are also frequently implicated. In Africans and African Americans, hypertension is an important precursor of HF,[2] and HF secondary to Chagas' disease is well recognized in South America.[3] In developing countries, HF more commonly develops as a result of rheumatic valvular heart disease and nutritional deficiencies.[4]

The prevalence of 'classical causes' of HF in the largest contemporary clinical trials and registries is shown in Table 4.2.[5–20] Whilst clinical trials often contain highly selective cohorts of patients, with reduced systolic function only, the large registries consistently demonstrate similar prevalences of the common aetiologies. Thus, the prevalence of the common causes of heart failure in real-life heart failure populations can be extrapolated from these studies, with coronary heart disease being the major cause in approximately two-thirds of patients. However, this has not always been the case. The original Framingham Heart Study, one of the earliest cardiovascular epidemiological studies, recorded hypertension as the most common cause of HF.[21] During the subsequent decades of follow-up, the proportion of cases of HF attributable to hypertension and valvular heart disease decreased, and those secondary to coronary artery disease rose (Fig. 4.1). The changing aetiology of HF in recent decades is multifactorial. Improvements in survival post myocardial infarction[22] and wider availability of techniques for diagnosing coronary artery disease are plausible reasons for the increasing prevalence of HF secondary to CHD. The declining role of hypertension as the primary cause of HF may be explained by advances in antihypertensive therapy preventing longer-term complications.[23]

At present, genetic and mitochondrial abnormalities are thought to be less frequent causes of HF, although increasingly it is apparent that many forms of 'idiopathic' dilated cardiomyopathy have a familial link. HF may also result from less common aetiologies, such as metabolic conditions, infiltrative processes, infective conditions, and iatrogenic causes. These rarer causes will be addressed in subsequent chapters of this section. The rest of this chapter will focus on the 'classical' causes of HF in Western countries.

The importance of establishing an aetiology

The appropriate management of the HF patients relies on establishing its aetiology, particularly with regard to the selection of investigations and the most suitable treatment strategies. Many of the robust evidence-based therapies available for the treatment of HF are derived from cohorts of patients with specific causes of HF. Determining the cause of HF, and identifying potential secondary contributing factors, is also important for targeting ways to avoid future episodes of acute decompensation. Examples of this include addressing risk factors for myocardial infarction and enrolling patients with alcoholic cardiomyopathy in rehabilitation programmes to attempt to alleviate their addiction. Identifying the genetic abnormality in familial conditions is also important, as it may give prognostic information as well as having an impact on

Table 4.1 Causes of heart failure and the common modes of presentation

Cause	Examples of presentations
CHD	Myocardial infarction Chronic ischaemia Arrhythmias
Hypertension	Heart failure with preserved systolic function 'Burnt out' hypertensive cardiomyopathy Malignant hypertension/acute pulmonary oedema
Valve disease	Primary valvular disease e.g. endocarditis Secondary valvular disease e.g. functional regurgitation Congenital valvular disease
Arrhythmias	Incessant atrial arrhythmias Ventricular arrhythmias
Dilated cardiomyopathy	Idiopathic Inherited (familial) Peripartum Toxins: alcohol, cocaine, iron, copper
Congenital heart disease	Corrected transposition of great arteries Repaired tetralogy of Fallot Ebstein's anomaly
Infective	Viral myocarditis Chagas' disease HIV Lyme disease
Iatrogenic	Anthracyclines Abstruzimab
Infiltrative	Amyloid Sarcoid Neoplastic
Storage disorders	Haemochromatosis Fabry's disease Glycogen storage diseases
Endomyocardial disease	Radiotherapy Endomyocardial fibrosis Carcinoid
Pericardial disease	Calcification Infiltrative
Metabolic	Endocrine disease Nutritional disease (thiamine deficiency, selenium deficiency) Autoimmune disease
Neuromuscular disease	Friedreich's ataxia Muscular dystrophy
High-output	Anaemia Thyrotoxicosis A-V fistulae Paget's disease

the lives of other members of an individual patient's family. Finally, establishing the cause of HF can be curative. An example of this is radiofrequency ablation (RFA) for tachycardiomyopathy.

Challenge of attributing aetiology

Although establishing the aetiology of HF is important, it is often challenging for the clinician. Several causes of HF frequently coexist and determining the primary aetiology can be difficult: one cause may obviously dominate, but commonly a patient may have multiple contributing causes. An example of this is the hypertensive diabetic patient with confirmed coronary artery disease on angiography who consumes excess alcohol. Secondary causes may contribute to the progression of HF and may be the primary reason for episodes of acute decompensation, although not the original primary cause of HF.

Coronary artery disease can be challenging to attribute as the primary cause of HF. Although coronary angiography may reveal the presence of atherosclerotic disease, this does not confirm an ischaemic cause for any cardiac dysfunction. Conversely, a myocardial infarction may result from plaque rupture in the context of otherwise unobstructed coronary arteries. Cardiac magnetic resonance imaging (CMR) can help to clarify the underlying diagnosis by characterizing the myocardium, with late gadolinium-enhanced images useful in identifying areas of previous myocardial infarction. In the absence of a definite clinical myocardial infarction, or evidence of such from coronary angiography/CMR, coronary artery disease can only be suspected as a possible cause of HF.

A further challenge in accurately ascribing the primary aetiology of HF may be when the condition is no longer present. Patients with HF secondary to long-standing hypertension may have normal or low blood pressure at the time of their HF presentation. A subset of patients with hypertrophic cardiomyopathy develop progressive left ventricular dilation with systolic dysfunction and thinning of the previously hypertrophied myocardium. This condition is often referred to as 'burnt out' hypertrophic cardiomyopathy and patients presenting at this stage of the disease may be incorrectly diagnosed as having primary dilated cardiomyopathy.

Coronary heart disease

Coronary artery disease is the commonest cause of HF in the Western world (Table 4.2). It may present in several different ways; acute myocardial infarction, chronic ischaemia, arrhythmia, and asymptomatic (occult) disease.

Acute physiological responses

An acute myocardial infarction initiates acute physiological mechanisms–the same processes that are used to enhance cardiac output in normal circumstances.[24] Activation of the sympathetic nervous system causes an increase in heart rate and cardiac output. Activation of systemic neurohumoral pathways leads to increases in circulating volume, enhancing venous return, and the effective maintenance of preload. Ultimately, these pathways act to preserve cardiac output via the Frank–Starling mechanism. Other physiological changes following myocardial infarction include systemic vasoconstriction, which maintains blood pressure at the expense of increasing the workload of the heart by increasing afterload. Often the outcome of the adaptive responses is the maintenance of normal cardiac output at rest but reduced reserve for any further demands in cardiac output. The consequence clinically is a reduction in exercise capacity and symptoms of HF on exertion for some patients. However, initially, many patients remain asymptomatic in response to these compensatory adjustments.[24]

Chronic remodelling and progressive cardiac injury

After myocardial infarction, cardiac structure changes occur in parallel with, and are linked to, physiological changes in activated

Table 4.2 Aetiology of heart failure in contemporary randomized clinical trials and major registries

Study	RCT/ REG	Size	Age[a]	Male (%)	Ischaemic (%)	Nonischaemic (%)	HT (%)	IDCM (%)	Valve[b] (%)	Other (%)	Unknown (%)
SOLVD[5]	RCT	2569	61	80	71	–	–	18	–	–	–
DIG[6]	RCT	6800	64	78	70	30	9	15	–	6	–
MERIT-HF[7]	RCT	3991	64	78	66	34	–	–	–	–	–
CIBIS-II[8]	RCT	2647	61	81	50	–	–	12	–	–	38
ATLAS[9]	RCT	3192	64	79	64	35	20	28	–	6	–
RALES[10]	RCT	1663	65	73	54	46	–	–	–	–	–
Val-HeFT[11]	RCT	5010	62	80	57	–	7	31	–	5	–
COPERNICUS[12]	RCT	2289	63	80	67	–	–	–	–	–	–
COMET[13]	RCT	3029	62	80	53	–	18	–	–	–	–
COMPANION[14]	RCT	1520	67	68	56	44	–	–	–	–	–
CARE-HF[15]	RCT	813	67	73	38	–	–	–	–	–	62
GISSI-HF[16]	RCT	4574	68	77	40	–	18	34	–	3	5
SOLVD[17]	REG	6273	62	74	69	31	7	13	–	11	–
SPICE[18]	REG	9580	66	74	63	–	4	17	5	–	6
ADHERE[19]	REG	105 388	72	48	57	–	–	–	–	–	–
OPTIMIZE-HF[20]	REG	48 612	73	48	46	–	23	–	–	–	–

HT, hypertension; IDCM, idiopathic dilated cardiomyopathy; RCT, randomized clinical trial; REG, registry.
[a] Mean age in years.
[b] Valvular heart failure.

neurohormonal systems. Activation of the sympathetic nervous system and renin–angiotensin–aldosterone system (RAAS) lead to the release of cytokines and growth factors that stimulate structural alterations at the cellular and extracellular level. The alterations include cardiac myocyte hypertrophy and extracellular matrix changes which lead to regional alterations in ventricular wall and chamber sizes in order to preserve cardiac output.[25]

Although initially protective, compensatory mechanisms that maintain cardiac output may ultimately be deleterious. Chronic activation of compensatory neurohormonal processes can lead to the development of HF in the absence of any further ischaemic injury.[26]

Chronic catecholamine secretion promotes myocyte hypertrophy and interstitial fibrosis.[27] It also interferes with inter- and intracellular signalling pathways by inducing down-regulation of adrenoreceptors and causing hyperphosphorylation of intracellular proteins. The consequence is hindrance of the ability of the adrenergic compensatory mechanisms to maintain cardiac output during future times of acute haemodynamic stress. Sympathetic nervous system activation also leads to further myocardial dysfunction by inducing the transcription of fetal genes and inducing cardiac myocyte death by promoting apoptosis and necrosis (see Chapter 12).

Chronic activation of the renin–angiotensin–aldosterone system occurs in response to a variety of triggers including renal hypoperfusion, myocardial production of angiotensin and aldosterone in response to increased wall stress, and sympathetic nervous system activation stimulating renal renin release[28]. Although activation

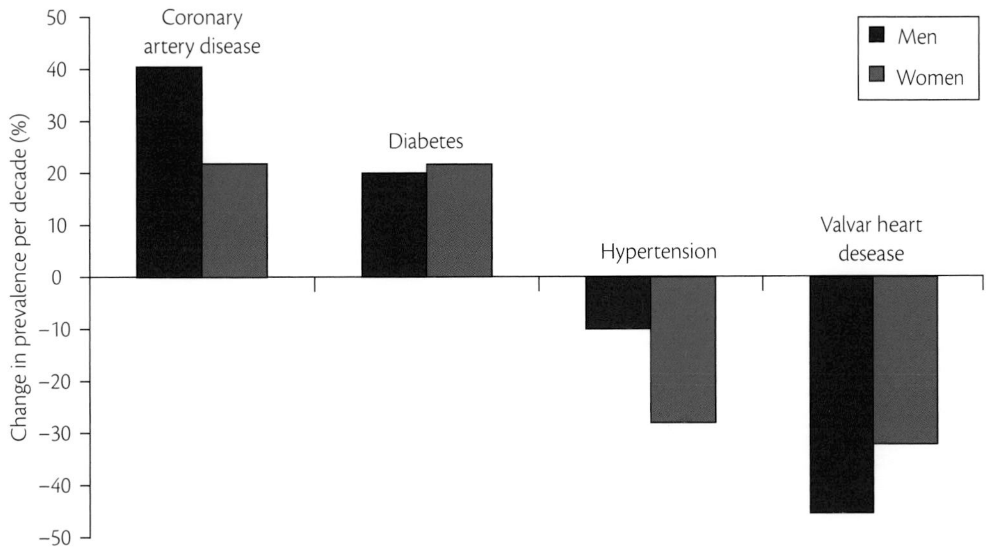

Fig. 4.1 The changing pattern of aetiology of CHF in the Framingham study with time.
From McMurray JJ, Stewart S. Epidemiology, aetiology, and prognosis of heart failure. *Heart* 2000;**83**:596–602.

of the RAAS maintains blood pressure and enhances preload by stimulating vasoconstriction and renal sodium retention, harmful consequences arise from the effects of angiotensin and aldosterone on cardiac myocytes. These effects include enhancing myocardial fibrosis by promoting collagen deposition, cardiac myocyte hypertrophy, and cellular apoptosis and necrosis.

Ultimately, chronic activation of the compensatory response damages cardiac structure and function.[24] Structural changes lead to ventricular dilatation, and the heart remodels to a more globular shape (Fig. 4.2), thereby altering atrioventricular valvular function, resulting in functional regurgitation and an increase in ventricular preload. A vicious cycle ensues. Furthermore, increases in cardiac load which increase myocardial oxygen requirements may precipitate subendocardial ischaemia, exacerbating further reductions in cardiac contractility.

Acute complications post myocardial infarction

Acute myocardial infarction may cause acute HF. Particular complications include acute mitral valve incompetence secondary to papillary muscle rupture, hibernation and stunning of the left ventricle, ventricular septal rupture, ventricular free wall rupture, right ventricular infarct syndrome, and cardiogenic shock.

Cardiogenic shock usually results from severe cardiac dysfunction, although the acute mechanical complications of myocardial infarction may contribute. It is defined as evidence of end-organ hypoperfusion and characterized by reduced blood pressure (systolic <90 mmHg) with raised ventricular filling pressure (pulmonary capillary wedge pressure >18 mmHg) and low cardiac output.[29]

Acute HF due to stunning or hibernation may completely return to normal when appropriately treated.[30] Stunning may occur following a prolonged ischaemic episode and can persist in the short term even after restoration of normal coronary blood flow. The amount and duration of stunning depends on the severity and duration of the preceding ischaemic event. Hibernation describes the state when cardiomyocytes fail to contract normally but remain structurally intact despite a significant reduction in coronary blood flow. Improving blood flow and oxygenation allows hibernating myocytes to return to normal function.

Hypertensive heart disease

Hypertension affects around one-quarter of the population of the Western world. It is an important cause of chronic HF in Western societies,[1,4] and remains the most common cause in developing countries.[31] It is particularly prevalent in Africans and African Americans.[2,32] Hypertension is proportionately more common in patients with HF and normal LVEF.[33]

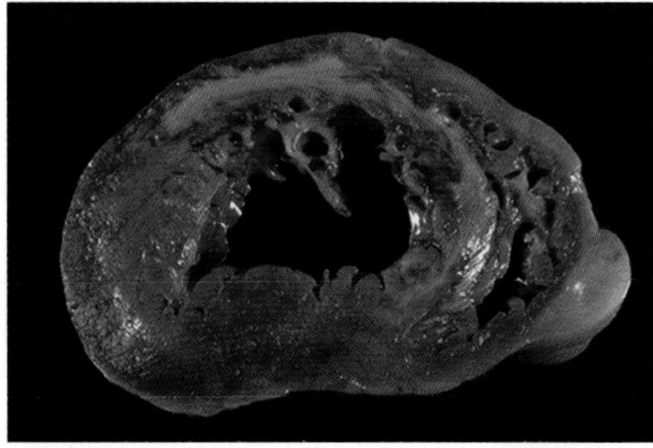

Fig. 4.2 The gross pathological appearance of myocardial infarction at post-mortem.

Hypertension leads to an increase in afterload which consequently leads to concentric left ventricular hypertrophy (Fig. 4.3). This compensatory mechanism preserves contractile function by recruiting additional sarcomere units of the muscle fibres to share the additional ventricular wall tension generated by the increased afterload, enabling higher forces and greater pressures to be generated.[34] The more hypertrophied the ventricular wall, the less tension experienced by each individual muscle fibre and consequently systolic function is not initially compromised. However, with progressive hypertrophy the compliance of the left ventricle reduces, producing a 'stiff' ventricle. This interferes with ventricular filling, leading to a reduction in end-diastolic volumes and increase in left ventricular end-diastolic pressure (LVEDP). Rises in LVEDP lead to increased left atrial and pulmonary venous pressures. A consequence may be atrial arrhythmias and reduced exercise tolerance.

As left ventricular hypertrophy progresses, sarcomeres are added in parallel to established sarcomeres, leading to ventricular dilatation and systolic dysfunction. The progression from left ventricular hypertrophy to HF is complex, involving multiple pathophysiological processes including altered cellular signalling processes, myocyte apoptosis and increased collagen deposition.[35] As progressive pump failure develops, blood pressure may normalize, known as 'burnt out' hypertensive HF.

Malignant hypertension is an important cause of acute HF.[36] Malignant hypertension is the sudden development of severe high blood pressure with diastolic measurements often in excess of 130 mmHg. Characteristics of this condition include fundal changes (retinal haemorrhages, exudates, and papilloedema), central nervous system involvement (headache, confusion, seizures, and coma) and renal impairment (oliguria and uraemia). Malignant hypertension may present as 'flash pulmonary oedema' with very rapid onset of symptoms and signs. Flash pulmonary oedema is often seen in patients with normal LVEF. Malignant hypertension affects almost 1% of all people with essential hypertension[36] and is more common in younger adults (particularly those with secondary hypertension) and African American men.[35,36] Although any cause of secondary hypertension may be a precursor to malignant hypertension, recurrent episodes of flash pulmonary oedema in the presence of significant hypertension is a classic presentation of renal artery stenosis. Other causes include phaeochromocytoma and Conn's syndrome.[36]

Valvular heart disease

Valvular dysfunction can be a cause (primary) or effect (secondary) of HF, with acquired valvular heart disease accounting for the majority of cases. There is a geographical variation in valvular pathology; for example, rheumatic valvular heart disease is a common cause of HF in the developing world.[4]

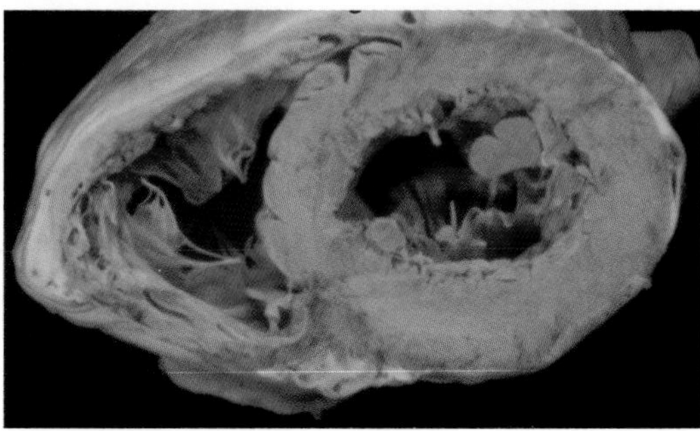

Fig. 4.3 The gross pathological appearance of concentric left ventricular hypertrophy at post-mortem.

Primary valvular pathology causing heart failure

Aortic valve disease

Aortic stenosis and regurgitation are common causes of valvular disease. Both can have long latent asymptomatic stages but progression in severity will ultimately lead to HF if left untreated.

Aortic stenosis is the most common valvular heart disease in developed countries and a frequent cause of HF internationally.[38] The three main causes are congenital, rheumatic, and degenerative. Degenerative aortic stenosis is more common in Western societies and tends to present in elderly populations (Fig. 4.4), and as a result, the prevalence of this valvular pathology is increasing as the average life expectancy increases.[38] A chronic inflammatory process involving deposition of lipids in the valve leaflets is followed by calcification of the valve annulus and subsequently the valve leaflets, limiting the circulatory flow across the aortic valve.[39,40] Rheumatic aortic valve disease is more common in developing countries[38] and leads to stenosis by causing inflammatory mediated fusion of the commissures and a reduction in the valve orifice area. Aortic stenosis causes HF by obstructing left ventricular outflow, resulting in an increased afterload, lower stroke volume, and reduced ejection fraction, with advanced disease suspected by the presence of symptoms. The severity of aortic stenosis is best assessed by calculating valve orifice area and using dobutamine stress echocardiography.[41]

Aortic regurgitation may be acute or chronic. Acute severe aortic regurgitation (e.g. secondary to infective endocarditis, aortic dissection, or trauma) is potentially life threatening by causing extremely elevated left ventricular filling pressures, severe pulmonary oedema, and inadequate cardiac output.[42] Chronic aortic regurgitation shares the same three main causes as aortic stenosis–congenital, rheumatic, and degenerative. Other less common causes include infective endocarditis, connective tissue or inflammatory diseases, antiphospholipid syndrome, anorectic drugs, and trauma.[43] Untreated, chronic aortic regurgitation slowly progresses from volume overload and left ventricular hypertrophy to left ventricular dilatation, then contractile dysfunction.[43] Patients are often asymptomatic in the early stages of this disease and may remain so after the left ventricle has begun to dilate. LVSD is potentially reversible if valve repair/replacement is undertaken soon after the onset of contractile dysfunction.

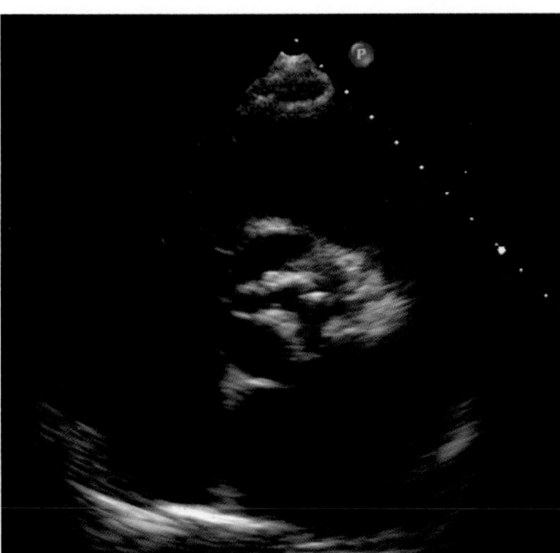

Fig. 4.4 Short axis parasternal view on transthoracic echocardiogram showing a calcified tricuspid aortic valve.

Mitral valve disease

Mitral regurgitation may be caused by primary (e.g. rheumatic heart disease, infective endocarditis, mitral valve prolapse, and connective tissue disease) or secondary valve disease.[44] Most patients with mitral regurgitation have a slow, insidious progression of their valve disease. Many are asymptomatic in the early stage, although the presentation may be more acute in cases of infective endocarditis. Progression to severe mitral regurgitation usually results in the development of symptoms of left-sided HF and pathophysiological consequences of left ventricular remodelling, left ventricular dysfunction, and pulmonary hypertension.[44] Sudden symptomatic deterioration is often seen with the subsequent development of atrial fibrillation secondary to left atrial dilatation.

Mitral stenosis is a primary valve disease, most commonly caused by rheumatic fever and persistent inflammatory valve disease in developing countries, and by degenerative disease with calcification of the annulus in developed countries.[45] As with mitral regurgitation, the early stages of this valve disease may be asymptomatic. As the severity of the stenosis progresses, a series of pathological changes ensues ultimately leading to a rise in left atrial pressure with dilatation of the atrium and consequently development of pulmonary hypertension,[45] leading to symptoms of exertional breathlessness. Left ventricular systolic function is usually preserved in severe mitral stenosis.

Tricuspid valve disease

Tricuspid stenosis is a more prevalent valvular pathology in developing countries, as the vast majority of cases are caused by rheumatic heart disease,[46] and usually coexists with mitral stenosis. The main causes of solitary tricuspid stenosis are congenital heart disease and carcinoid syndrome.[46,47] Tricuspid stenosis may be detected by the auscultation of a diastolic murmur, loudest in inspiration. Clinical signs of HF are those of right HF.

Tricuspid regurgitation is most commonly functional. However, primary tricuspid regurgitation may be caused by infective endocarditis (particularly in intravenous drug users), or rheumatic valve disease, as well as carcinoid syndrome.[48] Symptoms and signs of tricuspid regurgitation are those of right-sided HF with a classic pansystolic murmur accentuated by inspiration.

Pulmonary valve disease

Pulmonary stenosis is exclusively a form of congenital heart disease. Most cases of pulmonary regurgitation also occur in patients with congenital heart disease, the causes of which are outlined below. Acquired cases of pulmonary regurgitation are rare and include infective endocarditis or carcinoid syndrome.

Secondary valvular dysfunction causing heart failure

Valvular dysfunction may be the consequence of many other causes of HF. Any cause of left ventricular dilation can result in regurgitation of the aortic, mitral, and tricuspid valves, known as functional regurgitation: the valve dysfunction is related to abnormal ventricular shape and function. Functional mitral regurgitation is common in ischaemic cardiomyopathy, where dilatation of the valve annulus prevents coaptation of the valve leaflets[49] (Fig. 4.5). Secondary mitral valve dysfunction can also result from failure of the valve apparatus following acute myocardial infarction if there is rupture or stretching of the chordae or papillary muscle,[49] often presenting with the sudden onset of pulmonary oedema. Functional tricuspid regurgitation may be caused by several pathologies including; right ventricular dysfunction, left-sided valvular disease

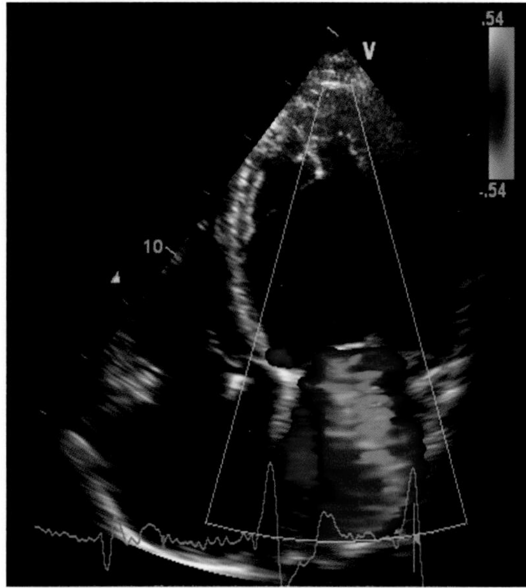

Fig. 4.5 Four-chamber apical view on transthoracic echocardiogram showing a jet of severe mitral regurgitation.

causing pulmonary hypertension, left ventricular dysfunction, or chronic pulmonary disease.[48]

Adult congenital valvular heart disease

A detailed account of congenital heart disease as a cause of HF is given in Chapter 7. A brief summary of congenital valve disease follows.

Pulmonary valve disease is usually congenital and detected early in childhood. Pulmonary stenosis may occur as an isolated congenital abnormality or as a feature of Noonan's syndrome or tetralogy of Fallot.[50] The symptomatic presentation is usually breathlessness with chronic progression to right HF.

Clinically significant pulmonary regurgitation occurs almost exclusively in patients with congenital heart disease. It may be a long-term complication of the repair of tetralogy of Fallot[51] and occur secondary to transannular patching, commissurotomy of the pulmonary valve, or failure of a pulmonary conduit. Progression in the severity of pulmonary regurgitation leads to right ventricular dilatation and subsequent right ventricular systolic dysfunction, reduced exercise tolerance and ventricular arrhythmias.[51] Sudden death may be a sequela of this condition.

Congenital tricuspid valve disease most commonly occurs as part of Ebstein's anomaly,[52] a condition characterized by apical displacement of the septal and posterior valve leaflets, leading to atrialization of a portion of the right ventricle. The structural deformity of the valve leads to tricuspid regurgitation and, although often detected in childhood, Ebstein's anomaly may present in adulthood with symptoms of fatigue, exercise intolerance, palpitations, and dyspnoea. Signs include cyanosis, a tricuspid regurgitant murmur, and right-sided HF. Arrhythmias are common, with supraventricular tachycardias occurring in approximately one-third. Ventricular arrhythmias are due to the presence of accessory pathways and sudden death may occur.

Arrhythmias

Arrhythmias are common in patients with HF, and may be either a cause or a consequence of it. Defining the cause and effect relationship can be difficult, particularly when tachycardia and cardiomyopathy present at the same time. HF predisposes to arrhythmias due to structural and electrical remodelling (see Chapter 36).

Sustained tachycardias may lead to HF (a tachycardiomyopathy, or tachycardia-related cardiomyopathy). Tachycardiomyopathy is systolic or diastolic (or both) dysfunction that usually results in ventricular dilatation and HF, and is caused by an uncontrolled ventricular rate.[53] Tachyarrhythmias may lead to a reduction in LVEF, an increase in end-diastolic and end-systolic volumes, and an increase in end-diastolic and pulmonary artery pressures. The degree of LVSD does not necessarily correlate with the duration or rate of the tachycardia.[54] Making the diagnosis is crucial, as treatment can be potentially curative (Fig. 4.6).[55–57]

The most common causes of tachycardiomyopathy are incessant atrial arrhythmias. The cardiomyopathy and tachycardia often present simultaneously. Potential causes include atrial tachycardias, reentrant tachycardias, and atrial fibrillation (AF).[58]

Atrial fibrillation is common in HF, with each condition predisposing to the other.[59] Some 10–50% of patients with LVSD have AF,[60] although AF is also common in patients with HF and normal LVEF.[61] Haemodynamic disturbances associated with AF include the loss of atrial contraction (and subsequent contribution to ventricular filling), an irregular and often uncontrolled ventricular rhythm, and activation of the deleterious neurohumoral systems. These all contribute to a reduction in cardiac output.[62]

Ventricular tachyarrhythmias are also common in chronic HF (see Chapter 36). Although more commonly a consequence of HF, ventricular tachycardia can potentially cause a tachycardiomyopathy if there are frequent paroxysms or the tachycardia is incessant.[63] The likely focus of ventricular tachycardia that is stable enough to cause a tachycardiomyopathy is the right ventricular outflow tract.[64] This form of ventricular tachycardia is recognized by the pattern of left bundle branch block with an inferior axis. Recognition is extremely important as it can be potentially cured by RFA.[64]

Alcohol

Alcohol excess is one of the commonest causes of a dilated cardiomyopathy and accounts for at least one-third of all cases.[65] There are no pathognomonic signs or specific tests for diagnosing alcoholic cardiomyopathy. It is impossible to differentiate it pathologically from other causes of dilated cardiomyopathy, and nonspecific pathological findings include interstitial fibrosis, myocytolysis, small-vessel coronary artery disease, and myocyte hypertrophy.[65] The diagnosis depends on a history of excessive alcohol consumption and the absence of other causes of cardiomyopathy. Two distinct phases and modes of clinical presentation of alcoholic heart disease are recognized: asymptomatic and symptomatic. The latter may be further divided into acute and chronic stages. Consumption of more than 90 g of alcohol per day for at least 5 years increases the risk of asymptomatic alcoholic cardiomyopathy.[64,65] The asymptomatic phase is often associated with diastolic dysfunction, whereas continual consumption of excess alcohol increases the risk of developing symptomatic HF which is frequently associated with LVSD (Fig. 4.7).[65] Importantly, in contrast with many other causes of cardiomyopathy, disease progression can be terminated or even reversed by complete abstinence from alcohol. However, the prognosis for patients with alcoholic cardiomyopathy who continue to consume excess alcohol is poor.[67]

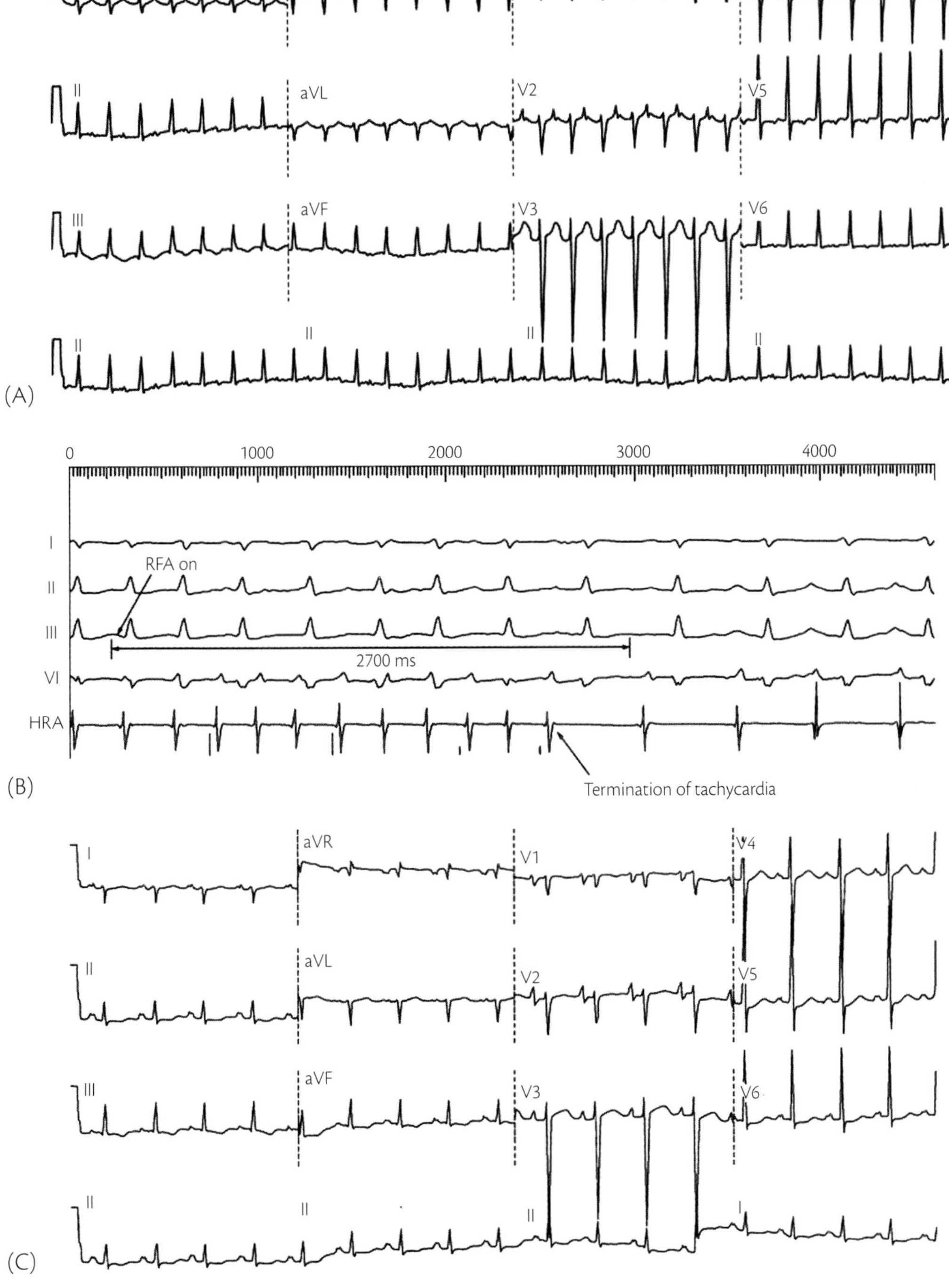

Fig. 4.6 ECG on admission for patient with tachycardiomyopathy (A). Electrophysiological studies subsequently demonstrated an incessant right atrial tachycardia (B). Echocardiography showed a dilated, poorly contracting left ventricle. Radiofrequency ablation (RFA) was curative for the atrial tachycardia and resulted in restoration of normal ventricular size and a significant improvement in ventricular function. ECG post RFA is displayed (C).
From Walker NL, Cobbe SM, Birnie DH. Tachycardiomyopathy: a diagnosis not to be missed. *Heart* 2004;**90**:e7.

Alcohol and its metabolites have direct toxic effects on cardiac myocytes, including disruption of: calcium transport and binding, mitochondrial respiration, lipid metabolism, myocardial protein synthesis, and cellular signal transduction[68] as well as apoptosis[64]. Alcohol excess may have other indirect toxic effects on the myocardium such as those derived from nutritional deficiencies (e.g. vitamin B_1 deficiency). Myocardial impairment due to cobalt sulphate (used as an additive) no longer occurs as this substance is no longer used in beer manufacturing.

Symptomatic alcoholic cardiomyopathy may present with any of the symptoms or signs of dilated cardiomyopathy of any aetiology, either as acute pulmonary oedema or more commonly with chronic HF. AF is a frequent finding in alcoholic cardiomyopathy (more so than other arrhythmias), and a paroxysm of AF is a common initial presenting sign. Stigmata of chronic liver disease may also be evident.

Approximately one-third of all alcoholics have evidence of LVSD. However, not all alcoholics develop a dilated cardiomyopathy and the reason for this is likely to be multifactorial. There is a genetic predisposition to alcohol cardiomyopathy. The DD genotype of the angiotensin converting enzyme (ACE) gene polymorphism increases the risk of developing cardiomyopathy by 16 times in those who consume excess alcohol.[69]

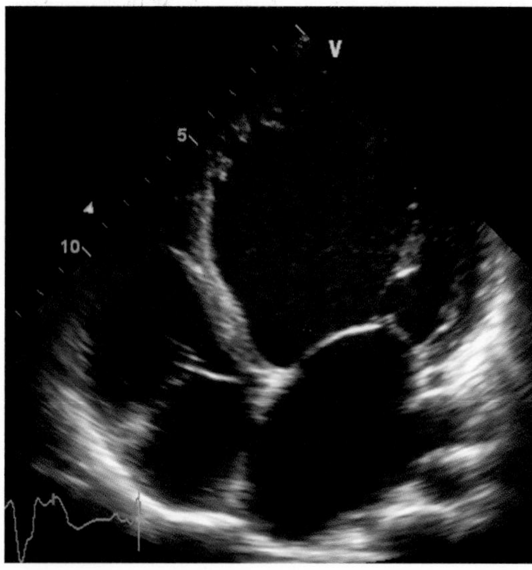

Fig. 4.7 Four-chamber apical view on transthoracic echocardiogram showing a dilated cardiomyopathy in a 40-year-old alcoholic.

Peripartum cardiomyopathy

Peripartum cardiomyopathy (PPCM) is a rare but devastating complication of pregnancy, associated with heart failure, malignant arrhythmias, thromboembolism, and death. Until recently it was defined as heart failure due to LV systolic dysfunction occurring between the last month of pregnancy and five months postpartum in women with no pre-existing heart disease.[70] However, a recent position statement by the working group on PPCM of the Heart Failure Association of the European Society of Cardiology proposed a more simplified definition with time constraints removed: 'Peripartum cardiomyopathy is an idiopathic cardiomyopathy presenting with HF secondary to left ventricular (LV) systolic dysfunction towards the end of pregnancy or in the months following delivery, where no other cause of HF is found. It is a diagnosis of exclusion. The LV may not be dilated but the ejection fraction (EF) is nearly always reduced below 45%'.[71]

Relatively little is known about the incidence and prevalence of PPCM, and the pathogenesis is also poorly understood. Multiple causes have been proposed, including myocarditis, auto-immune disease, oxidative stress, and the uncovering of existing cardiac disease by the haemodynamic stresses of pregnancy. Although definitive evidence for a disease-specific culprit is lacking, there is considerable interest in the putative role of the shorter 16-kDa form of prolactin in the progression of PPCM.[72]

Presentation and diagnosis

The clinical presentation of PPCM is very variable, from exertional dyspnoea and peripheral oedema to cardiogenic shock. Cases that present in the prepartum period are typically delayed because symptoms of worsening dyspnoea and ankle oedema are frequently attributed to the pregnant state itself. Common complications of PPCM include malignant arrhythmias and mural thrombus formation, as well as both systemic and pulmonary thromboembolism.

The diagnosis of PPCM is currently one of exclusion[70–71] that requires both the clinical confirmation of symptoms and signs of heart failure and objective evidence of LV systolic dysfunction. The electrocardiogram may be normal or display non-specific ST or T wave abnormalities and the chest radiograph may display cardiomegaly with varying degrees of pulmonary venous congestion. However, in some younger patients clinical and radiographic evidence of congestion may be absent whilst the pulmonary wedge pressure is high.

Prognosis and predictors of outcome

Studies of varying sizes and populations have reported mortality rates ranging from 0-30%,[73–76] and full recovery in 23-66% in patients on contemporary therapy.[74–77] Predictors of an adverse prognosis include increasing maternal age,[73] higher parity,[78] later onset of symptoms following delivery,[78] non-caucasian,[73, 79] and a delay in diagnosis.[79] Various echocardiographic parameters have been associated with poorer outcome including reduced LVEF,[76, 79] increased LVEDD,[73, 78, 80] reduced fractional shortening,[80] and presence of LV thrombus.[73] More recently, NT-proBNP,[77] Fas/APO-1,[75] and troponin T (cTnT)[81] have been shown to predict patients whose LV function subsequently fails to improve.

There are few data describing the outcome for subsequent pregnancies in PPCM, but there is a higher reported incidence of HF in those with previous PPCM compared to mothers with no previous history of PPCM. Varying incidences of recurrence of LV dysfunction and heart failure as well as mortality have been reported.[81–83] Therefore women with PPCM who previously presented with LV ejection fraction of <25%, or in whom LV function has not recovered completely, should be advised against future pregnancy.[71]

Treatment

The management of PPCM should reflect the clinical presentation. Patients should be managed in a specialist heart failure unit with multidisciplinary input from a team that includes a cardiologist, cardiac anaesthetist, obstetrician, and neonatologist. Emergency delivery of the baby should be an early aim when PPCM is diagnosed prenatally.[71] Where possible, patients should be established on standard disease-modifying therapy, but advanced treatments including intra-aortic balloon pump, ventricular assist devices (as bridge to recovery, or bridge to transplantation) and transplantation are occasionally necessary.[71]

In Murine models of enhanced oxidative stress, the increased expression and activity of cathepsin-D led to an increase in the 16kDa fragment of prolactin. This possesses vasoconstrictor, anti-angiogenic, and pro-inflammatory apoptotic properties, and resulted in a dilated cardiomyopathy. However, mice treated with the prolactin antagonsist bromocriptine did not develop cardiomyopathy. Following this finding and the subsequent publication of numerous case reports of recovery of LV function following bromocriptine therapy,[84,85] a small single-centre pilot-study has recently been published.[86] PPCM patients randomised to receive bromocriptine had a higher incidence of recovery of LV function ($p=0.012$), a lower mortality, and a significant reduction in the composite end point of poor outcome (death, New York Heart Association functional class III/IV, or left ventricular ejection fraction <35% at 6 months) compared with the group on standard therapy (10% vs 80%; $p=0.006$). The size of this study prevents robust and definitive conclusions about the benefits of bromocriptine therapy in PPCM, but larger studies are on-going.

Summary

HF is the common endpoint of a wide range of cardiovascular and noncardiovascular conditions. The list of potential causes continues to expand as our knowledge of the pathophysiology of

HF increases. In Western societies, CHD and hypertension remain the commonest causes of HF. The prevalence of HF secondary to CHD has increased in recent years, due in part to improved survival following acute myocardial infarction. In addition to coronary disease and hypertension, valvular heart disease, arrhythmias and alcohol are other common causes of HF in developed countries. Peripartum cardiomyopathy should also be considered in women developing symptoms and signs of heart failure towards the end of pregnancy, or in the months following delivery.

References

1. McMurray JJ, Stewart S. Epidemiology, aetiology, and prognosis of heart failure. *Heart* 2000;**83**:596–602.
2. Kalinowski L, Dobrucki IT, Malinski T. Race-specific differenc...es in endothelial function. Predisposition of African Americans to vascular diseases. *Circulation* 2004;**109**:2511–17.
3. Cubillos-Garzon LA, Casas JP, Morillo CA, Bautista LE. Congestive heart failure in Latin America: the next epidemic. *Am Heart J* 2004;**147**:412–17.
4. Cowie MR, Mosterd A, Wood DA, *et al.* The epidemiology of heart failure. *Eur Heart J* 1997;**18**:208–25.
5. The SOLVD Investigators. Effect of enalapril in survival in patients with reduced left ventricular ejection fractions and congestive heart failure. *N Engl J Med* 1991;**325**:293–302.
6. The Digitalis Investigation Group. The effect of digoxin on mortality and morbidity in patients with heart failure. *N Engl J Med* 1997;**336**:525–33.
7. MERIT Investigators. Effect of metoprolol CR/XL in chronic heart failure: metoprolol CR/XL randomised intervention trial in congestive heart failure (Merit-HF). *Lancet* 1999;**353**:2001–7.
8. CIBIS-II Investigators and Committees. The Cardiac Insufficiency Bisoprolol Study II (CIBIS-II): a randomised trial. *Lancet* 1999;**353**:9–13.
9. Packer M, Poole-Wilson PA, Armstrong PW, *et al.* Comparative effects of low and high doses of the angiotensin-converting enzyme inhibitor, lisinopril, on morbidity and mortality in chronic heart failure. *ATLAS Study Group. Circulation* 1999;**100**:2312–18.
10. Pitt B, Zannad F, Remme WJ, *et al.* The effect of spironolactone on morbidity and mortality in patients with heart failure. Randomized aldactone evaluation study investigators. *N Engl J Med* 1999;**341**:709–17.
11. Cohn J, Tognoni G; for the Valsartan Heart Failure Trial Investigators. A randomized trial of the angiotensin-receptor blocker valsartan in chronic heart failure. *N Engl J Med* 2001;**345**:1667–75.
12. Packer M, Coats AJ, Fowler MB, *et al.* Carvedilol Prospective Randomized Cumulative Survival Study Group. Effect of carvedilol on survival in severe chronic heart failure. *N Engl J Med* 2001;**344**:1651–8.
13. Poole-Wilson PA, Swedberg K, Cleland JG, *et al.*; Carvedilol Or Metoprolol European Trial Investigators. Comparison of carvedilol and metoprolol on clinical outcomes in patients with chronic heart failure in the Carvedilol Or Metoprolol European Trial (COMET): randomized controlled trial. *Lancet* 2003;**362**:7–13.
14. Bristow MR, Saxon LA, Boehmer J, *et al.*; Comparison of Medical Therapy, Pacing, and Defibrillation in Heart Failure (COMPANION) Investigators. Cardiac-Resynchronization Therapy with or without an Implantable Defibrillator in Advanced Chronic Heart Failure. *N Engl J Med* 2004;**350**:2140–50.
15. Cleland JGF, Daubert JC, Erdmann E, *et al.*; for the Cardiac Resynchronization – Heart Failure (CARE-HF) Study Investigators. The effect of cardiac resynchronization on morbidity and mortality in heart failure. *N Engl J Med* 2005;**352**:1539–49.
16. GISSI-HF Investigators, Tavazzi L, Maggioni AP, Marchioli R, *et al.* Effect of rosuvastatin in patients with chronic heart failure (the GISSI-HF trial): a randomised, double-blind, placebo-controlled trial. *Lancet* 2008;**372**:1231–39.
17. SOLVD Investigators. Natural history and patterns of current practice in heart failure. *J Am Coll Cardiol* 1993;**4A**:14A–19A.
18. Bart BA, Ertl G, Held P, *et al.* Contemporary management of patients with left ventricular systolic dysfunction. Results from the study of patients intolerant of converting enzyme inhibitors (SPICE) registry. *Eur Heart J* 1999;**20**:1182–90.
19. Adams KF Jr, Fonarow GC, Emerman CL, *et al.*; ADHERE Scientific Advisory Committee and Investigators. Characteristics and outcomes of patients hospitalized for heart failure in the United States: Rationale, design, and preliminary observations from the first 100,000 cases in the Acute Decompensated Heart Failure National Registry (ADHERE). *Am Heart J* 2005;**149**:209–16.
20. Fonarow GC, Abraham WT, Albert NM, *et al.*; OPTIMIZE-HF Investigators and Hospitals. Influence of a performance-improvement initiative on quality of care for patients hospitalized with heart failure. *Arch Intern Med* 2007;**167**:1493–502.
21. Kannel WB, Ho KK, Thom T. Changing epidemiological features of cardiac failure. *Eur Heart J* 1994;**72**:S3–9.
22. Velagaleti RS, Pencina MJ, Murabito JM, *et al.* Long-term trends in the incidence of heart failure after myocardial infarction. *Circulation* 2008;**118**:2057–62.
23. Furberg CD, Yusuf S. Effect of drug therapy on survival in chronic heart failure. *Adv Cardiol* 1986;**34**:124–30.
24. Mann DL, Bristow MR. Mechanisms and models in heart failure. *The Biomechanical model and beyond. Circulation* 2005;**111**:2837–49.
25. Jessup M, Brozena S. Heart failure. *N Engl J Med* 2003;**348**:2007–18.
26. Pfeffer MA, Braunwald E. Ventricular remodelling after myocardial infarction: experimental observations and clinical implications. *Circulation* 1990;**81**:1161–72.
27. Bristow MR. β-Adrenergic receptor blockade in chronic heart failure. *Circulation* 2000;**101**:558–69.
28. Francis GS, Goldsmith SR, Levine TB, Olivari MT, Cohn JN. The neurohumoral axis in congestive heart failure. *Ann Intern Med* 1984;**101**:370–7.
29. Nieminen MS, Böhm M, Cowie MR, *et al.*; ESC Committe for Practice Guideline (CPG). Executive summary of the guidelines on the diagnosis and treatment of acute heart failure: the Task Force on Acute Heart Failure of the European Society of Cardiology. *Eur Heart J* 2005;**26**:384–416.
30. Dutka DP, Camici PG. Hibernation and congestive heart failure. *Heart Fail Rev* 2003;**8**:167–73.
31. Amoah AG, Kallen C. Aetiology of heart failure as seen from a National Cardiac Referral Centre in Africa. *Cardiology* 2000;**93**:11–18.
32. Kahn DF, Duffy SJ, Tomasian D, *et al.* Effects of black race on forearm resistance vessël function. *Hypertension* 2002;**40**:195–201.
33. Hogg K, Swedberg K, McMurray JJ. Heart failure with preserved left ventricular systolic function: epidemiology, clinical characteristics, and prognosis. *J Am Coll Cardiol* 2004;**43**:317–27.
34. James MA, Saadeh AM, Jones JV. Wall stress and hypertension. *J Cardiovasc Risk* 2000;**7**:187–90.
35. Lips DJ, deWindt LJ, van Kraaij DJW, Doevendans PA. Molecular determinants of myocardial hypertrophy and failure: alternative pathways for beneficial and maladaptive hypertrophy. *Eur Heart J* 2003;**24**:883–896.
36. Kitiyakara C, Guzman N. Malignant hypertension and hypertensive emergencies. *J Am Soc Nephrol* 1998;**9**:133–42.
37. Lip GY, Beevers M, Beevers G. The failure of malignant hypertension to decline: a survey of 24 years' experience in a multi-racial population in England. *J Hypertens* 1994;**12**:1297–1305.
38. Carabello B, Paulus W. Aortic stenosis. *Lancet* 2009;**373**:956–66.
39. Otto CM, Kuusisto J, Reichenbach DD, Gown AM, O'Brien KD. Characterization of the early lesion of degenerative valvular aortic stenosis: histological and immunohistochemical studies. *Circulation* 1994;**90**:844–53.
40. Aronow WS, Ahn C, Kronzon I, Goldman ME. Association of coronary risk factors and use of statins with progression of mild valvular aortic stenosis in older persons. *Am J Cardiol* 2001;**88**:693–95.
41. deFilippi CR, Willett DL, Brickner ME, *et al.* Usefulness of dobutamine echocardiography in distinguishing severe from nonsevere valvular aortic stenosis in patients with depressed left ventricular function and low transvalvular gradients. *Am J Cardiol* 1995;**75**:191–4.

42. Cohn LH, Birjiniuk V. Therapy of acute aortic regurgitation. *Cardiol Clin* 1991;**9**:339–52.
43. Bekeredjian R, Grayburn PA. Valvular heart disease: aortic regurgitation. *Circulation* 2005;**112**:125–34.
44. Carabello B. The current therapy for mitral regurgitation. *J Am Coll Cardiol* 2008;**52**:319–26.
45. Chandrashekhar Y, Westaby S, Narula J. Mitral stenosis. *Lancet* 2009;**374**:1271–83.
46. Waller BF, Howard J, Fess S. Pathology of tricuspid valve stenosis and pure tricuspid regurgitation–Part 1. *Clin Cardiol* 1995;**18**:97–102.
47. Gustafsson BI, Hauso O, Drozdov I, Kidd M, Modlin IM. Carcinoid heart disease. *Int J Cardiol* 2008;**129**:318–24.
48. Shah P, Raney A. Tricuspid valve disease. *Curr Probl Cardiol* 2008;**33**:47–84.
49. Marwick TH, Lancellotti P, Pierard L. Ischaemic mitral regurgitation: mechanisms and diagnosis. *Heart* 2009;**95**:1711–18.
50. Bonow RO, Carabello BA, Chatterjee K, *et al.* ACC/AHA 2006 Guidelines for the Management of Patient With Valvular Heart Disease: A Report of the American College of Cardiology/American Heart Association Task Force on Practice Guidelines. *Circulation* 2006;**114**: e84–e231.
51. Apitz C, Webb GD, Redington AN. Tetralogy of Fallot. *Lancet* 2009;**374**:1462–71.
52. Paranon S, Acar P. Ebstein's anomaly of the tricuspid valve: from fetus to adult: congenital heart disease. *Heart* 2008;**94**:237–43.
53. Brugada P, Andries E. Tachycardiomopathy. The most frequently unrecognized cause of heart failure? *Acta Cardiol* 1993;**2**:165–9.
54. Packer DL, Bardy GH, Worley SJ, *et al.* Tachycardia-induced cardiomyopathy: a reversible form of LV dysfunction. *Am J Cardiol* 1986;**57**:563–70.
55. Rabbani LE, Wang PJ, Couper GL, Friedman PL. Time course of improvement in ventricular function after ablation of incessant automatic atrial tachycardia. *Am Heart J* 1991;**121**:816–19.
56. Tavernier R, De Pauw M, Trouerbach J. Incessant automatic atrial tachycardia: a reversible cause of tachycardiomyopathy. *Acta Cardiol* 1999;**54**:227–9.
57. Walker NL, Cobbe SM, Birnie DH. Tachycardiomyopathy: a diagnosis not to be missed. *Heart* 2004;**90**:e7.
58. Shinbane JS, Wood MA, Jensen DN, Ellenbogen KA, Fitzpatrick AP, Scheinman MM. Tachycardia-induced cardiomyopathy: a review of animal models and clinical studies. *J Am Coll Cardiol* 1997;**29**: 709–15.
59. Wang TJ, Larson MG, Levy D, *et al.* Temporal relations of atrial fibrillation and congestive heart failure and their joint influence on mortality: the Framingham Heart Study. *Circulation* 2003;**107**:2920–5.
60. The AF-CHF Trial Investigators. Rationale and design of a study assessing treatment strategies of atrial fibrillation in patients with heart failure: the Atrial Fibrillation and Congestive Heart Failure (AF-CHF) trial. *Am Heart J* 2002;**144**:597–607.
61. Olsson LG, Swedberg K, Ducharme A, *et al.*; CHARM Investigators. Atrial fibrillation and risk of clinical events in chronic heart failure with and without left ventricular systolic dysfunction: results from the Candesartan in Heart failure-Assessment of Reduction in Mortality and morbidity (CHARM) program. *J Am Coll Cardiol* 2006;**47**:1997–2004.
62. Efremidis M, Pappas L, Sideris A, Filippatos G. Management of atrial fibrillation in patients with heart failure. *J Cardiac Fail* 2008;**14**:232–7.
63. Umana E, Solares CA, Alpert MA. Tachycardia-induced cardiomyopathy. *Am J Med* 2003;**114**:51–5.
64. Jaggarao NS, Nanda AS, Daubert JP. Ventricular tachycardia induced cardiomyopathy: improvement with radiofrequency ablation. *Pacing Clin Electrophysiol* 1996;**19**:505–8.
65. Piano MR. Alcoholic cardiomyopathy: Incidence, clinical characteristics, and pathophysiology. *Chest* 2002;**121**(5):1638–50.
66. Laonigro I, Correale M, Di Biase M, Altomare E. Alcohol abuse and heart failure. *Eur J Heart Failure* 2009;**11**:453–462.
67. Lazarevic AM, Nakatani S, Neskovic AN, *et al.* Early changes in left ventricular function in chronic asymptomatic alcoholics: Relation to the duration of heavy drinking. *J Am Coll Cardiol* 2000;**35**:1599.
68. Duan J, McFadden GE, Borgerding AJ, *et al.* Overexpression of alcohol dehydrogenase exacerbates ethanol-induced contractile defect in cardiac myocytes. *Am J Physiol* 2002;**282**:H1216.
69. Fernandez-Sola J, Nicolas JM, Oriola J, *et al.* Angiotensin-converting enzyme gene polymorphism is associated with vulnerability to alcoholic cardiomyopathy. *Ann Intern Med* 2002;**137**:321.
70. Pearson GD, Veille JC, Rahimtoola S, *et al.* Peripartum ardiomyopathy: National Heart, Lung, and Blood Institute and Office of Rare Diseases (National Institutes of Health) workshop recommendations and review. *JAMA. 2000*;**283**(9):1183–8.
71. Sliwa K, Hilfiker-Kleiner D, Petrie MC, *et al.* Current state of knowledge on aetiology, diagnosis, management, and therapy of peripartum cardiomyopathy: a position statement from the Heart Failure Association of the European Society of Cardiology Working Group on peripartum cardiomyopathy. *Eur J Heart Fail.* 2010;**12**:767–78.
72. Hilfiker-Kleiner D, Kaminski K, Podewski E, *et al.* A cathepsin D-cleaved 16 kDa form of prolactin mediates postpartum cardiomyopathy. *Cell.* 2007;**128**:859–600.
73. Amos AM, Jaber WA, Russell SD, *et al.* Improved outcomes in peripartum cardiomyopathy with contemporary. *Am Heart J.* 2006;**152**:109–13.
74. Sliwa K, Förster O, Libhaber E, Fett JD, Sundstrom JB, Hilfiker-Kleiner D, Ansari AA. Peripartum cardiomyopathy: inflammatory markers as predictors of outcome in 100 prospectively studied patients. *Eur Heart J.* 2006;**27**:441–6.
75. Sliwa K, Skudicky D, Bergemann A, Candy G, Puren A, Sareli P. Peripartum cardiomyopathy: analysis of clinical outcome, left ventricular function, plasma levels of cytokines and Fas/APO-1. *J Am Coll Cardiol.* 2000;**35**:701–5.
76. Duran N, Günes H, Duran I, Biteker M, Ozkan M. Predictors of prognosis in patients with peripartum cardiomyopathy. *Int J Gynaecol Obstet.* 2008;**101**:137–40.
77. Forster O, Hilfiker-Kleiner D, Ansari AA, Sundstrom JB, Libhaber E, Tshani W, Becker A, Yip A, Klein G, Sliwa K. Reversal of IFN-gamma, oxLDL and prolactin serum levels correlate with clinical improvement in patients with peripartum cardiomyopathy. *Eur J Heart Fail. 2008*;**10**:861–8.
78. Ravikishore AG, Kaul UA, Sethi KK, Khalilullah M. Peripartum cardiomyopathy: prognostic variables at initial evaluation. *Int J Cardiol. 1991*;**32**:377–80.
79. Goland S, Modi K, Bitar F, Janmohamed M, Mirocha JM, Czer LS, Illum S, Hatamizadeh P, Elkayam U. Clinical profile and predictors of complications in peripartum cardiomyopathy. *J Card Fail.* 2009;**15**:645–50.
80. Chapa JB, Heiberger HB, Weinert L, Decara J, Lang LM, Hibbard JU. Prognostic value of echocardiography in peripartum cardiomyopathy. *Obstet Gynecol.* 2005;**105**:1303–8.
81. Habli M, O'Brien T, Nowack E, Khoury S, Barton JR, Sibai B. Peripartum cardiomyopathy: prognostic factors for long-term maternal outcome. *Am J Obstet Gynecol.* 2008;**199**:415.e1–5.
82. Fett JD, Christie LG, Murphy JG. Brief communication: Outcomes of subsequent pregnancy after peripartum cardiomyopathy : a case series from Haiti. Ann Intern Med. 2006;**145**:30–4.
83. Fett JD, Fristoe KL, Welsh SN, . Risk of heart failure relapse in subsequent pregnancy among peripartum cardiomyopathy mothers. 2010;109:34-6. *Int J Gynaecol Obstet.* 2010;**109**:34–6.
84. Hilfiker-Kleiner D, Meyer GP, Schieffer E, Goldmann B, Podewski E, Struman I, Fischer P, Drexler H. Recovery from postpartum cardiomyopathy in 2 patients by blocking prolactin release with bromocriptine. *J Am Coll Cardiol.* 2007;**50**:2354–5.
85. Habedank D, Kühnle Y, Elgeti T, Dudenhausen JW, Haverkamp JW, Dietz R. Recovery from peripartum cardiomyopathy after treatment with bromocriptine. *Eur J Heart Fail.* 2008;**10**:1149–51.
86. Sliwa K, Blauwet L, Tibazarwa K, Libhaber E, Smedema JP, Becker A, McMurray J, Yamac H, Labidi S, Struman I, Hilfiker-Kleiner D, . Evaluation of bromocriptine in the treatment of acute severe peripartum cardiomyopathy: a proof-of-concept pilot study. *Circulation.* 2010;**121**:1465–73.

5

The genetics of heart failure

Giuseppe Limongelli and Perry M. Elliott

Introduction

Heart failure (HF), defined in its broadest sense as a syndrome characterized by symptoms and signs of ventricular dysfunction in the presence of structural and or functional abnormalities of heart function, affects millions of people worldwide; in addition, a substantial number of individuals have asymptomatic abnormalities of heart function that predispose them to symptomatic HF in later life. Coronary artery disease and hypertension are by far the most common causes of HF, but a substantial minority of cases are caused by a heterogeneous group of heart muscle diseases, the cardiomyopathies. These disorders differ in several important respects from other causes of HF in that they are often familial and present throughout life. With recent advances in the understanding of the molecular genetics of cardiomyopathies,[1–10] cardiologists are having to adapt diagnostic and treatment protocols in order to optimize management of individual patients and their families. In this chapter we review the clinical presentation and pathophysiology of the most common monogenic cardiomyopathies and the cardiovascular manifestations of mutations in the genes controlling the respiratory chain (mitochondrial diseases).

Cardiomyopathies

Definitions and nomenclature

It was Wallace Brigden in 1957 who observed that when describing heart muscle disorders,

> adjectives such as isolated, idiopathic, nonspecific, specific, interstitial, diffuse, and circumscribed abound in the literature; others, such as acute, subacute, chronic pernicious, and malignant, relate to the clinical picture; while still others, such as eosinophilic, allergic, idiosyncratic, and granulomatous hint at aetiology, as does familial cardiomegaly.[11]

His contribution to the resolution of this nosological confusion was to use the term cardiomyopathy to denote 'isolated noncoronary myocardial disease'. In 1961, John Goodwin promulgated this concept by defining cardiomyopathies as disorders of heart muscle 'of unknown or obscure aetiology, often with endocardial, and sometimes with pericardial involvement, but not atherosclerotic in origin'.[12] Subtypes of cardiomyopathy were defined using specific morphological and physiological features.[13]

This scheme for classifying heart muscle disorders survived largely unchanged until a review by a joint World Health Organization/International Society and Federation of Cardiology panel in 1995,[14] in which the rigid distinction between primary and secondary disease was blurred and a new entity, arrhythmogenic right ventricular caridomyopathy, was formally recognized. In 2007, the Working Group on Myocardial and Pericardial Diseases of the European Society of Cardiology proposed an update of the WHO/ISFC classification, defining cardiomyopathy as 'a myocardial disorder in which the heart muscle is structurally and functionally abnormal in the absence of coronary artery disease, hypertension, valvular disease and congenital heart disease sufficient to explain the observed myocardial abnormality'.[15] Cardiomyopathies were still grouped into specific morphological and functional phenotypes, but each phenotype was subclassified into familial/genetic and nonfamilial/nongenetic forms; the distinction between primary and secondary forms was abandoned.

Cardiomyopathy subtypes

Four major types of cardiomyopathy are recognized: dilated cardiomyopathy (DCM), hypertrophic cardiomyopathy (HCM), restrictive cardiomyopathy (RCM), and arrhythmogenic right ventricular cardiomyopathy (ARVC).

Dilated cardiomyopathy

DCM is defined by the presence of left ventricular dilatation and systolic impairment in the absence of abnormal loading conditions (e.g. hypertension, valve disease) or coronary artery disease sufficient to cause systolic dysfunction.[9,10,15] It often coexists with right ventricular dilation and dysfunction. The prevalence of DCM is estimated to be around 1 in 2500 adults, with an annual incidence of between 5 and 8 per 100 000 [16]. In children, the incidence is much lower (0.5–0.8 per 100 000 per year), but DCM is the commonest cardiomyopathy in the paediatric population.[17,18]

Some 20–30% of adult patients with DCM have a familial predisposition.[19] The reported prevalence of familial DCM in paediatric studies is lower (up to 17%).[20,21] More than 30 genes encoding a variety of proteins expressed within the cardiomyocyte, ranging from the cardiac sarcomere, the nuclear envelope, transcription factors, and the dystrophin-associated cytoskeletal complex have been identified as causes of DCM.[1,9,10] Most are transmitted as an autosomal dominant trait, but other forms of inheritance, including autosomal recessive, X-linked, and matrilinear are described.[1,9,10,15] DCM with a typical phenotype comprising bradycardia, conduction disorders, and atrial fibrillation has been associated with *SCN5A* mutations.[16,22] However, the clinical importance of these findings and the mechanism by which such mutations cause ventricular dysfunction remain to be determined.

Hypertrophic cardiomyopathy

HCM is defined as left ventricular hypertrophy in the absence of abnormal loading conditions (valve disease, hypertension, congenital heart defects) sufficient to explain the degree of hypertrophy.[1,5,15] Studies in North America, Europe, Japan, and China consistently report the prevalence of unexplained left ventricular hypertrophy to be approximately 1 in 500 adults.[16,23–27] The prevalence of HCM in children is unknown, but two population studies report an annual incidence of 0.3–0.5 per 100 000.[17,18]

In most adolescents and adults, HCM is an autosomal dominant trait caused by mutations in cardiac sarcomere protein genes.[28–30] Mutations in genes encoding Z-disc proteins–myozenin (*MYOZ2*), telethonin (*TCAP*) and phospholamban (PLN)–are also reported.[31, 32] Other genetic disorders that mimic the phenotypic expression of sarcomeric HCM include metabolic or storage disorders (mutations in the genes encoding the γ-2 regulatory subunit of AMP-activated protein kinase (PRKAG2); lysosome-associated membrane protein 2 (LAMP2); or GLA-encoded α-galactosidase A), neuromuscular disorders (mutations in frataxin gene causing Friedreich's ataxia), chromosome abnormalities (Down's syndrome, trisomy 18), and genetic syndromes such as cardiofacial disorders (Noonan's syndrome, LEOPARD syndrome, cardiofaciocutaneous syndrome, Costello's syndrome) or phakomatoses (neurofibromatosis, tuberous sclerosis).[4,5,33–38]

Restrictive cardiomyopathy

RCM, the least common of all the cardiomyopathies, is characterized by increased stiffness of the myocardium that causes ventricular pressure to rise steeply with small increases in ventricular volume. This pathophysiology occurs in a number of different diseases, including HCM and DCM, but by convention, the term RCM should only be used when systolic and diastolic volumes of one or both ventricles are normal or reduced and there is no increase in ventricular wall thickness.[15]

RCM can be idiopathic, familial, or result from various systemic disorders, in particular amyloidosis, sarcoidosis, carcinoid heart disease, scleroderma, and anthracycline toxicity.[39] Familial disease is described in approximately 30% of patients with idiopathic restrictive cardiomyopathy.[40] Autosomal dominant RCM is commonly caused by sarcomeric gene defects (particularly cardiac troponin I).[41] Desmin gene defects cause RCM associated with atrioventricular block and skeletal myopathy.[42] Rarely, familial disease is associated with autosomal recessive inheritance (such as haemochromatosis caused by mutations in the HFE gene, or glycogen storage disease), or with X-linked inheritance (Anderson–Fabry disease).[39]

Arrhythmogenic right ventricular cardiomyopathy

ARVC is a disorder characterized clinically by ventricular arrhythmia, HF, and sudden death, and histologically by cardiomyocyte loss and replacement with fibrous or fibro-fatty tissue.[43] The estimated prevalence of ARVC is 1 in 5000 of the population.[43] Systematic family studies have shown that ARVC is inherited in approximately 50% of cases.[43] The mode of transmission is usually autosomal dominant with variable penetrance, but rare autosomal recessive forms are well recognized.[7,8,43] To date, most mutations occur in genes encoding proteins of the desmosome and adherens junction: specifically, plakoglobin (JUP), desmoplakin (DSP), plakophilin 2 (PKP2), desmoglein (DSG2), and desmocollin (DSC2).[7,8,43] Two nondesmosomal genes have been associated with ARVC–ryanodine receptor (RYR2) and transforming growth factor β 3 (TGFβ3)–but their association with ARVC remains controversial.[7,8,43] Recently, a mutation in the transmembrane protein 43 (TNEM43) has been described (ARVD5).[44] TNEM43 is predicted to be a cytoplasmic membrane protein without a cadherin domain; the *TNEM43* gene also contains a response element for an adipogenic transcription factor.

Left ventricular noncompaction

Left ventricular noncompaction (LVNC) is a myocardial disorder defined by the presence of prominent trabeculations on the luminal surface of the left ventricle associated with deep intertrabecular recesses that extend into the ventricular wall.[15,45] LVNC often occurs in association with other congenital heart abnormalities, such as atrial and ventricular septal defects, congenital aortic stenosis, and coarctation of the aorta. Isolated LVNC was thought to be extremely rare with a prevalence between 0.05 and 0.24%, but with improvements in diagnostic imaging, the frequency of the diagnosis has increased.[15,45] However, there is controversy with respect to the diagnostic criteria for LVNC and it is not clear whether it is a distinct cardiomyopathy, or merely a congenital or acquired morphological trait shared by phenotypically distinct cardiomyopathies.[15,45,46]

Several genes have been implicated in LVNC.[7,45] These include TAZ/G4.5 located on the X chromosome which encodes for tafazzin, a protein involved in the maintenance of cardiolipin levels expressed at high levels in cardiac and skeletal muscle cells.[15,45] Mutations in this gene cause Barth's syndrome. Other genes implicated in isolated LVNC include *ZASP* encoding the LIM domain binding protein 3, a protein belonging to the Z-disc structure; α-dystrobrevin, a protein of the glycoprotein complex that interacts with other components of the complex conferring stability to the plasma membrane during the process of contraction and relaxation of the muscles; *lamin A/C* encoding a ubiquitously expressed protein found in the inner surface of the nuclear envelope; and sarcomeric genes encoding β-myosin heavy chain (*MYH7*), α-cardiac actin (*ACTC*) and cardiac troponin T (*TNNT2*).[45,46]

Pathophysiology

Most of the genes implicated in the pathophysiology of the cardiomyopathies are involved in force generation and propagation, energy production and regulation, calcium signalling or transcription regulation.[3–10,28–38,41–45] (Table 5.1, Fig. 5.1, Fig. 5.2).

Sarcomeric proteins

Genetic mutations in sarcomeric protein genes are implicated in a number of cardiomyopathy subtypes including HCM, RCM, DCM, and LVNC.[1–5,9,10,28–30,41,45,46] In HCM, more than 400 different sarcomeric mutations are known, the greatest number occuring in the genes encoding for β-myosin heavy chain (*MYH7*) and myosin-binding protein C (*MYBPC3*).[4,28–30] Most mutations are missense mutations, but nonsense, frameshift, and in-frame insertion/deletion mutations are well described, particularly in *MYBPC3*.[4,28–30]

Table 5.1 Genes involved in cardiomyopathies. For each gene is reported the symbol, the inheritance pattern, the correspondent genotype/phenotypes and the frequency of the mutations. If there are multiple possible phenotypes the different patterns of inheritance and frequency are indicated.

Sarcomeric proteins				
Gene	**Symbol**	**Inheritance**	**Phenotype**	**Frequency**
Cardiac β-Myosin Heavy chain	MYH7	AD	Variable: moderate to severe prognosis (apical HCM and LVNC), DCM and DCM in Laing distal myopathy	HCM 30% to 40%; DCM 4–6%
Cardiac Troponin T	TNNT2	AD	HCM: Worse prognosis and a high percentage of sudden deaths. DCM	HCM 5%; DCM 3%
Cardiac Troponin I	TNNI3	HCM AD DCM AR RCM AD	It has been related to restrictive physiology/cardiomyopathy, biventricular hypertrophy and apical hypertrophy, DCM	HCM 5%, DCM <1% RCM?
Cardiac Troponin C	TNNC	AD	DCM	<1%
Cardiac Myosin Binding Protein C	MYBPC3	AD	Later onset of the disease and has generally a good prognosis; cases of children with a severe hypertrophy have also been reported, DMC	HCM 30% to 40%; DCM?
Cardiac α-Myosin Heavy Chain	MYH6	AD	DCM, HCM	DCM? 2–3%; HCM <1%
Titin	TTN	AD	DCM, HCM	DCM?; HCM rare
Cardiac actin	ACTC	DCM and HCM AD	DCM, LVNC, HCM	DCM <1%; HCM 1%
Essential Myosin Light Chain	MYL3	AD	HCM	NA
Regulatory Myosin Light Chain	MYL2	AD	HCM	1%
α-Tropomyosin	TPM1	AD	HCM, DCM	HCM 1% to 2%; DCM <1%
Z-disc proteins				
Gene	**Symbol**	**Inheritance**	**Phenotype**	**Frequency**
Cypher/ZASP	LDB3		LVNC	
Metavinculin	VCL	AD	DCM, HCM	DCM <1%–1%; HCM rare
LIM binding domain 3	LDB3	AD	DCM, HCM	DCM <1%–1%; HCM rare
Titin-cap or telethonin	TCAP	AD	DCM, HCM	DCM <1%–1%; HCM <1%
Myozenin 2	MYOZ2	AD	HCM	<1%
Muscle LIM protein	CSRP3	AD	DCM, HCM	DCM <1%; HCM rare
Cytoskeletal proteins				
Gene	**Symbol**	**Inheritance**	**Phenotype**	**Frequency**
Desmin	DES	AD	DCM	<1%–1%
α- and β-dystroglycans	DAG1	NA	DCM	NA
α-, β-, γ- and δ-sarcoglycans	SGCA, SGCB, SGCG, SGCD	SGCD AD	DCM	SGCD <1%
Caveolin-3	CAV3	AD	DCM, HCM	HCM rare

AD, *autosomic dominant*, AR, *autosomic recessive*, XL, *X-linked*, NA, not available.

Data from Tester DJ, Ackerman MJ. Cardiomyopathic and channelopathic causes of sudden unexplained death in infants and children. *Annu Rev Med.* 2009;60:69–84 and Hershberger RE, Cowan J, Morales A, Siegfried JD. Progress with genetic cardiomyopathies: screening, counseling, and testing in dilated, hypertrophic, and arrhythmogenic right ventricular dysplasia/cardiomyopathy. *Circ Heart Fail* 2009;**2:**253–61.

Table 5.1 *(Cont'd)* Genes involved in cardiomyopathies. For each gene is reported the symbol, the inheritance pattern, the correspondent genotype/phenotypes and the frequency of the mutations. If there are multiple possible phenotypes the different patterns of inheritance and frequency are indicated.

Cytoskeletal proteins				
Gene	**Symbol**	**Inheritance**	**Phenotype**	**Frequency**
Lamin A/C	LMNA	DCM AD; EMD2, AD; EMD3, AR; LGMD1B, AD	LVNC, DCM, DCM in Emery-Dreifuss muscular Dystrophy types 2 and 3 (EMD2 and EMD3), DCM in limb girdle muscular dystrophy (LGMD) 1B	DCM 4-8%
Syntrophin	SNT	NA	DCM	NA
Dystrobrevin	DTN	NA	DCM	NA
Dystrophin	DMD	XL	DCM in Duchenne muscular dystrophy (DMD), Becker muscular dystrophy (BMD)	NA
Desmosomal proteins				
Gene	**Symbol**	**Inheritance**	**Phenotype**	**Frequency**
Plakoglobin	JUP	Naxos syndrome, AD	ARVC/D, ARVC/D in Naxos syndrome	Rare
Desmoplakin	DSP	Carvajal syndrome, AR	ARVC/D, DCM in Carvajal syndrome	ARVC/D 6% to 16%
Desmoglein 2	DSG2	AD	ARVC/D	ARVC/D 12% to 40%
Desmocollin 2	DSC2	AD	ARVC/D	Rare
Plakophilin-2	PKP2	AD, AR	ARVC/D	AD 11% to 43%, AR rare
Sarcoplasmic reticulum				
Gene	**Symbol**	**Inheritance**	**Phenotype**	**Frequency**
Ryanodine receptor-2	RYR-2	AD	ARVD	Rare
Phospholamban	PLN	AD	DCM, HCM	DCM?; HCM rare
Sodium channel mutations				
Gene	**Symbol**	**Inheritance**	**Phenotype**	**Frequency**
α-subunit of the cardiac sodium channel	SCN5A	AD	DCM	2–3%
Metabolic proteins				
Gene	**Symbol**	**Inheritance**	**Phenotype**	**Frequency**
Protein kinase, AMP-activated, gamma 2 non-catalytic subunit	PRKAG2	AD	HCM in Wolf-Parkinson White syndrome	NA
α-galactosidase A	GLA	XL	HCM in Fabry disease	NA
Lysosomal-associated membrane protein 2	LAMP2	XL	HCM in Danon disease	NA
Others				
Gene	**Symbol**	**Inheritance**	**Phenotype**	**Frequency**
Hereditary haemochromatosis	HFE	AR	DCM and RCM in Hereditary haemochromatosis	NA
Hereditary amyloidosis	TTR	AD	HCM and RCM in Hereditary amyloidosis	NA
RAS-MAPK pathway genes	PTPN11/ RAF1/SOS1/ KRAS/ HRAS/ BRAF/ MEK1-2	AD	HCM in Noonan (NS)/ Leopard (LS) syndromes	NA
Frataxin	FRDA	AR	HCM in Friedreich ataxia	NA

AD, *autosomic dominant*, AR, *autosomic recessive*, XL, *X-linked*, NA, not available.

Data from Tester DJ, Ackerman MJ. Cardiomyopathic and channelopathic causes of sudden unexplained death in infants and children. *Annu Rev Med.* 2009;60:69–84 and Hershberger RE, Cowan J, Morales A, Siegfried JD. Progress with genetic cardiomyopathies: screening, counseling, and testing in dilated, hypertrophic, and arrhythmogenic right ventricular dysplasia/cardiomyopathy. *Circ Heart Fail* 2009;**2:**253–61.

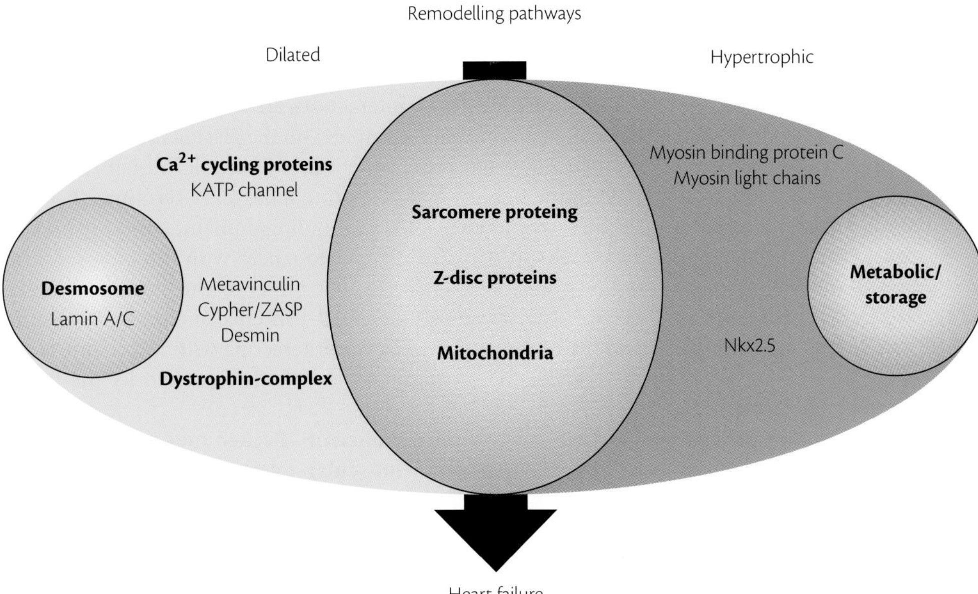

Fig. 5.1 Human gene mutations and pathways causing inherited cardiomyopathies.
From Morita H, *et al. J Clin. Invest* 2005;**115**:518–26.

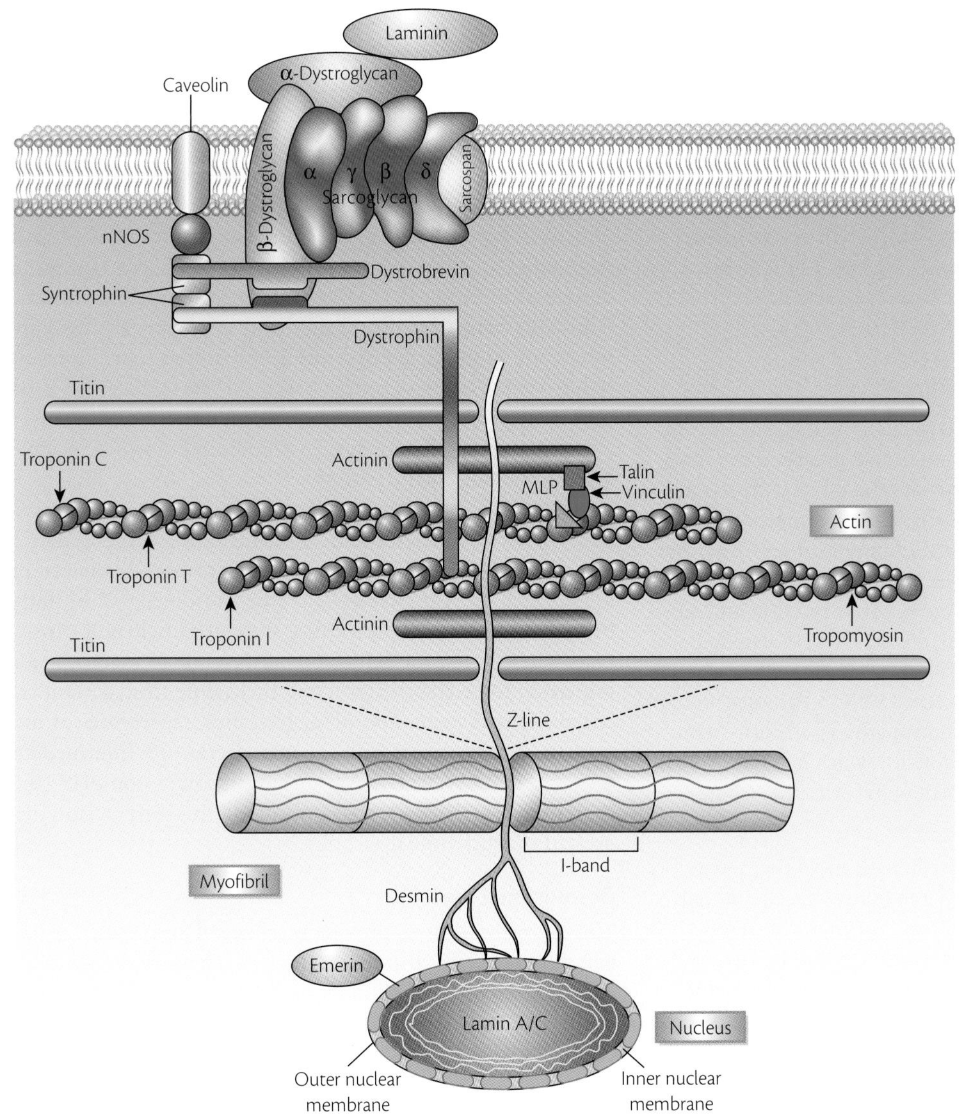

Fig. 5.2 Diagram showing proteins implicated in human inherited cardiomyopathies.
From Towbin JA, Bowles NE. The failing heart. *Nature* 2002; **415**:227–233.

In general, sarcomeric protein gene mutations are characterized by incomplete penetrance and variable clinical expression, the explanation for which includes locus heterogeneity and the variable effect of mutations at different locations within the same gene on the structure and function of the encoded peptide (allelic heterogeneity).[4,5,28,30] It is thought that the majority of sarcomeric protein gene mutations have a dominant negative effect on sarcomere function, i.e. the mutant protein is incorporated into the sarcomere, but its interaction with the normal (wild-type) protein disrupts normal sarcomeric assembly and function; haploinsufficiency (i.e. when there is only a single functional copy of a gene, the other being inactivated by the mutation) may also be important.[4,5,28,30]

In HCM, it is suggested that hypertrophy results from reduced contractile function, but studies of myocyte function in patients with mutations in sarcomere protein genes are inconsistent.[48] Murine models of sarcomeric mutations show increased calcium sensitivity and altered calcium cycling between the sarcomere and the sarcoplasmic reticulum. *In vitro* studies using purified myosin filaments and skinned papillary muscle have demonstrated increased calcium sensitivity of force development, predicted to result in impaired ventricular relaxation *in vivo*.[49–51]

Sarcomere mutations that cause DCM occur in the same genes implicated in HCM, but the predominant mechanism that leads to the phenotype seems to be the impairment of the transmission of contractile force.[30,52,53] The molecular basis of RCM phenotype arising from mutant sarcomeric proteins is unknown, but impaired ATP-mediated dissociation of myosin from actin (causing impaired myocardial relaxation and restrictive physiology), titin disregulation by the mutant proteins, and phosphorylation of sarcomeric proteins have been suggested.[52,54] The recent discovery of sarcomeric mutations (*MYH7*, *ACTC*, *TNNT*) in patients with LVNC indicates that sarcomere proteins may also have a role in myocardial development.[45,47]

Z-disc proteins

Z-discs are the lateral boundaries of the sarcomere and their role is fundamental in mechanical stretch sensing.[55] Mutations in genes encoding Z-disc proteins have been implicated in dilated cardiomyopathy (e.g. metavinculin, which provides the direct connection to the plasma membrane, and MLP, which forms a complex with titin and telethonin) and in hypertrophic cardiomyopathies (α-actinin, which mediates the interaction between actin and titin, telethonin, which interacts with muscle LIM protein, MLP, and titin and has a structural function, and ZASP, which interacts with α-actinin-2 and interferes with PKC-mediated signalling).[30–32,55,56] Mutations in ZASP and actin have been found to cause LVNC.[57] Another protein involved in the development of cardiomyopathies is melusin (a muscle-specific integrin β1-interacting protein), which has a key role in mechanotransduction and development of hypertrophy.[55,56]

Cytoskeletal proteins

Cytoskeletal proteins act as an intracellular scaffold that passes on the contractile force from the sarcomere to the extracellular matrix and protects the cardiomyocyte from mechanical stress.[55,56] Mutations that compromise the cytoskeleton can increase ventricular stiffness and impair contractility of myocytes by reducing force transmission and resistance to stress.[55,56]

The dystrophin–glycoprotein complex is composed of dystrophin, sarcoglycans, dystroglycans, syntrophins, and sarcospan.[55,56] Mutations in genes that encode the various components of this complex are associated with dilated cardiomyopathy and neuromuscular disorders (dystrophinopathies).[55–58] Dystrophin itself is a large cytoskeletal protein expressed in skeletal, cardiac, and smooth muscle cells. Its interactions are with actin and dystrophin-associated glycoprotein complex (on the plasma membrane), while its function is force transduction, intracellular organization, and membrane stability.[55,56] The protein has an N-terminus that binds to the sarcomere via an actin-binding domain, a rod region composed of spectrin-like repeat sequences with interspersed hinge regions, and a C-terminus that binds to the sarcolemma via a group of dystrophin-associated proteins, including syntrophin and β-dystrogylycan, as well as interacting with ion channels such as Nav 1.5, the cardiac sodium channel encoded by the *SCN5A* gene.[56]

When dystrophin is deficient (Becker muscular dystrophy) or absent (Duchenne muscular dystrophy), normal levels of mechanical stress result in increased cell membrane permeability, loss of membrane integrity, and progressive cell destruction.[56] Progressive myocyte destruction, whether in skeletal or cardiac muscle, results in a loss of muscle mass, fibrosis, and muscle weakness.[56] Dystrophin has also been associated to an X-linked dilated cardiomyopathy in which there is little or no clinical evidence of skeletal muscle weakness.[57,58] Interestingly, a similar pathology occurs when dystrophin is disrupted by acquired disease such as viral-induced myocarditis or coronary artery disease.[59] It may be that dystrophin disruption represents a 'final common pathway' of ventricular remodelling and failure.[59]

Genetic mutations in δ-sarcoglycan, one of the four proteins (α, β, γ, δ) that associate to form the sarcoglycan complex, cause sporadic and familial dilated cardiomyopathy.[57,58] The δ component is expressed in striated and smooth muscles, with higher expression in the skeletal and cardiac muscles. The mutations described in human DCM are missense substitution (autosomal dominant transmission and sudden death at an early age) and two other mutations that delete the 238th codon corresponding to a lysine residue (no signs of HF before 20 years of age) .[55,56] Absence of δ-sarcoglycan has been demonstrated to result in the loss of the entire complex.[56] δ-Sarcoglycan mutations are also associated with limb-girdle muscular dystrophy.[55–58]

Intermediate filaments connect the Z-disc to the sarcolemma.[55,56] Desmin is a muscle-specific intermediate filament that forms connections between Z-discs and myofibrils and between plasma membrane, nuclear envelope, and desmosomes.[42,56] Mutations in the gene encoding desmin cause skeletal muscle and cardiac disease by rendering the cells more susceptible to mechanical stress, impairing force transmission and by leading to structural changes because of the formation of 'aggresomes' (aggregates of mutated proteins that associate with the sarcomere).[42,56] Intermediate filaments are linked to dystrophin-glycoprotein complex (through α-dystrobrevin) and interruption of this interaction may be present in Duchenne dystrophy.[56]

Desmosomal proteins

The intercalated discs provide mechanical and electrical coupling between adjacent cardiomyocytes.[55,56] They are made up of three distinct structures: gap junctions, adherens junctions, and desmosomes.[56] The *gap junction* mediates the transfer of ions between cells, whereas the *adherens junction*, composed of cadherins, β-catenin, and γ-catenin (plakoglobin), mediates the transmission of force between cells.[56] The *desmosome* provides mechanical attachment between cells by linking the desmosomal cadherins, desmocollin, and desmoglein with the intermediate filament cytoskeleton.[56] The intracellular components of the desmosomal cadherins interact with plakoglobin and plakophilin, which in turn bind to the N-terminal domain of a plakin protein, desmoplakin.[56] The C-terminal of desmoplakin anchors desmin intermediate filaments to the cell surface. Plectin, another member of the plakin family, is also present in desmosomes and contributes to the mechanical strength of cells.[56] In addition to providing cells with mechanical strength, the desmosome also plays an important role in tissue morphogenesis and differentiation.[55,56]

Mutations in desmosomal proteins cause ARVC and DCM.[1,2,7,8,61] More than 50 individual mutations have been identified to date, but the mechanism by which mutations result in disease is unclear.[2,7,8] Mutations may increase the susceptibility of the myocardium to the damaging effects of mechanical stress, thereby predisposing to cardiomyocyte detachment, death, and eventual replacement by fibro-fatty tissue.[8] In ARVC, the predilection for the right ventricle has been explained by its thin wall and greater distensibility, but desmosomal proteins interact with many other proteins including components of the cellular cytoskeleton and intermediate filaments and it is possible that dysfunction of either ventricle is the result of reduced cytoskeletal integrity and impaired force transduction.[7,43,55,56] Some desmosomal proteins (in particular plakoglobin) are also important signalling molecules.[7]

Inner nuclear membrane proteins

Lamin A/C and emerin are nuclear matrix proteins involved in different myopathies.[6,55,56] Lamin A and C are encoded by the same gene (*LMNA*) and are located on the nuclear surface of the inner nuclear membrane; their expression is confined to heart and skeletal muscle.[56] Lamins are predicted to have a structural role in maintaining the integrity of the nuclear envelope.[56] Mutations in lamin A/C and emerin genes cause skeletal muscle diseases (Emery–Dreifuss muscular dystrophy) and isolated dilated cardiomyopathy.[6,55,56] About 19 mutations (mostly missense, deletions, and frameshift mutations) especially in the central rod domain in the *LMNA* gene have been described in patients affected by dilated cardiomyopathy.[56] Studies on transgenic lamin A/C mice have shown increased nuclear deformation, fragmentation of the chromatin and impairment of mechanotransduction, suggesting a possible role of the proteins of the nuclear envelope as mechanosensors.[56]

Calcium homeostasis

Calcium exchange between cytoplasm and extracellular matrix and between cytoplasm and storage organelles is fundamental to the regulation of the contraction-relaxation cycle in muscle cells.[56] Contraction of the sarcomere starts when calcium in released by sarcoplasmic reticulum; this step is regulated by a set of proteins localized within and on the membrane of the organelle, the most important of which are calsequestrin, which binds calcium into the sarcoplasmic reticulum, and the ryanodine-2 receptor, which allows calcium exit into the cytoplasm (stimulated by the entry of calcium ions in the myocyte through L-type calcium channels).[56] Calcium ions diffuse into the cytoplasm and to bind troponin C molecules in the sarcomere, triggering contraction; relaxation of the sarcomere is facilitated by the removal of calcium from the cytoplasm into the sarcoplasmic endoreticulum by calcium ATPase (SERCA 2a) and via the plasma membrane sodium/calcium exchanger.[56]

Dysregulation of calcium homeostasis has been described in hypertrophic cardiomyopathy.[55,56,62] Calreticulin is a calcium-binding protein that acts as a chaperone in the sarcoplasmic reticulum. It is present in two forms, but its role in the cardiac tissue remains unknown.[56,62] Mutations in the calreticulin gene have been found in two patients to date: one had a unique mutation, while the other also had two mutations in *MYBPC3*.[62] Mutations in calsequestrin (*CASQ2*) are also described in association with *MYBPC3* mutations but their pathogenicity (if any) is unclear.[62] Phospholamban mutations have been found both in dilated cardiomyopathy (homozygous) and hypertrophic cardiomyopathy (heterozygous).[62] One of the identified mutations (Arg9Cys) causes abnormal interaction between PKA and phospholamban, so affecting the phosphorylation pattern of the regulator which results in a constitutive inhibition of SERCA2a.

Mutations in the ryanodine receptor gene (*RYR2*), more typically associated with catecholaminergic polymorphic ventricular tachycardia, have been reported in association with a localized form of ARVC. However mutations in this gene are no longer classified as a subtype of ARVC.[1,2,7,8]

Genetic modifiers

A number of attempts have been made to investigate the effect of likely polymorphisms on disease expression in cardiomyopathies. Probably the best studied are genes important in the renin–angiotensin–aldosterone system (RAAS). The deletion/insertion (D/I) polymorphism in the angiotensin converting enzyme (ACE) has been associated with several cardiovascular disorders including left ventricular hypertrophy in untreated hypertension and atherosclerosis.[63] Patients with HCM and the DD genotype have increased tissue levels of ACE, and small cohort studies have found that the D allele is overrepresented in HCM patients.[63]

Chronic β-adrenergic receptor (ADBR) activation is implicated in the pathogenesis of HF and β-blockers have been demonstrated to improve survival in ischaemic and nonischaemic left ventricular systolic dysfunction.[64] Common functional polymorphisms in β-adrenergic receptor genes have been associated with diverse clinical features (such as functional status and exercise capacity) and outcome in HF patients, and with pharmacogenetic interaction with β-blockers.[64] A recent meta-analysis analysing the effect of ADRB1 Arg389Gly polymorphism on left ventricular remodelling with the use of β-blockers demonstrated a 5% improvement in left ventricular ejection fraction in Arg389 homozygotes.[64] There is accumulating molecular evidence for a different functional response to β-blockers associated with this polymorphism.

MicroRNAs are a new class of RNA that have a basic role in regulating gene expression.[65] They are about 22 nucleotides long and are not translated into proteins. They inhibit the expression of target mRNA, binding in a sequence-specific manner. Some studies provide evidence for reactivation of a fetal microRNA program that can substantially contribute to alterations of gene expression in the failing human heart.[65] Microarray technology analysis has provided evidence that the pattern of expression of microRNAs is altered in stress/overload hypertrophy and HF.[65,66] These results argue for miRNAs having a fundamental role in the development of heart disease and, as such, being potential targets and/or agents of future novel therapies.

Clinical aspects of genetic cardiomyopathies

In routine clinical practice, the approach to the diagnosis of cardiomyopathies is relatively crude, with little emphasis given to the detection of specific disorders that cause heart muscle disease. However, a systematic approach to the assessment of family pedigree, symptoms and physical examination in combination with a detailed cardiac evaluation and in some cases biochemical testing, can be helpful in identifying and managing some uncommon but clinically important forms of familial cardiomyopathy (Fig. 5.3).

Diagnosis

Age of onset

Age at diagnosis or presentation is an important clue to the differential diagnosis in all cardiomyopathies. In neonates and infants, the frequency of inborn errors of metabolism and congenital syndromes is much greater than in older children or adults. For example, in children presenting with HCM below the age of 18 years in a US paediatric registry, 8.7% had inborn errors of metabolism, 9% had inherited syndromes, and 7.5% had neuromuscular disorders.[67] One exception is Anderson–Fabry disease, a lysosomal storage disorder that accounts for 1–4% of HCM in individuals over the age of 40 but rarely if ever causes HCM in children and young adults.[33] Sarcomeric protein gene mutations represent the most common cause of HCM in individuals who present from adolescence onwards, although recent cohort studies have shown that sarcomeric gene mutations do occur in infants and children with otherwise unexplained left ventricular hypertrophy.[59,68] Children with HCM associated with inborn errors of metabolism and inherited syndromes have significantly worse survival.[67]

DCM is more likely to present in the first year of life than in older children or adolescents; most cases are idiopathic or caused by inborn errors of metabolism and malformation syndromes.[17,18,20,21] The most frequently reported causes of DCM in older children are myocarditis (46%) and neuromuscular disease (26%).[21] The 1- and 5-year rates of death or transplantation are 31% and 46%, respectively.[21] Most deaths or transplantation occurs within 2 years of DCM presentation, except with neuromuscular disease.[18,21] In adults, left ventricular systolic impairment is more likely to be caused by coronary artery disease (50–70%), hypertension (2–4%), and valve disease (1.5–4%).[68] Other important differentials include alcohol and drug abuse.[68] The relative contribution of myocarditis and genetic disease in adults with DCM remains controversial. Studies have shown that up to 64% of patients have an inflammatory cardiomyopathy and 67% inflammatory endothelial activation.[68] There is also at least circumstantial evidence that some of the inflammation relates to an autoimmunity; in others it is suggested that the inflammation is caused by viral persistence, but the prevalence in adults varies from 0% to as much as 80% of patients in different series.[68] Against this viral hypothesis are the numerous studies that find a familial predisposition to DCM in 20–50% of cases.[68]

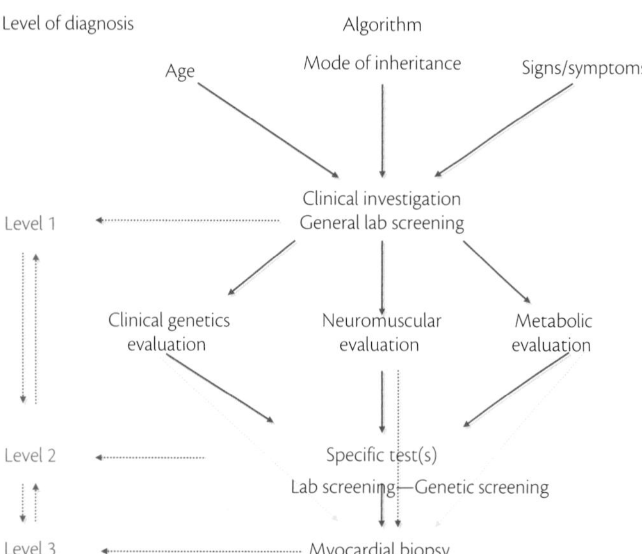

Fig. 5.3 Clinical algorithm for the diagnosis of inherited cardiomyopathies.
Level 1. Age of onset (infants, children, adolescents, adults); inheritance (autosomal dominant, autosomal recessive, X-linked, matrilinear); cardiac signs or symptoms (dyspnoea, presyncope–syncope, palpitations, angina). Clinical investigations (anamnesis, ECG, echocardiography with new technologies, cardiopulmonary stress test, ECG Holter, cardiac MRI); general lab investigation (haemocrome, glycaemia, cardiac enzymes and isozymes, lipid profile, liver function, renal function, uric acid, Ca^{2+}, Mg^{2+}, K^+, Na^+, selenium, thyroid function, proteinuria, blood lactate and pyruvate, ammonemia, ketonuria).
Level 2. Clinical genetics evaluation (dysmorphisms, including short stature or overgrowth; cutaneous anomalies as lentigines, café au lait spots, cutis laxa, lipodystrophy, angiokeratomas; facial dysmorphia, coarse face, distinctive face, or face hypotonia; webbed neck, macroglossia, epicanthus, hypertelorism, ptosis, retinitis pigmentosa, cataract; cryptorchidism; encephalopaty, mental retardation; specific orthopaedic, endocrinologic, radiologic, metabolic examinations; Karyotype and tailored genetic screening); neuromuscular evaluation (congenital hypotonia; muscle weakness beginning in infancy or after infancy; ataxia; myotonia; electroencephalogram, electromyography, muscle biopsy with histology, immunoistochemistry, biochemical study, and genetics); metabolic evaluation (some include: carnitine, acylcarnitine, fasting plasma fatty acids, aminoacids, insulinaemia, hypoparathyroidism (PTH), deficiency of coagulation factors, α-1,4-glucosidase (acid maltase), amylo-1,6-glucosidase deficiency, α-galactosidase A deficiency, 3-methylglutaconic aciduria, others).[73]
Level 3. Endomyocardial biopsy is indicated in specific conditions (eg. suspect of giant cell myocarditis or infiltrative disorders or unexplained heart muscle disorders).[81]

Family history

A three- to four-generation family history should be obtained in all patients with a new diagnosis of cardiomyopathy.[1,69] This helps to determine the probability of familial disease and its mode of inheritance and may elicit clues to the possible aetiology. For example, the presence of male-to-male transmission effectively confirms autosomal dominant inheritance, whereas a pedigree in which there is female-to-male transmission with affected males and healthy affected mothers suggests X-linked recessive disease. Common pitfalls in pedigree interpretation include X-linked disorders (such as Anderson–Fabry disease and dystrophinopathies) in which female 'carriers' develop the same disease as affected males (albeit later in life) and autosomal dominant disorders with low clinical penetrance in some family members that give the appearance of sporadic disease. Disease caused by *de novo* mutations can also be misattributed to environmental or acquired conditions.

A common finding is the presence of different cardiomyopathy phenotypes within the same family.[1,15,41,45,47,52,69] A dilated, failing heart may be the late evolution of different diseases such as familial dilated cardiomyopathy, arrhythmogenic cardiomyopathy with left ventricular involvement and hypertrophic cardiomyopathy.[1,9,15,43,69,70] Restrictive ventricular physiology can also occur in a number of different pathologies, including HCM

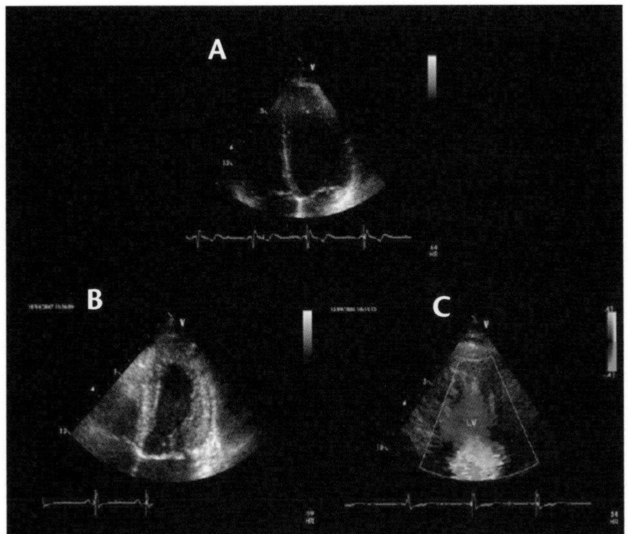

Fig. 5.4 Genotype–phenotype correlation in inherited cardiomyopathies. The figure shows three apical four chamber echocardiographic views from individuals within the same family: (A) normal subject without mutation; (B) patient with MYBPC3 mutation and classic hypertrophic cardiomyopathy; (C) patient with the same MYBPC3 mutation and apical left ventricular noncompaction (intrafamilial heterogeneity).
From Frisso, *et al. Clin Genet* 2009;**76**(1):91–101.

and DCM.[1,39,40,41,52,69] Left ventricular hypertrabeculation/noncompaction has been associated with HCM and DCM, and has been recently found to share a common genetic background (sarcomeric gene mutations)[1,45,47,69] (Fig. 5.4).

Other examples of diagnostic clues that may be elicited from the family history include early onset supraventricular or ventricular arrhythmias; progressive atrioventricular block requiring pacemaker implantation; multiple sudden deaths, suggesting laminopathy;[6,70] and a family history of sensorineural deafness and/or diabetes mellitus and/or retinitis pigmentosa, consistent with mitochondrial disorders.[71]

Clinical examination

Many cardiomyopathies are associated with congenital dysmorphic syndromes.[1,15,17,18,20,21,37,67,72] One of the most common is Noonan's syndrome which is characterized by short stature, variable degrees of developmental delay, cutaneous abnormalities (café au lait spots), and other features such as hypertelorism, ptosis, low-set posteriorly rotated ears, and a webbed neck.[72] Noonan's syndrome shares many features with the less common LEOPARD syndrome (lentigines, deafness), Costello's syndrome (coarse face, redundant skin of hands and feet, curly hair), and cardiofaciocutaneous syndrome (distinctive craniofacial appearance, hyperkeratosis).[15,17,18,72] Recently, the term 'neurocardio-facial-cutaneous syndrome' has been introduced for all these conditions. Many are caused by germ-line mutations in some of the key components of the highly conserved RAS-MAPK cascade.[73,74] Missense *PTPN11*, *KRAS*, *SOS1*, *RAF1*, *MEK1*, and *BRAF* gene mutations have been associated with hypertrophic cardiomyopathy in the context of different neurocardio-facial-cutaneous syndromes.[73,74] Pulmonary stenosis and other valve dysplasias, septal and other congenital heart defects, hypertrophic cardiomyopathy, and rhythm disturbances are typically seen in patients with neurocardio-facial-cutaneous syndromes.[37,72] Somatic mutations in the *RAS-MAPK* gene pathway may also predispose patients to various neoplastic and lymphoproliferative disorders.[73,74]

Macroglossia, frequent respiratory infections or respiratory failure, hypotonia or proximal muscle weakness, hearing loss, hepatomegaly, splenomegaly, and cardiac failure (dilated or hypertrophic cardiomyopathy with systolic dysfunction) are almost pathognomonic of Pompe's disease (α-1,4-glucosidase deficiency).[72] Untreated, this disorder is fatal in infancy with rapid cardiac and respiratory failure.

Angiokeratomas, anhidrosis (less commonly, hyperhidrosis), Raynaud's-like symptoms with neuropathy (burning extremity pain), cutaneous angiokeratomata, ocular manifestations (cornea verticillata and retinal vascular dilation), tinnitus, diarrhoea, and proteinuria are typical features of Anderson–Fabry disease.[33]

Skeletal muscle weakness may indicate a primary neuromuscular disorder (cardioskeletal myopathy associated with creatine kinase elevation as in dystrophinopathy or motor ataxia as in Friedreich's ataxia), a mitochondrial disease (particularly if encephalopathy, ocular myopathy, or retinitis are present), a storage disorder (progressive exercise intolerance, cognitive impairment, and retinitis pigmentosa, as in Danon's disease), or metabolic disorders (generally associated with hypoglycaemia, metabolic acidosis, hyperammoniaemia or specific biochemical abnormalities).[72] In such patients, skeletal muscle weakness usually precedes cardiomyopathies and dominates the clinical picture. Occasionally, however, skeletal myopathy is subtle, and the first symptom of disease may be cardiac failure.

Cardiac features

ECG conduction abnormalities, including right branch block, are reported in Noonan's and LEOPARD syndrome, particularly when pulmonary stenosis or other congenital anomalies are present.[72] Supraventricular tachycardia, especially chaotic atrial rhythm/multifocal atrial tachycardia or ectopic atrial tachycardia, is common in patients with Costello's syndrome.

Ventricular pre-excitation on standard ECG is a common feature of storage diseases (Pompe's disease, Anderson–Fabry disease, *PRKAG2* mutations, Danon's disease), and mitochondrial disorders (MELAS, MERFF).[33,34,35,72,75] Progressive atrioventricular conduction delay is a cardinal feature of nuclear envelope disorders (laminopathy and emerinopathy, in which the fibrosis often involves the myocardium around the atrioventricular node and the branches)[6] and in DCM and RCM associated with desmin accumulation (desminopathy).[42]

There are few if any disease-specific changes on echocardiography, but in context a number of features can point to a specific diagnosis. Concentric hypertrophy, often associated with a noncompaction with or without progressive systolic dysfunction, is common in metabolic/storage and mitochondrial disorders.[72] The coexistence of left ventricular noncompaction and localized inferobasal left ventricular akinesia is reported in dystrophinopathies (Fig. 5.5).[76] Pericardial effusion associated with biatrial dilation, restrictive physiology, and an abnormal texture of the interventricular septum ('granular sparkling') is very suggestive of amyloid, although other infiltrative or storage diseases should be considered.[72,77] Finally, in HCM it has been suggested that septal morphology is preferentially sigmoidal in patients with Z-disc mutation, in contrast to myofilament HCM, which generally has a reverse-curve contour.[78]

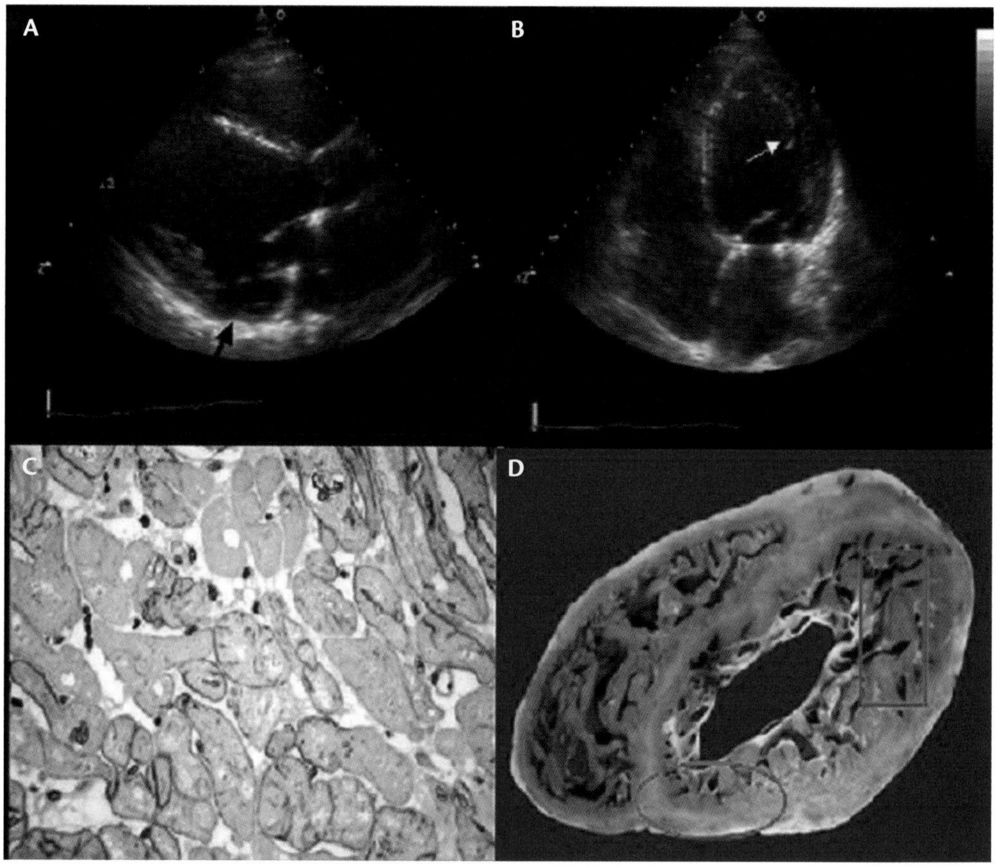

Fig. 5.5 Clinical and pathological 'hallmarks' of dystrophin cardiomyopathy. (A) Localized inferobasal left ventricular akinesia and thinning. (B) Noncompaction appearance of the apicolateral left ventricular wall. (C) Immunostaining of myocardial tissue for detection of N-terminal domain of dystrophin (monoclonal antibody NCL-DYSB, clone 34C5, Novocastra) revealed discontinuous and partially disrupted positive myocytes (of varying intensity) interspersed with negative myocytes. (D) Macroscopic examination shows a localized inferobasal left ventricular thinning. From Rapezzi C, *et al. Heart* 2007;**93**;10.

Particular patterns of focal myocardial late gadolinium enhancement on cardiac magnetic resonance imaging have been reported in different cardiomyopathies (Fig. 5.6).[79] Examples include papillary muscles (sarcoid); the mid-myocardium in the posterolateral left ventricle (Anderson–Fabry disease, glycogen storage disease, myocarditis, Becker muscular dystrophy); subendocardium (systemic sclerosis, Loeffler's endocarditis, amyloid, Churg–Strauss syndrome); and diffuse myocardial (cardiac amyloidosis).

Endomyocardial biopsy/autopsy

Endomyocardial biopsy may be diagnostic for myocarditis and for some metabolic or mitochondrial disorders. Recent guidelines recommend that endomyocardial biopsy should be performed in the setting of new onset HF of less than 2 weeks duration with normal or enlarged left ventricular dimensions and haemodynamic compromise, or between 2 weeks and 3 months in the presence of left ventricular dilation and ventricular arrhythmias or higher degree heart block.[80] Occasionally, clinically unsuspected cardiomyopathy is diagnosed at necropsy or by molecular autopsy, and prompts investigation in family members at risk.[72]

Genetic counselling

Genetic counselling is an essential component of the diagnostic process and management of inherited cardiomyopathies.[1] The process involves ascertainment of a three-generation family pedigree that includes information on individuals that have the same diagnosis as the index case or other phenotypes that could represent expression of the same underlying genetic abnormality. This provides information on the heritability of the disease, including mode of transmission and its clinical manifestations, and informs recommendations for clinical screening of at-risk-relatives and discussion of the benefits, risks, limitations, and possible outcomes of genetic testing in the patient and their relatives.

The most important rationale for genetic testing in cardiomyopathy is to identify a disease-causing mutation in an index case in order to provide presymptomatic diagnosis of family members and thereby offer clinical surveillance, early medical intervention, and reproductive advice.[1] In selected cases, genetic testing can influence management (e.g. laminopathies, storage and infiltrative diseases).[1,6,33–35] Whenever genetic testing is considered, individuals should be informed about the purpose of the test, the most probable mode of inheritance, its reliability, and the potential hazards and limitations including the psychological and social impact of the test result on the patient and their family. Rules on confidentiality of the result, especially in relation to insurance and employers, should be discussed.

Disease-specific management

Although over the last two decades major advances have been made in both our understanding of the molecular basis and capability to treat cardiomyopathies, the real impact of genetic testing in the clinical setting is still unknown. Medication and device indications are mainly based on cardiac phenotype, and are generally independent of genotype. As yet, there are few disease-specific treatments in inherited heart muscle disorders. Examples of diseases in which

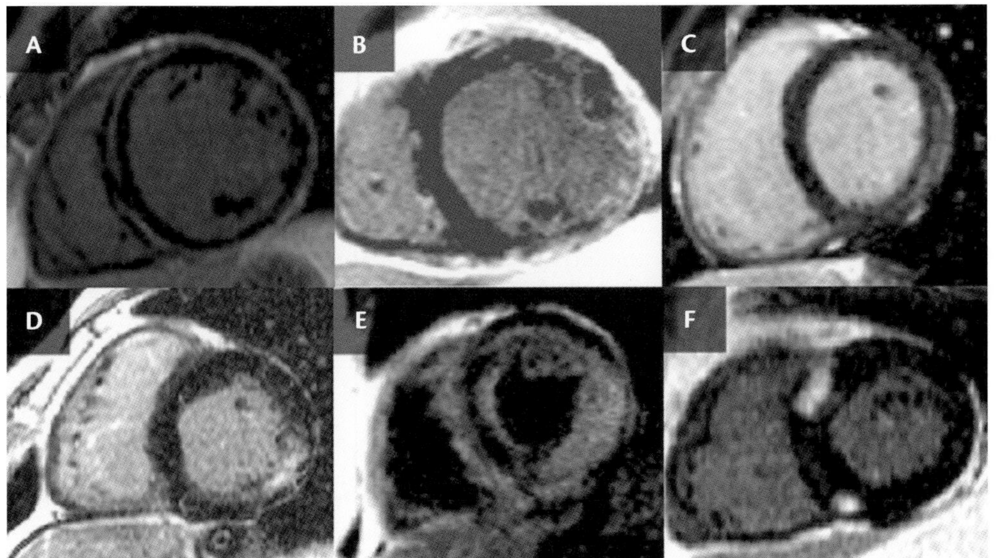

Fig. 5.6 Cardiac magnetic resonance imaging (cMRI) with late gadolinium enhancement (LGE). Focal myocardial interstitial expansion may be visualized as LGE. The LGE extent and pattern may provide a clue to the underlying disease aetiology and stage. Characteristic cases here are from patients with (A) dilated cardiomyopathy; (B) dystrophinopathy; (C) left ventricular involvement in arrhythmogenic right ventricular cardiomyopathy; (D) Anderson–Fabry disease; (E) transthyretin amyloid, and (F) sarcomeric hypertrophic cardiomyopathy.
Courtesy of Dr James Moon, University College London.

there are disease modifying interventions include lamininopathies, lysosomal storage diseases, and Friedreich's ataxia.

Lamininopathies

DCM associated with *LMNA* mutations seems to be a highly penetrant, age-dependent, malignant disease characterized by high rates of major cardiac events.[6] In particular, many patients die suddenly even after pacing.[81] The current consensus recommendation is that when these patients require permanent pacing for bradycardia indications, an implantable defibrillator (ICD) should be recommended.[81] Guidance on prophylactic ICD implantation in the absence of pacing indications is less certain, but should probably be considered in individuals with clear phenotypic expression.[82] Highly competitive sports should be discouraged in patients with laminopathies.[82]

Lysosomal storage diseases

Two different recombinant enzyme preparations have been developed for the treatment of Pompe's disease patients: α-glucosidase, produced in rabbit milk, and α-glucosidase, produced in Chinese hamster ovary (CHO) cell lines. The CHO enzyme received marketing approval in 2006 after it was proven to be effective in ameliorating muscle strength and improving heart function. Recombinant enzyme replacement in the infantile and childhood forms appears to cause regression of left ventricular hypertrophy and is associated with improved survival.[83] Enzyme replacement therapy has its limitations, however, due to unsatisfactory access of recombinant α-glucosidase to the muscle cells and due to the formation of antibodies. Preclinical gene therapy experiments have shown that antibody formation limits long-term efficacy. Immunomodulatory gene therapy with a very low vector dose might enhance the efficacy of enzyme therapy in Pompe's disease and other lysosomal storage disorders.[84]

In Anderson–Fabry disease, treatment with recombinant α-galactosidase A improves renal and neurological manifestations as well as quality of life, and probably retards the progression of cardiac manifestations.[85]

Friedreich's ataxia

Friedreich's ataxia is an autosomal recessive congenital ataxia caused by a defect in the gene that encodes for a mitochondrial protein named frataxin located on chromosome 9.[36] This protein is essential for proper functioning of mitochondria. The loss of frataxin is caused by a large GAA trinucleotide expansion in the first intron of the gene (by gene silencing through induction of heterochromatic structure).[36] This results in mitochondrial iron accumulation, which causes toxic free-radical generation and oxidative cellular damage. These mechanisms lead to deficiency of the Krebs cycle enzyme aconitase and the mitochondrial respiratory chain complexes I–III.[36] The most frequent cardiac finding is concentric or asymmetric left ventricular hypertrophy, but clinical signs of cardiac involvement typically occur late in the course of the disease.[86] Idebenone, a short-chain benzoquinone and synthetic analogue of coenzyme Q, is a potent free-radical scavenger.[36] Several open-label, non-placebo-controlled trials, indicated that treatment with idebenone (5–10 mg/kg/day) might ameliorate left ventricular mass in patients with the disease.[36] A well-designed phase II trial suggested concentration-dependent functional improvements in non-wheelchair-bound children and adolescents.[36]

Respiratory chain disorders

Mitochondrial DNA

Mitochondria are the principal site of energy production in most eukaryotic cells.[71] Each cell contains more than one mitochondrion (the number is variable among cell types) and every mitochondrion contains between two and ten copies of a circular DNA molecule (mitochondrial DNA or mtDNA). Cardiomyocytes contain about 10 000 copies of mtDNA.

MtDNA is composed of approximately 16 500 base pairs coding for 37 genes encoding 13 subunits of respiratory complexes I, III, IV, and V; 22 mitochondrial transfer RNAs (20 standard amino acids, plus an extra gene for leucine and serine); and 2 ribosomal RNAs.[71,87] With each cell division, mitochondria (and therefore mtDNA) are randomly distributed to daughter cells.

Mitochondria can also replicate their DNA independent of the cell cycle in response to the energy needs of the cell. In humans, mitochondria are inherited exclusively from the mother.[71,87] After fertilization, sperm mitochondria are tagged with ubiquitin and actively destroyed.[71,87] This uniparental derivation means that recombination events are rare, a phenomenon that is exploited in the study of population genetics.

In healthy individuals, mtDNA copies are usually identical at birth (homoplasmy), but during life the mitochondrial genome is particularly prone to somatic mutation because, unlike nuclear DNA, mtDNA is continuously replicated, even in nondividing tissues such as myocardium. This can lead to the propagation of somatic mutations within single cells by a process called clonal expansion.[88] In addition, mtDNA lacks an extensive DNA repair mechanism and histonic 'protection'. Deletions and duplications of mtDNA become pathogenic if they fall within genes involved in the respiratory chain or RNA genes.[71,87]

mtDNA and nDNA mutations

Many rearrangements (single deletions, duplications, large rearrangements) and point mutations of the mitochondrial genome have been described.[71,87] Patients with pathogenic mutations in mtDNA disease have cells that contain a mixture of mutated and wild-type (normal) mtDNA (heteroplasmy).[89] Unlike nuclear gene mutations (which are homozygous or heterozygous), the 'mtDNA mutation load' transmitted to offspring can vary from 1% to 100%. The development of disease in a specific tissue or organ is dependent on the so called 'threshold' effect, determined by the proportion of mutated copies compared to wild-type copies of mtDNA.[89] The threshold varies with the energy requirements of different tissues and cells and on local factors influencing the effect of the genetic mutation. Tissues with high energy requirement such as heart, skeletal muscles, or central nervous system are particularly predisposed to develop disease.[89] The threshold at which pathogenic mutations become important may reduce over time with the accumulation of other functionally important somatic mutations in mtDNA increase with ageing, a sort of 'second hit' mechanism.[71,87,89]

A large number of nuclear genes is involved in the synthesis of respiratory chain subunits and essential cofactors required in the normal assembly of respiratory chain function.[71,87] The transcription and translation of mtDNA is also dependent on a number of nuclear genes.[71,87] Other critical nuclear genes relevant for mitochondrial cardiomyopathies include *TAZ*, which codes for the membrane protein tafazzin, and is disrupted in Barth syndrome,[90] and the various components of the coenzyme Q_{10} biosynthetic pathway.[91] Respiratory chain disease caused by nuclear gene mutations is transmitted as an autosomal dominant trait.[71,87]

Cardiac disease in respiratory chain defects

Mitochondrial disorders are clinically and genetically heterogeneous diseases. The same genetic defect may cause multisystem disorder with cardiac involvement, or an isolated cardiomyopathy with or without conduction disorders.[71,87] Conversely, a similar clinical syndrome can be caused by different genetic defects affecting nDNA or mtDNA.[71] An example of this extreme variability is the m.3243A→G mutation in the leucine (UUR) tRNA (*MTTL1*) gene, first described in a patient with mitochondrial encephalomyopathy with lactic acidosis and stroke-like episodes (MELAS).[92–94] Some families harbouring m.3243A→G have predominantly diabetes and deafness, whereas others have chronic progressive external ophthalmoplegia or hypertrophic cardiomyopathy.[92–96] A summary of some of the more well-defined clinical syndromes is shown in Table 5.2.

Cardiovascular involvement is a common feature in adults and children with respiratory chain disease, with ECG abnormalities representing the most common abnormality.[95,96] Cardiac conduction defects are a defining feature of the Kearns–Sayre syndrome[95,96] and may occur in association with a cardiomyopathy in patients with m.3243A→G.[95,96] Accessory pathways and the Wolff–Parkinson–White (WPW) syndrome are also described in patients with Leber hereditary optic neuropathy (LHON) and in patients with m.3243A→G.[95,96]

Echocardiographic evidence for cardiomyopathy is present in about one-third to two-thirds of patients, and in the majority is of the hypertrophic type.[95–97] ^{31}P-magnetic resonance spectroscopy studies have shown that the myocardial bioenergetic defect precedes the hypertrophic phase.[98] Pure dilated cardiomyopathy is rarer, although progression to systolic impairment is frequently seen during follow-up.[95] The association between LVNC and respiratory chain disease is relatively frequent, and left ventricular hypertrabeculation/noncompaction in association with progressive systolic impairment are an 'echocardiographic hallmark' of the disease.[45,95] Mutations associated with LVNC are the mtDNA mutations 3243A→G, 8381A→G, and various ND1 and cytb mutations.[99]

Diagnosis

The presence of exclusively maternal inheritance or multisystem disease (visual problems, hearing loss, alopecia, muscle weakness, language disorders, seizures, endocrine abnormalities) in a family with a cardiomyopathy is always suspicious of respiratory chain disease.[95,99] The coexistence of left ventricular hypertrophy (or left ventricular dilation/noncompaction, with increased left ventricular mass on MRI) and systolic dysfunction is typical.[95,99] Physical examination should look for clinical signs of multisystem involvement. The ECG can show signs of left ventricular hypertrophy and/or conduction disorders.[95,96] When respiratory chain disease is suspected, endocrine assessment (oral glucose tolerance test, thyroid function tests, alkaline phosphatase, fasting calcium, and parathyroid hormone levels) is mandatory.[95] The presence of an elevated serum creatine kinase and high levels of lactate in blood are also suggestive.[72,95,97] Additional metabolic investigations including urinary organic and amino acids are usually only necessary in neonates and young children.[72,95,97]

Peripheral neurophysiological investigations (electromyogram and nerve conduction studies) may identify a myopathy or neuropathy which is usually axonal and mixed sensorimotor.[100] Electroencephalography may reveal diffuse slow-wave activity consistent with subacute encephalopathy, or it may reveal a predisposition to seizures.[100] Brain imaging can be normal, but may show atrophy, abnormal basal ganglia (including calcification), or a leukoencephalopathy.[100]

Once a diagnosis is strongly suspected on clinical grounds, a skeletal muscle biopsy (or skin biopsy or fibroblast culture in children) is often performed to confirm and characterize the pattern of respiratory chain enzyme activity because some mtDNA defects (particularly mtDNA deletions) are not detectable

Table 5.2 Mitochondrial and nuclear defects leading to cardiomyopathies. Numbers relate to base position in the mitochondrial genome.

Genome affected	Gene	Site of defect	Cardiac Manifestation	Associated features
Mitochondrial	**tRNA leucine**	**3260 A>G**	**HCM, Wolff- Parkinson- White**	**MIMyCa, MELAS**
		3303 C>T	Fatal infantile cardiomyopathy, HCM	Skeletal Myopathy with Ragged-red fibers.
		3243 A>G	HCM, Wolff- Parkinson- White	The commonest mtDNA mutation: MELAS, Diabetes, deafness, renal failure
	tRNA isoleucine	4269 A>G	Infantile DCM	Multisystem disorder (including: encephalom yopathy,epilepsy,short stature,deafness, focal glomerulosclerosis)
		4284 G>A	DCM	Multisystem disorder (including mental retard, deafness and diabetes)
		4295 A>G	HCM	Isolated cardiomyopathy
		4300 A>G	HCM	Isolated cardiomyopathy
		4317 A>G	Fatal infantile cardiomyopathy	MELAS
		4320 A>G	HCM	Encephalopathy
	tRNA lysine	8348 A>G	HCM > DCM	Isolated, progressive cardiomyopathy
		8363 G>A	HCM > DCM	Cardiomyopathy and deafness
		8344 A>G	HCM	MERFF
		8361 G>A	HCM	MERFF
		8356 T>C	HCM	MERFF-MELAS overlap
	MTND1 (Complex I)	3460 G>A	HCM, WPW?	Leber Optic Atrophy
	MTND4 (Complex I)	11778G>A		
	MTND6 (Complex I)	14484 T>C		
Nuclear	SCO2	Different mutations	HCM	Fatal infantile cardioencephalomyopathy
	NDUFS2 (Complex I)	Different mutations	HCM	Leigh syndrome
	NDUFS4 (Complex I)			
	TAZ	Different mutations	LVNC	Barth syndrome

MiMyca: Maternally Inherited Myopathy and Cardiomyopathy
MELAS: Mitochondrial myopathy, encephalopathy, lactic acidosis, and stroke-like episode
MERFF: Myoclonic epilepsy associated with ragged-red fibers
HCM: Hypertrophic cardiomyopathty
DCM: Dilated cardiomyopathy
MTDNA: Mitochondrial DNA encoded subunits
SCO2: Synthesis of cytochrome c oxidase
NDUFS: NADH dehydrogenase (ubiquinone) Fe-S
TAZ: Tafazzin
2003 Feb;24(3):221–4
Modified from Bindoff L. *Mitochondria and the heart. Eur Heart J.*

in a DNA sample extracted from blood. Analysis of DNA extracted from muscle (or cardiac biopsy) is essential to establish the diagnosis.[71,87,100] Typical histological findings include the sub-sarcolemmal accumulation of mitochondria beneath the muscle cell membrane ('ragged-red' fibres) and cytochrome *c* oxidase (COX) deficiency.[100] Electron microscopy may identify paracrystalline inclusions in the intermembrane space (also seen in other nonmitochondrial disorders such as myotonic and other muscular dystrophies).[100] A mosaic histochemical defect generally points towards a primary mtDNA defect.[71,87,100] Multiple respiratory chain defects usually points to a disorder of intramitochondrial protein synthesis, which can be of mtDNA or nuclear DNA in origin. Specific isolated complex involvement suggests particular mtDNA genes, a nuclear structural subunit gene or a nuclear-encoded respiratory chain assembly factor.[71,87,100]

The first step for molecular genetic analysis is Southern blot to look for mtDNA rearrangements or mtDNA depletion, followed by polymerase chain reaction (PCR) and restriction fragment length polymorphism analysis for common point mutations, and then the entire sequencing of mtDNA.[71,87] Since mtDNA is highly polymorphic, a mutation can only be considered to be pathogenic if it has arisen independently several times in the population, is not present in controls, and has been associated with a specific disease mechanism.[71,87,100] Family, tissue segregation, and single-cell studies may show that higher levels of the mutation are associated with mitochondrial dysfunction and disease, which strongly suggests that the mutation is causing the disease.[71,87,100]

Some of the common nuclear genes are screened as part of standard procedures on blood samples, but a genetic diagnosis is not possible in many patients either because comprehensive screening is not possible, or because the underlying gene defects have not yet been identified.[71,87,100,101]

Management

There is currently no definitive treatment for patients with mitochondrial disease, except for patients with deficiency of coenzyme Q_{10}.[102] Management is aimed at minimizing disability, preventing cardiac and systemic complications, and genetic counselling. Patients with mitochondrial disorders should undergo careful and repeated clinical assessment to diagnose and manage cardiovascular involvement.

The prognosis of cardiovascular disease differs between children and adults.[95–97] In paediatric patients with respiratory chain disease, survival is poorer in patients with cardiomyopathy compared to patients with noncardiac disease, particularly in those with COX (complex IV) deficiency.[97] In contrast, the incidence of severe cardiovascular complications seems relatively low in adults[95,96] and most deaths are related to noncardiac causes (mainly respiratory failure).[95] There many be a slightly higher mortality in adults with central nervous system manifestations.[95,97,103]

Stringent glycaemic control in diabetes associated with m.3243A→G is imperative, as well as treatment of the cardiomyopathy with cardioprotective agents (such as ACE inhibitors) at an early stage.[95] Heart transplantation can be considered in mitochondrial cardiomyopathy in cases where the clinical expression of respiratory enzyme deficiency is limited to the myocardium.[104]

Summary

Inherited forms of heart muscle disease are a heterogenoeus group of disorders characterized by substantial genetic and phenotypic heterogeneity. Evidence suggests that clinical phenotypes and outcome vary according to the disease gene and type of mutations. If this is correct, then there is the potential for condition-specific management strategies to delay disease progression and prevent complications such as sudden death. Even in the absence of specific therapies, cardiologists should be alert to symptoms and signs suggestive of genetic disease and need to become familiar with the general issues related to genetic counselling, screening and genetic testing of families.

References

1. Hershberger RE, Lindenfeld J, Mestroni L, Seidman CE, Taylor MR, Towbin JA. Genetic evaluation of cardiomyopathy: a Heart Failure Society of America Practice Guideline. *J Cardiac Fail* 2009;**15**:83–97.
2. Lambiase PD, Elliott PM. Genetic aspects and investigation of sudden death in young people. *Clin Med* 2008;**8**:607–10.
3. van Spaendonck-Zwarts KY, van den Berg MP, van Tintelen JP. DNA analysis in inherited cardiomyopathies: current status and clinical relevance. *Pacing Clin Electrophysiol* 2008;**31** Suppl 1:S46–9.
4. Alcalai R, Seidman JG, Seidman CE. Genetic basis of hypertrophic cardiomyopathy: from bench to the clinics. *J Cardiovasc Electrophysiol* 2008;**19**:104–10.
5. Keren A, Syrris P, McKenna WJ. Hypertrophic cardiomyopathy: the genetic determinants of clinical disease expression. *Nat Clin Pract Card Med* 2008;**5**:158–68.
6. Mestroni L, Taylor M. Lamin A/C gene and the heart: how genetics may impact clinical care. *J Am Coll Cardiol* 2008;**52**:1261e2.
7. Awad MM, Calkins H, Judge DP. Mechanisms of disease: molecular genetics of arrhythmogenic right ventricular dysplasia/cardiomyopathy. *Nat Clin Pract Cardiovasc Med* 2008;**5**:258–67.
8. Sen-Chowdhry S, Syrris P, McKenna WJ. Role of genetic analysis in the management of patients with arrhythmogenic right ventricular dysplasia/cardiomyopathy. *J Am Coll Cardiol* 2007;**50**:1813–21.
9. Burkett EL, Hershberger RE. Clinical and genetic issues in familial dilated cardiomyopathy. *J Am Coll Cardiol* 2005;**45**:969–81.
10. Mestroni L, Maisch B, McKenna WJ, *et al.* Guidelines for the study of familial dilated cardiomyopathies. Collaborative Research Group of the European Human and Capital Mobility Project on Familial Dilated Cardiomyopathy. *Eur Heart J* 1999;**20**:93–102.
11. Brigden W. Uncommon myocardial diseases: the non-coronary cardiomyopathies. *Lancet* 1957 Dec 14;**273**:1179–84.
12. Goodwin JF, Gordon H, Hollman A, *et al.* Clinical aspects of cardiomyopathy. *Br Med J* 1961;**i**:69–79.
13. Report of the WHO/ISFC Task Force on the Definition and Classification of Cardiomyopathies. *Br Heart J* 1980; **44**:672–3.
14. Richardson P, McKenna W, Bristow M, *et al.* Report of the 1995 World Health Organization/International Society and Federation of Cardiology Task Force on the Definition and Classification of cardiomyopathies. *Circulation* 1996;**93**:841–2.
15. Elliott P, Andersson B, Arbustini E, *et al.* Classification of the cardiomyopathies: a position statement from the European Society Of Cardiology Working Group on Myocardial and Pericardial Diseases. *Eur Heart J* 2008;**29**:270–6.
16. Codd MB, Sugrue DD, Gersh BJ, Melton LJ 3rd. Epidemiology of idiopathic dilated and hypertrophic cardiomyopathy. A population-based study in Olmsted County, Minnesota, 1975–1984. *Circulation* 1989;**80**:564–572.
17. Nugent AW, Daubeney PE, Chondros P, *et al.* The epidemiology of childhood cardiomyopathy in Australia. *New Engl J Med* 2003;**348**:1639–46.
18. Lipshultz SE, Sleeper LA, Towbin JA, *et al.* The incidence of pediatric cardiomyopathy in two regions of the United States. *New Engl J Med* 2003;**348**:1647–55.
19. Grunig E, Tasman JA, Kucherer H, Franz W, Kubler W, Katus HA (). Frequency and phenotypes of familial dilated cardiomyopathy. *J Am Coll Cardiol* 1998;31:186–94.
20. Daubeney PE, Nugent AW, Chondros P, *et al.* Clinical features and outcomes of childhood dilated cardiomyopathy: results from a national population-based study. *Circulation* 2006;**114**:2671–8.
21. Towbin JA, Lowe AM, Colan SD, *et al.* Incidence, causes, and outcomes of dilated cardiomyopathy in children. *JAMA* 2006;**296**:1867–76.
22. Remme CA, Wilde AA, Bezzina CR. Cardiac sodium channel overlap syndromes: different faces of SCN5A mutations. *Trends Cardiovasc Med* 2008;**18**:78–87.
23. Morita H, Larson MG, Barr SC, *et al.* Single-gene mutations and increased left ventricular wall thickness in the community: the Framingham Heart Study. *Circulation* 2006;**113**:2697–705.
24. Zou Y, Song L, Wang Z, *et al.* Prevalence of idiopathic hypertrophic cardiomyopathy in China: a population-based echocardiographic analysis of 8080 adults. *Am J Med* 2004;**116**:14–18.
25. Maron BJ, Gardin JM, Flack JM, Gidding SS, Kurosaki TT, Bild DE. Prevalence of hypertrophic cardiomyopathy in a general population

of young adults. Echocardiographic analysis of 4111 subjects in the CARDIA Study. Coronary Artery Risk Development In (Young) Adults. *Circulation* 1995;**92**:785–9.

26. Maron BJ, Peterson EE, Maron MS, Peterson JE. Prevalence of hypertrophic cardiomyopathy in an outpatient population referred for echocardiographic study. *Am J Cardiol* 1994;**73**:577–80.
27. Hada Y, Sakamoto T, Amano K, *et al.* Prevalence of hypertrophic cardiomyopathy in a population of adult Japanese workers as detected by echocardiographic screening. *Am J Cardiol* 1987;**59**:183–4.
28. Marian AJ, Roberts R. The molecular genetic basis for hypertrophic cardiomyopathy. *J Mol Cell Cardiol* 2001;**33**:655–70.
29. Richard P, Charron P, Carrier L, *et al.* Hypertrophic cardiomyopathy: distribution of disease genes, spectrum of mutations, and implications for a molecular diagnosis strategy. *Circulation* 2003;**107**:2227–32.
30. Seidman JG, Seidman C. The genetic basis for cardiomyopathy: from mutation identification to mechanistic paradigms. *Cell* 2001;**104**:557–67.
31. Bos JM, Poley RN, Ny M, *et al.* Genotype-phenotype relationships involving hypertrophic cardiomyopathy-associated mutations in titin, muscle LIM protein, and telethonin. *Mol Genet Metab* 2006;**88**:78–85.
32. Osio A, Tan L, Chen SN, *et al.* Myozenin 2 is a novel gene for human hypertrophic cardiomyopathy. *Circ Res* 2007;**100**:766–8.
33. Sachdev B, Takenaka T, Teraguchi H, *et al.* Prevalence of Anderson-Fabry disease in male patients with late onset hypertrophic cardiomyopathy. *Circulation* 2002;**105**:1407–11.
34. Murphy RT, Mogensen J, McGarry K, *et al.* Adenosine monophosphate-activated protein kinase disease mimicks hypertrophic cardiomyopathy and Wolff-Parkinson-White syndrome: natural history. *J Am Coll Cardiol* 2005;**45**:922–30.
35. Maron BJ, Roberts WC, Arad M, *et al.* Clinical outcome and phenotypic expression in LAMP2 cardiomyopathy. *JAMA* 2009;**301**:1253–9.
36. Schulz JB, Boesch S, Bürk K, *et al.* Diagnosis and treatment of Friedreich ataxia: a European perspective. *Nat Rev Neurol* 2009;**5**: 222–34.
37. Limongelli G, Sarkozy A, Pacileo G, *et al.* Genotype-phenotype analysis and natural history of left ventricular hypertrophy in LEOPARD syndrome. *Am J Med Genet* 2008;**146A**:620–8.
38. Limongelli G, Pacileo G, Melis D, *et al.* Trisomy 18 and hypertrophy cardiomyopathy in an 18-year-old woman. *Am J Med Genet* 2008;**146A**:327–9.
39. Kushwaha SS, Fallon JT, Fuster V. Restrictive cardiomyopathy. *N Engl J Med* 1997;**336**:267–76.
40. Denfield SW. Restrictive cardiomyopathy and constrictive pericarditis. In: Chang AC, Towbin JA (eds.) *Heart failure in children and young adults: from molecular mechanisms to medical and surgical strategies*, pp. 264–277. Saunders Elsevier, Philadelphia, 2006.
41. Mogensen J, Kubo T, Duque M, *et al.* Idiopathic restrictive cardiomyopathy is part of the clinical expression of cardiac troponin I mutations. *J Clin Invest* 2003;**111**: 209–16.
42. Dalakas MC, Park KY, Semino-Mora C, *et al.* Desmin myopathy, a skeletal myopathy with cardiomyopathy caused by mutations in the desmin gene. *N Engl J Med* 2000;**342**:770–80.
43. Basso C, Corrado D, Marcus FI, Nava A, Thiene G. Arrhythmogenic right ventricular cardiomyopathy. *Lancet* 2009;**373**:1289–300.
44. Merner ND, Hodgkinson KA, Haywood AF, *et al.* Arrhythmogenic right ventricular cardiomyopathy type 5 is a fully penetrant, lethal arrhythmic disorder caused by a missense mutation in the TMEM43 gene. *Am J Hum Genet* 2008;**82**:809–21.
45. Sen-Chowdhry S, McKenna WJ. Left ventricular noncompaction and cardiomyopathy: cause, contributor, or epiphenomenon? *Curr Opin Cardiol* 2008;**23**:171–5.
46. Kohli SK, Pantazis AA, Shah JS, *et al.* Diagnosis of left-ventricular non-compaction in patients with left-ventricular systolic dysfunction: time for a reappraisal of diagnostic criteria? *Eur Heart J* 2008;**29**: 89–95.
47. Klaassen S, Probst S, Oechslin E, *et al.* Mutations in sarcomere protein genes in left ventricular noncompaction. *Circulation* 2008;**117**:2893–901.
48. Redwood C, Lohmann K, Bing W, *et al.* Investigation of a truncated cardiac troponin T that causes familial hypertrophic cardiomyopathy: Ca^{2+} regulatory properties of reconstituted thin filaments depend on the ratio of mutant to wild-type protein. *Circ Res* 2000;**86**:1146–52.
49. Blanchard E, Seidman C, Seidman JG, *et al.* Altered crossbridge kinetics in the alphaMHC403/+ mouse model of familial hypertrophic cardiomyopathy. *Circ Res* 1999;**84**:475–83.
50. Miller T, Szczesna D, Housmans PR, *et al.* Abnormal contractile function in transgenic mice expressing a familial hypertrophic cardiomyopathy-linked troponin T (I79N) mutation. *J Biol Chem* 2001;**276**:3743–55.
51. Prabhakar R, Petrashevskaya N, Schwartz A, *et al.* A mouse model of familial hypertrophic cardiomyopathy caused by a alpha-tropomyosin mutation. *Mol Cell Biochem* 2003;**251**:33–42.
52. Marian AJ. Phenotypic plasticity of sarcomeric protein mutations. *J Am Coll Cardiol* 2007;**49**:2427–1429.
53. Senthil V, Chen SN, Sidhu JS, Roberts R, Marian AJ. Differences in protein-protein interactions as a basis for the contrasting phenotypes of hypertrophic and dilated cardiomyopathies resulting from different mutations in the same sarcomeric protein. *J Am Coll Cardiol* 2006;**47** Suppl A:62A–3A.
54. Cazorla O, Freiburg A, Helmes M, *et al.* Differential expression of cardiac titin isoforms and modulation of cellular stiffness. *Circ Res* 2000;**86**:59–67.
55. Liew CC, Dzau VJ. Molecular genetics and genomics of heart failure. *Nat Rev Genet* 2004;**5**:811–25.
56. Fatkin D, Graham RM. Molecular mechanisms of inherited cardiomyopathies. *Physiol Rev* 2002;**82**:945–80.
57. Vatta M, Mohapatra B, Jimenez S, *et al.* Mutations in Cypher/ZASP in patients with dilated cardiomyopathy and left ventricular non-compaction. *J Am Coll Cardiol* 2003;**42**:2014–27.
58. Palmieri B, Sblendorio V. Duchenne muscular dystrophy: an update, part I (review). *J Clin Neuromusc Dis* 2006;**8**:53–9.
59. Palmieri B, Sblendorio V. Duchenne muscular dystrophy: an update, part II (review). *J Clin Neuromusc Dis* 2007;**8**:122–51.
60. Towbin JA, Vatta M. Myocardial infarction, viral infection, and the cytoskeleton final common pathways of a common disease? *J Am Coll Cardiol* 2007;**50**:2215–17.
61. Posch MG, Posch MJ, Geier C, *et al.* A missense variant in desmoglein-2 predisposes to dilated cardiomyopathy. *Mol Genet Metab* 2008;**95**:74–80.
62. Chiu C, Tebo M, Ingles J, *et al.* Genetic screening of calcium regulation genes in familial hypertrophic cardiomyopathy. *J Mol Cell Cardiol* 2007;**43**:337–43.
63. Marian AJ, QT Yu, R Workman, G Greve, R Roberts. Angiotensin-converting enzyme polymorphism in hypertrophic cardiomyopathy and sudden cardiac death. *Lancet* 1993;**342**:1085–6.
64. Muthumala A, Drenos F, Elliott PM, Humphries SE. Role of beta adrenergic receptor polymorphisms in heart failure: systematic review and meta-analysis. *Eur J Heart Fail* 2008;**10**:3–13.
65. Care A, Catalucci D, Felicetti F, *et al.* MicroRNA-133 controls cardiac hypertrophy. *Nat Med* 2007;**13**:613–18.
66. Marian AJ. Genetic determinants of cardiac hypertrophy. *Curr Opin Cardiol* 2008;**23**:199–205.
67. Colan SD, SE Lipshultz, AM Lowe, *et al.* Epidemiology and cause-specific outcome of hypertrophic cardiomyopathy in children: findings from the Pediatric Cardiomyopathy Registry. *Circulation* 2007;**115**:773–81.
68. Morita H, Rehm HL, Menesses A, *et al.* Shared genetic causes of cardiac hypertrophy in children and adults. *N Engl J Med* 2008;**358**:1899–908.

69. Frisso G, Limongelli G, Pacileo G, *et al.* A child cohort study from southern Italy enlarges the genetic spectrum of hypertrophic cardiomyopathy. *Clin Genet* 2009;**76**(1):91–101.
70. Taylor MR, Carniel E, Mestroni L. Cardiomyopathy, familial dilated. *Orphanet J Rare Dis 2006*;**1**:27.
71. DiMauro S, Schon EA. Mitochondrial respiratory-chain diseases. *N Engl J Med* 2003;**348**:2656–68.
72. Schwartz ML, Cox GF, Lin AE, *et al.* Clinical approach to genetic cardiomyopathy in children. *Circulation* 1996;**94**:2021–38.
73. Bentires-Alj M, Kontaridis MI, Neel BG: Stops along the RAS pathway in human genetic disease. *Nat Med* 2006;**12**:283–5.
74. Tidyman WE, Rauen KA. The RASopathies: developmental syndromes of Ras/MAPK pathway dysregulation. *Curr Opin Genet Dev* 2009;**19**:230–6.
75. Nikoskelainen EK, Savontaus ML, Huoponen K, Antila K, Hartiala J. Pre-excitation syndrome in Leber's hereditary optic neuropathy. *Lancet* 1994;**344**:857–8.
76. Rapezzi C, Leone O, Biagini R, *et al.* Echocardiographic clues to diagnosis of dystrophin related dilated cardiomyopathy. *Heart* 2007;**93**:10.
77. Cueto-Garcia L, Reeder GS, Kyle RA, *et al.* Echocardiographic findings in systemic amyloidosis: spectrum of cardiac involvement and relation to survival. *J Am Coll Cardiol* 1985;**6**:737–43.
78. Binder J, Ommen SR, Gersh BJ, *et al.* Echocardiography-guided genetic testing in hypertrophic cardiomyopathy: septal morphological features predict the presence of myofilament mutations. *Mayo Clin Proc* 2006; **81**:459–67.
79. Silva C, Moon JC, Elkington AG, *et al.* Myocardial late gadolinium enhancement in specific cardiomyopathies by cardiovascular magnetic resonance: a preliminary experience. *J Cardiovasc Med (Hagerstown)* 2007;**8**:1076–9.
80. Cooper LT, Baughman KL, Feldman AM, *et al.* The role of endomyocardial biopsy in the management of cardiovascular disease: a scientific statement from the American Heart Association, the American College of Cardiology, and the European Society of Cardiology. *Circulation* 2007;**116**:2216–33.
81. Meune C, Van Berlo JH, Anselme F, *et al.* Primary prevention of sudden death in patients with lamin A/C Gene mutations. *New Engl J Med* 2006;**354**:209–10.
82. Pasotti M, Klersy C, Pilotto A, *et al.* Long-term outcome and risk stratification in dilated cardiolaminopathies. *J Am Coll Cardiol* 2008;**52**:1250–60.
83. Beck M. Alglucosidase alfa: Long term use in the treatment of patients with Pompe disease. *Ther Clin Risk Manag* 2009;**5**:767–72.
84. Koeberl DD, Kishnani PS. Immunomodulatory gene therapy in lysosomal storage disorders. *Curr Gene Ther* 2009;**9**:503–10.
85. Linhart A, Kampmann C, Zamorano JL, *et al.* Cardiac manifestations of Anderson-Fabry disease: results from the international Fabry outcome survey. *Eur Heart J* 2007;**28**:1228–35.
86. Child JS, Perloff JK, Bach PM, Wolfe AD, Perlman S, Kark RA. Cardiac involvement in Friedreich's ataxia: a clinical study of 75 patients. *J Am Coll Cardiol* 1986;**7**:1370–8.
87. Taylor RW, Turnbull DM. Mitochondrial DNA mutations in human disease. *Nat Rev Genet* 2005;**6**:389–402.
88. Brierley EJ, Johnson MA, Lightowlers RN, James OF, Turnbull DM. Role of mitochondrial DNA mutations in human aging: implications for the central nervous system and muscle. *Ann Neurol* 1998;**43**:217–23.
89. Chinnery PF, Thorburn DR, Samuels DC, *et al.* The inheritance of mitochondrial DNA heteroplasmy: random drift, selection or both? *Trends Genet* 2000;**16**:500–5.
90. Barth PG, Valianpour F, Bowen VM, *et al.* X-linked cardioskeletal myopathy and neutropenia (Barth syndrome): an update. *Am J Med Genet A* 2004;**126A**:349–54.
91. Quinzii C, Naini A, Salviati L, *et al.* A mutation in para-hydroxybenzoate-polyprenyl transferase (COQ2) causes primary coenzyme Q10 deficiency. *Am J Hum Genet* 2006;**78**:345–9.
92. Goto Y, Nonaka I, Horai S. A mutation in the tRNA(Leu)(UUR) gene associated with the MELAS subgroup of mitochondrial encephalomyopathies. *Nature* 1990;**348**:651–3.
93. Zeviani M, Gellera C, Antozzi C, *et al.* Maternally inherited myopathy and cardiomyopathy: association with mutation in mitochondrial DNA $tRNA^{Leu(UUR)}$. *Lancet* 1991;**338**:143–7.
94. Reardon W, Ross RJ, Sweeney MG, *et al.* Diabetes mellitus associated with a pathogenic point mutation in mitochondrial DNA. *Lancet* 1992;**340**:1376–9.
95. Limongelli G, Tome-Esteban M, Dejthevaporn C, *et al.* Prevalence and natural history of heart disease in adults with primary mitochondrial respiratory chain disease. *Eur J Heart Fail* 2010;**12**:114–21.
96. Anan R, Nakagawa M, Miyata M, *et al.* Cardiac involvement in mitochondrial diseases. A study on 17 patients with documented mitochondrial DNA defects. *Circulation* 1995;**91**:955–61.
97. Scaglia F, Towbin JA, Craigen WJ, *et al.* Clinical spectrum, morbidity, and mortality in 113 pediatric patients with mitochondrial disease. *Pediatrics* 2004;**114**:925–31.
98. Lodi R, Rajagopalan B, Blamire AM, *et al.* Abnormal cardiac energetics in patients carrying the A3243G mtDNA mutation measured in vivo using phosphorus MR spectroscopy. *Biochim Biophys Acta* 2004;**1657**:146–50.
99. Finsterer J. Cardiogenetics, neurogenetics, and pathogenetics of left ventricular hypertrabeculation/noncompaction. *Pediatr Cardiol* 2009;**30**:659–81.
100. Morris AA, Jackson MJ, Bindoff LA, Turnbull DM. The investigation of mitochondrial respiratory chain disease. *J Roy Soc Med* 1995;**88**:217P–22P.
101. Longley MJ, Clark S, Yu Wai Man C, *et al.* Mutant POLG2 disrupts DNA polymerase gamma subunits and causes progressive external ophthalmoplegia. *Am J Hum Genet* 2006;**78**:1026–34.
102. Chinnery P, Majamaa K, Turnbull D, Thorburn D. Treatment for mitochondrial disorders. *Cochrane Database Syst Rev* 2006: CD004426.
103. Arpa J, Cruz-Martínez A, Campos Y, *et al.* Prevalence and progression of mitochondrial diseases: a study of 50 patients. *Muscle Nerve* 2003;**28**:690–5.
104. Robbins RC, Bernstein D, Berry GJ, *et al.* Cardiac transplantation for hypertrophic cardiomyopathy associated with Sengers syndrome. *Ann Thorac Surg* 1995;**60**:1425–7.

6

Metabolic heart failure

Stanley H. Korman and Andre Keren

Inherited metabolic disorders are an important cause of heart failure (HF), particularly because many of them are amenable to treatment. It is therefore important that metabolic disorders are recognized and accurately diagnosed. The heart is dependent on normal metabolic function to provide a continuous source of energy at rest and even more so during exertion or stress. Many disorders of metabolism therefore affect cardiac function and may have devastating consequences (Table 6.1).

Cardiac failure in metabolic disorders is most commonly a consequence of cardiomyopathy. Hypertrophic cardiomyopathy is typical of the glycogen and lysosomal storage diseases as well as the disorders of mitochondrial energy production. Dilated cardiomyopathy is a feature of some of the organic acidurias, disorders of carnitine metabolism, and some mitochondrial disorders. Often the distinction is unclear, with a transition from hypertrophic to dilated cardiomyopathy as the disease progresses.

Additional mechanisms leading to cardiac failure in metabolic disorders include valvular disease, arrhythmias and conduction disturbances, coronary artery disease, and pulmonary hypertension.

Biochemical basis

Fatty acid oxidation disorders: the carnitine shuttle and mitochondrial β-oxidation

The energy metabolism of the heart before birth relies more on glycolysis than on aerobic fatty acid metabolism. After birth there is a transition to predominantly aerobic metabolism, with oxidation of long-chain free fatty acids as the preferred substrate.

Following their uptake from the blood, free fatty acids are activated by the acyl-CoA synthetase system. The entry of long-chain fatty acyl-CoA esters into the mitochondrion for subsequent β-oxidation is dependent upon the carnitine transport shuttle, using intracellular carnitine provided by the plasma membrane carnitine transporter (OCTN2). Fatty acids activated at the outer mitochondrial membrane are transesterified to their equivalent acylcarnitines by carnitine palmitoyl-transferase I (CPT1), translocated into the mitochondrial matrix by carnitine/acylcarnitine translocase (CACT), and reconverted to the original acyl-CoA ester by CPT2.

Within the mitochondrial matrix, chain-shortening by oxidative removal of two-carbon (acetyl) units occurs via repeated cycles of four sequential reactions catalysed by enzymes with varying and overlapping chain length specificities. The first reaction is an acyl-CoA dehydrogenation catalysed by very-long-chain, long-chain, medium-chain, or short-chain acyl-CoA dehydrogenases (VLCAD, LCAD, MCAD, and SCAD, respectively). These homologous enzymes use FAD as a cofactor which transfers electrons via the electron transfer flavoprotein (ETF) and its dehydrogenase (ETFDH) to the respiratory chain. Next, a hydration step catalysed by long-chain or short-chain 2-enoyl-CoA hydratase produces an L-3-hydroxyacyl-CoA which undergoes dehydrogenation by long-chain or short-chain L-3-hydroxyacyl-CoA. Finally, cleavage by long-chain (LKAT) or short-chain (SKAT) 3-ketoacyl-CoA thiolases generates an acyl-CoA ester shortened by two carbons and an acetyl-CoA which is available for ketogenesis (only in the liver) or oxidation in the Krebs cycle.

For long-chain oxidation, the last three reactions of the cycle are performed by a single multienzyme complex, the mitochondrial trifunctional protein (MTP), composed of four α-subunits performing the long-chain hydratase and hydroxyacyl-CoA dehydrogenase (LCHAD) activities, and four β-subunits performing the thiolase activity.

Defects in most of these enzymes have been identified. Cardiac disease (cardiomyopathy and/or arrhythmias) is a feature of the carnitine transporter defect and CPT2, CACT, VLCAD, and LCHAD/MTP deficiencies. Cardiomyopathy is not a feature of CPT1 and MCAD deficiencies. Defects in ETF or ETFDH produce a combined deficiency of multiple acyl-CoA dehydrogenases (MAD), with impaired oxidation of fatty acids of all chain lengths as well as organic acids (including glutaric and isovaleric). The pathogenesis of these disorders may be related to both deficiency of energy production and accumulation of toxic acyl-CoAs.

Table 6.1 Classification and summary of metabolic disorders with cardiovascular manifestations

Disease[a]	Abbreviation	OMIM[b]	Enzyme deficiency	Gene symbol	Major cardiovascular manifestations	Diagnostic approach	Treatment strategy
Disorders of the carnitine shuttle							
Carnitine deficiency, systemic primary (carnitine uptake defect)	CUD	#212140	OCTN2 (organic cation/carnitine transporter)	*SLC22A5*	DCM/HCM, TA	Plasma carnitine ↓↓ Urine carnitine ↑↑; AC; transport assay; gene	Carnitine ++
Carnitine/acylcarnitine translocase deficiency	CACT	+212138		*SLC25A20*	DCM/HCM, TA	AC; enzyme; gene	Low-fat, high CHO diet; MCT; carnitine?
Carnitine palmitoyl-transferase II deficiency	CPT2	*600650		*CPT2*	HCM/other, TA	AC; enzyme; gene	Low fat, high CHO diet; MCT; carnitine?
Mitochondrial fatty acid β-oxidation disorders							
Very long-chain acyl-CoA dehydrogenase deficiency	VLCAD	#201475		*ACADVL*	HCM/other, TA	OA; AC; gene; enzyme	Low fat, high CHO diet; MCT; carnitine?
Long-chain 3-hydroxyacyl-CoA dehydrogenase deficiency	LCHAD	#609016		*HADHA*	HCM/other, TA	OA; AC; gene; enzyme	Low fat, high CHO diet; MCT; carnitine?
Mitochondrial trifunctional protein deficiency	MTP or TFP	#609015		*HADHA* *HADHB*	HCM/other, TA	OA; AC; gene; enzyme	Low-fat, high CHO diet; MCT; carnitine?
Multiple acyl-CoA dehydrogenase def. (glutaric aciduria type II)	MAD	#231680	Electron transfer flavoprotein (ETF), ETF dehydrogenase	*ETFA* *ETFB* *ETFDH*	HCM/other	OA; AC; gene; enzyme	Low fat, high CHO diet; carnitine? Riboflavin
Disorders of organic acid metabolism							
Propionic acidaemia	PA	#606054	Propionyl-CoA carboxylase	*PCCA* *PCCB*	DCM	OA; AC; gene; enzyme	E.R.; Protein-modified diet; carnitine
Methylmalonic acidemia	MMA	#251000	Methylmalonyl-CoA mutase	*MUT*	DCM	OA; AC; gene	E.R.; Protein-modified diet; carnitine; OH-cobalamin; metronidazole
β-Ketothiolase deficiency	T2	*607809	Acetoacetyl-CoA thiolase	*ACAT1*	HCM/DCM	OA; AC; gene; enzyme	E.R.; carnitine;
Malonic aciduria	MA	#248360	Malonyl-CoA decarboxylase	*MLYCD*	HCM	OA; AC; gene;	Low fat, high CHO diet; carnitine
D-2-Hydroxyglutaric aciduria	D2HGA	#600721	D-2-Hydroxyglutarate dehydrogenase	*D2HGDH*	DCM	OA; gene; enzyme	
Methylmalonic acidaemia and homocystinuria, cblC type	cblC	#277400	Homocysteine methyltetrahydrofolate methyltransferase	*MMACHC*	Hypercoagulability	Total homocysteine; OA; AC; gene	OH-cobalamin, carnitine, diet
Barth syndrome (3-methyl-glutaconic aciduria type 2) (X-linked)	BTHS	#302060		*TAZ*	DCM/ noncompaction, TA	OA; monolysocardiolipin/ cardiolipin; gene	
Hyperoxaluria, primary, type I		#259900	Alanine-glyoxylate aminotransferase	*AGXT*	DCM, heart block, vascular	Urine oxalic, glycolic acids; enzyme; gene	pyridoxine, liver/kidney transplant

Glycogen storage diseases							
Pompe disease	GSD II	#232300	Acid maltase	*GAA*	HCM, TA, short PR	Enzyme; gene	Enzyme RT
Glycogen debrancher enzyme def. (Cori disease)	GSD III	#232400	Amylo-1,6-glucosidase, 4-α-glucanotransferase	*AGL*	HCM	Enzyme; gene	high CHO, high protein diet; cornstarch
Glycogen branching enzyme def. (Andersen disease)	GSD IV	#232500	Glucan (1,4-α-), branching enzyme 1	*GBE1*	HCM/DCM	Enzyme; gene	
Glycogen storage disease of heart, lethal congenital; familial HCM with WPW	CMH6	#261740 #600858	AMP-activated protein kinase, γ2 non-catalytic subunit	*PRKAG2*	HCM, WPW	Gene	
Danon disease (X-linked vacuolar CM and myopathy)		#300257		*LAMP2*	HCM DCM in advanced stage, WPW	Gene	
Lysosomal storage diseases							
Fabry disease (X-linked)		#310500	α-Galactosidase	*GLA*	HCM, valves, coronary, hypertension, heart block	Enzyme (unreliable in carrier females); gene	Enzyme RT
Hurler syndrome Hurler–Scheie syndrome Scheie syndrome	MPS IH IH/S MPS IS	#607014 #607015 #607016	α-L-Iduronidase	*IDUA*	HCM, valves, coronary	GAGs: dermatan sulphate, heparan sulphate; enzyme; gene	Enzyme RT/HSCT
Hunter syndrome (X-linked)	MPS II	+309900	Iduronate 2-sulphatase	*IDS*	valves, HCM, coronary	GAGs: dermatan sulphate, heparan sulphate; enzyme; gene	Enzyme RT
Sanfilippo syndrome A Sanfilippo syndrome B Sanfilippo syndrome C Sanfilippo syndrome D	MPS IIIA MPS IIIB MPS IIIC MPS IIID	#252900 #252920 #252930 #252940	Heparan *N*-sulphatase *N*-Acetyl-α-glucosaminidase Heparin acetyl-CoA: α-Glucosaminide *N*-Acetyltransferase *N*-Acetylglucosamine-6-sulphatase	*SGSH* *NAGLU* *HGSNAT* *GNS*	valves, HCM	GAGs: heparan sulphate; enzyme; gene	
Maroteaux–Lamy syndrome	MPS VI	#253200	Arylsulphatase B	*ARSB*	valves, DCM	GAGs: dermatan sulphate; enzyme; gene	Enzyme RT
Pompe disease	GSD II	#232300	Acid maltase	*GAA*	HCM, TA, short PR	Enzyme; gene	Enzyme RT
Congenital disorders of glycosylation[c]							
Congenital disorder of glycosylation, type Ia	CDG1a	#212065	Phosphomannomutase 2	*PMM2*	HCM/DCM, pericardial effusion; hyper-coagulability	Serum transferrin electrophoresis; enzyme; gene	

[a] Inheritance is autosomal recessive except where X-linked inheritance is indicated.

[b] Online Mendelian Inheritance in Man: http://www.ncbi.nlm.nih.gov/omim/.

[c] CDG type 1A only is presented, as the prototype and most common of this group of disorders.

AC, bloodspot or plasma acylcarnitines; CHO, carbohydrate; DCM, dilated cardiomyopathy; enzyme RT, enzyme replacement therapy; ER, emergency regimen; GAGs, urine glycosaminoglycans; HCM, hypertrophic cardiomyopathy; HSCT, haematopoietic stem cell transplantation; MCT, medium-chain triglycerides; OA, urine organic acids; TA, tacharrhythmia.

Disorders of amino and organic acid metabolism

The organic acidaemias are disorders of small-molecule intermediary metabolism, most of which result from defects in the degradation of amino acids. Of particular importance are the pathways of catabolism of the three branched-chain amino acids—leucine, isoleucine and valine. Cardiomyopathy has been reported as a feature of the following organic acid disorders:

- Propionic acidaemia
- Methylmalonic acidaemia
- β-Ketothiolase (T2) deficiency
- Malonic aciduria
- D-2-Hydroxyglutaric aciduria
- cblC (combined homocystinaemia and methylmalonic aciduria)
- Barth syndrome
- Hyperoxaluria.

Disorders of glycogen and carbohydrate metabolism

Glycogen is the storage form of glucose used as a source of energy particularly in skeletal and cardiac muscle and brain. Glycogen is composed of glucose residues joined in a straight chain by α-1,4 linkages, with branch points every 4–10 residues formed by α-1,6 linkages. The branching of the molecule gives it a compact spherical shape and confers solubility in water. Defects in the pathways of glycogen synthesis and degradation result in storage of abnormal amounts and/or forms of glycogen. The glycogen storage disorders (GSD) with cardiac involvement are GSD II, GSD III, GSD IV, and Danon disease.

GSD II (Pompe disease)

This is discussed under lysosomal disorders in the next section.

GSD III (debranching enzyme deficiency)

Debranching enzyme eliminates the branch points in glycogen during its degradation by performing two sequential activities, each with its own separate catalytic site on the enzyme. Following the shortening of the outer glycogen straight chain by the enzyme phosphorylase to within four glucosyl units of the α-1,6 branch point, the transferase activity of debranching enzyme transfers three outer units to the end of another chain into α-1,4 linkage, and the amylo-1,6-glucosidase activity then hydrolyses the remaining glucose residue at the branch point. Absence of debranching enzyme results in interruption of glycogen breakdown at branch points in the molecule and accumulation of abnormal glycogen (limit dextran) in affected tissues. As a result of differential splicing, the *AGL* gene encodes four major isoenzymes which are variably expressed in liver and muscle. The majority of patients have the type IIIa variant affecting both liver and muscle; type IIIb disease is confined to the liver and has been associated specifically with mutations in exon 3 of the 35-exon *AGL* gene.[1]

GSD IV (branching enzyme deficiency)

Branching enzyme, as its name suggests, forms the branch points in the glycogen molecule by transferring a segment of six or more glucosyl units from the outer end of a glycogen chain to an α-1,6-linkage branch point on the same or neighbouring chain. In its absence, glycogen contains fewer branch points and longer straight chains, resulting in storage of a poorly soluble molecule resembling amylopectin in cytoplasmic inclusion.

Danon disease

This was formerly believed to be a variant of Pompe disease, 'GSD IIB', but with normal acid maltase activity. It is now known to be caused by mutations in the *LAMP2* gene encoding the lysosome-associated membrane protein-2.

Mitochondrial respiratory chain disorders

Disorders of the mitochondrial respiratory chain, which is the final common pathway of aerobic fuel oxidation, are discussed in Chapter 5.

Lysosomal storage disorders

These disorders are characterized by the accumulation of complex macromolecules normally degraded in lysosomes.

GSD II (Pompe disease)

GSD II results from deficiency of the lysosomal enzyme α-glucosidase which degrades lysosomal glycogen to completion by cleavage of both α-1,4 and α-1,6 (branchpoint) glucosidic linkages. In contrast to other glycogen-metabolizing enzymes, it functions optimally at an acidic pH and hence is commonly known as acid maltase. Its deficiency results in lysosomal storage of structurally normal glycogen in periodic acid–Schiff (PAS)-positive vacuoles in all tissues. It is therefore classified as both a lysosomal and a glycogen storage disorder. In the most severe form with <1% residual enzyme activity, there is massive accumulation of glycogen in cardiac and skeletal muscle and liver, whereas in milder forms with higher residual activity, there is more moderate storage confined to skeletal muscle. The enzyme encoded by the *GAA* gene undergoes extensive post-translational modification in the endoplasmic reticulum by glycosylation at seven sites, followed by phosphorylation of mannose residues enabling its targeting to lysosomal mannose-6-phosphate receptors. The enzyme may be most reliably assayed in muscle or fibroblasts, showing good correlation of residual enzyme activity with age of onset and clinical severity. Blood lymphocytes or leucocytes may also be used, but the assay is complicated by the presence of α-glucosidases active at neutral pH.

Mucopolysaccharidoses (MPS)

Defects in the pathway of lysosomal degradation of mucopolysaccarides (glycosaminoglycans, or GAGs) lead to the accumulation of dermatan sulphate, heparan sulphate, keratan sulphate, chondroitin sulphate, or hyaluronan, depending on the specific enzyme deficiency. Cardiac involvement secondary to accumulation of GAGs in the myocardium, valves and coronary arteries is most severe in:

- Hurler syndrome (MPS I)
- Hunter syndrome (MPS II)
- Sanfilippo syndrome (MPS III)
- Maroteaux–Lamy syndrome (MPS VI).

Anderson–Fabry disease (α-galactosidase)

This disorder is discussed in Chapter 5.

Congenital disorders of glycosylation

The congenital disorders of glycosylation (CDG) are a relatively recently recognized diverse group of inherited defects of protein glycosylation whereby oligosaccharides are linked to proteins, an essential step for ensuring their normal biological functioning. This is a complex process involving many steps in the synthesis of specific glycans, their linkage to the amide group of asparagine (*N*-glycosylation) or hydroxyl group of serine or threonine (*O*-glycosylation) residues in the protein backbone and their subsequent remodelling. Cardiomyopathy has been reported in type I CDG disorders involving the early assembly pathway and type II defects in the later remodelling pathway of *N*-glycosylation. Readers are referred to Haeuptle and Hennet[2] for a detailed review of the *N*-glycosylation pathway and the clinical and molecular features of the 15 different reported defects.

Clinical presentation

Cardiac involvement may be the dominant clinical feature of metabolic disorders or may be a relatively minor facet of a multisystem phenotype. A thorough history and complete physical examination may reveal important diagnostic clues (see Table 6.2).

Disorders of the carnitine shuttle and mitochondrial fatty acid β-oxidation

In general, the severity and clinical presentations of these disorders fall into three distinct phenotypes according to age of onset:

- In the newborn period, with prominent cardiomyopathy, multiorgan failure and high mortality.
- In later infancy or childhood, when fasting or a minor febrile or gastrointestinal illness in an apparently healthy child may precipitate a 'Reye-like' episode with acute encephalopathy, hepatic insufficiency, hypoketotic hypoglycaemia, hyperammonaemia, arrhythmias, and even sudden death.
- In later childhood or adulthood, with episodic rhabdmyolysis and myoglobinuria.

CPT2, VLCAD, and MAD deficiency

These presentations conform to the above phenotypes, with good correlation between severity of the mutation and clinical phenotype.[3, 4] In their most severe forms, CPT2 and MAD deficiencies may be recognized on antenatal ultrasound examination due to multiple malformations including multicystic kidneys and cerebral dysplasia.[5]

CACT deficiency

This usually presents in the newborn period with cardiomyopathy and multiorgan failure or as sudden death, presumably due to arrhythmia. Most of the reported *SCL25A20* gene mutations are private.[6]

Generalized MTP deficiency

This results from mutations in the genes encoding either the α-subunit or β-subunit, leading to deficiency of all three enzyme activities. The clinical spectrum ranges from severe neonatal-onset disease with cardiomyopathy and early death, to mild, late-onset disease with peripheral neuropathy and/or intermittent rhabdomyolysis. There is good correlation between clinical severity and the biochemical phenotype in fibroblasts.[7]

Table 6.2 Diagnostic clues to metabolic cardiovascular disease

Clinical feature	Possible diagnoses
Psychomotor retardation	Lysosomal, mitochondrial, Danon, CDG, malonic, D-2-hydroxyglutaric;
Coarse facies	Lysosomal
Corneal clouding	MPS
Pigment retinopathy	LCHAD/MTP
Macroglossia	Pompe, lysosomal
Angiokeratomata	Fabry
Tachyarrhythmia	Fatty acid oxidation, Barth, Pompe
WPW	Danon, PRKAG2
Sudden death	Fatty acid oxidation, MPS
Heart block	hyperoxaluria, Fabry, MPS II, MPS VI
Valvular disease	MPS, Fabry
Pericardial effusion	CDG
Hepatosplenomegaly	Lysosomal, GSD IV
Hepatomegaly without splenomegaly	GSD II, III, CDG
Nephrolithiais	Hyperoxaluria
Impaired renal function	Methylmalonic, hyperoxaluria
Cystic renal disease	CPT2, MAD
Hypotonia, myopathy	Fatty acid oxidation, Pompe, GSD III, GSD IV, mitochondrial, Barth, Danon
Rhabdomyolysis	Fatty acid oxidation, mitochondrial
Skeletal dysplasia	MPS (stiff joints, dysostosis multiplex), CDG
X-linked inheritance	Danon, Fabry, Barth, MPS II (Hunter)
Reye-like episode	Fatty acid oxidation
Odour of sweaty feet	MAD deficiency
Thromboembolic	cblC, homocystinuria,
Hypoglycaemia	Fatty acid oxidation, GSD III, CDG
Neutropenia	Barth syndrome, methylmalonic, propionic
Thrombocytopenia	cblC, methylmalonic, propionic
Metabolic acidosis	Methylmalonic, propionic, mitochondrial
Maternal pregnancy syndromes (HELLP, AFLP)	LCHAD/MTP, sometimes other fatty acid oxidation

See text and Table 6.3 for abbreviations.

Isolated LCHAD deficiency

This deficiency, with relative preservation of the hydratase and thiolase activities, is caused by mutations in the α-subunit at the LCHAD catalytic site, in particular the prevalent c.G1528C (p.Glu510Gln) mutation.[8] It causes moderate to severe disease, usually with cardiomyopathy.

Additional manifestations unique to LCHAD/MTP deficiency are pigmentary chorioretinopathy,[9] peripheral neuropathy,[10] neonatal cholestasis, and lactic acidosis.

AFLP (acute fatty liver of pregnancy) and HELLP (hemolysis, elevated liver enzymes, low platelets) syndromes may develop in pregnant mothers with a fetus affected by LCHAD/MTP deficiency.[11]

Systemic primary carnitine deficiency

This may present early with a Reye-like hypoglycaemic episode, or later in the first year of life with progressive cardiomyopathy and myopathy leading to death by 3 or 4 years of age unless diagnosed and appropriately treated. The cardiomyopathy may be hypertrophic or dilated, sometimes with features of endocardial fibroelastosis. Milder defects may remain asymptomatic despite significantly low plasma carnitine levels. Apparently asymptomatic adult females have been diagnosed after their newborn infants were found on newborn screening to have low blood carnitine levels secondary to the primary carnitine deficiency in their mothers.[12,13]

Disorders of amino and organic acid metabolism

Cardiomyopathy may be an uncommon or relatively minor feature of these disorders but may occasionally assume primary importance.

Propionic acidaemia

This most commonly presents with life-threatening episodes of metabolic ketoacidosis. Dilated cardiomyopathy (DCM) develops in later childhood in approximately one in four patients who survive the first year of life, independent of the age of onset of the disorder, number of episodes of metabolic decompensation, or degree of metabolic control.[14] DCM is one of the most significant long-term complications of propionic acidaemia, sometimes with fatal outcome. It appears to be reversible following orthotopic liver transplantation.

Malonic aciduria

The major clinical manifestations of this relatively rare disorder are HCM and psychomotor retardation, in addition to seizures, hypotonia, and hypoglycaemia.[15,16]

D-2-hydroxyglutaric aciduria

This neurometabolic disorder is characterized by epilepsy, psychomotor retardation, hypotonia, and characteristic neuroimaging findings. Cardiomyopathy, most commonly dilated, develops in about half of the patients with the more severe early-onset phenotype.[17]

Hyperoxaluria

Type I hyperoxaluria is characterized by urolithiasis and nephrocalcinosis leading to renal failure and deposition of oxalate crystals in extrarenal tissues, including the myocardium and conduction system, resulting in DCM and heart block. Type II is milder and only rarely associated with cardiomyopathy.

Barth syndrome

This X-linked disorder is caused by mutations in the *TAZ* gene encoding taffazin[18] and presenting in boys with the following symptoms:

- Dilated cardiomyopathy, often with left ventricular trabeculations or true noncompaction. Presentation is soon after birth or in the first months of life, but about 10% of patients have no evidence of cardiomyopathy. Mean ejection fraction is about 50%. Most respond to standard HF therapy, but severe cardiomyopathy may lead to death or require transplantation. Ventricular arrhythmias become more common in older patients.[19]
- Skeletal myopathy leading to delayed motor milestones, positive Gower sign, and waddling gait.
- Neutropenia with susceptibility to severe infections.
- Poor growth and weight gain.

The biochemical phenotype includes:

- Abnormal urine organic acids: increased 3-methylglutaconic/3-methylglutaric acids and 2-ethylhydracrylic acid. Why these metabolites of the leucine and isoleucine degradation pathways, respectively, are increased in Barth syndrome is not understood.
- Hypocholesterolaemia.
- Abnormal mitochondrial respiratory chain complex activities.
- Decreased levels of the mitochondrial phospholipid cardiolipin, increased monolysocardiolipin, and a lower degree of unsaturation of the monolysocardiolipin acyl chains, reflecting the role of the inner mitochondrial membrane protein taffazin in cardiolipin remodelling.

The cblC cobalamin metabolism defect

This defect, resulting in combined methymalonic aciduria with homocystinaemia, is associated with risk of thrombus formation as well as structural heart defects.[20]

Glycogen storage disorders

GSD III

This presents in early childhood as marked hepatomegaly without splenomegaly, and short stature. Fasting hypoglycaemia is variable, although when present is less severe than in GSD I and is not accompanied by lactic acidaemia. Patients with type IIIa disease have muscle involvement manifesting as skeletal muscle weakness and elevated plasma creatine kinase (CK) levels. Whereas the hepatomegaly, hypoglycaemia, and elevation of liver transaminases tend to improve with age, the myopathy may progressively worsen in later childhood and adulthood. About half of the patients develop a cardiomyopathy that resembles idiopathic HCM, although there is no correlation between the severity of the skeletal myopathy and the extent of cardiac involvement. The cardiomyopathy appears to progress with age but in most patients appears to be of little or no clinical significance,[21,22] although progression to HF or sudden death from arrhythmias have been reported. There is a suggestion that dietary management with cornstarch and a high protein intake may be effective in this context.[23]

GSD IV

This disease is clinically variable. The hepatic form is most typical, presenting before age 2 years with hepatosplenomegaly and failure to thrive progressing to cirrhosis, portal hypertension, liver failure and death by age 5 years. Fasting hypoglycemia is rare. An uncommon variant presents in later childhood, predominantly as dilated cardiomyopathy with myopathy and hepatosplenomegaly.[24] Cardiac and muscle biopsies reveal massive accumulation of polyglucosan bodies. The most severe form is the congenital neuromuscular variant which can present during pregnancy with reduced fetal movements, polyhydramnios, and hydrops fetalis. At birth there is profound hypotonia with contractures and respiratory muscle failure leading to early death; cardiomyopathy is an inconsistent feature of this presentation. The adult-onset variant (adult polyglucosan body disease) may present with an isolated myopathy or combined central and peripheral nervous system involvement.

PRKAG2

Heterozygous mutations in this gene were identified in five unrelated patients with congenital onset and fatal outcome of massive nonlysosomal deposition of glycogen in the myocardium. As in previously reported infants with a similar phenotype, phosphorylase kinase deficiency limited to the heart was identified in autopsy specimens. However, this appears to be a secondary or artifactual deficiency, as no mutations were identified in any of the eight genes encoding phosphorylase kinase subunits.[25] Milder mutations in the same gene are associated with dominantly inherited familial hypertrophic cardiomyopathy with WPW syndrome [26]. Glycogen-filled vacuoles are evident in myocytes.

Danon disease

This X-linked dominant inherited disorder is characterized by the triad of HCM, skeletal myopathy, and mental retardation. HCM appears in affected males in childhood or teenage years with death before 30 years, whereas heterozygous females have milder cardiomyopathy, usually dilated, with later onset. Myopathy is usually mild in males with proximal limb and neck weakness and five- to tenfold elevation of CK level, and IQ varies from 60 to 90. About one-third of patients have WPW syndrome. Muscle histology reveals numerous intracytoplasmic autophagic vacuoles with glycogen particles and cytoplasmic debris.[27]

Lysosomal storage disorders

Pompe disease

Severe and progressive HCM together with generalized hypotonia, muscle weakness, and paucity of movement are the cardinal manifestations of infantile-onset Pompe disease. Hepatomegaly and macroglossia may be present. Massive cardiomegaly is evident on chest radiograph and the ECG characteristically reveals a short PR interval and very tall QRS complexes. Additional cardiac complications include left ventricular outflow obstruction and conduction system abnormalities. Cardiorespiratory failure or ventricular arrhythmias usually lead to death by the age of 1 year. Late-onset Pompe disease is predominantly a disorder of skeletal muscle weakness, without significant myocardial involvement.

Mucopolysaccharidoses

HCM is only one of many manifestations of the multisystem MPS disorders and may be masked by more obvious clinical features such as coarse facies, corneal clouding, hearing loss, developmental delay, short stature, hepatosplenomegaly, skeletal dysplasia (dysostosis multiplex), and stiff joints. Additional contributing factors to the cardiac dysfunction are coronary artery stenoses, and aortic and mitral valve thickening leading to progressive insufficiency and/or stenosis. Pulmonary hypertension and cor pulmonale may develop secondary to obstructive upper airway disease. Typical storage cells are found in the myocardial interstitium, the intima of the coronary arteries and the thickened valves. Cardiomyopathy may occasionally be the presenting feature of MPS, but the majority of patients have normal systolic function. The conductive system may be histologically affected and arrhythmias are occasionally observed. Despite significant stenosis of the extramural coronary arteries, ischaemic events are uncommonly documented. Nevertheless, sudden and unexpected death occurs in a significant number of patients, suggesting an arrhythmia or acute ischaemic event.

MPS I

Hurler, Hurler–Scheie, and Scheie syndromes are the severe, intermediate and mild variants of the phenotypic spectrum of MPS type I with onset of symptoms in infancy, early childhood and adolescence to adulthood, respectively. Cardiovascular involvement is limited to valvular disease in Scheie syndrome.

MPS II (Hunter syndrome)

This differs from MPS IH (Hurler syndrome) by virtue of X-linked inheritance, later onset and milder severity of disease, and the absence of corneal clouding.

MPS III (Sanfilippo syndrome)

This is a predominantly neurological disorder with relatively mild somatic features.

MPS VI (Maroteaux–Lamy syndrome)

Patients with this syndrome resemble those with Hurler syndrome, with the exception of having normal intelligence (as dermatan sulphate, unlike heparan sulphate, is not a component of the central nervous system).

Congenital disorders of glycosylation

Cardiac involvement in CDG may be in the form of DCM or HCM, in addition to pericardial effusion occasionally leading to cardiac tamponade, and sometimes structural heart defects. Presentation is usually in early life, or even prenatally with hydrops fetalis. These are multisystem disorders, with additional features including dysmorphism, hepatomegaly, psychomotor retardation, cerebellar hypoplasia, failure to thrive, skeletal dysplasia, inverted nipples, hypoglycaemia, coagulopathy, hepatic dysfunction, and protein-losing enteropathy. Because of the multiple subtypes of CDG type I and II and their phenotypic heterogeneity, a high index of clinical suspicion is required leading to screening for these disorders by transferrin electrophoresis.[2,28]

Diagnostic evaluation

Clinical suspicion

A high index of suspicion is essential if the possibility of a metabolic disorder is not to be missed. Acute presentations of metabolic disorders are often wrongly attributed to sepsis or asphyxia. Samples taken during crisis presentation are often the most informative. In cases of sudden or unexplained death, a metabolic diagnosis may be established retrospectively from samples collected post-mortem, including skin and tissue biopsies.

Routine laboratory investigations

Readily available laboratory tests can provide important diagnostic information:

- Hypoglycaemia with absent urine ketones in Reye-like presentation of FAOD
- Metabolic acidosis and increased anion gap in organic acidaemias
- Lactic acidosis in mitochondrial disorders
- Hyperammonaemia in Reye-like presentation of FAOD
- CPK elevation in GSD and in rhabdomyolysis due to FAOD
- Elevated liver transaminases and coagulopathy in Reye-like presentation of FAOD

- Elevated uric acid and triglycerides in GSD
- Neutropenia and hypocholesterolaemia in Barth syndrome
- Neutropenia and/or thrombocytopenia in acute presentations of organic acidurias

Urine organic acids

Organic acids are extracted from a random urine sample, derivatized and analysed by gas chromatography–mass spectrometry (GC-MS). The following findings are of diagnostic significance (Table 6.3).

- Hypoketonuric dicarboxylic aciduria is characteristic of FAOD. The normal ketone body formation during fasting or hypoglycaemia is impaired in patients with deficient mitochondrial β-oxidation of fatty acids, whereas dicarboxylic acids can still be formed via the alternative pathway of fatty acid ω-oxidation in microsomes. This results in a significant dicarboxylic aciduria with relative paucity of ketones, although this may only be evident during stress or fasting. Hypoketonuric dicarboxylic aciduria with a relative predominance of long-chain 3-hydroxydicarboxylic acids is suggestive of LCHAD/MTP deficiency.
- Specific organic acidurias have their own diagnostic pattern, including propionic, methylmalonic, malonic and D-2-hydroxyglutaric acidurias (see Table 6.3).
- 3-Methylglutaconic aciduria together with increased 2-ethylhydracrylate is characteristic of Barth syndrome;[18] 3-methylglutaconic aciduria is also a feature of the HCM associated with mitochondrial ATP synthase deficiency due to *TMEM70* mutations.[29]
- The combination of some or all of the following metabolites is suggestive of a mitochondrial respiratory chain defect: increased lactate, ketones, Krebs cycle intermediates, ethylmalonic acid, 3-methylglutaconic acid.

Table 6.3 Abnormal findings on acylcarnitine and organic acid analysis[a]

Disease	Abbreviation	Urine organic acids	Blood/plasma acylcarnitine
Disorders of the carnitine shuttle			
Carnitine deficiency, systemic primary (carnitine uptake defect)	CUD		↓↓C0; Plasma carnitine ↓↓ Urine carnitine ↑↑
Carnitine/acylcarnitine translocase deficiency	CACT		C16, C16:1, C18, C18:1, C14, C14:1
Carnitine palmitoyl transferase II deficiency	CPT2		C16, C16:1, C18, C18:1, C14, C14:1
Mitochondrial fatty acid β-oxidation disorders			
Very long-chain acyl-CoA dehydrogenase deficiency	VLCAD	DC, ↓ketones	C14:1
Long-chain 3-hydroxyacyl-CoA dehydrogenase deficiency	LCHAD	OH-DC, DC, ↓ketones	C16OH, C18:1OH
Mitochondrial trifunctional protein deficiency	MTP or TFP	OH-DC, DC, ↓ketones	C16OH, C18:1OH
Multiple acyl-CoA dehydrogenase def. (glutaric aciduria type II)	MAD	Glutaric, 2-OH-glutaric, ethylmalonic & dicarboxylic acids; isovaleryl-, isobutyryl- and hexanoyl- glycines	C4, C5, C5DC, C8, C12, C14
Disorders of organic acid metabolism			
Propionic acidaemia	PA	3-OH-propionic, methylcitric, tiglyl- and propionyl- glycines	C3, C3/C2
Methylmalonic acidaemia	MMA	Methylmalonic, 3-OH-propionic, methylcitric, tiglyl- and propionyl- glycines	C3
β-Ketothiolase deficiency	T2	Ketones, tiglylglycine, 2-methyl-3-OH-butyric, 2-methylacetoacetic	C5OH, C5:1
Malonic aciduria	MA	Malonic, methylmalonic	C3DC
D-2-Hydroxyglutaric aciduria	D2HGA	D-2-OH-glutaric	
Methylmalonic acidaemia and homocystinuria, cblC type	cblC	Methylmalonic total homocysteine	C3
Barth syndrome (3-methylglutaconic aciduria type 2)	BTHS	3-Methylglutaconic, 3-methylglutaric, 2-ethylhydracrylic	
Hyperoxaluria, primary, type I		Oxalic, glycolic	

[a] Metabolite levels are increased unless otherwise indicated.

Acylcarnitines: C0, free carnitine; C16, acylcarnitine with 16-carbon chain length (palmitoylcarnitine); C16:1, monounsaturated C16 carnitine; C16OH, hydroxy-C16 carnitine; C5DC, C5-dicarboxylic carnitine, etc.

Organic acids: DC, dicarboxylic acids; OH-DC, long-chain hydroxydicarboxylic acids.

Carnitine, free and total

Although plasma carnitine levels are not necessarily an accurate reflection of tissue carnitine levels, their determination is important for assessment of primary or secondary carnitine deficiency. Total carnitine is made up of esterified carnitine (the sum of individual acylcarnitine species) and free carnitine. In carnitine transporter defect, both free and total plasma carnitine levels are extremely low, whereas urine carnitine excretion is inappropriately high. This is best assessed by simultaneous determination of carnitine and creatinine levels in paired plasma and urine samples and calculation of the carnitine excretion index. In the organic acidurias and disorders of fatty acid β-oxidation, free carnitine is low while the ratio of esterified carnitine (the difference between total and free carnitine) to free carnitine is increased.

Acylcarnitines

By application of tandem mass spectrometry (TMS), individual acylcarnitine species can be quantified (not just total esterified carnitine as above), allowing recognition of specific diagnostic patterns (see Table 6.2). Long-chain (C16 and C18) acylcarnitines are elevated in CPT2 and translocase deficiencies (Fig. 6.1d), long-chain hydroxyacylcarnitines in MTP/LCHAD deficiency (Fig. 6.1f), C14:1 in VLCAD deficiency Fig. 6.1e), and short-, medium-, and long-chain acylcarnitine species in MAD deficiency (Fig. 6.1c). In the organic acidurias, C3 carnitine is elevated in propionic acidaemia (Fig. 6.1b), C3-dicarboxylic in malonic acidaemia. Determination of acylcarnitines by TMS is highly sensitive, rapid and relatively cheap, making it eminently suitable for universal screening of newborns by analysis of dried blood spots on filter paper (Guthrie) cards.[30] Analysis of plasma and urine samples is used for diagnostic testing. *In vitro* acylcarnitine profiling of cultured fibroblasts fed with deuterated fatty acid substrates is a highly sensitive technique for identifying the defect in patients with borderline or equivocal results.[31]

Transferrin electrophoresis

Initial screening for CDG involving defects in *N*-glycosylation is by evaluation of transferrin glycosylation pattern in serum or dried blood spots. This is most commonly performed by isoelectric focusing, but capillary electrophoresis and TMS methods are also available.[32] Normal transferrin contains four sialic acid residues. Abnormal patterns reveal a reduced intensity of the normal tetrasiolatransferrin band, with the appearance of di- and asialotransferrin bands in type I CDG, and tri-, di-, mono- and asialotransferrin bands in type II CDG disorders. Transferrin isoelectrophoresis may give a false-negative result in the first months of life and should be repeated if there is clinical suspicion. CDG must be differentiated from abnormal patterns of transferrin glycosylation due to galactosaemia, hereditary fructose intolerance, and chronic alcoholism. Definitive diagnosis of the precise subtype is based on analysis of the specific enzyme and gene.[33]

Cardiolipin analysis

Abnormal cardiolipin remodelling in Barth syndrome patients is used as a diagnostic test based on demonstration of an increase in the ratio of monolysocardiolipin to cardiolipin, as determined by HPLC-MS. This assay can be performed on fibroblasts, muscle, lymphocytes,[34] or dried blood spots.[35]

Specific enzyme assay

In many disorders the diagnosis may already be established on the basis of a characteristic profile of metabolites as described above, in which case confirmation of the diagnosis by enzyme assay may be superfluous. There may still, however, be a role for enzyme assay in this situation when the degree of residual enzyme activity is known to be a predictor of clinical severity and outcome. In other disorders, particularly the lysosomal storage disorders, enzyme assay remains the gold standard for diagnosis.

In contrast to metabolite and molecular testing which are becoming increasingly available and cheaper as a result of technological advances and automation, enzyme assays for diagnosing metabolic disorders are for the most part manually performed, time-consuming, and expensive procedures. They must be individually developed and validated and require special reagents and a high degree of expertise. Their availability is therefore often limited to national or international reference laboratories, creating logistic difficulties in shipment of samples under appropriate conditions.

Selection of the appropriate tissue for assay is an important issue and is determined by the expression profile of the specific enzyme. Peripheral blood is the most practical and is appropriate when the enzyme can be assayed in serum or in isolated erythrocytes or leucocytes. Many enzymes are expressed in fibroblasts cultured from a skin biopsy. Although it can take several weeks until the fibroblast culture is established, fibroblasts provide an unlimited source of cells for testing, are easily shipped, and can be permanently cryopreserved. In some cases, however, diagnosis of an enzyme deficiency can only be established in the target organ for the disease, necessitating a liver, skeletal, or even myocardial biopsy.

Lysosomal enzymes have traditionally been assayed in peripheral blood leucocytes or fibroblasts, either individually or as a panel of enzymes. Recently, methodologies have been developed for assay of lysosomal enzymes in dried blood spots on standard cards used for newborn screening. This approach requires only small volumes of blood and the cards can be easily mailed to the laboratory under ambient conditions. The lysosomal enzyme activities remain stable during storage in this format. The use of TMS technology allows multiple enzymes to be assayed in a single analysis.[36] With the advent of enzyme replacement therapy for lysosomal disorders, this creates the very real prospect of including lysosomal storage disorders in newborn screening programmes, enabling early diagnosis and institution of treatment before irreparable damage has occurred.[37]

Mutation analysis

The causative genes for each disorder are listed in Table 6.1. Molecular testing is becoming increasingly available and is a powerful diagnostic tool for diagnosing metabolic disorders. However, there are numerous pitfalls in performing and interpreting molecular studies and it should not be used routinely simply because it exists. It is of particular value in the following circumstances:

- There is no available or reliable biochemical test, or when biochemical testing requires an invasive procedure.
- A single or limited number of pathogenic mutations are known to be responsible for the disease in a given family or community.

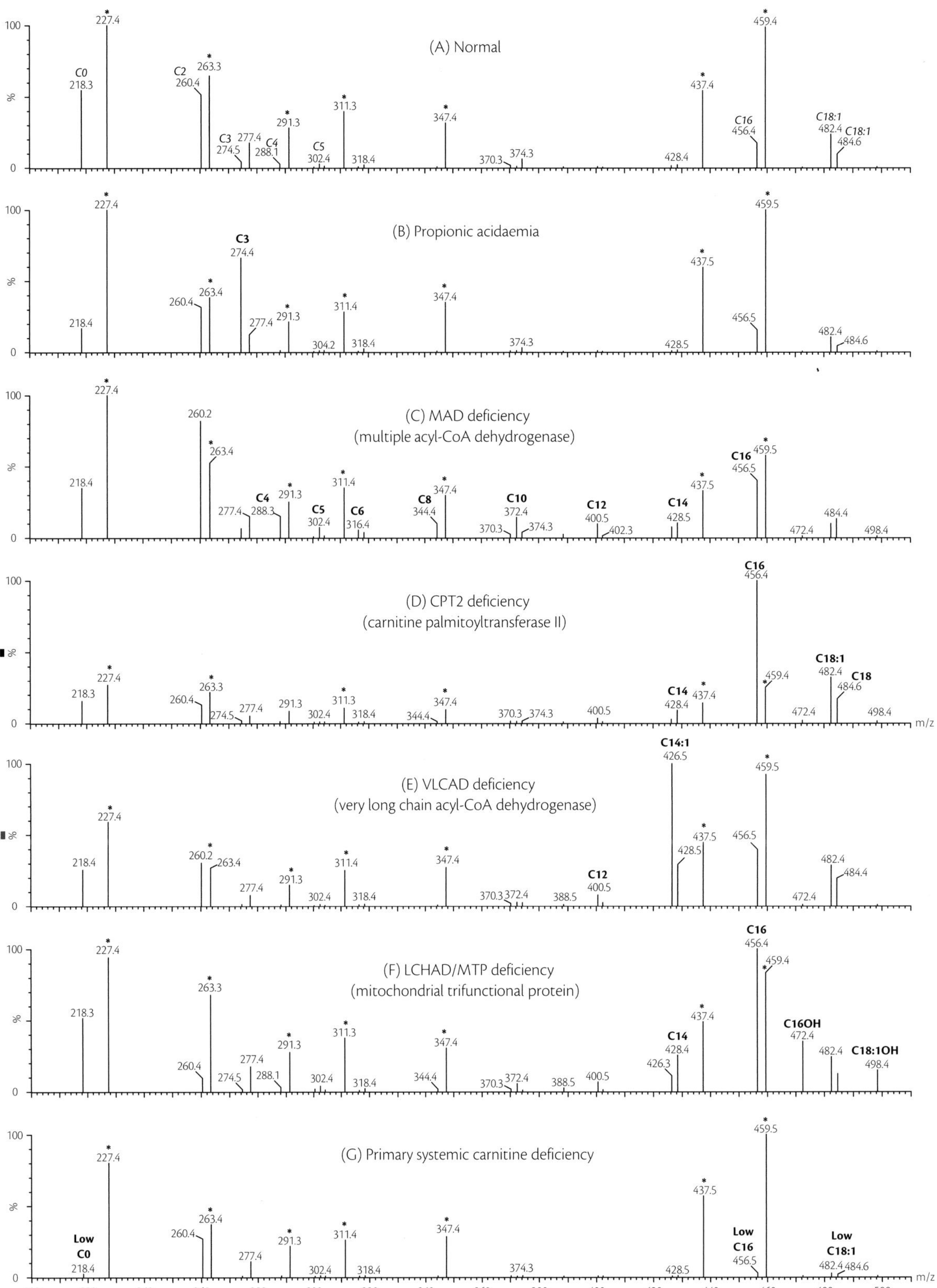

Fig. 6.1 Dried blood spot acylcarnitine profiles by tandem mass spectrometry. Panel A illustrates a normal profile. * indicates deuterated internal standard peaks; from left to right: free carnitine, C2, C3, C4, C5, C8, C14, C16 deuterated internal standards. The major acylcarnitine peaks are labelled in italics. C0, free carnitine. Panels B–F are from patients with organic acid and fatty acid oxidation disorders. Abnormally increased acylcarnitine peaks are labelled in bold.

- There is a clear correlation between genotype and phenotype, allowing prediction of expected disease course and severity (e.g. VLCAD deficiency).
- Prenatal diagnosis is requested, as molecular testing for a known mutation is often more rapid and reliable than biochemical testing.
- Carrier testing of relatives is requested.

Treatment

In contrast to many genetic disorders for which there are few or no therapeutic options, effective treatment is available for many of the inherited metabolic disorders. Development of an effective treatment depends on accurate diagnosis of the specific biochemical defect together with an understanding of its metabolic consequences and mechanism of disease pathogenesis. Some disorders have specific therapies, but general guidelines are applicable to many of these conditions.

Emergency management

Many metabolic disorders, especially those of fatty acid oxidation, organic and amino acid metabolism, and some of the GSDs, are characterized by acute episodes of decompensation on a background of relative well-being. These acute exacerbations can be life-threatening or lead to permanent sequelae. They are often precipitated by catabolic stress such as acute febrile illness, vomiting and/or diarrhoea, extended fasting, and surgery or other trauma. Management of these episodes therefore aims to:

- Reduce the dietary sources and endogenous production of toxic metabolites.
- Promote the elimination of toxic metabolites.
- Reverse the catabolic process by provision of high energy intake.

The basic principles are to:

- Give clear explanations to the family in advance, including a printed summary with a brief description of the illness and a list of instructions outlining the protocol for investigation and management of an acute crisis.
- Stop oral intake of precursors of toxic metabolites, i.e. protein in organic acidurias, long-chain fats in disorders of fatty acid oxidation.
- Use intravenous glucose as the primary energy source, given as a 10% infusion (or higher concentration through a central line) to provide at least 8–10 mg/kg per min, with monitoring for hyperglycsemia, which is managed by addition of continuous insulin infusion (this has the added benefit of promoting the switch from a catabolic to anabolic state).
- Use intravenous lipid infusion as an additional energy source, except in disorders of long-chain fatty acid oxidation, where MCT oil (medium-chain triglycerides) is an option.
- Give carnitine (preferably intravenously) in organic acid disorders, but with extreme caution in long-chain fatty acid oxidation disorders (FAOD).
- Increase fluid intake above standard maintenance levels to facilitate clearance of toxic metabolites.
- Treat aggressively any precipitating febrile illness with antipyretics, with or without antibiotics as appropriate.
- Treat significant metabolic acidosis and hyperammonaemia.

'Emergency regimen' for initial home management

Early institution of home treatment at the very first signs of an acute intercurrent illness can often abort an acute decompensation crisis and avoid the need for hospital management as described above.[38] The emergency regimen is based on:

- Clear instructions and training given to the parents in advance.
- Cessation of regular feeds.
- Use of an oral glucose polymer solution, thereby providing a large amount of rapidly absorbed calories in a relatively low osmolarity solution. Suitable products include Polycose

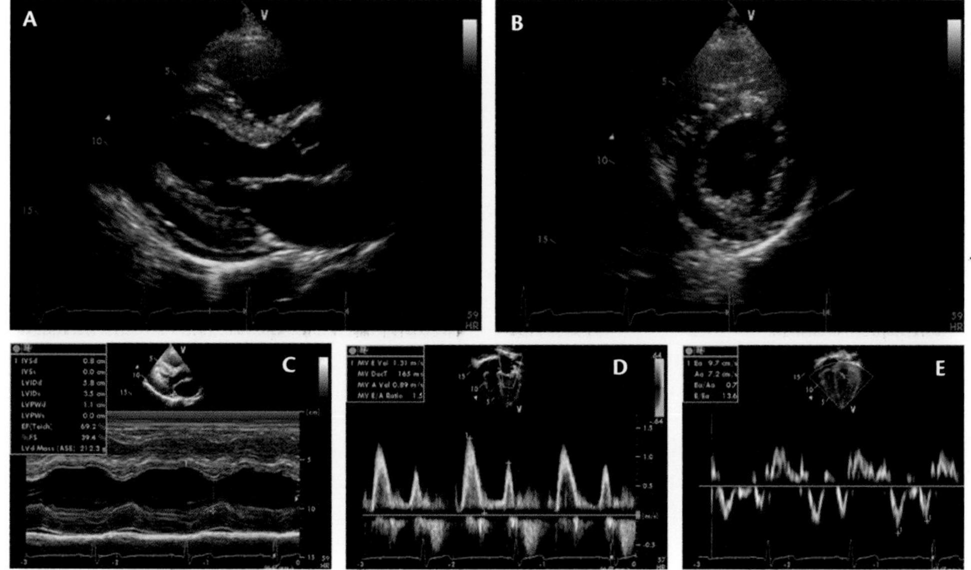

Fig. 6.2 Typical echocardiographic findings in a 38-year-old patient with Anderson–Fabry disease who receives enzyme replacement therapy. Parasternal long axis view (A), short axis view (B), and M-mode recording (C) show concentric left ventricular hypertrophy (more pronounced in this case in the posterior wall) and small amount of posterior pericardial effusion. Pseudonormal E/A ratio on mitral Doppler (D) and low relaxation velocities on mitral annular tissue Doppler (E) are compatible with stage II diastolic dysfunction with elevated filling pressure.

(Abbott Nutrition), Caloreen (Nestlé), or Polyjoule (Nutricia). A 15–30% solution is used, depending on age.

- Administration of small amounts at frequent intervals around the clock, thereby ensuring substantial absorption between episodes of vomiting.
- Immediate referral to hospital if there is persistent vomiting or deterioration in conscious state.
- Otherwise, reintroduction of regular feeds within 24 h.

High caloric intake and avoidance of fasting

A high caloric intake is essential to maintain patients in an anabolic rather than catabolic state. However, many factors make it difficult to achieve a high caloric intake, including recurrent vomiting, anorexia related to metabolic acidosis, unpalatable special diets, and feeding difficulties related to cardiac disease.

Fasting should be assiduously avoided. Even a normal overnight fast may be poorly tolerated in patients with metabolic disorders. Management approaches to avoid fasting and achieve a high caloric intake may include the following.

Frequent diurnal and nocturnal feeds

PEG (percutaneous endoscopic gastrostomy)

This procedure can often resolve many of the feeding issues in severe patients, by allowing for:

- 'Top-up' of oral feeds
- Continuous drip feedings which may be better tolerated than bolus feedings
- Nocturnal feeds, without the need to wake the child
- Emergency home administration of glucose during hypoglycaemia.

Uncooked cornstarch

This undergoes prolonged hydrolysis by amylase in the intestine, providing a relatively continuous source of glucose for absorption for 4–6 h. Cornstarch was originally introduced as treatment for GSD type I, where it replaced the requirement for overnight continuous intragastric glucose infusion. It has found wider application in patients with metabolic disorders as a source of 'slow release' glucose. One dose before bedtime and possibly a second during the night resolves the issue of overnight fasting.

Special diet

Manipulation of the content of the diet according to the specific metabolic defect can have a major therapeutic impact.

Substrate restriction

Restriction of the dietary source of substrate preceding the metabolic block reduces the production and accumulation of toxic metabolic intermediates.

- Natural protein intake is restricted in the organic acidurias to limit the intake of the amino acid(s) whose metabolism is blocked. The diet may be supplemented with an otherwise nutritionally complete special formula devoid of the specific amino acids (e.g. methionine-, threonine-, valine- and isoleucine-free for propionic and methylmalonic acidaemia). Over-restriction of protein intake must be avoided, as this can exacerbate decompensation by inducing muscle protein catabolism to supply deficient essential amino acids.
- Long-chain fats are restricted in defects of the carnitine shuttle and long-chain fatty acid defects. Essential fatty acids must be supplemented when on a low-fat diet.

Use of alternative metabolic pathways

Functionally intact metabolic pathways can be exploited as an alternative metabolic route, e.g. a high-carbohydrate diet metabolized via glycolysis for patients with FAOD on a low-fat diet.

Bypassing the metabolic block

This can be achieved by providing an exogenous source of a distal metabolite.

- MCT oil contains medium-chain triglycerides which enter the mitochondrion directly for β-oxidation without requiring the carnitine shuttle. MCT is therefore used in patients with defects of the carnitine shuttle as well as long-chain fatty acid oxidation defects (VLCAD and LCHAD/MTP).[39]
- Triheptanoin has been proposed as an alternative to MCT in long-chain fatty acid disorders on the basis that medium-odd-chain rather than medium-even-chain fatty acids would supply both acetyl-CoA and anapleurotic propionyl-CoA and restore disturbed Krebs cycle dysfunction. Significant improvement of cardiomyopathy and rhabdomyolysis was reported in patients with VLCAD deficiency,[40] but confirmation of these initially promising results has not been forthcoming.
- 3-Hydroxybutyrate. In FAOD, ketone body production by the liver is impaired. Ketones exported from the liver normally serve as an important energy source for the myocardium and other tissues during fasting. Oral administration of the ketone sodium-D,L-3-hydroxybutyrate to two infants with MAD deficiency and critical cardiomyopathy unresponsive to other therapies resulted in progressive and sustained improvement.[41]

L-Carnitine

Carnitine is essential for the transport of long-chain fatty acids into the mitochondrion for subsequent β-oxidation.

Primary carnitine deficiency

In this disorder, administration of pharmacological doses of carnitine is life saving.

Fatty acid β-oxidation disorders and organic acidurias

In these inherited disorders, carnitine has an essential function in the reverse direction, binding and enabling the removal from the mitochondrion of the accumulating toxic acyl-CoA compounds and the regeneration of essential free coenzyme A. The acylcarnitines thus formed are excreted into the urine, resulting in secondary carnitine depletion. Correction of carnitine deficiency is essential in the management of the organic acidurias, the usual starting dose being 100 mg/kg per day. However, in the long-chain fatty acid β-oxidation disorders such as LCHAD and VLCAD deficiency, use of carnitine supplementation is controversial. Although carnitine has been used to correct secondary carnitine depletion in these disorders, there is concern that its administration during acute metabolic crises may lead to sudden death due to the potentially toxic effects of long-chain acylcarnitines.

Supplementation of vitamins and cofactors

General supplementation of vitamins and minerals

This is important in patients with poor intake or restricted diets. When cornstarch is used as described above it may constitute a significant proportion of the caloric intake but is devoid of essential nutrients.

Specific vitamins in pharmacological doses

These may restore enzyme activity in vitamin-responsive defects or disorders of cofactor metabolism, e.g.:

- Vitamin B_{12}-responsive methylmalonic acidemia
- Vitamin B_{12} (hydroxocobalamin) in the cblC cobalamin metabolism defect
- Riboflavin (vitamin B_2)-responsive multiple acyl-CoA dehydrogenase deficiency.[42]

Bezafibrate

Bezafibrate is a PPAR (peroxisomal proliferator-activated receptor) agonist widely used for its hypolipidaemic action; it increases gene expression, residual enzyme activity, and fatty acid oxidation capacity in fibroblast lines from patients with CPT2[43] and VLCAD deficiency.[44] A pilot trial in CPT2 deficiency patients produced encouraging results.[45] These effects were only apparent, however, in patients with significant residual enzyme activity in fibroblasts and a milder (predominantly muscular) clinical presentation. It is unlikely to benefit patients with cardiomyopathy, as they have severe enzyme deficiency.

Enzyme replacement therapy (ERT)

ERT has revolutionized the management of patients with lysosomal storage disorders, for whom previously there was little to offer beyond symptomatic and supportive treatment. ERT was initially achieved for Gaucher disease. The two major breakthroughs allowing the development of ERT were the ability to produce large quantities of recombinant enzyme, and recognition of the critical importance of the mannose-6-phosphate (M6P) recognition marker for receptor-mediated uptake of lysosomal enzymes. The recombinant enzyme is modified by addition of mannose-6-phosphate (M6P) moieties for recognition by plasma membrane M6P receptors which sequester modified enzyme into lysosome-targeted transport vesicles, allowing delivery to and uptake by the lysosome.

ERT requires intravenous infusion of the recombinant enzyme every 1–2 weeks and involves a significant commitment by both the medical team and the patient. Common reactions include local irritation and infusion-related hypersensitivity responses. Treatment is usually initiated in a hospital outpatient setting, with the aim of eventual transfer to home infusion therapy. The high cost of this lifelong treatment programme is a major issue in terms of insurance coverage, particularly where therapeutic benefit is only limited or where clinical manifestations are relatively minor. Enzyme infused intravenously does not cross the blood–brain barrier, limiting its use in treatment of lysosomal storage disorders with progressive neurological involvement.[46]

Pompe disease (GSD II)

ERT was initially performed using recombinant human enzyme derived from transgenic rabbit milk, and subsequently from genetically engineered CHO cells. Myozyme (alglucosidealfa, Genzyme Corporation, Cambridge MA) has been approved for clinical use by the US Food and Drug Authority since 2006. Targeting muscle is problematic, as most of the infused enzyme is taken up by liver and spleen, with only a small amount reaching heart and even less skeletal muscle. High doses are therefore required to achieve a therapeutic effect. Current recommended dosage is 20 mg/kg body weight administered every 2 weeks, although up to 40 mg/kg has been used in individual patients. Clinical studies in patients with the severe infantile form reveal that the most dramatic effect is on the heart, with significant improvement in cardiac hypertrophy and function as well as prolonged survival beyond the expected age of 1 year in untreated infants. Serial muscle biopsies show clearing of glycogen, with good correlation between extent of glycogen clearance and clinical response. Many achieve motor milestones such as sitting, standing, and walking, which are not expected in the natural course of the disease. However a significant proportion of treated infants in the initial studies died or remained ventilator dependent due to respiratory muscle failure. The most favourable results have been achieved in patients treated early, before irreversible muscle damage has occurred.[47–49]

The feasibility of newborn screening for Pompe disease has created the possibility of initiating ERT before clinical deterioration has occurred. Indeed, a recently published study reported an encouraging outcome for ERT in six infants identified in a newborn screening programme in Taiwan. Five of the six, despite being still clinically asymptomatic in the first month of life, had the severe early-onset form of the disease as evidenced by significant cardiomyopathy, abnormal muscle histology, and severe enzyme deficiency in fibroblasts. Following early institution of ERT and follow-up for 14–32 months, all survived with normalization of cardiac size and muscle histology, normal growth, and normal age-appropriate motor development.[50]

MPS

Recombinant enzyme products are available for ERT of MPS I, II, and VI and can be of benefit in reducing the severity of the somatic manifestations including cardiac disease, but cannot affect the progression of central nervous system disease. In contrast, haematopoietic stem cell transplantation (HSCT) with bone marrow or umbilical cord stem cells can arrest or even reverse CNS and somatic manifestations. The choice between these two therapeutic approach depends on the age of the patient, extent of disease, and predicted rate of progression.[51]

References

1. Shen JJ, Chen YT. Molecular characterization of glycogen storage disease type III. *Curr Mol Med* 2002;**2**(2):167–75.
2. Haeuptle MA, Hennet T. Congenital disorders of glycosylation: an update on defects affecting the biosynthesis of dolichol-linked oligosaccharides. *Hum Mutat* 2009;**30**(12):1628–41.
3. Thuillier L, Rostane H, Droin V, *et al.* Correlation between genotype, metabolic data, and clinical presentation in carnitine palmitoyltransferase 2 (CPT2) deficiency. *Hum Mutat* 2003;**21**(5):493–501.
4. Andresen BS, Olpin S, Poorthuis BJ, *et al.* Clear correlation of genotype with disease phenotype in very-long-chain acyl-CoA dehydrogenase deficiency. *Am J Hum Genet* 1999;**64**(2):479–94.
5. Meir K, Fellig Y, Meiner V, *et al.* Severe infantile carnitine palmitoyltransferase II (cpt ii) deficiency in 19-week fetal sibs. *Pediatr Dev Pathol* 2009;12(6):481–6.

6. Korman SH, Pitt JJ, Boneh A, *et al.* A novel SLC25A20 splicing mutation in patients of different ethnic origin with neonatally lethal carnitine-acylcarnitine translocase (CACT) deficiency. *Mol Genet Metab* 2006;**89**(4):332–8.
7. Olpin SE, Clark S, Andresen BS, *et al.* Biochemical, clinical and molecular findings in LCHAD and general mitochondrial trifunctional protein deficiency. *J Inherit Metab Dis* 2005;**28**(4):533–44.
8. Tyni T, Pihko H. Long-chain 3-hydroxyacyl-CoA dehydrogenase deficiency. *Acta Paediatr* 1999;**88**(3):237–45.
9. Tyni T, Paetau A, Strauss AW, Middleton B, Kivela T. Mitochondrial fatty acid beta-oxidation in the human eye and brain: implications for the retinopathy of long-chain 3-hydroxyacyl-CoA dehydrogenase deficiency. *Pediatr Res* 2004;**56**(5):744–50.
10. Tein I, Vajsar J, MacMillan L, Sherwood WG. Long-chain L-3-hydroxyacyl-coenzyme A dehydrogenase deficiency neuropathy: response to cod liver oil. *Neurology* 1999;**52**(3):640–3.
11. Browning MF, Levy HL, Wilkins-Haug LE, Larson C, Shih VE. Fetal fatty acid oxidation defects and maternal liver disease in pregnancy. *Obstet Gynecol* 2006;**107**(1):115–20.
12. Lee NC, Tang NL, Chien YH, *et al.* Diagnoses of newborns and mothers with carnitine uptake defects through newborn screening. *Mol Genet Metab* 2010;**100**(1):46–50.
13. El Hattab AW, Li FY, Shen J, *et al.* Maternal systemic primary carnitine deficiency uncovered by newborn screening: clinical, biochemical, and molecular aspects. *Genet Med* 2010;**12**(1):19–24.
14. Romano S, Valayannopoulos V, Touati G, *et al.* Cardiomyopathies in propionic aciduria are reversible after liver transplantation. *J Pediatr* 2010;**156**(1):128–34.
15. Ficicioglu C, Chrisant MR, Payan I, Chace DH. Cardiomyopathy and hypotonia in a 5-month-old infant with malonyl-CoA decarboxylase deficiency: potential for preclinical diagnosis with expanded newborn screening. *Pediatr Cardiol* 2005;**26**(6):881–3.
16. Salomons GS, Jakobs C, Pope LL, *et al.* Clinical, enzymatic and molecular characterization of nine new patients with malonyl-coenzyme A decarboxylase deficiency. *J Inherit Metab Dis* 2007;**30**(1):23–8.
17. van der Knaap MS, Jakobs C, Hoffmann GF, *et al.* D-2-hydroxyglutaric aciduria: further clinical delineation. *J Inherit Metab Dis* 1999;**22**(4):404–13.
18. Barth PG, Valianpour F, Bowen VM, *et al.* X-linked cardioskeletal myopathy and neutropenia (Barth syndrome): an update. *Am J Med Genet A* 2004;**126A**(4):349–54.
19. Spencer CT, Bryant RM, Day J, *et al.* Cardiac and clinical phenotype in Barth syndrome. *Pediatrics* 2006;**118**(2):e337–e346.
20. Profitlich LE, Kirmse B, Wasserstein MP, Diaz GA, Srivastava S. High prevalence of structural heart disease in children with cblC-type methylmalonic aciduria and homocystinuria. *Mol Genet Metab* 2009;**98**(4):344–8.
21. Carvalho JS, Matthews EE, Leonard JV, Deanfield J. Cardiomyopathy of glycogen storage disease type III. *Heart Vessels* 1993;**8**(3):155–9.
22. Lee PJ, Deanfield JE, Burch M, Baig K, McKenna WJ, Leonard JV. Comparison of the functional significance of left ventricular hypertrophy in hypertrophic cardiomyopathy and glycogenosis type III. *Am J Cardiol* 1997;**79**(6):834–8.
23. Dagli AI, Zori RT, McCune H, Ivsic T, Maisenbacher MK, Weinstein DA. Reversal of glycogen storage disease type IIIa-related cardiomyopathy with modification of diet. *J Inherit Metab Dis* 2009; DOI: 10.1007/s10545-009-1088-x.
24. Nase S, Kunze KP, Sigmund M, Schroeder JM, Shin Y, Hanrath P. A new variant of type IV glycogenosis with primary cardiac manifestation and complete branching enzyme deficiency. In vivo detection by heart muscle biopsy. *Eur Heart J* 1995;**16**(11):1698–704.
25. Burwinkel B, Scott JW, Buhrer C, *et al.* Fatal congenital heart glycogenosis caused by a recurrent activating R531Q mutation in the gamma 2-subunit of AMP-activated protein kinase (PRKAG2):not by phosphorylase kinase deficiency. *Am J Hum Genet* 2005;**76**(6):1034–49.
26. Arad M, Benson DW, Perez-Atayde AR, *et al.* Constitutively active AMP kinase mutations cause glycogen storage disease mimicking hypertrophic cardiomyopathy. *J Clin Invest* 2002;**109**(3):357–62.
27. Sugie K, Yamamoto A, Murayama K, *et al.* Clinicopathological features of genetically confirmed Danon disease. *Neurology* 2002;**58**(12):1773–8.
28. Footitt EJ, Karimova A, Burch M, *et al.* Cardiomyopathy in the congenital disorders of glycosylation (CDG): a case of late presentation and literature review. *J Inherit Metab Dis* 2009; DOI: 10.1007/s10545-009-1262-1.
29. Cizkova A, Stranecky V, Mayr JA, *et al.* TMEM70 mutations cause isolated ATP synthase deficiency and neonatal mitochondrial encephalocardiomyopathy. *Nat Genet* 2008;**40**(11):1288–90.
30. Chace DH. Mass spectrometry in newborn and metabolic screening: historical perspective and future directions. *J Mass Spectrom* 2009;**44**(2):163–70.
31. Law LK, Tang NL, Hui J, *et al.* A novel functional assay for simultaneous determination of total fatty acid beta-oxidation flux and acylcarnitine profiling in human skin fibroblasts using (2)H(3)(1)-palmitate by isotope ratio mass spectrometry and electrospray tandem mass spectrometry. *Clin Chim Acta* 2007;**382**(1–2):25–30.
32. Babovic-Vuksanovic D, O'Brien JF. Laboratory diagnosis of congenital disorders of glycosylation type I by analysis of transferrin glycoforms. *Mol Diagn Ther* 2007;**11**(5):303–11.
33. Marklova E, Albahri Z. Screening and diagnosis of congenital disorders of glycosylation. *Clin Chim Acta* 2007;**385**(1–2):6–20.
34. Houtkooper RH, Rodenburg RJ, Thiels C, *et al.* Cardiolipin and monolysocardiolipin analysis in fibroblasts, lymphocytes, and tissues using high-performance liquid chromatography-mass spectrometry as a diagnostic test for Barth syndrome. *Anal Biochem* 2009;**387**(2):230–7.
35. Kulik W, van Lenthe H, Stet FS, *et al.* Bloodspot assay using HPLC-tandem mass spectrometry for detection of Barth syndrome. *Clin Chem* 2008;**54**(2):371–8.
36. Gelb MH, Turecek F, Scott CR, Chamoles NA. Direct multiplex assay of enzymes in dried blood spots by tandem mass spectrometry for the newborn screening of lysosomal storage disorders. *J Inherit Metab Dis* 2006;**29**(2–3):397–404.
37. Zhang XK, Elbin CS, Chuang WL, *et al.* Multiplex enzyme assay screening of dried blood spots for lysosomal storage disorders by using tandem mass spectrometry. *Clin Chem* 2008;**54**(10):1725–8.
38. Van Hove JL, Myers S, Kerckhove KV, Freehauf C, Bernstein L. Acute nutrition management in the prevention of metabolic illness: a practical approach with glucose polymers. *Mol Genet Metab* 2009;**97**(1):1–3.
39. Jones PM, Butt Y, Bennett MJ. Accumulation of 3-hydroxy-fatty acids in the culture medium of long-chain L-3-hydroxyacyl CoA dehydrogenase (LCHAD) and mitochondrial trifunctional protein-deficient skin fibroblasts: implications for medium chain triglyceride dietary treatment of LCHAD deficiency. *Pediatr Res* 2003;**53**(5):783–7.
40. Roe CR, Sweetman L, Roe DS, David F, Brunengraber H. Treatment of cardiomyopathy and rhabdomyolysis in long-chain fat oxidation disorders using an anaplerotic odd-chain triglyceride. *J Clin Invest* 2002;**110**(2):259–69.
41. Van Hove JL, Grunewald S, Jaeken J, *et al.* D,L-3-hydroxybutyrate treatment of multiple acyl-CoA dehydrogenase deficiency (MADD). *Lancet* 2003;**361**(9367):1433–5.
42. Olsen RK, Olpin SE, Andresen BS, *et al.* ETFDH mutations as a major cause of riboflavin-responsive multiple acyl-CoA dehydrogenation deficiency. *Brain* 2007;**130**(8):2045–54.
43. Djouadi F, Bonnefont JP, Thuillier L, *et al.* Correction of fatty acid oxidation in carnitine palmitoyl transferase 2-deficient cultured skin fibroblasts by bezafibrate. *Pediatr Res* 2003;**54**(4):446–51.
44. Djouadi F, Aubey F, Schlemmer D, *et al.* Bezafibrate increases very-long-chain acyl-CoA dehydrogenase protein and mRNA expression in

deficient fibroblasts and is a potential therapy for fatty acid oxidation disorders. *Hum Mol Genet* 2005;**14**(1)(8):2695–703.
45. Bonnefont JP, Bastin J, Behin A, Djouadi F. Bezafibrate for an inborn mitochondrial beta-oxidation defect. *N Engl J Med* 2009;**360**(8):838–40.
46. Lim-Melia ER, Kronn DF. Current enzyme replacement therapy for the treatment of lysosomal storage diseases. *Pediatr Ann* 2009;**38**(8):448–55.
47. Schoser B, Hill V, Raben N. Therapeutic approaches in glycogen storage disease type II/Pompe Disease. *Neurotherapeutics* 2008;**5**(4):569–78.
48. van der Ploeg AT, Reuser AJ. Pompe disease. *Lancet* 2008;**372**(9646):1342–53.
49. Chen LR, Chen CA, Chiu SN, *et al.* Reversal of cardiac dysfunction after enzyme replacement in patients with infantile-onset Pompe disease. *J Pediatr* 2009;**155**(2):271–5.
50. Chien YH, Lee NC, Thurberg BL, *et al.* Pompe disease in infants: improving the prognosis by newborn screening and early treatment. *Pediatrics* 2009;**124**(6):e1116–e1125.
51. Muenzer J, Wraith JE, Clarke LA. Mucopolysaccharidosis I: management and treatment guidelines. *Pediatrics* 2009;**123**(1):19–29.

7

Adult congenital heart disease

L. Swan

Introduction

Over the last 20 years, the face of congenital heart disease has changed beyond all recognition. Early death in childhood has been replaced by late death in adulthood (Fig. 7.1). With increasing longevity, long-term sequelae of congenital disease corrected in early life are being recognized. In a sizeable proportion the consequences include ventricular dysfunction and heart failure (HF).

The inclusion of congenital heart disease as an important aetiology of adult HF is a demonstration of changing demographics. Indeed, there are now more adults with congenital heart lesions than children.[1] It is estimated that there are 185 000 adults with significant congenital heart disease in the United Kingdom.[2] Many of the long-term consequences of congenital heart disease were not appreciated in the early era of paediatric cardiac surgery. Many patients (such as those with repaired coarctation of the aorta) were discharged, resulting in only a minority of the patients now being under specialist cardiology follow-up. When an adult patient presents with HF, it is important to exclude a pre-existing congenital aetiology.

It is difficult to define HF in adults with congenital heart disease. Early definitions ('A clinical syndrome caused by an abnormality of the heart and recognized by a characteristic pattern of haemodynamic, renal, neural and hormonal responses', Poole-Wilson, 1985) could encompass every congenital cardiac lesion. Even the modern European Society of Cardiology definition[3] ('Symptoms of HF at rest or exercise and objective evidence of cardiac dysfunction ± response to treatment', ESC Task Force 2005) captures a very wide and divergent range of congenital lesions. For the purpose of this chapter we will concentrate on disorders where ventricular function is the predominant lesion (Fig. 7.2).

Differential diagnosis

Caution needs to be applied when diagnosing HF in patients with complex lesions. For example, an elevated jugular venous pressure (JVP) is a normal finding in a patient with a healthy Fontan circulation (a right atrial to pulmonary artery anastomosis) where the JVP is a marker of the pulmonary artery pressure and not a manifestation of an elevated right ventricular end-diastolic pressure. Accurate interpretation of imaging also requires expert knowledge of the underlying anatomy and physiology. For example, imaging may reveal diffuse interstitial lung changes in a breathless patient with an elevated JVP. In the setting of a patient with a Mustard repair (atrial baffle operation to treat transposition of the great arteries) these findings are equally likely to be due to pulmonary vein obstruction as pulmonary oedema. An accurate diagnosis is crucial, as aggressive treatment with angiotensin converting enzyme (ACE) inhibition and diuretics may lead to an important clinical deterioration.

Prevalence of heart failure in adult congenital heart disease

Age is an important contributor to HF and as the population with adult congenital heart disease (ACHD) ages, endstage HF will become an increasing burden. With the exclusion of those with late repair, or those from a pioneering surgical centre, the oldest Mustard and Fontan patients are likely to be in their late 30s. Most of these patients will have a degree of ventricular pathology.

There are no robust data to determine the true prevalence of HF in congenital heart disease. Piran *et al.*[4] examined a consecutive cohort of 188 patients with single-ventricle physiology or systemic right ventricles: 22% of transposition patients with an atrial switch, 32% of the congenitally corrected transpositions, and 40% of the Fontan patients had HF. The mortality of the symptomatic HF patients was 47% over 15 years of follow-up. Although the mortality slopes are more gradual than those with acquired HF, it should be remembered that these are young patients.

Oechslin *et al.*[5] described a cross-sectional study of 2600 ACHD patients followed in a single centre. In this cohort, the mean age of death was 37 years. Chronic HF accounted for 21% of deaths. It was

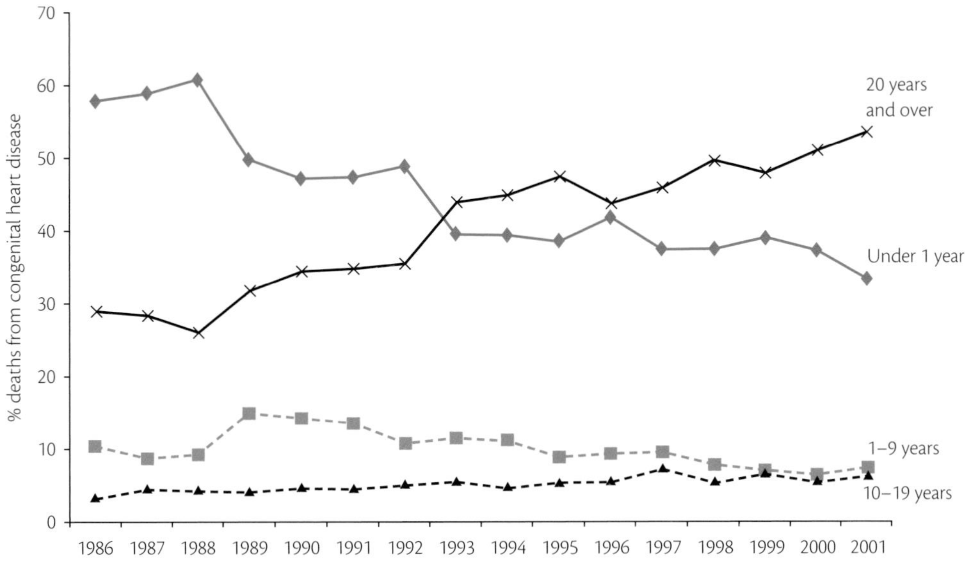

Fig. 7.1 Percentage of deaths from congenital heart disease by age group, 1986–2001, England and Wales.
From Petersen S, Peto V, Rayner M. British Heart Foundation Health Promotion Research Group; www.heartstats.org.

A Mustard

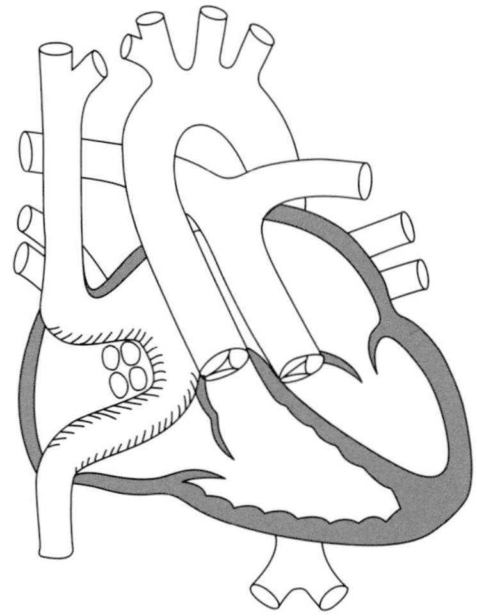

B Congenitally corrected transposition of the great arteries (CCTGA)

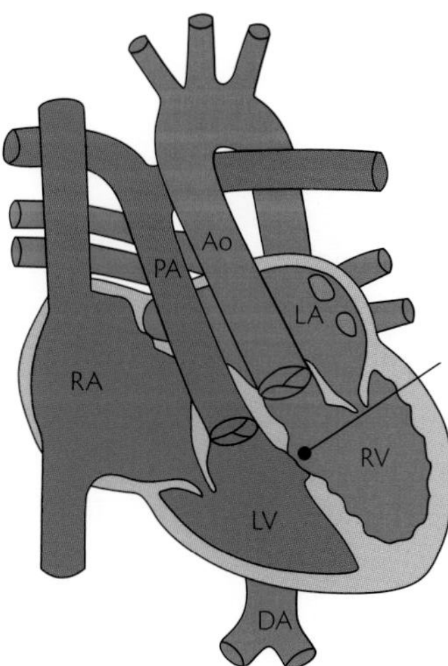

C Fontan (tricuspid atresia)

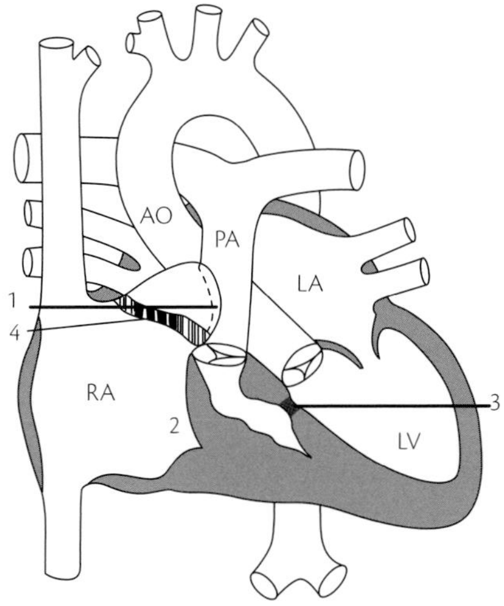

D Univentricular heart (double inlet left ventricle)

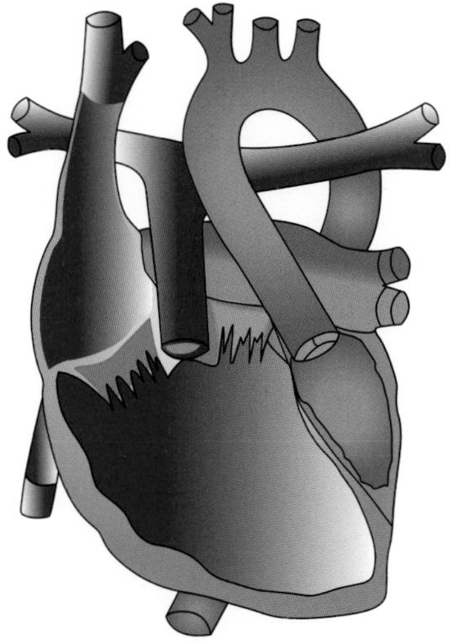

Fig. 7.2 Anatomical drawings of common complex congenital heart lesions:
(A) Mustard; (B) congenitally corrected transposition of the great arteries (CCTGA); (C) Fontan (tricuspid atresia); (D) univentricular heart (double-inlet left ventricle).

also presumably a cause of a high proportion of the sudden cardiac deaths (26% of all deaths) and of the perioperative deaths (18% of all deaths). There is thus a need for effective therapy that will add both quantitatively and qualitatively to long-term outcome.

The wider prevalence of systolic or diastolic ventricular dysfunction in patients with ACHD is unknown. In most units, HF is the third commonest cause of emergency admission in ACHD patients (behind arrhythmia and suspected endocarditis). Lesions at particular risk of HF will be described more fully late in this chapter.

The features of heart failure in adult congenital heart disease

The clinical features of HF in this group have many similarities with the general HF population. There are, however, a few important differences.

Symptoms

The presence of symptoms is a very late manifestation of ventricular disease in the ACHD population. Life-long 'acclimatization' to a cardiac lesion results in a high threshold for presenting with symptoms of effort intolerance and lethargy. In addition, patients will often accept palpitation as a normal finding as it has been present since childhood. When ACHD patients are formally exercised, there is little correlation between degree of symptoms and peak oxygen update.[6]

It is often unclear from objective testing what finally triggers the reporting of symptoms. The reporting of symptoms is, however, associated with an increased cardiothoracic ratio, an increased risk of frank decompensation and an increased risk of nonsinus rhythm. [4] The presence of limiting symptoms (NYHA class>2) also identifies those with an increased mortality.

Effort tolerance

Formal cardiopulmonary exercising testing is highly informative in patients with ACHD. A simple Bruce protocol exercise test will highlight multiple predictors of prognosis and may help identify the cause of effort limitation (Box 7.1). Serial cardiopulmonary effort testing is often used to time intervention and to chart the progression of ventricular pathology. Of those with very significant effort limitation, a six-minute walk test (6MWT) may also be informative. In those with severe disease, there is a strong correlation between 6MWT distance and peak oxygen uptake.[7] The 6MWT distance is also a prognostic marker in several subgroups of patient.

Cardiomegaly

The presence of cardiomegaly on a plain chest radiograph is a strong and robust predictor of mortality in patients with congenital heart disease.[8] A cardiothoracic ratio of greater than 55% is associated with an approximately eightfold increase in mortality. Although a very simple marked of disease severity, it is a potential 'flag' identifying patients at increased risk.

Broad QRS on ECG

A broad QRS complex on a 12-lead ECG may be a manifestation of ventricular disease. In patients with tetralogy of Fallot, a QRS duration in excess of 180 ms (broad right bundle branch block) is associated with significant pulmonary regurgitation, right ventricular pathology and the risk of ventricular tachycardia.[9] Sudden death risk stratification is difficult in many subgroups of patients with congenital heart disease. QRS duration, prior atrial arrhythmia and ventricular disease are all recognized risk factors. Ventricular stimulation at electrophysiological study may also be informative, but a negative study does not exclude future malignant arrhythmias. The insertion of a defibrillator for primary prevention will be appropriate in those at highest risk.

The value of QRS duration in guiding the appropriateness of cardiac resynchronization therapy (CRT) is unclear.

Box 7.1 Prognostic indicators in adults with congenital heart disease

Blood tests
- Creatinine

Liver function
- Plasma ANP
- Plasma BNP
- Serum sodium level
- Haemoglobin

Exercise variables
- NYHA class
- Exercise time (cardiopulmonary testing) and exercise distance (6-min walk test)
- Peak oxygen uptake (MVo_2)
- V_E/Vco_2 slope
- Heart rate reserve

Rhythm
- Paced
- QRS duration
- Arrhythmia (atrial and ventricular)

Imaging
- Ejection fraction (systemic ventricle)
- Deceleration time
- Right ventricular volumes
- Left ventricular volumes
- Pulmonary artery pressure

Miscellaneous
- Aetiology of heart failure/lesion type

Neurohormonal activiation

Renin, endothelin, pro-BNP, atrial natriuretic peptide (ANP) and noradrenaline are all increased in patients with ACHD. The degree of activation is related to ventricular function and NYHA (New York Heart Association) class.[10] Plasma B-type natriuretic peptide (BNP) levels are also informative regarding outcome for perioperative patients.

There is also a similar cytokine pattern in this population compared with other forms of dilated cardiomyopathy.[11]

Other manifestations of heart failure

Cachexia is a concerning finding in this subgroup of HF patients. It is associated with an increased metabolic rate, increased symptoms, and an elevated neurohormonal profile.[12] Although not fully understood, there are multiple similar pathogenic features linking the cachexia found in ACHD patients with that found in patients with acquired heart disease.

An unusual feature of advanced congenital heart disease is the phenomenon of protein-losing enteropathy (PLE). It occurs particularly in the setting of a chronically elevated right-sided pressure such as occurs in the Fontan circulation.[13] The most common features are ascites, lower limb oedema, pleural effusions, and gastrointestinal upset. Diuretics alone are often ineffective in preventing further accumulation of fluid. Atrial pacing, fenestration, steroids, octreotide, unfractionated heparin, and ACE inhibitors are some of the other treatment modalities that have been suggested.[14–17] When a patient with right heart disease presents with fluid overload a serum albumin and stool α_1-antitrypsin should be measured to exclude concomitant PLE.

Prognostication

As adult congenital heart disease is a very heterogenous group of conditions, it is very difficult to identify an 'ACHD Heart Failure Survival Score'. There are, however, multiple known prognostic indicators. Many of these overlap with the prognostic factors associated with acquired HF and dilated cardiomyopathy (Box 7.1).

The presence of ventricular dysfunction increases cardiovascular mortality for almost every congenital heart lesion. Although many lesions are a complex interaction between several different haemodynamic components, the addition of ventricular dysfunction (particularly when affecting the systemic ventricle) is associated with deterioration in functional class and increased mortality. For example, in patients with tetralogy of Fallot, traditionally thought to be a right heart lesion, the addition of left ventricular dysfunction is associated with a significant increase in the risk of sudden cardiac death.[18]

Causes of ventricular dysfunction in congenital heart disease

In patients with congenital heart disease, the cause of ventricular dysfunction is often multifactorial, particularly so for the adult patient who has had decades of abnormal haemodynamics and several cardiopulmonary bypass procedures.

Volume-dependent lesions

The simplest model of 'congenital' HF is that associated with acute or chronic volume overload. A well patient who suddenly ruptures a sinus of Valsalva (SOV) aneurysm into the right ventricle will develop an acute left-to-right intracardiac shunt. This will volume load the left ventricle and, depending on the size of the shunt, lead to ventricular dysfunction ± dilatation. A similar pathology arises in very young children with a large ventricular septal defect (VSD). Although drug therapy can lead to an improvement in symptoms, the definitive treatment in these scenarios is to close the shunt. e.g. by device closing the ruptured SOV aneurysm or operating on the VSD.

In the more complex patient, volume overload is usually a chronic insult to the ventricle. It may be due to a variety of lesions but is most commonly due to regurgitant valves, intracardiac shunts, or arterial shunts (including a Blalock–Taussig shunt).

HF and a reduction in systemic cardiac output may also occur as a result of inadequate delivery of volume to the systemic ventricle. This mechanism may occur in patients with a Fontan circulation, severe Ebstein anomaly, or an atrial switch procedure (Mustard or Senning repair).

Pressure-dependent lesions

Significant left and right ventricular outflow tract obstruction will eventually lead to ventricular disease. This is usually a very slow process and often interrupted by surgical or catheter intervention. Hypertension (arterial or pulmonary) and aortic pathology such as coarctation may also be detrimental. Although the left ventricle will cope for many years with a volume load, the right ventricle appears to be less adaptable. The addition of significant impairment of the right ventricle adds considerable to the morbidity and mortality in 'right heart pressure lesions' such as idiopathic pulmonary arterial hypertension.

Rhythm and conduction issues

Atrial arrhythmias are common in patients with congenital heart disease. A large arrhythmia burden may lead to a chronic impairment of ventricular function. Particular in those with complex lesions, an acute arrhythmia (even when occurring with reasonable rate control) can have a dramatic impact on ventricular efficiency. The loss of atrioventricular synchrony is often poorly tolerated. Many patients have reduced ventricular filling times and therefore even a 'slowish' tachycardia (e.g. with a heart rate of 100–120) can lead to an important fall in cardiac output.

Conduction defects and dyssynchrony are also common in patients with congenital heart disease. The benefits of cardiac resynchronization are actively being investigated. QRS duration is a risk factor for sudden cardiac death in several subgroups including those with tetralogy of Fallot and Eisenmenger's syndrome.[19]

Intrinsic myocardial issues

For many lesions, there appears to be an intrinsic abnormality of ventricular function. In a subset, there may be features of either non-compaction (in up to 10%) or endomyocardial fibroelastosis. In others, the degree of ventricular disease is not explained by the haemodynamic lesion. This is particularly true for patients with left heart lesions (e.g. patients with coarctation) or VSD. With advances in imaging, particularly late gadolinium cardiac magnetic resonance (CMR), it is becoming increasingly recognized that myocardial fibrosis is common in such patients. Previous surgical scars, cardiopulmonary bypass, and ischaemia are also implicated in the process.

The importance of multiple cardiopulmonary bypass procedures on ventricular function should not be underestimated, particularly in patients operated on in the early days of cardiac surgery when optimal myocardial protection techniques were not well established.

Ischaemia

Atherosclerotic coronary disease is rare in adults with congenital heart disease. However, coronary anomalies and even coronary embolism may occur. Ischaemia may also occur due to the effect of profound hypoxia. Patients with Eisenmenger's syndrome or single ventricles may have resting oxygen saturations in the mid 70% range, which may again be detrimental to myocyte function.

Ventricular interaction

Abnormal right ventricular–left ventricular interaction is common. A very large and dyskinetic RV in the closed pericardium (e.g. in Ebstein's anomaly or tetralogy) may impair left ventricular filling, synchrony, and relaxation.

As with acquired heart disease, there are additional compounding factors that may be detrimental, including thyroid disease (often amiodarone induced), pericardial pathology, anaemia, and pregnancy.

The systemic right ventricle

The systemic right ventricle occurs when the morphological RV is supporting the systemic circulation, i.e. the RV is in a subaortic position. Although this arrangement often offers excellent short-term palliation for complex lesions (such as in transposition with an atrial switch), it is a flawed circulation.

The structure and geometry of the RV copes less well with pressure overload than with volume overload. As the RV hypertrophies, it is prone to a reduction in myocardial capillary density and to demand ischaemia. Compliance, coronary filling, and cellular receptor expression are different when compared to a subaortic systemic left ventricle. The tricuspid valve is also not adapted to cope with systemic pressures and often becomes regurgitant. All of these features help explain the progressive deterioration in right ventricular function seen in many patients with a systemic right ventricle.

Heart failure in specific lesions

Systemic right ventricle

The right ventricle operates as the systemic ventricle in patients with congenitally corrected transposition of the great arteries (CCTGA), transposition with a previous atrial switch, in a proportion of patients with double-outlet right ventricle, and in some single-ventricle conditions. Eventual HF is almost inevitable. There are however many unanswered mysteries: for example, one CCTGA patient may present with refractory HF at the age of 30, whilst another may remain undiagnosed until the age of 70. Why some systemic ventricles cope well and why some decompensate early is unknown.

A rather speculative therapeutic option for the treatment of HF in this setting is to band the pulmonary artery (effectively creating moderate pulmonary stenosis) and render the subpulmonary left ventricle 'hypertensive'. Originally done as a staging procedure towards a late arterial switch (the plan being to train the left ventricle prior to its becoming the systemic ventricle), the results of late switch operations were disappointing in adults. It was found incidentally that a few patients with simple PA banding alone reported symptomatic improvement. The mechanism was that banding resulted in the interventricular septum moving towards the (systemic) right ventricle with consequent changes in right ventricular volumes and geometry. The degree of tricuspid regurgitation was also reduced.[20] The technique has not been widely adopted and the long-term role for such procedures is unknown.

Tetralogy of Fallot

Left ventricular dysfunction is a late consequence of tetralogy. It is often associated with endstage disease, multiple previous surgical procedures, and ventricular scarring. Aortic root dilation and aortic regurgitation may also contribute. The presence of left ventricular dysfunction in tetralogy is a risk for ventricular tachycardia and may be as a criterion for the insertion on a defibrillator.[21]

Single-ventricle physiology (univentricular hearts)

The term 'single-ventricle physiology' encompasses a heterogenous group of some of the most complex congenital heart disorders. There is usually a circulation where one of the ventricles is either small or has a very abnormal inlet valve and is unable to function in a sequential series circuit.[22] There is usually a ventricular septal defect and the ventricular mass is described as being 'single', i.e. working essentially as one unit. The subpulmonary ventricle is often at systemic pressure.

The majority of patients with a univentricular circulation will have a degree of cyanosis. Chronic cyanosis, ventricular overload, and an innately abnormal ventricular geometry eventually lead to systolic and diastolic ventricular dysfunction. The presence of atrioventricular valve regurgitation will exacerbate the situation. Furthermore, reduced pulmonary blood flow in the absence of a normal subpulmonary ventricle further compromises an already impaired systemic cardiac output leading to complications of 'right heart congestion'.

Table 7.1 ACE inhibitor and angiotensin receptor blocker studies in ACHD

Study	Drug	Design	Subjects	Outcome
Hopkins *et al.*[26] *Am J Cardiol* 1996	ACEI	Retrospective study 1 year of therapy	10 cyanotic patients	Improved symptoms
Kouatli *et al.*[27] *Circulation* 1997	Enalapril	Randomized Cross-over, 10 wks	18 Fontan patients	No change in exercise or cardiac index
Ohuchi *et al.*[28] *Circulation* 2001	ACEI	1.8 years follow-up	10 Fontan patients	No change in neurohormones, baroreceptor profile or function
Hechter *et al.*[29] *Am J Cardiol* 2001	ACEI	Non-randomized 6 months	14 systemic RV patients	No change in MVo_2 or ejection fraction
Lester *et al.*[30] *Am J Cardiol* 2001	Losartan	Cross-over study	7 systemic RV patients	Improvements in exercise and ejection fraction
Robinson *et al.*[31] *Pediatr Cardiol* 2002	Enalapril	Mustard 12 months	9 systemic RV patients	No change in MVO_2
Dore *et al.*[32] *Circulation* 2005	Losartan	Systemic RV 16 weeks	29 systemic RV patients	No change in exercise or BNP

ACEI, angiotensin converting enzyme inhibitor; BNP, B-type natriuretic peptide.

Hypoplastic left heart syndrome (HLS) is the most common type of single-ventricle physiology, but at present there are few adult survivors. With advances in care, many ACHD units expect to see increasing numbers of HLS patients in the next few years. Adult survivors of HLS will have been palliated with multiple operations including a Fontan-type procedure. The long-term outlook remains poor.[24]

Right ventricular failure

Right ventricular failure (in a normally sited, subpulmonary right ventricle) is common in congenital heart disease. Atrial septal defects, atrioventricular septal defects, right ventricular outflow tract/pulmonary valve disease, and pulmonary hypertension are common causes. The optimal treatment of right HF (subpulmonary) has not been established in any setting, either congenital or acquired. There is little evidence base regarding therapies and few clinical guidelines. Optimizing fluid balance and minimizing the effect of chronic venous congestion of the gut and liver are key features.

Treatment of chronic heart failure in adult congenital heart disease

Medication

The use of HF drugs is common in ACHD. In the most recent European Survey study, 39% of Fontan patients and 33% of transposition patients receive ACE inhibitors. The corresponding values for β-blockers were 26% and 17%. The scientific rationale behind some prescribing is unclear. Despite a very weak evidence base, most ACHD specialists adopt a pragmatic approach and extrapolate data from the acquired HF studies. The trials of medical therapy (e.g. ACE inhibitors) in patients with ACHD have, with a few exceptions, been poorly designed or underpowered. The use of inappropriate surrogate endpoints further clouds the issues (Table 7.1).

Given the lack of evidence base, there is also a tendency to 'half-treat' patients with low doses of medication on the premise of 'first doing no wrong'. In addition, there is a historic (paediatric) preference for the use of diuretics, spironolactone (predating recent mortality studies), and digoxin. Prescribing is rarely in measured response to NYHA status as for acquired heart disease. The lack of HF specialist input and the supporting infrastructure of HF nurses also contribute to underprescribing. Overriding all of these issues is the reluctance of young patients to take medication, especially for 'asymptomatic' ventricular disease when a beneficial effect cannot be guaranteed.

As mentioned previously, there are potential dangers in prescribing HF therapies in subsets of these patients, e.g. in the patient with a Fontan circulation. A careful review of anatomy and physiology should be performed before embarking on a commitment to lifelong treatment.

Nondrug therapies

There are case series of the use of CRT in patients with ACHD. To date, CRT appears to improve morbidity and to have an impact on softer endpoints such as cardiothoracic ratio and ventricular dimensions (Fig. 7.3). As in the wider population of patients receiving CRT, those with significant systemic left ventricular disease and whose with chronic subpulmonary ventricular pacing appear to benefit the most.[25] It will be some time before there are sufficiently powered studies to assess any potential mortality benefit.

Transplantation is still an attractive option for a subset of deteriorating ACHD patients. Complex anatomy, multiple previous sternotomies/thoracotomies, and a high level of panel-reactive antibodies are additional hurdles. For certain disease groups, transplantation is unlikely ever to meet the need for life-prolonging therapy. The Fontan patient and hypoplastic left heart patient represent components of the ACHD cohort that are particularly difficult to transplant.

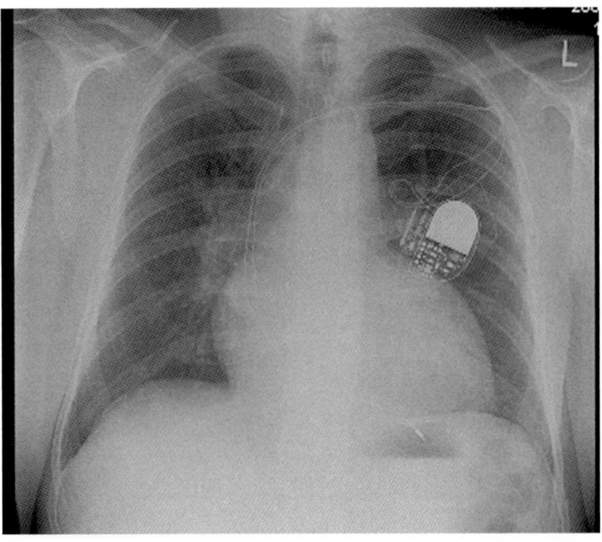

A

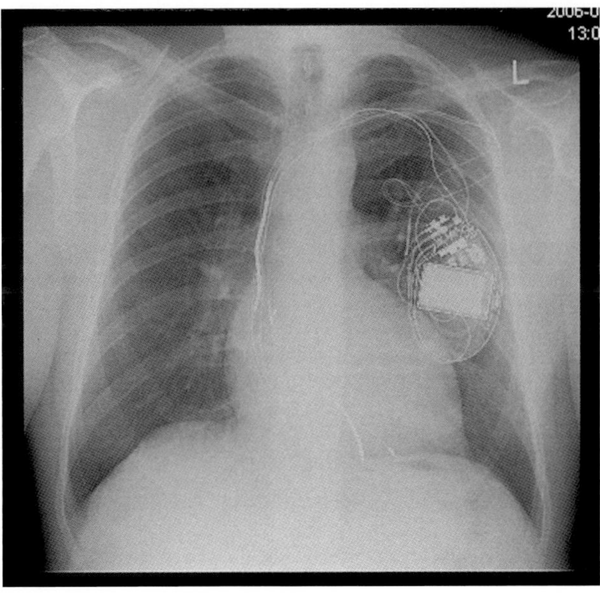

B

Fig. 7.3 Case example of a 41-year-old man with congenitally corrected transposition of the great arteries (CCTGA). The patient was chronically paced (subpulmonary ventricle) for AV block (chest radiograph A). The patient had NYHA III symptoms despite maximal heart failure medication. Upgrade to CRT resulted in an improvement in functional class and a reduction in cardiothoracic ratio (chest radiograph B).

Conclusion

Congenital heart disease will become an increasingly important cause of HF in adults. Although many of the principles of management are similar to those of acquired HF, important differences remain. Optimal treatment of ACHD patients requires close cooperation between the adult congenital team and HF physicians. ACHD is an area of HF that is ripe for research and provides novel haemodynamic models for further study.

References

1. Opotowsky AR, Omar SK, Webb GD. Trends in hospitalizations for adults with congenital heart disease in the U.S. *J Am Coll Cardiol* 2009;**54**:460–7.
2. Petersen S, Peto V, Rayner M. *Congenital heart disease statistics 2003.* British Heart Foundation Health Promotion Research Group. www.heartstats.org.
3. Guidelines for the diagnosis and treatment of chronic heart failure (update 2005). *Eur Heart J* 2005;**26**:1115–40.
4. Piran S, Veldtman G, Siu S, Webb GD, Liu PP. Heart failure and ventricular dysfunction in patients with single or systemic right ventricles. *Circulation* 2002;**105**:1189–94.
5. Oechslin EN, Harrison DA, Connelly MS, Webb GD, Siu SC. Mode of death in adults with congenital heart disease. *Am J Cardiol* 2000;**86**(10):1111–16.
6. Diller GP, Dimopoulos K, Okonko D, *et al.* Exercise intolerance in adult congenital heart disease: comparative severity, correlates and prognostic implication. *Circulation* 2005;**112**:828–35.
7. Cahalin LP, Mathier MA, Semigran MJ, Dec GW, DiSalvo TG. The six-minute walk test predicts peak oxygen uptake and survical in patients with advances heart failure. *Chest* 1996;**110**:325–32.
8. Dimopoulos K, Giannakoulas G, Petracco R, [*et al*]. The cardiothoracic ratio: a simple, strong and reproducible marker of disease severity and outcome in adults with congenital heart disease. In press.
9. Gatzoulis MA, Balaji S, Webber SA, Siu SC, Hokanson JS, Poile C. Risk factors for arrhythmia and sudden cardiac death late after repair of tetralogy of Fallot: a multicentre study. *Lancet* 2000;**356**:975–81.
10. Bolger AP, Sharma R, Li W, *et al.* Neurohormonal activation and the chronic heart failure syndrome in adults with congenital heart disease. *Circulation* 2002;**106**(1):92–9.
11. Sharma R, Bolger AP, Li W, *et al.* Elevated circulating levels of inflammatory cytokines and bacterial endotoxin in adults with congenital heart disease. *Am J Cardiol* 2003;**92**(2):188–93.
12. Vonder Muhll I, Cholet A, Stehr K, Gatzoulis MA. Prevalence and predictors of cachexia in adults with congenital heart disease. Canadian Cardiovascular Congress 2003 (abstract). *Can J Cardiol* 2003;**19** Suppl A:49A–295A.
13. Hess J, Kruizinga K, Bijleveld CM, Hardjowijono R, Eygelaar A. Protein-losing enteropathy after Fontan operation. *J Thorac Cardiovasc Surg* 1984;**88**(4):606–9.
14. Rothman A, Snyder J. Protein-losing enteropathy following the Fontan operation: resolution with prednisone therapy. *Am Heart J* 1991;**121**:618–19.
15. Mertens L, Dumoulin M, Gewillig M. Effect of percutaneous fenestration of the atrial septum on protein-losing enteropathy after the Fontan operation. *Br Heart J* 1994;**72**:591–2.
16. Ryerson L, Goldberg C, Rosenthal A, Armstrong A. Usefulness of heparin therapy in protein-losing enteropathy associated with single ventricle palliation. *Am J Cardiol.* 2008;**101**:248–51.
17. Cohen MI, Rhodes LA, Wernovsky G, Gaynor JW, Spray TL, Rychik J. Atrial pacing: an alternative treatment for protein-losing enteropathy after the Fontan operation. *J Thorac Cardiovasc Surg* 2001;**121**: 582–3.
18. Ghai A, Silversides C, Harris L, Webb GD, Siu SC, Therrien J. Left ventricular dysfunction is a risk factor for sudden cardiac death in adults late after repair of tetralogy of Fallot. *J Am Coll Cardiol* 2002;**40**:1675–80.
19. Diller GP, Dimopoulos K, Broberg CS, *et al.* Presentation, survival prospects and predictors of death in Eisenmenger syndrome: a combined retrospective and case-control study. *Eur Heart J* 2006;**27**:1737–42.
20. Poirier NC, Yu JH, Brizard CP, Mee RB. Long-term results of left ventricular reconditioning and anatomic correction for systemic right ventricular dysfunction after atrial switch procedures. *J Thorac Cardiovasc Surg.* 2004;**127**(4):975–81.
21. Khairy P, Harris L, Landzberg MJ, *et al.* Implantable cardioverter-defibrillators in tetralogy of Fallot. *Circulation* 2008;**117**: 363–70.
22. Khairy P, Poirier N, Mercier L. Univentricular hearts. *Circulation* 2007;**115**:800–812.
23. Engelfriet P, Boersma E, Oechslin E, *et al.* The spectrum of adult congenital heart disease in Europe: morbidity and mortality in a 5 year follow-up period. The Euro Heart Survey on adult congenital heart disease. *Eur Heart J* 2005;**26**:2325–33.
24. Mahle WT, Spray TL, Wernovsky G, Gaynor JW, Clark BJ. Survival after reconstructive surgery for hypoplastic left heart syndrome: A 15-year experience from a single institution. *Circulation* 2000;**102**(III):136–41.
25. Janousek J. Cardiac resynchronization in congenital heart disease. *Heart* 2009;**95**:940–7.
26. Hopkins WE, Kelly DP. Angiotensin-converting enzyme inhibitors in adults with cyanotic congenital heart disease. *Am J Cardiol* 1996;**77**:439–40.
27. Kouatli AA, Garcia JA, Zellers TM, Weinstein EM, Mahony L. Enalapril does not enhance exercise capacity in patients after Fontan procedure. *Circulation* 1997;**96**:1507–12.
28. Ohuchi H, Hasegawa S, Yasuda K, Yamada O, Ono Y, Echigo S. Severely impaired cardiac autonomic nervous activity after the Fontan operation. *Circulation.* 2001;**104**:1513–8.
29. Hechter SJ, Fredriksen PM, Liu P, *et al.* Angiotensin-converting enzyme inhibitors in adults after the Mustard procedure. *Am J Cardiol.* 2001;**87**:660–3.
30. Lester SJ, McElhinney DB, Viloria E, *et al.* Effects of losartan in patients with a systemically functioning morphologic right ventricle after atrial repair of transposition of the great arteries. *Am J Cardiol.* 2001;**88**:1314–16.
31. Robinson B, Heise CT, Moore JW, *et al.* Afterload reduction therapy in patients following intraatrial baffle operation for transposition of the great arteries. *Pediatr Cardiol* 2002;**23**(6):618–23.
32. Dore A, Houde C, Chan KL, *et al.* Angiotensin receptor blockade and exercise capacity in adults with systemic right ventricles: a multicenter, randomized, placebo-controlled clinical trial. *Circulation.* 2005;**112**:2411–16.

8

Infective and infiltrative causes of heart failure

Roy S. Gardner and Andrew L. Clark

Heart failure (HF) can result from any form of cardiac injury. Infective and infiltrative causes are rare, but important to identify, as many are potentially reversible.

Infective causes of heart failure

Myocarditis

Myocarditis is inflammation of myocardium due to one of a large number of causes (Table 8.1, 8.2). In developed countries, a viral aetiology—currently parvovirus B19—is most commonly implicated, but the principle offender changes with time.[1–3] Less commonly, myocarditis can be caused by systemic disease, hypersensitivity drug reactions, and toxins.

Myocardial inflammation may be focal or diffuse, involving any or all cardiac chambers. The clinical course is also variable—from full recovery to sudden death, or the need for urgent cardiac transplantation or implantation of a ventricular assist device (VAD). The variability appears, in part, to be due to the underlying aetiology. The major long-term consequence of myocarditis is chronic heart failure (CHF) due to dilated cardiomyopathy.

Pathogenesis

The viruses that frequently cause myocarditis are parvovirus B19, Coxsackie B, and adenoviruses 2 and 5. They appear to enter cardiac myocytes or macrophages through specific receptors and co-receptors[4] triggering an innate immune response through several mechanisms, as well as causing a proinflammatory cytokine release.[5] However, it is poorly understood why the vast majority of infections with these viruses do not lead to myocarditis or a dilated cardiomyopathy.

A clinical and pathological classification by Lieberman *et al.*[6] gives prognostically useful information:[7, 8]

- Fulminant—preceding flu-like illness, with a distinct onset of cardiac symptoms and rapid deterioration. Patients present with shock or symptoms and signs of severe left ventricular systolic dysfunction (LVSD). The clinical course is variable and patients either recover over the space of a few weeks or deteriorate rapidly requiring consideration of cardiac transplantation. Endomyocardial biopsy shows active myocarditis. Immunosuppressive therapy is ineffective.
- Acute—unclear onset with gradual decline in cardiac function. Patients present with symptoms of progressive HF and ventricular dilatation with LVSD. There is active or borderline myocarditis on biopsy, which resolves with time. Patients either respond to congestive heart failure (CHF) therapy or progress to dilated cardiomyopathy.
- Chronic active—onset indistinct with progressive deterioration, present with CHF with LVSD. Initial biopsy shows active or borderline myocarditis, and subsequent biopsy shows continued inflammation, fibrosis, giant cells, with eventual development of a dilated cardiomyopathy.
- Chronic persistent—no distinct onset of symptoms (primarily chest pain or palpitations) characterized by a persistent infiltrate on biopsy, often with foci of myocyte necrosis, but without ventricular dysfunction. Immunosuppressive therapy does not affect myocardial infiltrate or clinical outcome.

Clinical features

Although myocarditis is classically associated with a prodromal viral illness with fever, myalgia, fatigue, and respiratory or gastrointestinal symptoms, reported symptoms are highly variable.[9] In the European Study of the Epidemiology and Treatment of Inflammatory Heart Disease,[10] 72% had dyspnoea, 32% chest pain, and 18% arrhythmias. Chest pain is particularly common in myopericarditis, but myocarditis can also mimic myocardial ischaemia (from coronary artery spasm) and therefore should be considered in patients with an acute coronary syndrome and unobstructed coronary arteries.[11]

Investigation and diagnosis

Biomarkers of cardiac injury, particularly the cardiac troponins (I or T), may be raised in acute myocarditis, but have limited

Table 8.1 Infective causes of myocarditis

Infecting agent	Examples
Viral	Adenovirus, arbovirus (dengue fever, yellow fever), arenavirus (lassa fever), coxsackievirus, cytomegalovirus, echovirus, Epstein–Barr virus, hepatitis B, herpesvirus, HIV-1, influenza virus, mumps virus, poliomyelitis virus, rabies, respiratory syncytial virus, rubella virus, rubeola virus, vaccinia virus, varicella virus, variola virus
Bacterial	Brucella, campylobacter, clostridia, diphtheria, franciella, gonococcus, haemophilus, legionella, meningococcus, mycobacteria, mycoplasma, pneumococcus, psittacosis, salmonella, staphylococcus, streptococcus, *Tropheryma whippelii* (Whipple's disease)
Fungal	actinomycetes, aspergillus, blastomyces, candida, coccidioides, cryptococcus, histoplasma, nocardia, sporothrix
Rickettsial	Rocky Mountain spotted fever, Q fever, scrub typhus, typhus
Spirochetal	Borrelia (Lyme disease), leptospira, syphilis
Helminthic	Cysticercus, echinococcus, schistosoma, toxocara (visceral larva migrans), trichinella
Protozoal	Entamoeba, leishmania, trypanosoma (Chagas' disease), toxoplasmosis

Adapted from Pisani B, Taylor DO, Mason JW. Inflammatory myocardial diseases and cardiomyopathies. *Am J Med* 1997;**102:**459–469.

Table 8.2 Noninfectious causes of myocarditis

Cause	Subgroup	Examples
Drug induced	Toxic myocarditis	Amphetamines, anthracyclines*, arsenic, catecholamines, chloroquine, cocaine*, cyclophosphamide*, emetine, 5-flouracil, α-interferon, Interleukin-2*, lithium, paracetamol, thyroid hormone
	Hypersensitivity myocarditis	Acetazolamide, allopurinol, amitriptyline, amphotericin B, ampicillin*, carbamazepine, cephalothin, chlorthalidone, colchicine, diclofenac, diphenhydramine, furosemide, hydrochlorothiazide*, Indomethacin, Isoniazid, lidocaine, methyldopa*, methysergide, oxphenbutazone, para-aminosalicyclic acid, penicillins*, phenindione, phenylbutazone, phenytoin, procainamide, pyribenzamine, reserpine, spironolactone, streptomycin, sulfadiazine*, sulfamethoxizole*, sulfisoxazole*, sulfonylureas, tetracycline, trimethaprim
Toxins		Arsenic, carbon monoxide, copper, iron, lead, mercury, phosphorus, scorpion stings, snake venom, spider bites, wasp sting
Systemic diseases		Arteritis (giant cell, Takayasau), β-thalassaemia major, Churg–Strauss vasculitis, Crohn's disease, cryoglobulinemia, dermatomyositis, diabetes mellitus, Hashimoto's thyroiditis, Kawasaki's disease*, mixed connective tissue disorder, myaesthenia gravis, periarteritis nodosa, pernicious anemia, pheochromocytoma, polymyositis, rheumatoid arthritis, sarcoidosis*, scleroderma, Sjogren's syndrome, systemic lupus erythematosis*, thymoma, ulcerative colitis, Wegener's granulomatosis
Other		Cardiac rejection*, eosinophilic myocarditis, genetic, giant cell myocarditis*, granulomatous myocarditis, head trauma, hypothermia, hyperpyrexia, ionizing radiation, mononuclear myocarditis, peripartum myocarditis*

* denotes more common causes.

Adapted from Pisani B, Taylor DO, Mason JW. Inflammatory myocardial diseases and cardiomyopathies. *Am J Med* 1997;**102:**4594–69

diagnostic sensitivity.[12,13] Raised troponin indicates recent onset or ongoing myocardial necrosis. Markers of inflammation, such as white cell count and C-reactive protein (CRP), may also be raised.

The ECG often shows sinus tachycardia and nonspecific ST/T wave abnormalities. Occasionally, changes consistent with an acute ST elevation myocardial infarction are seen, and may reflect pericarditis or coronary artery spasm.[14]

The chest radiograph may be normal, or show evidence of cardiomegaly and/or pulmonary oedema. Echocardiography reveals global, but variable degrees of cardiac dysfunction. Mitral and tricuspid regurgitation are common. Fulminant myocarditis may be differentiated from acute myocarditis by a smaller left ventricular cavity size and increased wall thickness.[15] Loss of right ventricular function is a powerful predictor of adverse outcome.[16]

Cardiac MRI (CMR) is increasingly used in suspected myocarditis as it is useful in myocardial characterization, particularly with the use of gadolinium-DTPA contrast enhancement.[17] Identifying areas of active myocarditis with CMR may also be helpful in localizing sites for endomyocardial biopsy (Fig. 8.1), although the role of endomyocardial biopsy remains contentious.[18] However, in cases where fulminant myocarditis or giant cell myocarditis (Fig. 8.2) are suspected, biopsy has a class I recommendation in the guidelines. In other forms of myocarditis, biopsy may reveal a lymphocytic infiltrate with or without myocardial necrosis, but the sensitivity of may be as low as 35% due to transient and patchy myocardial involvement. The Dallas histopathological criteria were devised in 1986:[19]

- Active myocarditis—an inflammatory infiltrate of the myocardium with necrosis and/or degeneration of adjacent myocytes 'not typical of the ischaemic damage associated with coronary heart disease'. The infiltrates are usually mononuclear, but may be neutrophilic or, occasionally, eosinophilic.
- 'Borderline myocarditis' is the term used when the inflammatory infiltrate is too sparse, or myocyte injury is not demonstrated, and a repeat biopsy may be indicated.

Treatment

Patients who present with an acute dilated cardiomyopathy due to myocarditis should be treated with rest and established HF therapy, including angiotensin converting enzyme (ACE) inhibitors, β-adrenoreceptor antagonists (when euvolaemic), and diuretics where needed. Although most patients will improve, some patients will require supportive therapy for cardiogenic shock including intra-aortic balloon pump (IABP), inotropes, and

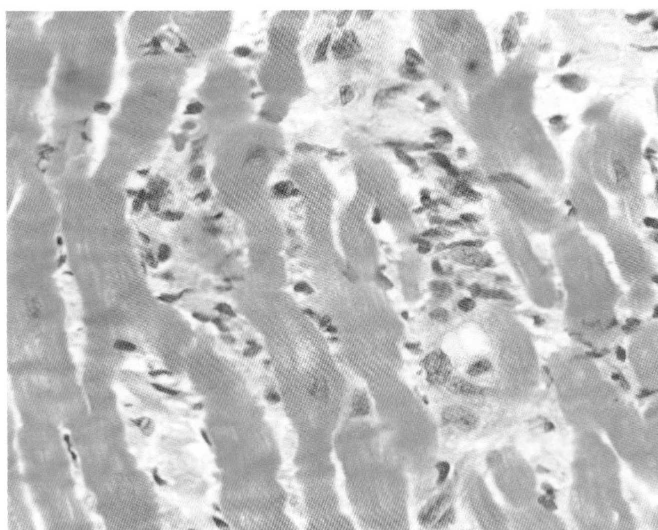

Fig. 8.1 Viral myocarditis. The myocardium contains focal intertstitial infiltration by mononuclear cells with associated cardiac myocyte degeneration. Haematoxylin and eosin ×400.
Courtesy of Dr Allan McPhaden, Glasgow Royal Infirmary.

consideration of a ventricular assist device (VAD) or urgent cardiac transpantation.[20,21] Patients with sustained or symptomatic ventricular arrhythmias may need to be treated with amiodarone or an implantable cardioverter-defibrillator (ICD),[22] although acute myocarditis could be considered a transient and reversible cause. There is currently no evidence of significant benefit from immunosuppressive therapy.[23,24]

Giant cell myocarditis

Giant cell myocarditis is a rare form of myocarditis that presents with rapidly deteriorating cardiac function and arrhythmias.[25] Approximately 20% of patients have coexisting autoimmune disease, and the great majority of affected individuals (~90%) are white. Endomyocardial biopsies reveal widespread necrosis and inflammation with the presence of lymphocytes, histiocytes, and eosinophils, as well as the characteristic multinucleated giant cells (Fig. 8.2).

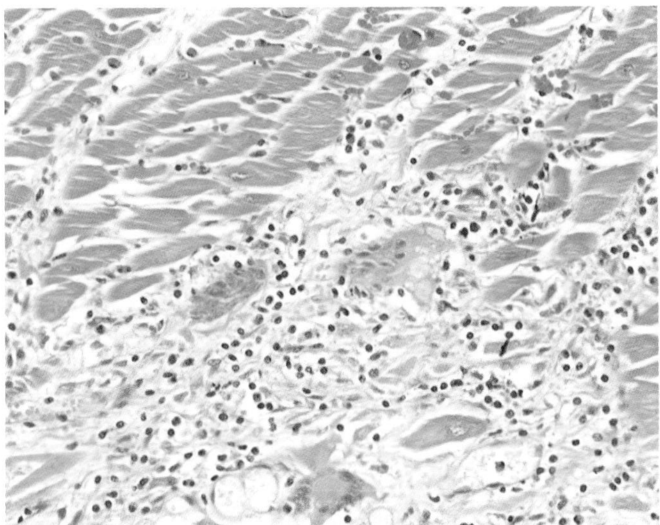

Fig. 8.2 Giant cell myocarditis. The myocardium is being damaged by a marked chronic inflammatory infiltrate that includes prominent multinucleated giant cells in the bottom half of the image. Haematoxlin and eosin ×200.
Courtesy of Dr Allan McPhaden, Glasgow Royal Infirmary.

The prognosis of giant cell myocarditis is very poor (<6 months) and identifying such patients early will allow the immediate administration of multidrug immunosuppressive therapy—a combination of prednisolone, ciclosporin, azathioprine, or muromonab-CD3 (OKT3). Due to the rapid deterioration of myocardial function, patients may require IABP or VAD therapy as a bridge to recovery, or a bridge to transplantation. It should be noted that a recurrence of giant cells occurs in 25% of transplanted hearts, but usually several years after surgery, and appears to respond to an increase in immunosuppression.

HIV cardiomyopathy

The survival of patients with HIV infection has improved dramatically with the use of highly active antiretroviral therapy (HAART) and the incidence of AIDS-defining events has significantly fallen.[26]

Cardiac involvement occurs in around 50% of patients with HIV, although it is frequently asymptomatic. HIV itself can cause a myocarditis, although most cases are clinically silent.[27] The pathogenesis of HIV cardiomyopathy is not fully established but thought to include infection of myocardial cells with HIV type 1 (HIV-1),[28] as HIV-1 genomic material has been demonstrated within cardiac myocytes in patients with cardiomyopathy at autopsy. Other possible causes for cardiovascular problems include subsequent opportunistic infection, neoplasia, and cardiotoxicity from pharmacologic agents, e.g. nucleoside analogues and pentamidine (Table 8.3). HF (principally right-sided) can also result from endocarditis in intravenous drug abusers. It should also be borne in mind that antiretroviral therapy can lead to premature coronary artery disease by inducing a syndrome akin to the metabolic syndrome.[29]

In a 5-year echocardiographic follow-up study of 952 asymptomatic HIV patients, 8% developed a dilated cardiomyopathy. The incidence was higher if the CD4 count was <400 cells/mm^3 and a histological diagnosis of myocarditis was made in 83%. HIV nucleic acid sequences were found in 76% and inflammatory infiltrates were predominantly composed of CD3 and CD8 lymphocytes. In those with active myocarditis, patients were also infected with: Coxsackie B (17%), cytomegalovirus (6%), and Epstein–Barr virus (3%).[30] Although this study was published in the *New England Journal of Medicine*, the work was later retracted by the journal's editors[31] and therefore the validity of the data is uncertain.

A rare but important differential diagnosis of HIV cardiomyopathy is infective myocarditis (e.g. myocardial toxoplasmosis, aspergillosis, tuberculosis, cryptococcosis, histoplasmosis, candidosis, herpes simplex, and cytomegalovirus).

Treatment

Conventional HF treatment may help improve cardiac function, even in asymptomatic HIV-positive patients. Physicians should also be aware of the possible interaction between protease inhibitors and β-adrenoreceptor antagonists, digoxin, or nondihydropyridine calcium antagonists due to possible prolongation of atrioventricular (AV) conduction. Protease inhibitors should be used with caution in patients with pre-existing conduction system disease.

Table 8.3 Cardiovascular problems in HIV infection

	Aetiology	Comment
Pericardium and effusions	Pericarditis	Pericardial effusion frequent, although tamponade is rare; tuberculosis effusion (may be associated with myocarditis) frequent in developing countries; other causes: bacterial pericarditis, Kaposi's sarcoma, and lymphoma
	Kaposi's sarcoma	Often disseminated; cardiac problems are infrequent
Myocardium	Cardiomyopathy	LVSD usually clinically silent; complex pathogenesis (direct virus effect, inflammatory response, autoantibodies)
	Myocarditis	Specific cause in <20% of patients; rare causes: toxoplasmosis, tuberculosis, cryptococcosis, histoplasmosis, aspergillosis, candidosis, cytomegalovirus, and herpes simplex; HIV itself can cause myocarditis
	Lymphoma	Non-Hodgkin's B-cell lymphoma; primary cardiac lymphoma is extremely rare
	Drug toxicity	Drug toxicity: amphotericin B, doxorubicin, foscarnet, interferon-α, zidovudine
Pulmonary hypertension	Inflammation and genetic factors	Possibly leading to right HF; histologically plexogenic arteriopathy is most commonly similar to the immunocompetent patient
Endocardium and valves	Infective endocarditis	Bacterial aetiology in intravenous drug abusers, is most often *Staph. aureus* and *Strep. viridans*; HIV infection itself is not associated with bacterial endocarditis
	Nonbacterial/ marantic	Tricuspid valve often involved; embolization of thrombus (frequently clinically silent)
Atherosclerosis	HAART	HAART may cause metabolic syndrome and lipodystrophy; premature atherosclerosis of coronary, cerebral, and peripheral arteries
Arrhythmia	No specific association with HIV infection	Arrhythmia caused by cardiomyopathy or myocarditis, myocardial infiltration in cardiac lymphoma; HIV itself does not cause rhythm disturbances
	Drug toxicity	Ganciclovir (against cytomegalovirus) may induce ventricular tachycardia; interferon-α can cause AV block and sudden death; pentamidine and pyrimethamine (for toxoplasmosis) cause QT prolongation, torsade de pointes; trimethoprim-sulfomethoxazole (*Pneumocystis carinii* prophylaxis) causes QT prolongation, torsade de pointes
Aneurysmal vascular disease	Inflammation	Premature aortic and cerebrovascular aneurysms described in patients with HIV infection

From Sudano I, Spieker LE, Noll G, Corti R, Weber R, Lüscher TF. Cardiovascular disease in HIV infection. *Am Heart J* 2006;**151:**11475–5.

Cardiovascular risk factors should be addressed,[32] but caution should be employed when initiating lipid-lowering therapy, because of interactions between HIV protease inhibitors (e.g. ritonavir, atazanavir, and saquinavir) and statins affecting cytochrome P450 function.[33] For this reason, simvastatin, atorvastatin, and lovastatin should be avoided, and pravstatin used with careful dose adjustment.

Although HIV is not a contra-indication for cardiac transplantation, few patients ultimately receive a new heart. Immunosuppressive agents such as ciclosporin and tacrolimus appear to slow virus replication and interleukin-2-induced T-cell replication,[34] and the incidence of opportunistic infections is not increased by pharmacological immunosuppression in HIV patients. However, there are pharmacological interactions between HAART and both ciclosporin and tacrolimus, with the need for careful dose adjustment.

Chagas' disease

Chagas' disease is a protozoal myocarditis endemic to South and Central America, caused by the parasite *Trypanosoma cruzi*. Between 16 million and 18 million people are infected with *T. cruzi* in Latin America; 70–90% of those infected are asymptomatic carriers and never develop any symptoms.

Acute Chagas' disease tends to be diagnosed most frequently in children, although individuals of all ages can be infected. It can cause a severe myocarditis, particularly in the young, resulting in HF and a high risk of mortality.[35] However, if chronic disease occurs, the manifestations are usually delayed and typically do not arise until 20 years later. Whether chronic disease is due directly to parasite invasion or to secondary autoimmune mechanisms is not clear.

Transmission and pathophysiology

The major route of transmission of *T. cruzi* is directly from the reduviid bug. However, the infection can also arise from other routes, including blood transfusion, organ transplantation, and vertical transmission. Organs involved show chronic inflammatory changes and diffuse fibrosis due antibody and cell-mediated immunity against *T. cruzi* antigens.

Clinical features

Chagas' disease can be associated with progressive cardiac dysfunction, conduction system disease, ventricular arrhythmias, and sudden death. Thromboembolic disease may also be a feature, as are the usual symptoms and signs of HF.

Investigation

Echocardiography may reveal either global LVSD or regional wall motion abnormality. In advanced disease there may be posterior hypokinesis with relative sparing of the septal wall. A left ventricular apical aneurysm is also frequently a feature. A Machado–Guerreiro complement fixation test or indirect immunofluorescence or enzyme-linked immunosorbent assay (ELISA) may aid the diagnosis.

Treatment

Antiparasitic agents (e.g. benznidazole) reduce parasitaemia, but have not been shown to eradicate the disease. Although not evidence-based, standard HF therapy, the control of ventricular arrhythmias with antiarrhythmic drugs (e.g. amiodarone), and anticoagulation to reduce the risk of thromboembolic disease should be considered.

Lyme disease

Lyme disease is a multisystem disease caused by infection from a tick-borne spirochete (*Borrelia burgdorferi*). Early features include erythema migrans and constitutional upset, but the development of cardiac, neurological, and joint involvement may follow after weeks to months. In the USA, cardiac involvement occurs in up to 10% of untreated adults during the early disseminated phase of the disease—usually within the first two months after infection. Lyme carditis is less common in Europe, possibly relating to infection by different organisms. Interestingly, although Lyme disease itself has a slight female predominance, the cardiac manifestations are much more common in males (3:1).

Clinical features

Erythema migrans is found in approximately 90% of people with Lyme disease. The early disseminated features occur days to months later, with myocarditis, lymphocytic meningitis, cranial nerve palsies, and migratory polyarthritis.

Myocarditis most commonly manifests as conduction system disease—often progressing rapidly from first degree to higher degrees of block over a relatively short period of time, this frequently requires temporary transvenous pacing.[36] Myopericarditis, and cardiomyopathy may also develop, but these are generally mild and self-limiting. Late features occur weeks to years later, and include chronic arthritis and neurological problems (e.g. dementia). Lyme myocarditis should be suspected in patients with a history of a tick bite, particularly if they have conduction system abnormalities. Serological studies with ELISA and western blot help to confirm the diagnosis.

Treatment

Lyme disease should generally be treated by those experienced in its management. Doxycycline is currently the antibacterial of choice for early disease, and intravenous ceftriaxone is recommended for Lyme disease associated with moderate to severe cardiac or neurological abnormalities, late Lyme disease, and Lyme arthritis. The duration of treatment is generally 2–4 weeks, although Lyme arthritis requires longer treatment with oral antibacterial drugs.

Infiltrative causes of heart failure

Infiltrative cardiomyopathies are characterized by the deposition of abnormal material into the ventricular myocardium, causing it to become increasingly stiff, with reduced ventricular compliance.[37] The restrictive physiology impedes ventricular filling, leading to impaired diastolic function. However, systolic function usually remains normal, at least early in the disease process.

Infiltrative cardiac diseases either increase ventricular wall thickness (Table 8.4), or cause chamber enlargement with secondary wall thinning (Table 8.5). However, infiltrative conditions can be mistaken for other cardiac conditions. A good example is cardiac amyloidosis, where the increased wall thickness, small ventricular volume, and occasional dynamic left ventricular outflow obstruction can mimic conditions with true myocyte hypertrophy such as hypertrophic cardiomyopathy and hypertensive heart disease.

Infiltrative cardiac conditions often result in a restrictive cardiomyopathy (Table 8.6), although this is uncommon in Western countries. However, in certain geographical locations (particularly the tropics—Africa, India, South and Central America, and Asia), restrictive cardiomyopathy is a more important cause of HF and death due to a higher incidence of endomyocardial fibrosis. Here we concentrate on the acquired causes of myocardial and endocardial infiltration.

Clinical features

Patients with restrictive cardiomyopathy often complain of exercise intolerance due to a fixed stroke volume limiting any increase in cardiac output. Elevated filling pressures and Kussmaul's sign (inspiratory increase in jugular venous pressure, JVP) may be apparent. Other clinical features include an impalpable apex beat (unlike constrictive pericarditis), third or fourth heart sound, peripheral oedema, hepatomegaly, and ascites.

Investigations

The ECG may show P mitrale/pulmonale, low precordial QRS amplitudes, and atrial arrhythmias. Echocardiography may initially appear unremarkable, with normal ventricular dimensions and systolic function. However, there is often marked biatrial enlargement secondary to elevated atrial pressures and a restrictive inflow pattern seen on mitral Doppler. Features that may help differentiate restrictive cardiomyopathy from constrictive pericarditis are shown in Table 8.7. On cardiac catheterization, left ventricular and right ventricular pressure tracings are in phase and right ventricular peak pressure is frequently in excess of 40 mmHg. CMR is very useful in the assessment of patients with infiltrative myocardial and endomyocardial disease, and may help identify areas likely to have a high diagnostic yield on endomyocardial biopsy.

Treatment

The mainstay of therapy for restrictive cardiomyopathy is diuretics, although caution should be taken to avoid underfilling patients, as a drop in filling pressure will have a marked adverse impact on cardiac output. Avoidance of atrial fibrillation (AF) or optimal rate control of AF will help maintain ventricular filling time. It is also of significant importance to identify and treat the underlying cause.

Prognosis

The prognosis of restrictive cardiomyopathy is generally poor and some patients will ultimately need cardiac transplantation if appropriate.

Cardiac sarcoidosis

Sarcoidosis is a multisystem, noncaseating, granulomatous disease of unknown aetiology. It is estimated to affect 1 in 10 000 people, with marked geographical and racial variation, being 3–4 times more common in black people. It typically affects young adults, and most commonly affects the lung (90%), presenting with either evidence of bilateral hilar lymphadenopathy or pulmonary infiltrates. Pulmonary hypertension carries an ominous prognosis. Skin, joint, or eye involvement is also common. However, clinical cardiac involvement is uncommon, affecting only around 2–5% of

Table 8.4 Infiltrative cardiac conditions that present with increased LV mass and thick ventricular walls

Condition	Age at presentation	History and clinical presentation	Echocardiography	ECG profile	CMR LGE	Biopsy
Cardiac amyloid	>30 yrs	Heart failure symptoms, nephrotic syndrome, idiopathic peripheral neuropathy, unexplained hepatomegaly	Symmetrical increase in LV and RV wall thickness, dilated LA and RA, granular appearance of myocardium, pericardial effusion, decreased EF in advanced cases	Decreased or normal QRS complex voltage, pseudoinfarction in inferolateral leads	Global, diffuse, pronounced in subendocardium; RV and LV walls	Myocyte atrophy, amyloid replaces normal cardiac tissue
Fabry's disease	Male: 11 ± 7 yrs; female: 23 ± 16 yrs	Neuropathic pain, impaired sweating, skin rashes	Symmetrical increase in LV and RV wall thickness, normal EF	Increased or normal QRS complex voltage, short or prolonged PR interval	Focal, midwall, inferolateral wall	Enlarged myocytes with clusters of concentric glycolipid (rnyelinoid bodies) within lysosomes
Danon's disease	<20 yrs	Heart failure, skeletal myopathy, mental retardation	Very thick LV (20–60 mm), RV may or may not be thick, decreased EF	Increased or normal QRS complex voltage, short PR interval (delta wave)	Subendocardial, does not correspond to perfusion territory	Sarcoplasmic vacuolization, focal storage of PAS-positive material, myofibrillar disarray
Friedreich's ataxia	25 yrs (range 2–51 yrs)	Gait abnormality	Increase in LV septal and posterior wall thickness, normal EF	Normal QRS complex voltage, ventricular tachycardia		Nonspecific
Cardiac oxalosis	>20 yrs	Juvenile urolithiasis and nephrocalcinosis	Symmetrical increase in LV and RV wall thickness; patchy, echodense speckled reflection; normal EF	Increased or normal QRS complex voltage, complete heart block	Increased myocardium attenuation on CT	Intra- and extracellular deposition of oxalate crystals without concomitant inflammation and necrosis
Mucopolysaccharidoses	12–4 yrs (median, 10 yrs)	Variable depending on subtype, coarse facial features, delayed mental development, skeletal deformities, corneal clouding, hepatosplenomegaly	Asymmetrical septal hypertrophy, mitral and/or aortic valve stenosis or insufficiency, normal EF	Increased or decreased QRS complex voltage, malignant arrhythmia		Swollen myocytes with clear cytoplasm due to accumulation of mucopolysaccharides within lysosomes
Differential diagnosis						
Hypertrophic cardiomyopathy	17–18 yrs	Maybe asymptomatic, dyspnoea, angina, syncope, sudden death	Asymmetrical hypertrophy small LV cavity, LVOT obstruction, normal EF	Increased QRS complex voltage pseudo-delta wave, giant T-wave inversion	Patchy, midwall, junctions of the ventricular septum and RV	Myocyte hypertrophy, myofibrillar disarray, and interstitial fibrosis
Hypertensive heart disease	Adults	History of hypertension	Symmetrical increase in LV wall thickness, mild LV dilation, normal EF	Increased QRS complex, nonspecific ST-T-wave changes	No pattern, predominantly subendocardial	Enlarged myocytes with enlarged or replicated nuclei

EF, ejection fraction; LA, left atrium; LV, left ventricle; RA, right atrium; RV, right ventricle. Adapted from Seward JB, Casaclang-Verzosa G. Infiltrative cardiovascular diseases: cardiomyopathies that look alike. *J Am Coll Cardiol* 2010;**55:**17697–9.

patients with sarcoidosis, although autopsy studies suggest that subclinical cardiac involvement is more common. Cardiac sarcoidosis generally affects the basal septum, conduction system, papillary muscles, and patchy regions on the ventricular free wall.

Pathophysiology

The aetiology of sarcoidosis is not clear, and several potential antigens have been suggested as triggers, including *Mycobacterium tuberculosis*, mycoplasma, aluminium, and pollen. T-helper cell

Table 8.5 Infiltrative cardiac conditions that present with dilated left ventricle and infarct pattern

Condition	Age at presentation	History	Echocardiography	ECG	CMR LGE	Cardiac biopsy
Sarcoidosis	Young adults	Congestive heart failure	Variable wall thickness, focal or global hypokinesia, LV aneurysm	Infrahisian block, atypical infarction pattern	Patchy, basal and lateral LV walls	Noncaseating, multinucleated giant cell granuloma surrounded by band of dense collagen fibres
Wegener's disease	Young adults	Chronic upper and lower respiratory tract infections	Regional hypokinesis pericardial effusion, mild, MR, LV systolic dysfunction	Atrial fibrillation, atrioventricular block, atypical infarction pattern	Diffuse, midwall	Vasculitis with necrotizing granulomatous inflammation
Haemochromatosis	Hereditary haemochromatosis: >30 yrs in men, older in women; secondary haemochromatosis: any age	Hereditary haemochromatosis: liver function abnormalities, weakness and lethargy, skin hyperpigmentation, diabetes mellitus, arthralgia, impotence in men; secondary haemochromatosis: haemolytic anemia, multiple blood transfusions	Dilated LV with global systolic dysfunction	Supraventricular arrhythmia, ventricular conduction abnormality is rare	$T2^*$ values substantially reduced	Iron deposits within the myocyte
Differential diagnoses						
Ischaemic cardiomyopathy	Adult	Coronary artery disease, congestive heart failure	Dilated LV, regional hypokinesis corresponding to perfusion territory, decreased systolic function	Multiform premature ventricular complexes, nonsustained ventricular tachycardia	Subendocardial, different degrees of transmural extension, corresponds to perfusion territory	
Idiopathic dilated cardiomyopathy	Adult	Congestive heart failure, no known cardiovascular disease	Dilated LV with global systolic dysfunction	Atrial fibrillation	No LGE, or if present, midwall and patchy	

Adapted from Seward JB, Casaclang-Verzosa G. Infiltrative cardiovascular diseases: cardiomyopathies that look alike. *J Am Coll Cardiol* 2010;**55:**17697–9.

activation leads to the formation of granuloma lesions and interleukin-6 is thought to be involved in the maintenance of inflammation by inducing T-cell proliferation. A positive association with cardiac sarcoidosis has been reported with HLA-DQB1∗0601.

Table 8.6 Causes of a restrictive cardiomyopathy

Myocardial	Infiltrative (e.g. amyloid, sarcoid, Gaucher's disease)
	Noninfiltrative (e.g. scleroderma)
	Storage diseases (e.g. haemochromatosis, glycogen and lysosomal storage disease)
Endomyocardial	Endomyocardial fibrosis
	Hypereosinophilic syndrome (Löffler's endocarditis)
	Carcinoid and metastatic disease
	Radiation
	Anthracycline therapy

Clinical features

The clinical consequences of cardiac sarcoidosis range from asymptomatic conduction abnormalities to fatal ventricular arrhythmias, depending upon the location and extent of granulomatous inflammation. Complete heart block is frequently seen, and patients are at risk of both supraventricular and ventricular tachycardias. HF symptoms may also develop due initially to restrictive physiology, although left ventricular dilatation and systolic dysfunction can develop. Cardiac imaging in sarcoidosis frequently demonstrates dyskinetic or akinetic segments interspersed with normal segments.[38] Pericardial effusions can occur, but rarely cause tamponade. There may also be valve dysfunction, including mitral valve prolapse. Most patients with cardiac sarcoidosis ultimately die from ventricular tachyarrhythmia, conduction disturbances, or progressive HF.

Investigations

The clinical findings of cardiac sarcoidosis are largely nonspecific. As a result, diagnostic tests such as endomyocardial biopsy (Fig. 8.3)

Table 8.7 Features differentiating constrictive pericarditis from restrictive cardiomyopathy

Feature	Constrictive pericarditis	Restrictive cardiomyopathy
Past medical history	Previous pericarditis, cardiac surgery, trauma, radiotherapy, connective tissue disease	These items rare
Jugular venous waveform	X and Y dips brief and 'flicking', not conspicuous positive waves	X and Y dips less brief, may have conspicuous A wave or V wave
Extra sounds in diastole	Early S_3, hjgh pitched 'pericardial knock'. No S_4	Later S3, low pitched, 'triple rhythm', S_4 in some cases
Mitral or tricuspid regurgitation	Usually absent	Often present
ECG	P waves reflect intra-atrial conduction delay Atrioventricular or intraventricular conduction defects rare	P waves reflect right or left atrial hypertrophy or overload. Atrioventricular or intraventricular conduction defects not unusual
Plain chest radiograph	Pericardial calcification in 20–30%	Pericardial calcification rare
Ventricular septal movement in diastole	Abrupt septal movement ('notch') in early diastole in most cases	Abrupt septal movement in early diastole seen only occasionally
Ventricular septal movement with respiration	Notable movement towards left ventricle in inspiration usually seen	Relatively little movement towards left ventricle in most cases
Atrial enlargement	Slight or moderate in most cases	Pronounced in most cases
Respiratory variation in mitral and tricuspid flow velocity	>25% in most cases	<15% in most cases
Equilibration of diastolic pressures in all cardiac chambers	Within 5 mmHg in nearly all cases, often essentially the same	Within 5 mmHg in a small proportion of cases
Dip-plateau waveform in the right ventricular pressure waveform	End-diastolic pressure more than one-third of systolic pressure in many cases	End-diastolic pressure often less than one-third of systolic
Peak right ventricular systolic pressure	Nearly always <60 mmHg, often <40 mmHg	Frequently >40 mmHg and occasionally >60 mmHg
Discordant respiratory variation of ventricular peak systolic pressures	Right and left ventricular peak systolic pressure variations are out-of-phase	Rjght and left ventricular peak systolic pressure variations are in-phase
Paradoxical pulse	Often present to a moderate degree	Rarely present
MR/CT imaging	Shows thick pericardium in most cases	Shows thick pericardium only rarely
Endomyocardial biopsy	Normal, or nonspecific abnormalities	Shows amyloid in some cases, rarely other specific infiltrative disease

From Hancock EW. *Heart* 2001;**86:**343–9.

may be required in patients without other manifestations of sarcoidosis, as usually the diagnosis has already been made from another system involvement (commonly lung).

The diagnosis of cardiac sarcoidosis is difficult (Box 8.1). Standard investigations include serum ACE and the Kveim–Siltzbach test. A chest radiograph is very important to identify lung involvement (e.g. hilar lymphadenopathy). A 12-lead ECG and 24-h Holter monitor will help to identify patients at risk of brady- or tachyarrhythmia. Echocardiography is not sensitive or specific enough to identify early or small areas of myocardial involvement, although is more useful in advanced disease.[39] The ventricular septum often appears hyperechogenic and there may be evidence of LVSD or left ventricular aneurysm. As mentioned above, dyskinetic or akinetic segments are commonly interspersed with normal segments. Nuclear imaging (particularly thallium-201 scintigraphy) has largely been superseded by contrast-enhanced CMR. Late gadolinium enhancement is patchy and typically involves the basal and lateral left ventricle walls.[40] This may help target subsequent endomyocardial biopsy, particularly as endomyocardial biopsy specimens are usually obtained from the apical septum.

Treatment

Corticosteroids are thought capable of halting or slowing the progression of inflammation and fibrosis in sarcoidosis. The initial starting dose is 60–80 mg of prednisone daily with a gradual tapering of the dose to a maintenance level of 10–15 mg per day over a period of 6 months. However, a possible association between corticosteroid treatment and formation of ventricular aneurysms has been described. Alternative agents such as chloroquine, hydroxychloroquine, and methotrexate may be given to patients who do not respond to corticosteroids or who cannot tolerate their side effects.

A permanent pacemaker is indicated in patients with complete heart block or other high-grade conduction system disease. An ICD is recommended in survivors of sudden death or patients with refractory ventricular tachyarrhythmias. Some also recommend an ICD for primary prevention because of the high rate of sudden death (presumed due to ventricular tachyarrhythmias) in cardiac sarcoidosis. Given the likely need for future pacing for bradycardia in many patients in the future, a dual-chamber ICD or CRT-D should be considered.

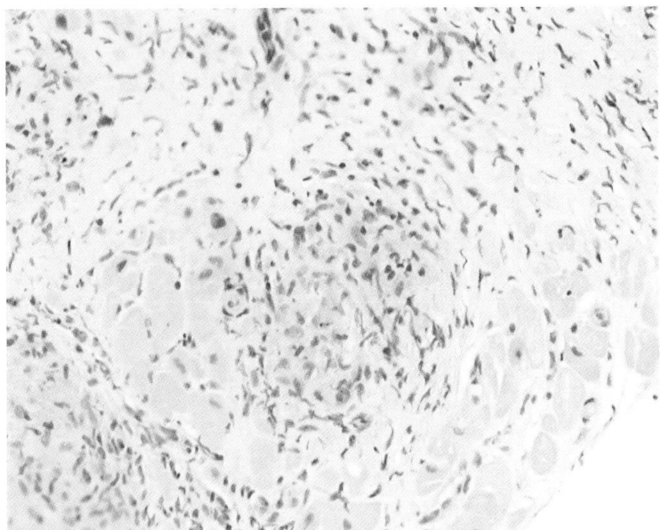

Fig. 8.3 Sarcoidosis. A central non–caseating granuloma is disrupting the myocardium with myocyte destruction and early replacement fibrosis. A second granuloma is present at the bottom left. Haematoxylin and eosin ×400.
Courtesy of Dr Allan McPhaden, Glasgow Royal Infirmary.

Cardiac transplantation for cardiac sarcoidosis is rare, but it remains a possibility for younger patients with severe endstage irreversible cardiac failure or resistant ventricular tachyarrhythmia, although disease can recur in the transplanted heart. Other types of surgery may be occasionally required such as correction of mitral valve disease or resection of ventricular aneurysms.

Box 8.1 Guidelines for the diagnosis of cardiac sarcoidosis

1. Histologic diagnosis group: endomyocardial biopsy demonstrates epithelioid granulomata without caseating granulomata.
2. Clinical diagnosis group: in patients with histologic diagnosis of extracardiac sarcoidosis, cardiac sarcoidosis is suspected when criterion (a) below and at least one of the criteria (b)–(e) is present and other aetiologies such as hypertension and coronary artery disease have been excluded:
   a) Complete RBBB, left axis deviation. AV block, VT, PVC, or pathological Q or ST-T change on resting or ambulatory ECG.
   b) Abnormal wall motion, regional wall thinning, or dilation of the left ventricle.
   c) Perfusion defect by ^{201}Tl-myocardial scintigraphy or abnormal accumulation by ^{67}Ga-citrate or ^{99}Tc-PYP myocardial scintigraphy.
   d) Abnormal intracardiac pressure, low cardiac output, or abnormal wall motion or depressed ejection fraction of the left ventricle.
   e) Interstitial fibrosis or cellular infiltration over moderate grade even if the findings are nonspecific.

From Hiraga, H, Yuwai, K, Hiroe, M, *et al. Guidelines for the diagnosis of cardiac sarcoidosis: study report of diffuse pulmonary diseases*, pp. 23–4. Japanese Ministry of Health and Welfare, Tokyo, 1993.

Haemochromatosis

Haemochromatosis is an autosomal recessive disorder in which mutations in the *HFE* gene (most commonly C282Y, on the short arm of chromosome 6) cause increased intestinal iron absorption. The clinical manifestations are related to excessive tissue iron deposition, particularly in the liver, pancreas, and pituitary, but also in the heart.

Clinical features

The clinical manifestations of iron accumulation include liver disease (ultimately leading to cirrhosis and an increased risk of hepatocellular carcinoma), skin pigmentation, diabetes mellitus, arthropathy, and hypogonadism. Cardiac effects can be the presenting manifestation in 15% of patients including HF, most commonly due to systolic rather than diastolic dysfunction, and conduction system disease.

Investigations

Investigation should begin with routine biochemistry including thyroid and liver function tests and iron studies (ferritin, transferrin saturation, serum iron, total iron binding concentration). Genetic testing for C282Y homozygosity can also be undertaken. Although the ECG can appear normal initially, the QRS complex can appear of low voltage with repolarization abnormalities.[41] CMR is the imaging modality of choice as echocardiography will be unable to distinguish haemochromatosis from a dilated cardiomyopathy. T_2* CMR can detect and quantify myocardial iron load and distribution.[42] Ultimately, a liver biopsy is the definitive test for iron overload, although with cardiac involvement, a right ventricular endomyocardial biopsy will show evidence of stainable sarcoplasmic iron (Fig. 8.4), where normally this should not be present.

Treatment

Venesection and chelation therapy are associated with an improvement of ventricular dysfunction.[43] However, irreversible myocardial dysfunction can occur with advanced disease. Some patients may require combined heart and liver transplantation, although

Fig. 8.4 Haemochromatosis. Granular intracellular cardiac myocyte deposits of haemosiderin are stained blue. Perls stain ×400.
Courtesy of Dr Allan McPhaden, Glasgow Royal Infirmary.

this is currently a rare occurrence because of the lack of available organs.

Wegener's granulomatosis

Wegener's granulomatosis is a multiorgan vasculitic condition characterized by necrotizing granulomatous inflammation which principally affects the lungs and the kidneys.[44] However, in a case series of 85 patients with confirmed Wegener's granulomatosis, 36% had cardiac abnormalities on echocardiography attributable to the disease.[45] Regional wall motion abnormalities were found in 65%, mild mitral regurgitation in 54%, LVSD in 50%, and pericardial effusion in 19%. Patients with cardiac abnormalities had a higher mortality rate than those without. Cardiac sarcoidosis should be suspected when regional wall motion abnormalities are not confined to a specific coronary artery territory. On CMR, late gadolinium enhancement in the midwall rather than the subendocardium is consistent with fibrosis rather than infarction.[46]

The management of Wegener's granulomatosis requires a multidisciplinary approach. Patients with cardiac involvement in Wegener's granulomatosis have 'severe', life-threatening disease.[47] Glucocorticosteroids and cyclophosphamide remain the standard of care for remission induction.

Endomyocardial disease

Endomyocardial fibrosis (EMF) is characterized by fibrous endocardial involvement of either or both ventricles, often with associated atrioventricular valvular regurgitation. EMF typically occurs in equatorial Africa, where it is a frequent cause of CHF. It is also recognized elsewhere, but generally within 15° of the equator.

Clinical features and investigation

EMF most frequently has biventricular involvement (50%), although single-chamber involvement does occur, either left ventricular (40%) or right ventricular (10%). Subsequently, atrial enlargement occurs, particularly where there is mitral or tricuspid regurgitation.

The symptoms and signs are primarily those of left/right ventricular failure. Eosinophilia may be present. The 12-lead ECG shows small QRS voltages with nonspecific ST/T wave abnormalities. Echocardiography may show apical obliteration of the involved ventricle, dilated atria, mitral or tricuspid regurgitation, and a pericardial effusion which may be large. Mural thrombi are common. An endomyocardial biopsy may be diagnostic.

Treatment

The mainstay of treatment is diuretics. Anticoagulation should be considered in view of the risk of mural thrombi, and particularly so if AF is present. AF can be rate-controlled with digoxin, although its occurrence heralds a poor prognosis. Surgical removal of fibrotic endocardium can lead to a significant improvement in symptoms, although recurrent fibrosis invariably occurs.

Löffler's endocarditis (the hypereosinophilic syndrome)

Hypereosinophilic syndrome (HES) is a clinical diagnosis where there is a sustained eosinophil count greater than 1500/mm^3 for at least 6 months, with multiorgan involvement. Most patients with HES have biventricular cardiac involvement (Löffler's endocarditis), with eosinophilic myocarditis, mural thrombosis, and fibrotic change, resulting in a restrictive cardiomyopathy. Associated involvement of the lungs, bone marrow, brain, and kidneys also occurs.

Clinical features and investigations

The syndrome is frequently heralded by systemic upset, including fever, weight loss, rash, and cough. Symptoms and signs of HF then develop, and AF and thromboembolic disease are common. The 12-lead ECG shows nonspecific T wave abnormalities, and the echocardiogram reveals localized thickening of the left ventricle basal posterior wall with restricted motion of the posterior mitral valve leaflet (Fig. 8.5). Left ventricular systolic function is invariably preserved, and atrial dilatation and apical thrombus are common.

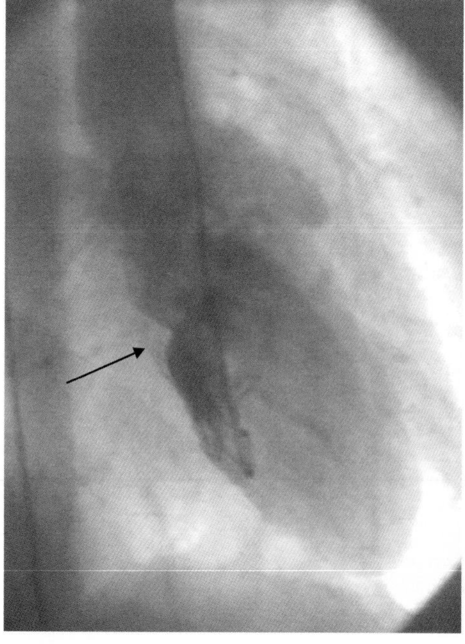
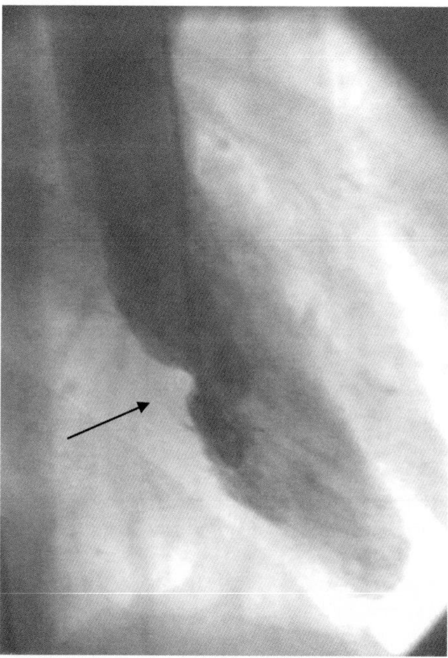

Fig. 8.5 End-diastolic and end-systolic frames from the left ventricular angiogram of a woman with hypereosinophilic cardiac disease. The arrows point to the dense material involving and immobilizing the posterior mitral valve leaflet.

Treatment

The treatment of Löffler's endocarditis is largely with diuretics and vasodilators, and anticoagulation should be considered. Other treatment strategies include corticosteroids ± hydroxyurea, and interferon may be tried in advanced cases. Attempts can also be made to surgically remove fibrotic endocardium.

Amyloidosis

Amyloid proteins are normal proteins which can become insoluble polymers forming β-pleated sheets in tissues. What leads to an amyloid precursor protein leading to amyloidosis depends upon circumstances: most commonly, it may be an intrinsically abnormal protein, as in inherited abnormalities of the transthyretin gene; or it may be a protein being produced in large quantities, as happens with AL and AA amyloidosis (see below).

As an amyloid protein is deposited in tissue, it is partly stabilized by serum amyloid P,[48] a normal circulating factor, which binds to amyloid proteins and makes them resistant to normal proteolytic mechanisms.[49] The systemic illness, amyloidosis, may develop, with the symptoms depending on the site of amyloid deposition. Not all types of amyloid affect the heart.

Classification of amyloidosis

The classification of amyloidosis has changed several times, and can be confusing. The modern system uses an abbreviation starting with A (for amyloid) followed by the abbreviation for the protein involved (Table 8.8). The most important from the perspective of the heart are AL and ATTR amyloid. In AL amyloid, an abnormal white cell clone produces large quantities of an inappropriate immunoglobulin light chain.

Presentation

The most common form of amyloid with important cardiac involvement is AL amyloid. It presents very insidiously and patients frequently give a long history of general malaise and weight loss and have often undergone a wide range of investigations before the correct diagnosis is reached. Overt HF can be a late presenting feature.

Suggestive features include periorbital purpura (so-called 'panda eyes') and macroglossia. Neuropathies, autonomic and sensory, can occur, as well as carpal tunnel syndrome. The autonomic neuropathy contributes to orthostatic hypotension and frequent syncope. Renal involvement is more or less constant and causes proteinuria, which is frequently in the nephrotic range.

Cardiac involvement

The heart is almost always involved histologically in patients with AL amyloid, but clinical involvement is present in around a third to half. In patients with cardiac involvement, death is commonly due to HF, or sudden, due to arrhythmia or pulseless electrical activity.

Amyloid can be deposited in small cardiac vessels, resulting in cardiac chest pain with apparently normal epicardial vessels.[50] More typically, patients have a restrictive cardiomyopathy in which the physical presence of the amyloid deposits prevents adequate diastolic relaxation of the ventricles. Interestingly, the light chains themselves may have a direct effect on the myocardium.[51, 52] The clinical picture is dominated by right-sided clinical signs with raised JVP and fluid retention. A gallop rhythm or loud third sound is frequent. Patients often have a low cardiac output state with very limited exercise capacity and marked fatigue. Patients may also present with a dilated cardiomyopathy, presumably reflecting late disease.

The atria dilate in response to the rise in ventricular filling pressures, making AF very common in amyloid heart disease. Thromboembolic complications are very common, even in patients in sinus rhythm. Sudden death occurs, presumably due to more complex arrhythmia, at least in some patients.[53]

Investigations

The ECG is typically abnormal and shows low-voltage complexes (Fig. 8.6), and commonly AF. The echocardiogram is extremely helpful. There is usually concentric left ventricular thickening (often labelled 'hypertrophy' but due to infiltration). The combination of left ventricular hypertrophy with small-voltage complexes on the ECG is characteristic.[54] The atrial walls are often thickened, together with the interatrial septum (Fig. 8.7). The texture of myocardium is abnormal and frequently 'speckled'. Diastolic flow across the mitral valve is grossly abnormal with a tall E wave and very short E wave deceleration time. The patient may be in sinus rhythm, but with no atrial mechanical activity.[55]

Cardiac catheterization shows a restrictive filling pattern in both ventricles with a dip-and-plateau pattern in diastole. In contrast to the pathophysiology of pericardial disease, the ventricular traces are often not identical (Fig. 8.8).

Imaging for amyloidosis itself is now possible using radiolabelled serum amyloid P (SAP) scanning and is helpful for assessing the burden of extracardiac deposits, but cannot be used to image the heart because of blood pool uptake.[56,57] The findings on CMR are characteristic in advanced disease, with subendocardial late gadolinium enhancement together with abnormal gadolinium kinetics.[58] Less is known about CMR earlier in the progress of the disease.

Ultimately, the diagnosis has to be made by tissue histology. Abdominal fat aspiration is said to be sensitive, and is certainly a safe first site for biopsy.[59] Other sites include rectal and gingival biopsies. Cardiac biopsy, usually from the right ventricle, may be necessary (see Figs 24.17 and 24.18, p. 263) but it is worth remembering to stain any other available tissue for amyloid as it is widely deposited (see Fig. 8.9). Amyloid takes up Congo red dye very readily and shows apple-green birefringence under polarized light.

Table 8.8 Types of amyloidosis

Abbreviation	Amyloid protein	Source of protein	Clinical tissue deposition
AL	Immunoglobulin light chains	White cell dyscrasias	Heart, kidneys
AA	Serum amyloid protein A; acute phase reactants	Chronic inflammation	Kidneys, spleen, adrenal glands, liver, and gut (heart involvement rare)
ATTR	Transthyretin	Abnormal gene	Heart, neurological
ATTR	Transthyretin	Age	Heart

There are other forms of amyloidosis, e.g. those associated with renal dialysis (β_2-microglobulin), prion disease, and Alzheimer's disease.

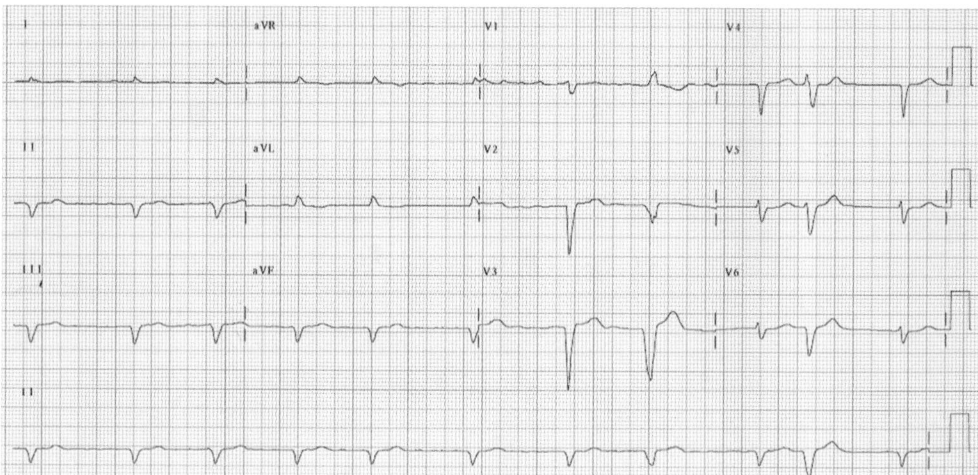

Fig. 8.6 12-lead ECG in patient with AL amyloidosis, showing atrial fibrillation, left axis deviation, and broad low-voltage complexes.

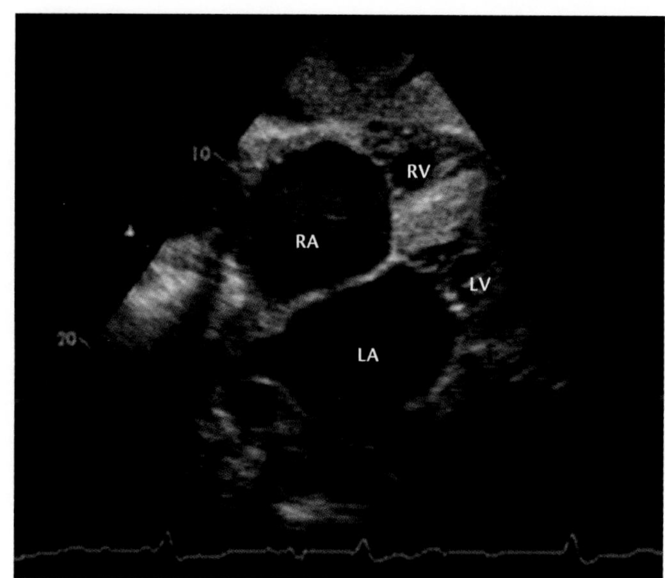

Fig. 8.7 Subcostal echocardiographic view of the heart in the same patient as in Fig. 8.6. Note the greatly dilated atria and relatively small, apparently hypertrophied ventricles. The interatrial septum is thickened.

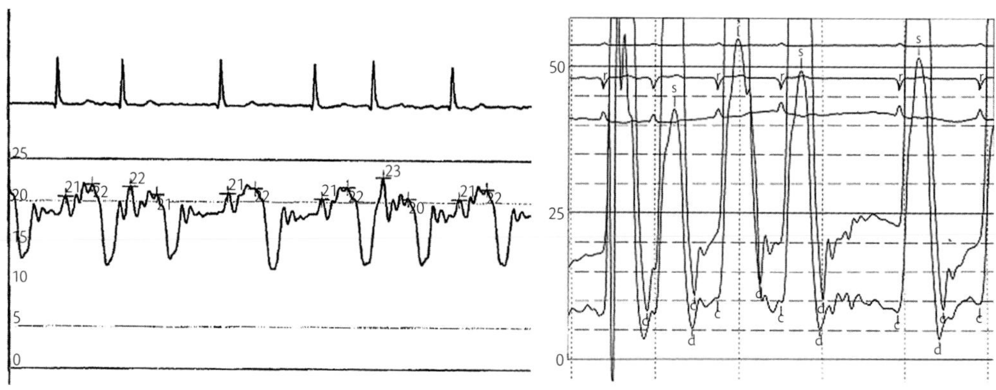

Fig. 8.8 Pressure trace from the right atrium (left panel) showing raised mean atrial pressure and a striking *y* descent. The patient is in atrial fibrillation. Simultaneous pressure traces from left and right ventricles (right panel). The diastolic pressures are widely separated, but show the features of restrictive filling. There is pulmonary hypertension.

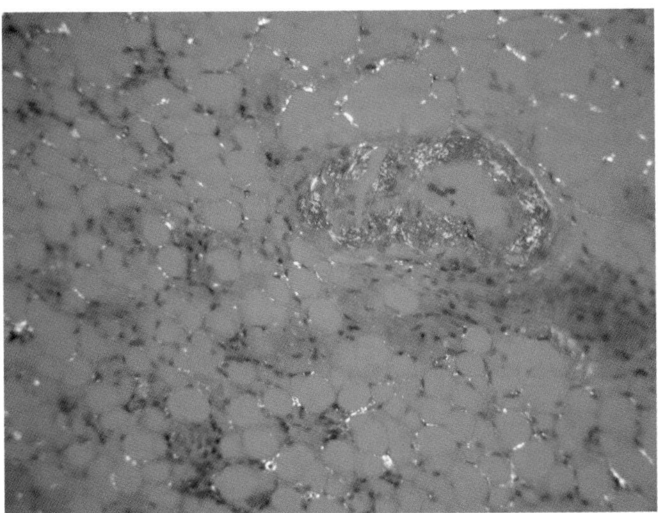

Fig. 8.9 Amyloid detected as apple-green birefringence on a pleural biopsy specimen. The biopsy had been taken as part of a diagnostic work up for pleural effusion some 2 years prior to presentation with a restrictive cardiomyopathy.

Other investigations in AL amyloid should include serum and urine protein electrophoresis for a paraprotein and free light chains (more commonly λ than κ). Bone marrow biopsy may be necessary. Urine protein estimation is important to assess renal involvement. Early involvement of expert haematologists is vital.

ATTR amyloid may be restricted to the heart and myocardial biopsy is often necessary to make the diagnosis.

Treatment

The prognosis in AL amyloid is bleak, with death within 2 years being usual.[60]

The presence of HF reduces median survival to months.[61] Cardiac involvement in amyloidosis is not treatable specifically. The HF syndrome itself is treated symptomatically with diuretics, but there is no evidence to suggest other therapy helps. Patients are particularly prone to develop hypotension with standard treatment, perhaps in part due to autonomic and small-vessel involvement. Digoxin should only be used with great caution as it binds avidly to amyloid protein and can be dangerous. It may help control heart rate in some patients. There is no clear role for an ICD in patients with amyloid, despite the high frequency of sudden death.[62]

Any successful treatment is aimed at the underlying cause, a white cell malignancy, and high-dose chemotherapy followed by autologous bone marrow transplant can in some cases be successful in treating underlying myeloma.[63] The treatment is toxic and only around half of patients may be suitable. Toxicity seems to be worse in patients with cardiac involvement.

Treatment of the myeloma may not successfully restore organ function, and for a very few patients, chemotherapy followed by bone marrow transplant and then heart transplant may be appropriate.

An intriguing possibility exploits the fact that serum amyloid P is always involved in amyloid formation. There is some evidence that reducing serum amyloid P can remove amyloid P from tissue deposits, exposing the amyloid itself to proteolysis.[64]

Patients with transthyretin amyloidosis, although clinically very similar to patients with AL amyloidosis, have a much better prognosis.[65] In some forms of familial disease, liver transplantation may be successful by removing the source of abnormal protein. In senile amyloidosis, there is no specific therapy available. There is some evidence that the nonsteroidal anti-inflammatory drug diflusinal may be helpful by stabilizing the native transthyretin structure and preventing tissue deposition.[66] Senile amyloidosis tends to be a disease of elderly men, making transplantation inappropriate for most. In this form of the disease, conduction system disturbance is common, and permanent pacing may be needed.

References

1. Mahrholdt H, Wagner A, Deluigi CC, *et al.* Presentation, patterns of myocardial damage, and clinical course of viral myocarditis. *Circulation* 2006;**114**:1581–90.
2. Kühl U, Pauschinger M, Noutsias M, *et al.* High prevalence of viral genomes and multiple viral infections in the myocardium of adults with 'idiopathic' left ventricular dysfunction. *Circulation* 2005;**111**:887–93.
3. Kindermann I, Kindermann M, Kandolf R, *et al.* Predictors of outcome in patients with suspected myocarditis. *Circulation* 2008;**118**:639–48.
4. Coyne CB, Bergelson JM. Virus-induced Abl and Fyn kinase signals permit coxsackie virus entry through epithelial tight junctions. *Cell* 2006;**124**:119–31.
5. Fairweather D, Frisancho-Kiss S, Rose NR. Viruses as adjuvants for autoimmunity: evidence from Coxsackie virus-induced myocarditis. *Rev Med Virol* 2005;**15**:17–27.
6. Lieberman EB, Hutchins GM, Herskowitz A, Rose NR, Baughman KL. Clinicopathologic description of myocarditis. *J Am Coll Cardiol* 1991;**18**:1617–26.
7. Hare JM, Baughman KL. Fulminant and acute lymphocytic myocarditis: the prognostic value of clinicopathological classification. *Eur Heart J* 2001;**22**:269–70.
8. McCarthy RE III, Boehmer JP, Hruban RH, *et al.* Long-term outcome of fulminant myocarditis as compared with acute (nonfulminant) myocarditis. *N Engl J Med* 2000;**342**:690–5.
9. Magnani JW, Dec GW. Myocarditis: current trends in diagnosis and treatment. *Circulation* 2006;**113**:876–90.
10. Hufnagel G, Pankuweit S, Richter A, Schönian U, Maisch B. The European Study of Epidemiology and Treatment of Cardiac Inflammatory Diseases (ESETCID): first epidemiological results. *Herz* 2000;**25**:279–85.
11. McCully RB, Cooper LT, Schreiter S. Coronary artery spasm in lymphocytic myocarditis: a rare cause of acute myocardial infarction. *Heart* 2005;**91**:202.
12. Smith SC, Ladenson JH, Mason JW, Jaffe AS. Elevations of cardiac troponin I associated with myocarditis: experimental and clinical correlates. *Circulation* 1997;**95**:163–8.
13. Lauer B, Niederau C, Kühl U, *et al.* Cardiac troponin T in patients with clinically suspected myocarditis. *J Am Coll Cardiol* 1997;**30**:1354–9.
14. Morgera T, Di Lenarda A, Dreas L, *et al.* Electrocardiography of myocarditis revisited: clinical and prognostic significance of electrocardiographic changes. *Am Heart J* 1992;**124**:455–67.
15. Felker GM, Boehmer JP, Hruban RH, *et al.* Echocardiographic findings in fulminant and acute myocarditis. *J Am Coll Cardiol* 2000;**36**:227–32.
16. Mendes LA, Dec GW, Picard MH, Palacios IF, Newell J, Davidoff R. Right ventricular dysfunction: an independent predictor of adverse outcome in patients with myocarditis. *Am Heart J* 1994;**128**:301–7.
17. Friedrich MG, Strohm O, Schulz-Menger J, Marciniak H, Luft FC, Dietz R. Contrast media-enhanced magnetic resonance imaging visualizes myocardial changes in the course of viral myocarditis. *Circulation* 1998;**97**:1802–9.
18. Cooper LT, Baughman KL, Feldman AM, *et al.* The role of endomyocardial biopsy in the management of cardiovascular disease: a scientific statement from the American Heart Association, the American College of Cardiology, and the European Society of Cardiology. *Circulation* 2007;**116**:2216–33.

19. Aretz HT, Billingham ME, Edwards WD, *et al.* Myocarditis: a histopathologic definition and classification. *Am J Cardiovasc Pathol* 1987;**1**:3–14.
20. Topkara VK, Dang NC, Barili F, *et al.* Ventricular assist device use for the treatment of acute viral myocarditis. *J Thorac Cardiovasc Surg* 2006;**131**:1190–1.
21. Moloney ED, Egan JJ, Kelly P, Wood AE, Cooper LT Jr. Transplantation for myocarditis: a controversy revisited. *J Heart Lung Transplant* 2005;**24**:1103–10.
22. Zipes D, Camm A, Borggrefe M, *et al.* ACC/AHA/ESC 2006 guideline for management of patients with ventricular arrhythmias and the prevention of sudden cardiac death: a report of the American College of Cardiology/American Heart Association Task Force and the European Society of Cardiology Committee for Practice Guidelines. *Circulation* 2006;**114**:e385–e484.
23. Wojnicz R, Nowalany-Kozielska E, Wojciechowska C, *et al.* Randomized, placebo-controlled study for immunosuppressive treatment of inflammatory dilated cardiomyopathy: two-year follow-up results. *Circulation* 2001;**104**:39–45.
24. Parrillo JE, Cunnion RE, Epstein SE, *et al.* A prospective, randomized, controlled trial of prednisone for dilated cardiomyopathy. *N Engl J Med* 1989;**321**:1061–8.
25. Cooper LT Jr, Berry GJ, Shabetai R. Idiopathic giant-cell myocarditis—natural history and treatment. *N Engl J Med* 1997;**336**:1860–6.
26. d'Arminio Monforte A, Sabin CA, Phillips A, *et al.* The changing incidence of AIDS events in patients receiving highly active antiretroviral therapy. *Arch Intern Med* 2005;**165**:416–23.
27. Pugliese A, Isnardi D, Saini A, *et al.* Impact of highly active antiretroviral therapy in HIV-positive patients with cardiac involvement. *J Infect* 2000;40:282 -4.
28. Chen F, Shannon K, Ding S, *et al.* HIV type 1 glycoprotein 120 inhibits cardiac myocyte contraction. *AIDS Res Hum Retroviruses* 2002;**18**: 777–84.
29. Sudano I, Spieker LE, Noll G, Corti R, Weber R, Luscher TF. Cardiovascular disease in HIV infection. *Am Heart J* 2006;**151**:1147–55.
30. Barbaro G, Di Lorenzo G, Grisorio B, Barbarini G. Incidence of dilated cardiomyopathy and detection of HIV in myocardial cells of HIV-positive patients. Gruppo Italiano per lo Studio Cardiologico dei Pazienti Affetti da AIDS. *N Engl J Med* 1998;**339**:1093–9.
31. Drazen JM, Curfman GD. Retraction: Barbaro, *et al.* Incidence of dilated cardiomyopathy and detection of HIV in myocardial cells of HIV-positive patients. *N Engl J Med* 1998;**339**:1093–9. *N Engl J Med* 2002;**347**:140.
32. Friis-Moller N, Weber R, Reiss P, *et al.* Cardiovascular disease risk factors in HIV patients—association with antiretroviral therapy. Results from the DAD study. *AIDS* 2003;**17**:1179–93.
33. Hulgan T, Sterling TR, Daugherty J, *et al.* Prescribing of contraindicated protease inhibitor and statin combinations among HIV infected persons. *J Acquir Immune Defic Syndr* 2005;**38**:277–82.
34. Sekigawa I, Koshino K, Hishikawa T, *et al.* Inhibitory effect of the immunosuppressant FK506 on apoptotic cell death induced by HIV-1 gp120. *J Clin Immunol* 1995;**15**:312 –7.
35. Rassi A Jr, Rassi A, Little WC, *et al.* Development and validation of a risk score for predicting death in Chagas' heart disease. *N Engl J Med* 2006;**355**:799–808.
36. McAlister HF, Klementowicz PT, Andrews C, Fisher JD, Feld M, Furman S. Lyme carditis: an important cause of reversible heart block. *Ann Intern Med* 1989;**110**:339–45.
37. Seward JB, Casaclang-Verzosa G. Infiltrative cardiovascular diseases: cardiomyopathies that look alike. *J Am Coll Cardiol* 2010;**55**:1769–79.
38. Yazaki Y, Isobe M, Hiramitsu S, *et al.* Comparison of clinical features and prognosis of cardiac sarcoidosis and idiopathic dilated cardiomyopathy. *Am J Cardiol* 1998;**82**:537–40.
39. Doughan AR, Williams BR. Cardiac sarcoidosis. *Heart* 2006;**92**:282–8.
40. Smedema JP, Snoep G, van Kroonenburgh MP, *et al.* Evaluation of the accuracy of gadolinium-enhanced cardiovascular magnetic resonance in the diagnosis of cardiac sarcoidosis. *J Am Coll Cardiol* 2005;**45**:1683–90.
41. Hoffbrand AV. Diagnosing myocardial iron overload. *Eur Heart J* 2001;**22**:2140–1.
42. Masci PG, Dymarkowski S, Bogaert J. The role of cardiovascular magnetic resonance in the diagnosis and management of cardiomyopathies. *J Cardiovasc Med* 2008;**9**:435–49.
43. Alexander J, Kowdley KV. Hereditary hemochromatosis: genetics, pathogenesis, and clinical management. *Ann Hepatol* 2005;**4**:240–7.
44. Hoffman GS, Kerr GS, Leavitt RY, *et al.* Wegener granulomatosis: an analysis of 158 patients. *Ann Intern Med* 1992;**116**:488–98.
45. Oliveira GH, Seward JB, Tsang TS, Specks U. Echocardiographic findings in patients with Wegener granulomatosis. *Mayo Clin Proc* 2005;**80**:1435–40.
46. Edwards NC, Ferro CJ, Townend JN, Steeds RP. Myocardial disease in systemic vasculitis and autoimmune disease detected by cardiovascular magnetic resonance. *Rheumatology* 2007;**46**:1208–9.
47. Seo P, Min YI, Holbrook JT, *et al.* Damage caused by Wegener's granulomatosis and its treatment: prospective data from the Wegener's Granulomatosis Etanercept Trial (WGET). Arthritis Rheum 2005; 52:2168–78.
48. Cathcart ES, Shirahama T, Cohen AS. Isolation and identification of a plasma component of amyloid. *Biochim Biophys Acta* 1967;**147**:392–393.
49. Tennent GA, Lovat LB, Pepys MB. Serum amyloid P component prevents proteolysis of the amyloid fibrils of Alzheimer disease and systemic amyloidosis. *PNAS* 1995;**92**:4299–4303.
50. Al Suwaidi J, Velianou JL, Gertz MA *et al.* Systemic amyloidosis presenting with angina pectoris. *Ann Intern Med* 1999;**131**:838–41.
51. Liao R, Jain M, Teller P, *et al.* Infusion of light chains from patients with cardiac amyloidosis causes diastolic dysfunction in isolated mouse hearts. *Circulation* 2001;**104**:1594–7.
52. Brenner DA, Jain M, Pimentel DR, *et al.* Human amyloidogenic light chains directly impair cardiomyocyte function through an increase in cellular oxidant stress. *Circ Res* 2004;**94**:1008–10.
53. Reisinger J, Dubrey SW, Lavalley M, Skinner M, Falk RH. Electrophysiologic abnormalities in AL (primary) amyloidosis with cardiac involvement. *J Am Coll Cardiol* 1997;**30**:1046–51.
54. Dubrey SW, Cha K, Skinner M, LaValley M, Falk RH. Familial and primary (AL) cardiac amyloidosis: echocardiographically similar diseases with distinctly different clinical outcomes. *Heart* 1997;**78**:74–82.
55. Dubrey S, Pollak A, Skinner M, Falk RH. Atrial thrombi occurring during sinus rhythm in cardiac amyloidosis: evidence for atrial electromechanical dissociation. *Br Heart J* 1995;**74**:541–544.
56. Hawkins PN, Pepys MB. Imaging amyloidosis with radiolabelled SAP. *Eur J Nucl Med* 1995;**22**:595–9.
57. Hazenberg BP, van Rijswijk MH, Piers DA, *et al.* Diagnostic performance of 123I-labeled serum amyloid P component scintigraphy in patients with amyloidosis. *Am J Med* 2006;**119**: 355.e15–355.e24.
58. Maceira AM, Joshi J, Prasad SK, *et al.* Cardiovascular magnetic resonance in cardiac amyloidosis. *Circulation* 2005;**111**:195–202.
59. Arbustini E, Verga L, Concardi M, Palladini G, Obici L, Merlini G. Electron and immuno-electron microscopy of abdominal fat identifies and characterizes amyloid fibrils in suspected cardiac amyloidosis. *Amyloid* 2002;**9**:108–14.
60. Kyle RA, Gertz MA, Greipp PR, *et al.* A trial of three regimens for primary amyloidosis: colchicine alone, melphalan and prednisone, and melphalan, prednisone, and colchicine. *N Engl J Med* 1997;**336**:1202–1207.

61. Kyle RA, Gertz MA: Primary systemic amyloidosis: clinical and laboratory features in 474 cases. *Semin Hematol* 1995;**32**:45–59.
62. Kristen AV, Dengler TJ, Hegenbart U, *et al.* Prophylactic implantation of cardioverter-defibrillator in patients with severe cardiac amyloidosis and high risk for sudden cardiac death. *Heart Rhythm* 2008;**5**:235–240.
63. Dember LM, Sanchorawala V, Seldin DC, *et al.* Effect of dose-intensive intravenous melphalan and autologous blood stem-cell transplantation on AL amyloidosis-associated renal disease. *Ann Intern Med* 2001;**134**:746–53.
64. Pepys MB, Herbert J, Hutchinson WL, *et al.* Targeted pharmacological depletion of serum amyloid P component for treatment of human amyloidosis. *Nature* 2002;**417**:254–9.
65. Grogan M, Gertz MA, Kyle RA, Tajik AJ. Five or more years of survival in patients with primary systemic amyloidosis and biopsy-proven cardiac involvement. *Am J Cardiol* 2000;**85**:664–5.
66. Sekijima Y, Dendle MA, Kelly JW: Orally administered diflunisal stabilizes transthyretin against dissociation required for amyloidogenesis. *Amyloid* 2006;**13**:236–49.

9

Iatrogenic heart failure

Martin Denvir

Introduction

Heart failure (HF) can result from adverse or unwanted effects of treatment for unrelated conditions. Iatrogenic literally means an illness or condition generated by the physician (from the Greek *iatros*, a physician, and *genic* meaning 'induced by'). In the acute setting, the physician can induce HF—in a patient without any clinically overt cardiac disease—by the inadvertent use of high volumes of fluid, or drugs known to depress cardiac function; or during cardiac surgery when the left ventricle experiences injury (either directly or indirectly) while on cardiopulmonary bypass. Chronic HF, on the other hand, is more common in patients treated for lymphoma, breast cancer, or more rarely lung cancer. In this clinical setting, the patient may present many months or years after the initial injury to the heart resulting from chemotherapeutic agents and/or radiotherapy. This chapter outlines the main causes of HF induced by the physician in the acute setting, and focuses on the epidemiology, presentation, and treatment of chronic HF syndromes resulting from treatment of childhood and adult cancers.

Iatrogenic heart failure in the acute setting

Occurrences of acute HF resulting from treatment or management are generally quite common scenarios in the hospital setting, and yet these are poorly described and documented in the published literature. A typical clinical example is the overzealous use of fluid in the perioperative period in elderly patients undergoing surgery for acute events such as traumatic hip fracture or abdominal sepsis. In these settings, it is common for the medical team caring for the patient to attempt to maintain tissue perfusion by infusing large quantities of crystalloid or colloid, particularly if the patent is shocked or hypotensive. Even in a patient with no previous clinical history of cardiac disease, this can result in volume overload and a clinical picture of acute HF with breathlessness, elevated venous pressure, pulmonary rales, and chest radiograph evidence of pulmonary oedema. Such adverse outcomes may now become increasingly rare as anaesthetists adopt strategies for careful preoperative planning of fluid management,[1] and implement the routine use of echocardiography for monitoring left ventricular performance during noncardiac surgery.[2]

Acute HF may also result from the use of drugs that are recognized to depress cardiac contractility. Thankfully, many drugs that are known to produce profound cardiac contractile depression are now rarely used. However, myocardial depression sufficient to result in clinical HF may result from the use of some evidence-based drugs at accepted clinical doses where the patient appears sensitive to the drug or where there is concomitant liver or renal impairment resulting in accumulation and subsequent toxicity. Such drugs include calcium antagonists, β-blockers, anaesthetic agents, and antiarrhythmic drugs (Table 9.1). HF may also result when using these drugs where the patient is systemically compromised for other reasons such as in severe sepsis. Careful consideration and clinical assessment is required when using these drugs in the intensive care unit. Acute severe left ventricular systolic dysfunction (LVSD) may also result from long-term use of intravenous inotropic agents such as noradrenaline or adrenaline in this setting, although these drugs are reserved for patients in a precarious haemodynamic situation. The mechanisms for this are thought to relate to progressive down-regulation of β-adrenoreceptor responsiveness due to chronic overstimulation of cardiomyocytes,[4] or direct cardiomyocyte cell death due to necrosis and apoptosis resulting from high-dose catecholamine exposure.[5,6]

Heart failure resulting from cancer therapy

Survival following treatment of many solid and haemopoetic tumours has improved dramatically over the last 20 years, mainly due to better pharmacological agents given in well-tested regimens. However, the trade-off for better survival has been the long-term consequences of therapies containing highly toxic systemic agents, frequently combined with radiotherapy. The toxic effects of chemotherapeutic agents on the heart are well described in the basic and clinical scientific literature,[7,8] although there are differences in the

Table 9.1 Iatrogenic causes of heart failure

Surgical	Drugs
Fluid overload	Calcium antagonists: Nifedipine Verapamil Amlodipine
Acute or chronic prosthetic heart valve regurgitation	β-blockers
Iatrogenic AV fistula formation	Antiarrhythmic drugs: Quinidine Procanamide Lignocaine
	Anaesthetic induction agents: Etomidate Propofol Fentanyl
	Centrally acting sympatholytic drugs: Clonidine α-methyl DOPA
	Adrenaline Noradrenaline
	Chemotherapeutic and immunosuppressant agents: Cytarabine arabinoside Gemcitabine Interleukin Methotrexate Mitomycin Muromonab-CD3 Pentostatin Tretinoin

Adapted from Zausig YA, Busse H, Lunz D, Sinner B, Zink W, Graf BM. Cardiac effects of induction agents in the septic rat heart. *Crit Care* 2009;**13**(5):R144.

epidemiology of long-term cardiotoxicity in the treatment of adult and childhood cancers. Table 9.2 summarizes some of the long-term sequelae of cancer therapy in which HF features strongly.

Anthracyclines and the heart

Clinical pharmacology of anthracyclines

Anthracyclines were initially isolated from the bacteria *Streptomyces peucetius,* and the compound first used in humans for the treatment of cancer was daunorubicin. Subsequently, the 14-hydroxy version was developed and named doxorubicin (also known as adriamycin or hydroxydaunorubicin; Fig. 9.1). It is used for the treatment of a number of solid tumours including gastric, breast and ovarian cancer, non-Hodgkin's and Hodgkin's lymphoma, thyroid carcinoma, neuroblastoma, small cell carcinoma of the lung, and Wilms' tumour. It is also extremely effective in the treatment of acute lymphoblastic leukaemia in children.

Doxorubicin is administered intravenously as a series of slow, single-dose, single-agent boluses no more than 60–75 mg/m^2 every 3–4 weeks, or 30 mg/m^2 every 2 weeks, up to a total cumulative dose not exceeding 550 mg/m^2. Early studies suggested that the incidence of congestive HF with doxorubicin was approximately 5% at this dose and that this represented the balance point for oncological efficacy versus cardiotoxicity. A reduction of the cumulative total dose is recommended in patients at higher risk of

Table 9.2 Relative risk of developing secondary health conditions among cancer survivors, as compared to siblings

Condition	Survivors (N = 10 397) (%)	Siblings (N = 3034) (%)	Relative risk (95% CI)
Major joint replacement	1.61	0.03	54.0 (7.6–386.3)
Congestive heart failure	1.24	0.10	15.1 (4.8–47.9)
Second malignant neoplasm	2.38	0.33	14.8 (7.2–30.4)
Cognitive dysfunction, severe	0.65	0.10	10.5 (2.6–43.0)
Coronary artery disease	1.11	0.20	10.4 (4.1–25.9)
Cerebrovascular accident	1.56	0.20	9.3 (4.1–21.2)
Renal failure or dialysis	0.52	0.07	8.9 (2.2–36.6)
Hearing loss not corrected by aid	1.96	0.36	6.3 (3.3–11.8)
Legally blind or loss of an eye	2.92	0.69	5.8 (3.5–9.5)
Ovarian failure	2.79	0.99	3.5 (2.7–5.2)

Adapted from Oeffinger KC, Mertens AC, Sklar CA, *et al.* Childhood Cancer Survivor Study. Chronic health conditions in survivors of childhood cancer. *N Engl J Med* 2006;**355**(15):1572–82, with permission.

cardiotoxicity. Risk factors for the development of cardiotoxicity are summarized in Box 9.1.

Cellular mechanism of anthracycline cardiotoxicity

Cardiomyocyte mitochondrial injury is a key feature of the cardiotoxicity induced by anthracyclines. Numerous studies in animal models and cell culture have suggested that free-radical formation by cardiomyocyte mitochondria causes widespread cellular damage due to the production of reactive oxygen species, including superoxide.[10–13] The mitochondria subsequently undergo structural changes including vacuolation, swelling, and fragmentation of cristae.[13] A number of other ultrastructural changes typically occur in the myocyte including loss of myofibrils, deformation of the nucleus, and dilatation of the sarcoplasmic reticulum.[14] Apoptosis also plays a role in myocyte cell loss and appears to be stimulated by free-radical production.[15,16]

Cardiotoxicity of anthracyclines in childhood

Cardiotoxic drugs used in childhood cancers are broadly similar to those used in adults. Anthracyclines, with a cumulative dose used of up to 550 mg/m^2, have played a significant therapeutic role in

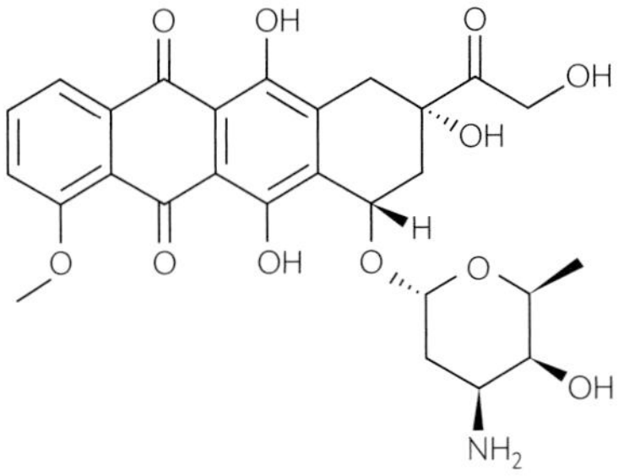

Fig. 9.1 Chemical structure of doxorubicin.

Box 9.1 Risk factors for the development of anthracycline cardiotoxicity

Demographic factors

- Age (elderly people and children more susceptible)
- Female gender

Clinical factors

- Ischaemic heart disease (angina, previous myocardial infarction)
- Hypertension
- Clinically significant valvular heart disease
- Congenital heart disease
- Cardiomyopathy and/or CHF

Therapeutic factors

- Cumulative dose >400 mg/m^2
- Previous treatment with anthracyclines
- Radiotherapy to the heart or mediastinum[9]
- Coadministration of other chemotherapeutic agents (including cyclophosphamide, trastuzumab, mitomycin C)

improving the 5-year survival in acute lymphoblastic leukaemia from less than 10% to over 80% in the last 30 years.[17] A number of long-term follow-up studies of children treated for haematological malignancies demonstrate a range of systolic, diastolic, and wall thickness abnormalities, as assessed by echocardiography or radionuclide ventriculography, in at least half of all subjects treated with anthracyclines during childhood.[18] However, these are almost exclusively retrospective cross-sectional studies and so there is considerable variation in reported subclinical cardiac toxicity. The incidence of clinically apparent CHF varies from as low as 0% to 16% in 30 studies published between 1966 and 2000.[19] In a single site study, clinical CHF was reported in 8% of children at 1 year[20] and in another 2.8% at 6 years.[21] This group estimated the risk in their cohort of 5% after 15 years for children treated with a cumulative dose of doxorubicin greater than 300 mg/m^2 between 1976 and 1997. A more recent study of 116 children treated for acute lymphoblastic leukaemia with doses of doxorubicin less than 300 mg/m^2 provided follow-up for a mean of 8.2 years. This study suggested that even at these apparently 'safe' cumulative doses the incidence of significantly reduced left ventricular wall thickness and increased left ventricular end-diastolic diameter was increased compared with age-matched controls.[22]

The variation in incidence of clinical CHF is also partly due to differing durations of follow-up, the heterogeneous populations studied and possibly due to the different ways in which CHF was defined in these studies. However, with an estimated 20 000 children now surviving cancer into adulthood in the United Kingdom, the potential for a substantial burden of cardiac disease, including HF, requiring future clinical care is evident.

Cardiotoxicity of anthracyclines in adults

There are many studies reported in the literature of follow-up of patients after treatment with cardiotoxic drugs, mainly anthracyclines. It would be fair to say that many of these studies are reports of a small number of patients being followed up after treatment in a clinical setting where the authors have carefully documented the clinical details and correlated these with the findings on echocardiography. While these are valuable studies there are a number of questions that arise in terms of their validity. First, the patients included represent survivors and exclude patients dying before any cardiac assessment was reported. Few studies give an indication of the total number from which their published population is derived. Secondly, many of the reported studies fail to state how many survivors were excluded and for what reasons. For example, patients with recurrence of their primary disease or metastases or with other comorbidities may have been excluded. Hence, the rigour in defining the population being assessed and presented within the published article is uncertain. Thirdly, and related to the first and second points above, very few studies have performed prospective longer-term follow-up studies in a large enough cohort to examine true incidence of clinical HF and associated mortality. Throughout the literature it is clear that while cumulatively many patients are followed up, the heterogeneity of the patients and uncertainty of methods used in follow-up make a true prediction of echocardiographic and clinical outcomes difficult. However, in adults treated with doxorubicin the earliest reports suggested that 4% of patients receiving a dose of 500–550 mg/m^2 developed cardiotoxicity, rising to 18% at doses between 551–600mg/m^2.[23]

More recent studies have indicated that the risk of cardiotoxicity may be higher than previously estimated at lower total cumulative doses. After doses of 240 mg/m^2 there is evidence for significant reductions in left ventricular function[24] and at 400 mg/m^2 the incidence of congestive HF may actually be closer to that previously thought to occur at 550 mg/m^2, namely 5%.[25] Overall, low cumulative doses appear to be associated with a lower risk of cardiotoxicity, but once above 450 mg/m^2 then the incidence of CHF starts to rise and probably rises exponentially above 500 mg/m^2. There is some evidence that infusions of doxorubicin rather than bolus injections may result in less cardiotoxicity[26] although some studies have not confirmed this.[27] A more recent systematic review suggested that infusions of 6 h or more duration may be associated with reduced cardiotoxicity in adults.[28] These authors strongly recommend further studies in children to assess the potential to reduce cardiotoxicity using infusion rather than bolus dosing.

Liposomal preparations of doxorubicin may also be associated with a reduced incidence of cardiotoxicity,[29] although long-term follow-up studies comparing free doxorubicin with pegylated versions are awaited. Epirubicin, a derivative of doxorubicin, has also been reported to have a low incidence of cardiotoxicity. After a median of 7 years follow-up (range 1 month to 15 years), Fumoleau *et al.*[30] reported a combined early and late occurrence of LVSD in 1.4% of patents treated with epirubicin compared to 0.2% in patients not treated with epirubicin. Clinical CHF developed in only 0.2% of patients treated with epirubicin. This compares with an expected incidence of CHF, if treated with equivalent doses of doxorubicin, of over 7%.

Diastolic dysfunction resulting from anthracyclines

Various echocardiographic measurements of relaxation change during acute infusion of anthracyclines including increased end-diastolic wall thickness, prolonged isovolumic relaxation time, and decreased E:A ratio.[31] Doppler tissue measurements also change following administration of cardiotoxic chemotherapeutic agents with a rise in E:A ratio and a lengthening of isovolumic relaxation time.[32]

A number of studies have examined long-term changes in diastolic function in survivors of childhood cancers treated with anthracyclines. Diastolic abnormalities, as measured by changes in inflow patterns and isovolumic relaxation times, can be identified in up to 50% of survivors.[19] However, longer-term follow-up studies of children with a variety of malignancies failed to suggest any significant longer-term diastolic abnormalities in survivors followed up for an average of almost 14 years after diagnosis.[33,34] Furthermore, a further study of diastolic abnormalities found both increases and decreases in E:A ratio compared with controls but showed no specific association with the development of clinically overt HF or mortality.[35] Some caution should be used in interpreting cross-sectional retrospective follow-up data of survivors as the impact of early and medium-term diastolic abnormalities on longer-term symptoms and development of clinical HF is unknown. The prevalence of diastolic abnormalities in nonsurvivors is also unknown.

Strategies to avoid anthracycline cardiotoxicity

Clinical strategies to avoid cardiotoxicity associated with anthracyclines include using the minimum efficacious dose for oncological response, and delivering the drug as an infusion rather than as a bolus thus reducing the peak dose of the drug. Currently doxorubicin is commonly given in doses of approximately 60–70 mg/m^2 repeated every 3 weeks on 4–6 occasions. This approach to administration is now widely used although there is some evidence that it makes little difference to the risk of developing cardiac dysfunction and HF compared to doses exceeding 45 mg/m^2 per week.[27]

The use of the antioxidant drug dexrazoxane indicated reductions in troponin release up to 180 days after treatment with doxorubicin in children with acute lymphoblastic leukaemia.[36] Disappointingly, this reduction in myocardial injury in the short term did not result in any difference in clinical endpoints over a 3-year follow-up period. Longer-term follow-up of these patients to assess development of chronic left ventricular dysfunction and clinical HF is not yet reported.

Careful clinical assessment before and during treatment are also important aspects to help reduce the risk of anthracycline cardiotoxicity. Interestingly, none of the clinical guidelines for treatment of breast cancer recommend simple baseline cardiac investigations before starting chemotherapy unless the patient is thought to be at high risk. The minimum investigation recommended by most cardiologists would be an ECG, but additionally an echocardiogram or multiple gated acquisition (MUGA) scan to assess left ventricular function should also be done. Baseline assessment provides a comparison with any future investigations in the event that complications arise during or after treatment. Table 9.3 shows a suggested algorithm for guiding management of patients with breast cancer. Although there is no guaranteed way of avoiding cardiotoxicity, the clinician should explain to the patient that some degree of judgement is required in assessing the risk–benefit ratio for efficacy of cancer treatment balanced against cardiotoxicity. Such discussions are clearly more important where the patient has a pretreatment risk of cardiotoxicity which is deemed to be medium or high or where the selected cumulative dose of anthracycline is high.

ECG

The ECG has largely been overlooked as a potential screening tool for either baseline cardiac disease prior to starting chemotherapy or as a method of monitoring for cardiotoxicity. However, given its powerful negative predictive value in the diagnosis of HF in breathless patients presenting with suspected HF, there is certainly scope for further research.[37] One study of children with cancer suggested that the QT interval may help in the assessment of cardiotoxicity in conjunction with echo-derived shortening fraction in identifying reduced ejection fraction following chemotherapy.[38] A more recent study suggested that an abnormal ECG was a powerful predictor of cardiotoxicity in patients treated for a variety of cancers and after adjustment for confounders was as predictive as the biomarkers B-type natriuretic peptide (BNP) and troponin.[39] Further large-scale prospective trials are needed.

Echocardiography

Echocardiography has been widely used to monitor cardiac function before during and after chemotherapy in both adults and children. The advantages are that it is cheap, does not involve ionizing radiation, and provides additional information regarding cardiac

Table 9.3 Clinical algorithm for guiding management and monitoring of cardiac risk associated with use of anthracyclines

Clinical risk level[a]	Example	Total cumulative dose of doxorubicin		
		<300 mg/m^2	**300–450 mg/m^2**	**>450 mg/m^2**
Low	No cardiovascular history, middle aged, no previous anthracycline exposure	ECG and echo/MUGA at baseline	ECG and echo/MUGA at baseline + 3 months after completion of chemotherapy	ECG and Echo/MUGA at baseline and after every cycle of chemotherapy + 3 months after completion + yearly thereafter
Medium	Stable hypertension or ischaemic heart disease managed with medication	ECG and echo/MUGA at baseline + every 1–2 cycles of chemotherapy + 3 months after completion of chemotherapy	ECG and echo/MUGA at baseline and after every cycle of chemotherapy + 3 months after completion + yearly thereafter	Avoid anthracyclines
High	Previous anthracycline therapy, hypertension, elderly	ECG and echo/MUGA at baseline and after every cycle of chemotherapy + 3 months after completion + yearly thereafter	Avoid anthracyclines	Avoid anthracyclines

[a] For assessment of clinical risk see Box 9.1.

structure and function over and above ejection fraction. Increasingly, with modern technology the quality of imaging has improved substantially and limitations related to body shape and size are less problematic.

Radionuclide ventriculography

This technique, commonly referred to as a MUGA scan, is widely used to measure ejection fraction in patients being treated for cancer. Technetium-99 is commonly used as the radioactive tracer, and the radioactivity over the heart is collected throughout a number of cardiac cycles. The ejection fraction is estimated from the difference between the radioactive counts in end-diastole and end-systole. Although the technique has limitations it is acknowledged to be a reasonably accurate and highly reproducible way to assess the systolic function. However, contemporary data suggest that with modern equipment there is no significant difference between methods of assessing ejection fraction.[40] Therefore, variations in the use of different imaging modalities probably reflects differences in clinical opinions, availability of techniques, and expertise from one region or one country to another.

Biomarkers (BNP and troponins)

Plasma biomarkers are a potentially valuable method of identifying cardiotoxicity in patients undergoing chemotherapy. In particular, the use of BNP to diagnose and monitor LVSD in patients with non-chemotherapy-related HF has is now widely accepted.[41] In patients with chemotherapy-related cardiotoxicity there have been numerous studies but to date these have been small, and few have provided long-term outcomes.

In children, one study identified elevated NT-proBNP, but not troponin, in 13% of survivors followed up for an average of 14 years after treatment for various childhood cancers using anthracyclines.[33] However, another study found no elevation in natriuretic peptide levels despite the presence of detectable echocardiographic abnormalities of systolic and diastolic function.[42] Our current understanding of the value of biomarkers in assessing cardiotoxicity in childhood cancers is poor.[43] This is mainly because the studies published to date have been predominantly observational cohort studies (with the exception of one study using troponin T),[36] with small numbers, no clear inclusion criteria, considerable variation in types of cancers, inconsistencies in the control groups used, and no long-term follow-up data. Further studies addressing these inconsistencies are clearly needed.

In the adult, there are also few studies with sufficient power to address the value of biomarkers in identifying and monitoring for cardiotoxicity. One study, involving 54 breast cancer patients, suggested that 2.5–6.5 years after treatment with higher doses of doxorubicin, patients had increased levels of plasma natriuretic peptides compared with those receiving lower doses.[44] However, only 2 patients developed clinical HF during follow-up in this study. In a more recent study, 5 patients (from 70 treated for breast cancer) developed clinical CHF during follow-up and BNP remained elevated in these patients while in other patients that developed a rise and then a fall in BNP levels there was no clinically overt CHF after a mean follow-up of 880 days.[45] In terms of long-term monitoring of cardiac function there is still little evidence that BNP/NT-proBNP can replace measurement of ejection fraction, as a recent study suggested that there was no correlation between fall in ejection fraction during treatment for breast cancer and associated changes in plasma BNP.[46]

Plasma troponin has been assessed prospectively as a potential marker of acute cardiac injury during chemotherapy and radiotherapy. In a series of over 700 patients with a variety of cancer types, Cardinale, *et al*,[47] identified a sub-population with no elevation of troponin during and after chemotherapy who were very unlikely to develop cardiac events, principally an asymptomatic reduction in ejection fraction of 25%, or more, during a mean of 20 months follow-up. Despite these important findings, there remains uncertainty regarding the optimal timing of troponin sampling and the longer term prediction of cardiac outcomes. In addition, further prospective studies are required to assess modern high sensitivity troponin assays in oncology patients. Troponin may, however, be emerging as a potentially more useful test than natriuretic peptides for identifying early cardiac injury associated with chemotherapy.

Trastuzumab

Trastuzumab (Herceptin) is a monoclonal antibody that blocks the human epithelial growth factor receptor 2 (HER2). The receptor protein is overexpressed or the gene is amplified in the tumour tissue of 15–25% of women with breast cancer and tends to be associated with more aggressive disease. When used in combination with other chemotherapy regimes, trastuzumab reduces the risk of relapse by approximately 50% and reduces the risk of death by 30% when given in conjunction with cytotoxic chemotherapy.[48,49] Therefore, trastuzumab is currently recommended as a treatment option for early-stage HER2-positive breast cancer following surgery, when combined with a sequential regimen of chemotherapy (neoadjuvant or adjuvant) and radiotherapy (if applicable). Patients should have a baseline assessment of left ventricular ejection fraction (LVEF) and only those above 55% should receive the drug.[50] This has caused considerable concern among the oncology and cardiology communities since 55% is well above the normal cut-off range for many cardiology departments. The consequences of applying this rigorously is that many women who are suitable for treatment would not receive it because their ejection fraction is normal but measures below 55%. The sensible clinical approach to this issue is for cardiologists and oncologists in centres treating breast cancer to agree the normal range for their locally agreed method of assessing LVEF. These agreed cut-off values rather than a fixed lower limit of 55% should guide both initiation and monitoring of cardiac function associated with trastuzumab therapy.[51]

The concerns regarding cardiac status stem from an unexpectedly high incidence of HF in early trials in using trastuzumab. Symptoms of HF were particularly common when trastuzumab was administered concurrently with chemotherapy. In the pivotal trial, paclitaxel monotherapy was associated with a 1% incidence of CHF, concurrent use of trastuzumab with paclitaxel was associated with a 13% incidence of CHF, and patients receiving the combination of anthracycline and trastuzumab concurrently had a 27% incidence of HF including 16% with NYHA class III or IV symptoms.[52]

A later series of trials published as a single study of open-label trastuzumab plus chemotherapy versus chemotherapy alone was designed more cautiously. The adjuvant chemotherapy was administered before starting trastuzumab and patients developing symptoms or signs of cardiotoxicity or a fall in ejection fraction during initial cytotoxic chemotherapy were excluded from receiving trastuzumab.[53] Although, trastuzumab was given in conjunction with paclitaxel, the resulting incidence of NYHA III or

IV HF in the trastuzumab treatment group was 4.1% compared with 0.8% in the control group after 3 years follow-up. A second trial designed to include a drug-free time period between finishing cytotoxic chemotherapy (including doxorubicin and cyclophosphamide) and starting a 1-year regime of trastuzumab infusions every 3 weeks resulted in a much lower incidence of HF of 1.7% compared with less than 0.1% in the control group.[49]

Cellular mechanisms of trastuzumab cardiotoxicity

The HER2 receptor is one of a family of four receptors linked to a signalling pathway that protects the cardiomyocyte from a variety of stresses including anthracycline toxicity, hypertension, ischaemia, and hypertension. Blocking this pathway results in a loss of this protective mechanism. This is supported by work using a mouse model with a cardiac ventricle specific knockout of the HER2 (ERbB2) receptor. These mice initially develop normally, but as adults they develop dilated cardiomyopathy and isolated cardiomyocytes are more susceptible to anthracycline toxicity.[54]

This pathway clearly represents an important potential therapeutic target for cardiac protection and possibly treatment of HF. However, a recent study of pacing induced cardiomyopathy in dogs suggested that while there was activation of the ErbB2 (HER2) receptor and its ligand (neuregulin) during development of HF, other downstream messengers in the pathway, ERK1 and 2, remained inactivated.[55] Further studies assessing changes in the ligands and receptors in this pathway in human HF are needed.

Reducing the risk of trastuzumab cardiotoxicity

In order to reduce the risk of cardiotoxicity, as well as not being recommended in those with a baseline LVEF of less than 55%, trastuzumab is contraindicated in the following patient groups: patients with angina treated with medication, history of myocardial infarction or HF, evidence of transmural myocardial infraction (Q waves) on resting ECG, high-risk uncontrolled arrhythmias, clinically significant valvular disease, and poorly controlled hypertension.[50] One further recommendation is that there is a period of at least 2 weeks between completing cytotoxic chemotherapy and starting trastuzumab.

Monitoring cardiac function during trastuzumab therapy

Monitoring cardiac function during treatment and identifying early subclinical declines in ejection fraction is one way to potentially reduce the incidence of serious adverse cardiac events resulting from trastuzumab therapy (Fig. 9.2). The current recommendation in the United Kingdom is that LVEF is assessed by either echocardiography or radionuclide ventriculography (MUGA) every 3 months during treatment and 3 months after treatment has concluded.[50] If there is no significant reduction in ejection fraction during treatment then no further follow-up is required. However, if ejection fraction falls by 10% or more during the course of treatment, then therapy should be withheld for 4–6 weeks. Following this, a further assessment of cardiac function and review by a cardiologist should occur before restarting the drug. If ejection fraction returns to pretreatment levels then trastuzumab treatment can be restarted with a further assessment of ejection fraction after 1 month. If ejection fraction remains reduced then a discussion with the patient regarding risk–benefit ratio should allow a balanced decision to be reached on whether treatment should be stopped completely. However, this approach has generated a considerable number of referrals to cardiologists of women with no symptoms of HF and where the ejection fraction, despite apparently falling by 10%, remains within the normal range. This high level of concern for potential cardiotoxicity is appropriate and understandable when using a new class of drug but has resulted in some clinicians calling for a more pragmatic approach to monitoring.[51,56]

Long-term outcomes following trastuzumab cardiotoxicity

In the case of trastuzumab the reduction in cardiac function, at least in the early phase, appears to be reversible. It is estimated that over 80% of patients who develop trastuzumab cardiotoxicity show significant symptomatic recovery after treatment is withdrawn.[57] In a series of 38 patients who were referred to a cardiology service after treatment with trastuzumab caused a mean fall in ejection fraction of 18%, 37 demonstrated a significant recovery of ejection fraction from 43% to 56% 1.5 months after withdrawal of treatment. Although 6 patients recovered without any treatment, the majority required temporary HF medication: 25 patients were retreated with trastuzumab and only 3 of these developed recurrent ventricular dysfunction.[59] Therefore, in most patients, treatment withdrawal combined with standard HF medications such as angiotensin converting enzyme (ACE) inhibitors and

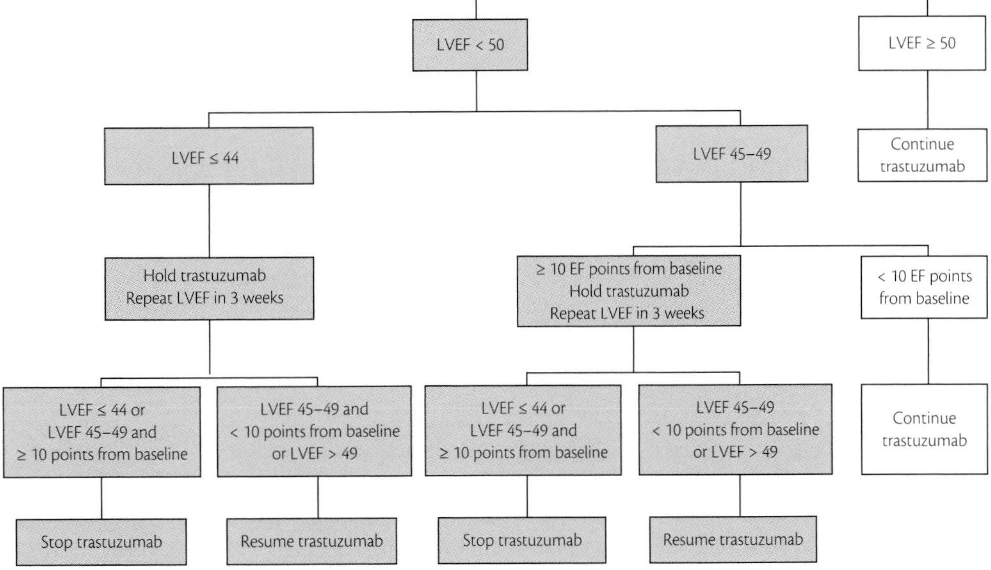

Fig. 9.2 A method for cardiac monitoring of patients during treatment with trastuzumab. Adapted from Suter TM, Procter M, van Veldhuisen DJ, *et al.* Trastuzumab-associated cardiac adverse effects in the herceptin adjuvant trial. *J Clin Oncol* 2007;**25**:3859–65.

β-adrenoreceptor antagonists is effective in restoring normal cardiac function and improving symptoms. Furthermore, at least half of patients that develop a fall in ejection fraction with trastuzumab and then recover can go on to complete the full treatment schedule, with HF medication used as a precautionary measure throughout the period of trastuzumab treatment.

Reversible versus nonreversible cardiotoxicity

Better understanding of the mechanisms and the clinical patterns of cardiac dysfunction that result from cancer-based chemotherapy has clarified our understanding of clinical management. Ewer and Lippman[60] proposed two types of cardiac damage that can result during and in the months and years after cancer treatment. Type 1 damage typically results from doxorubicin chemotherapy and is usually chronic and irreversible. Type 1 is typically cumulative, dose dependent and results in ultrastructural changes within cardiomyocytes involving myofibrils and mitochondria. In contrast, type 2 damage, caused by Trastuzumab, is unrelated to dose, produces no ultrastructural changes and is reversible in the majority of cases. While this paradigm of myocardial injury types in cancer therapy is appealing, recent studies have indicated that trastuzumab cardiotoxicity can result in small elevations of troponin[58] suggesting that there must be some direct cardiomyocyte injury possibly not yet identified by biopsy studies.

Management of chemotherapy-related cardiomyopathy

Diagnosis

The diagnosis of HF in the cancer patient should be made with standard approaches but with careful consideration given to the details of which cancer therapies have been used and when. This may seem obvious, but it is not uncommon to see a patient many years after treatment for cancer where the clinical case record is unavailable for a number of reasons. Previous use of anthracyclines may be likely if the patient remembers being given a bright red coloured injection or infusion. Tattoos on the precordium may indicate previous mantle radiotherapy in the case of lymphoma.

In a cancer patient, the detection of cardiac involvement may occur in a number of ways. Asymptomatic LVSD may be picked up by routine follow-up in the outpatient setting by echocardiography or radionuclide imaging. However, symptoms of breathlessness on exertion together with objective evidence of LVSD on echocardiography are highly suggestive of the diagnosis of cardiomyopathy. Where these features are combined with clinical signs of fluid overload including peripheral oedema, lung crepitations, and raised jugular venous pressure then the diagnosis of clinical HF may be made. Acute severe HF with symptoms of breathlessness and fluid retention may occur rarely either during chemotherapy or shortly afterwards,[61] although it is important to exclude other causes of breathlessness commonly found in cancer patients such as pulmonary embolism and pericardial effusion.

It is also important to consider the possibility of coronary heart disease as a cause for cardiac dysfunction. The absence of any risk factors for coronary heart disease and the absence of an obvious regional wall motion abnormality on cardiac imaging make this diagnosis unlikely, although a number of chemotherapeutic agents can produce coronary spasm or predispose to coronary thrombotic events including 5-fluorouracil and new agents such as capecitabine.[62–64] Modern evaluation with cardiac magnetic resonance imaging (CMR) and CT are also likely to provide important useful information about diagnosis and aetiology.[65]

Treatment of cancer therapy related cardiomyopathy and heart failure

There are no large randomized trials of standard HF therapy in patients with anthracycline or trastuzumab cardiomyopathy. However, there are a few reports of improved cardiac function following treatment using standard HF medications in children.[66,67] There are also recent reports of improvements with device therapy.[68] In the most severe form, anthracycline cardiomyopathy can be treated with cardiac transplantation[69] or left ventricular assist devices.[70]

The largest preventive study reported is a double-blind randomized trial of enalapril in 135 long-term survivors of childhood cancer with an identified baseline abnormality in cardiac systolic function following anthracycline chemotherapy. No patients had evidence of clinical HF at enrolment. Mean age at diagnosis of cancer was 8 years old and all had completed cancer therapy at least 2 years previously. Patients were randomized to placebo or enalapril and followed up for a mean of 2.9 years. There was no difference in the primary outcome measure which was rate of change of maximal cardiac index and left ventricular end-systolic wall stress assessed by echocardiography.[71]

Despite the lack of direct evidence for use of standard HF medications in cancer patients, there are pragmatic reasons and a general consensus among experts that ACE inhibitors and β-blockers should be used in the treatment of anthracycline-induced cardiomyopathy with or without clinically overt HF.[51,72,73]

Conclusions

Iatrogenic HF may appear to be an inevitable consequence of modern approaches to cancer therapy and cardiac surgery. However, careful assessment of patients prior to these interventions and modification of management based on the associated risks is an important way of reducing the incidence of this condition. With increasingly aggressive management of many cancers it is likely that there will be new challenges in dealing with the potential cardiotoxicity of such therapies. There is a need for careful and continuous assessment of patients receiving cancer therapy and for adverse cardiovascular outcomes to be clearly identified within all clinical trials of new treatment modalities.

References

1. Yeager MP, Spence BC. Perioperative fluid management: current consensus and controversies. *Semin Dial* 2006;**19**(6):472–9.
2. Subramaniam D, Talmor D. Echocardiography for management of hypotension in the intensive care unit. *Crit Care Med* 2007;**35**: S401–7.
3. Zausig YA, Busse H, Lunz D, Sinner B, Zink W, Graf BM. Cardiac effects of induction agents in the septic rat heart. *Crit Care* 2009;**13**(5):R144.
4. Reithmann C, Hallström S, Pilz G, Kapsner T, Schlag G, Werdan K. Desensitization of rat cardiomyocyte adenylyl cyclase stimulation by plasma of noradrenaline-treated patients with septic shock. *Circ Shock* 1993;**41**(1):48–59.

5. Fu YC, Chi CS, Yin SC, Hwang B, Chiu YT, Hsu SL. Norepinephrine induces apoptosis in neonatal rat cardiomyocytes through a reactive oxygen species-TNF alpha-caspase signaling pathway. *Cardiovasc Res* 2004 Jun 1;**62**(3):558–67.
6. Goldspink DF, Burniston JG, Ellison GM, Clark WA, Tan LB. Catecholamine-induced apoptosis and necrosis in cardiac and skeletal myocytes of the rat in vivo: the same or separate death pathways? *Exp Physiol* 2004;**89**(4):407–16.
7. Oeffinger KC, Mertens AC, Sklar CA, *et al.* Childhood Cancer Survivor Study. Chronic health conditions in survivors of childhood cancer. *N Engl J Med* 2006;**355**(15):1572–82.
8. Ewer MS, Yeh ETH. *Cancer and the heart.* BC Decker Inc., Hamilton, Ontario, 2006.
9. Myrehaug S, Pintilie M, Tsang R, *et al.* Cardiac morbidity following modern treatment for Hodgkin lymphoma: supra-additive cardiotoxicity of doxorubicin and radiation therapy. *Leuk Lymphoma* 2008;**49**(8):1486–93.
10. Gille L, Nohl H. Analyses of the molecular mechanism of adriamycin-induced cardiotoxicity. *Free Radic Biol Med* 1997;**23**(5):775–82.
11. Yen HC, Oberley TD, Gairola CG, Szweda LI, St Clair DK. Manganese superoxide dismutase protects mitochondrial complex I against adriamycin-induced cardiomyopathy in transgenic mice. *Arch Biochem Biophys* 1999;**362**(1):59–66.
12. Doroshow JH. Effect of anthracycline antibiotics on oxygen radical formation in rat heart. *Cancer Res* 1983;**43**(2):460–72.
13. Yen HC, Oberley TD, Vichitbandha S, Ho YS, St Clair DK. The protective role of manganese superoxide dismutase against adriamycin-induced acute cardiac toxicity in transgenic mice. *J Clin Invest* 1996;**98**(5):1253–60. Erratum in: *J Clin Invest* 1997;**99**(5):1141.
14. Herman EH, Zhang J, Hasinoff BB, Clark JR Jr, Ferrans VJ. Comparison of the structural changes induced by doxorubicin and mitoxantrone in the heart, kidney and intestine and characterization of the Fe(III)-mitoxantrone complex. *J Mol Cell Cardiol* 1997;**29**:2415–2430.
15. Gilleron M, Marechal X, Montaigne D, Franczak J, Neviere R, Lancel S. NADPH oxidases participate to doxorubicin-induced cardiac myocyte apoptosis. *Biochem Biophys Res Commun* 2009;**388**(4):727–31.
16. Kumar D, Kirshenbaum L, Li T, Danelisen I, Singal P. Apoptosis in isolated adult cardiomyocytes exposed to adriamycin. *Ann N Y Acad Sci* 1999;**874**:156–68.
17. Seibel NL. Treatment of acute lymphoblastic leukemia in children and adolescents: peaks and pitfalls. *Hematology Am Soc Hematol Educ Program* 2008:374–80.
18. Lipshultz SE, Colan SD, Gelber RD, *et al.* Late cardiac effects of doxorubicin therapy for acute lymphoblastic leukemia in childhood. *N Engl J Med* 1991;**324**:808–15.
19. Kremer LC, van der Pal HJ, Offringa M, *et al.* Frequency and risk factors of subclinical cardiotoxicity after anthracycline therapy in children: a systematic review. *Ann Oncol* 2002;**13**:819–29.
20. Lipshultz SE, Colan SD, Gelber RD, *et al.* Late cardiac effects of doxorubicin therapy for acute lymphoblastic leukemia in childhood. *N Engl J Med* 1991;**324**(12):808–15.
21. Kremer LC, van Dalen EC, Offringa M, *et al.* Anthracycline-induced clinical heart failure in a cohort of 607 children: long-term follow-up study. *J Clin Oncol* 2001;**19**:191–6.
22. Rathe M, Carlsen NL, Oxh j H, Nielsen G. Long-term cardiac follow-up of children treated with anthracycline doses of 300 mg/m^2 or less for acute lymphoblastic leukemia. *Pediatr Blood Cancer* 2010;**54**(3):444–8.
23. Lefrak EA, Pitha J, Rosenheim S, Gottlieb JA. A clinicopathologic analysis of Adriamycin cardiotoxicity. *Cancer* 1973;**32**:302–14.
24. Perez EA, Suman VJ, Davidson NE, *et al.* Effect of doxorubicin plus cyclophosphamide on left ventricular ejection fraction in patients with breast cancer in the North Central Cancer Treatment Group N9831 Intergroup Adjuvant Trial. *J Clin Oncol* 2004;**22**:3700–4.
25. Swain SM, Whaley FS, Ewer MS. Congestive heart failure in patients treated with doxorubicin: a retrospective analysis of three trials. *Cancer* 2003;**97**(11):2869–79.
26. Hortobagyi GN, Frye D, Buzdar AU, *et al.* Decreased cardiac toxicity of doxorubicin administered by continuous intravenous infusion in combination chemotherapy for metastatic breast carcinoma. *Cancer* 1989;**63**: 37–45.
27. Lipshultz SE, Giantris AL, Lipsitz SR, *et al.* Doxorubicin administration by continuous infusion is not cardioprotective: the Dana-Farber 91–01 Acute Lymphoblastic Leukemia protocol. *J Clin Oncol* 2002;**20**(6):1677–82.
28. van Dalen EC, van der Pal HJ, Caron HN, Kremer LC. Different dosage schedules for reducing cardiotoxicity in cancer patients receiving anthracycline chemotherapy. *Cochrane Database Syst Rev* 2009;(4) CD005008.
29. Safra T, Muggia F, Jeffers S, *et al.* Pegylated liposomal doxorubicin (doxil): reduced clinical cardiotoxicity in patients reaching or exceeding cumulative doses of 500 mg/m^2. *Ann Oncol* 2000;**11**(8):1029–33.
30. Fumoleau P, Roché H, Kerbrat P, *et al.*; French Adjuvant Study Group. Long-term cardiac toxicity after adjuvant epirubicin-based chemotherapy in early breast cancer: French Adjuvant Study Group results. *Ann Oncol* 2006;**17**(1):85–92.
31. Ganame J, Claus P, Eyskens B, *et al.* Acute cardiac functional and morphological changes after anthracycline infusions in children. *Am J Cardiol* 2007;**99**(7):974–7.
32. Pudil R, Horacek JM, Strasova A, Jebavy L, Vojacek J. Monitoring of the very early changes of left ventricular diastolic function in patients with acute leukemia treated with anthracyclines. *Exp Oncol* 2008;**30**(2):160–2.
33. Mavinkurve-Groothuis AM, Groot-Loonen J, Bellersen L, Pourier MS, Feuth T, Bökkerink JP, Hoogerbrugge PM, Kapusta L. Abnormal NT-pro-BNP levels in asymptomatic long-term survivors of childhood cancer treated with anthracyclines. *Pediatr Blood Cancer* 2009;**52**(5):631–6.
34. Santin JC, Deheinzelin D, Junior SP, Lopes LF, de Camargo B. Late echocardiography assessment of systolic and diastolic function of the left ventricle in pediatric cancer survivors after anthracycline therapy. *J Pediatr Hematol Oncol* 2007;**29**(11):761–5).
35. Bu'Lock FA, Mott MG, Oakhill A, Martin RP. Left ventricular diastolic filling patterns associated with progressive anthracycline-induced myocardial damage: A prospective study. *Pediatr Cardiol* 1999;**20**(4):252–63.
36. Lipshultz SE, Rifai N, Dalton VM, *et al.* The effect of dexrazoxane on myocardial injury in doxorubicin-treated children with acute lymphoblastic leukemia. *N Engl J Med* 2004;**351**(2):145–53.
37. Shah S, Davies MK, Cartwright D, Nightingale P. Management of chronic heart failure in the community: role of a hospital based open access heart failure service. *Heart* 2004;**90**(7):755–9.
38. Jakacki RI, Larsen RL, Barber G, Heyman S, Fridman M, Silber JH. Comparison of cardiac function tests after anthracycline therapy in childhood. Implications for screening. *Cancer* 1993;**72**(9):2739–45.
39. Lee HS, Son CB, Shin SH, Kim YS. Clinical correlation between brain natriutetic peptide and anthracyclin-induced cardiac toxicity. *Cancer Res Treat* 2008;**40**(3):121–6.
40. Godkar D, Bachu K, Dave B, Megna R, Niranjan S, Khanna A. Comparison and co-relation of invasive and noninvasive methods of ejection fraction measurement. *J Natl Med Assoc* 2007;**99**(11):1227–8, 1231–4.
41. McDonagh TA, Holmer S, Raymond I, Luchner A, Hildebrant P, Dargie HJ. NT-proBNP and the diagnosis of heart failure: a pooled analysis of three European epidemiological studies. *Eur J Heart Fail* 2004;**6**(3):269–73.
42. Kantar M, Levent E, Cetingul N, *et al.* Plasma natriuretic peptides levels and echocardiographic findings in late subclinical anthracycline toxicity. *Pediatr Hematol Oncol* 2008;**25**(8):723–33.

43. Bryant J, Picot J, Baxter L, Levitt G, Sullivan I, Clegg A. Use of cardiac markers to assess the toxic effects of anthracyclines given to children with cancer: a systematic review. *Eur J Cancer* 2007;**43**(13):1959–66.
44. Perik PJ, De Vries EG, Boomsma F, *et al.* Use of natriuretic peptides for detecting cardiac dysfunction in long-term disease-free breast cancer survivors. *Anticancer Res* 2005;**25**(5):3651–7.
45. Pichon MF, Cvitkovic F, Hacene K, *et al.* Drug-induced cardiotoxicity studied by longitudinal B-type natriuretic peptide assays and radionuclide ventriculography. *In Vivo* 2005;**19**(3):567–76.
46. Daugaard G, Lassen U, Bie P, *et al.* Natriuretic peptides in the monitoring of anthracycline induced reduction in left ventricular ejection fraction. *Eur J Heart Fail* 2005;**7**(1):87–93.
47. Cardinale D, Sandri MT, Colombo A, Colombo N, Boeri M, Lamantia G, Civelli M, Peccatori F, Martinelli G, Fiorentini C, Cipolla CM. Prognostic value of troponin I in cardiac risk stratification of cancer patients undergoing high-dose chemotherapy. *Circulation* 2004 Jun 8; **109**(22):2749–54.
48. Romond EH, Perez EA, Bryant J, *et al.* Trastuzumab plus adjuvant chemotherapy for operable HER2-positive breast cancer. *N Engl J Med* 2005;**353**:1673–84.
49. Piccart-Gebhart MJ, Procter M, Leyland-Jones B, *et al.* Trastuzumab after adjuvant chemotherapy in HER2-positive breast cancer. *N Engl J Med* 2005;**353**:1659–1672.
50. NICE technology appraisal. http://guidance.nice.org.uk/TA107/Guidance/pdf/English
51. Jones AL, Barlow M, Barrett-Lee PJ, *et al.* Management of cardiac health in trastuzumab-treated patients with breast cancer: updated United Kingdom National Cancer Research Institute recommendations for monitoring. *Br J Cancer* 2009;**100**(5):684–92.
52. Slamon DJ, Leyland-Jones B, Shak S, *et al.* Use of chemotherapy plus a monoclonal antibody against HER2 for metastatic breast cancer that overexpresses HER2. *N Engl J Med* 2001;**344**(11):783–92.
53. Romond EH, Perez EA, Bryant J, *et al.* Trastuzumab plus adjuvant chemotherapy for operable HER2-positive breast cancer. *N Engl J Med* 2005;**353**:1673–84.
54. Crone SA, Zhao YY, Fan L, *et al.* ErbB2 is essential in the prevention of dilated cardiomyopathy. *Nat Med* 2002;**8**:459–65.
55. Doggen K, Ray L, Mathieu M, Mc Entee K, Lemmens K, De Keulenaer GW. Ventricular ErbB2/ErbB4 activation and downstream signalling in pacing-induced heart failure. *J Mol Cell Cardiol* 2009;**46**(1):33–8.
56. Suter TM, Procter M, van Veldhuisen DJ, *et al.* Trastuzumab-associated cardiac adverse effects in the herceptin adjuvant trial. *J Clin Oncol* 2007;**25**:3859–65.
57. Suter TM, Cook-Bruns N, Barton C. Cardiotoxicity associated with trastuzumab (Herceptin) therapy in the treatment of metastatic breast cancer. *Breast* 2004;**13**(3):173–83.
58. Cardinale D, Colombo A, Torrisi R, Sandri MT, Civelli M, Salvatici M, Lamantia G, Colombo N, Cortinovis G, Dessanai MA, Nolè F, Veglia F, Cipolla CM. Trastuzumab-induced cardiotoxicity: clinical and prognostic implications of troponin I evaluation. *J Clin Oncol* 2010; **28**(25):3910–6.
59. Ewer MS, Vooletich MT, Durand JB, *et al.* Reversibility of trastuzumab-related cardiotoxicity: new insights based on clinical course and response to medical treatment. *J Clin Oncol* 2005;**23**: 7820–6.
60. Ewer MS, Lippman SM. Type II chemotherapy-related cardiac dysfunction: time to recognize a new entity. *J Clin Oncol* 2005;**23**(13):2900–2.
61. Bristow MR, Thompson PD, Martin RP, Mason JW, Billingham ME, Harrison DC. Early anthracycline cardiotoxicity. *Am J Med* 1978;**65**(5):823–32.
62. To AC, Looi KL, Damianovich D, Taylor GB, Sidebotham D, White HD. A case of cardiogenic shock caused by capecitabine treatment. *Nat Clin Pract Cardiovasc Med* 2008;**5**(11):725–9.
63. Scott PA, Ferchow L, Hobson A, Curzen NP. Coronary spasm induced by capecitabine mimicks ST elevation myocardial infarction. *Emerg Med J* 2008;**25**(10):699–700.
64. Sentürk T, Kanat O, Evrensel T, Aydinlar A. Capecitabine-induced cardiotoxicity mimicking myocardial infarction. *Neth Heart J* 2009;**17**(7–8):277–80.
65. McCrohon JA, Moon JC, Prasad SK, *et al.* Differentiation of heart failure related to dilated cardiomyopathy and coronary artery disease using gadolinium-enhanced cardiovascular magnetic resonance. *Circulation* 2003;**108**(1):54–9.
66. Hauser M, Wilson N. Anthracycline induced cardiomyopathy: successful treatment with angiotensin converting enzyme inhibitors. *Eur J Pediatr* 2000;**159**(5):389.
67. Lipshultz SE, Lipsitz SR, Sallan SE, *et al.* Long-term enalapril therapy for left ventricular dysfunction in doxorubicin-treated survivors of childhood cancer. *J Clin Oncol* 2002;**20**:4517–22.
68. Ahlehoff O, Gall e AM, Hansen PR. Anthracycline-induced cardiomyopathy: Favourable effects of cardiac resynchronization therapy. *Int J Cardiol* 2010;**142**(2):e23–4.
69. Dorent R, Pavie A, Nataf P, *et al.* Heart transplantation is a valid therapeutic option for anthracycline cardiomyopathy. *Transplant Proc* 1995;**27**(2):1683.
70. Freilich M, Stub D, Esmore D, *et al.* Recovery from anthracycline cardiomyopathy after long-term support with a continuous flow left ventricular assist device. *J Heart Lung Transplant* 2009;**28**(1): 101–3.
71. Silber JH, Cnaan A, Clark BJ, *et al.* Enalapril to prevent cardiac function decline in long-term survivors of pediatric cancer exposed to anthracyclines. *J Clin Oncol* 2004;**22**:820–8.
72. Cardinale D, Colombo A, Cipolla CM. Prevention and treatment of cardiomyopathy and heart failure in patients receiving cancer chemotherapy. *Curr Treat Options Cardiovasc Med* 2008;**10**(6): 486–95.
73. Ewer MS, Vooletich MT, Durand JB, *et al.* Reversibility of trastuzumab-related cardiotoxicity: new insights based on clinical course and response to medical treatment. *J Clin Oncol* 2005;**23**(31):7820–6.

PART IV

Pathophysiology of heart failure: cellular and molecular changes

10

Intracellular calcium handling in heart failure

Godfrey L. Smith and Rachel C. Myles

Introduction

Heart failure (HF) is a heterogeneous clinical syndrome which may be characterized by a variety of phenotypic changes, many of which have been linked to abnormalities in the intracellular calcium (Ca^{2+}) signal. These range from mechanical dysfunction, usually characterized by reduced systolic contractile function, to electrophysiological dysfunction including QT interval prolongation, an increased incidence of ventricular premature beats (VPBs) and arrhythmic sudden cardiac death (SCD). In ventricular myocardial cells, intracellular Ca^{2+} ion fluxes govern the translation of the depolarizing signal into mechanical contraction, a process termed excitation–contraction (E-C) coupling. Abnormalities of intracellular Ca^{2+} handling are thought to underlie both mechanical and electrophysiological dysfunction in failing myocardium. This chapter summarizes the events involved in normal E-C coupling and describes the changes observed in HF, with particular focus on the changes reported in remodelled ventricular myocardium. Changes in intracellular Ca^{2+} signalling in other cardiac cell types, such as atrial cardiomyocytes and Purkinje fibre cells, may also be crucial to the final HF phenotype, but less is known about pathological changes in these tissues, and therefore these will only be mentioned briefly.

Cellular anatomy of the ventricular cardiomyocyte

Cellular dimensions

Ventricular myocardium is a functional syncytium of individual cardiomyocytes approximately 0.12 mm long, 0.02 mm wide, and 0.01 mm thick. A diagrammatic representation of a single cardiomyocyte is shown in Fig. 10.1. The individual cellular dimensions do not change significantly across mammalian species (e.g. mice to whales); instead, the number of cells varies, with the human ventricles being made up of around 10^8 cardiomyocytes.

Intercalated discs

The structural integrity and electrical homogeneity of ventricular muscle is maintained by a specialized end-to-end connection between myocytes termed the intercalated disc. In adult hearts this consists of highly interdigitating membrane surfaces containing three types of functional links: the zona adherens, desmosomes, and gap junctions. Gap junctions provide the electrical link between myocytes by forming pore structures that produce a pathway of low electrical resistance, thus providing efficient electrical coupling between cells. In ventricular myocytes these pore structures are formed by two connexin units of the connexin 43 type. The intercalated disc protein complex known as the zona adherens provides strong mechanical linkage between cells. It consists of two proteins, cadherin and catenin, which link the internal cytoskeleton of adjacent cells.

The near simultaneous activation of the large numbers of cardiomyocytes during each heartbeat occurs because the electrical signal that triggers contraction propagates from cell to cell via gap junctions at a relatively high velocity (~50 cm/s). The strong mechanical linkage between cells provided by the zona adherens and desmosomes ensures that the contraction of individual cardiomyocytes is summed to produce coordinated mechanical systole.

Transverse-axial tubular system

Ventricular myocytes have a sarcotubular system running transversely across the diameter of the cell, which is continuous with the surface membrane (sarcolemma). These invaginations of the surface membrane normally occur approximately every 2 μm (0.002 mm). Both electron and light microscopy have revealed that this transverse tubular system contains a considerable number of tubules running in the axial direction within the cell (see Fig. 10.1), leading to the use of the more accurate description 'transverse-axial tubular' (TAT) system.[1, 2] As in skeletal muscle, the major function of the TAT system in cardiac muscle is the rapid propagation of electrical excitation to the cell interior.[3] Recent studies have

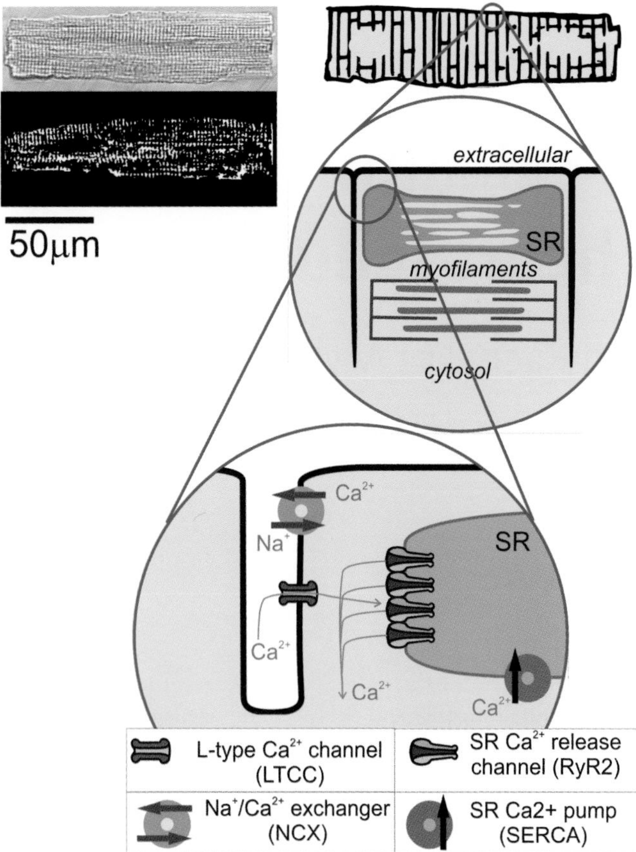

Fig. 10.1 Cellular anatomy of a ventricular cardiomyocyte. The left panel shows a widefield microscopy image of an isolated ventricular cardiomyocyte, with a corresponding confocal image of the cell in which the extracellular membranes have been tagged with a fluorescent dye, in order to show the extent of the transverse-axial tubular (TAT) system. The right panel shows a diagrammatic representation of an isolated ventricular cardiomyocyte with the TAT system indicated. The expanded segments show (i) the close relationship of the sarcoplasmic reticulum to the surface membrane and TAT system, and (ii) the dyadic cleft with the major constituent pumps and channels involved in cardiac E-C coupling.

provided functional evidence that a number of proteins directly involved in E-C coupling are located in the TAT system.[4, 5] The expression of L-type Ca^{2+} (LTCC) channels within the TAT system ensures that these extracellular Ca^{2+} channels in the surface membrane are brought into close proximity (10–20 nm) to the intracellular Ca^{2+} channels associated with the intracellular Ca^{2+} store, the sarcoplasmic reticulum (SR). The Na^{2+}/Ca^{2+} exchanger (NCX) is also located predominately in the TAT system.[5] This protein is the main route of Ca^{2+} efflux from the cell, therefore its TAT system location ensures efficient Ca^{2+} efflux to the extracellular space across the diameter of the myocyte. There is also functional and immunohistochemical evidence that the inward rectifying K^+ channel (I_{K1}) is expressed in the TAT system.[6] This channel plays an essential role in stabilizing the resting membrane potential and shaping the cardiac action potential and thus contributes to overall cardiac excitability.[7]

Normal cardiac excitation–contraction coupling

Mechanism of systolic Ca^{2+} increase

Contraction of individual ventricular myocytes is initiated by the action potential (AP). An initial rapid depolarization, mediated by opening of sarcolemmal voltage-gated Na^+ channels, causes the opening of sarcolemmal voltage-gated LTCC. The resultant influx of Ca^{2+} triggers the release of a larger amount of Ca^{2+} from the SR by a process known as Ca^{2+}-induced Ca^{2+}-release (CICR).[8] Ca^{2+} binding to the intracellular Ca^{2+} channel, the ryanodine receptor (RyR), causes it to open and release the Ca^{2+} stored within the SR. On the face of it, this mechanism would generate a positive feedback loop for intracellular Ca^{2+} release resulting in an 'explosive' Ca^{2+} release event that emptied the SR on each beat. Yet E-C coupling is associated with an increase in intracellular Ca^{2+} concentration ($[Ca^{2+}]i$) from approximately 200 nM during diastole to a peak that varies from around 700 nM to nearly 2000 nM during systole depending on various factors. The ability to generate this range of peak systolic Ca^{2+} values is a vital feature of normal cardiac function; it allows the strength of the heartbeat to vary, allowing the heart to respond to various challenges including altered mechanical load and heart rate. Fine control over the peak systolic Ca^{2+} and the subsequent force of contraction can be reconciled with an 'all-or-none' CICR mechanism as this type of release occurs only in a limited volume of the cell, which acts as a functional Ca^{2+} release unit (CRU) and not the whole cytosol. Variable systolic Ca^{2+} can therefore be achieved by activation of variable numbers of independent CRUs within a single cell.[9] Evidence for CRUs emerged with the observation of discrete Ca^{2+} release events (Ca^{2+} sparks) occurring infrequently and asynchronously during diastole but occurring synchronously during systole.[10] Anatomical evidence for the existence of CRUs comes from electron micrography showing that surface membranes containing LTCCs come into close (10–20 nm) apposition to discrete clusters of RyRs in the intracellular SR membrane.[11,12] This is shown diagrammatically in Fig. 10.1.

Regulation of SR Ca^{2+} release channel

As described above, the SR Ca^{2+} release channels are clustered into arrays on the junctional SR membrane, such that each channel contacts up to four of its neighbours. The size of these clusters is under debate, but estimates range from 4 to 30 channels.[13–15] In addition to cytosolic Ca^{2+}, other endogenous ions and small molecules (e.g. Mg^{2+}, ATP and cADP-ribose) modulate the activity of RyR.[16,17] Phosphorylation of RyR via either Ca^{2+}-calmodulin activated kinase (CaM kinase) or cAMP-activated kinase (A-kinase) are thought to alter the Ca^{2+} sensitivity of the channel.[18,19] Furthermore, auxiliary proteins are associated with the Ca^{2+} release channel and have been shown to modulate its activity. These include: FK506-binding protein,[19] sorcin,[20] calmodulin,[21] and S100A1[22] on the cytosolic side and calsequestrin, junctin, and triadin on the luminal side.[23] Most of these regulatory pathways have been found to be altered in HF, making the overall picture of the activity of the RyR in HF complex.

Mechanism of diastolic Ca^{2+} decrease

Intracellular Ca^{2+} is restored to diastolic levels by several mechanisms. The dominant fraction of the intracellular Ca^{2+} (85–90%) is pumped back into the SR via the activity of the sarcoendoplasmic reticulum Ca^{2+}-ATPase (SERCA) pump. A significant proportion of Ca^{2+} (5–10%) is extruded across the plasma membrane by the sodium-calcium exchanger (NCX). Ca^{2+} is also removed from the cytosol by extrusion across the sarcolemma by the Ca^{2+}-ATPase, although its contribution on a beat-to-beat basis is thought to be quantitatively small (1–2%). The major flux pathways are illustrated in Fig. 10.1. The rate at which diastolic Ca^{2+} is restored dictates the rate at which the heart relaxes during diastole and depends on the relative activity of these extrusion mechanisms. Recently, another factor has been uncovered that influences the kinetics and final level of intracellular Ca^{2+} during diastole, namely the 'leak' of Ca^{2+} from the SR, which occurs mainly via the SR Ca^{2+} release channel. Normally the contribution of this mechanism to diastolic Ca^{2+} is minor, but as described later, a larger than normal Ca^{2+} SR leak may contribute to the HF phenotype. This leak can take two forms: (1) continuous loss of Ca^{2+} and (2) spontaneous Ca^{2+} waves. Continuous loss of Ca^{2+} is assumed to occur across the complete SR network via dysfunctional RyR and may cause a limited increase in diastolic Ca^{2+} without local gradients of intracellular Ca^{2+}. As yet, although this pathway has been identified in animal models of HF,[24] the contribution that continuous Ca^{2+} leak makes to systolic and diastolic function in human HF is uncertain. Under some circumstances, local SR Ca^{2+} release within a region of a heart cell can trigger a spontaneous wave (i.e. not dictated by an AP) of SR Ca^{2+} release that propagates throughout the cell at speeds of around 0.1 mm/s. At each point in the cell, as the wave occurs, the magnitude of SR Ca^{2+} release is comparable to that occurring during systole, but because propagation is much slower (up to 1 s for the wave to travel throughout the cell), meaning that the activation of the contractile proteins is asynchronous and therefore ineffective. The high intracellular Ca^{2+} stimulates Ca^{2+} extrusion from the cell by the normal mechanisms, including SERCA and NCX. This spontaneous SR Ca^{2+} release tends to occur when the heart cell is experiencing higher than normal intracellular Ca^{2+}, and the Ca^{2+} wave is an efficient mechanism of stimulating Ca^{2+} efflux from the cell.[25] However, the extrusion of this intracellular Ca^{2+} on NCX generates a large inward current which can depolarize the membrane potential causing so called 'after-depolarizations' which arise during the repolarization phase of the AP (early after-depolarizations or EADs) or in diastole (delayed after-depolarizations or DADs). These depolarizations may be of sufficient amplitude to trigger an AP, thus producing a VPB. This is not part of the normal E-C coupling process and EADs and DADs are not common in healthy hearts. As described later in this chapter, changes in the SR function in HF may make spontaneous Ca^{2+} release more common and this may be the cellular basis for increased incidence of EADs, DADs, VPBs, and possibly arrhythmias in HF.

Changes in heart failure

Abnormal cell shape and structure in heart failure

Adult cardiac myocytes are incapable of mitosis, so the adaptive response to myocyte loss or mechanical stress in HF is hypertrophy of the surviving cells. In addition to gross changes in cell shape, recent work using confocal microscopy suggests that there is a relative loss of the TAT system in myocytes from animal models of HF[26] and in human HF.[1] A reduction in the amount of functional TAT membrane is also indicated by a reduction in the ratio of membrane surface area to volume.[27,28] Disruption of the TAT system structure in such a way as to prevent a significant amount of expressed protein (e.g. LTCC, NCX, and I_{K1}) access to the surface membrane would have pronounced effects on cardiac excitability and E-C coupling and may therefore be an important cause of the poor contractility observed in HF. This 'structural' hypothesis for dysfunction is in contrast other studies that suggest altered expression of Ca^{2+} handling proteins as the primary cause of dysfunctional E-C coupling.[29] It is almost certainly the case that changes in cellular structure, the expression of the major Ca^{2+} handling proteins, and altered regulation of these channels, pumps, and exchangers all contribute to the complex HF phenotype.

Intracellular Ca^{2+} signals in failing hearts

Studies on human myocardium are difficult for a number of reasons including: (1) access to viable samples of normal and failing myocardium; (2) variation in age, medication, and underlying pathology in the available tissue which likely produces significant heterogeneity; and (3) selection bias meaning that samples are unlikely to be truly representative of human HF. Thus, animal models of HF are commonly used to study subcellular changes. For technical reasons, most of these studies have been carried out in single isolated ventricular myocardial cells, although confirmation in multicellular preparations and whole hearts is available in some cases. Human E-C coupling in HF has been studied in cells isolated from hearts explanted at the time of cardiac transplantation, and therefore reflects changes seen in endstage HF, usually due either to ischaemic cardiomyopathy or to nonischaemic dilated cardiomyopathy. It is important to note that experimental animal models are rarely allowed to develop endstage HF and that the experimental techniques used to achieve a HF-like phenotype in animals (e.g. chronic rapid pacing or combined pressure and volume overload) are not the common causes of HF in humans. In addition to this, most experimental animals are smaller and have naturally higher resting heart rates than do humans and many animals display significant differences from humans in their underlying cardiac electrophysiology, Ca^{2+} handling mechanisms and contractile protein properties. These differences means that extrapolation of data from animal models to the situation found in failing human myocardium should be undertaken with caution.

Changes in E-C coupling in heart failure

As suggested above, the changes in E-C coupling that accompany hypertrophy in failing hearts are complex and may depend on the duration, extent and underlying aetiology of HF (e.g. dilated or ischaemic cardiomyopathy). The amplitude and time course of intracellular Ca^{2+} transients are altered in both animal models of HF and in failing human myocardium. In general, systolic $[Ca^{2+}]i$ is lower than normal, and the duration of the Ca^{2+} transient is prolonged in myocytes from failing myocardium (illustrated in Fig. 10.2).[30–33] These changes are thought to be the predominant cause of the contractile dysfunction observed in HF. Despite pronounced electrophysiological changes in myocytes from failing hearts, changes in the amplitude and time course of the L-type Ca^{2+} current are not commonly observed indicating that, in general, the trigger for Ca^{2+} release from the SR is not altered in failing hearts.[29] Early studies suggested that the principal basis for reduced intracellular Ca^{2+} in HF was depressed SR function.[29] While SERCA mRNA measurements in failing hearts almost always show a significant reduction, a series of reports show no difference in SERCA protein expression or activity in HF.[22,34,35] In failing human hearts, a wide range of SERCA protein levels were measured, from 33% to 100% of normal values.[36] This variability may be related to differences in the underlying pathology, since a greater decrease in SR Ca^{2+} ATPase expression/activity was observed in myocardium from patients with ischaemic cardiomyopathy compared to dilated cardiomyopathy.[37] The functional impact of reduced SERCA expression is difficult to predict, in

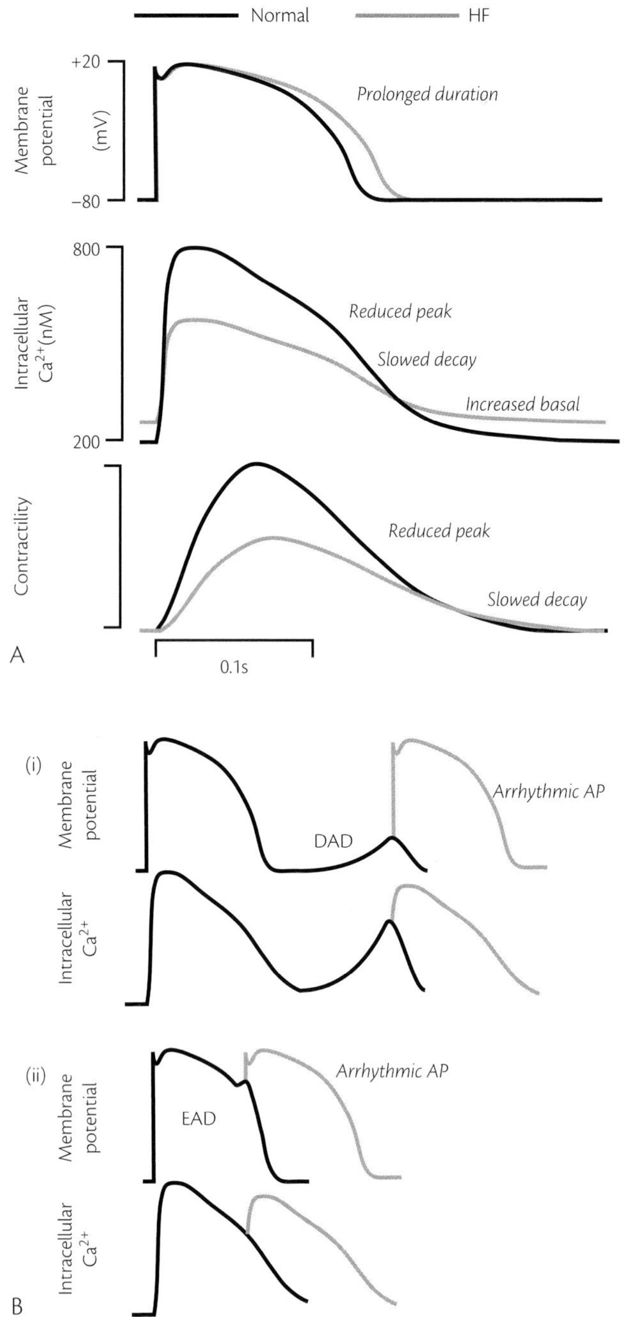

Fig. 10.2 Changes in cellular calcium handling in heart failure. (A) Typical changes observed in the ventricular action potential (AP), intracellular Ca^{2+} transient, and contraction profile of isolated human ventricular myocytes from patients with heart failure compared with those from normal hearts. (B) Membrane potential and intracellular Ca^{2+} transient traces showing (i) a delayed afterdepolarization (DAD), which occurs during diastole and is triggered by SR Ca^{2+} release, as indicated by the preceding rise in intracellular Ca^{2+}, and results in a spontaneous arrhythmic AP; (ii) an early afterdepolarization (EAD), which occurs during the AP and can also trigger a spontaneous arrhythmic AP.

several studies involving animal models of HF, reduced systolic [Ca^{2+}] was accompanied by unchanged SR Ca^{2+} content.[38–40] This has led to the suggestion that reduced ability of normal Ca^{2+} influx to trigger Ca^{2+} release from the SR is an important aspect of the pathology of HF. Direct evidence for this has been provided by the technique of linescan confocal imaging. This technique allows the rapid (every 1–2 ms) scanning of the intracellular [Ca^{2+}] within a thin (*c.*1 μm section) of a cardiac cell. This technique has indicated that, under normal circumstances, depolarization produces a synchronous Ca^{2+} release along the length of a ventricular myocyte.[41] However, measurements on myocytes from failing hearts indicate a heterogeneous activation pattern, suggesting that SR Ca^{2+} release does not occur to the same extent at every intracellular site.[38] One explanation for this result is a reduction in the TAT system in failing cells diminishing the number of LTCC in close proximity to RyR. However, no study to date has correlated defects in the SR Ca^{2+} release with the disrupted TAT system structure in HF. An alternative explanation is that the ability of LTCC to trigger release from the RyR cluster is reduced to a subset of RyR clusters heterogeneously distributed throughout the cardiomyocyte.

Factors that alter RyR function in heart failure

Recent work revealing the complex modulation of RyR function via association/dissociation of regulatory proteins or phosphorylation/dephosphorylation has lead to the discovery that the pattern of regulation is significantly altered in HF. Initial work on human myocardium indicated that the 12.6-kDa member of the family of FK-506 binding proteins (FKBP12.6) was lost from RyR in failing hearts, and that this altered RyR function in such a way as to increase the Ca^{2+} sensitivity of the RyR and increase leak of Ca^{2+} from the SR. Later work showed that the dissociation of FKBP12.6 from RyR in HF was the result of hyperphosphorylation of RyR by an associated A-kinase. However, the link between A-kinase, FKBP12.6, and RyR dysfunction in HF is not a universal finding, and other work suggests that RyR dysfunction in HF occurs independently of A-kinase.[42] Other regulatory proteins, such as sorcin and S100A1 have been implicated,[43] as has CaM kinase. Increased CaM kinase activity is observed in HF and is associated with RyR dysfunction, increased leak from the SR and increased frequency of spontaneous Ca^{2+} release.

However, several studies have established that modification of the Ca^{2+} sensitivity of RyR alone cannot give rise to sustained effects on intracellular Ca^{2+} and contractility, as autoregulatory processes ensure that the Ca^{2+} transient is similar in amplitude despite large changes in RyR Ca^{2+} sensitivity.[44] Thus poor contractility cannot be simply addressed by a drug acting purely on the RyR, and it is likely that drugs with more than one intracellular action will be required for effective positive inotropy.

The link between intracellular Ca^{2+} and arrhythmias

Postulated mechanisms for arrhythmogenesis in HF have focused either on single-cell arrhythmic mechanisms, particularly triggered activity (due to early or late after-depolarizations) or on heterogeneity of electrophysiological properties between cells (conduction velocity or refractoriness, predisposing to re-entry). EADs are defined as depolarizing potentials that occur before the action potential repolarizes completely. EADs are facilitated by prolongation of action potential duration, whether by delayed inactivation of either Na^{+} or Ca^{2+}currents or by reduction in repolarizing outward current. EADs may be caused by a depolarizing current generated either by premature recovery from inactivation and reactivation of LTCC or by an inward current activated by a rise of intracellular Ca^{2+} (e.g. the forward mode NCX). However, there is no consensus as to whether EADs are triggered by, or are dependent upon spontaneous SR Ca^{2+} release. Late EADs occur during phase 3 of the AP and are thought to be due to Ca^{2+}-activated inward currents (NCX or the nonselective current or Ca^{2+} activated Cl^- current) generated by spontaneous Ca^{2+} SR release in a similar fashion to DADs.[45]

DADs are caused by spontaneous Ca^{2+} release from local regions of the SR which give rise to a transient inward current during the diastolic period. Conditions of intracellular Ca^{2+} overload, such as are produced by catecholamine administration or digitalis toxicity, predispose to DADs. Whereas early EADs are common during bradycardia, the amplitude and frequency of DADs increases with increasing heart rate. Interestingly, the changes in RyR function observed in HF are also thought to predispose the SR to spontaneous release and therefore to the generation of a late EAD or DAD. The increased incidence of these potential arrhythmic triggers, manifest as increased VPBs, substantially increase the risk of arrhythmic SCD. Thus pharmacological therapy designed to (amongst other things) normalize the behaviour of RyR could potentially reduce the incidence of SCD.

Paradoxical changes in NCX abundance and activity in heart failure

In cardiac muscle, sarcolemmal NCX plays an essential role in regulating intracellular [Ca^{2+}]i. Changes in the activity of NCX modulate the force of contraction,[33, 46] and may contribute to the poor mechanical function in HF. Furthermore, NCX activity is electrogenic and may generate proarrhythmic currents in normal and hypertrophic myocardium.[47] In many animal models of cardiac hypertrophy and HF, both NCX expression and activity are increased.[47–51] However, other studies have reported contrary findings.[52] The most difficult results to reconcile are those from a mouse aortic banding model of cardiac hypertrophy; in this study NCX protein and RNA levels were increased but NCX current was decreased.[53] When considering NCX expression pattern, these findings raise two interesting possibilities to explain the changes in NCX activity and abundance:

NCX expression pattern is altered in HF; the increased expression is the result of increases in NCX protein in the remaining TAT system and surface membrane. This NCX would be less effective at extruding Ca^{2+} since the disrupted TAT system would prevent Ca^{2+} within the centre of the cell having immediate access to the extracellular space.

NCX expression pattern in similar to normal, the increased NCX is within the TAT system, but a fraction of the TAT system has limited access to the extracellular space. Recently, a similar situation was created experimentally by detubulating isolated rat cardiac myocytes.[5] This acute treatment markedly reduced the rate of Ca^{2+} extrusion but did not alter NCX expression levels. If a similar disconnection of the TAT system developed in the failing myocytes, the increased NCX expression would not be reflected in an increased Ca^{2+} extrusion from the cell.

Contributions of non-ventricular tissue to the heart failure phenotype

Potentially, Ca^{2+} signalling disturbances in atrial cardiomyocytes and Purkinje cells may also contribute to the poor contractility and proarrhythmic status associated with HF.

Atrial cells are smaller in diameter (*c*.0.01 mm) and length (*c*.0.1 mm) than ventricular cardiomyocytes and some measurements suggest that there is a less developed TAT system. The intracellular Ca^{2+} transient is smaller and slower in atrial myocytes from failing hearts in an analogous way to that observed in failing ventricular cardiomyocytes. Few human studies exist, but animal models of HF indicate that changes in Ca^{2+} signalling is associated with a reduction of the already poorly developed TAT system.[54] The E-C coupling process in atria is thought to rely more on propagation of the Ca^{2+} signal from the periphery to the central region of the cell rather than action potential propagation into the cell diameter via the TAT system. Interestingly, several studies suggest that Ca^{2+} signalling within atrial cells is influenced by inositol-tris-phosphate activated receptors (IP^3R) on the SR membrane as well as RyR.[55] The relative expression of IP^3R versus RyR channels is thought to be altered in failing hearts which may predispose the atrial cell to either initiate or sustain arrhythmic activity. In humans, HF is associated with an increased risk of atrial fibrillation (AF), but the cellular basis for this is unknown and further work is required to establish whether the modification of Ca^{2+} signalling may predispose to or sustain AF activity.

The Purkinje fibre network is made up of modified cardiomyocytes and is responsible for the rapid activation of the endocardial surface. The cells are wider (*c*.0.03 mm) than ventricular cardiomyocytes with a less dense TAT system and fewer myofibrils and mitochondria. As with atrial cells, propagation of the surface depolarization to the centre of these cells is thought to occur via regenerative SR Ca^{2+} release. Complex patterns of Ca^{2+} release have been observed in Purkinje cells involving both central and peripheral sections of the SR network.[56] Analogous to atrial cells, IP^3R are thought to play a key role in regulating spontaneous Ca^{2+} release in Purkinje fibre cells. Several lines of evidence indicate that the trigger for sustained arrhythmias may arise within the Purkinje network, particularly those resulting from an ischaemia/reperfusion cycle.[57] The role of intracellular Ca^{2+} in generation of EAD- or DAD-based arrhythmias in Purkinje cells is an active area of research. Surviving Purkinje cells within the infarct are more prone to spontaneous Ca^{2+} release and arrhythmic activity.[56] Modification of RyR is thought to contribute to this effect since this pro-arrhythmic activity can be normalized by the drug JTV 519[56] and lends support to the concept that Purkinje fibre based triggers for arrhythmic behaviour in HF may be amenable to specific pharmacological suppression by drugs acting to normalize intracellular Ca^{2+} handling.

Summary

Abnormalities of Ca^{2+} release and reuptake occur in the remodelled myocardium of failing hearts. These changes are thought to mediate both the poor inotropic and the proarrhythmic state of the failing heart. The molecular and structural basis for these changes appears to be multifactorial, and includes abnormal subcellular structure and altered regulation of Ca^{2+} signalling proteins. Basic research on failing human myocardium and animal models of the disease has suggested novel therapeutic approaches to normalize Ca^{2+} signalling in failing hearts which promise more effective pharmacological therapies in the near future.

References

1. Soeller C, Cannell MB. Examination of the transverse tubular system in living cardiac rat myocytes by 2-photon microscopy and digital image-processing techniques. *Circ Res* 2002;**84**(3):266–75.
2. Forbes MS, Hawkey LA, Sperelakis N. The transverse-axial tubular system (TATS) of mouse myocardium: its morphology in the developing and adult animal. *Am J Anat* 1984;**170**:143–62.
3. Cheng H, Cannell MB, Lederer WJ. Propagation of excitation-contraction coupling into ventricular myocytes. *Pflügers Archiv* 1994;**428**:415–17.
4. Kawai M, Hussain M, Orchard CH. Excitation-contraction coupling in rat ventricular myocytes after formamide-induced detubulation. *Am J Physiol* 1999;**277**:H603–H609.
5. Yang Z, Pascarel C, Steele DS, Komukai K, Brette F, Orchard CH. Na^+-Ca^{2+} exchange activity is localized in the T-tubules of rat ventricular myocytes. *Circ Res* 2002;**91**:315–22.
6. Gotoh Y, Imaizumi Y, Watanabe AM, Shibata EF, Clark RB, Giles WR. Inhibition of transient outward K^+ current by DHP Ca^{2+} antagonists and agonists in rabbit cardiac myocytes. *Am J Physiol* 1991;**260**:H1737–42.
7. McLerie M, Lopatin A. Dominant-negative suppression of I(K1) in the mouse heart leads to altered cardiac excitability. *J Mol Cell Cardiol* 2003;**35**:367–78.
8. Fabiato A. Calcium-induced release of calcium from the sarcoplasmic reticulum. *J Gen Physiol* 1985;**85**:189–320.
9. Stern MD. Theory of excitation-contraction coupling in cardiac muscle. *Biophys J* 1992;**63**:497–517.
10. Cannell MB, Cheng H, Lederer WJ. The control of calcium release in heart muscle. *Science* 1995;**268**:1045–9.
11. Franzini-Armstrong C, Protasi F, Ramesh V. Shape, size and distribution of Ca^{2+} Release units and couplons in skeletal and cardiac muscles. *Biophys J* 1999;**77**:1528–39.
12. Gathercole DV, Colling DJ, Skepper JN, Takagishi Y, Levi AJ, Severs NJ. Immunogold-labeled L-type calcium channels are clustered in the surface plasma membrane overlying junctional sarcoplasmic reticulum in guinea-pig myocytes-implications for excitation-contraction coupling in cardiac muscle. *J Mol Cell Cardiol* 2000;**32**:1981–94.
13. Keizer J, Smith GD, Ponce-Dawson S, Pearson JE. Saltatory propagation of Ca^{2+} waves by Ca^{2+} sparks. *Biophys J* 1998;**75**:595–600.
14. Izu LT, Mauban RH, Balke CW, Wier WG. Large currents generate cardiac Ca^{2+} sparks. *Biophys J* 2000;**80**:88–102.
15. Cannell MB, Soeller C. Sparks of interest in cardiac excitation–contraction coupling. *TiPS* 1998;**19**:16–20.
16. Kermode H, Williams AJ, Sitsapesan R. The interactions of ATP, ADP and inorganic phosphate with the sheep cardiac ryanodine receptor. *Biophys J* 1998;**74**:1296–304.
17. Rakovic S, Galione A, Ashamu GA, Potter BVL, Terrar DA. A specific cyclic ADP-ribose antagonist inhibits cardiac excitation-contraction coupling. *Curr Biol* 1996;**6**:989–96.
18. Bowling N, Walsh RA, Song G, *et al.* Increased protein kinase C activity and expression of Ca^{2+}-sensitive isoforms in the failing human heart. *Circulation* 1999;**99**:384–91.
19. Marx SO, Reiken S, Hisamatsu Y, *et al.* PKA phosphorylation dissociates FKB12.6 from the calcium release channel (ryanodine receptor): defective regulation in failing hearts. *Cell* 2000;**101**:365–76.
20. Lokuta AJ, Meyers MB, Sander PR F. G. I. a. V. H. H. Modulation of cardiac ryanodine receptors by sorcin. *J Biol Chem* 1997;**272**:25333–8.
21. Balshaw DM, Xu L, Yamaguchi N, Pasek DA, Meissner G. Calmodulin binding and inhibition of cardiac muscle calcium release channel (ryanodine receptor). *J Biol Chem* 2001;**276**:20144–53.
22. Naqvi RU, Tweedie D, MacLeod KT. Evidence for the action potential mediating the changes to contraction observed in cardiac hypertrophy in the rabbit. *Int J Cardiol* 2000;**77**:189–206.
23. Gyorke I, Hester N, Jones LR, Gyorke S. The role of calsequestrin, triadin, and junctin in conferring cardiac ryanodine receptor responsiveness to luminal calcium. *Biophys J* 2004;**86**:2121–8.
24. Shannon TR, Pogwizd SM, Bers DM. Elevated sarcoplasmic reticulum Ca^{2+} leak in intact ventricular myocytes from rabbits in heart failure. *Circ Res.* 2003;**93**:592–4.
25. Diaz ME, Trafford AW, ONeill SC, Eisner DA. Measurement of sarcoplasmic reticulum Ca^{2+} content and sarcolemmal Ca^{2+} fluxes in isolated rat ventricular myocytes during spontaneous Ca^{2+} release. *J Physiol* 1997;**501**(1):3–16.
26. He JQ, Foell JD, Wolff M, *et al.* Reduction in density of transverse tubules in L-type Ca^{2+} channels in canine tachycardia-induced heart failure. *Cardiovasc Res* 2002;**49**:298–307.
27. Gomez AM, Schwaller B, Porzig H, Vassort G, Niggli E, Egger M. Increased exchange current but normal Ca^{2+} transport via Na^+-Ca^{2+} exchange during cardiac hypertrophy after myocardial infarction. *Circ Res* 2002;**91**:323–30.
28. Quinn FR, Currie S, Duncan AM, *et al.* Myocardial infarction causes increased expression but decreased activity of the myocardial Na^+-Ca^{2+} exchanger in the rabbit. *J Physiol* 2003;**553**:229–42.
29. Hasenfuss G, Meyer M, Schillinger W, Preuss M, Pieske B, Just H. Calcium handling proteins in the failing human heart. *Basic Res Cardiol* 1997;**92**:87–93.
30. Gwathmey JK, Copelas L, MacKinnon R, *et al.* Abnormal intracellular calcium handling in myocardium from patients with end-stage heart failure. *Circ Res* 1987;**61**:70–6.
31. Beuckelmann DJ, Nabauer M, Erdmann E. Intracellular calcium handling in isolated ventricular myocytes from patients with terminal heart failure. *Circulation* 1992;**85**:1046–55.
32. Piacentino V III, Weber CR, Chen X, *et al.* Cellular basis of abnormal calcium transients of failing human ventricular myocytes. *Circ Res* 2003;**92**:651–8.
33. Ranu HK, Terracciano CM, Davia K, *et al.* Effects of Na^+/Ca^{2+}-exchanger overexpression on excitation- contraction coupling in adult rabbit ventricular myocytes. *J Mol Cell Cardiol* 2002;**34**:389–400.
34. Schwinger RHG, Bohm M, Schmidt U, *et al.* Unchanged protein levels of SERCAII and phospholamban but reduced Ca^{2+} uptake and Ca^{2+}-ATPase activity of cardiac SR from dilated cardiomyopathy patients compared with patients with non-failing hearts. *Circulation* 1995;**92**:3220–8.
35. Movsesian MA, Bristow MR, Krall J. Ca^{2+} uptake by cardiac SR from patients with idiopathic cardiomyopathy. *Circ Res* 1989;**65**:1141–4.
36. Hasenfuss G, Reinecke H, Studer R, *et al.* Relation between myocardial function and expression of sacroplasmic reticulum Ca^{2+}-ATPase in failing and nonfailing human myocardium. *Circ Res* 1994;**75**:434–42.
37. Sen L, Cui G, Fonarow GC, Laks H Differences in mechanisms of SR dysfunction in ischemic vs. idiopathic dilated cardiomyopathy. *Am J Physiol* 2000;279:709–18.
38. Litwin SE, Zhang D, Bridge JH B. Dyssynchronous Ca^{2+} sparks in myocytes from infarcted hearts. *Circ Res* 2000;**87**:1040–7.
39. Pogwizd SM, Schlotthauer K, Li L, Yuan W, Bers DM. Arrhythmogenesis and contractile dysfunction in heart failure: roles of sodium-calcium exchange, inward rectifier potassium current, and residual -adrenergic responsiveness. *Circ Res* 2001;**88**:1159–67.
40. Gomez AM, Valdivia HH, Cheng H, *et al.* Defective excitation-contraction coupling in experimental cardiac hypertrophy and heart failure. *Science* 1997;**276**:800–6.
41. Cheng H, Cannell MB, Lederer WJ. Propagation of excitation-contraction coupling into ventricular myocytes. *Pflugers Arch* 1994;**428**:415–17.
42. Ikemoto N, Yamamoto T. Postulated role of inter-domain interaction within the ryanodine receptor in Ca^{2+} channel regulation. *Trends Cardiovasc Med* 2000;**10**:310–16.
43. Most P, Bernotat J, Ehlermann P, *et al.* S100A1: a regulator of myocardial contractility. *Proc Natl Acad Sci U S A* 2001;**98**:13889–94.

44. Eisner DA, Choi HS, Diaz ME, O'Neill SC, Trafford AW. Integrative analysis of calcium cycling in cardiac muscle. *Circ Res* 2000;**87**:1087–94.
45. Choi B-R, Burton, Salama G. Cytolsolic Ca^{2+} triggers early after depolarizations and torsade de pointes in rabbits with type-2 long QT syndrome. *J Physiol* 2002;**543**:615–631.
46. Schillinger W, Janssen PML, Emami S, *et al.* Impaired contractile performance of cultured rabbit ventricular myocytes after adenoviral gene transfer of Na^+-Ca^{2+} exchanger. *Circ Res* 2000;**87**:581–7.
47. Pogwizd SM, Yuan MQ, Samarel AM, Bers DM. Upregulation of Na/Ca exchanger expression and function in an arrhythmogenic rabbit model of heart failure. *Circ Res* 1999;**85**:1009–19.
48. Hatem SN, Sham JSK, Morad M. Enhanced Na^+-Ca^{2+} exchange activity in cardiomyopathic syrian hamster. *Circ Res* 1994;**74**:253–61.
49. Studer R, Reinecke H, Bilger J, Eschenhagen T, Bohm M, Hasenfuss G. Gene expression of the Na^+-Ca^{2+} exchanger in end stage human heart failure. *Circ Res* 1994;**75**:443–53.
50. Hasenfuss G. Alterations of calcium-regulatory proteins in heart failure. *Cardiovasc Res* 1997;**37**:279–89.
51. Hasenfuss G, Schillinger W, Lehnart SE, *et al.* Relationship between Na^+-Ca^{2+}-exchanger protein levels and diastolic function of failing human myocardium. *Circulation* 1999;**99**:641–8.
52. Sipido KR, Volders PG, Vos MA, Verdonck F. Altered Na/Ca exchange activity in cardiac hypertrophy and heart failure: a new target for therapy? *Cardiovasc Res* 2002;**53**:782–805.
53. Wang Z, Nolan B, Kutschke W, Hill JA. Na^+-Ca^{2+} exchanger remodeling in pressure overload cardiac hypertrophy. *J Biol Chem* 2001;**276**:17706–11.
54. Dibb KM, Clarke JD, Horn MA, *et al.* Characterization of an extensive transverse tubular network in sheep atrial myocytes and its depletion in heart failure. *Circ.Heart Fail* 2009;**2**:482–9.
55. Berridge MJ, Bootman MD, Lipp P. Calcium a life and death signal. *Nature* 1998;**395**:645–8.
56. Boyden PA, Barbhaiya C, Lee T, ter Keurs HE. Nonuniform Ca^{2+} transients in arrhythmogenic Purkinje cells that survive in the infarcted canine heart. *Cardiovasc Res* 2003;**57**:681–93.
57. Janse MJ, Wit AL. Electrophysiological mechanisms of ventricular arrhythmias resulting from myocardial ischemia and infarction. *Physiol Rev* 1989;**69**:1049–169.

11

Myocardial energetics

Peter H. Sugden and Stephen J. Fuller

Introduction

The heart is an example of a specialized type I ('red') striated muscle in that it is continuously active and reliant principally on aerobic metabolism for its energy supply. In normal humans at rest, the heart extracts 60–65% of O_2 available in the coronary circulation. This corresponds to an O_2 utilization rate of about 4.5μmol/min per gram wet weight, which may increase by three- to fourfold during exercise. This maximal physiological O_2 uptake is probably higher than any other organ. The majority of O_2 is utilized by the ventricles, particularly by the left ventricle because of its greater mass and pressure–volume product than the right ventricle. Although the heart (like all organs) is composed of several different cell types, ventricular cardiac myocytes (the contractile cells of the heart) constitute about 75% of the heart mass. These myocytes possess a well-developed myofibrillar apparatus and a capacity for aerobic metabolism that fit them for their major role *in vivo*, namely the rhythmic contraction which provides the force needed for the ejection of blood from the ventricles.

Although much of the myocyte volume is taken up by myofibrils, the mitochondria constitute about 30%. In the heart, these subcellular organelles regenerate the bulk of ATP from ADP and inorganic phosphate (P_i). ATP is an 'energy transducing molecule' which couples the energy available from fuel metabolism into external work (principally myofibrillar contraction but also processes involved in ion transport and biosynthetic pathways). Mitochondria possess an outer (OMM) and an inner (IMM) mitochondrial membrane, and the latter encloses the mitochondrial matrix into which multiple invaginations of the IMM (the cristae) protrude. The division of the mitochondria into the matrix and intermembrane space is functionally important in ATP regeneration.

The ATP content of the heart is only sufficient to allow contraction for a few beats, and its supplies of endogenous fuels (e.g. glycogen, triglycerides) are limited given the amount of work it has to perform. Thus, in order to maintain fuel oxidation, ATP regeneration, and muscle contraction, a highly developed coronary circulation and uninterrupted coronary blood flow are necessary to ensure adequate delivery of O_2 and fuels, and to remove the product of aerobic metabolism, CO_2. However, like all tissues, the heart contains phosphocreatine (PCr or creatine phosphate) which acts as a short-term ATP buffer during rapid increases in the rate of ATP utilization. Thus, under 'stressed' conditions, PCr transphosphorylates ADP to ATP in an equilibrium reaction catalysed by creatine kinase (Equation 11.1):

$$\text{PCr} + \text{ADP} + \text{H}^+ \rightleftharpoons \text{creatine} + \text{ATP} \qquad \text{(Equation 11.1)}$$

Even so, the concentration of PCr is only about twice that of ATP, and the utility of the creatine kinase reaction is limited to short-term buffering of ATP concentrations.

Metabolism in the healthy heart

Energy for contraction

The heart is omnivorous and utilizes any metabolic fuel presented to it, within the constraints of metabolic regulation. The major substrates for oxidation in humans are lipid-derived fuels (principally long-chain fatty acids (LCFAs) such as palmitate, but also triglycerides and ketone bodies (acetoacetate and its reduction product, 3-hydroxybutyrate) in specialized circumstances) and the carbohydrate-derived fuels (glucose, lactate, and pyruvate). Although the heart can oxidize amino acids, these are of minor importance. The accepted dogma is that the human heart relies predominantly (70%) on lipid-derived fuels for its energy supply,[1] but the majority of investigations have involved postabsorptive subjects where lipid metabolism is generally more favoured than in the immediately postprandial state.

Glucose metabolism

The initial stages of glucose metabolism are exclusively cytoplasmic (Fig. 11.1). Glucose is transported across the cardiac myocyte plasma membrane by two carriers, namely the type 1 and type 4 glucose transporters (GLUT1 and GLUT4).[2] GLUT1 provides

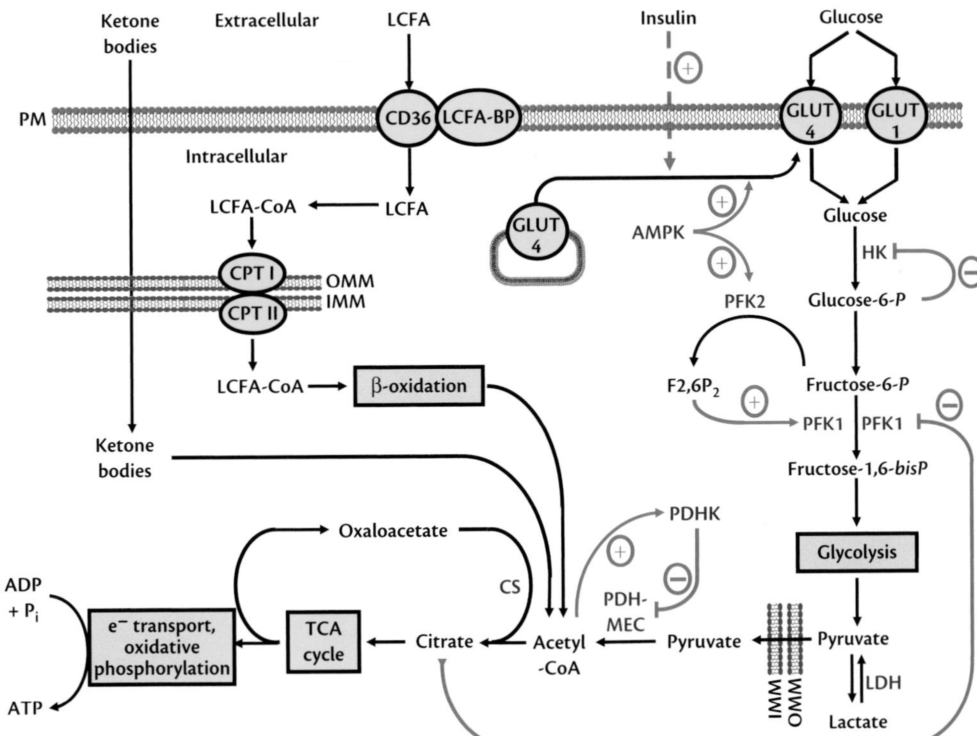

Fig. 11.1 Fuel inter-relationships. The major part of this diagram shows how utilization of lipid fuels restricts utilization of glucose (the Randle cycle). For full details, see the text. Processes are in light blue, membrane-bound proteins are in yellow, enzymes are in dark blue, metabolic intermediates are in black, regulatory steps are red lines. AMPK, AMP-activated protein kinase; CPT, carnitine palmitoyl transferase; CS, citrate synthase; e^-, electron; $F2,6P_2$, fructose 2,6-bisphosphate; GLUT, glucose transporter; HK, hexokinase; IMM, inner mitochondrial membrane; LCFA(-BP), long-chain fatty acid (binding protein); LDH, lactate dehydrogenase; OMM, outer mitochondrial membranes; PDHK, pyruvate dehydrogenase kinase; PDH-MEC, PDH multienzyme complex; PFK, phosphofructokinase; PM, plasma membrane.

a basal constitutive component whereas GLUT4 mediates inducible glucose uptake. Insulin increases glucose uptake by recruiting intracellular endosomal GLUT4 to the plasma membrane. Intracellular glucose is mainly used to provide energy for contraction but, in addition, can be polymerized to the intracellular storage carbohydrate glycogen. Although the heart has a limited capacity to store glycogen and its breakdown may not be quantitatively significant under normal conditions, it may provide energy for a limited period in pathological conditions (e.g. during myocardial infarction, when the supplies of exogenous fuels and O_2 are disrupted).

Each molecule of glucose is degraded through the glycolytic pathway to pyruvate, the chemical energy released allowing the net regeneration of two molecules of ATP (from ADP) per glucose molecule utilized. This so-called 'substrate-level phosphorylation' occurs at the phosphoglycerate kinase and pyruvate kinase steps. Additionally, two molecules of the electron acceptor nicotinamide adenine dinucleotide (NAD^+) are reduced to NADH. Glycolysis can occur anaerobically (see below) but this is inefficient in terms of the quantity of ATP regenerated compared with that available from complete oxidation of glucose. Under the aerobic conditions normally existing in the heart, pyruvate is transported into the mitochondria, and the glycolytically derived electrons (as NADH) enter on a 'shuttle mechanism' (the malate/aspartate shuttle) regenerating cytoplasmic NAD^+.

The heart can metabolize circulating lactate formed from anaerobic metabolism in other tissues. Lactate is first oxidized to pyruvate by the cytoplasmic enzyme, lactate dehydrogenase (Equation 11.2):

$$\text{lactate} + NAD^+ \rightleftharpoons \text{pyruvate} + NADH + H^+ \qquad \text{(Equation 11.2)}$$

The pyruvate thus formed and the reducing equivalents enter oxidative metabolism in the same way as glycolytically derived pyruvate and NADH. Under anaerobic or hypoxic conditions where oxidative metabolism is reduced, the lactate dehydrogenase reaction is reversed, leading to formation of lactate and regeneration of cytoplasmic NAD^+.

Mitochondrial pyruvate metabolism

In the mitochondria, pyruvate is oxidized by the pyruvate dehydrogenase multienzyme complex (PDH-MEC) to acetyl-coenzyme A (acetyl-CoA) and CO_2, with reduction of NAD^+ to NADH.[3] This is a critical regulatory step in humans and many other organisms since it is physiologically irreversible and commits pyruvate (hence glucose) to oxidation. Before the PDH-MEC stage, glucose can be hepatically or renally resynthesized from lactate or pyruvate by gluconeogenesis. The activity of PDH-MEC is therefore subject to stringent regulation that couples its activity to the nutritional state of the animal. Thus, in the postabsorptive or fasted state, its activity is decreased to allow glucose conservation for tissues with an obligatory requirement for exogenous glucose, and this is brought about by increased reliance on lipid-derived fuels, with the converse occurring on feeding. This is one of the facets of the so-called glucose–fatty acid cycle or Randle cycle[4–6] in which utilization of lipid fuels during fasting suppresses glucose utilization (see Fig. 11.1).

Acetyl-CoA then enters the nine-stage tricarboxylic (TCA) cycle (also known as the citric acid or Krebs cycle) by condensing with oxaloacetate to form citrate (the citrate synthase step) and CoA (Figs 11.1 and 11.2). By decarboxylation and oxidation (Fig. 11.2), two carbons of citrate are lost as CO_2, and the electrons are used to reduce O_2 to H_2O. The intermediate steps in the TCA cycle oxidations involve principally NAD^+ as the initial e^- acceptor, and these reducing equivalents are used to drive ATP regeneration. The CO_2 lost originates from the oxaloacetate moiety of citrate rather than acetyl-CoA. The carbons donated by acetyl-CoA become part of the oxaloacetate backbone after the first turn of the TCA cycle and

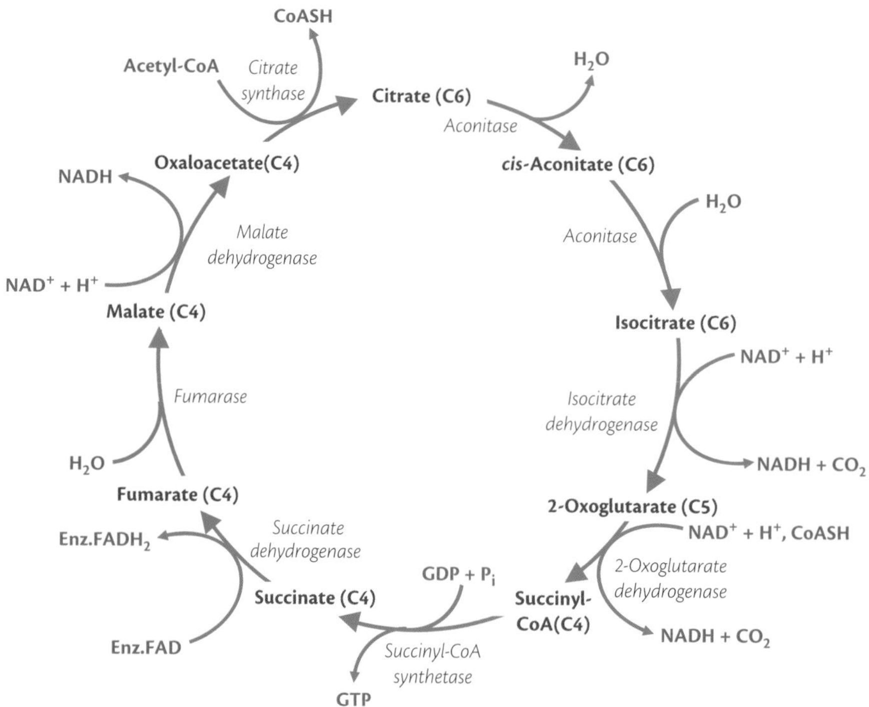

Fig. 11.2 The tricarboxylic acid (TCA) cycle. The TCA cycle is exclusively mitochondrial and in effect oxidizes the acetyl moiety of acetyl-CoA to CO_2 and H_2O. The enzymes involved are shown in blue, the intermediates of the cycle in dark red with the number of carbon atoms in their structures in parentheses, and the ancillary metabolites in red. CO_2 is lost at the isocitrate dehydrogenase and 2-oxoglutarate dehydrogenase steps. Reducing equivalents are removed as NADH at the isocitrate dehydrogenase, 2-oxoglutarate dehydrogenase, and malate dehydrogenase steps. Electrons in NADH pass down (regenerating NAD^+) the electron transport chain (a series of carriers) and the energy released is used to drive oxidative phosphorylation (reduction of molecular O_2 to H_2O and ATP resynthesis at a P/O ratio of about 3). Succinate dehydrogenase is a flavoprotein containing flavin adenine dinucleotide (FAD) which functions as an electron carrier in the electron transport chain, but is 'lower energy' than NADH and yields less ATP (P/O ratio of about 2). However, the succinyl-CoA synthetase step regenerates GTP from GDP + P_i, so the two steps combined are energetically equivalent to NADH.

thus complete loss of the 'acetyl-CoA carbon' as CO_2 may require several turns of the cycle. However, intermediates of the TCA cycle are often used in biosynthetic reactions, and so the carbon may be retained.

Metabolism of lipid fuels

Triglycerides, LCFAs, and ketone bodies are all capable of providing energy for the heart. LCFAs (principally palmitate) are present in the plasma either noncovalently bound to albumin or covalently bound as triglycerides which are in turn complexed with apolipoproteins. Ketone bodies are synthesized hepatically from LCFA but are present in the plasma only at low concentrations under 'normal' conditions. Compared with LCFA, they represent a relatively soluble, readily-diffusing, utilizable, nontoxic fuel and their concentrations increase during starvation or after exercise. Postexercise ketosis is effectively an 'overshoot phenomenon' whereby high plasma concentrations of LCFA used to fuel exercise continue to give rise to ketone bodies. In pathological conditions (e.g. untreated diabetes mellitus), their plasma concentrations rise to a much greater extent than in starvation. This results from the more extreme increases in plasma LCFA.

Like glucose, albumin-bound LCFAs enter the cardiac myocyte by a transporter-mediated process (principally the transmembrane CD36 protein in conjunction with a plasma membrane LCFA binding protein), and diffusion within the cytoplasm is facilitated by a cytoplasmic LCFA binding protein(s) (Fig. 11.1).[2] There are other pathways (diffusion through the plasma membrane, other LCFA transport proteins), but these are less important in the heart than CD36. Triglycerides are hydrolysed by the ecto-enzyme lipoprotein lipase on the capillary wall to form LCFAs (which then enter the myocyte) and glycerol, potentially a substrate for resynthesis of glucose by gluconeogenesis.

LCFAs and ketone bodies can only be catabolized aerobically, and their catabolism takes place exclusively in the mitochondria. LCFAs are first 'activated' in the cytoplasm by the formation of a covalent thioester bond with CoA (compare acetyl-CoA), and then cross the mitochondrial membranes. This involves the carnitine palmitoyl transferase I/carnitine palmitoyl transferase II system in the OMM and the IMM, respectively. The OMM transferase is an important point of control of LCFA metabolism. Once in the mitochondrial matrix, LCFA-CoA is reformed, and two-carbon fragments are successively removed as acetyl-CoA from LCFA (as LCFA-CoA) in a series of reactions known generically as β-oxidation. Ketone bodies, as acetoacetyl-CoA, are metabolized by a somewhat different process, to acetyl-CoA. Acetyl-CoA formed from β-oxidation or ketone body utilization is then oxidized through the TCA cycle (Figs 11.1 and 11.2). Because the commonest LCFAs contain even numbers of carbon residues which are 'lost' during the TCA cycle, these LCFAs generally cannot be utilized for net production of glucose.

Oxidative phosphorylation

The mechanism by which reduction of O_2 to H_2O by NADH is coupled to ATP resynthesis (electron transport and oxidative phosphorylation) remained a mystery long after the metabolic pathways of fuel metabolism had been elucidated. Initial work primarily attributed to Peter Mitchell led to the development of the 'chemiosmotic hypothesis'.[7,8] Here, the transport of e^- down an electrochemical gradient of carriers on the internal face of the IMM is coupled to electrogenic vectorial pumping of protons into the space between the IMM and OMM. This sets up a 'proton motive force' which is energized by both a pH gradient and a potential difference across the IMM. The electrons pass to the next carrier, and the protons are vectorially directed into the intermembrane space. The ultimate e^- acceptor is molecular O_2 which is reduced to H_2O. The energy of the proton motive force flowing back down the energy gradient across the IMM is utilized to drive the resynthesis of ATP from ADP and P_i by the IMM ATP synthase. One consequence of the chemiosmotic hypothesis is that a precise relationship between O_2 consumed and ATP resynthesized (the P/O ratio, ATP molecules resynthesized from ADP/oxygen atom reduced) does not necessarily exist. Previously, the P/O ratio was thought to be stoichiometrically fixed to 3. However, the P/O ratio would remain at about 3 under normal circumstances, simply because of the free energy available and the efficiency of the process. The bulk of the mitochondrially generated ATP then exchanges with ADP in the cytoplasm, providing the energy for myofibrillar contraction and other processes. This exchange is mediated by the adenine nucleotide translocase of the IMM, though there is evidence that PCr and creatine kinase are also involved in transferring so-called 'high-energy phosphate' from the mitochondria to the cytoplasm.[9]

Energy yields and O_2 consumption

The combined metabolism of glucose through anaerobic glycolysis and the TCA cycle allows a much greater release of free energy than metabolism through anaerobic glycolysis alone. Whereas metabolism of glucose to lactate results in the regeneration of 2 mol ATP/mol glucose, the complete oxidation of pyruvate to CO_2 and water yields about 18 mol ATP/mol pyruvate (assuming a P/O ratio of 3). Thus, the complete oxidation of 1 mol of glucose results in the regeneration of (2 + 18 + 18), i.e. 38 mol, ATP and is thus far more efficient in terms of chemical energy released than its metabolism to lactate. However, it is absolutely dependent on a well-developed blood supply to provide not only O_2 but also glucose. For the LCFA palmitic acid $[CH_3(CH_2)_{14}{\cdot}CO_2^-]$, 2 mol ATP equivalents are used in the activation of 1 mol palmitate to palmitoyl-CoA. Thereafter, seven rounds of β-oxidation will regenerate approximately 35 mol ATP/mol palmitate, and produce 8 mol acetyl-CoA. The ensuing eight turns of the TCA cycle will regenerate about 96 mol ATP/mol palmitate, a net resynthesis of about 129 mol of ATP/mol palmitate.

LCFA and glucose do not produce the same amount of ATP/O_2 reduced to H_2O (though we are assuming a P/O ratio of 3). For complete oxidation, glucose requires 6 mol O_2/mol glucose, thus providing 6.33 mol ATP/mol O_2. In contrast, the complete oxidation of palmitate requires 23 mol O_2/mol palmitate, thus providing 5.61 mol ATP/mol O_2. In other words, glucose offers an 'O_2 advantage' of about 10%. Whilst this may not be a significant factor in normal hearts, it might offer a significant advantage in situations where O_2 delivery is compromised (e.g. heart failure). In fact, experimental studies in pigs[10] suggest that glucose may offer as much as about a 50% advantage over LCFAs in terms of the myocardial O_2 uptake:left ventricle pressure–volume product because of factors additional to those conferred by simple energetic considerations. For example, 'uncoupling' of oxidative phosphorylation (reducing the proton motive force but maintaining O_2 consumption) by known endogenous uncouplers (for example, LCFAs, LCFA-CoA, and LCFA-carnitine, which are detergents and disrupt membrane structure) could reduce the P/O ratio.

Acute changes in cardiac energetics in hypoxia and ischaemia

Hypoxia

Although the terms 'hypoxia' (inadequate O_2 supply) and 'ischaemia' (inadequate blood supply) are used interchangeably, they are not necessarily synonymous. Hypoxia may occur in the absence of ischaemia, whereas ischaemia inevitably involves an element of hypoxia. *Ex vivo*, the glucose-perfused heart can survive a degree of hypoxia,[11] and this is presumably also true *in vivo*. However, the heart cannot survive total anaerobiosis because anaerobic carbohydrate metabolism would have to increase about 20-fold to satisfy cardiac energy requirements. This is impossible given the maximal activity of the glycolytic pathway. As O_2 tension falls, glucose uptake and glycolytic flux are increased, and glucose is increasingly metabolized anaerobically. Glycolytic pyruvate is reduced by NADH to lactate by lactate dehydrogenase, and the NAD^+ originating from glycolysis is regenerated (i.e. Equation 11.2 is reversed, being driven towards lactate production by the increased pyruvate, NADH, and H^+ concentrations). Lactate production increases but, assuming it can be released into the perfusion medium, this does not present a major problem. The same is probably true *in vivo* where lactate can be released into the coronary circulation if perfusion is maintained. Two mechanisms operate in the short term to maintain ATP. First, ATP is buffered by the creatine kinase equilibrium (Equation 11.1). Any intracellular acidification through lactate production drives the equilibrium to the right, favouring ATP resynthesis. However, as stated above, the operation of the creatine kinase equilibrium is probably only important in short term ATP buffering. Secondly, glycolytic flux is increased. Here, the adenylate kinase equilibrium (Equation 11.3) plays a central role:

$$\text{ATP} + \text{AMP} \rightleftharpoons 2\text{ADP} \qquad \text{(Equation 11.3)}$$

Numerous NMR studies have shown that the concentration of ATP in muscle cytoplasm is about 8–10 mM. The total concentration of ADP is about a tenth of this (though much of the ADP pool exists in a protein-bound state in muscle). From mass action considerations, a small percentage fall in ATP and the necessarily larger percentage increase in free ADP will be 'amplified' in terms of percentage increases in AMP concentrations. The situation is not as simple as this because AMP concentrations are additionally affected by changes in pH, PCr, free Mg^{2+}, and P_i. At physiological ATP concentrations, AMP is a powerful activator of 6-phosphofructo-1-kinase (PFK1), an important rate-controlling step of glycolysis, leading to an increase in glycolytic rate.

Glycogen breakdown is also increased by AMP (and catecholamine release) by activation of the glycogen phosphorylase step. The phosphorylated monosaccharidic glucose subunits enter glycolysis as glucose 6-phosphate (Fig. 11.1). Although each glycogen-derived 'glucose molecule' produces three molecules of ATP, one

ATP per glucose molecule is expended in glycogen synthesis, so the net production of ATP per glucose molecule remains at two (as in simple glycolysis).

Ischaemia

The most obvious pathological manifestation of cardiac hypoxia occurs during coronary artery disease and myocardial ischaemia. Myocardial infarction may totally deprive part of the heart of its blood supply, especially if there is no developed collateral circulation. In total ischaemia, the only intracellular metabolically available fuels are the limited free intracellular glucose and the glucose stored as glycogen. Essentially the same mechanisms operate to maintain ATP concentrations as those operating in hypoxia.

However, because lactate cannot be removed effectively from the myocyte, intracellular pH (pH_i) falls, and NADH accumulates. These eventually produce a profound inhibition of glycolysis because the 3-phosphoglyceraldehyde dehydrogenase step is inhibited by low pH and by product inhibition by NADH. In addition, binding of Ca^{2+} to the protein regulating myofibrillar contraction (the 'Ca^{2+} sensor', troponin C) is pH-sensitive and is disfavoured at lower pH_i values. Thus, a higher Ca^{2+} concentration is required to maintain an equivalent contractile force. This has energetic consequences for the ATP-consuming Ca^{2+} pumping involved in contraction, in that increased ATP consumption is necessary. Maintenance of ATP regeneration is impossible, ATP concentrations eventually fall, and contractile activity ceases.

Production of reactive oxygen species by mitochondria

Although complete four e^- reduction of O_2 to H_2O is the norm in oxidative phosphorylation, a small proportion of O_2 may be incompletely reduced by a single e^- to form superoxide anion radicals ($O_2{\bullet}^-$) even under normal aerobic conditions.[12] This potentially exposes tissues to cytotoxic oxidative stress from $O_2{\bullet}^-$ and $O_2{\bullet}^-$-derived reactive oxygen species (ROS). The proportion of O_2 reduced to $O_2{\bullet}^-$ *in vivo* is difficult to estimate, but, in isolated mitochondria, it may be as high as 1–2%.[12] This is probably a maximum figure because of the optimal experimental conditions used and, *in vivo*, $O_2{\bullet}^-$ formation is probably much less. However, given that cardiac myocytes contain abundant mitochondria that are continuously respiring, it is unlikely to be negligible. Furthermore, production of ROS rises during ischaemia and is increased further in any subsequent reperfusion.[12,13]. There are two major fates of $O_2{\bullet}^-$. First, although it is not a particularly reactive species itself, $O_2{\bullet}^-$ can react very rapidly with NO, which is itself a radical (more accurately $NO{\bullet}$), to form highly reactive peroxynitrite anions ($ONOO^-$) which damages macromolecules. Secondly, $O_2{\bullet}^-$ spontaneously dismutes into H_2O_2 and O_2. Dismutation (step (1) in Equation 11.4 below) is enhanced by superoxide dismutase (SOD), of which there are two isoforms, mitochondrial Mn^{2+}SOD or SOD2 and cytoplasmic Cu^{2+}/Zn^{2+}SOD or SOD1, thereby reducing formation of peroxynitrite. The importance of SOD2 is demonstrated by the finding that globally null SOD2 mice die in the early postnatal period, one of the pathological findings being a cardiomyopathy with clear fibrosis of the endocardium.[14] H_2O_2 is less reactive than $O_2{\bullet}^-$, and is rapidly decomposed into H_2O, and O_2 by catalase (step (2) in Equation 11.4):

$$\underset{\text{(Step 1)}}{2O_2{\bullet}^- + 2H^+ \rightarrow O_2 + H_2O_2} \underset{\text{(Step 2)}}{\rightarrow \tfrac{1}{2}O_2 + H_2O} \quad \text{(Equation 11.4)}$$

Even though it is rapidly destroyed, production of H_2O_2 may still be cytotoxic because, in the presence of transition metal ions (such as Fe^{2+} present within the myocyte), it will produce highly reactive hydroxyl radicals by the nonenzymic Fenton reaction. These species will damage macromolecules and react with metabolites.

Energetics in heart failure (HF)

The reasons underlying the transition of the heart into failure are probably manifold and multifactorial, but one aspect of the process involves cardiac energetics. Some of the changes seen in acute hypoxia and ischaemia contribute but there are additional changes, notably the long-term 'metabolic remodelling' of the heart. Partly because of ATP yield/O_2 (see above), the failing heart favours utilization of carbohydrates over lipid fuels and this involves changes in patterns of gene expression over the longer term.

Chronic changes in oxidative metabolism

In human HF, the levels of expression of genes associated with β-oxidation (medium-chain acyl-CoA dehydrogenase, long-chain acyl-CoA dehydrogenase), mitochondrial membrane fatty acid transport (the carnitine palmitoyl transferases), the TCA cycle (citrate synthase) and mitochondrial uncoupling protein 2 decline and, where examined, these changes are reflected at the protein level.[15,16] This suggests that the failing heart is less able to metabolize oxidatively. For carbohydrate metabolism, transcripts for the PDH kinases (the regulatory enzymes involved in the inhibition of PDH-MEC) and the GLUTs decline.[16] Assuming that these changes are reflected at the protein level, the latter will disfavour carbohydrate utilization whereas the former should favour oxidative metabolism of glucose. It is impossible to predict changes in biochemical processes simply on the basis of transcript abundances. Leaving these findings aside, the mechanisms by which oxidative capacity of the heart is regulated are becoming clearer, and here the peroxisome proliferator-activated receptors (PPARs) and the PPAR coactivators (PGCs) are important.

PPARs and PGCs

The PPARs, i.e. PPARα, PPARβ/δ, and the alternatively spliced forms of PPARγ ($PPAR\gamma_1$, $PPAR\gamma_2$, $PPAR\gamma_3$)[17] and PGCs (PGC-1α, PGC-1β, and PERC)[18–20] are central to the chronic regulation of oxidative metabolism. PPARs are nuclear receptors and transcription factors that act as 'lipid sensors', being activated by LCFAs and the products of their metabolism (Fig. 11.3). PPARγ is also the 'receptor' for the insulin-sensitizing thiazolidinedione drugs that are extensively used in the treatment of type 2 diabetes. PGC-1α acts as the master regulator of transcription by coactivating PPARs, and other transcription factors (nuclear respiratory factors, oestrogen-related receptors, retinoid X receptors) (Fig. 11.3). It is induced either at the level of transcription or is activated (either directly by post-translational modification or by release from repressor proteins) to promote a shift towards oxidative metabolism.

Therapeutic modulation of fuel utilization

Whether metabolic remodelling is detrimental or beneficial is still debated,[21] though the majority opinion believes that it is beneficial. The question of whether pharmacological agents that increase reliance of the early-stage failing heart on carbohydrate metabolism are beneficial then arises—or would a reversion to the normal

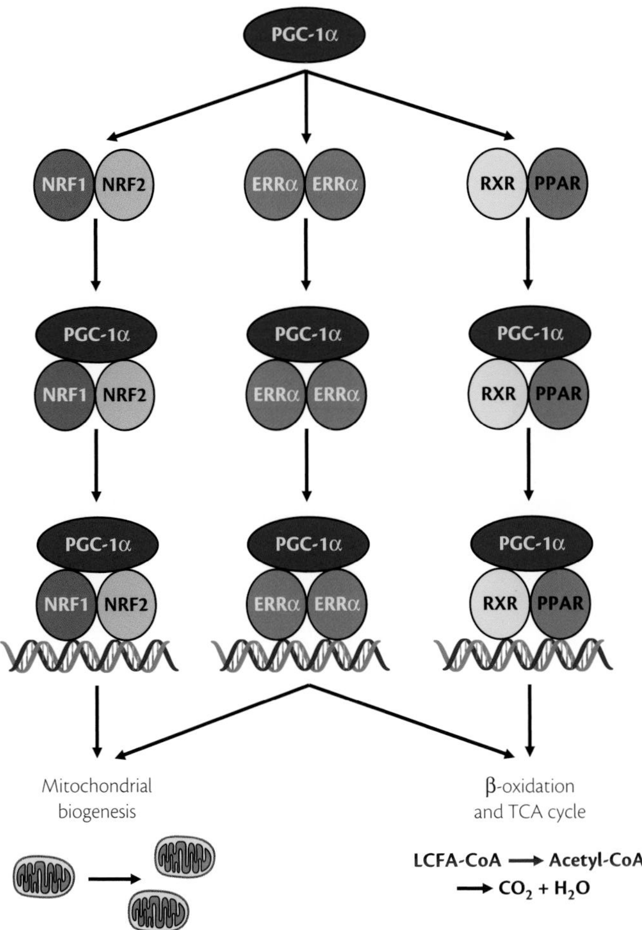

Fig. 11.3 Peroxisome proliferator-activated receptors (PPARs) and PPARs coactivators (PGCs). PGCs are master regulators at the level of gene expression of pathways involved in oxidative metabolism. They themselves are induced trancriptionally, and are activated under conditions where oxidative metabolism is enhanced (e.g. aerobic exercise). They bind to dimers of transcription factors such as nuclear respiratory factors (NRFs), oestrogen-related receptors (ERRs), retinoid X receptors (RXRs) and PPARs. PPARs are also receptors for LCFAs and their metabolites, which increase their ability to activate transcription. The trimers binds to the promoter regions of genes and, with ancillary proteins, increase the transcription of those genes. The genes are those concerned with promoting oxidative metabolism.

state of greater reliance on fatty fuels be preferable? This has been the focus of many reviews,[18,21–24] though it is probably too early to draw definite conclusions. The general approach involves inhibition of LCFA metabolism either by reduction of LCFA uptake into the mitochondria through inhibition of the carnitine palmitoyl transferases (Fig. 11.1) (etomoxir, oxfenicine, perhexiline) or inhibition of β-oxidation itself (Fig. 11.1) (ranolazine, trimetazidine).[22] There have been a few small-scale clinical trials of these reagents which appear hopeful, but a clear correlation of benefit with reduced LCFA metabolism is not always apparent. This is clearly an area where more data are required. The β-blocker carvedilol, which is of proven benefit in HF patients, may reduce LCFA metabolism[25] and this may contribute to its superiority over some other β-blockers. Apart from drug-based therapies, increased cardiac oxidative metabolism and energy transfer from exercise training may also contribute to its beneficial effects in HF.[26]

The lipotoxicity hypothesis

In partial or intermittent ischaemia, LCFA-CoA, and LCFA-carnitine accumulate because they cannot be oxidized. These are powerful detergents and they disrupt membranes to the detriment of cellular integrity. Triglycerides are synthesized because accumulating LCFA-CoA re-esterifies glycerol-3-phosphate (formed from the reduction of the glycolytic intermediate 3-phosphoglyceraldehyde by NADH):

$$\text{glycerol-3-phosphate} + 3\text{LCFA-CoA} \rightarrow \text{triglyceride} + P_i + 3\text{CoA} \qquad \text{(Equation 11.5)}$$

In cardiomyopathies that develop in genetic conditions which interfere with lipid oxidation, triglyceride accumulation is evident.[18] Furthermore, a reduced ability to oxidize lipids when they may be readily available (e.g. in diabetes) in early-stage HF may lead to 'lipotoxicity', a condition in which the accumulation of the intermediates of lipid oxidation and triglyceride is cytotoxic.[18,27,28]

Adenine nucleotide and creatine pools

ATP, total adenine nucleotides (TAN; ATP + ADP + AMP) and total creatine (PCr + creatine) pools are progressively lost in the failing heart.[29,30] As the metabolic pools diminish, oxidative stress increases. In the experimental setting—a pacing-induced (volume overload) canine model of HF—the transition point from the initial compensatory phase to the maladaptive phase corresponds to a 30% loss of TAN.[31] This transition point is also influenced by the total exchangeable phosphate pools (TEP; 2ATP + ADP + P_i + PCr + mitochondrial matrix GTP) and total creatine pool (PCr + creatine). Thus, at given values of TAN and TEP, the total creatine pool is adjusted to obtain the maximum available free energy from ATP hydrolysis and any changes (increases or decreases) in the total creatine pool will result in diminished performance unless accompanied by adjustments in TAN and TEP.[31]

The central role of AMP-activated protein kinase (AMPK)

At constant values of TAN, etc., proportionally small decreases in ATP concentrations are amplified as proportionally much larger increases in AMP concentrations by the adenylate kinase equilibrium (Equation 11.3). AMPK senses changes in AMP concentrations and functions as a 'cellular fuel gauge',[32–35] and it may represent a therapeutic target in cardiovascular disease.[36] Activation of AMPK (by AMP) shifts tissues from an anabolic state, in which protein, glycogen and fatty acid synthesis are favoured, to a catabolic state in which glucose uptake, glycolysis, fatty acid oxidation, and mitochondrial biogenesis are favoured (Fig. 11.4). This is achieved by AMPK-mediated phosphorylation of target proteins to modify their biological activity.[32–35] For example, AMPK phosphorylates the 6-phosphofructo-2-kinase/fructose-2,6-bisphosphatase bifunctional regulatory enzyme to stimulate the 6-phosphofructo-2-kinase activity (Fig. 11.1). Fructose 2,6-bisphosphate concentrations increase to activate the 'rate-controlling' PFK-1 step in glycolysis, thereby stimulating glycolytic flux.

Structure and regulation of AMPK

AMPK is a heterotrimer composed of an α (α_1 or α_2), β (β_1 or β_2), and a γ (γ_1, γ_2, or γ_3) subunit (Fig. 11.4). The α subunit is the catalytic subunit (the major species in heart is α_2), the β subunit is

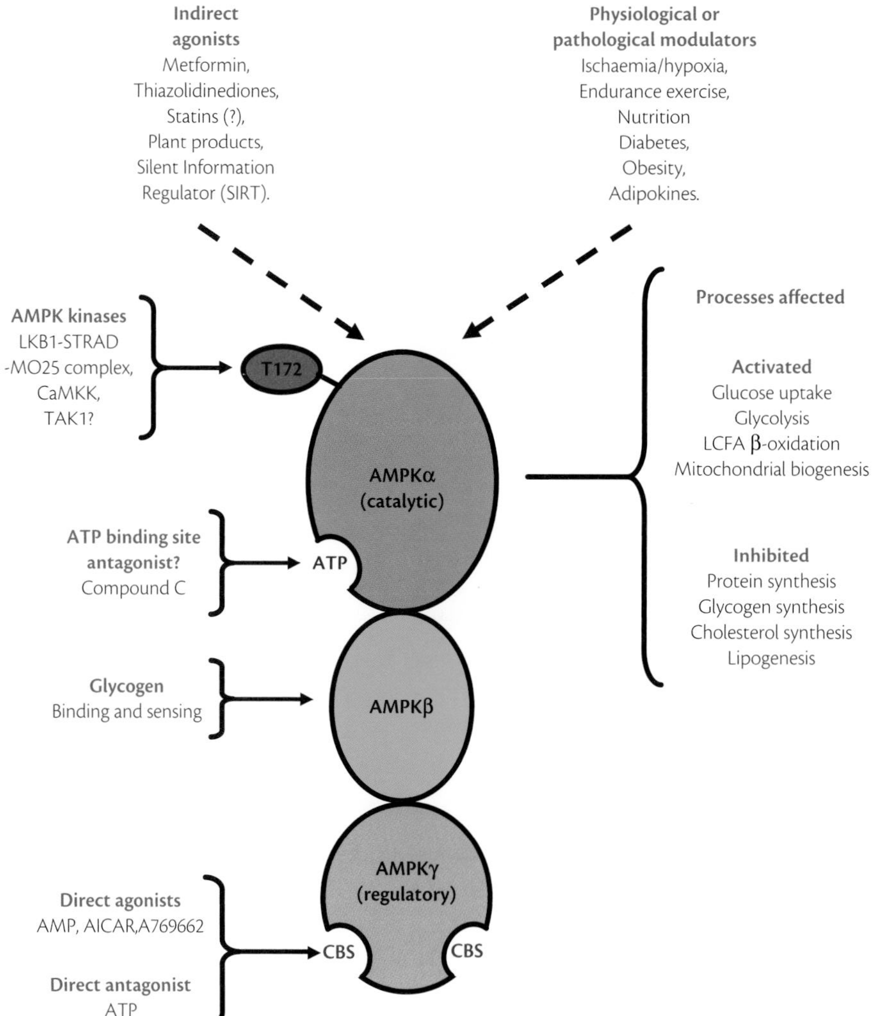

Fig. 11.4 AMP-activated protein kinase (AMPK). AMPK is the intracellular 'energy sensor' and is activated when ATP pools are depleted and AMP levels are increased. Activation of AMPK increases catabolism and decreases anabolism. As described in the text, it is a heterotrimer. The γ subunit contains two binding sites for AMP, the cystathionine β-synthase (CBS) domains, and this binding is antagonized by ATP. The β subunit is the glycogen binding/sensing subunit. The α subunit is the catalytic subunit and phosphorylates substrate proteins. It therefore has an ATP binding site. AMPK is itself activated by phosphorylation of threonine-172 (T172) in the α subunit and this is particularly favoured when the γ subunit is ligated to AMP. The best-characterized AMPK kinase is the tumour suppressor LKB1. AICAR, 5-amino-4-imidazolecarboxamide riboside; CaMKK, Ca^{2+}/calmodulin-dependent kinase; LCFA, long-chain fatty acid; TAK1, transforming growth factor β-activated kinase 1.

a 'scaffold' which may be involved in binding to and quantitative sensing of glycogen, and the γ subunit is the regulatory adenine nucleotide binding subunit. AMPK activity is regulated in two ways. The γ subunit contains two adenine nucleotide binding sites (each composed of two 'cystathionine β-synthase' or 'Bateman' hemidomains) which may differ in their affinities for adenine nucleotides and in their relative effects. Binding of AMP activates AMPK whereas ATP competes with AMP to inhibit AMPK activity. Maximally, AMP binding increases AMPK activity by about 10-fold. In addition, phosphorylation of the α subunit (on a threonine residue, Thr-172) activates AMPK about 100-fold and this phosphorylation is favoured when AMPK is in its AMP-ligated state. There are a number of upstream protein kinases which reportedly effect this activation, but the best characterized is the tumour suppressor LKB1. Indeed, the tumour-suppressive properties of LKB1 probably involve an element of AMP-mediated inhibition of cell growth.

Ischaemia, heart failure, and AMPK

Ex vivo, AMPK is activated in both myocardial ischaemia and in ischaemia/reperfusion (AMP/ATP increased), and this increases fatty acid oxidation during reperfusion by inhibiting acetyl-CoA carboxylase (the first step in fatty acid synthesis).[37] Studies in experimental animals indicate that AMPK is activated in left ventricular hypertrophy and HF.[38,39] Whether activation of AMPK in acute stress (short-term ischaemia, ischaemia/reperfusion) or chronic (HF) stress is beneficial or detrimental is still debated.[40] Activation of AMPK is also seen in the heart following exercise[41] and presumably will lead to mitochondrial biogenesis during which, by analogy with skeletal muscle, AMPK activates PGC-1.[42] If this is the case, oxidative metabolism and mitochondrial biogenesis should be favoured during failure, quite the reverse of the demonstrated increased dependence of the failing heart on carbohydrate (and anaerobic?) metabolism.

Conversely, transgenic mice which cardiospecifically overexpress an inhibitory ('dominant-negative') form of the AMPK α_2 subunit (to limit activation of AMPK) have been engineered. Here, inhibition of AMPK activation is not detrimental and may even be beneficial in recovery from *ex vivo* ischaemia on reperfusion.[43] This conclusion concurs with an earlier study using hearts from AMPK α_2-null mice perfused *ex vivo*.[44] Here, although the ischaemic contracture in AMPK α_2-null hearts was more severe with an earlier onset than with wild-type hearts, the degree of functional recovery during reperfusion did not differ.

AMPK-directed therapies in heart failure?

Other than the studies described in the previous section, is there any evidence that modulation of AMPK activity or its downstream effectors is valuable in heart disease?[36] The biguanide metformin has been used extensively in type 2 diabetes, and there is evidence that it ameliorates any associated HF. Metformin appears to be beneficial in experimentally induced HF.[39] Metformin is a weak 'uncoupler' of oxidative phosphorylation (P/O ratio decreased), leads to decreased ATP/ADP ratios, and to increases in AMP concentrations and activation of AMPK (Fig. 11.4). The thiazolidinediones (also used in type 2 diabetes) may also have a beneficial effect, though their use in HF may be contraindicated because of increased water retention. Although the target for these drugs is PPARγ, PPARγ itself may upregulate release of the adipokine adiponectin from adipose tissue, leading to activation of AMPK in other tissues. Assuming that AMPK activation is beneficial in HF, direct activation of AMPK would seem desirable. In the laboratory setting, 5-amino-4-imidazolecarboxamide riboside (AICAR) is used, but this is unsuitable for clinical use. The AMPK activator A769662 has poor bioavailability, and effort is now being expended in synthesizing more useful derivatives.

Mutations in AMPK leading to heart failure

Mutations in the γ_2 subunit of AMPK (expressed in both cardiac and skeletal muscle) give rise to an autosomal-dominant cardiac phenotype (characterized by a Wolff–Parkinson–White type premature excitation arrhythmia and glycogen accumulation).[34,45] Although originally thought to be a 'cardiac hypertrophy', the increased size and weight of the heart is caused by glycogen accumulation and the bound water associated with it. The precise cause of the arrhythmia is not understood but the assumption is that glycogen accumulation introduces alternative atrioventricular conduction pathways. Eight of the 10 individual mutations associated with the disease map to the two AMPK (γ subunit adenine nucleotide binding sites. Two (spontaneous) mutations give rise to a particularly severe phenotype leading to early infant mortality, and these are therefore not heritable. The precise cause of the glycogen accumulation is unclear. If AMP is unable to activate AMPK, cardiac anabolism would be favoured with concurrent synthesis of glycogen and lipids. Equally, if ATP is unable to inhibit AMPK, its basal activity would increase, favouring glucose uptake, and LCFA oxidation. However, operation of the Randle cycle (Fig. 11.1) could suppress glycolysis at the 6-phosphofructo-1-kinase step, and cause accumulation of glucose 6-phosphate. This might drive synthesis of glycogen. Indeed, a transgenic mouse model in which the AMPK γ subunit is mutated displays the characteristics of the latter scenario, with increased glucose uptake and fatty acid oxidation, and accumulation of glycogen.[46]

References

1. Bing RJ. Cardiac metabolism. *Physiol Rev* 1965;**45**:171–213.
2. Shwenk RW, Luiken JJFP, Bonen A, Glatz JFC. Regulation of sarcolemmal glucose and fatty acid transporters in cardiac disease. *Cardiovasc Res* 2008;**79**:249–58.
3. Patel MS, Roche TE. Molecular biology and biochemistry of pyruvate dehydrogenase complexes. *FASEB J* 1990;**4**:3224–33.
4. Randle PJ, Garland PB, Hales CN, Newsholme EA. The glucose-fatty acid cycle. Its role in insulin sensitivity and the metabolic disturbances of diabetes mellitus. *Lancet* 1963;**i**(7285):785–789.
5. Sugden MC, Holness MJ. Mechanisms underlying regulation of the expression and activities of the mammalian pyruvate dehydrogenase kinases. *Arch Physiol Biochem* 2006;**112**:139–49.
6. Hue L, Taegtmeyer H. The Randle cycle revisited: a new head for an old hat. *Am J Physiol Endocrinol Metab* 2009;**297**: E578–91.
7. Harold FM. Gleanings of a chemiosmotic eye. *Bioessays* 2001;**23**: 848–55.
8. Nicholls DG. Forty years of Mitchell's proton circuit: from little grey books to little grey cells. *Biochim Biophys Acta* 2008;**1777**:550–6.
9. Walliman T, Dolder M, Schlattner U, *et al.* Some new aspects of creatine kinase (CK): compartmentation, structure, function and regulation for cellular and mitochondrial bioenergetics and physiology. *Biofactors* 1998;**8**:229–34.
10. Korvald C, Elvenes OP, Myrmel T. Myocardial substrate metabolism influences left ventricular energetics in vivo. *Am J Physiol Heart Circ Physiol* 2000;**278**:H1345–51.
11. Smith DM, Sugden PH. The effects of insulin and lack of effect of workload and hypoxia on protein degradation in the perfused working rat heart. *Biochem J* 1983;**210**:55–61.
12. Murphy MR. How mitochondria produce reactive oxygen species. *Biochem J* 2009;**417**:1–13.
13. Solaini G, Harris DA. Biochemical dysfunction in heart mitochondria exposed to ischaemia and reperfusion. *Biochem J* 2005;**390**:377–94.
14. Li Y, Huang T-T, Carlson EJ, *et al.* Dilated cardiomyopathy and neonatal lethality in mutant mice lacking manganese superoxide dismutase. *Nat Genet* 1995;**11**:376–81.
15. Sack MN, Rader TA, Park S, Bastin J, McCune SA, Kelly DP. Fatty acid oxidation enzyme gene expression is downregulated in the failing heart. *Circulation* 1996;**94**:2837–42.
16. Razeghi P, Young ME, Alcorn JL, Moravec CS, Frazier OH, Taegtmeyer H. Metabolic gene expression in fetal and failing human heart. *Circulation* 2001;**104**:2923–31.
17. Evans RM, Barish GD, Wang Y-X. PPARs and the complex journey to obesity. *Nat Med* 2004;**10**:351–61.
18. Huss JM, Kelly DP. Mitochondrial energy metabolism in heart failure: a question of balance. *J Clin Invest* 2005;**115**:547–55.
19. Finck BN, Kelly DP. PGC-1 coactivators: inducible regulators of energy metabolism in health and disease. *J Clin Invest* 2006;**116**:615–22.
20. Ventura-Clapier R, Garnier A, Veksler V. Transcriptional control of mitochondrial biogenesis: the central role of PGC-1 . *Cardiovasc Res* 2008;**79**:208–17.
21. van Bilsen M, van Nieuwenhoven FA, van der Vusse GJ. Metabolic remodelling of the failing heart: beneficial or detrimental?. *Cardiovasc Res* 2009;**81**:420–8.
22. Abozguia K, Clarke K, Lee L, Frenneaux M. Modification of myocardial substrate use as a therapy for heart failure. *Nat Clin Pract Cardiovasc Med* 2006;**3**:490–8.
23. Kodde IF, van der Stok J, Smolenski RT, de Jong JW. Metabolic and genetic regulation of cardiac energy substrate preference. *Comp Biochem Physiol A Mol Integr Physiol* 2007;**146**:26–39.
24. Fragasso G, Salerno A, Spoladore R, Basanelli G, Arioli F, Margonato A. Metabolic therapy of heart failure. *Curr Pharm Des* 2008;**14**:2582–91.
25. Wallhaus TR, Taylor M, DeGrado TR, *et al.* Myocardial free fatty acid and glucose use after carvedilol treatment in patients with congestive heart failure. *Circulation* 2001;**103**:2441–6.
26. Ventura-Clapier R. Exercise training, energy metabolism, and heart failure. *Appl Physiol Nutr Metab* 2009;**34**:336–9.
27. Borradaile NM, Schaffer JE. Lipotoxicity in the heart. *Curr Hypertens Rep* 2005;**7**:412–17.
28. Chess DJ, Stanley WC. Role of diet and fuel overabundance in the development and progression of heart failure. *Cardiovasc Res* 2008;**79**:269–78.
29. Ingwall JS, Weiss RG. Is the failing heart energy starved? On using chemical energy to support heart function. *Circ Res* 2004;**95**:135–45.
30. Ingwall JS. Energy metabolism in heart failure and remodelling. *Cardiovasc Res* 2009;**81**:412–19.
31. Wu F, Zhang J, Beard DA. Experimentally observed phenomena on cardiac energetics in heart failure emerge from simulations of cardiac metabolism. *Proc Natl Acad Sci U S A* 2009;**106**:7143–8.

32. Hardie DG. AMP-activated/SNF1 protein kinases: conserved guardians of cellular energy. *Nat Rev Mol Cell Biol* 2007;**8**:774–785.
33. Carling D, Sanders MJ, Woods A. The regulation of AMP-activated protein kinase by upstream kinases. *Int J Obes (Lond)* 2008;**32** (Suppl. 4):S55–9.
34. Hardie DG. Role of AMP-activated protein kinase in the metabolic syndrome and heart disease. *FEBS Lett* 2008;**582**:81–9.
35. Steinberg GR, Kemp BE. AMPK in health and disease. *Physiol Rev* 2009;**89**:1025–78.
36. Wong AKF, Howie J, Petrie JR, Lang CC. AMP-activated protein kinase pathway: a potential therapeutic target in cardiometabolic disease. *Clin Sci (Lond)* 2009;**116**:607–20.
37. Kudo N, Barr AJ, Barr RL, Desai S, Lopaschuk GD. High rates of fatty acid oxidation during reperfusion of ischemic hearts are associated with a decrease in malonyl-CoA levels due to an increase in 5′-AMP-activated protein kinase inhibition of acetyl-CoA carboxylase. *J Biol Chem* 1995;**270**:17513–20.
38. Tian R, Musi N, D'Agostino J, Hirshman MF, Goodyear LJ. Increased adenosine monophosphate-activated protein kinase activity in rat hearts with pressure-overload hypertrophy. *Circulation* 2001;**104**:1664–9.
39. Sasaki H, Asanuma H, Fujita M, *et al.* Metformin prevents progression of heart failure in dogs: role of AMP-activated protein kinase. *Circulation* 2009;**119**:2568–77.
40. Lopaschuk GD. AMP-activated protein kinase control of energy metabolism in the ischemic heart. *Int J Obes (Lond)* 2008;**32** (suppl.4):S29–35.
41. Coven DL, Hu X, Cong L, *et al.* Physiological role of AMP-activated protein kinase in the heart: graded activation during exercise. *Am J Physiol Endocrinol Metab* 2003;**285**:E629–36.
42. Zong H, Ren JM, Young LH, *et al.* AMP kinase is required for mitochondrial biogenesis in skeletal muscle in response to chronic energy deprivation. *Proc Natl Acad Sci U S A* 2002;**99**:15983–7.
43. Folmes CD, Wagg CS, Shen M, Clanachan AS, Tian R, Lopaschuk GD. Suppression of 5′-AMP-activated protein kinase activity does not impair recovery of contractile function during reperfusion of ischemic hearts. *Am J Physiol Heart Circ Physiol* 2009;**297**: H313–21.
44. Zarrinpashneh E, Carjaval K, Beauloye C, *et al.* Role of the α_2-isoform of AMP-activated protein kinase in the metabolic response of the heart to no-flow ischemia. *Am J Physiol Heart Circ Physiol* 2006;**291**:H2875–83.
45. Arad M, Seidman CE, Seidman JG. AMP-activated protein kinase in the heart: role during health and disease. *Circ Res* 2007;**100**:474–88.
46. Luptak I, Shen M, He H, *et al.* Aberrant activation of AMP-activated protein kinase remodels metabolic network in favor of cardiac glycogen storage. *J Clin Invest* 2007;**117**:1432–9.

12

The failing cardiomyocyte

Alexander Lyon and Sian Harding

Introduction

The human myocardium consists of a variety of different cell types. The cell that has been most extensively studied is the cardiomyocyte, which represents the single contracting unit of the myocardium. It has been estimated that there are 3 billion cardiomyocytes in the human ventricular myocardium, organized into the complex three-dimensional architecture of the ventricular myocardial tissue. Conceptually there are two underlying pathophysiological problems at the level of the cardiomyocyte which drive the functional deterioration of the failing heart. The first is numerical loss of cardiomyocytes, due both to the underlying causal disease process, such as acute myocardial infarction or chemotherapy, and to further loss secondary to apoptosis and necrosis triggered by the neurohormonal and inflammatory activation in the failing myocardium irrespective of the initial injury. Secondly, the remaining viable cardiomyocytes are required to provide sufficient contractile force to maintain an adequate cardiac output, despite loss of significant numbers and abnormal stress–strain relationships resulting from altered chamber geometry and extracellular matrix remodelling. The surviving cardiomyocytes compensate temporarily via transition to an adaptive hypertrophic state,[1, 2] which is associated with activation of fetal gene expression patterns.[3] However, the persistent drive from the neurohormonal activation to maintain cardiac output, and activation of systemic inflammatory systems secondary to tissue hypoperfusion and congestion, combined with reduced metabolic efficiency in the hypertrophied cardiomyocytes, results in the development of contractile dysfunction of the hypertrophied cardiomyocyte.[4] This is independent of the underlying cause of heart failure (HF), some of which cause further continuing impairment of cardiomyocyte function, such as familial dilated cardiomyopathy due to mutations in the cytoskeletal or sarcomeric proteins.[5]

The common endpoint for the failing heart, irrespective of underlying aetiology, is characterized at a cellular and molecular level by a distinctive failing signature. Cardiomyocytes isolated from failing human and animal hearts demonstrate impairment of both contraction (inotropy) and relaxation (lusitropy).[6] Mechanical dysfunction of failing cardiomyocytes is amplified at higher beating frequencies, increased calcium concentration or during catecholamine stimulation. The loss of the force-frequency response (the Treppe or Bowditch effect) is a hallmark characteristic of HF (Fig. 12.1).[6]

A variety of different pathophysiological factors have been proposed to underlie these mechanical alterations, including abnormal morphological and structural remodelling, and functional changes in signalling pathways, ionic fluxes, organelle function, and gene expression. It is becoming increasingly apparent that these are not independent processes; rather, crosstalk and interplay between the different pathophysiological processes serve to amplify the abnormalities and drive the deterioration of the failing cardiomyocyte phenotype.

Morphological changes

Cardiomyocyte size and shape

Healthy human cardiomyocytes are elongated, rod-shaped structures, typically 20–30 μm wide, approximately 100 μm in length, and 20–30 μm in depth.[7] Studies using micropipettes record a cardiomyocyte cell capacitance of ~100 pF, equating to a volume of ~30 pL.[8] A characteristic of failing cardiomyocytes is hypertrophy and enlargement (Fig. 12.2). The precise changes depend upon the underlying disease. For example, cardiomyocytes from ventricles with pressure overload, as in left ventricular hypertrophy secondary to hypertension or aortic stenosis, exhibit increases in width and length, whereas cells from ventricles experiencing volume overload, as in mitral regurgitation or advanced dilated cardiomyopathy, demonstrate increases predominantly in length.[4] Endstage failing hearts explanted at transplantation contain myocytes exhibiting a decompensated failing phenotype. These cells are larger than normal myocytes, but smaller than cells isolated from hearts with compensated left ventricular hypertrophy. Comparison of size changes with alteration in function concluded that the two were independent, and

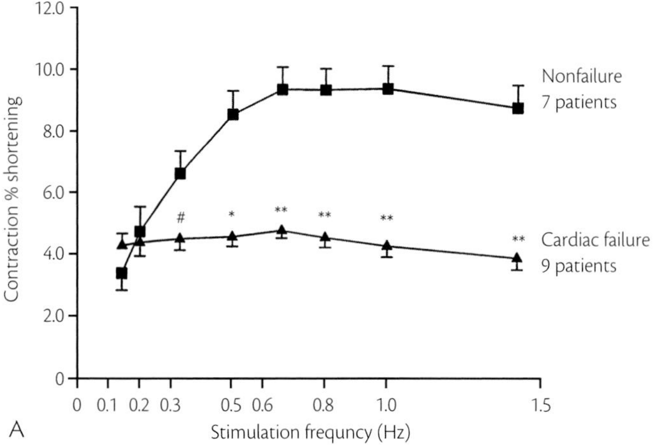

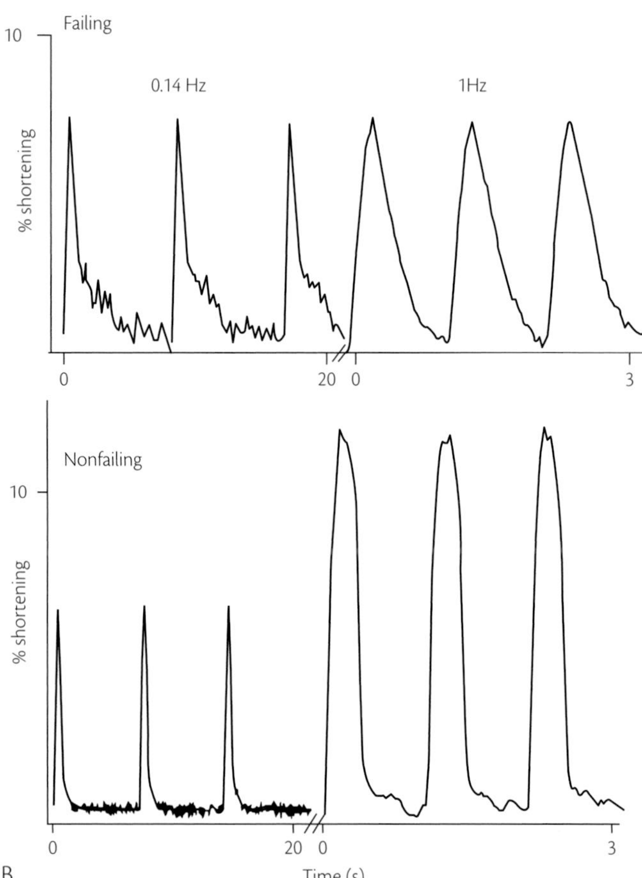

Fig. 12.1 Impaired force-frequency response and abnormal contraction and relaxation kinetics in failing human cardiomyocytes. (A) Plot of changes in cell length expressed in percentage shortening in response to increasing stimulation rate (maximally stimulating Ca^{2+} and 37°C). ANCOVA, failing vs nonfailing hearts, $P<.001$. #$P<.05$, *$P<.01$, **$P<.001$, by *t* test. (B) Tracings at high speed of cells from failing and nonfailing hearts at 0.14 and 1.0 Hz in maximal Ca^{2+}. At 0.14 Hz, there is prolongation of relaxation in the myocyte from the failing heart (top) compared with the nonfailing control heart (bottom). Although still evident at 1.0 Hz, this phenomenon becomes less prominent owing to an acceleration of relaxation in the myocyte from a failing heart. From Davies CH, Davia K, Bennett JG, Pepper JR, Poole-Wilson PA, Harding SE. Reduced contraction and altered frequency response of isolated ventricular myocytes from patients with heart failure. *Circulation* 1995;**92**:2540–9, with permission.

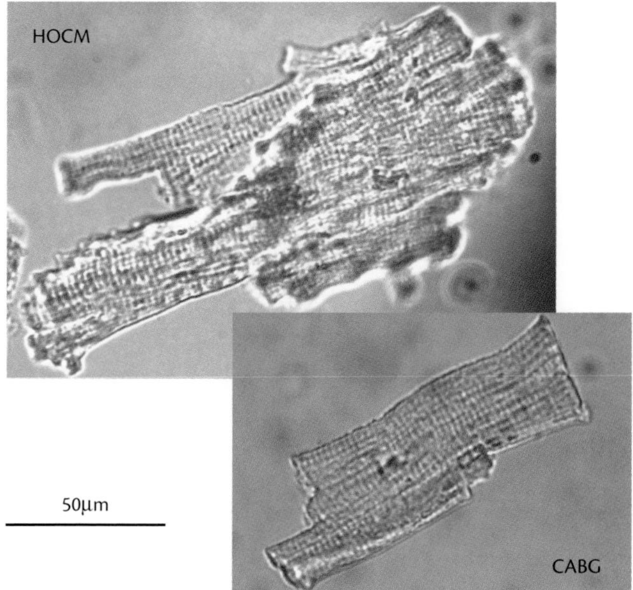

Fig. 12.2 Brightfield images of human ventricular myocytes from (A) a biopsy of nonfailing heart taken during the CABG procedure and (B) a sample taken from a DCM patient during cardiac transplantation.

that even those cells with normal dimensions from hypertrophied heart were compromised.[9]

Surface topology

Normal ventricular cardiomyocytes are characterized by extremely organized surface architecture, reflecting the intracellular organization of the sarcomeric units for optimal excitation–contraction (E-C) coupling. High-resolution scanning ion-conductance microscopy (SICM) and freeze-fracture electron microscopy reveal the regular pattern of indented grooves of the sarcolemma which overlie the Z line of the myofilament sarcomere (Fig. 12.3).[10] These Z grooves serve critical functional roles. They form an anatomical restraint for sarcolemmal ion channels and receptors, allowing spatial compartmentalization of cell surface signalling,[11] and also contain the origin of the transverse tubule (T-tubule) openings, which invaginate deep into the myocyte and underpin the spatial coupling of T-tubule and sarcoplasmic reticulum for efficient E-C coupling.[12] Between these surface Z grooves lies the crest region of the cardiomyocyte. Normal cells are identified by the regular alternating architecture of Z grooves and crest membrane.[10] In failing cardiomyocytes isolated from both endstage failing human hearts at transplantation, and animal models of chronic HF, this surface topology is severely disrupted, with loss of Z grooves, alteration of crest structures, and loss of T-tubule openings (see Fig. 12.3).[13] These changes have numerous functional consequences, such as spatial disruption and temporal delay in E-C coupling. Interestingly, these morphological changes appear independent of the underlying aetiology of the HF, and reflect the part of the common phenotype of endstage decompensated failing hearts.

Intercellular communication

Cardiomyocytes in healthy hearts are precisely integrated into the myocardial syncytium, with intercellular communication and passage of signalling molecules and electrical currents facilitated

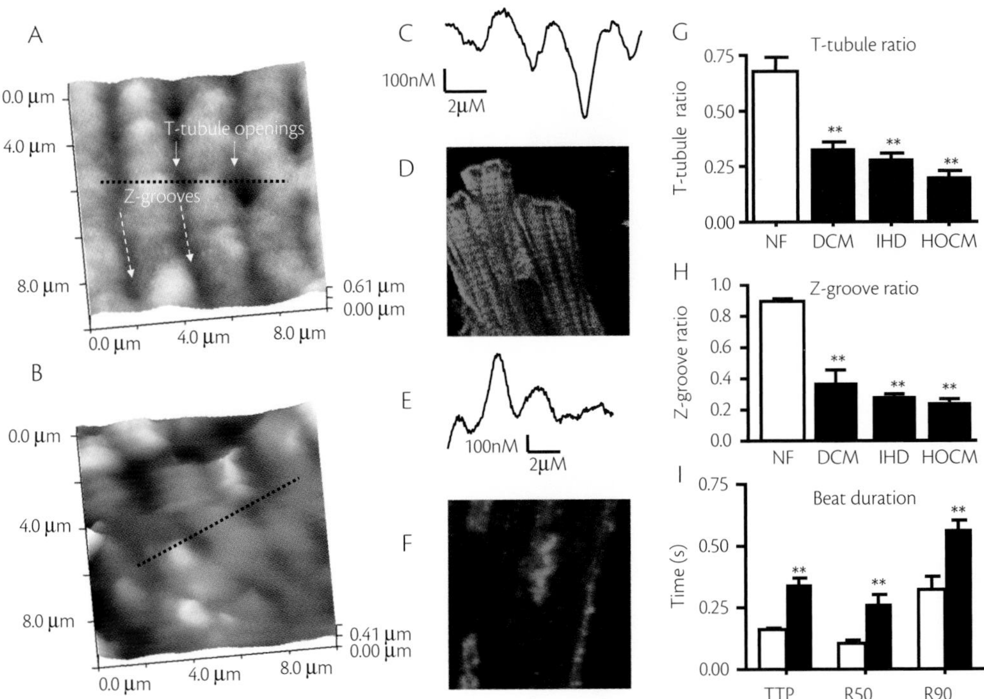

Fig. 12.3 Scanning ion-conductance microscopy images from the surface of cardiomyocytes isolated from nonfailing (A) and failing (B) human hearts. The black dotted line represents the linear selection presented as a one-dimensional surface contour map from nonfailing (C) and failing (E) human cardiomyocytes. Confocal images after staining with di-8-ANNEPPS in nonfailing (D) and failing cardiomyocytes (F).

From Lyon AR, MacLeod KT, Zhang Y, *et al.* Loss of T-tubules and other changes to surface topography in ventricular myocytes from failing human and rat heart. *Proc Natl Acad Sci U S A* 2009;**106**(16):6854–9, with permission of the National Academy of Sciences.

by gap junctions (GJs) located predominantly at intercalated discs. GJs are small macromolecular channels composed of channel-forming proteins known as connexins. One GJ is formed by two hemichannels, each consisting of six connexin molecules arranged in a hexagonal array around a central aqueous pore. The channels conduct ions between neighbouring cardiomyocytes, allowing current charge to flow between cells: the channels are thus critical in determining the efficacy of electrical wavefront conduction across the heart.[14] The transfer of charge between coupled cardiomyocytes depends upon the number of GJs, their location, and the conductivity of each GJ. GJ conductivity depends upon the connexin subtype, with connexin 43 (Cx43) being the major connexin isoform expressed in ventricular cardiomyocytes.[15] Other important factors regulating GJ function include post-translational modifications such as phosphorylation (e.g. protein kinase C), local $[Ca^{2+}]_i$, and interaction with a variety of other structural and regulatory proteins, such as N-cadherin, which determine Cx43 delivery and location within the intercalated disc.[16]

Cx43 expression, phosphorylation, and conductance are altered in ischaemic or failing human and animal myocardium, with Cx43 redistribution away from the intercalated discs and more even distribution across the cardiomyocyte surface [15,17–19] (Fig. 12.4). This impairs charge transfer between cardiomyocytes, reducing electrical and functional coupling, which may expose differences in action potential duration (APD) between uncoupled cardiomyocytes, and may predispose to conduction block.

Animal HF models have provided further insights into the role of connexins in the development of both contractile and electrical dysfunction in the failing heart. There is a uniform reduction in connexin expression in the canine tachycardia–cardiomyopathy model, which amplifies both the gradient for APD dispersion and the conduction slowing in the subepicardial border with the M cells.[20] The reduction of Cx43 levels precedes the development of reduced conduction velocity, and a relative increase in the unphosphorylated Cx43 correlates with the onset of significant left ventricular impairment in the pacing HF model.[21] The change in Cx43 phosphorylation status correlates with the shift in GJ distribution away from the intercalated discs and towards the lateral sarcolemmal membranes (see Fig. 12.4). Alterations in cellular Cx43 distribution have also been reported in models of left ventricular dysynchrony secondary to left bundle branch block with abnormal patterns of ventricular activation.[22] This compounds the mechanical and electrophysiological impairment resulting from dyssynchrony, and interestingly these changes in Cx43 distribution are normalized by biventricular pacing.

Extracellular matrix

In the failing heart, in addition to gap junction uncoupling between cardiomyocytes, there are significant changes in the extracellular matrix (ECM) and architecture of the myocardium leading to cell slippage and increased resistance between cardiomyocytes,[23–25] microscopic and/or macroscopic scar formation, and altered perfusion with generation of ischaemia. Cardiac fibroblasts in failing hearts increase in number, demonstrate increased metabolic activity, and increase interstitial matrix synthesis and deposition.[26,27] Fibroblast proliferation is driven by neurohormal activation.[28,29]

The ECM includes interstitial collagens, proteoglycans, glycoproteins, cytokines, growth factors, matrikines, and proteases. Increased deposition of extracellular matrix in the failing heart

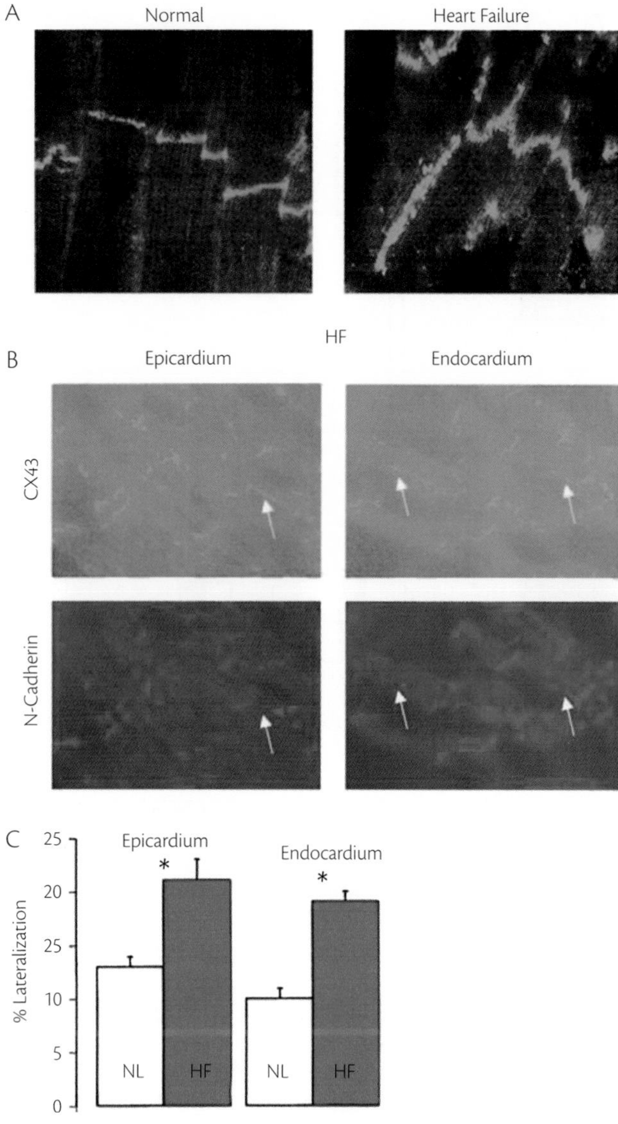

Fig. 12.4 Redistribution of connexin 43 to lateral cardiomyocyte membranes in ventricular myocardium from a canine model of tachycardia-induced HF. (A) Representative epicardial sections from a normal and failing heart showing lateralization of Cx43 in HF. (B) Colocalization of Cx43 and N-cadherin fluorescence in representative epicardial and endocardial tissue slices from a failing heart. (C) Bar plots quantifying the degree of lateralization (absence of colocalization with N-cadherin) of Cx43 in epicardial and endocardial layers of normal (NL) and failing (HF) hearts.

From Akar FG, Spragg DD, Tunin RS, Kass DA, Tomaselli GF. Mechanisms underlying conduction slowing and arrhythmogenesis in nonischemic dilated cardiomyopathy. *Circ Res* 2004;**95**(7):717–25.

has a number of important functional sequelae. At a cellular level, cardiomyocytes interact with the ECM via a number of adhesion proteins or anchors. In addition to providing structural support and transmitting mechanical forces from myofilament cross-bridging, these also serve to activate adverse intracellular secondary messenger pathways.[30] Interstitial matrix deposition also increases spatial uncoupling between adjacent cardiomyocytes. These changes reduce conduction velocity of the electrical depolarization wavefront, contributing to the arrhythmic substrate with focal points of conduction block [31]. Furthermore, fibroblasts within failing myocardium demonstrate increased connexin expression, and may form GJs with cardiomyocytes. The functional chemical and metabolic consequences of these *de novo* cell-to-cell contacts remain to be explored, but the potential adverse effects on myocardial electrical properties have been demonstrated.[32] Increased fibrosis is frequently noted around arterioles and capillaries, and contributes to the microvascular dysfunction and secondary myocardial ischaemia in the failing heart, irrespective of aetiology (Fig. 12.5).[33]

Functional changes

Impaired β-adrenoceptor signalling

Sympathetic stimulation of healthy ventricular muscle is predominantly achieved via activation of the β_1- and β_2-adrenoceptors (β_1AR, β_2AR) located on the cardiomyocyte sarcolemma. β_1AR is the commonest receptor subtype, accounting for about 80% of βAR protein in healthy ventricular tissue. β_1AR and β_2AR are G-protein coupled receptors, and are targets for both noradrenaline released from local sympathetic nerve endings, and circulating adrenaline diffusing from the coronary circulation. Under normal physiological conditions, agonist binding to either receptor induces activation of Gs protein secondary messenger system. Ligand binding to the βAR initiates a conformational change with release of the Gsα and Gβγ subunits. Gsα activates adenylyl cyclase, an enzyme which catalyses the production of cyclic 3′, 5′-AMP (cAMP) and activation of protein kinase A (PKA).

PKA phosphorylates of a number of critical proteins involved in the E-C coupling system, including the L-type Ca^{2+} channel (LTCC), increasing LTCC opening probability; the cardiac ryanodine receptor (RyR), increasing RyR opening probability and calcium release from the sarcoplasmic reticulum (SR) stores; troponin I, reducing the affinity of troponin I for troponin C; and phospholamban (PLB), reducing PLB-mediated inhibition of the SR calcium ATPase channel (SERCA2a).[34] These effects all increase the gain of the E-C coupling system during cardiomyocyte contraction and relaxation, leading to the positive inotropic and lusitropic response of ventricular myocardium to catecholamines after βAR activation.

A number of major and predominantly detrimental changes to this system occur in the failing heart. Firstly, there is chronically elevated sympathetic tone in patients with HF, driving chronic activation of the βAR system.[35] The effect is counterbalanced as βAR expression and density is reduced in cardiac failure.[36] Human myocytes from chronically failing hearts have a blunted contractile response to βAR stimulation, with a decreased β1AR:β2AR ratio[37] and an increased Gi:Gs ratio (Fig. 12.6).[38] The extent of the decrease correlates with the severity of cardiac impairment, and predominantly affects the β_1AR, whose levels can be reduced by up to 50%. β_2AR levels remain stable or are reduced only marginally, and as a result the β_1AR:β_2AR ratio is reduced from 4:1 towards 1:1 in failing hearts.

Levels of Giα increase, with a down-regulation of Gsα, and this change in the Gs:Gi protein ratio is critical in the failing cardiomyocyte as β_2ARs (relatively increased in the failing myocardium) couple additionally to Gi proteins.[39] Inhibition of Gi activation using pertussis toxin can reverse functional βAR desensitization in ventricular myocytes from human (and guinea-pig) heart.[40] Increased β_2AR-Giα signalling in response to catecholamine stimulation results in a negative inotropic response.[41] The precise

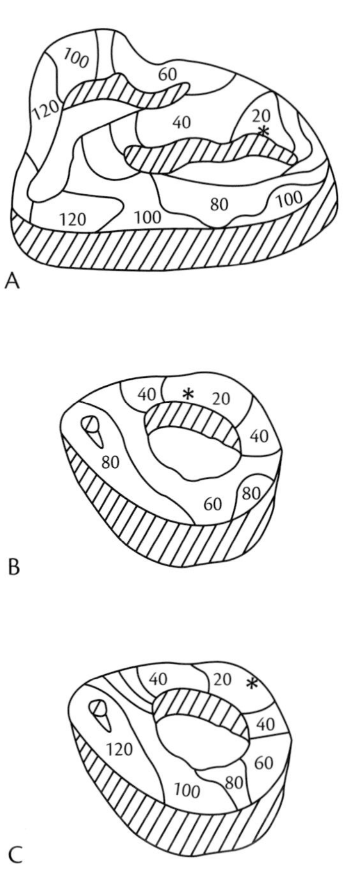

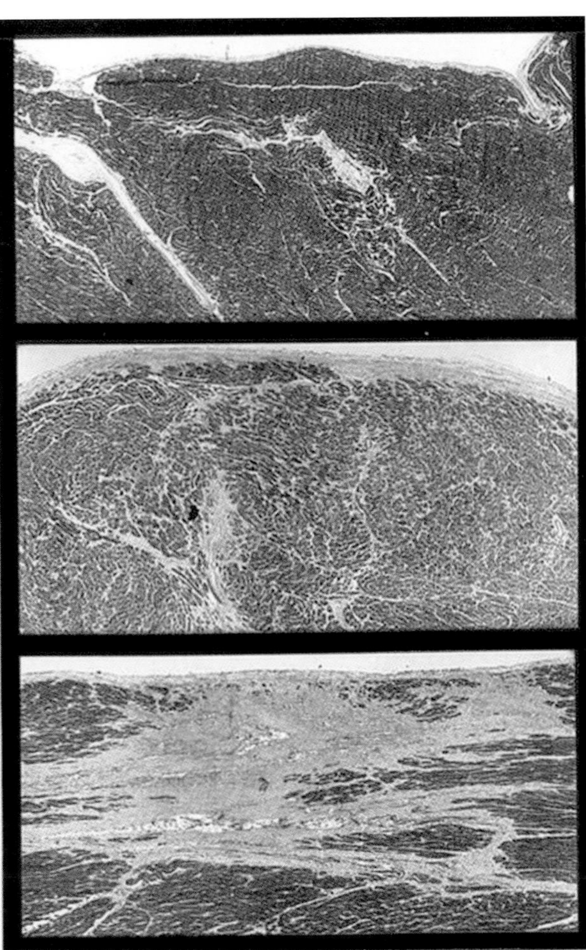

Fig. 12.5 Regional fibrosis is located in areas of increased focal triggered activity within failing human hearts. Left: Sections from activation maps showing sites of focal initiation of ventricular arrhythmias (*). (A) spontaneously occurring PVC (level I) from patient 2. (B) beat T_1 (level IV) of 3-beat VT from patient 1. (C) beat T_2 (level IV) of 3-beat VT from patient 2. Right: Corresponding photomicrographs of trichrome-stained sections of myocardium in vicinity of focal initiation sites demonstrating minimal (top), moderate (middle), and extensive (bottom) fibrosis.
From Pogwizd SM, McKenzie JP, Cain ME. Mechanisms underlying spontaneous and induced ventricular arrhythmias in patients with idiopathic dilated cardiomyopathy. *Circulation* 1998;**98**(22):2404–14.

mechanism(s) underlying this negative inotropic response remain to be elucidated, but proposed mechanisms include Giα-mediated inhibition of adenylyl cyclase, activation of the Na^+/Ca^{2+} exchanger, competitive inhibition of β_2AR-Gs coupling, increased buffering of activated Gαs by Gβγ released from activated Gi, and activation of the p38 mitogen activated protein kinase (p38MAP kinase) pathway. Interestingly, some β-blockers, including those used clinically, can activate the β_2AR-Gi negative inotropic pathways.[42]

A recent intriguing finding is that the location of βAR differs both between β1AR and β2AR subtypes in normal cardiomyocytes, and between healthy and failing cardiomyocytes. Using a combination of SICM, fluorescent reporter probes to cAMP, and nanoscale agonist application, the surface location of β1- and β2ARs have been mapped to specific cell surface structures of the cardiomyocyte.[43] In healthy ventricular myocytes, β1ARs are located across the entire surface of the cell, and pharmacological receptor stimulation results in cell-wide propagating cAMP signals, independent of the origin of the β1AR location. In contrast, β2ARs are restricted to the z-groove and T-tubule openings, and have spatially restricted (compartmentalized) cAMP signals. In cardiomyocytes from failing hearts, where the organized Z-groove and T-tubule structure is altered (see 'Surface topology'), the β2ARs are located across the entire cell surface, and agonist activation leads to cell-wide cAMP signals analogous to the β1AR of the normal (and failing) myocytes (Fig. 12.7). This could be relevant, as the Gi proteins are located in the intergroove crest membrane,[44] and therefore this physical β2AR redistribution may contribute to increased βAR-Gi coupling and the failing cardiomyocyte phenotype.

Chronic βAR activation results in cardiomyocyte apoptosis, which contributes to myocardial dysfunction.[45–47] However, the β_1AR and β_2AR exert differing effects on cardiomyocyte survival pathways. In double β_1AR/β_2AR (null) mice engineered to express a single 'pure' β_1AR phenotype, stimulation of β_1AR resulted in increased cardiomyocyte apoptosis and reduced survival.[48,49] In contrast, the null mice expressing a 'pure' β_2AR phenotype at levels up to 60-fold those of the wild type had a generally good survival despite increased basal cardiac function, and cardiomyopathy was seen only at higher expression levels.[50]

Chronic β1AR activation is harmful to isolated cardiomyocytes, and in HF patients the increased sympathetic activation and noradrenaline levels correlate inversely with survival.[51] Activation of β2AR-Gi coupled pathways is protective via activation of antiapoptotic pathways (Gβγi-PI3K-Akt pathway activation), but at the potential mechanical cost of negative inotropism. This may reflect an evolutionary response to protect the myocardium from the toxic effects of excessive catecholamine stimulation.[52]

Calcium pathophysiology

The abnormalities of calcium physiology in the failing cardiomyocyte are described in Chapter 11. A summary of the major changes is listed in Box 12.1.

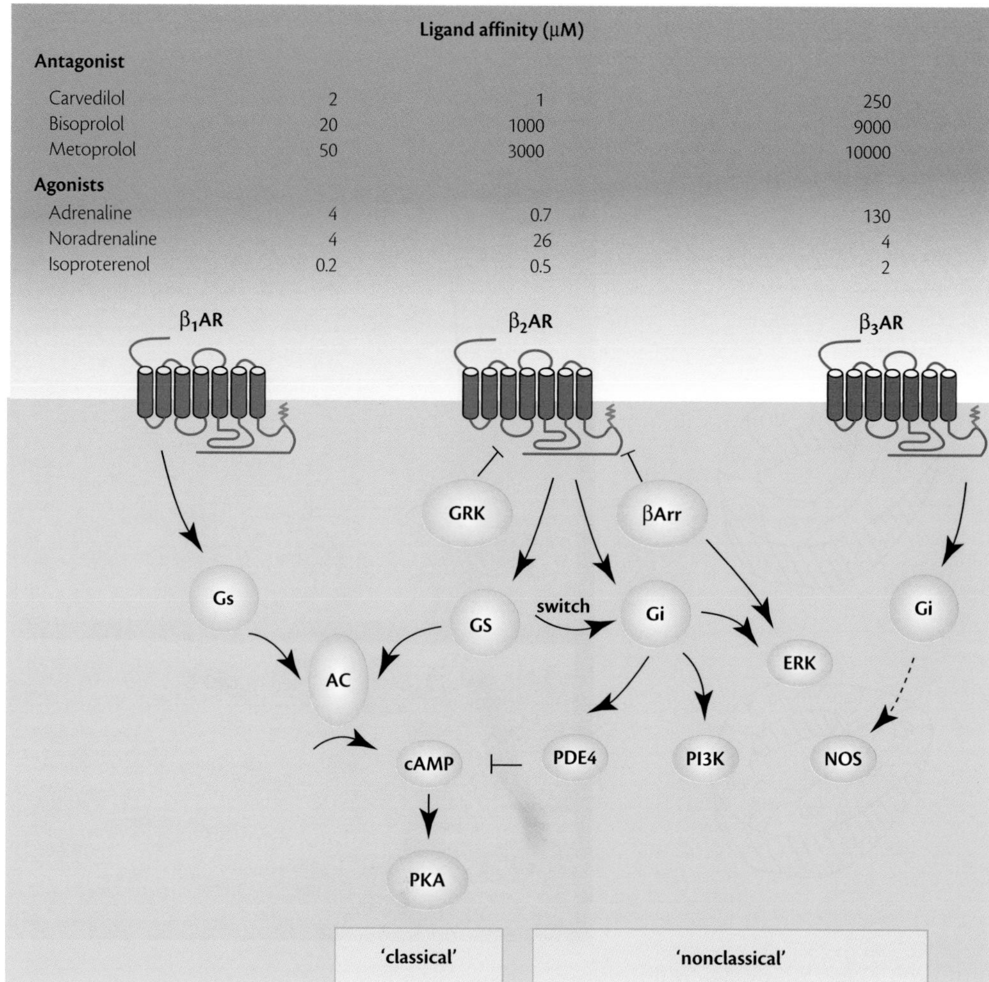

Ligand affinity (μM)	β_1AR	β_2AR	β_3AR
Antagonist			
Carvedilol	2	1	250
Bisoprolol	20	1000	9000
Metoprolol	50	3000	10000
Agonists			
Adrenaline	4	0.7	130
Noradrenaline	4	26	4
Isoproterenol	0.2	0.5	2

Fig. 12.6 Agonist activation and coupling/signalling properties of β-adrenergic receptor subtypes.
From Lohse MJ, Engelhardt S, Eschenhagen T. What is the role of beta-adrenergic signaling in heart failure? *Circ Res* 2003;**93**(10):896–906.

Sodium pathophysiology

Although cardiomyocyte calcium pathophysiology has been the focus of intense research over the last four decades, it is only relatively recently that the important role of sodium homeostasis in cardiomyocyte function has become apparent. In fact, the pathophysiology

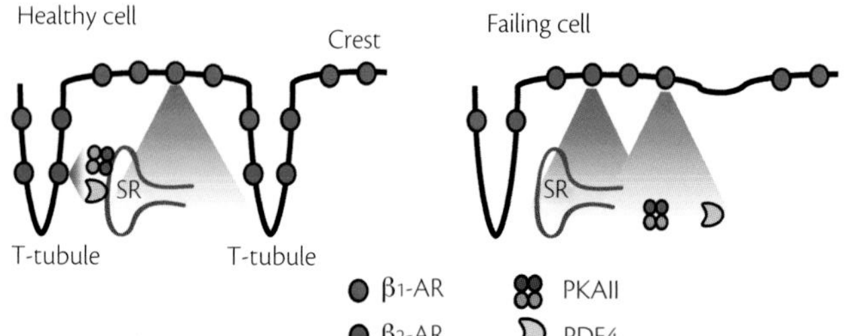

Fig. 12.7 Schematic describing how the cAMP signalling from β_1 and β_2ARs is organized in healthy and failing cardiomyoytes. In healthy cells the β_1AR is distributed throughout various membrane regions and induces propagating cAMP signals, whereas β_2AR signalling is locally confined via receptor localization in the T-tubules, cAMP interaction with PKAII molecules and local PDE4 activation. In HF β_2AR redistribution from the T-tubules to cell crest and loss of PKAII localization lead to cAMP propagation throughout the entire cytosol similar to the behaviour of the β_1AR.
From Nikolaev VO, Moshkov A, Lyon AR, *et al.* Beta2-adrenergic receptor redistribution in heart failure changes cAMP compartmentation. *Science* 2010 26;**327**(5973):1653–7.

Box 12.1 Major changes of calcium physiology in the failing cardiomyocyte

- Decreased SR calcium reuptake
- Increased SR calcium leak with increased calcium spark and wave frequency during diastole
- Reduced SR calcium content
- Increased extrusion by the sodium–calcium exchanger (NCX)
- Elevated resting (baseline) calcium concentration
- A reduction in peak amplitude of the stimulated calcium transient
- Increased time to peak amplitude
- Prolonged calcium transient decay kinetics
- Prolongation of action potential duration
- Increased calcium-dependent triggered activity (delayed after-depolarizations)
- Increased calcium sensor activity (calmodulin kinase II, calcineurin)

of these two important cations is intrinsically linked via the sodium-calcium exchange transporter (NCX) on the cardiomyocyte cell surface.

In the normal cardiomyocyte, $[Na^+]_i$ is kept at low levels (5–10 mM in large mammals, 10–15 mM in rodents) by the sarcolemmal Na^+/K^+-ATPase exchange protein. During the cardiac cycle, NCX functions predominantly in forward mode with calcium extrusion. In both hypertrophied and failing human and animal cardiomyocytes, $[Na^+]_i$ is elevated by around 3–6 mM.[53–55] The mechanisms underlying this are incompletely understood. It may be the result of reduced Na^+/K^+-ATPase gene expression[56–58] or activity,[59,60] increased sodium influx via the Na^+/H^+ exchanger (NHE) [61,62] and increased entry via the late Na^+ current.[63] Abnormal regulation of Na^+/K^+-ATPase activity may occur via two separate pathways in the failing heart. Phospholemman (PLM) is a small regulatory protein which inhibits Na^+/K^+-ATPase.[64] PKA-and PKC-mediated phosphorylation of PLM removes the inhibitory effect, in a manner analogous to PLB phosphorylation and SERCA2a. PLM phosphorylation is increased in failing rabbit and human hearts.[60]

A second mechanism responsible for down-regulation of Na^+/K^+-ATPase activity in HF is via redox modification. In failing hearts, increased PKC activity increases Na^+/K^+-ATPase glutathionylation, which impairs Na^+/K^+-ATPase activity, contributing to the accumulation of excessive intracellular Na^+ ions.[65]

Increased cellular $[Na^+]_i$ has a number of deleterious consequences which contribute to the development of the failing phenotype.

- Firstly, the increased $[Na^+]_i$ reduces the energy gradient for the forward mode operation of NCX, and stimulates an increase in NCX reverse mode activity. This effect is primarily during systole, when the higher $[Na^+]_{i,}$ lower peak calcium levels and prolonged APD promote reverse mode NCX function in the failing cardiomyocyte. In turn, calcium is driven into the failing cardiomyocyte, which may be a compensatory mechanism to raise cell and SR calcium stores and increase contractile force. However, because of SERCA2a down-regulation, the increased calcium entry via NCX during phases 1 and 2 of the action potential cannot be cleared into the SR. Instead, the increased calcium influx must be balanced by increased forward mode NCX activity during phase 4, which may contribute to increased cellular triggered activity via afterdepolarizations.[66]
- Secondly, NCX proteins are also present on the inner mitochondrial membrane. Increased $[Na^+]_i$ disrupts mitochondrial calcium uptake, and this contributes to energetic inefficiency of the failing cardiomyocyte via uncoupling of the calcium-sensitive energy supply–demand relationship.[67]
- Finally, increased $[Na^+]_i$ will potentially reduce the electrochemical gradient for clearance of H^+ by the NHE protein, impairing the buffering of intracellular acidosis in the failing cardiomyocyte.

Mitochondrial dysfunction and oxidative stress

Cardiomyocytes are highly metabolically active, in order to meet the energy demands of cardiac contraction 60–100 times per minute for the lifetime of an individual. Cardiomyocytes are designed to perform highly efficient aerobic respiration coordinated by an organized lattice network of thousands of mitochondria in a single cardiomyocyte.

Cardiomyocytes from failing hearts have impaired energetic efficiency,[68] reflected at both the cellular and intact organ level by a reduced phosphocreatine:ATP ratio, which has been demonstrated to directly correlate with the severity of HF.[69] The reduced ratio is indicative of impaired mitochondrial function in failing cardiomyocytes, which is a reflection of the combined effects of cellular calcium and sodium overload, and increased oxidative stress.

Oxidative stress is caused by mitochondrial dysfunction with increased production of reactive oxygen species (ROS). ROS levels are elevated in failing myocardium.[70, 71] They are generated by the leak of superoxide anions from the electron transport chain, or the production of hydrogen peroxide. Oxidative stress is a driver of the spiralling deterioration of cardiomyocyte function in HF, as ROS interacts to accelerate several pathophysiological pathways. These include increasing SR calcium leak via RyR2 oxidation,[72] impairing Na^+/K^+-ATPase and SERCA2a activity, mitochondrial membrane potential ($\Delta\psi m$) depolarization with uncoupling of ATP synthesis from oxidative phosphorylation, and self-generation of further ROS. A further critical outcome of increased mitochondrial oxidative stress is the predisposition to apoptosis (see 'Impaired cell survival and increased apoptosis').

Abnormal gene expression

One of the hallmarks of the common final pathway of HF, independent of aetiology, is the activation of fetal gene expression programmes. These have been demonstrated in human HF samples, both with respect to fetal myocyte protein expression and fetal microRNA profiles.[73,74] The precise mechanisms underlying the switches are unknown, but it is clearly established that the adult failing heart undergoes a number of functional adaptive changes which generate cellular physiology reminiscent of the fetal ventricular myocardium. The changes include switches in metabolic pathways from fatty acid to carbohydrate metabolism, changes in T-tubule and SR physiology, altered sarcolemmal ion channel expression, and alteration of myofilament myosin heavy chain isoforms.

All these changes result in physiology characteristic of fetal ventricular myocardium.[3] The switch to fetal gene expression profiles may reflect the myocyte response to stress and the impaired oxygen supply–demand relationship in the failing heart in an attempt to optimize energy utilization and contractile function. Indeed, fetal gene expression programmes are reactivated in chronically ischaemic hibernating myocardium.[75] Activation of fetal gene expression pathways have beneficial effects on cell survival, at least initially. However, the changes from adult to fetal physiology introduce numerous inefficiencies in the adult heart, e.g. in E-C coupling, which may ultimately contribute to the vicious circle of decline begetting decline for cardiomyocytes within the failing myocardium.

Impaired cell survival and increased apoptosis

Another hallmark of failing myocardium is a progressive reduction in the number of cardiomyocytes. This may be the direct result of the causative disease, as with myocardial infarction, but also results from progressive activation of cell death pathways (apoptosis). Infarction and other acute myocardial injury initially cause acute cell necrosis resulting from a sudden depletion of ATP. Necrosis is characterized by cell swelling, membrane lysis, and release of intracellular contents into the interstitial space, resulting in inflammation and secondary injury. In contrast, apoptosis is an energy-consuming process of programmed cell death via protein and chromatin fragmentation which does not trigger an immune response.

Adult mammalian cardiomyocytes rarely undergo apoptosis within healthy hearts, with only one apoptotic cell visible per 10 000–100 000 cardiomyocytes.[76] In contrast, the rates of apoptosis, as measured using TUNEL staining for DNA condensation and fragmentation, are significantly increased in chronically failing hearts irrespective of aetiology (Fig. 12.8).[77] The biological pathways underlying apoptosis are complex and will be summarized briefly below. For more detailed discussion of the pathways involved in apoptosis, readers are referred to two excellent recent reviews.[78,79]

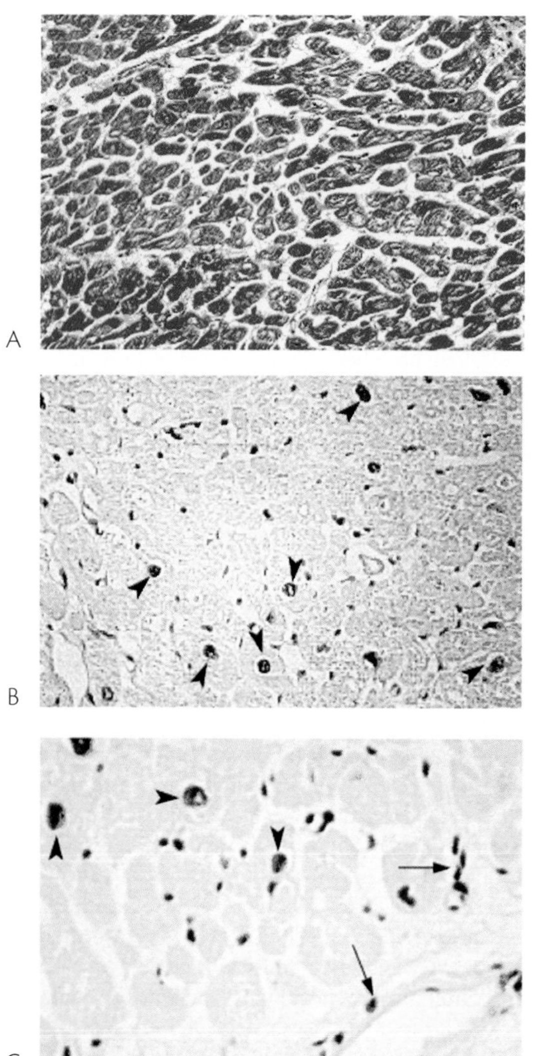

Fig. 12.8 Evidence of apoptosis in endstage idiopathic dilated cardiomyopathy. In panel A, a myocardial section from a patient with dilated cardiomyopathy (Patient 6) contains normal myocytes and no interstitial fibrosis (Masson's trichrome staining, ×75). Extensive apoptosis can be seen in myocytes in panel B (arrowheads). Apoptosis usually occurred in groups of cells, and the severity varied from extensive (panel B) to mild (panel C) to absent in different regions of the myocardium. In addition to its presence in myocytes (arrowheads) in panel C, apoptosis was also observed in vascular smooth-muscle cells of an intramyocardial arteriole as well as in rare interstitial cells (arrows). (Panels B and C, end-labelling for apoptotic nuclei and haematoxylin counterstaining, ×250.)

From Narula J, Haider N, Virmani R, *et al.* Apoptosis in myocytes in end-stage heart failure. *N Engl J Med* 1996;**335**(16):1182–9, with permission.

There are three major apoptotic pathways in ventricular cardiomyocytes: the death receptor pathway (also known as the extrinsic pathway), the mitochondrial death pathway (also known as the intrinsic pathway), and the ER-stress pathway (Fig. 12.9).[80] All three pathways converge upon a cascade of sequential activation of a family of 'suicide enzymes' known as caspases (cysteine and serine proteases).[81] These enzymes exist as prozymogens (inactive enzymes) and are cleaved by caspases upstream in the pathway to generate active enzymes, which catalyse cleavage of the downstream prozymogen. The ultimate effector caspases (particularly caspase 3) catalyse the breakdown of other target proteins in the cell which initiate irreversible protein degradation, DNA fragmentation, nuclear condensation, and cell death.

The death receptor pathways start with cell surface membrane receptors which respond to cytokine binding by activation of intracellular proapoptotic secondary messenger pathways. The receptors are predominantly members of the TNF membrane receptor superfamily, including the Fas receptors and tumour necrosis factor receptor 1 (TNFR1). On ligand binding, Fas receptors undergo oligomerization and recruit the Fas-associated death domain (FADD). The Fas–FADD complex binds to and activates procaspase 8. Active caspase 8 initiates an intracellular cascade of caspase activation which culminates in the cleavage of DNA and degradation of critical homeostatic proteins, resulting in apoptosis. A transgenic mouse model with cardiac-restricted overexpression of caspase 8 developed dilated cardiomyopathy without need for any additional insult.[82]

The mitochondrial pathway is initiated by excessive oxidative stress and accumulation of mitochondrial ROS. Mitochondrial ROS accumulation occurs as the result of electron leak from various complexes of the inner mitochondrial membrane electron transport chain, resulting in superoxide anion generation. ROS are increased beyond levels that can be effectively buffered by the antioxidant systems in ischaemic myocardium, after reperfusion following acute ischaemia, and in chronically failing myocardium. Once ROS levels rise, the permeability of the mitochondrial outer membrane increases via the assembly of the mitochondrial permeability transition pore (mPTP).[83] MPTP opening initiates an irreversible collapse of $\Delta\psi m$. In turn, the collapse of $\Delta\psi m$ leads to a range of effects including the cessation of ATP synthesis. The mitochondrial swell with focal rupture of the outer mitochondrial membrane, and the release of several proapoptotic factors such as cytochrome *c*, apoptosis inducing factor (AIF), endonuclease G (Endo G), and second mitochondria-derived activator of caspases (Smac/Diablo). The final result is the initiation of apoptosis. Cytochrome *c* binds to Apaf-1 and forms the apoptosome complex with activation of caspase 9. Caspase 9 cleaves and activates caspase 3, and the latter directly cleaves target proteins, including DNA polymerase, stimulating endonuclease activity and induction of apoptosis.

The mitochondrial death pathway has a number of regulatory systems, the most extensively investigated being the Bcl-2 protein family.[84] The Bcl-2 proteins are subdivided on structural classification into the 'multidomain' and 'BH3-only' subcategories. The proapoptotic multidomain Bcl-2 proteins, Bax and Bak, contribute to mPTP formation and activation of apoptosis. They are regulated by complementary antiapoptotic multidomain proteins (the prototypical ones being Bcl-2 and Bcl-xl) which bind and competitively inhibit the proapoptotic Bax and Bak. The BH3-only proteins act

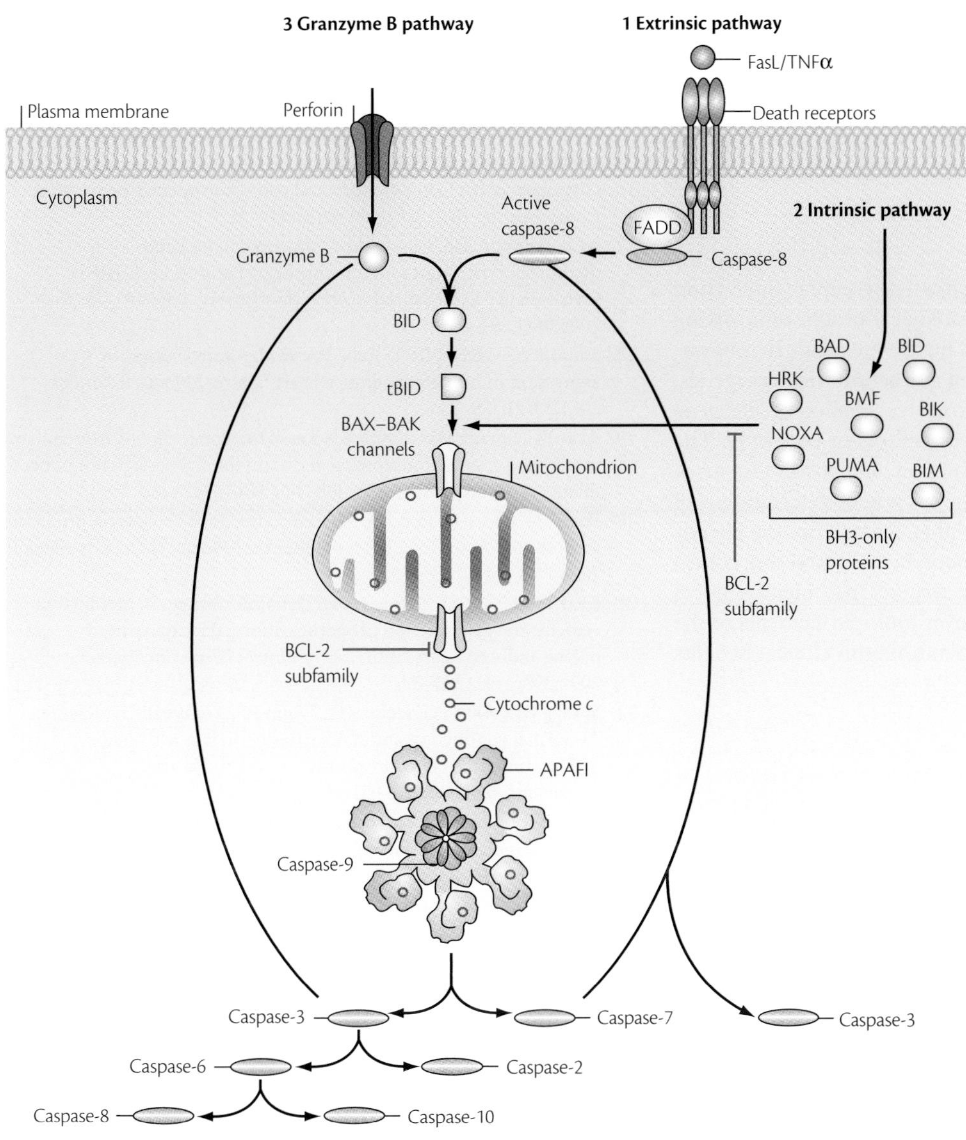

Fig. 12.9 Pathways leading to intracellular caspase activation and initiation of apoptosis.
From Taylor RC, Cullen SP, Martin SJ. Apoptosis: controlled demolition at the cellular level. *Nat Rev Mol Cell Biol* 2008;**9**(3):231–41, with permission.

as stress sensors, responding to increased levels of cellular stress including increased oxidative stress and growth factor deprivation. They mobilize to the mitochondria and regulate permeability transition. One example in cardiomyocytes is the Nix protein. Overexpression induces an apoptotic cardiomyopathy.[85]

The BH3-only proteins may indirectly activate the Bcl-2 pathways via sequestration of the antiapoptotic BH3-only proteins Bcl-2 and Bcl-xl. Therefore the balance of pro- and antiapoptotic proteins is key to determining cardiomyocyte fate in the failing heart. For example, the ratio of Bax:Bcl-xl significantly increases during the transition from compensated hypertrophy to decompensated HF in a rodent model, correlating with the increase in cytoplasmic cytochrome *c* and caspase 3 activation.[86]

The third apoptotic pathway is activated by increased endoplasmic reticulum (ER) stress. The ER is the site of protein synthesis, and in particular protein folding prior to export to the ultimate subcellular destination. Increased ER stress, secondary to abnormal calcium homeostasis, impaired energy utilization or abnormal ER protein transport, results in the accumulation of unfolded proteins in the ER lumen,[87,88] which activates the 'unfolded protein response' (UPR). The UPR initiates a transcriptional programme to increase ER protein folding capacity, degrade misfolded proteins, and reduce basal protein synthesis rates. Whilst the UPR is compensatory, if it is prolonged, it also initiates apoptosis via activation of caspase 12 and upregulation of the transcription factor CHOP/GADD 153. Caspase 12 activates caspase 3 and apoptosis directly, whereas CHOP/GADD 153 increases expression of proapoptotic genes including the BH3-only protein Puma.

Additional homeostatic systems which appear to interact with apoptosis are the autophagy pathways for recycling organelles and their proteins. Activity of autophagy pathways is dysregulated in HF models.[89] Examples of crosstalk between critical proteins in the regulation of autophagy and apoptosis have been reported.[90] For example, Atg5, an essential autophagy protein, activates apoptosis via both mitochondrial and death receptor pathways.

In summary, apoptosis is a highly regulated cell death system which is increased in failing hearts due to activation of a number of different proapoptotic pathways, with exhaustion of the counter-balancing antiapoptotic systems.[91] The result is the progressive loss of cardiomyocytes after an initial insult, which insidiously increases the demands on the remaining myocytes within the failing heart.

Summary

The biology of the failing cardiomyocyte is a complex interaction of a number of abnormal pathophysiological processes involving signalling pathways, intracellular ion fluxes, intercellular communications, oxidative stress, impaired mitochondrial energetics, altered structural morphology, abnormal reactivation of fetal gene expression patterns and activation of cell death pathways. The crosstalk between these pathways is complex, and positive feedback between the systems leads to the vicious cycle of deterioration of mechanical function and cell survival that characterize the phenotype of the failing cardiomyocyte. Identifying and targeting critical nodal points and master regulatory systems may identify novel therapeutic strategies which can recover multiple elements of the failing phenotype and translate into meaningful clinical benefits for patients with HF.

References

1. Diez J, Gonzalez A, Lopez B, Querejeta R. Mechanisms of disease: pathologic structural remodeling is more than adaptive hypertrophy in hypertensive heart disease. *Nat Clin Pract Cardiovasc Med* 2005;**2**(4):209–16.
2. Dorn GW, Robbins J, Sugden PH. Phenotyping hypertrophy: eschew obfuscation. *Circ Res* 2003;**92**(11):1171–5.
3. Rajabi M, Kassiotis C, Razeghi P, Taegtmeyer H. Return to the fetal gene program protects the stressed heart: a strong hypothesis. *Heart Fail Rev* 2007 **12**;(3–4):331–43.
4. Opie LH, Commerford PJ, Gersh BJ, Pfeffer MA. Controversies in ventricular remodelling. *Lancet* 2006;**367**(9507):356–67.
5. Burkett EL, Hershberger RE. Clinical and genetic issues in familial dilated cardiomyopathy. *J Am Coll Cardiol* 2005;**45**(7):969–81.
6. Davies CH, Davia K, Bennett JG, Pepper JR, Poole-Wilson PA, Harding SE. Reduced contraction and altered frequency response of isolated ventricular myocytes from patients with heart failure. *Circulation* 1995;**92**:2540–9.
7. Severs NJ. The cardiac muscle cell. *Bioessays* 2000;**22**(2):188–99.
8. Terracciano CMN, Harding SE, Adamson DL, *et al.* Changes in sarcolemmal Ca entry and sarcoplasmic reticulum Ca content in ventricular myocytes from patients with end-stage heart failure following myocardial recovery after combined pharmacological and ventricular assist device therapy. *Eur Heart J* 2003;**24**:1329–39.
9. del Monte F, O'Gara P, Poole-Wilson PA, Yacoub MH, Harding SE. Cell geometry and contractile abnormalities of myocytes from failing human left ventricle. *Cardiovasc Res* 1995;**30**:281–90.
10. Gorelik J, Yang LQ, Zhang Y, Lab M, Korchev Y, Harding SE. A novel Z-groove index characterizing myocardial surface structure. *Cardiovasc Res* 2006;**72**(3):422–9.
11. Gorelik J, Gu Y, Spohr HA, Shevchuk AI, *et al.* Ion channels in small cells and subcellular structures can be studied with a smart patch-clamp system. *Biophys J* 2002;**83**(6):3296–303.
12. Song LS, Sobie EA, McCulle S, Lederer WJ, Balke CW, Cheng H. Orphaned ryanodine receptors in the failing heart. *Proc Natl Acad Sci U S* 2006;**103**(11):4305–10.
13. Lyon AR, MacLeod KT, Zhang Y, *et al.* Loss of T-tubules and other changes to surface topography in ventricular myocytes from failing human and rat heart. *Proc Natl Acad Sci U S* 2009;**106**(16):6854–9.
14. Kleber AG, Rudy Y. Basic mechanisms of cardiac impulse propagation and associated arrhythmias. *Physiol Rev* 2004;**84**(2):431–88.
15. Peters NS, Green CR, Poole-Wilson PA, Severs NJ. Reduced content of connexin43 gap junctions in ventricular myocardium from hypertrophied and ischemic human hearts. *Circulation* 1993;**88**(3):864–75.
16. Giepmans BNG. Gap junctions and connexin-interacting proteins. *Cardiovascular Research* 2004;**62**(2):233–45.
17. Ai X, Pogwizd SM. Connexin 43 downregulation and dephosphorylation in nonischemic heart failure is associated with enhanced colocalized protein phosphatase type 2A. *Circ Res* 2005;**96**(1):54–63.
18. Dupont E, Matsushita T, Kaba RA, *et al.* Altered connexin expression in human congestive heart failure. *J Mol Cell Cardiol* 2001;**33**(2):359–71.
19. Akar FG, Spragg DD, Tunin RS, Kass DA, Tomaselli GF. Mechanisms underlying conduction slowing and arrhythmogenesis in nonischemic dilated cardiomyopathy. *Circ Res* 2004;**95**(7):717–25.
20. Poelzing S, Rosenbaum DS. Altered connexin43 expression produces arrhythmia substrate in heart failure. *Am J Physiol Heart Circ Physiol* 2004;**287**(4):H1762–770.
21. Akar FG, Nass RD, Hahn S, *et al.* Dynamic changes in conduction velocity and gap junction properties during development of pacing-induced heart failure. *Am J Physiol Heart Circ Physiol* 2007;**293**(2):H1223–30.
22. Spragg DD, Akar FG, Helm RH, Tunin RS, Tomaselli GF, Kass DA. Abnormal conduction and repolarization in late-activated myocardium of dyssynchronously contracting hearts. *Cardiovasc Res* 2005;**67**(1):77–86.
23. Lindsey ML, Mann DL, Entman ML, Spinale FG. Extracellular matrix remodeling following myocardial injury. *Ann Med* 2003;**35**(5):316–26.
24. Olivetti G, Capasso JM, Sonnenblick EH, Anversa P. Side-to-side slippage of myocytes participates in ventricular wall remodeling acutely after myocardial infarction in rats. *Circ Res* 1990;**67**:23–34.
25. Beltrami CA, Finato N, Rocco M, *et al.* Structural basis of end-stage failure in ischemic cardiomyopathy in humans. *Circulation* 1994;**89**:151–63.
26. Hein S, Arnon E, Kostin S, *et al.* Progression from compensated hypertrophy to failure in the pressure-overloaded human heart: structural deterioration and compensatory mechanisms. *Circulation* 2003;**107**(7):984–91.
27. Souders CA, Bowers SLK, Baudino TA. Cardiac fibroblast: the renaissance cell. *Circ Res* 2009;**105**(12):1164–76.
28. Kim J, Eckhart AD, Eguchi S, Koch WJ. Beta-adrenergic receptor-mediated DNA synthesis in cardiac fibroblasts is dependent on transactivation of the epidermal growth factor receptor and subsequent activation of extracellular signal-regulated kinases. *J BiolChem* 2002;**277**(35):32116–23.
29. Johar S, Cave AC, Narayanapanicker A, Grieve DJ, Shah AM. Aldosterone mediates angiotensin II-induced interstitial cardiac fibrosis via a Nox2-containing NADPH oxidase. *FASEB J* 2006;**20**(9):1546–8.
30. Kostin S, Hein S, Arnon E, Scholz D, Schaper J. The cytoskeleton and related proteins in the human failing heart. *Heart Fail Rev* 2000;**5**(3):271–80.
31. Pogwizd SM, McKenzie JP, Cain ME. Mechanisms underlying spontaneous and induced ventricular arrhythmias in patients with idiopathic dilated cardiomyopathy. *Circulation* 1998;**98**(22):2404–14.
32. Chilton L, Giles W, Smith GL. Evidence of intercellular coupling between co-cultured adult rabbit ventricular myocytes and myofibroblasts. *J Physiol* 2007;**583**(Pt 1):225–36.
33. Beltrami CA, Finato N, Rocco M, *et al.* The cellular basis of dilated cardiomyopathy in humans. *J Mol Cell Cardiol* 1995;**27**(1):291–305.
34. Lohse MJ, Engelhardt S, Eschenhagen T. What is the role of beta-adrenergic signaling in heart failure?. *Circ Res* 2003;**93**(10):896–906.

35. Cohn JN, Levine TB, Olivari MT, *et al.* Plasma norepinephrine as a guide to prognosis in patients with chronic congestive heart failure. *New Engl J Med* 1984;**311**:819–23.
36. Bristow MR, Hershberger RE, Port JD, *et al.* Beta-adrenergic pathways in nonfailing and failing human ventricular myocardium. *Circulation* 1990;**82**:I12–25.
37. Bristow MR, Ginsburg R, Umans V, *et al.* B1-and B2-adrenergic receptor subpopulations in nonfailing and failing human ventricular myocardium: Coupling of both receptor subtypes to muscle contraction and selective B1-receptor down-regulation in heart failure. *Circ Res* 1986;**59**:297–309.
38. Harding SE, Brown LA, Wynne DG, Davies CH, Poole-Wilson PA. Mechanisms of beta-adrenoceptor desensitisation in the failing human heart. *Cardiovasc Res* 1994;**28**:1451–60.
39. Davies CH, Davia K, Bennett JG, Pepper JR, Poole-Wilson PA, Harding SE. Reduced contraction of isolated human ventricular myocytes in ischaemic cardiomyopathy. *Circulation* 1994;**90**:1397.
40. Brown LA, Harding SE. The effect of pertussis toxin on β-adrenoceptor responses in isolated cardiac myocytes from noradrenaline-treated guinea-pigs and patients with cardiac failure. *Br J Pharmacol* 1992;**106**:115–22.
41. Heubach JF, Ravens U, Kaumann AJ. Epinephrine activates both Gs and Gi pathways, but norepinephrine activates only the Gs pathway through human beta2-adrenoceptors overexpressed in mouse heart. *Mol Pharmacol* 2004;**65**(5):1313–22.
42. Gong H, Sun H, Koch WJ, *et al.* The specific β_2AR blocker, ICI 118,551, actively decreases contraction through a Gi-coupled form of the β_2AR in myocytes from failing human heart. *Circulation* 2002;**105**:2497–503.
43. Nikolaev VO, Moshkov A, Lyon AR, *et al.* Beta2-adrenergic receptor redistribution in heart failure changes cAMP compartmentation. *Science* 2010 26;**327**(5973):1653–7.
44. Head BP, Patel HH, Roth DM, *et al.* G-protein-coupled receptor signaling components localize in both sarcolemmal and intracellular caveolin-3-associated microdomains in adult cardiac myocytes. *J Biol Chem* 2005;**280**(35):31036–44.
45. Geng YJ, Ishikawa Y, Vatner DE, *et al.* Apoptosis of cardiac myocytes in Gsalpha transgenic mice. *Circ Res* 1999;**84**(1):34–42.
46. Communal C, Singh K, Pimental D, Colucci W. Norepinephrine stimulates apoptosis in adult rat ventricular myocytes of the b-adrenergic pathway. *Circ* 1998;**98**:1329–34.
47. Shizukuda Y, Buttrick PM, Geenen DL, Borczuk AC, Kitsis RN, Sonnenblick EH. beta-adrenergic stimulation causes cardiocyte apoptosis: influence of tachycardia and hypertrophy. *Am J Physiol* 1998;**275**(3 Pt 2):H961–8.
48. Zhu WZ, Zheng M, Koch WJ, Lefkowitz RJ, Kobilka BK, Xiao RP. Dual modulation of cell survival and cell death by beta(2)-adrenergic signaling in adult mouse cardiac myocytes. *Proc Natl Acad Sci U S* 2001;**98**(4):1607–12.
49. Engelhardt S, Hein L, Wiesmann F, Lohse MJ. Progressive hypertrophy and heart failure in beta1-adrenergic receptor transgenic mice. *Proc Natl Acad Sci U S* 1999;**96**(12):7059–64.
50. Liggett SB, Tepe NM, Lorenz JN, *et al.* Early and delayed consequences of beta(2)-adrenergic receptor overexpression in mouse hearts: critical role for expression level. *Circulation* 2001;**101**(14):1707–14.
51. Packer M. Neurohormonal interactions and adaptations in congestive heart failure. *Circulation* 1988;**77**:721–30.
52. Lyon AR, Rees PS, Prasad S, Poole-Wilson PA, Harding SE. Stress (Takotsubo) cardiomyopathy—a novel pathophysiological hypothesis to explain catecholamine-induced acute myocardial stunning. *Nat Clin Pract Cardiovasc Med* 2008;**5**(1):22–9.
53. Pieske B, Maier LS, Piacentino V, III, Weisser J, Hasenfuss G, Houser S. Rate dependence of [Na+]i and contractility in nonfailing and failing human myocardium. *Circulation* 2002;**106**(4):447–53.
54. Despa S, Islam MA, Weber CR, Pogwizd SM, Bers DM. Intracellular Na^+ concentration is elevated in heart failure but Na/K pump function is unchanged. *Circulation* 2002;**105**(21):2543–8.
55. Gray RP, McIntyre H, Sheridan DS, Fry CH. Intracellular sodium and contractile function in hypertrophied human and guinea-pig myocardium. *Pflugers Arch* 2001;**442**(1):117–23.
56. Dixon IM, Hata T, Dhalla NS. Sarcolemmal Na^+-K^+-ATPase activity in congestive heart failure due to myocardial infarction. *Am J Physiol* 1992;**262**:C664–71.
57. Kim CH, Fan TH, Kelly PF, *et al.* Isoform-specific regulation of myocardial Na,K-ATPase alpha-subunit in congestive heart failure. Role of norepinephrine. *Circulation* 1994;**89**:313–20.
58. Shamraj OL, Grupp IL, Grupp G, *et al.* Characterisation of Na/K-ATPase, its isoforms, and the inotropic response to ouabain in isolated failing human hearts. *Cardiovasc Res* 1993;**27**:2229–37.
59. Ove Semb S, Lunde PK, Holt E, Tonnessen T, Christensen G, Sejersted OM. Reduced myocardial Na^+, K^+-pump capacity in congestive heart failure following myocardial infarction in rats. *J Mol Cell Cardiol* 1998;**30**(7):1311–28.
60. Bossuyt J, Ai X, Moorman JR, Pogwizd SM, Bers DM. Expression and phosphorylation of the na-pump regulatory subunit phospholemman in heart failure. *Circ Res* 2005;**97**(6):558–65.
61. Baartscheer A, Schumacher CA, van Borren MMGJ, Belterman CNW, Coronel R, Fiolet JWT. Increased Na^+/H^+-exchange activity is the cause of increased $[Na^+]$i and underlies disturbed calcium handling in the rabbit pressure and volume overload heart failure model. *Cardiovasc Res* 2003;**57**(4):1015–24.
62. Yokoyama H, Gunasegaram S, Harding SE, Avkiran N. Sarcolemmal Na^+/H^+ exchanger activity and expression in human ventricular myocardium. *J Am Coll Cardiol* 2000;**36**:534–40.
63. Undrovinas AI, Maltsev VA, Kyle JW, Silverman N, Sabbah HN. Gating of the late Na^+ channel in normal and failing human myocardium. *J Mol Cell Cardiol* 2002;**34**(11):1477–89.
64. Despa S, Bossuyt J, Han F, *et al.* Phospholemman-phosphorylation mediates the beta-adrenergic effects on Na/K pump function in cardiac myocytes. *Circ Res* 2005;**97**(3):252–9.
65. Figtree GA, Liu CC, Bibert S, *et al.* Reversible oxidative modification: a key mechanism of Na^+-K^+ pump regulation. *Circ Res* 2009 July 17;**105**(2):185–93.
66. Pogwizd SM, Sipido KR, Verdonck F, Bers DM. Intracellular Na in animal models of hypertrophy and heart failure: contractile function and arrhythmogenesis. *Cardiovasc Res* 2003 March 15;**57**(4):887–96.
67. Maack C, Cortassa S, Aon MA, Ganesan AN, Liu T, O'Rourke B. Elevated cytosolic Na^+ decreases mitochondrial Ca^{2+} uptake during excitation-contraction coupling and impairs energetic adaptation in cardiac myocytes. *Circ Res* 2006;**99**(2):172–82.
68. Ingwall JS, Weiss RG. Is the failing heart energy starved?: on using chemical energy to support cardiac function. *Circ Res* 2004;**95**(2):135–45.
69. Beer M, Seyfarth T, Sandstede JO, *et al.* Absolute concentrations of high-energy phosphate metabolites in normal, hypertrophied, and failing human myocardium measured noninvasively with 31P-SLOOP magnetic resonance spectroscopy. *J Am Coll Cardiol* 2002;**40**(7):1267–74.
70. Ide T, Tsutsui H, Kinugawa S, *et al.* Direct evidence for increased hydroxyl radicals originating from superoxide in the failing myocardium. *Circ Res* 2000;**86**(2):152–7.
71. Ide T, Tsutsui H, Kinugawa S, *et al.* Mitochondrial electron transport complex I is a potential source of oxygen free radicals in the failing myocardium. *Circ Res* 1999;**85**(4):357–63.
72. Yan Y, Liu J, Wei C, Li K, Xie W, Wang Y, Cheng H. Bidirectional regulation of Ca^{2+} sparks by mitochondria-derived reactive oxygen species in cardiac myocytes. *Cardiovasc Res* 2008;**77**(2):432–41.

73. Razeghi P, Young ME, Alcorn JL, Moravec CS, Frazier OH, Taegtmeyer H. Metabolic gene expression in fetal and failing human heart. *Circulation* 2001;**104**(24):2923–31.
74. Thum T, Galuppo P, Wolf C, *et al.* MicroRNAs in the human heart: a clue to fetal gene reprogramming in heart failure. *Circulation* 2007;**116**(3):258–67.
75. Depre C, Kim SJ, John AS, *et al.* Program of cell survival underlying human and experimental hibernating myocardium. *Circ Res* 2004;**95**(4):433–40.
76. Soonpaa MH, Field LJ. Survey of studies examining mammalian cardiomyocyte DNA synthesis. *Circ Res* 1998;**83**(1):15–26.
77. Narula J, Haider N, Virmani R, *et al.* Apoptosis in myocytes in end-stage heart failure. *N Engl J Med* 1996;**335**(16):1182–9.
78. Diwan A, Dorn GW, II. Decompensation of cardiac hypertrophy: cellular mechanisms and novel therapeutic targets. *Physiology* 2007;**22**(1):56–64.
79. Lee Y, Gustafsson AB. Role of apoptosis in cardiovascular disease. *Apoptosis* 2009;**14**(4):536–48.
80. Taylor RC, Cullen SP, Martin SJ. Apoptosis: controlled demolition at the cellular level. *Nat Rev Mol Cell Biol* 2008;**9**(3):231–41.
81. Communal C, Sumandea M de TP, Narula J, Solaro RJ, Hajjar RJ. Functional consequences of caspase activation in cardiac myocytes. *Proc Natl Acad Sci U S* 2002;**99**(9):6252–6.
82. Wencker D, Chandra M, Nguyen K, *et al.* A mechanistic role for cardiac myocyte apoptosis in heart failure. *J Clin Invest* 2003;**111**(10):1497–504.
83. Halestrap AP. What is the mitochondrial permeability transition pore?. *J Mol Cell Cardiol* 2009;**46**(6):821–31.
84. Kirshenbaum LA, de Moissac D. The bcl-2 gene product prevents programmed cell death of ventricular myocytes. *Circulation* 1997;**96**(5):1580–5.
85. Syed F, Odley A, Hahn HS, *et al.* Physiological growth synergizes with pathological genes in experimental cardiomyopathy. *Circ Res* 2004;**95**(12):1200–6.
86. Sharma AK, Dhingra S, Khaper N, Singal PK. Activation of apoptotic processes during transition from hypertrophy to heart failure in guinea pigs. *Am J Physiol Heart Circ Physiol* 2007;**293**(3):H1384–90.
87. Okada K, Minamino T, Tsukamoto Y, *et al.* Prolonged endoplasmic reticulum stress in hypertrophic and failing heart after aortic constriction: possible contribution of endoplasmic reticulum stress to cardiac myocyte apoptosis. *Circulation* 2004;**110**(6):705–12.
88. del Monte F., Hajjar RJ. Intracellular devastation in heart failure. *Heart Fail Rev* 2008;**13**(2):151–62.
89. Tannous P, Zhu H, Johnstone JL, *et al.* Autophagy is an adaptive response in desmin-related cardiomyopathy. *Proc Natl Acad Sci U S* 2008;**105**(28):9745–50.
90. Nishida K, Yamaguchi O, Otsu K. Crosstalk between autophagy and apoptosis in heart disease. *Circ Res* 2008;**103**(4):343–51.
91. Haider N, Arbustini E, Gupta S, *et al.* Concurrent upregulation of endogenous proapoptotic and antiapoptotic factors in failing human hearts. *Nat Clin Pract Cardiovasc Med* 2009;**6**(3):250–61.

PART V

Pathophysiology of heart failure

13

The pathophysiology of heart failure

Theresa A. McDonagh and Henry J. Dargie

Introduction

The classical definition of heart failure (HF) is fundamentally a pathophysiological one. It is the 'inability of the heart to provide sufficient oxygen to the metabolizing tissues despite and adequate filling pressure'.[1] Initially, the abnormalities found in the HF syndrome were described in terms of their haemodynamic effects. However, as the relationship between the pathophysiology of HF and its therapy has emerged over the last 20 years, it is now clear that the pathophysiology of HF is highly complex. It also involves neurohormonal and inflammatory adaptations which initially help the situation but chronically contribute to progression of the HF syndrome and adversely affect the structure and function of the heart itself. This chapter reviews the pathophysiology of HF by outlining what is known about its key players: haemodynamic abnormalities, ventricular remodelling, neurohormonal activation, and inflammatory responses.

Although any cardiac pathology can ultimately lead to HF, most is known about the pathophysiology of HF due to myocardial failure leading to left ventricular systolic dysfunction (LVSD), which concerns most of this chapter. Much work is needed to elucidate further the pathophysiology of HF when it occurs in the presence of normal systolic function.

Haemodynamic responses

In response to a reduction in myocardial contractility and/or in the presence of an excessive haemodynamic load, the heart employs a number of adaptive mechanisms to maintain cardiac output. The most important of these is the Frank–Starling mechanism whereby an increase in preload helps augment cardiac output (Fig. 13.1).[2] Secondly, myocardial hypertrophy begins to provide greater contractility.[3] Activation of neurohormonal systems, in particular the renin–angiotensin–aldosterone system (RAAS) and sympathetic nervous system, also stimulate contractility and increase preload by their effects on volume homeostasis and support of arterial pressure and perfusion.[4] These mechanisms initially improve cardiac performance: however, chronically, they become maladaptive.[1]

Adverse ventricular remodelling

Remodelling is the term most commonly used to describe the changes in size, shape, and function of the left ventricle that occur as a result of the initial cardiac pathology and its subsequent progression with the activation of the neurohormonal systems described in more detail below. Pathological changes occurring at cellular, organ, and systemic levels drive the process.[5]

The initial insult and its duration determine the broad category of remodelling. There are two distinct types. The first is concentric remodelling, when there is a generalized increase in LV wall thickness and mass. Ventricular dilatation does not occur initially but does subsequently with time. The second type is often referred to as eccentric remodelling, a hallmark of which is dilation of the ventricle, decreased systolic function, and consequent mitral, tricuspid, and aortic valve regurgitation. Eccentric remodelling is classically seen following myocardial infarction, in states of volume overload, valve regurgitation and dilated cardiomyopathies.[5,6]

In both kinds of remodelling, an important cellular change is myocyte hypertrophy, which can be triggered by increased load, neurohormonal driven signalling pathways, inflammation, and oxidative stress. Ultimately, these processes lead to well-described post-translational modifications which result in a myocyte phenotype similar to that seen during foetal development, consequent upon activation of the 'foetal gene programme'. The changes include the generation of new sarcomeres, an increase in the size of myocytes, and a change in their substrate preference from free fatty acids to glucose.[7] Initially whether these processes occur concentrically or eccentrically, they minimize ventricular wall stress. Over time, however, the changes lead to progressive contractile dysfunction and chamber dilation with a subsequent change in the shape of the left ventricle from elliptical to spherical.[8]

Other events at cellular level are also occurring during ventricular remodelling. There is on going cell death by both necrosis and

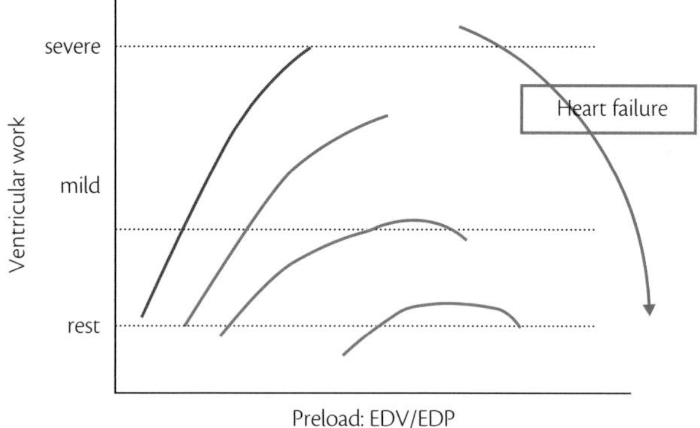

Fig. 13.1 Starling's law of the heart. In the normal heart (blue), ventricular work increases as a function of preload. The horizontal lines show the ventricular work required at rest, then for mild and finally severe exertion. With increasing severity of heart failure (brown lines), a greater preload is needed for a given level of activity. Note the 'descending limb' of the Starling curve for patients with severe heart failure: the implication is that a reduction in preload might (paradoxically) increase ventricular work. EDP, end-diastolic pressure; EDV, end-diastolic volume.

apoptosis (programmed cell death).[9] Apoptosis can be triggered by many of the same stimuli that lead to myocardial hypertrophy, i.e. load, neurohormonal driven signalling pathways, inflammation, and oxidative stress (see Chapter 12).[10] In addition, there are changes in the interstitial matrix with an increase in fibrosis and collagen turnover.[11] There is an increase in activity of matrix metalloproteinases (MMPs) and a decrease in their endogenous inhibitors, tissue metalloproteinases (TIMPS).[12] The end result is increasing ventricular dilatation (Table 13.1).

The alteration in the geometry of the left ventricle ultimately contributes to increased wall stress (by the law of Laplace) and leads to dilation of the mitral valve annulus and stretching and remodelling of the papillary muscles causing shortening of the posterior mitral valve leaflet thereby causing functional or ischaemic mitral regurgitation (Box 13.1, Table 13.2). The mitral regurgitation further exacerbates ventricular dilation by introducing an element of volume overload into the equation. The presence of mitral regurgitation in HF is, not surprisingly, associated with an adverse prognosis.[13,14]

Adverse left ventricular remodelling is associated with increased mortality rates irrespective of the underlying cardiac pathology and is a target for many of the therapeutic advances directed at HF due to LVSD. The remodelling that occurs following myocardial infarction, where there is initial infarct expansion at the border zone between infarcted and normal myocardium, is also a therapeutic target: perfusion strategies limit infarct size and the afterload reducing effects of angiotensin converting enzyme (ACE)

Table 13.1 Mechanisms of remodelling

Site of change	Mechanisms
Myocyte hypertrophy	Concentric Eccentric
Myocyte cell loss	Apoptosis Necrosis
Interstitial fibrosis	↑MMP, ↓TIMP ↑collagen turnover, fibrosis

MMP, matrix metalloproteinase; TIMP, tissue metalloproteinase.

Box 13.1 The law of Laplace

$$T = PR/h$$

where T is wall tension, P is pressure within the chamber, R is the radius of curvature of the chamber and h is wall thickness.

inhibitors reduce wall stress which can limit the remodelling process (Fig. 13.2).[15–17]

When coronary artery disease is the cause of the HF, further adverse remodelling can be exacerbated by intercurrent ischaemic events. Left ventricular dysfunction may have a component of hibernating myocardium where myocytes in poorly perfused areas shut down their metabolic activities and cease to contract. Hibernation is potentially reversible by restoring perfusion. This is possibly, in part, one of the mechanisms underlying the beneficial effects of β-blockers.[18]

The adverse remodelling process can lead to both electrical and mechanical dyssynchrony which then leads to a vicious cycle of a further reduction in cardiac output, augmented neurohormonal activation, reduction in left ventricular function, more severe mitral incompetence, and further ventricular remodelling. Dyssynchrony manifests as severe chronic heart failure (CHF) and has a poorer outlook and is now the target of cardiac resynchronization therapy.[19–21]

Heart failure with normal ejection fraction

It seems logical to discuss HF with normal ejection fraction (HeFNEF) under the heading of remodelling as the main differences between predominantly systolic dysfunction and HeFNEF seem to be related to the type of remodelling which the heart undergoes: in HeFNEF, the left ventricular hypertrophy phenotype predominates.

Up to 50% of patients presenting with HF have preserved (normal) left ventricle systolic ejection fraction. The syndrome has several other names: diastolic HF, and HF with preserved systolic function (see Chapter 26). The main abnormality occurs in diastole and is due to impaired relaxation or stiffness.

Less is known about the pathophysiology of this form of HF. A lot of work has focused on describing diastolic function in terms of haemodynamics by measuring left ventricular pressure–volume loops and trying to quantify relaxation, filling abnormalities, and chamber stiffness.[22]

Abnormalities of diastolic function happen in most patients with LVSD, but in patients with isolated diastolic HF, the only abnormality in the left ventricular pressure loops occurs in diastole, where

Table 13.2 Effect of ventricular dilation on wall stress. As the ventricle dilates, stroke volume is maintained but at a cost of ever greater wall tension

	Normal	DCM
LVEDV	90	400
LVESV	20	330
Stroke volume	70	70
LVEF (%)	78	18
Average wall tension (dyne/cm)	2.99×10^5	5.79×10^5

DCM, dilated cardiomyopathy.

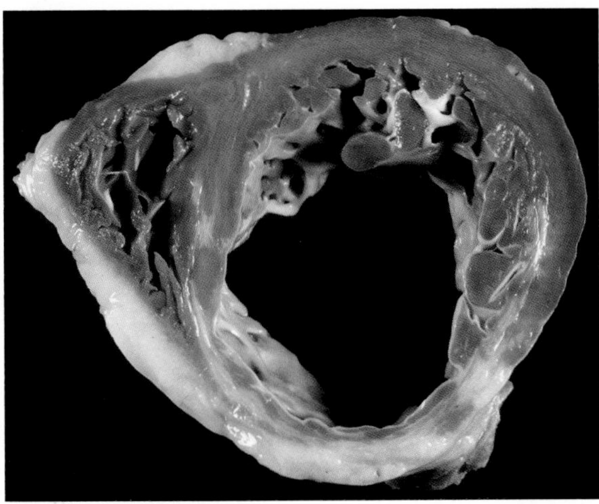

Fig. 13.2 Pathological specimen of an adversely remodelled left ventricle showing left ventricular hypertrophy, strands of fibrotic tissues, and an inferior myocardial infarct scar. The left ventricle is spherical.

the curve is shifted upwards and to the left (Fig. 13.3A), so that there is increased diastolic pressure with normal diastolic volumes. In patients with systolic HF (Fig. 13.3B), there are changes in the pressure volume loop that include a reduction in both LVEF and stroke volume. The diastolic portion is not normal either in that there is increased diastolic pressure. In mixed systolic and diastolic dysfunction (Fig. 13.3C), there is usually a modest decrease in LVEF, and an increase in end-diastolic volume and pressure, reflecting decreased chamber compliance.[22]

Noninvasive ways of assessing diastolic dysfunction are covered in Chapter 19. In diastolic HF, complex abnormalities occur at the level of the myofilaments, myocytes, matrix, and the heart.[23] In the myofilaments, abnormal stiffness and relaxation can be due to changes in the proteins within the contractile thick and thin filaments, myosin-binding protein C (MyBPC), and the linkage protein titin. Titin is a key player and changes in the PEVK region of its isoforms can alter stiffness and elastic recoil in the myocardium. At the myocyte level, calcium signalling and interaction with myofilaments play an important role. Expression and post-translational modifications of the sarcoplasmic reticulum calcium release channel (RyR), Ca^{2+} uptake proteins (PLB, SERCA), sarcolemma exchanger (NCX), and ion pumps can all occur. They are summarized in Fig. 13.4.[24]

Importantly, the neurohormonal changes seen in systolic HF (discussed in the next section. 'Neurohormonal activation') also occur in HeFNEF, although to a lesser extent (Fig. 13.5).[25]

As compared with patients with predominantly systolic dysfunction, patients with HeFNEF tend to be older, are more likely to be female, and often have hypertension as the main aetiology, although coronary artery disease (CAD) is a common finding as well.[26] It is, of course, the main type of HF found in hypertrophic cardiomyopathy and infiltrative cardiac diseases.

Neurohormonal activation

A variety of neurohormonal systems are activated in response to the alteration in cardiac function. These are well-developed evolutionary responses designed to protect against exsanguination. They therefore increase blood pressure and critical organ perfusion in

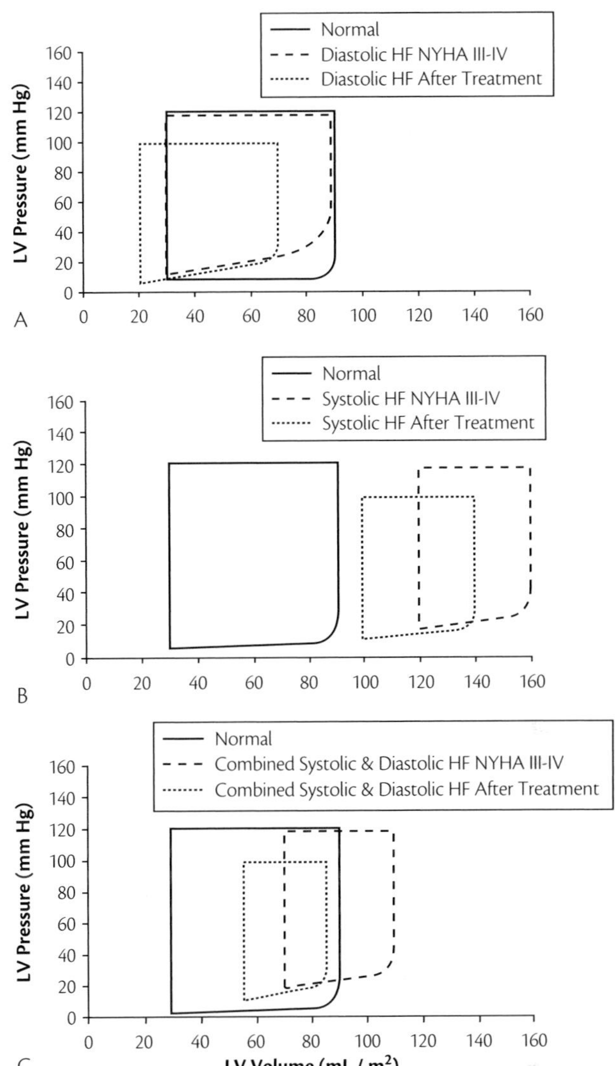

Fig. 13.3 Pressure–volume loops contrasting isolated diastolic heart failure (A) with systolic heart failure (B) and combined systolic and diastolic heart failure (C). A normal patient (solid line) is compared with a patient with heart failure before (dashed line) and after (dotted line) treatment. HF indicates heart failure.
From Zile MR, Brutsaert DL. New concepts in diastolic dysfunction and diastolic heart failure: Part II: causal mechanisms and treatment. *Circulation* 2002;**105**(12):1503–8.

the short term but ultimately also become maladaptive when chronically stimulated.

Sympathetic nervous system

Several mechanisms are involved in sympathetic nervous system activation, which occurs very early in HF, when the cardiac output drops. The fall in cardiac output (and blood pressure) is sensed by mechanoreceptors in the aortic arch, carotid sinus, left ventricular, and renal afferents leading to increased central sympathetic flow and raised circulating concentrations of noradrenaline. There is both increased neuronal release of noradrenaline and decreased reuptake. Initially the sympathetic activation supports the failing circulation by encouraging myocyte hypertrophy, an increased heart rate, vasoconstriction, and lusitropy.[27,28] However, the effects are ultimately deleterious. Both adrenaline and noradrenaline are directly toxic to the myocardium, promoting apoptosis and calcium overload.[29,30] Myocardial oxygen consumption is increased

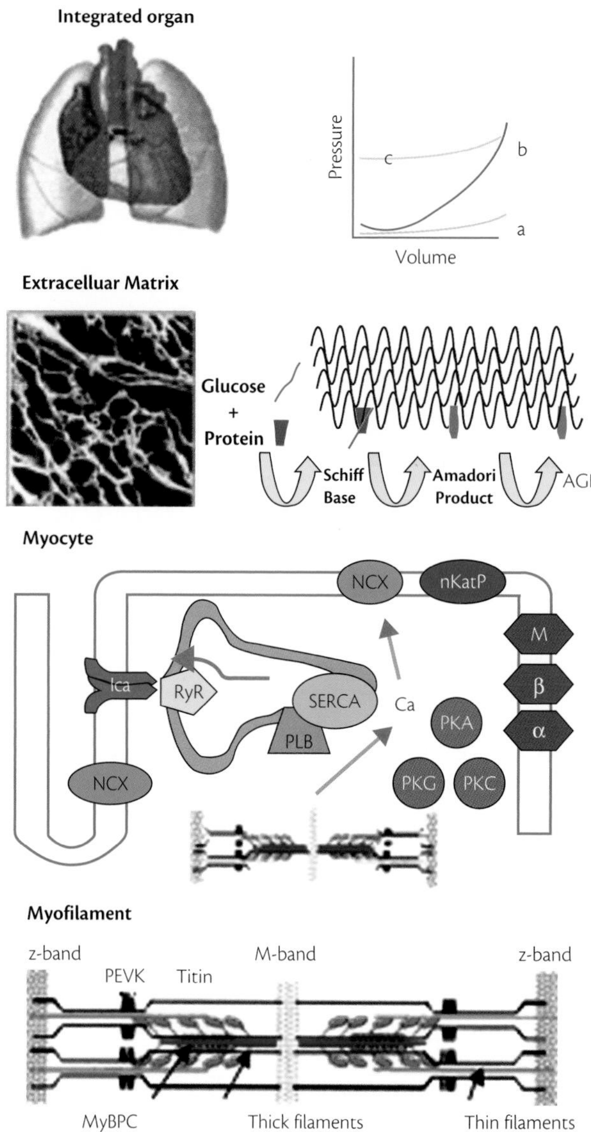

Fig. 13.4 The pathophysiology of diastolic heart failure. Mechanisms of diastolic dysfunction from the sarcomere through to the intact heart coupled with the vasculature. At the level of the myofilament, abnormal stiffness and relaxation can occur by modifications of proteins within the contractile thick and thin filaments, myosin-binding protein C, and the linkage protein titin. Changes in the PEVK region of titin among its isoforms can confer differential stiffness and elastic recoil to the myocardium. At the myocyte level, calcium signalling and interaction with myofilaments play an important role. Expression and post-translation modifications of the sarcoplasmic reticulum calcium release channel, Ca^{2+} uptake proteins (PLB, SERCA), sarcolemma exchanger, and ion pumps (Na^+,K^+-ATPase) by kinases all participate in this interaction. At the next level of integration, diastolic properties are coupled with an EC matrix that surrounds each myocyte and forms bundles among muscle fibres. The scanning electron micrograph (left) shows the connective tissue skeleton from a human heart, with perimysial fibres (P) enveloping groups of myocytes, smaller endomysial fibres supporting and connecting individual cells, and endomysial weave (W) enveloping individual myocytes, with cells linked to adjacent cells by lateral struts (S). Collagen is also post-translationally crosslinked to alter its properties (including generation of advanced glycation crosslinks) from protein/glucose interaction. At the integrated organ level, properties of the heart are impacted by the vascular loads imposed, by geometric factors, and external constraints (pericardium/ right heart). Measured DPVRs shifted upward in parallel (a vs c, top right) more commonly reflect such extrinsic influences, whereas intrinsic stiffness appears as a steeper relation (a vs b). AGE, advanced glycation cross-links; MyBPC, myosin-binding protein C; NCX, sarcolemma exchanger; NKATP, Na^+,K^+-ATPase; P, perimysial fibres; RyR, reticulum calcium release channel; S, lateral struts; W, endomysial weave.

From Kass DA, Bronzwaer JG, Paulus WJ. What mechanisms underlie diastolic dysfunction in heart failure? *Circ Res* 2004;**94**(12):1533–42.

and further adverse remodelling takes place. Down-regulation of β_1-adrenoreceptors occurs, which further inhibits the ability of the heart to respond to a catecholamine surge.[31,32]

The parasympathetic nervous system is also disturbed in HF. There is a reduction in vagal tone. The primary abnormality is though to be a reduction in baroreceptor sensitivity.[33]

This link between sympathetic activation and HF was described by Cohn's group, who noted that raised circulating concentrations of noradrenaline were associated with an adverse prognosis in HF.[28] The final endorsement of the deleterious effects of the SNS in HF came about with the β-blocker treatment trials that demonstrated improved outcomes for patients (Fig. 13.6).[34,35]

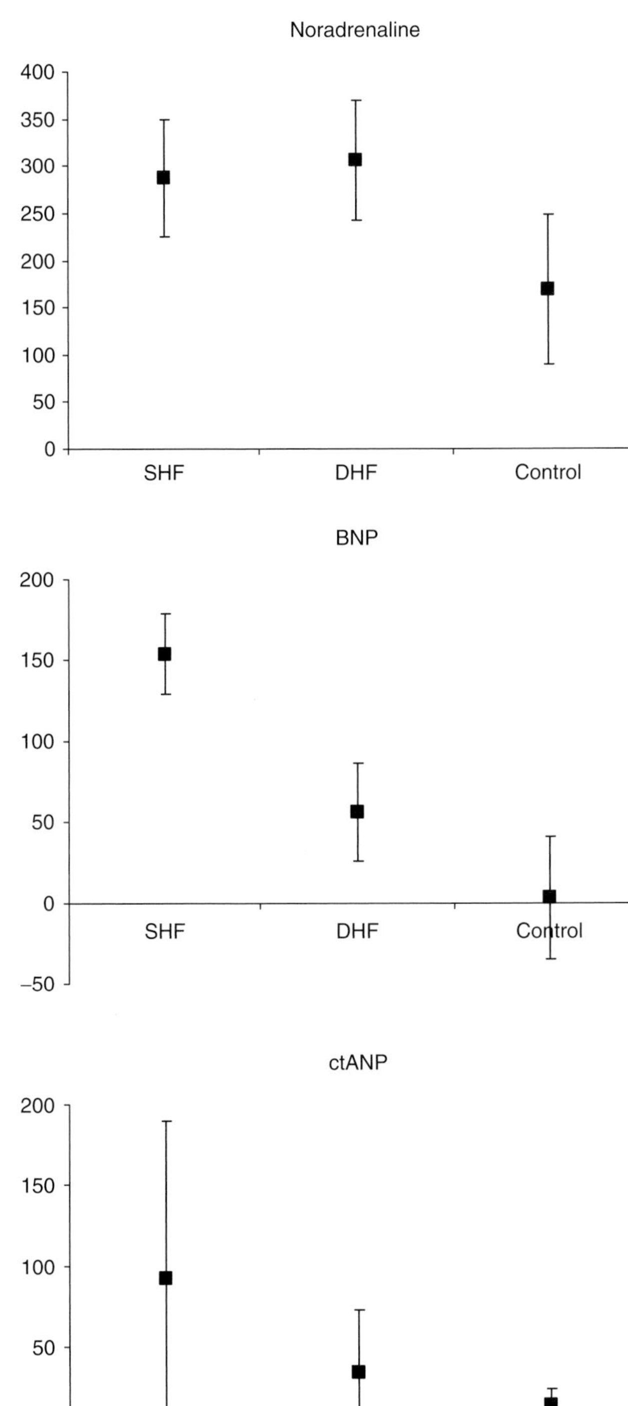

Fig. 13.5 Neuroendocrine activation in systolic and diastolic heart failure. Concentrations of noradrenaline, BNP, and the C-terminal of ANP on the y-axes. ANP, atrial ntrialuretic peptide; BNP, B-type natriuretic pepetide; DHF, diastolic heart failure; SHF, systolic heart failure.
Data from Kitzman DW, Little WC, Brubaker PH, *et al.* Pathophysiological characterization of isolated diastolic heart failure in comparison to systolic heart failure. *JAMA* 2002;**288**(17):2144–50.

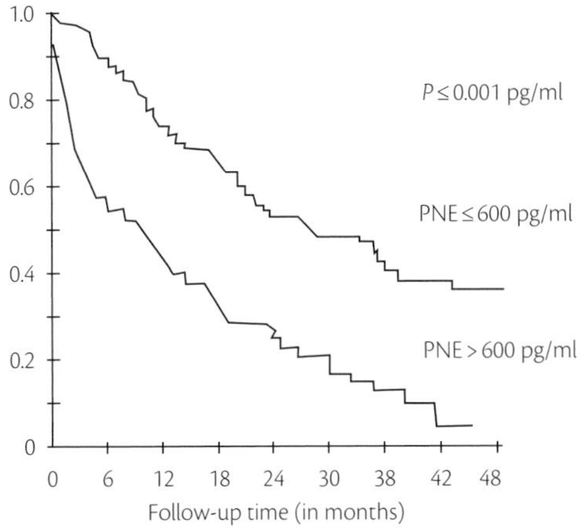

Fig. 13.6 Noradrenaline concentrations and prognosis in heart failure. Plasma PNE (noradrenaline concentrations above and below 600 pg/mL and survival.
From Rector TS, Olivari MT, Levine TB, Francis GS, Cohn JN. Predicting survival for an individual with congestive heart failure using the plasma norepinephrine concentration. *Am Heart J* 1987;**114**(1 Pt 1):148–52.

Renin–angiotensin–aldosterone system

The drop in cardiac output and blood pressure also stimulates the RAAS. This does not have the immediate effects of SNS activation. Indeed, there is little RAAS activation in patients with asymptomatic left ventricular dysfunction and more profound activation comes as the syndrome progresses (Fig. 13.7). The activation is also markedly increased by diuretic use.[36]

Release of renin from the juxtaglomerular apparatus in the kidney occurs through two main mechanisms: first, adrenergic stimulation of β-receptors and secondly, the decreased renal blood flow sensed by mechanoreceptors.[37] Renin circulates and converts angiotensinogen already in the circulation (synthesized by the liver) into angiotensin I. Angiotensin I is converted to angiotensin II principally through the action of ACE in the pulmonary circulation and other vascular beds (Fig. 13.8).[38] However, angiotensin II is also produced in numerous tissues (including myocytes) by non-ACE-dependent pathways via proteases such as chymase, kallikrein, and cathepsin. The alternative pathways are thought to be the routes by which 'ACE and aldosterone escape' occur when patients are treated with ACE inhibitors.[39]

Angiotensin II is the principal effector hormone of the RAAS. It causes vasoconstriction, myocyte and vascular hypertrophy, and aldosterone release. In addition, it is responsible for the release of other neurohormones such as vasopressin, endothelin and cathecholamines. It also causes thirst by a direct cerebral effect (Fig. 13.9).

The effects are mediated by activation of two receptors. The angiotensin II type 1 receptor (AT_1) is thought to be the one through which most of the deleterious effects occur. However, some adverse effects, such as apoptosis, can occur via stimulation of the type 2 (AT_2) receptor.

The importance of RAAS activation in the progression of HF has been greatly highlighted and further understood by the landmark treatment trials with ACE inhibitors, which were the first drugs to alter the mortality of HF.[40–42] More recent trials with angiotensin receptor blockers have emphasized the importance of RAAS activation.[43]

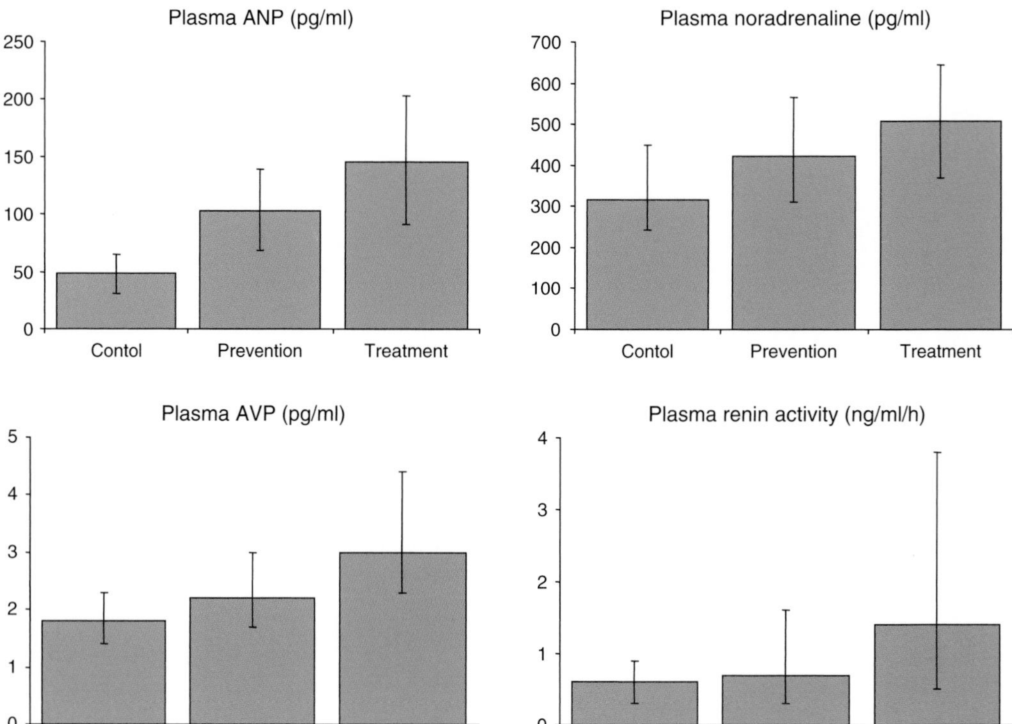

Fig. 13.7 Selected neurohormones in the SOLVD treatment programme. "Prevention" patients had asymptomatic left ventricular systolic dysfunction whereas those in the "treatment" trial had heart failure. ANP, atrial natriuretic peptide; AVP, arginine vasopressin. The median and interquartile ranges are shown. Data from Francis GS, Benedict C, Johnstone DE, *et al.* Comparison of neuroendocrine activation in patients with left ventricular dysfunction with and without congestive heart failure. A substudy of the Studies of Left Ventricular Dysfunction (SOLVD). *Circulation* 1990;**82**:1724–9.

Aldosterone

Angiotensin II causes release of the mineralocorticoid hormone aldosterone. Under normal conditions, its production is regulated via adrenocorticotropic hormone (ACTH) and serum potassium concentrations. Aldosterone encourages sodium retention and potassium excretion. The potassium loss contributes to the arrhythmia burden in HF. Aldosterone release is also stimulated by endothelin, cathecholamines, and vasopressin. Plasma concentrations rise in proportion to the severity of the disease.[44] More recently, its role in causing fibrosis in the myocardium by promoting collagen turnover has been highlighted by the beneficial effects of treatment with aldosterone antagonists both on survival in patients with HF and on reducing fibrosis in both human and animal models.[45–47]

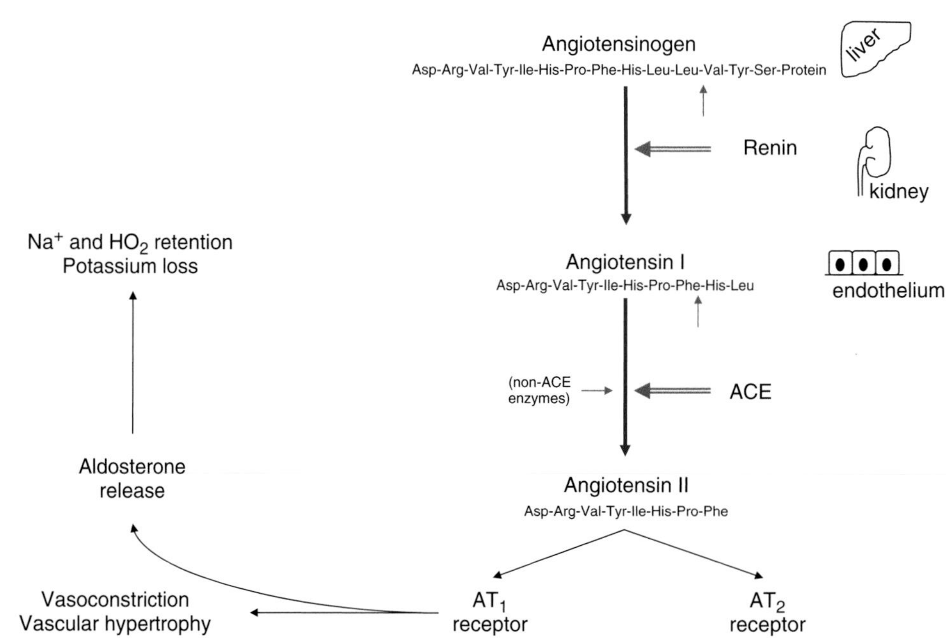

Fig. 13.8 The renin angiotensin aldosterone system. The amino acid sequences for angiotensinogen and angiotensins I and II are shown. ACE is angiotensin converting enzyme.

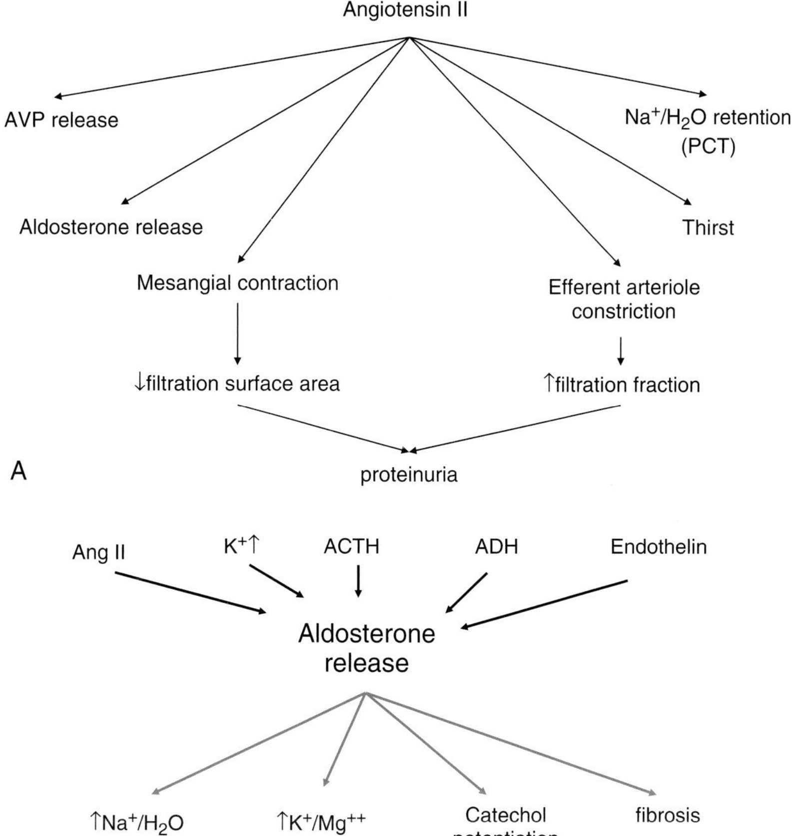

Fig. 13.9 (A) The effects of angiotensin II. (B) Factors triggering aldosterone release and its subsequent effects.

Endothelin

In a similar fashion to angiotensin, endothelin is produced as a pre-pro-peptide that is cleaved by a furin protease into Big Endothelin. Further cleavage by endothelin converting enzyme (a neutral endopeptidase) occurs to produce a family of three endothelins. Endothelin 1 is the predominant isoform expressed in humans. It is mainly produced in endothelial cells. It acts via two receptors, A and B. The receptors are G-protein coupled and activate phospholipase C, eventually leading to calcium release from the sarcoplasmic reticulum. Endothelin's principal effects are potent vasoconstriction, growth promotion, inotropy, and aldosterone and angiotensin II release.[48–51]

Circulating concentrations of endothelin are elevated two- to threefold in HF patients in proportion to haemodynamic and functional disease severity (Fig. 13.10).[51,52] It is thought to be a key player in the remodelling process. High plasma concentrations are independently associated with an adverse outcome in HF. They also track closely with the degree of pulmonary hypertension.[53,54]

Despite the early promise of endothelin A receptor blockade, which improved myocyte hypertrophy, and mixed A and B receptor blockade with bosentan, which favourably altered haemodynamics, larger clinical trials with endothelin antagonists have been disappointing [55–57].

Vasopressin

Vasopressin, also known as arginine vasopressin (AVP—in contrast to lysine vasopressin, found in pigs), or antidiuretic hormone (ADH), is a peptide released in response to a decrease in cardiac output, atrial stretch, and a drop in plasma osmolality. Angiotensin II and noradrenaline also augment its release in HF. Vasopressin's main site of action is the renal distal collecting tubule where it acts via the V_2 receptor to mobilize aquaporin-2 channels to the cell surface. Aquaporin-2 allows water reabsorption from the urine in the collecting duct down the osmotic concentration gradient in the renal medulla. Vasopressin also acts via V_1 and V_2

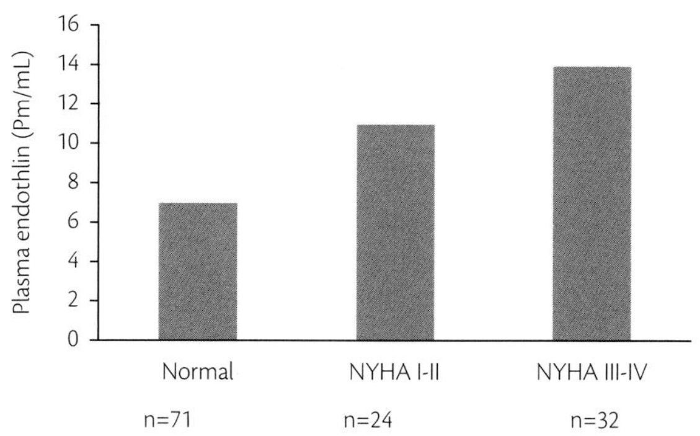

Fig. 13.10 Plasma concentrations of endothelin in heart failure according to the NYHA classification.

Adapted from Rodeheffer RJ, Lerman A, Heublein DM, Burnett JC, Jr. Increased plasma concentrations of endothelin in congestive heart failure in humans. *Mayo Clin Proc* 1992;**67**(8):719–24.

receptors to cause vasoconstriction in the pulmonary and peripheral circulation.

Although AVP is normally released in response to an increase in plasma osmolality, it is paradoxically raised in patients in proportion to the severity of HF[36] despite such patients often having hyponatraemia (which might be expected to reduce AVP). Nonosmotic stimuli to AVP release, such as angiotensin II and prostaglandins, become dominant in these circumstances.

Short treatments with the AVP antagonists conivapatan and tolvaptan improve haemodynamics, fluid removal, and electrolyte balance, but a recent long-term trial has not shown any conclusive effects on HF morbidity and mortality.[58,59] It may be that the AVP antagonists are of particular benefit in patients with hyponatraemia, but such a proposal has not been specifically tested.

Natriuretic peptides

The natriuretic peptides (NP), hormones produced by the heart, are also activated in HF. The most important ones in HF are atrial natriuretic peptide (ANP), mainly produced in the atria, and B-type natriuretic peptide (BNP), which is predominantly found in the ventricular myocardium.[60] Their release is stimulated by increased wall stress and stretch as well as by the circulating neurohormones, endothelin, angiotensin II, aldosterone, vasopressin, and noradrenaline. They act as counter-regulatory hormones and have a major role in controlling cardiovascular homeostasis via their key effector functions: natriuresis, diuresis, and vasodilation. Plasma concentrations of the NPs are raised in proportion to the severity of HF and are powerful predictors of a poor prognosis.[61–64] Although the counter-regulatory system is ultimately too weak to prevent progression of HF, the NPs have become very useful biomarkers to aid in diagnosis and assignment of prognosis, and as potential tools for monitoring therapy in HF. Manipulation of the system either by inhibiting of NP breakdown with neutral endopeptidase inhibitors or by augmenting their effects by use of intravenous exogenous recombinant BNP has not proved very successful to date, although further trials of these strategies are under way.[65,66]

Inflammatory activation

Potentially, inflammation may play an important role in the pathophysiology of HF (see Chapter 8). As in other phases of cardiac pathology, there is a nonspecific indication of underlying generalized inflammation given by a raised CRP concentration.[67]

The key inflammatory players investigated to date are the inflammatory mediators, cytokines. Initial work in patients with advanced HF and cardiac cachexia showed that plasma concentrations of tumour necrosis factor α (TNFα) were elevated.[68,69] Since then, many studies have shown increases in other cytokines such as interleukin-1β (IL-1β), IL-2, IL-6, Fas ligand, monocyte chemoattractant protein-1 (MCP-1) and macrophage inflammatory protein α (MIP-1α).[70] In a similar manner to neurohormonal activation, prolonged inflammatory activation with an imbalance between pro- and anti-inflammatory cytokines is ultimately deleterious.

TNFα is, to date, the most studied cytokine in HF. It is predominantly released from macrophages, although neutrophils, lymphocytes, platelets, mast cells, and endothelial cells can all produce it. In addition, it can be released by myocytes subject to stretch.

It is increased, as are its soluble receptors, in proportion to the severity of HF (Fig. 13.11).[71] Both TNFα and IL-6 have been shown to be independent predictors of prognosis in HF.[72] TNFα has a negatively inotropic action as well as toxic effects on the myocardium that lead to apoptosis, myocyte hypertrophy, and matrix remodelling, contributing to progressive adverse ventricular remodelling. Similarly, both IL-1 and IL-6 are negatively inotropic *in vitro* and their circulating concentrations are increased in proportion to the clinical and haemodynamic severity in HF patients.[73,74]

Less is known about the role of other chemokines in HF. The production of MCP-1 is stimulated by IL-1, IL-6, TNFα, and angiotensin II. Levels of MCP-1 are increased in animal models of HF.[75] More recently, MCP-1, MIP-1α, and RANTES (regulated upon activation, normal T cell expressed and secreted) have been shown to be elevated in human HF patients and correlated with traditional markers of disease severity such as NYHA class and

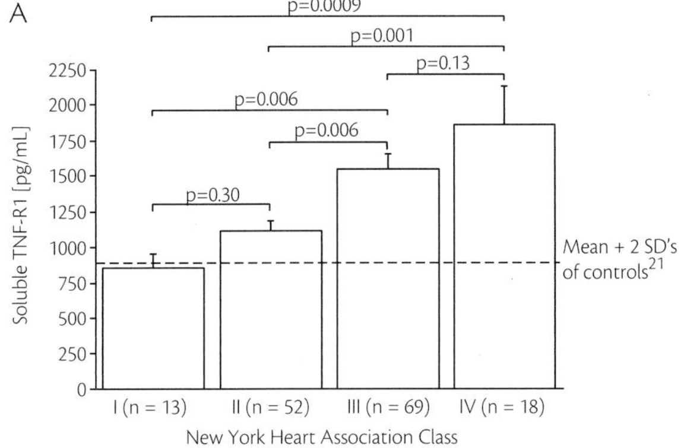

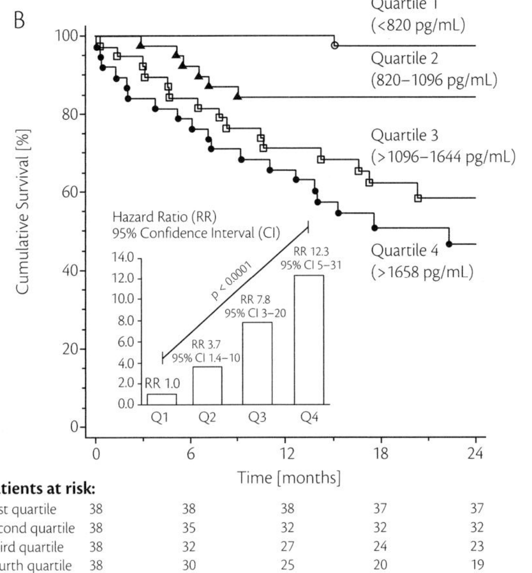

Patients at risk:

	0	6	12	18	24
First quartile	38	38	38	37	37
Second quartile	38	35	32	32	32
Third quartile	38	32	27	24	23
Fourth quartile	38	30	25	20	19

Fig. 13.11 Plasma soluble tumour necrosis factor (sTNF) receptors, NYHA class, and survival in heart failure. (A) Relationship between sTNF-R1 and NYHA functional class. Upper limit of normal concentrations of sTNF-R1 of healthy control subjects of similar age (mean±2 SD) is indicated, based on data published elsewhere. (B) Kaplan–Meier survival curves for sTNF-R1 quartiles at 24 months. Cutoff values and corresponding hazard ratios (small bar plots) are given. *P* value refers to Cox proportional hazards analysis.

From Rauchhaus M, Doehner W, Francis DP, *et al.* Plasma cytokine parameters and mortality in patients with chronic heart failure. *Circulation* 2000;**102**(25):3060–7.

Table 13.3 Novel biomarkers in heart failure: peptides, soluble receptors, cytokines, and chemokines which are raised in circulating concentrations in heart failure

MMPs	Apelin
TIMPs	Troponin
CRP	Interleukin 6
TenascinC	TNF
Galectin 3	Endothelin
Ghrelin	Resistin
Osteopontin	Relaxin
PCIP	RAGE
ICTP	Leptin
ST2	MCP1
Adiponectin	GDF-15
Copeptin	Myeloperoxidase

ejection fraction.[76] Furthermore, chemokines and their receptors are found in biopsies taken from failing myocardium.[77] They may well play an important role in the pathogenesis of the condition.

To date, however, modulation of inflammatory mediators in HF by statins, TNFα receptor blockers or monoclonal antibodies directed to TNFα has failed to demonstrate beneficial effects in large studies in HF patients.[78,79]

Other novel biomarkers

Many other biomarkers are elevated in patients with HF (Table 13.3). Whether these are mere epiphenomena or whether they are involved in the pathophysiology of the syndrome is as yet unclear. Some seem to be obvious candidates for a major role: for example, ST2, the soluble receptor for IL-33, seems to be linked to early fibrosis in the heart,[80,81] and apelin, the endogenous ligand of the APJ receptor, is a potent inodilator produced in the heart but down regulated in HF and up-regulated in models of reverse remodelling.[82–84] Manipulation of these systems will unravel their roles.

Systemic consequences of heart failure

The HF syndrome does not just affect the heart. As a result of the extensive compensatory activity, structural changes take place in vascular arterioles with increasing stiffness of vessels and endothelial dysfunction. Morphological and functional changes occur in skeletal muscle and respiratory function is affected with an increase in physiological dead space and airways obstruction.[85–87]

Conclusion

The pathophysiological processes at play in the HF syndrome combine to produce a progressive state of reduced left ventricular function, left ventricular adverse remodelling, and dilatation which leads to death from progressive pump failure or ventricular arrhythmia. Except in cases where the myocardial function returns to normal or near normal, neurohormonal blockade leads to some reverse remodelling, associated with an improved outlook for patients. However, the natural history for many patients is that treatment merely delays deterioration in left ventricular function which is then associated with many comorbidities (particularly renal dysfunction) which ultimately lead to progressive multiorgan dysfunction and death.

References

1. Braunwald E. Heart failure: pathophysiology and treatment. *Am Heart J* 1981;**102**(3 Pt 2):486–90.
2. Katz AM. The descending limb of the Starling curve and the failing heart. *Circulation* 1965;**32**(6):871–5.
3. Katz AM. Cellular mechanisms in congestive heart failure. *Am J Cardiol* 1988;**62**(2):3–8A.
4. Francis GS, Cohn JN, Johnson G, Rector TS, Goldman S, Simon A. Plasma norepinephrine, plasma renin activity, and congestive heart failure. Relations to survival and the effects of therapy in V-HeFT II. The V-HeFT VA Cooperative Studies Group. *Circulation* 1993;**87** (6 Suppl):VI40–8.
5. Mann DL. Basic mechanisms of left ventricular remodeling: the contribution of wall stress. *J Card Fail* 2004;**10**(6 Suppl):S202–6.
6. Frey N, Olson EN. Cardiac hypertrophy: the good, the bad, and the ugly. *Annu Rev Physiol* 2003;**65**:45–79.
7. Opie LH, Commerford PJ, Gersh BJ, Pfeffer MA. Controversies in ventricular remodelling. *Lancet* 2006;**367**(9507):356–67.
8. St John Sutton M, Pfeffer MA, Moye L, *et al.* Cardiovascular death and left ventricular remodeling two years after myocardial infarction: baseline predictors and impact of long-term use of captopril: information from the Survival and Ventricular Enlargement (SAVE) trial. *Circulation* 1997;**96**(10):3294–9.
9. Narula J, Hajjar RJ, Dec GW. Apoptosis in the failing heart. *Cardiol Clin* 1998;**16**(4):691–710, ix.
10. Kitsis RN, Mann DL. Apoptosis and the heart: a decade of progress. *J Mol Cell Cardiol* 2005;**38**(1):1–2.
11. Mann DL, Bristow MR. Mechanisms and models in heart failure: the biomechanical model and beyond. *Circulation* 2005;**111**(21): 2837–49.
12. Polyakova V, Hein S, Kostin S, Ziegelhoeffer T, Schaper J. Matrix metalloproteinases and their tissue inhibitors in pressure-overloaded human myocardium during heart failure progression. *J Am Coll Cardiol* 2004;**44**(8):1609–18.
13. Mehra MR, Griffith BP. Is mitral regurgitation a viable treatment target in heart failure? The plot just thickened. *J Am Coll Cardiol* 2005;**45**(3):388–90.
14. Trichon BH, Felker GM, Shaw LK, Cabell CH, O'Connor CM. Relation of frequency and severity of mitral regurgitation to survival among patients with left ventricular systolic dysfunction and heart failure. *Am J Cardiol* 2003;**91**(5):538–43.
15. Pfeffer MA, Pfeffer JM. Ventricular enlargement following a myocardial infarction. *J Cardiovasc Pharmacol* 1987;**9** Suppl 2:S18–20.
16. Pfeffer MA, Pfeffer JM. Ventricular enlargement and reduced survival after myocardial infarction. *Circulation* 1987;**75**(5 Pt 2):IV93–7.
17. Pfeffer JM, Pfeffer MA. Angiotensin converting enzyme inhibition and ventricular remodeling in heart failure. *Am J Med* 1988;**84**(3A):37–44.
18. Cleland JG, Pennell DJ, Ray SG, *et al.* Myocardial viability as a determinant of the ejection fraction response to carvedilol in patients with heart failure (CHRISTMAS trial): randomised controlled trial. *Lancet* 2003;**362**(9377):14–21.
19. Spragg DD, Leclercq C, Loghmani M, *et al.* Regional alterations in protein expression in the dyssynchronous failing heart. *Circulation* 2003;**108**(8):929–32.
20. Spragg DD, Kass DA. Pathobiology of left ventricular dyssynchrony and resynchronization. *Prog Cardiovasc Dis* 2006;**49**(1):26–41.
21. Cleland JG, Daubert JC, Erdmann E, *et al.* The effect of cardiac resynchronization on morbidity and mortality in heart failure. *N Engl J Med* 2005;**352**(15):1539–49.

22. Zile MR, Brutsaert DL. New concepts in diastolic dysfunction and diastolic heart failure: Part I: diagnosis, prognosis, and measurements of diastolic function. *Circulation* 2002;**105**(11):1387–93.
23. Zile MR, Brutsaert DL. New concepts in diastolic dysfunction and diastolic heart failure: Part II: causal mechanisms and treatment. *Circulation* 2002;**105**(12):1503–8.
24. Kass DA, Bronzwaer JG, Paulus WJ. What mechanisms underlie diastolic dysfunction in heart failure? *Circ Res* 2004;**94**(12):1533–42.
25. Kitzman DW, Little WC, Brubaker PH, *et al.* Pathophysiological characterization of isolated diastolic heart failure in comparison to systolic heart failure. *JAMA* 2002;**288**(17):2144–50.
26. Zile MR, Baicu CF, Bonnema DD. Diastolic heart failure: definitions and terminology. *Prog Cardiovasc Dis* 2005;**47**(5):307–13.
27. Kaye DM, Lefkovits J, Jennings GL, Bergin P, Broughton A, Esler MD. Adverse consequences of high sympathetic nervous activity in the failing human heart. *J Am Coll Cardiol* 1995;**26**(5):1257–63.
28. Cohn JN, Levine TB, Olivari MT, *et al.* Plasma norepinephrine as a guide to prognosis in patients with chronic congestive heart failure. *N Engl J Med* 1984;**311**(13):819–23.
29. Mann DL, Kent RL, Parsons B, Cooper GT. Adrenergic effects on the biology of the adult mammalian cardiocyte. *Circulation* 1992;**85**(2):790–804.
30. Singh K, Communal C, Sawyer DB, Colucci WS. Adrenergic regulation of myocardial apoptosis. *Cardiovasc Res* 2000;**45**(3):713–19.
31. Bristow MR. Myocardial beta-adrenergic receptor downregulation in heart failure. *Int J Cardiol* 1984;**5**(5):648–52.
32. Bristow MR. The adrenergic nervous system in heart failure. *N Engl J Med* 1984;**311**(13):850–1.
33. Binkley PF, Nunziata E, Haas GJ, Nelson SD, Cody RJ. Parasympathetic withdrawal is an integral component of autonomic imbalance in congestive heart failure: demonstration in human subjects and verification in a paced canine model of ventricular failure. *J Am Coll Cardiol* 1991;**18**(2):464–72.
34. Packer M, Bristow MR, Cohn JN, *et al.* The effect of carvedilol on morbidity and mortality in patients with chronic heart failure. U.S. Carvedilol Heart Failure Study Group. *N Engl J Med* 1996;**334**(21):1349–55.
35. Dargie HJ. Effect of carvedilol on outcome after myocardial infarction in patients with left-ventricular dysfunction: the CAPRICORN randomised trial. *Lancet* 2001;**357**(9266):1385–90.
36. Francis GS, Benedict C, Johnstone DE, *et al.* Comparison of neuroendocrine activation in patients with left ventricular dysfunction with and without congestive heart failure. A substudy of the Studies of Left Ventricular Dysfunction (SOLVD). *Circulation* 1990;**82**(5):1724–9.
37. Francis GS. The relationship of the sympathetic nervous system and the renin-angiotensin system in congestive heart failure. *Am Heart J* 1989;**118**(3):642–8.
38. Francis GS, Goldsmith SR, Levine TB, Olivari MT, Cohn JN. The neurohumoral axis in congestive heart failure. *Ann Intern Med* 1984;**101**(3):370–7.
39. Struthers AD. The clinical implications of aldosterone escape in congestive heart failure. *Eur J Heart Fail* 2004;**6**(5):539–45.
40. Effects of enalapril on mortality in severe congestive heart failure. Results of the Cooperative North Scandinavian Enalapril Survival Study (CONSENSUS). The CONSENSUS Trial Study Group. *N Engl J Med* 1987;**316**(23):1429–35.
41. Effect of enalapril on survival in patients with reduced left ventricular ejection fractions and congestive heart failure. The SOLVD Investigators. *N Engl J Med* 1991;**325**(5):293–302.
42. Effect of enalapril on mortality and the development of heart failure in asymptomatic patients with reduced left ventricular ejection fractions. The SOLVD Investigators. *N Engl J Med* 1992;**327**(10):685–91.
43. Pfeffer MA, Swedberg K, Granger CB, *et al.* Effects of candesartan on mortality and morbidity in patients with chronic heart failure: the CHARM-Overall programme. *Lancet* 2003;**362**(9386):759–66.
44. Swedberg K, Eneroth P, Kjekshus J, Wilhelmsen L. Hormones regulating cardiovascular function in patients with severe congestive heart failure and their relation to mortality. CONSENSUS Trial Study Group. *Circulation* 1990;**82**(5):1730–6.
45. Struthers AD. Aldosterone: cardiovascular assault. *Am Heart J* 2002;**144**(5 Suppl):S2–7.
46. Weber KT. Aldosterone in congestive heart failure. *N Engl J Med* 2001;**345**(23):1689–97.
47. Pitt B, Zannad F, Remme WJ, *et al.* The effect of spironolactone on morbidity and mortality in patients with severe heart failure. Randomized Aldactone Evaluation Study Investigators. *N Engl J Med* 1999;**341**(10):709–17.
48. Miller WL, Redfield MM, Burnett JC Jr. Integrated cardiac, renal, and endocrine actions of endothelin. *J Clin Invest* 1989;**83**(1):317–20.
49. Neubauer S, Ertl G, Haas U, Pulzer F, Kochsiek K. Effects of endothelin-1 in isolated perfused rat heart. *J Cardiovasc Pharmacol* 1990;**16**(1):1–8.
50. Cowburn PJ, Cleland JG, McArthur JD, MacLean MR, McMurray JJ, Dargie HJ. Pulmonary and systemic responses to exogenous endothelin-1 in patients with left ventricular dysfunction. *J Cardiovasc Pharmacol* 1998;**31** Suppl 1:S290–3.
51. Iwanaga Y, Kihara Y, Hasegawa K, *et al.* Cardiac endothelin-1 plays a critical role in the functional deterioration of left ventricles during the transition from compensatory hypertrophy to congestive heart failure in salt-sensitive hypertensive rats. *Circulation* 1998;**98**(19):2065–73.
52. McMurray JJ, Ray SG, Abdullah I, Dargie HJ, Morton JJ. Plasma endothelin in chronic heart failure. *Circulation* 1992;**85**(4):1374–9.
53. Pousset F, Isnard R, Lechat P, *et al.* Prognostic value of plasma endothelin-1 in patients with chronic heart failure. *Eur Heart J* 1997;**18**(2):254–8.
54. Pacher R, Bergler-Klein J, Globits S, *et al.* Plasma big endothelin-1 concentrations in congestive heart failure patients with or without systemic hypertension. *Am J Cardiol* 1993;**71**(15):1293–9.
55. Anand I, McMurray J, Cohn JN, *et al.* Long-term effects of darusentan on left-ventricular remodelling and clinical outcomes in the EndothelinA Receptor Antagonist Trial in Heart Failure (EARTH): randomised, double-blind, placebo-controlled trial. *Lancet* 2004;**364**(9431):347–54.
56. Torre-Amione G, Young JB, Colucci WS, *et al.* Hemodynamic and clinical effects of tezosentan, an intravenous dual endothelin receptor antagonist, in patients hospitalized for acute decompensated heart failure. *J Am Coll Cardiol* 2003;**42**(1):140–7.
57. McMurray JJ, Teerlink JR, Cotter G, *et al.* Effects of tezosentan on symptoms and clinical outcomes in patients with acute heart failure: the VERITAS randomized controlled trials. *JAMA* 2007;**298**(17):2009–19.
58. Udelson JE, Smith WB, Hendrix GH, *et al.* Acute hemodynamic effects of conivaptan, a dual V(1A) and V(2) vasopressin receptor antagonist, in patients with advanced heart failure. *Circulation* 2001;**104**(20):2417–23.
59. Konstam MA, Gheorghiade M, Burnett JC Jr, *et al.* Effects of oral tolvaptan in patients hospitalized for worsening heart failure: the EVEREST Outcome Trial. *JAMA* 2007;**297**(12):1319–31.
60. Wei CM, Heublein DM, Perrella MA, *et al.* Natriuretic peptide system in human heart failure. *Circulation* 1993;**88**(3):1004–9.
61. Davis M, Espiner E, Richards G, *et al.* Plasma brain natriuretic peptide in assessment of acute dyspnoea. *Lancet* 1994;**343**(8895):440–4.
62. Maisel AS, Krishnaswamy P, Nowak RM, *et al.* Rapid measurement of B-type natriuretic peptide in the emergency diagnosis of heart failure. *N Engl J Med* 2002;**347**(3):161–7.
63. Tsutamoto T, Wada A, Maeda K, *et al.* Attenuation of compensation of endogenous cardiac natriuretic peptide system in chronic heart failure: prognostic role of plasma brain natriuretic peptide concentration in patients with chronic symptomatic left ventricular dysfunction. *Circulation* 1997;**96**(2):509–16.

64. Gardner RS, Ozalp F, Murday AJ, Robb SD, McDonagh TA. N-terminal pro-brain natriuretic peptide. A new gold standard in predicting mortality in patients with advanced heart failure. *Eur Heart J* 2003;**24**(19):1735–43.
65. Rouleau JL, Pfeffer MA, Stewart DJ, *et al.* Comparison of vasopeptidase inhibitor, omapatrilat, and lisinopril on exercise tolerance and morbidity in patients with heart failure: IMPRESS randomised trial. *Lancet* 2000;**356**(9230):615–20.
66. Sackner-Bernstein JD, Kowalski M, Fox M, Aaronson K. Short-term risk of death after treatment with nesiritide for decompensated heart failure: a pooled analysis of randomized controlled trials. *JAMA* 2005;**293**(15):1900–5.
67. Anand IS, Latini R, Florea VG, *et al.* C-reactive protein in heart failure: prognostic value and the effect of valsartan. *Circulation* 2005;**112**(10):1428–34.
68. Levine B, Kalman J, Mayer L, Fillit HM, Packer M. Elevated circulating levels of tumor necrosis factor in severe chronic heart failure. *N Engl J Med* 1990;**323**(4):236–41.
69. McMurray J, Abdullah I, Dargie HJ, Shapiro D. Increased concentrations of tumour necrosis factor in 'cachectic' patients with severe chronic heart failure. *Br Heart J* 1991;**66**(5):356–8.
70. Adamopoulos S, Parissis JT, Kremastinos DT. A glossary of circulating cytokines in chronic heart failure. *Eur J Heart Fail* 2001;**3**(5):517–26.
71. Rauchhaus M, Doehner W, Francis DP, *et al.* Plasma cytokine parameters and mortality in patients with chronic heart failure. *Circulation* 2000;**102**(25):3060–7.
72. Maeda K, Tsutamoto T, Wada A, *et al.* High levels of plasma brain natriuretic peptide and interleukin-6 after optimized treatment for heart failure are independent risk factors for morbidity and mortality in patients with congestive heart failure. *J Am Coll Cardiol* 2000;**36**(5):1587–93.
73. Torre-Amione G, Vooletich MT, Farmer JA. Role of tumour necrosis factor-alpha in the progression of heart failure: therapeutic implications. *Drugs* 2000;**59**(4):745–51.
74. MacGowan GA, Mann DL, Kormos RL, Feldman AM, Murali S. Circulating interleukin-6 in severe heart failure. *Am J Cardiol* 1997;**79**(8):1128–31.
75. Shioi T, Matsumori A, Kihara Y, *et al.* Increased expression of interleukin-1 beta and monocyte chemotactic and activating factor/monocyte chemoattractant protein-1 in the hypertrophied and failing heart with pressure overload. *Circ Res* 1997;**81**(5):664–71.
76. Aukrust P, Ueland T, Muller F, *et al.* Elevated circulating levels of C-C chemokines in patients with congestive heart failure. *Circulation* 1998;**97**(12):1136–43.
77. Damas JK, Eiken HG, Oie E, *et al.* Myocardial expression of CC- and CXC-chemokines and their receptors in human end-stage heart failure. *Cardiovasc Res* 2000;**47**(4):778–87.
78. Mann DL. Targeted anticytokine therapy and the failing heart. *Am J Cardiol* 2005;**95**(11A):9–16C; discussion 38–40C.
79. Mann DL, McMurray JJ, Packer M, Swedberg K, Borer JS, Colucci WS, *et al.* Targeted anticytokine therapy in patients with chronic heart failure: results of the Randomized Etanercept Worldwide Evaluation (RENEWAL). *Circulation* 2004;**109**(13):1594–602.
80. Januzzi JL, Jr., Peacock WF, Maisel AS, *et al.* Measurement of the interleukin family member ST2 in patients with acute dyspnea: results from the PRIDE (Pro-Brain Natriuretic Peptide Investigation of Dyspnea in the Emergency Department) study. *J Am Coll Cardiol* 2007;**50**(7):607–13.
81. Rehman SU, Mueller T, Januzzi JL Jr. Characteristics of the novel interleukin family biomarker ST2 in patients with acute heart failure. *J Am Coll Cardiol* 2008;**52**(18):1458–65.
82. Chong KS, Gardner RS, Ashley EA, Dargie HJ, McDonagh TA. Emerging role of the apelin system in cardiovascular homeostasis. *Biomark Med* 2007;**1**(1):37–43.
83. Chong KS, Gardner RS, Morton JJ, Ashley EA, McDonagh TA. Plasma concentrations of the novel peptide apelin are decreased in patients with chronic heart failure. *Eur J Heart Fail* 2006;**8**(4):355–60.
84. Chen MM, Ashley EA, Deng DX, *et al.* Novel role for the potent endogenous inotrope apelin in human cardiac dysfunction. *Circulation* 2003;**108**(12):1432–9.
85. Mancini DM, Walter G, Reichek N, *et al.* Contribution of skeletal muscle atrophy to exercise intolerance and altered muscle metabolism in heart failure. *Circulation* 1992;**85**(4):1364–73.
86. Sullivan MJ, Higginbotham MB, Cobb FR. Increased exercise ventilation in patients with chronic heart failure: intact ventilatory control despite hemodynamic and pulmonary abnormalities. *Circulation* 1988;**77**(3):552–9.
87. Bank AJ, Lee PC, Kubo SH. Endothelial dysfunction in patients with heart failure: relationship to disease severity. *J Card Fail* 2000;**6**(1):29–36.

14

Cardiac natriuretic peptides and heart failure

Theresa A. McDonagh

The natriuretic peptide system

The natriuretic peptide (NP) family, to date, consists of four structurally similar hormones, A, B, C, and D, each sharing a 17 amino acid disulphide ring structure (Fig. 14.1). They are counter-regulatory hormones in heart failure (HF) and have a major role in controlling cardiovascular homeostasis via their key effector functions: natriuresis, diuresis, and vasodilatation.

The first to be discovered was atrial natriuretic peptide (ANP). Early experiments demonstrated that dilatation of the cardiac atria could induce natriuresis. Secretary granules were then identified in the atria using electron microscopy. The significance of these became apparent when de Bold and colleagues subsequently injected atrial myocyte extracts into rats and observed both natriuresis and vasodilatation. The product of the secretory granules was therefore named ANP.[1,2]

B-type natriuretic peptide (BNP) was discovered in 1988. It was isolated first from porcine brain, and hence originally known as brain natriuretic peptide.[3] Active BNP is a 32 amino acid structure. In contrast to ANP, in HF, it is mainly secreted from the left ventricle in response to increased left ventricular pressure, wall stress, and stretch.[4–8] Other stimuli also lead to its secretion, notably ischaemia, the neurohormone endothelin, and the growth factor TGFβ.

Figure 14.2 depicts the main actions of ANP and BNP which include natriuresis, vasodilatation, antiproliferative effects, and inhibition of the sympathetic and renin–angiotensin systems which are in overdrive in HF.[9–13]

Two further NPs have since been identified: C-type natriuretic peptide (CNP) and D (dendroaspis)-type natriuretic peptide (DNP). CNP is principally found in the central nervous system (CNS) and vascular endothelium.[14] It has limited natriuretic and diuretic effects but it is a potent vasodilator. DNP was initially isolated from the venom of the green mamba snake *Dendroaspis augusticeps*, and has been shown to be potent in relaxing isolated precontracted rodent aorta and canine coronary arteries.[15]

The genes encoding human ANP and BNP are located on the short arm of chromosome 1. The BNP gene is a rapid response gene; BNP is synthesized *de novo* in response to stimuli. ANP, in contrast, is stored in secretory granules and can be released into the circulation in response to an increase in left atrial pressure. The postprocessing of both peptides is similar and is shown for BNP in Fig. 14.3. BNP is produced as the pre-pro hormone (pre-proBNP), processed to proBNP, and then cleaved by furin to mature 32 amino acid BNP, which is biologically active, and 76 amino acid N-terminal (NT)-proBNP, which is not biologically active.[16] These are produced in a 1:1 ratio. ProBNP is synthesized by myocytes and fibroblasts principally in the ventricles (but also to a lesser degree in the atria) in response to an increase in left ventricular filling pressure and wall stress. Picomolar concentrations are detectable in the plasma of normal individuals.[17]

The NPs exert their action by binding to three different receptors, A, B, and C, which are located in the kidneys, vascular endothelium, adrenal glands, and the CNS, as well as in the heart (Fig. 14.4).[18] Interaction of NPs with the A and B receptors leads to intracellular production of cGMP. The positive lusitropic effects of the hormones are thought to be due to an increase in calcium entry into the myocytes. CNP acts via the NPR-B receptor: it does not cause natriuresis or diuresis but vasodilatation, and exerts paracrine effects on vascular growth.

Clearance of the NPs from the circulation is by two main mechanisms. First, via receptor-mediated endocytosis and lysosomal degradation; and secondly, by enzymatic degradation by neutral endopeptidase (Fig. 14.4).[19] The half-lives of the active hormones are shorter than that of the inactive N-terminal fragments, so the mean half-life of BNP is 20 min whereas NT-proBNP, which is cleared passively, in part by the kidneys, has a longer half-life of between 60 and 120 min.

Plasma concentrations of the NP hormones in humans are affected by several factors independent of the presence of cardiovascular pathology. They are higher in women than in men, they

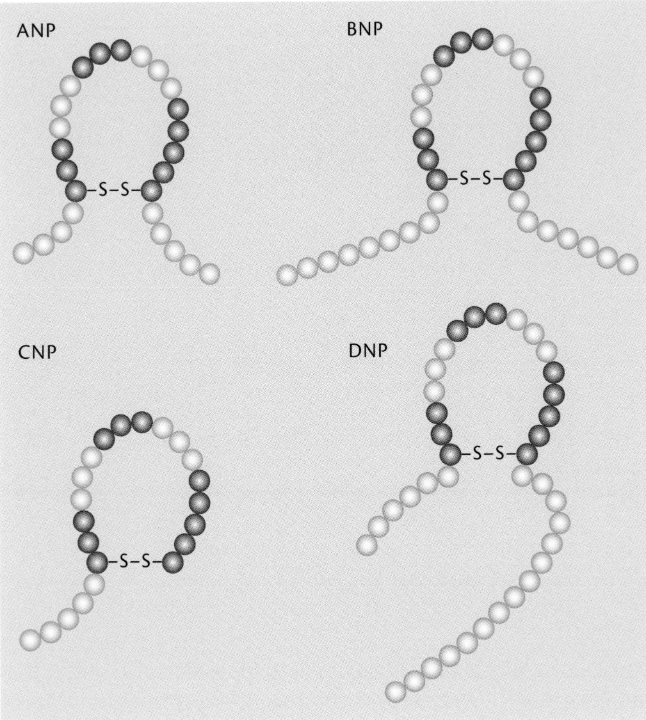

Fig. 14.1 Schematic demonstrating the similar 17 amino acid disulphide ring structure in the A-, B-, C-, and D-type natriuretic peptides. Identical amino acid sequences are marked in black.
From Gardner RS, Chong KS, McDonagh TA. B-type natriuretic peptides in heart failure. *Biomark Med* 2007;**1**(2):243–50.

are lower in obese subjects, and their values increase with age, a phenomenon which is thought to be associated with progressive nephron loss.[4,20–22] The circulating concentrations of both ANP and BNP are raised in a myriad of cardiovascular conditions affecting either cardiac structure or function, as well as being increased by renal dysfunction.

Undoubtedly, the main focus of research interest for both ANP and BNP has been in HF. There are four main areas in which measuring the plasma concentrations of NPs may be of use clinically: diagnosis, screening for asymptomatic cardiac dysfunction, assessing prognosis, and therapy monitoring for HF. A potential fifth use of NPs as therapeutic agents for HF is covered in Chapter 44.

Diagnosis

We have known for a considerable time now that the circulating concentrations of the NPs are raised in patients with HF.[23–25] Importantly, their concentrations are also elevated in the known precursor phase of HF—asymptomatic left ventricular systolic dysfunction (LVSD).[24,26] Levels of NPs are raised whether HF results from systolic dysfunction or whether it occurs in the presence of preserved systolic function.[27] NPs also circulate in higher concentrations in patients with post myocardial infarction (MI) left ventricular dysfunction.[28–30] In considering their usefulness as diagnostic tests for HF, we need to comment on their sensitivity and specificity in determining the presence of HF as it presents clinically, e.g. in the acute setting, in the coronary care unit post myocardial infarction, in primary care, and in the clinic setting for chronic HF.

Acute heart failure

Davis *et al.* first reported on the usefulness of BNP in distinguishing whether breathlessness was due to HF or an exacerbation of chronic obstructive pulmonary disease in patients presenting acutely breathless to the accident and emergency department. A BNP concentration of 22 pg/mL or more predicted the presence of HF with 93% sensitivity and 90% specificity.[31] This was subsequently confirmed in a much larger US study where the area under the curve (AUC) for BNP diagnosing breathless due to HF in this setting was 0.97.[32] BNP is therefore an accurate means to diagnose HF presenting to the emergency department and to distinguish it accurately from other causes of acute breathlessness.

Chronic heart failure presenting in primary care and in outpatient clinics

Cowie *et al.* described the utility of the NP hormones in diagnosing incident HF cases assessed at a HF clinic in West London.[33] The gold standard diagnosis was a panel of three cardiologists reviewing the clinical and echocardiographic information. BNP was the most accurate of the peptides in diagnosing HF, superior to both ANP and N-terminal proatrial natriuretic peptide (N-ANP). A BNP concentration of 22 pmol/L or more diagnosed HF with a sensitivity of 97%, a specificity of 84%, a positive predictive accuracy of 70%, and a negative predictive accuracy of 97%. Interestingly in this study, BNP was a far better method for detecting HF than

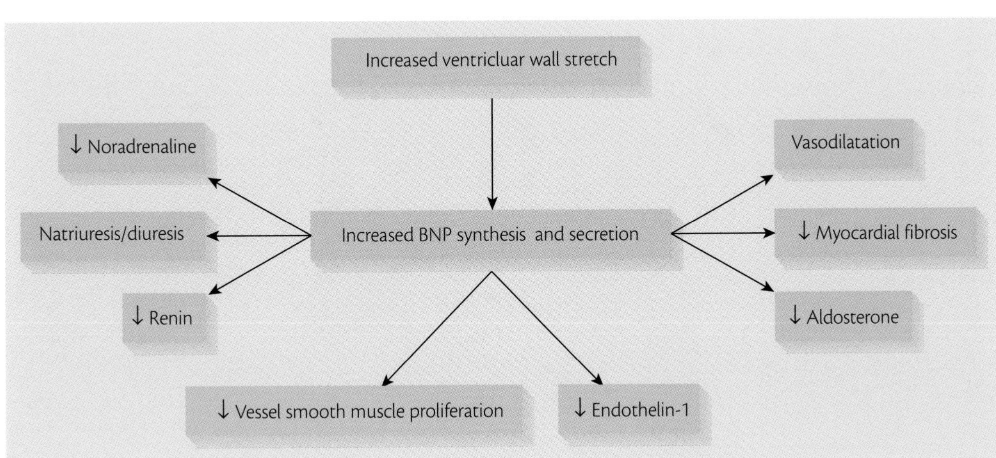

Fig. 14.2 The action of B-type natriuretic peptides.
From Gardner RS, Chong KS, McDonagh TA. B-type natriuretic peptides in heart failure. *Biomark Med* 2007;**1**(2):243–50.

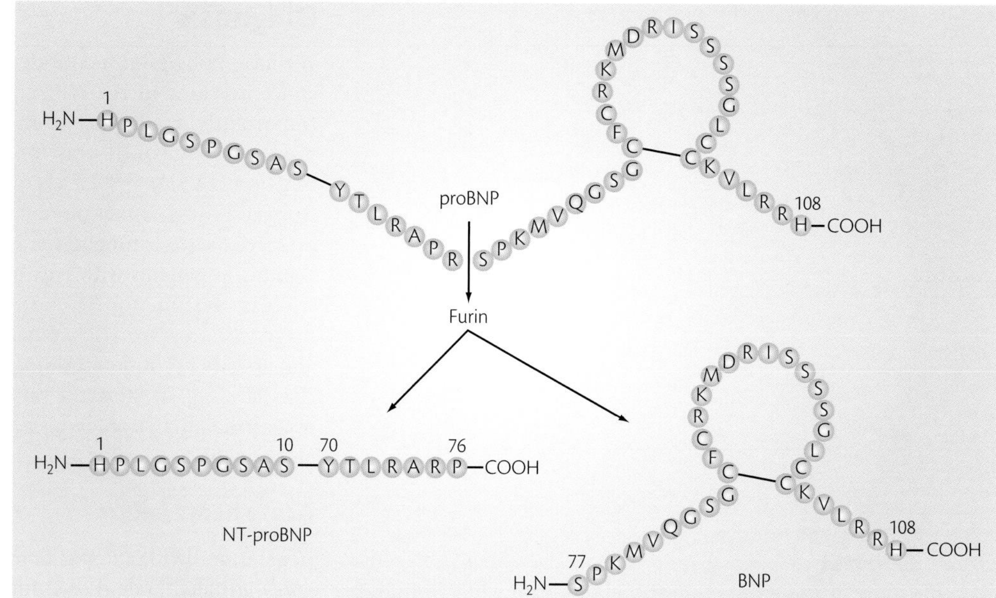

Fig. 14.3 The enzymatic cleavage of proBNP into inactive NT-proBNP and biologically active BNP. A, alanine; BNP, B-type natriuretic peptide; C, cysteine; D, aspartic acid; F, phenylalanine; G, glycine; H, histidine; I, isoleucine; K, lysine; L, leucine; M, methionine; N, asparagine; NT-proBNP, N-terminal prohormone BNP; P, proline; ProBNP, prohormone BNP; Q, glutamine; R, arginine; S, serine; T, threonine; V, valine; Y, tyrosine.
From Gardner RS, Chong KS, McDonagh TA. B-type natriuretic peptides in heart failure. *Biomark Med* 2007;**1**(2):243–50.

use of an increased cardiothoracic ratio on the chest radiograph. This work was later confirmed in a larger UK multicentre trial using BNP and NT-pro-BNP which showed that both peptides have a similar diagnostic accuracy for the exclusion of HF in patients being referred from primary care suspected of having HF (Fig. 14.5).[34]

Post myocardial infarction

Struther's group first demonstrated that a raised BNP concentration was the most sensitive method of detecting a left ventricular ejection fraction (LVEF) of 40% or less post MI when compared to ANP, various clinical scoring systems, and qualitative echocardiography.[35] Richards *et al.* subsequently compared many possible forms of the NPs in their ability to detect HF after a MI. Both BNP and NT-proBNP were superior to the atrial peptides in terms of both their sensitivity and negative predictive accuracies. BNP itself was highly accurate at diagnosing HF, with a sensitivity of 85% and a negative predictive accuracy of 93%.[28]

NPs can thus diagnose HF precisely. Early studies used complex radioimmunoassays. More recent studies have used more user-friendly ELISAs for BNP and NT-proBNP, and point-of-care tests for BNP are now available in clinical practice. Simple cut-point concentrations have been described for the two commonly used assays (BNP and NT-proBNP) and are shown in Table 14.1.

Most published work demonstrates that the B-type peptides are superior to ANP in diagnosing HF, but more recent work

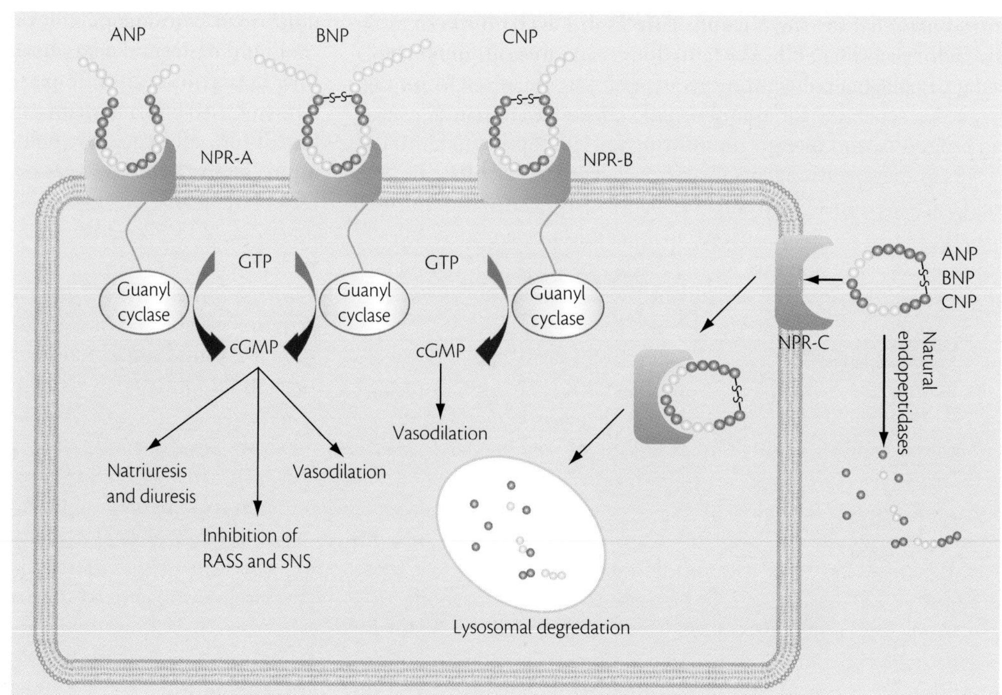

Fig. 14.4 Action and clearance of natriuretic peptides. NP, natriuretic peptide; NPR, natriuretic peptide receptor.
From Gardner RS, Chong KS, McDonagh TA. B-type natriuretic peptides in heart failure. *Biomark Med* 2007;**1**(2):243–50.

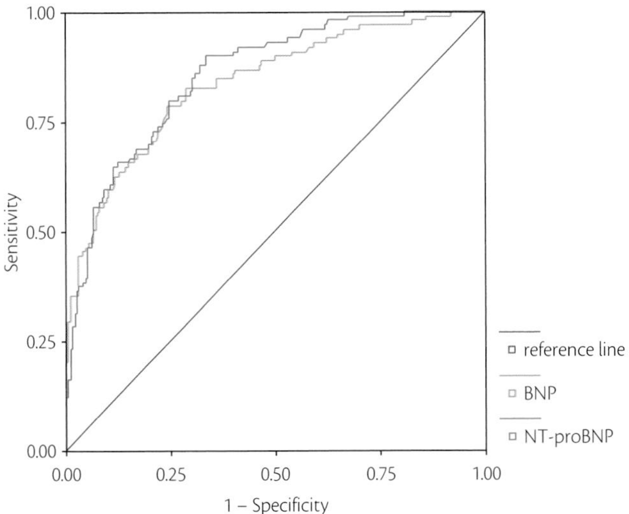

Fig. 14.5 Receiver operating curves (ROC) for BNP and NT-proBNP.
From Zaphiriou A, Robb S, Murray-Thomas T, *et al.* The diagnostic accuracy of plasma BNP and NTproBNP in patients referred from primary care with suspected heart failure: results of the UK natriuretic peptide study. *Eur J Heart Fail* 2005;**7**(4):537–41.

using assays directed at the mid region of the pro-ANP molecule (which are more stable than previous assays of the C-terminal and N-terminal fragments of ANP) shows similar accuracy to the BNP studies.[36] The striking feature of NPs diagnostically is their high negative predictive value—in other words, if the concentration of NP is low, HF or left ventricular dysfunction is highly unlikely. High concentrations are not, however, diagnostic of HF, but simply flag up the need for further detailed cardiorenal investigation to determine the cause of increase. As such, their most important diagnostic role is in helping to diagnose suspected HF in breathless patients and allowing more cost-effective use of detailed cardiology imaging and expertise. Their diagnostic use is now well established in clinical practice and is emphasized in both European and US clinical guidelines.[37,38]

Screening

The second possible role for NPs in screening for asymptomatic disease is much less well studied. Screening for left ventricular dysfunction lies under the diagnostic umbrella of 'HF' but refers to uncovering disease which is asymptomatic; HF by definition, although difficult to diagnose, is nevertheless a symptomatic condition. What is the evidence that NPs can screen for the most studied and treatable precursor phase of HF, asymptomatic LVSD?

The first evidence to be published was from the North Glasgow MONICA study, where a population of 2000 men and women aged 25–74 were screened by echocardiography; 3.1% had LVSD defined as a LVEF of 30% or less, and 1.4% of the population had asymptomatic LVSD. BNP gave an AUC of 0.884, which was superior to N-ANP.[26] The concentration of BNP used in this study was in excess of 17.9 pg/mL with the Peninsula radioimmunoassay. It would not be cost-effective to screen the entire population by this method but better to target those most likely to have the disease: i.e. in those over 55 years with some manifestation of ischaemic heart disease, where the AUC is 0.88. This compares very well with other established screening tests such as prostate specific antigen (PSA) for prostatic cancer (AUC 0.92), mammography for breast cancer (AUC 0.85), and cervical cytology for cervical cancer (AUC 0.70).

Table 14.1 Suggested cut-points for BNP and BT-proBNP for the exclusion of heart failure

Clinical setting	BNP	NT-proBNP
Acute heart failure	100 pg/mL	300 pg/mL
Chronic heart failure	50 pg/mL	<60 years 50 pg/mL 60–75 years 100 pg/mL >75 years 250 pg/mL

Adapted from Cowie MR *et al. Br J Cardiol* 2010;**17**:76–80.

A more recent study from the US screened for asymptomatic LVSD in the Olmsted County population (1869 subjects >45 years) using the more modern, rapid assays for BNP (Biosite) and NT-proBNP (Roche).[39] They have found similar results, this time for detecting LVEF of 40% or less. Interestingly, BNP and NT-proBNP performed similarly. The test was also effective in older individuals and women: this is important, as there had been concerns that the normal rise in the peptides with age and the higher values in women might limit their usefulness as screening tools. The cut-points used in the total population were 66 pg/mL for BNP and 228 pg/mL for NT-proBNP. The study also showed that left ventricular systolic or diastolic function could be detected to similar degrees. Hobbs *et al.* have also compared the two peptides in an English population, reporting similar results.[40] BNP therefore seems to provide an accurate means of excluding left ventricular dysfunction in the general population, with AUCs of more than 0.85 and negative predictive values in excess of 0.90.

There is controversy as to whether BNP should be used alone or in combination with the ECG as a screening tool. Most groups have found in population-based studies of screening or in the detection of HF that the ECG does not add anything to the pick-up rate of LVSD. However, in a recent large study of 1360 subjects, aged 45–80, Ng *et al.*[41] reported that using a history of ischaemic heart disease and an ECG abnormality reduced the number of cases needing to be screened to detect one case of LVSD (identified by subsequent echocardiogram) to 7, from 44 with BNP alone. Hedberg *et al.*[42] also looked at screening with BNP/ECG or both in an elderly population of 407 individuals aged over 75 years. Both were highly efficient at excluding left ventricular dysfunction. The ECG alone yielded fewer false positives, leading to the conclusion that in older individuals BNP added value only in those with an abnormal ECG. The argument about including the ECG with BNP as a screening test is largely academic, as in clinical practice both would be carried out. However, in general practice, where confidence in declaring an ECG truly normal is lower than in hospital practice, a BNP test would be easier to interpret as the first step in a screening strategy.

The vast majority of studies examining BNP as a screening test have measured plasma BNP. However, one study has found that urinary N-BNP gives similar AUCs to plasma N-BNP.[43] The accuracy of the diagnosis may also be improved by combining a blood and urinary strategy, but further work is needed in this area before it could challenge a single blood value at present.[44]

Most of the studies using BNP to screen for asymptomatic LVSD have been very positive, but this is not universally the case. In particular, in the Framingham study offspring cohort, AUCs for 'any left ventricular dysfunction' were only 0.76 for men and 0.56 for women.

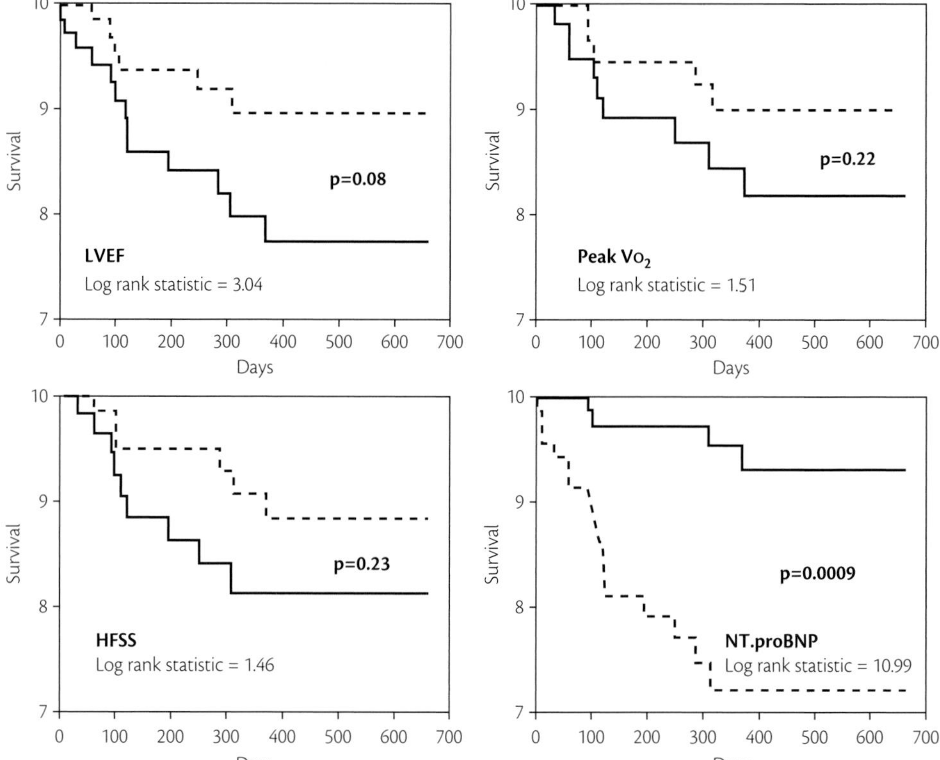

Fig. 14.6 Kaplan–Meier survival curves for left ventricular ejection fraction (LVEF), maximum oxygen uptake (peak Vo_2),heart failure survival score (HFSS) and NT-proBNP stratified above (broken line) and below (solid line) the median value against all-cause mortality.
From Gardner RS, Chong V, Morton I, McDonagh TA. N-terminal brain natriuretic peptide is a more powerful predictor of mortality than endothelin-1, adrenomedullin and tumour necrosis factor-alpha in patients referred for consideration of cardiac transplantation. *Eur J Heart Fail* 2005;**7**(2):253–60.

For systolic dysfunction (defined as LVEF ≤40% and/or a fractional shortening <22%), the AUC was 0.79 for men and 0.85 for women.[45,46] Of note, in this study LVEF was estimated visually rather than measured meticulously using the Simpson's bi-plane rule method employed in other population-based studies which reported more favourable results.

An important question to be addressed under the heading of screening is its cost-effectiveness. Little work is available in this area. In a retrospective analysis from the North Glasgow MONICA study, Nielsen *et al.* reported that screening high-risk subjects (those with hypertension and/or those with an abnormal ECG) would reduce the cost per detected case of LVSD by 26% for the cost ratio of 1/20 (BNP/echocardiogram).[46] Heidenreich[47] also addressed the issue in a meta-analysis of all population-based studies which have used BNP and echocardiography to detect LVSD in the general population. He concluded that in populations with a prevalence of LVSD of at least 1%, it would be cost-effective to screen with BNP followed by echocardiography, thereby improving outcome at a cost of $50 000 per QALY gained.

In general, we can conclude that BNP can detect, with acceptable accuracy, asymptomatic left ventricular dysfunction (systolic or otherwise) in the general population and in high-risk subgroups. The question that therefore remains is, 'Why are we not screening in this manner?' There are potentially several reasons. The first is economic and varies in different health care systems. Many systems are overwhelmed by detecting and treating the manifest stage of the condition—overt HF—never mind going looking for asymptomatic disease. Another stated reason is that we do not yet have enough information about how to screen for asymptomatic LVSD, what concentrations of BNP we should use, and whether age- and sex-specific cut-points are required. There is also the issue that in screening for asymptomatic LVSD we will also pick up other diseases, as an increased BNP concentration is a nonspecific marker of cardiac structural and functional disease and of renal impairment. However, the added value of BNP as a prognostic marker undoubtedly means that we would be uncovering important abnormalities by using this strategy. But perhaps the principal reason we are not doing this yet is philosophical—maybe we are not yet convinced that screening will really improve patient outcomes.

Prognosis

There is now a wealth of data indicating that NPs are excellent prognostic markers in HF. Numerous studies confirm they are independent predictors of a poor prognosis in all grades of HF ranging from asymptomatic left ventricular dysfunction through to NYHA class IV.[48–51] Indeed, they appear to be the best single prognostic markers we have to date, when we examine studies that have used multivariable models including established and novel markers of poor outcome including NYHA class, LVEF, peak Vo_2, serum sodium concentration, QRS duration, and plasma catecholamines and endothelin.

In addition to their role in predicting all-cause and cardiovascular mortality in HF, NPs also seem to be effective in predicting sudden cardiac death. In a study by Berger *et al.*, a BNP concentration greater than the median was the only independent predictor of sudden death in 452 patients with LVSD.[52]

The prognostic role of NPs has also been examined in patients being considered for cardiac transplantation. A recent study demonstrated that an NT-proBNP concentration greater than the median value at baseline was the single best predictor of mortality in these patients (Fig. 14.6).[53] How we use the information gained clinically is as yet unclear. Should we take a single baseline value, or a concentration which fails to fall on follow-up, or should we

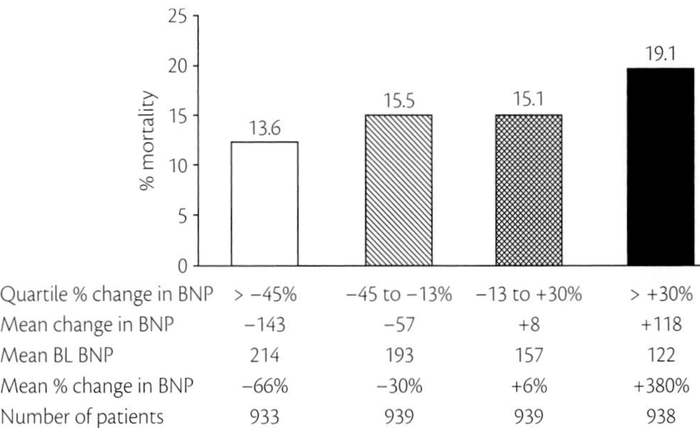

Quartile % change in BNP	> −45%	−45 to −13%	−13 to +30%	> +30%
Mean change in BNP	−143	−57	+8	+118
Mean BL BNP	214	193	157	122
Mean % change in BNP	−66%	−30%	+6%	+380%
Number of patients	933	939	939	938

Fig. 14.7 Change in BNP concentrations and mortality.
From Anand IS, Fisher LD, Chiang YT, *et al.* Changes in brain natriuretic peptide and norepinephrine over time and mortality and morbidity in the Valsartan Heart Failure Trial (Val-HeFT). *Circulation* 2003;**107**(9):1278–83.

incorporate BNP/NT-proBNP concentrations into our clinical scoring models for assessing prognosis?

Therapy monitoring

The concept of monitoring patients using NPs arises out their prognostic ability and can be thought about in three different, yet related, ways. First, we could use BNP concentrations in a general sense to help us risk-stratify patients we are reviewing, with the aim of trying to intensify the therapy of those we perceive to be at highest risk. Secondly, BNP could be used to aid discharge planning in patients admitted to hospital with decompensated HF. The third potential role concerns using BNP concentrations *per se* serially to monitor patients with HF and to use the values in clinical decision-making, including the titration of therapy.

Some information from studies in acute HF is helping to clarify the usefulness of single or serial BNP measurements.

Cheng *et al.*, in a study of 72 patients admitted to hospital with decompensated HF, demonstrated that the clinical endpoints of death or readmission to hospital with HF occurred in those whose BNP concentrations increased during the admission.[54] There were no clinical endpoints in those whose BNP concentrations fell. A single predischarge BNP concentration was also an accurate determinant of readmission. Hence, in the patient with decompensated HF serial monitoring of BNP looking for a fall is helpful clinically.

Logeart *et al.*, in an elegant study involving a derivation and validation cohort, reported that the predischarge BNP concentration was the best independent predictor of readmission in patients with decompensated HF, with those with a value of less than 300 pg/mL having the lowest readmission rates.[55] However, those patients with the greatest decrease in BNP had a better outcome than those with a more modest reduction (HR = 0.18 [0.07–0.48], p = 0.001). Hence in patients with decompensated HF, serially measuring BNP and aiming for a discharge BNP of less than 300 pg/mL seems important for discharge planning. Serial BNP testing has also been shown to be of more value in this situation that repeated examination by Doppler echocardiography.[56]

In chronic heart failure (CHF), fewer data are available on serial measurements. In Val-HeFT, those patients with the greatest reduction in their BNP concentration had the lowest mortality over the course of the study (Fig. 14.7).[57] More recently, the Val-HeFT Group published results using NT-proBNP from the placebo arm of the trial. A single determination of NT-proBNP had higher prognostic discrimination than continuous changes of concentrations, expressed as either an absolute or a percentage change. However, in the Cox proportional hazards model, stratification of patients into four categories depending on NT-proBNP levels (relative to a threshold value) at two time points, 4 months apart, provided prognostic information beyond that of a single determination.[58] In chronic but more advanced HF, Gardner *et al.* have shown that NT-proBNP concentrations greater than the median on follow-up also predict a poor outcome, as does an increase in NT-proBNP over 4 months of follow-up.[59] It therefore appears that serial monitoring of concentrations in CHF patients gives more information than merely looking at baseline values.

Titration of therapy

This use of NPs as an HbA_{1c} or 'biochemical Swan–Ganz catheter' depends to some extent on what happens to their concentrations with the drug and device therapies we give for HF. Diuretics reduce NP concentrations,[60,61] whereas there are reports suggesting that digoxin increases their levels.[62,63] However, it is the actions of disease-modifying drugs that are perhaps the most interesting. There is good evidence that both angiotensin converting enzyme (ACE) inhibitors and angiotensin II receptor blockers (ARBs) decrease BNP.[64,65] Tsutamoto reported in 37 patients with CHF that treatment with spironolactone for 4 months significantly reduced BNP concentrations compared to placebo.[66] The information regarding β-adrenoreceptor antagonists and BNP is a little more confusing to date. Data from the RESOLVD study with metoprolol versus placebo treatment for 24 weeks reported a rise in BNP despite the expected improvement in left ventricular function, reduction in mortality, and fall in angiotensin II and renin concentrations with metoprolol.[67] However, in a nonrandomized Japanese study looking at 52 patients with CHF, again comparing metoprolol with placebo, both ANP and BNP concentrations fell with the β-blocker.[68] More recent work shows that β-blockers may increase BNP concentrations initially but chronically they seem to reduce it, which fits with their effects on long-term reverse remodelling.[69]

There are thus two speculative schools of thought at the moment. The first presumes that initially the β-adrenoreceptor antagonists increase BNP due to their negatively inotropic and chronotropic properties, but that as the beneficial effect of the drugs on left ventricular function emerge, the peptide concentrations fall. The second school proposes that the improvement seen with the drugs could be explained, at least in part, by their ability to increase NP levels.

Irrespective of the effect of β-blockade, evidence is now emerging suggesting that when we optimize therapy in patients with HF, be that increasing ACE inhibitors, adding spironolactone, or up-titrating β-adrenoreceptor antagonists (which is, after all what we do when dealing clinically with HF patients), BNP concentrations fall.[70] Cardiac resynchronization therapy (biventricular pacing) also reduces BNP concentrations.[71] The real question is, however, 'Can we use NP concentrations to target our drug and device therapies for HF?'

There are now several randomized studies of BNP-driven care versus usual care which address the question. Murdoch *et al.* randomized a small group of 20 patients attending a HF clinic to usual care or optimization of HF drugs according to BNP-driven care, where the BNP target was to be within the normal range. The study showed a greater suppression of markers of the renin–angiotensin–aldosterone system in those receiving BNP-driven care.[72] Subsequently, Richard's group published a small study of 69 patients attending a HF clinic[73] randomized either to care according to their NT-BNP concentration or to usual care. Those allocated to NT-proBNP-driven care had a significantly lower incidence of death or readmission to hospital at 6 months (p = 0034), suggesting that the approach may give better patient outcomes.

Since then, several larger studies have reported. In the STARS-BNP study, patients were randomized to either optimal medical therapy or therapy guided to drive BNP below 100 pg/ml.[34] Mean doses of ACE inhibitors and β-adrenoreceptor antagonists were higher in the BNP-driven group, and the combined endpoint of HF-related death or hospitalization was significantly lower (24% vs 52%, p <0.001) at the median follow-up of 15 months.

The multicentre TIME-HF study examined the use of NT-proBNP-guided therapy versus usual care in 499 patients with systolic HF. After 18 months, the hazard ratio (95% CI) for standard therapy versus NT-proBNP-guided therapy for the primary endpoint, survival free of any hospitalization, was 0.92 (0.73–1.15), and for survival it was 0.68 (0.46–1.01), both nonsignificant. Survival free of HF hospitalization was significantly reduced. The results were much more striking in individuals aged less than <75 years, although the primary endpoint was still not significantly reduced.[74]

The Battlescarred Study also recently reported similar results in a three-way randomization of 364 patients with HF to NT-proBNP-guided care, usual care, or intensive medical care. Both systolic and nonsystolic HF patients were included. One-year mortality was lower in both the hormone-guided (9.1%) and intensive clinically guided (9.1%) groups compared with usual care (18.9%; p = 0.03). However, 3-year mortality was reduced in patients 75 years of age or less receiving hormone-guided treatment (15.5%) compared with their peers receiving either intensive clinically managed treatment (30.9%; p = 0.048) or usual care (31.3%; p = 0.021).[75]

So, to date, there is no convincing evidence that titrating HF therapies to try to drive down NP concentrations consistently improves outcomes for patients. It may be that the studies performed to date are insufficiently powered to prove the concept conclusively: a recent meta-analysis by Felker *et al.*, which takes into account the above studies plus others presented, but as yet unpublished, reported a significant mortality advantage for biomarker-guided therapy (hazard ratio 0.69, 95% CI 0.55–0.86) compared to controls.[76]

However, it should also be pointed out that titrating therapy to reduce NP concentrations may be a bridge too far. Lewin *et al.* used BNP concentrations and serial weight changes to try to predict clinical deterioration in patients attending a HF clinic,[77] and found that neither was accurate. They pointed out that as yet we know little about the day-to-day, month-to-month variability of BNP in CHF patients, and thus cannot know whether the changes we are looking for can be used. Wu recently showed that many short-term therapeutic studies of inpatients have largely resulted in statistically significant declines in BNP and NT-proBNP with clinical evidence of patient improvements.[78] In contrast, however, many therapeutic studies involving long-term outpatient monitoring have produced changes in BNP/NT-proBNP that do not exceed the biological variance.[79] More work clearly needs to be done and we will need larger studies of NP treatment titration before we can use NP-guided treatment routinely in clinical practice.

Conclusions and the future for natriuretic peptides

The last 30 years have seen a huge transformation in the field of cardiac natriuretic peptide hormones. NPs have moved from being merely of research interest to being established biomarkers for HF. To date, they have a well-defined role in the diagnosis of HF and their prognostic abilities are beginning to be used. Under the diagnostic umbrella, their true role in screening for precursor phases of HF needs to be determined. Their prognostic utility requires further applied research to work out their role in risk stratification and treatment monitoring in HF. We need to study how they should be used to aid selection for more complex advanced HF therapies including CRT implantation and selection for transplantation. Of particular importance is any potential role they have in identifying those at risk of sudden death in HF so as to prioritize defibrillator therapy. We also have much to learn about the potential role of NPs in the area of chemotherapy-induced cardiotoxicity as a cause of HF and monitoring for cancer therapies. In addition, we have to unravel how NPs should be used with other more novel biomarkers which also predict an adverse outcome in HF.

References

1. de Bold AJ, Borenstein HB, Veress AT, Sonnenberg H. A rapid, potent natriuretic response to intravenous injection of atrial myocardial extract in rats. *Life Sci* 1981;**28**(1):89–94.
2. de Bold AJ. Tissue fractionation studies on the relationship between an atrial natriuretic factor and specific atrial granules. *Can J Physiol Pharmacol* 1982;**60**(3):324–30.
3. Sudoh T, Kangawa K, Minamino N, Matsuo H. A new natriuretic peptide in porcine brain. *Nature* 1988;**332**(6159):78–81.
4. Wei CM, Heublein DM, Perrella MA, *et al.* Natriuretic peptide system in human heart failure. *Circulation* 1993;**88**(3):1004–9.
5. Yasue H, Yoshimura M, Sumida H, *et al.* Localization and mechanism of secretion of B-type natriuretic peptide in comparison with those of A-type natriuretic peptide in normal subjects and patients with heart failure. *Circulation* 1994;**90**(1):195–203.
6. Yoshimura M, Yasue H, Okumura K, *et al.* Different secretion patterns of atrial natriuretic peptide and brain natriuretic peptide in patients with congestive heart failure. *Circulation* 1993;**87**(2):464–9.
7. Edwards BS, Zimmerman RS, Schwab TR, Heublein DM, Burnett JC Jr. Atrial stretch, not pressure, is the principal determinant controlling the acute release of atrial natriuretic factor. *Circ Res* 1988;**62**(2):191–5.
8. Kinnunen P, Vuolteenaho O, Ruskoaho H. Mechanisms of atrial and brain natriuretic peptide release from rat ventricular myocardium: effect of stretching. *Endocrinology* 1993;**132**(5):1961–70.
9. Kurtz A, Della BR, Pfeilschifter J, Taugner R, Bauer C. Atrial natriuretic peptide inhibits renin release from juxtaglomerular cells by a cGMP-mediated process. *Proc Natl Acad Sci U S A* 1986;**83**(13):4769–73.
10. Kawaguchi H, Sawa H, Yasuda H. Effect of atrial natriuretic factor on angiotensin converting enzyme. *J Hypertens* 1990;**8**(8):749–53.
11. Oelkers W, Kleiner S, Bahr V. Effects of incremental infusions of atrial natriuretic factor on aldosterone, renin, and blood pressure in humans. *Hypertension* 1988;**12**(4):462–7.
12. Ebert TJ, Cowley AW Jr. Atrial natriuretic factor attenuates carotid baroreflex-mediated cardioacceleration in humans. *Am J Physiol* 1988;**254**(4 Pt 2):R590–4.
13. Kohno M, Yasunari K, Yokokawa K, Murakawa K, Horio T, Takeda T. Inhibition by atrial and brain natriuretic peptides of endothelin-1 secretion after stimulation with angiotensin II and thrombin of cultured human endothelial cells. *J Clin Invest* 1991;**87**(6):1999–2004.

14. Hunt PJ, Richards AM, Espiner EA, Nicholls MG, Yandle TG. Bioactivity and metabolism of C-type natriuretic peptide in normal man. *J Clin Endocrinol Metab* 1994;**78**(6):1428–35.
15. Lee CY, Burnett JC Jr. Natriuretic peptides and therapeutic applications. *Heart Fail Rev* 2007;**12**(2):131–42.
16. McKie PM, Burnett JC, Jr. B-type natriuretic peptide as a biomarker beyond heart failure: speculations and opportunities. *Mayo Clin Proc* 2005;**80**(8):1029–36.
17. Hunt PJ, Yandle TG, Nicholls MG, Richards AM, Espiner EA. The amino-terminal portion of pro-brain natriuretic peptide (Pro-BNP) circulates in human plasma. *Biochem Biophys Res Commun* 1995;**214**(3):1175–83.
18. Nakao K, Ogawa Y, Suga S, Imura H. Molecular biology and biochemistry of the natriuretic peptide system. I: Natriuretic peptides. *J Hypertens* 1992;**10**(9):907–12.
19. Kenny AJ, Bourne A, Ingram J. Hydrolysis of human and pig brain natriuretic peptides, urodilatin, C-type natriuretic peptide and some C-receptor ligands by endopeptidase-24.11. *Biochem J* 1993;**291** (Pt 1):83–8.
20. Redfield MM, Rodeheffer RJ, Jacobsen SJ, Mahoney DW, Bailey KR, Burnett JC Jr. Plasma brain natriuretic peptide concentration: impact of age and gender. *J Am Coll Cardiol* 2002;**40**(5):976–82.
21. McDonagh TA, Holmer S, Raymond I, Luchner A, Hildebrant P, Dargie HJ. NT-proBNP and the diagnosis of heart failure: a pooled analysis of three European epidemiological studies. *Eur J Heart Fail* 2004;**6**(3):269–73.
22. McCullough PA, Duc P, Omland T, *et al.* B-type natriuretic peptide and renal function in the diagnosis of heart failure: an analysis from the Breathing Not Properly Multinational Study. *Am J Kidney Dis* 2003;**41**(3):571–9.
23. Francis GS, McDonald KM, Cohn JN. Neurohumoral activation in preclinical heart failure. Remodeling and the potential for intervention. *Circulation* 1993;**87**:IV90–6.
24. Lerman A, Gibbons RJ, Rodeheffer RJ, *et al.* Circulating N-terminal atrial natriuretic peptide as a marker for symptomless left-ventricular dysfunction [see comments]. *Lancet* 1993;**341**:1105–9.
25. Motwani JG, McAlpine H, Kennedy N, Struthers AD. Plasma brain natriuretic peptide as an indicator for angiotensin- converting-enzyme inhibition after myocardial infarction [see comments]. *Lancet* 1993;**341**:1109–13.
26. McDonagh TA, Robb SD, Murdoch DR, *et al.* Biochemical detection of left-ventricular systolic dysfunction [see comments]. *Lancet* 1998;**351**(9095):9–13.
27. Lubien E, DeMaria A, Krishnaswamy P, *et al.* Utility of B-natriuretic peptide in detecting diastolic dysfunction: comparison with Doppler velocity recordings. *Circulation* 2002;**105**(5):595–601.
28. Richards AM, Nicholls G, Yandle TG, *et al.* Plasma N-Terminal Pro-Brain Natriuretic peptide and adrenomedullin: new neurohormonal predictors of left ventricular function and prognosis after myocardial infarction. *Circulation* 1998;**97**:1921–1929.
29. Talwar S, Squire IB, Downie PF, *et al.* Profile of plasma N-terminal proBNP following acute myocardial infarction; correlation with left ventricular systolic dysfunction. *Eur Heart J* 2000;**21**(18):1514–21.
30. Luchner A, Hengstenberg C, Lowel H, *et al.* N-terminal pro-brain natriuretic peptide after myocardial infarction: a marker of cardio-renal function. *Hypertension* 2002;**39**(1):99–104.
31. Davis M, Espiner E, Richards G, *et al.* Plasma brain natriuretic peptide in assessment of acute dyspnoea. *Lancet* 1994;**343**:440–4.
32. Morrison LK, Harrison A, Krishnaswamy P, Kazanegra R, Clopton P, Maisel A. Utility of a rapid B-natriuretic peptide assay in differentiating congestive heart failure from lung disease in patients presenting with dyspnea. *J Am Coll Cardiol* 2002;**39**(2):202–9.
33. Cowie MR, Struthers AD, Wood DA, *et al.* Value of natriuretic peptides in assessment of patients with possible new heart failure in primary care. *Lancet* 1997;**350**:1349–53.
34. Zaphiriou A, Robb S, Murray-Thomas T, *et al.* The diagnostic accuracy of plasma BNP and NTproBNP in patients referred from primary care with suspected heart failure: results of the UK natriuretic peptide study. *Eur J Heart Fail* 2005;**7**(4):537–41.
35. Choy AM, Darbar D, Lang CC, *et al.* Detection of left ventricular dysfunction after acute myocardial infarction: Comparison of clinical, echocardiographic, and neurohormonal methods. *Br Heart J* 1994;**72**:16–22.
36. von HS, Jankowska EA, Morgenthaler NG, *et al.* Comparison of midregional pro-atrial natriuretic peptide with N-terminal pro-B-type natriuretic peptide in predicting survival in patients with chronic heart failure. *J Am Coll Cardiol* 2007;**50**(20):1973–80.
37. Dickstein K, Cohen-Solal A, Filippatos G, *et al.* ESC Guidelines for the diagnosis and treatment of acute and chronic heart failure 2008: the Task Force for the Diagnosis and Treatment of Acute and Chronic Heart Failure 2008 of the European Society of Cardiology. Developed in collaboration with the Heart Failure Association of the ESC (HFA) and endorsed by the European Society of Intensive Care Medicine (ESICM). *Eur Heart J* 2008;**29**(19):2388–442.
38. Hunt SA, Abraham WT, Chin MH, *et al.* ACC/AHA 2005 Guideline Update for the Diagnosis and Management of Chronic Heart Failure in the Adult: a report of the American College of Cardiology/American Heart Association Task Force on Practice Guidelines (Writing Committee to Update the 2001 Guidelines for the Evaluation and Management of Heart Failure): developed in collaboration with the American College of Chest Physicians and the International Society for Heart and Lung Transplantation: endorsed by the Heart Rhythm Society. *Circulation* 2005;**112**(12):e154–235.
39. Costello-Boerrigter LC, Boerrigter G, Redfield MM, *et al.* Amino-terminal pro-B-type natriuretic peptide and B-type natriuretic peptide in the general community: determinants and detection of left ventricular dysfunction. *J Am Coll Cardiol* 2006;**47**(2):345–53.
40. Hobbs FD, Davis RC, Roalfe AK, Hare R, Davies MK. Reliability of N-terminal proBNP assay in diagnosis of left ventricular systolic dysfunction within representative and high risk populations. *Heart* 2004;**90**(8):866–70.
41. Ng LL, Loke I, Davies JE, *et al.* Identification of previously undiagnosed left ventricular systolic dysfunction: community screening using natriuretic peptides and electrocardiography. *Eur J Heart Fail* 2003;**5**(6):775–82.
42. Hedberg P, Lonnberg I, Jonason T, Nilsson G, Pehrsson K, Ringqvist I. Electrocardiogram and B-type natriuretic peptide as screening tools for left ventricular systolic dysfunction in a population-based sample of 75-year-old men and women. *Am Heart J* 2004;**148**(3):524–9.
43. Vasan RS, Benjamin EJ, Larson MG, *et al.* Plasma natriuretic peptides for community screening for left ventricular hypertrophy and systolic dysfunction: the Framingham heart study. *JAMA* 2002;**288**(10):1252–9.
44. Ng LL, Loke IW, Davies JE, *et al.* Community screening for left ventricular systolic dysfunction using plasma and urinary natriuretic peptides. *J Am Coll Cardiol* 2005;**45**(7):1043–50.
45. Vasan RS, Benjamin EJ, Larson MG, *et al.* Plasma natriuretic peptides for community screening for left ventricular hypertrophy and systolic dysfunction: the Framingham heart study. *JAMA* 2002;**288**(10):1252–9.
46. Nielsen OW, McDonagh TA, Robb SD, Dargie HJ. Retrospective analysis of the cost-effectiveness of using plasma brain natriuretic peptide in screening for left ventricular systolic dysfunction in the general population. *J Am Coll Cardiol* 2003;**41**(1):113–20.
47. Heidenreich PA, Gubens MA, Fonarow GC, Konstam MA, Stevenson LW, Shekelle PG. Cost-effectiveness of screening with B-type natriuretic peptide to identify patients with reduced left ventricular ejection fraction. *J Am Coll Cardiol* 2004;**43**(6):1019–26.
48. Tsutamoto T, Wada A, Maeda K, *et al.* Attenuation of compensation of endogenous cardiac natriuretic peptide system in chronic heart failure - Prognostic role of brain natriuretic peptide concentration in patients

with chronic symptomatic left ventricular dysfunction. *Circulation* 1997;96:509–16.

49. McDonagh TA, Cunningham AD, Morrison CE, *et al.* Left ventricular dysfunction, natriuretic peptides, and mortality in an urban population. *Heart* 2001;**86**(1):21–6.
50. Gardner RS, Chong V, Morton I, McDonagh TA. N-terminal brain natriuretic peptide is a more powerful predictor of mortality than endothelin-1, adrenomedullin and tumour necrosis factor-alpha in patients referred for consideration of cardiac transplantation. *Eur J Heart Fail* 2005;**7**(2):253–60.
51. Gardner RS, Ozalp F, Murday AJ, Robb SD, McDonagh TA. N-terminal pro-brain natriuretic peptide. A new gold standard in predicting mortality in patients with advanced heart failure. *Eur Heart J* 2003;**24**(19):1735–43.
52. Berger R, Huelsmann M, Strecker K, *et al.* Neurohormonal risk stratification for sudden death and death owing to progressive heart failure in chronic heart failure. *Eur J Clin Invest* 2005;**35**(1):24–31.
53. Gardner RS, Chong V, Morton I, McDonagh TA. N-terminal brain natriuretic peptide is a more powerful predictor of mortality than endothelin-1, adrenomedullin and tumour necrosis factor-alpha in patients referred for consideration of cardiac transplantation. *Eur J Heart Fail* 2005;**7**(2):253–60.
54. Cheng V, Kazanagra R, Garcia A, *et al.* A rapid bedside test for B-type peptide predicts treatment outcomes in patients admitted for decompensated heart failure: a pilot study. *J Am Coll Cardiol* 2001;**37**(2):386–91.
55. Logeart D, Thabut G, Jourdain P, *et al.* Predischarge B-type natriuretic peptide assay for identifying patients at high risk of re-admission after decompensated heart failure. *J Am Coll Cardiol* 2004;**43**(4):635–41.
56. Gackowski A, Isnard R, Golmard JL, *et al.* Comparison of echocardiography and plasma B-type natriuretic peptide for monitoring the response to treatment in acute heart failure. *Eur Heart J* 2004;**25**(20):1788–96.
57. Anand IS, Fisher LD, Chiang YT, *et al.* Changes in brain natriuretic peptide and norepinephrine over time and mortality and morbidity in the Valsartan Heart Failure Trial (Val-HeFT). *Circulation* 2003;**107**(9):1278–83.
58. Masson S, Latini R, Anand IS, Barlera S, Angelici L, Vago T *et al.* Prognostic value of changes in N-terminal pro-brain natriuretic peptide in Val-HeFT (Valsartan Heart Failure Trial). *J Am Coll Cardiol* 2008;**52**(12):997–1003.
59. Gardner RS, Chong KS, Morton JJ, McDonagh TA. A change in N-terminal pro-brain natriuretic peptide is predictive of outcome in patients with advanced heart failure. *Eur J Heart Fail* 2007;**9**(3):266–71.
60. Anderson JV, Woodruff PW, Bloom SR. The effect of treatment of congestive heart failure on plasma atrial natriuretic peptide concentration: a longitudinal study. *Br Heart J* 1988;**59**(2):207–11.
61. Tsutsui T, Tsutamoto T, Maeda K, Kinoshita M. Comparison of neurohumoral effects of short-acting and long-acting loop diuretics in patients with chronic congestive heart failure. *J Cardiovasc Pharmacol* 2001;**38** Suppl 1:S81–5.
62. Tsutamoto T, Wada A, Maeda K, *et al.* Digitalis increases brain natriuretic peptide in patients with severe congestive heart failure. *Am Heart J* 1997;**134**:910–16.
63. Kobusiak-Prokopowicz M, Swidnicka-Szuszkowska B, Mysiak A. [Effect of digoxin on atrial natriuretic peptide (ANP), brain natriuretic peptide (BNP) and cyclic 3′, 5′-guanosine monophosphate (cGMP) in patients with chronic congestive heart failure]. *Pol Arch Med Wewn* 2001;**105**(6):475–82.
64. Yoshimura M, Yasue H, Tanaka H, *et al.* Responses of plasma concentrations of A type natriuretic peptide and B type natriuretic peptide to alacepril, an angiotensin- converting enzyme inhibitor, in patients with congestive heart failure. Br Heart J 1994;**72**:528–33.
65. Tsutamoto T, Wada A, Maeda K, *et al.* Relationship between plasma levels of cardiac natriuretic peptides and soluble Fas: plasma soluble Fas as a prognostic predictor in patients with congestive heart failure. *J Card Fail* 2001;**7**(4):322–8.
66. Tsutamoto T, Wada A, Maeda K, *et al.* Effect of spironolactone on plasma brain natriuretic peptide and left ventricular remodeling in patients with congestive heart failure. *J Am Coll Cardiol* 2001;**37**(5):1228–33.
67. The RESOLVD Investigators. Effect of metoprolol CR in patients with ischaemic and dilated cardiomyopathy. *Circulation* 2002;**101**:378–84.
68. Hara Y, Hamada M, Shigematsu Y, *et al.* Effect of beta-blocker on left ventricular function and natriuretic peptides in patients with chronic heart failure treated with angiotensin-converting enzyme inhibitor. *Jpn Circ J* 2000;**64**(5):365–9.
69. Fung JW, Yu CM, Yip G, *et al.* Effect of beta blockade (carvedilol or metoprolol) on activation of the renin-angiotensin-aldosterone system and natriuretic peptides in chronic heart failure. *Am J Cardiol* 2003;**92**(4):406–10.
70. Maeda K, Tsutamoto T, Wada A, *et al.* High levels of plasma brain natriuretic peptide and interleukin-6 after optimized treatment for heart failure are independent risk factors for morbidity and mortality in patients with congestive heart failure. *J Am Coll Cardiol* 2000;**36**(5):1587–93.
71. Yu CM, Fung JW, Zhang Q, *et al.* Improvement of serum NT-ProBNP predicts improvement in cardiac function and favorable prognosis after cardiac resynchronization therapy for heart failure. *J Card Fail* 2005;**11**(5 Suppl):S42–6.
72. Murdoch DR, McDonagh TA, Byrne J, *et al.* Titration of vasodilator therapy in chronic heart failure according to plasma brain natriuretic peptide concentration: randomized comparison of the hemodynamic and neuroendocrine effects of tailored versus empirical therapy [see comments]. *Am Heart J* 1999;**138**(6 Pt 1):1126–32.
73. Troughton RW, Frampton CM, Yandle TG, Espiner EA, Nicholls MG, Richards AM. Treatment of heart failure guided by plasma aminoterminal brain natriuretic peptide (N-BNP) concentrations [see comments]. *Lancet* 2000;**355**(9210):1126–30.
74. Pfisterer M, Buser P, Rickli H, *et al.* BNP-guided vs symptom-guided heart failure therapy: the Trial of Intensified vs Standard Medical Therapy in Elderly Patients With Congestive Heart Failure (TIME-CHF) randomized trial. *JAMA* 2009;**301**(4):383–92.
75. Lainchbury JG, Troughton RW, Strangman KM, *et al.* N-terminal pro-B-type natriuretic peptide-guided treatment for chronic heart failure: results from the BATTLESCARRED (NT-proBNP-Assisted Treatment To Lessen Serial Cardiac Readmissions and Death) trial. *J Am Coll Cardiol* 2009;**55**(1):53–60.
76. Felker GM, Hasselblad V, Hernandez AF, O'Connor CM. Biomarker-guided therapy in chronic heart failure: a meta-analysis of randomized controlled trials. *Am Heart J* 2009;**158**(3):422–30.
77. Lewin J, Ledwidge M, O'Loughlin C, McNally C, McDonald K. Clinical deterioration in established heart failure: what is the value of BNP and weight gain in aiding diagnosis?. *Eur J Heart Fail* 2005;**7**(6):953–7.
78. Wu AH. Serial testing of B-type natriuretic peptide and NTpro-BNP for monitoring therapy of heart failure: the role of biologic variation in the interpretation of results. *Am Heart J* 2006;**152**(5): 828–34.
79. O'Hanlon R, O'Shea P, Ledwidge M, *et al.* The biologic variability of B-type natriuretic peptide and N-terminal pro-B-type natriuretic peptide in stable heart failure patients. *J Card Fail* 2007;**13**(1):50–5.

15

Vasopressin

Benjamin R. Szwejkowski, Sushma Rekhraj, and Allan Struthers

Anatomy and physiology

Synthesis of vasopressin

Arginine vasopressin (AVP; also known as antidiuretic hormone, ADH) is a polypeptide hormone synthesized by the neurosecretory cells of the supraoptic nucleus located within the hypothalamus. Vasopressin is packaged into secretory vesicles and transported by fast axons through the pituitary stalk to the posterior pituitary gland. The posterior pituitary gland acts as a supporting structure for the axonal nerve endings which lie on the surfaces of capillaries and it is here that vasopressin is secreted directly into the bloodstream. Oxytocin is also released by nerves in the posterior pituitary gland, but synthesized within a different nucleus of the hypothalamus called the paraventricular nucleus. Vasopressin contains nine amino acids and is similar in structure to oxytocin except that in vasopressin the isoleucine and leucine of oxytocin are replaced by phenylalanine and arginine.

Regulation of vasopressin release

The principle mechanism for the regulation of vasopressin release is high osmotic pressure, low blood volume, and decreased arterial pressure. Osmoreceptors (modified neuron receptors) are located in the hypothalamus and activate the neurosecretory cells of the supraoptic nucleus to synthesize and release vasopressin. There is negative feedback, with vasopressin release falling in response to a fall in osmotic pressure and a rise in blood volume. When blood volume increases, atrial stretch receptors are activated and this in turn leads to inhibited vasopressin secretion. There are baroreceptors in the carotid, aortic, and pulmonary vessels which also stimulate vasopressin secretion via the vagus and glossopharyngeal nerves. The secretion of vasopressin is more sensitive to osmolality than blood volume; for instance, a change in plasma osmolality of 1% is enough to increase vasopressin secretion whereas as much as a 10% change in blood volume is needed to increase vasopressin secretion. Other exogenous substances affect vasopressin production, such as nicotine and morphine which stimulate vasopressin release and alcohol which inhibits vasopressin release.

Actions of vasopressin

Vasopressin regulates osmotic pressure and circulating blood volume by causing water retention in the kidney and peripheral vasoconstriction (Fig. 15.1). Vasopressin acts via the three known vasopressin receptors throughout the body, V_{1A}, V_{1B}, and V_2. The V_2 receptor is found in the collecting duct and distal convoluted tubule within the kidney and it is the direct stimulatory action of vasopressin mediated by intracellular cAMP which causes water-permeable pores called aquaporin-2 to be synthesized.[1] Aquaporin-2 is inserted into the apical cell membranes to make the ducts and tubules more permeable to water reabsorption through osmosis, conserving water within the body and making the urine more concentrated. Circulating levels of vasopressin correlate directly with aquaporin-2 expression. V_{1A} receptors are found on the coronary smooth muscle cells and peripheral arterial cells, and mediate platelet aggregation. Stimulation of the V_{1A} receptor causes G proteins to activate phospholipase C-β and increase intracellular calcium, causing peripheral vasoconstriction, leading to a corresponding rise in blood pressure. Vasopressin may play a role in myocardial hypertrophy and remodelling in rats and this is discussed in detail below. The V_{1B} receptor modulates adrenocorticotropic hormone (ACTH) from the anterior pituitary.

Potential future treatments: vasopressin antagonists

Pathophysiology of vasopressin in heart failure

In patients with heart failure (HF) and hyponatraemia, a consistent finding is high levels of vasopressin in the circulating blood volume, which is paradoxical and inappropriate.[2] In low-output cardiac failure there is underfilling of the arterial circulation that leads to baroreceptor-mediated increase in sympathetic tone. It is this increased sympathetic tone that causes nonosmotic vasopressin release and triggers the other neurohormonal adaptations discussed in this chapter. This inappropriate vasopressin release leads to further water retention in an already oedematous state.[2] There is

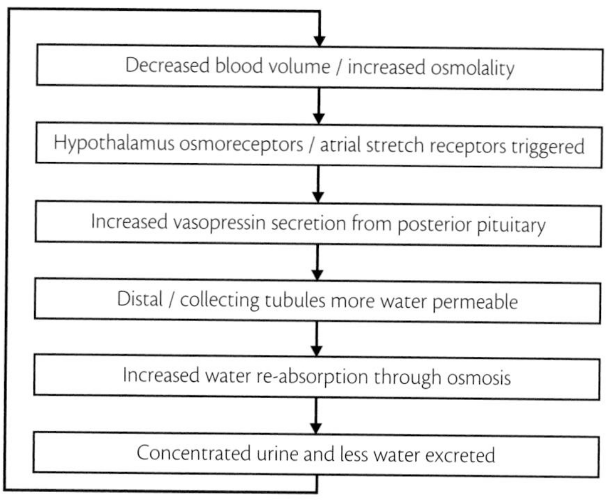

Fig. 15.1 Vasopressin regulation.

the loss of the baroreflex suppression in response to vasopressin in HF patients, which may also contribute to high circulating vasopressin levels as this overrides the left atrial stretch receptors and osmoreceptor response to excess vasopressin.[3,4] The Studies of Left Ventricular Dysfunction (SOLVD) population investigated whether these neurohormonal adaptations occur in patients with left ventricular dysfunction before the onset of pulmonary congestion.[5] The SOLVD study design was a multicentre study comparing 56 control subjects, 151 patients with ejection fractions of 35% or less with no symptoms of HF, and 81 patients with overt HF. There is a statistically significant increase in plasma vasopressin, noradrenaline and atrial naturiuretic factor in the asymptomatic group. This study therefore showed that patients who have ejection fractions of 35% or less who are on no treatment (including digoxin, vasodilators, or diuretics) but have no symptoms of HF have neurohormonal activation, and it may be the case that neurohormonal adaptations are not solely due to decompensation and pulmonary congestion. In rats with HF induced by left coronary artery ligation there was a significant increase in aquaporin-2 expression that correlated with high levels of vasopressin.[6,7] Again in rat models, quantative analysis of urinary aquaporins have correlated with high levels of serum vasopressin.[2] This method could be a potential marker for HF in the future.

As far back as the 1980s infused vasopressin was found to cause adverse haemodynamic effects in HF patients by causing increased systemic vascular resistance and increased afterload.[4,8] Vasopressin may also have detrimental affects on myocardial cells causing their hypertrophy. In rats, vasopressin stimulates cardiac hypertrophy via the V_{1A} receptor.[9–13] Elevated vasopressin levels in the Survival and Ventricular Enlargement (SAVE) population were associated with adverse cardiovascular outcomes in the setting of left ventricular dysfunction after myocardial infarction.[14]

Fluid overload and its associated symptoms, such as peripheral oedema and dyspnoea, are the most common reason for hospitalization in HF patients. Hyponatraemia and impaired renal function in this patient population carries a poor prognosis. Loop diuretics have limitations as they may make hyponatraemia worse and can impair renal function. Therefore drugs that antagonize either V_{1A} and/or V_2 receptors have been developed in the hope that they would promote water excretion, maintain renal function, and normalize hyponatraemia. However, these vasopressin receptor antagonists have not been shown to improve long-term mortality and are hence not yet licensed in the United Kingdom.

Vasopressin antagonism in animal models

The first wave of V_2 receptor antagonists (OPC 31260, OPC 21268) showed that they can increase diuresis, decrease urinary osmolality, and increase plasma osmolality in rats with experimental HF.[7] Since then two main vasopressin antagonists have emerged for clinical study; YM087 (conivaptan),which is a V_{1A} and V_2 receptor antagonist, and OPC-41061 (tolvaptan) which is a V_2 receptor antagonist.

Tolvaptan is highly selective (29:1) for V_2 receptors over V_{1A} receptors.[15] The initial studies using tolvaptan were in rats and dogs with induced HF.[15–17] A consistent finding in these initial trials was that tolvaptan produced an increase in urine volume with both single and multiple dosing; it also improved serum sodium with no changes in plasma urea or creatinine. In rats, tolvaptan has proven additive affects over and above furosemide on urine volume, electrolyte free water clearance, urine osmolality, and serum sodium. Unlike furosemide, tolvaptan does not seem to affect the angiotensin system in animal models, highlighting an obvious potential clinical advantage. Dogs with pacing-induced HF given tolvaptan significantly decreased pulmonary capillary wedge pressure and, as shown in rat models, increased urine volume without changing sodium excretion, peripheral vascular resistance, renal blood flow, or glomerular filtration rate.[17]

Conivaptan is a nonpeptide, orally active V_{1A} and V_2 receptor antagonist with a 10:1 selectivity for the V_{1A} receptor.[18] Conivaptan has the same positive effects as tolvaptan in rats and dogs,[18,19] but in addition, because conivaptan also has an effect on the V_{1A} receptor, it also decreases peripheral vasoconstriction and may reduce cardiac hypertrophy. Conivaptan reduces blood pressure, left ventricular end-diastolic pressure, and right ventricular systolic pressure in rat models.[20,21] It also inhibits vasopressin-induced hyperplasia and hypertrophy in rat cultured smooth muscle cells.[10] V_{1A} receptor antagonism also has been shown to prevent HF when given to rats on days 1 to 21 after induced myocardial infarction.[22] Conivaptan therefore has a potential added benefit over tolvaptan because of its dual receptor antagonism and its added effects against vasoconstriction and cardiac hypertrophy.

Tolvaptan trials in humans

Tolvaptan has been developed for oral use in humans. Two key studies have been published by Gheorghiade *et al.*[23,24] In the first study, tolvaptan was given in 254 patients in a double-blind trial where the patients continued their current HF therapy and were not fluid restricted.[23] Patients were randomized to receive 30, 60, or 90 mg of tolvaptan or placebo once daily for 25 days. In the second study, the Acute and Chronic Therapeutic Impact of a Vasopressin Antagonist in Congestive Heart Failure (ACTIV in CHF), tolvaptan was assessed in a phase II feasibility trial in addition to standard HF therapies.[24] This later study was the first trial to assess the acute and chronic effects of an oral vasopressin antagonist in patients hospitalized with HF. The design of this latter study was a randomized double-blind trial with 319 hospitalized HF patients and follow-up lasted 60 days after 30, 60, or 90 mg of tolvaptan or placebo once daily. Both of these initial trials showed tolvaptan to be well tolerated, albeit with minor side effects such as urinary frequency, thirst, and dry mouth. Importantly, tolvaptan

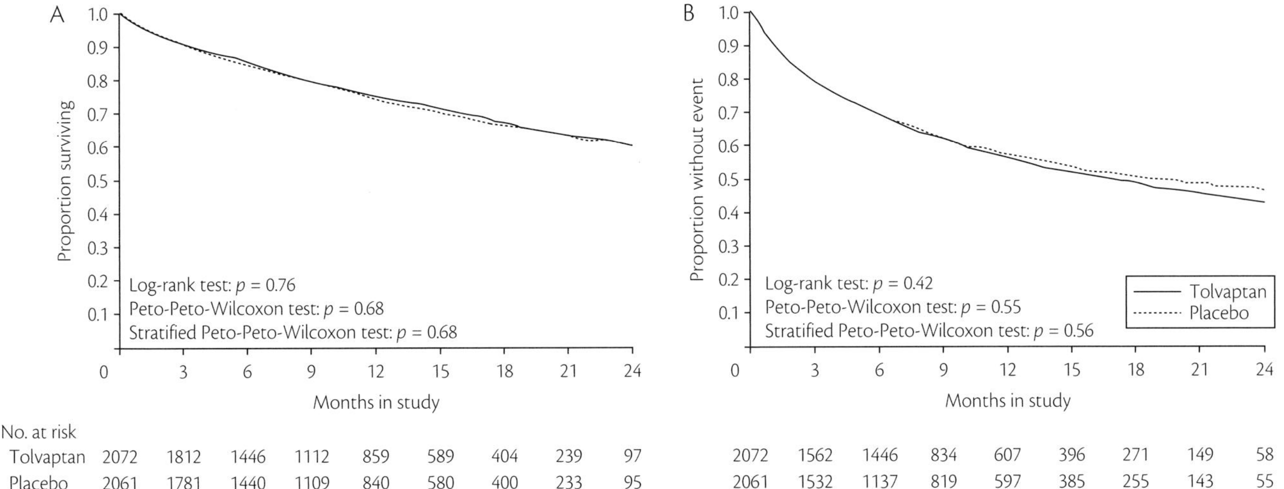

Fig. 15.2 Kaplan–Meier analyses of (A) all-cause mortality and (B) cardiovascular mortality or hospitalization for heart failure.
From Konstam MA *et al.*, Effects of oral tolvaptan in patients hospitalized for worsening heart failure: the EVEREST outcome trial. *JAMA* 2007;**297**(12):1319–1331.

significantly reduced body weight and oedema. It also increased urine volumes and decreased urine osmolality with no changes in heart rate, blood pressure, renal function, or potassium. In the subgroup of patients who had hyponatraemia, tolvaptan normalized serum sodium. Thus tolvaptan is associated with significant weight reduction on top of diuretics. Compared with placebo, the use of tolvaptan was not associated with any significant worsening in HF at 60 days. These two studies did not look at mortality nor any longer-term effects; however, there was a trend towards lower mortality in tolvaptan-treated patients with renal dysfunction or severe systemic congestion.

The Efficacy of Vasopressin Antagonism in Decompensated Heart Failure (EVEREST) trial was then designed to answer the questions of long-term effects of tolvaptan and the effect of mortality in hospitalized patients with acute decompensated HF.[25,26] It was a phase III double-blind randomized placebo-controlled trial involving 4133 patients with NYHA III–IV and left ventricular ejection fraction of less than 40%. Patients received either tolvaptan 30 mg/day or placebo within 48 h of their hospital admission. This study again showed oral tolvaptan in addition to standard treatment for HF in hospitalized patients improved serum sodium without harming renal function. Tolvaptan achieved short-term symptom benefit including early and sustained weight reduction and improvement in oedema and dyspnoea as assessed by changes in patient assessed dyspnoea and Kansas City Cardiomyopathy Questionnaire (KCCQ). Tolvaptan was safe and well tolerated. Long-term tolvaptan treatment did not have any effect on long-term mortality or on HF morbidity in this trial. It also did not meet its primary endpoint of reducing hospitalizations with HF or cardiac deaths (Fig. 15.2). Future studies are needed to see if higher doses and follow-up over a longer period of time have an impact on mortality.

A remodelling study was also performed with tolvaptan. The Multicentre Evaluation of Tolvaptan Effect on Remodelling (METEOR) trial[27] randomized 240 people to either 30 mg/day of tolvaptan or placebo in a double-blind randomized placebo-controlled trial. The patients had HF and systolic dysfunction and were given the drug for 1 year. They failed to show any benefit from tolvaptan on left ventricular volumes and remodelling.

Conivaptan trials in humans

Conivaptan has been developed for both oral and intravenous use in humans. Udelson *et al.* studied the additive affects of conivaptan to standard HF therapy in patients with NYHA III/IV.[28] The study design was a randomized placebo-controlled trial where the patients received either 10, 20, or 40 mg of intravenous conivaptan or placebo short term. Thirty-five patients were recruited into each group with 140 patients in total. Pulmonary capillary wedge pressure and right atrial pressure were significantly reduced in both the 20-mg and 40-mg conivaptan groups. As with the tolvaptan studies urine output was significantly higher in the conivaptan-treated groups but serum osmolality, serum sodium, serum potassium, blood pressure, and heart rate levels did not differ significantly compared with placebo. Conivaptan was associated with headache but there were no serious adverse events. Further studies are needed to see if oral conivaptan given long term has favourable benefits on morbidity and mortality.

In 2005 the Food and Drug Admistration (FDA) approved the use of conivaptan for hospitalized patients with euvolaemic hyponatraemia (not including HF) in the United States. It is not approved for use in HF patients at present.

Conclusion

Vasopressin antagonists have been developed and in clinical studies have shown some beneficial effects on urine output, renal function, and occasionally symptoms. Future studies are needed to see if they favourably alter harder endpoints such as morbidity and mortality. It is also unclear as yet which patients will benefit most; will a benefit be seen in all fluid-overloaded HF patients or only those with demonstrated hyponatraemia as well?

References

1. Nielsen S, Kwon T-H, Christensen BM, *et al.* Physiology and pathophysiology of renal aquaporins. *J Am Soc Nephrol* 1999;**10**(3):647–63.
2. Sanghi P, Uretsky BF, Schwarz ER. Vasopressin antagonism: a future treatment option in heart failure. *Eur Heart J* 2005;**26**(6):538–43.

3. Goldsmith SR. Baroreflex loading maneuvers do not suppress increased plasma arginine vasopressin in patients with congestive heart failure. *J Am Coll Cardiol* 1992;**19**(6):1180–4.
4. Uretsky BF, Verbalis JG, Generalovich T, Valdes A, Reddy PS. Plasma vasopressin response to osmotic and hemodynamic stimuli in heart failure. *Am J Physiol Heart Circ Physiol* 1985;**248**(3):H396–402.
5. Francis G, Benedict C, Johnstone D, *et al.* Comparison of neuroendocrine activation in patients with left ventricular dysfunction with and without congestive heart failure. A substudy of the Studies of Left Ventricular Dysfunction (SOLVD). *Circulation* 1990;**82**(5):1724–9.
6. Nielsen S, Terris J, Andersen D, *et al.* Congestive heart failure in rats is associated with increased expression and targeting of aquaporin-2 water channel in collecting duct. *Proc Natl Acad Sci U S A* 1997;**94**(10):5450–5.
7. Xu DL, Martin PY, Ohara M, *et al.* Upregulation of aquaporin-2 water channel expression in chronic heart failure rat. *J Clin Invest* 1997;**99**(7):1500–5.
8. Goldsmith SR, Francis GS, Cowley AW Jr, Goldenberg IF, Cohn JN. Hemodynamic effects of infused arginine vasopressin in congestive heart failure. *J Am Coll Cardiol* 1986;**8**(4):779–83.
9. Nakamura Y, Haneda T, Osaki J, Miyata S, Kikuchi K. Hypertrophic growth of cultured neonatal rat heart cells mediated by vasopressin V1A receptor. *Eur J Pharmacol* 2000;**391**(1–2):39–48.
10. Tahara A, Tomura Y, Wada K, *et al.* Effect of YM087, a potent nonpeptide vasopressin antagonist, on vasopressin-induced hyperplasia and hypertrophy of cultured vascular smooth-muscle cells. *J Cardiovasc Pharmacol* 1997;**30**(6):759–66.
11. Tahara A, Tomura Y, Wada K-I, *et al.* Effect of YM087, a potent nonpeptide vasopressin antagonist, on vasopressin-induced protein synthesis in neonatal rat cardiomyocyte. *Cardiovasc Res* 1998;**38**(1):198–205.
12. Xu Y, Hopfner RL, McNeill JR, Gopalakrishnan V. Vasopressin accelerates protein synthesis in neonatal rat cardiomyocytes. *Mol Cell Biochem* 1999;**195**(1):183–90.
13. Fukuzawa J, Haneda T, Kikuchi K. Arginine vasopressin increases the rate of protein synthesis in isolated perfused adult rat heart via the V1 receptor. *Mol Cell Biochem* 1999;**195**(1):93–8.
14. Rouleau JL, Packer M, Moye L, *et al.* Prognostic value of neurohumoral activation in patients with an acute myocardial infarction: effect of captopril. *J Am Coll Cardiol* 1994;**24**(3):583–91.
15. Yamamura Y, Nakamura S, Itoh S, *et al.* OPC-41061, a highly potent human vasopressin V2-receptor antagonist: pharmacological profile and aquaretic effect by single and multiple oral dosing in rats. *J Pharmacol Exp Ther* 1998;**287**(3):860–7.
16. Hirano T, Yamamura Y, Nakamura S, Onogawa T, Mori T. Effects of the V2-receptor antagonist OPC-41061 and the loop diuretic furosemide alone and in combination in rats. *J Pharmacol Exp Ther* 2000;**292**(1):288–94.
17. Miyazaki T, Fujiki H, Yamamura Y, Nakamura S, Mori T. Tolvaptan, an orally active vasopressin V(2)-receptor antagonist—pharmacology and clinical trials. *Cardiovasc Drug Rev* 2007;**25**(1):1–13.
18. Yatsu T, Tomura Y, Tahara A, *et al.* Cardiovascular and renal effects of conivaptan hydrochloride (YM087), a vasopressin V1A and V2 receptor antagonist, in dogs with pacing-induced congestive heart failure. *Eur J Pharmacol* 1999;**376**(3):239–46.
19. Yatsu T, Tomura Y, Tahara A, *et al.* Pharmacological profile of YM087, a novel nonpeptide dual vasopressin V1A and V2 receptor antagonist, in dogs. *Eur J Pharmacol* 1997;**321**(2):225–30.
20. Wada K-i, Tahara A, Arai Y, *et al.* Effect of the vasopressin receptor antagonist conivaptan in rats with heart failure following myocardial infarction. *Eur J Pharmacol* 2002;**450**(2):169–77.
21. Wada K-i, Fujimori A, Matsukawa U, *et al.* Intravenous administration of conivaptan hydrochloride improves cardiac hemodynamics in rats with myocardial infarction-induced congestive heart failure. *Eur J Pharmacol* 2005;**507**(1–3):145–51.
22. Van Kerckhoven R, Lankhuizen I, van Veghel R, Saxena PR, Schoemaker RG. Chronic vasopressin V1A but not V2 receptor antagonism prevents heart failure in chronically infarcted rats. *Eur J Pharmacol* 2002;**449**(1–2):135–41.
23. Gheorghiade M, Niazi I, Ouyang J, *et al.* Vasopressin V2-receptor blockade with tolvaptan in patients with chronic heart failure: results from a double-blind, randomized trial. *Circulation* 2003;**107**(21):2690–6.
24. Gheorghiade M, Gattis WA, O'Connor CM, *et al.* Effects of tolvaptan, a vasopressin antagonist, in patients hospitalized with worsening heart failure: a randomized controlled trial. *JAMA* 2004;**291**(16):1963–71.
25. Konstam MA, Gheorghiade M, Burnett JC Jr, *et al.* Effects of oral tolvaptan in patients hospitalized for worsening heart failure: the EVEREST outcome trial. *JAMA* 2007;**297**(12):1319–31.
26. Gheorghiade M, Konstam MA, Burnett JC Jr, *et al.* Short-term clinical effects of tolvaptan, an oral vasopressin antagonist, in patients hospitalized for heart failure: the EVEREST clinical status trials. *JAMA* 2007;**297**(12):1332–43.
27. Udelson JE, McGrew FA, Flores E, *et al.* Multicenter, randomized, double-blind, placebo-controlled study on the effect of oral tolvaptan on left ventricular dilation and function in patients with heart failure and systolic dysfunction. *J Am Coll Cardiol* 2007;**49**(22):2151–9.
28. Udelson JE, Smith WB, Hendrix GH, *et al.* Acute hemodynamic effects of conivaptan, a dual V1A and V2 vasopressin receptor antagonist, in patients with advanced heart failure. *Circulation* 2001;**104**(20):2417–23.
29. Nielsen S, Frokiar J, Marples D, Kwon T-H, Agre P, Knepper MA. Aquaporins in the kidney: from molecules to medicine. *Physiol Rev* 2002;**82**(1):205–44.
30. Robertson GL, Athar S. The interaction of blood osmolality and blood volume in regulating plasma vasopressin in man. *J Clin Endocrinol Metab* 1976;**42**(4):613–20.
31. Kozono D, Yasui M, King LS, Agre P. Aquaporin water channels: atomic structure molecular dynamics meet clinical medicine. *J Clin Invest* 2002;**109**(11):1395–9.
32. Dunn FL, Brennan TJ, Nelson AE, Robertson GL. The role of blood osmolality and volume in regulating vasopressin secretion in the rat. *J Clin Invest* 1973;**52**(12):3212–9.
33. Stricker EM, Sved AF. Controls of vasopressin secretion and thirst: similarities and dissimilarities in signals. *Physiol Behav* 2002;**77**(4–5):731–6.

16

Cytokines and inflammatory markers

Stamatis Adamopoulos, Panagiota Georgiadou, and Vassilios Voudris

Introduction

The expression of classic neurohormones, such as angiotensin II and noradrenaline, plays an important role in disease progression in chronic heart failure (HF). This so-called neurohormonal activation seems to be involved in the cardiomyopathic process of adverse left ventricular remodelling and dysfunction, via both direct and indirect effects.[1,2] Therapies blocking the excessive activation of the renin–angiotensin system and the adrenergic system have become the mainstay of pharmacological treatment of chronic HF.[3]

Another important pathway in chronic HF progression is inflammatory activation.[4,5] Experimental studies have shown that proinflammatory cytokines may induce many aspects of the syndrome of chronic HF, such as left ventricular dysfunction, pulmonary oedema, and the process of left ventricular remodelling, including myocyte hypertrophy, progressive myocyte loss through apoptosis, and endothelial dysfunction. Although the cause of the inflammation is unknown, both infectious (e.g.endotoxins) and noninfectious (e.g. oxidative stress, haemodynamic overload) events could be operating, including interaction with the neurohormone system. Inflammatory markers have emerged as potential indicators of the evolution of HF, ranging from their use for screening, diagnosis, determining prognosis, and guiding treatment.[6]

The emerging association of inflammatory mediators with the pathogenesis and progression of chronic HF has already resulted in the development of new anti-inflammatory strategies, which might be used as adjunctive therapy in patients with chronic HF.[7,8] Moreover, there is accumulating evidence that a critical network of interactions is formed by inflammatory and the classic neurohormonal mediators, and that many of the conventional therapies for HF may, at least partially, modulate the proinflammatory cytokine milieu. However, therapies tested so far have been largely disappointing.

The 'cytokine hypothesis'

In the early 1980s, cytokines were first characterized as a new group of peptides. They are secreted by different cell types and mediate cell-to-cell interactions via specific cell-surface receptors. They regulate key aspects of various cellular functions, such as activation, expansion, differentiation, and death.[9,10] The best-studied of these cytokines is tumour necrosis factor (TNF). Comparatively less is known about the interleukins (IL) IL-1, IL-2, IL-6, and interferon (IFN)-γ in the setting of chronic HF.

The chronic HF syndrome seems to progress, at least in part, as a result of the toxic effects exerted by endogenous cytokine cascades on the cardiac and skeletal muscle and on the peripheral circulation. So far, the origin of inflammatory mediators remains unclear and has been the subject of controversy. Several hypotheses have been described with respect to the source of proinflammatory cytokines in HF. One is endotoxin-induced immune activation secondary to bowel oedema (Fig. 16.1). Persistent immunological stimulation by microbial antigens, which translocate into the body from the oedematous gastrointestinal tract, may lead to cytokine production by monocytes in the bloodstream and possibly other tissues.[11] Lipopolysaccharide is a bacterial endotoxin which strongly induces the production of TNFα and other proinflammatory mediators.[12,13] However, this 'infectious hypothesis' fails to account for several clinical and experimental observations. The beneficial effects of antimicrobial therapy are not clear so far. Patients with chronic HF and no peripheral oedema also have elevated plasma cytokines, whereas patients with right heart failure, although oedematous, do not have elevations of plasma cytokines.

Nevertheless, the 'cytokine hypothesis' for disease progression in chronic HF (Fig. 16.2) does not depend only on the infectious hypothesis. Other factors may lead to the the tissue injury ('tissue injury hypothesis') and the myocardial cytokine production. Mechanical overload and shear stress may induce the myocardial production of cytokines, growth factors and stress proteins.[14,15] Hypoxia and ischaemia result in the expression of inflammatory cytokines such as TNFα, monocyte chemoattractant protein (MCP)-1, and IL-8 via activation of the transcription nuclear factor NF-κB.[14] Oxidized low-density lipoprotein cholesterol is a potent inducer of cytokine expression.

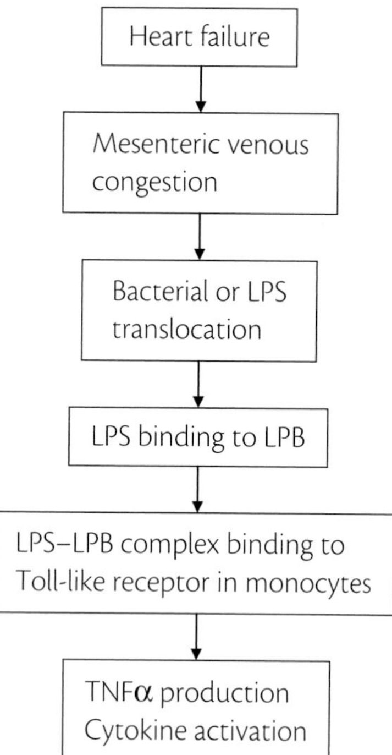

Fig. 16.1 The 'infectious' hypothesis for cytokine activation in chronic heart failure. LPB, lipopolysaccharide-binding protein; LPS, lipopolysaccharide (endotoxin).
Adapted from *Lancet* 1999;**353**:1838–42

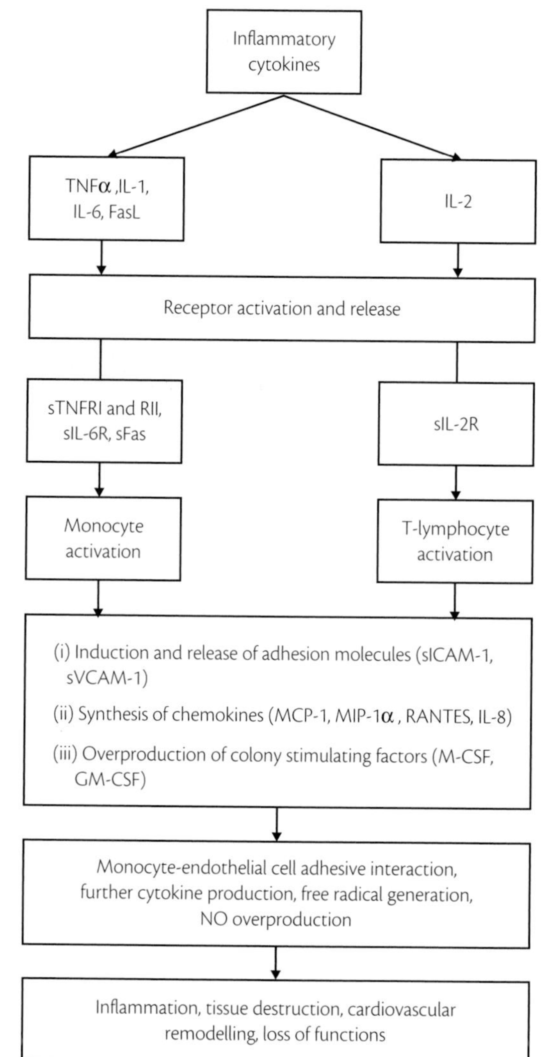

Fig. 16.2 Schematic representation of the inflammatory cascade implicated in the pathophysiology of chronic heart failure.
From *Eur J Heart Fail* 2001;**3**:517–526, with permission.

Recent studies have suggested that a group of receptors named Toll-like receptors (TLRs) may be involved in immunological and inflammatory activation within the myocardium not only in response to microbes but also to molecules released from injured and stressed cells. Ligand binding leads to the activation of several kinases and NF-κB.[15] Enhanced monocyte and macrophage expression of stimulatory molecules, including proinflammatory cytokines, follow as downstream effects. In this way, a powerful immune response is possible even in the absence of infection.

The chronic HF syndrome may cause tissue hypoxia and free-radical production, in turn leading to NF-κB-mediated production of cytokines. Elevated plasma cytokines further reduce impaired vasodilator reserve, triggering a vicious circle of more severe tissue underperfusion.

Chronic β-adrenergic stimulation induces myocardial, but not systemic, elaboration of the major proinflammatory cytokines TNFα, IL-1β, and IL-6. There is thus a biological 'cross-talk' between the two cardinal neurohumoral systems in the myocardium.[16]

The deleterious effects of cytokines are mediated by reduced protein synthesis and increased protein degradation leading to muscle atrophy of the central (cardiac) and, perhaps more importantly, peripheral (skeletal) muscles. Proinflammatory cytokines and oxidative stress cause insulin resistance and downregulation of gene expression for the anabolic peptide IGF-I and reduce phosphorylation of the phosphatidyinositol-3-OH kinase (PI-3K), which in turn lowers the activation of the protein kinase B (Akt).[17,18] Reduced Akt activation in both skeletal muscle and heart (1) decreases protein synthesis via reduced phosphorylation of the 'mammalian target of rapamycin' (known as mTOR) and glucogen synthase kinase (GSK)[19] and (2) up-regulates activity of forkhead box O (FOXO) transcription factors, which in turn activates the ubiquitin–proteasome pathway, resulting in protein degradation.[20,21] In addition, both reduced tissue IGF-1 and insulin resistance activate caspase 3, resulting in further myofibrillar protein breakdown and degradation through the ubiquitin-proteasome pathway.[22]

Whether activated caspase 3 results in muscle apoptosis remains controversial.[23] 'Skeletal myopathy', resulting from the imbalance between increased muscle catabolism and attenuated muscle anabolism, plays a leading role in the genesis of symptoms of exercise limitation and, through the exaggerated muscle ergoreflex,[24] dyspnoea.

TNFα

TNFα is one of the best-characterized proinflammatory mediators in chronic HF. It was first described in 1975 and named cachectin. TNFα is now recognized as a pleiotropic cytokine which can be expressed by almost all nucleated cells and has multiple actions on both local and systemic inflammation.

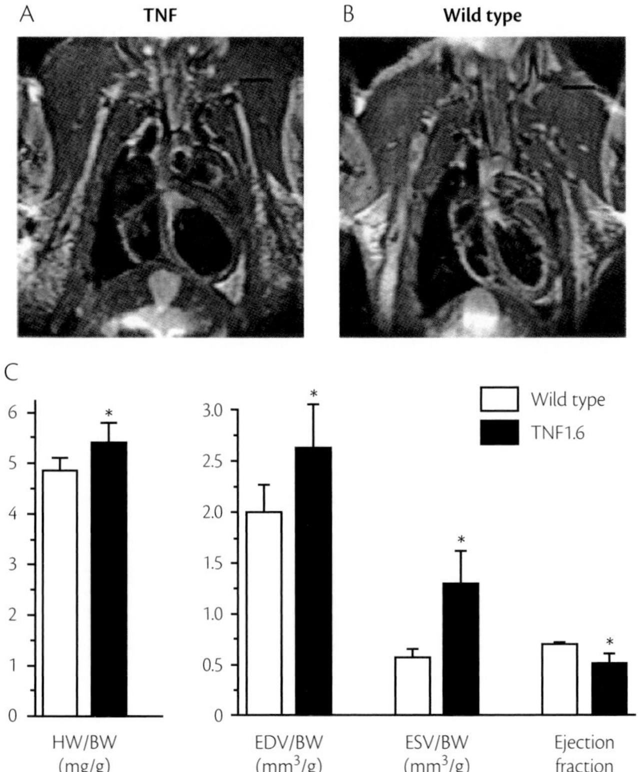

Fig. 16.3 Transgenic mice with cardiac-specific overexpression of TNFα develop dilated cardiomyopathy. MRI (coronal view) from (A) transgenic mice and (B) 24-week-old wild type. (C) Transgenic animals have cardiac hypertrophy with chamber dilation and decreased ejection fraction. BW, body weight; EDV, end-diastolic volume; ESV, end-systolic volume; HW, heart weight. Open bar, wild type; solid bar, TNF *$p < 0.05$.
From *Circulation Res* 1997;**81**:627–35, with permission.

TNFα is increased in relation to the severity of chronic HF and correlates with the degree of sympathetic and renin–angiotensin system activation.[25] TNF is elevated not only in the circulation, but also in the myocardium of patients with chronic HF.[26] Recent research has shown that while TNFα rises in the serum of deteriorating patients who require left ventricular assist devices (LVADs), myocardioal expression of TNFα falls after mechanical circulatory support.[27,28]

TNF levels are particularly elevated in cachectic chronic HF patients and these levels have been found to be the strongest predictors of the degree of previous weight loss.[29]

TNFα may contribute directly to the evolution and progression of HF (Fig. 16.3) and is a predictor of worse outcome. In a substudy of the SOLVD study, patients with TNFα plasma levels above 6.5 pg/mL had worse survival.[30] In a large population of advanced chronic HF patients, circulating TNFα was an independent predictor of mortality.[31]

Although TNF is usually thought of as being harmful, some studies have suggested that TNF has a protective, inotropic action on the failing heart as a stress response protein.[32] Further, injection of TNF improves survival of TNF knockout mice with viral myocarditis in a dose-dependent manner by increasing viral clearance.[33]

TNFα has been implicated in the development of left ventricular dysfunction and remodelling. It increases cardiac myocyte apoptosis, via activation of cytokine-induced nitric oxide (NO) synthase, ceramidase and sphingomyelin pathways, NF-κB activation, and the eventual uncoupling of β-adrenergic signalling[34] as well as via mitochondrial DNA damage. TNFα can mediate cardiac myocyte mitochondrial DNA damage and, therefore, dysfunction in cardiac myocytes via enhanced oxidative stress (overproduction of reactive oxygen species).[35]

TNFα is capable of inducing endothelial dysfunction and skeletal muscle wasting, leading to 'skeletal myopathy' through chronic tissue underperfusion, enhanced muscle catabolism, and possibly myocyte apoptosis. Serum TNFα is inversely correlated with skeletal muscle blood flow and exercise capacity, in both stable and decompensated patients with chronic HF.[36] It may also contribute to elevated insulin and leptin levels and the development of anorexia and cachexia.[34]

TNF receptors

The effects of TNFα on the heart are initiated by two specific receptors on myocytes: a lower affinity, 55-kDa receptor (TNFR1) and a higher affinity, 75-kDa receptor (TNFR2).[10] TNFR1 is more abundant and appears to mediate the deleterious effects of TNFα, whereas TNFR2 appears to have a more protective role. Both receptors are cleaved from the cell membrane and subsequently converted to their soluble forms, sTNFR1 and sTNFR2. The soluble receptors may not only neutralize TNFα, inhibiting its highly cytotoxic activities, but perhaps also stabilize TNFα, potentiating its detrimental long-term actions in lower concentrations.[37]

Like TNFα itself, sTNF receptors are highest in patients with severe decompensated chronic HF and in cachectic chronic HF patients, but are also increased in stable patients with mild chronic HF.[38] Plasma concentrations of sTNFR vary less than those of TNFα and are thought to indicate the history of inflammatory immune activation; therefore, they may be better markers of HF than serum levels of TNFα.

In patients with advanced chronic HF, sTNFR2 is a strong predictor of mortality, which may reflect its ability to act as a 'slow-release reservoir' of bioactive TNF into the circulation.[30] In the setting of acute myocardial infarction, which is a powerful trigger for cytokine activation, sTNFR1 is a better short- and long- term predictor of death and chronic HF.[38] The reasons for the discrepancy may relate to differences in clinical settings, study population sizes, and demographics. It is not yet clear whether circulating sTNFR is an epiphenomenon, simply indicative of a generalized inflammatory state and not a true causal mediator of disease progression. Recent evidence suggests that signalling through both receptors is required to induce the inflammatory and remodelling responses to TNF and the overall balance between opposing receptor-specific effects determines the ultimate impact of TNF.[39]

IL-6

Circulating IL-6 is elevated in patients with chronic HF in relation to disease severity.[40] Like TNF, IL-6 is a maladaptive protein, which participates in the development and progression of HF by exerting direct toxic effects on the heart and peripheral circulation. Its role is complex, as it has both proinflammatory and anti-inflammatory effects.[41] IL-6 may induce a hypertrophic response from myocytes and cause myocardial dysfunction by NO generation, but also appears to block cardiac myocyte apoptosis.[42] In the peripheral circulation, IL-6 production may contribute to abnormalities of endothelium-dependent vasodilation, vascular resistance, increased vascular permeability, or muscle wasting. IL-6 spillover in the peripheral circulation increases with the severity of chronic HF and is associated with sympathetic nervous system activity.[43]

Serum IL-6 is produced by many cell types, including leucocytes, endothelial cells, vascular smooth muscle cells, cardiomyocytes, and fibroblasts.[44] IL-6 may be more important in the development of chronic HF than other inflammatory markers, as it has effects on platelets, endothelium, the coagulation cascade, and metabolism factors. IL-6 is a central mediator of the acute-phase response and a primary determinant of the hepatic production of C-reactive protein (CRP) and TNF. IL-6 concentrations, not surprisingly, correlate with TNFα and CRP levels.

IL-6 is a strong predictor of new-onset heart failure in healthy populations[45,46] and in older patients with acute ischaemic heart disease.[47] Its prognostic power in patients with established chronic HF is not clear. Increased concentrations of IL-6 are independently associated with a poorer prognosis in chronic HF patients, but concentrations of its soluble receptor (IL-6R) are not.[10,43] Other reports have not found significant prognostic value of IL-6.[48] Because of a relatively high short-term variability and non-normal distribution of IL-6 concentrations, interpretation of results may vary between studies.[49] In addition, episodes of myocardial ischaemia may trigger IL-6 production, making interpretation of prognostic data more difficult. Notably, a small subunit within the IL-6 receptor, named gp130, is a potent inducer of cardiomyocyte hypertrophy.[50,51] The gp130-signalling pathway seems to mediate the expression and activation of IL-6, IL-6/IL-6R complex, and other IL-6- related cytokines, such as leukaemia inhibitory factor and cardiotrophin-1, playing a critical role in both adaptive and maladaptive responses within the myocardium. Ventricular-restricted gp130 knockout mice develop dilated cardiomyopathy and profound myocyte apoptosis.[51] However, the clinical significance of these findings in chronic HF remains uncertain.

IL-1

The IL-1 cytokine family has four main members: IL-1α, IL-1β, IL-1 receptor antagonist (IL-1Ra), and IL-18. IL-1β is the major extracellular form in humans and a major proinflammatory cytokine.[52,53] The expression of IL-1β is increased in the coronary arteries and myocardium of patients with dilated cardiomyopathy when compared to those with ischaemic HF.[54] It has negative inotropic effects on the myocardium by uncoupling β-adrenergic signalling in a dose-dependent fashion, and it depresses myocardial contractility by stimulating NO synthase and ceramidase pathways.[55] IL-1 β may also suppress cardiac function by increasing cyclooxygenase-2 and phospholipase A2 gene expression, and by phosphatidylinositol-3′ kinase activation, which results in NF-κB activation.[52,53] In addition, IL-1 is involved in myocyte apoptosis, hypertrophy, and arrhythmogenesis. IL-1β is elevated in the myocardium of patients with HF and is increased in deteriorating patients.[56]

There is still little information about endogenous IL-1Ra, a naturally occurring cytokine, which blocks the action of IL-1, attenuating its effects. IL-1Ra is often considered a more sensitive marker of IL-1 system activation than IL-1 levels.[57] However, given that IL-1Ra is a specific antagonist of IL-1, elevated levels of IL-1Ra could represent an appropriate response to counteract the inflammatory process caused by IL-1.[57]

IL-18 is a more recently identified member of the IL-1 family, initially identified for its role in inducing IFN-γ production.[58] IL-18 is produced by vascular endothelial cells and macrophages in the human heart. It is a proinflammatory cytokine with multiple biological functions and, like many cytokines, it acts synergistically with other similar proteins and mediators.[59] IL-18 is a strong predictor of future cardiovascular risk in stable and unstable angina[60] and is up-regulated in the myocardium of patients with chronic HF. Although ischaemic insult is a major trigger of IL-18 expression, enhanced IL-18 processing is seen in patients with chronic HF of either ischaemic or nonischaemic origin.[61] IL-18 may aggravate the inflammatory response via increased expression of endothelial cell adhesion molecules and secretion of proinflammatory mediators. It is a potent antiangiogenic cytokine and its inhibition might have beneficial effects on tissue remodelling.[58] IL-18 up-regulates membrane Fas ligand expression and may therefore contribute to Fas-mediated apoptosis of Fas-expressing cardiomyocytes.

Granulocyte-macrophage colony-stimulating factor (GM-CSF)

The glycoprotein GM-CSF stimulates the proliferation, differentiation, and activity of multiple myeloid cells including neutrophils, monocytes/macrophages, eosinophils, and dendritic cells. It belongs to the large family of haemopoietic cell colony-stimulating factors and stimulates a range of activities, including leucocyte adhesion, free-radical generation, and cytokine production.[44] It is implicated in myelosuppressive disorders, drug-induced agranulocytosis, and immunodeficiency syndromes. In atherosclerosis, GM-CSF has angiogenic properties and confers some protective effects.[62] In human tissue from endstage HF, GM-CSF is highly expressed. Elevated GM-CSF levels have been demonstrated in chronic HF, which were associated with both the neurohormonal activation and haemodynamic deterioration.[63]

IL-10

IL-10 was initially described as a cytokine synthesis inhibitory factor. It is produced by a variety of inflammatory cells, especially macrophages and T-cells, and is found in advanced atherosclerotic plaques, where it confers a protective effect: IL-10 levels predict outcome in acute coronary syndromes.[64] IL-10 inhibits monocyte adherence to human aortic endothelial cells *in vitro*. The ability of IL-10 to suppress certain CD40/CD40L ligand-mediated monocyte responses may account for some of its antiatherogenic effects.[65]

IL-10 is involved in the production of matrix metalloproteinases (MMP) and cytokines, activation of NF-κB, and apoptosis and cell death.[66] IL-10 down-regulates the secretion of TNFα, IL-1, and IL-6 but enhances the release of sTNFR, contributing to the reduction of TNFα activity. IL-10 also attenuates the production of macrophage-derived NO and oxygen free radicals. Circulating IL-10 levels can be elevated in patients with dilated cardiomyopathy and IL-10 mRNA can be detected in the failing myocardium, possibly as a counter-regulatory response.

One study indicated a differentiation in cytokine patterns with respect to HF aetiology; IL-10 was much lower in patients with dilated cardiomyopathy as compared to ischaemic cardiomyopathy.[67] On the other hand, other studies have shown decreased plasma levels of IL-10 with the lowest concentrations observed in advanced chronic HF. Administration of immunoglobulin to chronic HF patients increased plasma concentrations of IL-10 and improved left ventricular ejection fraction (LVEF).[68]

Transforming growth factor (TGF) β

TGFβ deactivates macrophages by suppressing inducible NO synthase protein expression. It is a potent negative regulator of inflammation in vascular cells by down-regulating cytokine-induced expression of adhesion molecules.[69] Members of the TGFβ superfamily are able to promote the differentiation of embryonic stem cells into cardiomyocytes.[70] Patients with idiopathic dilated cardiomyopathy have increased $TGF\beta_1$ gene expression in macrophages associated with increased plasma concentrations. Excessive production of $TGF\beta_1$ may reflect either an adaptive role of macrophages in tissue repair or impaired ventricular compliance with increased collagen deposition.[71]

Chemokines

Chemokines are a family of chemotactic cytokines and are important factors in the control and regulation of leucocyte trafficking into inflamed tissues.[72,73] The attraction of leucocytes is essential for inflammation and the host response to infection but may also play a critical role in the pathogenesis of chronic HF. Chemokines may promote myocardial failure both directly (e.g. modulation of apoptosis, fibrosis, and angiogenesis) and indirectly (e.g. recruitment and activation of infiltrating leucocytes). Chemokines are classified into three distinct families on the basis of structure and function: C-C (e.g. monocyte chemoattractant protein-1), CXC (e.g. IL-8), and CX3C (e.g. fractalkine).

Monocyte Chemoattractant Protein-1 (MCP-1)

MCP-1 belongs to the C-C subfamily, which lack an amino acid between the first two N-terminal cysteine residues.[73] It is produced by a variety of leucocytes, endothelial cells, and fibroblasts. MCP-1 is mainly characterized by its ability to induce directional migration of leucocytes, with a crucial role in controlling inflammation and immune responses. MCP-1 possesses chemotactic and activating effects for both monocytes and lymphocytes, and in particular, MCP-1 is a major signal for the accumulation of mononuclear leucocytes in disease.

The pathogenic role of MCP-1 (and its receptor CCR2) in atherosclerosis and its complications is via monocyte and neutrophil interactions with endothelium.[74] Raised levels of MCP-1 have been found in cardiac lymph and in the endothelium of small veins from ischaemic canine myocardium. Pressure overload induces myocardial expression of MCP-1, which attracts and activates monocytes and macrophages, and the recruited cells produce proinflammatory cytokines.[75,76] Hypoxia and ischaemia are also potent inducers of MCP-1, involving activation of NF-κB.

Myocardial overexpression of MCP-1 is associated with monocyte infiltration of the myocardium and cardiac hypertrophy, ventricular dilatation, and depressed contractile function. Serum MCP-1 correlates with the degree of left ventricular dysfunction and may also be involved in cardiomyocyte apoptosis in severe HF. Chronic exposure to MCP-1 favours myocardial apoptosis and ventricular dysfunction by inducing transcriptional factors: gene therapy directed against MCP-1 may slow the progression of HF.[77]

Macrophage inflammatory protein (MIP)-1

MIP-1 is a C-C chemokine produced by various types of inflammatory cells, exerting chemotactic activity for both monocytes and lymphocytes. MIP-1 is high in patients with chronic HF, with particularly high levels in patients with the most severe HF.[77] Abundant expression of MIP-1 may be an important factor in mediating the infiltration and activation of mononuclear leucocytes into the myocardium of chronic HF patients but may also have other functions, such as generating reactive oxygen species and cytokine production.

Regulated on activation normal T-cell expressed and secreted (RANTES)

RANTES is a member of the C-C chemokine group, produced by a variety of cell types including platelets. It is a potent chemoattractant for T cells and monocytes, and is implicated in inflammatory diseases including atherosclerosis. RANTES may also modulate free-radical generation and the production of other cytokines.[78] It is highly expressed within atheroma and is up-regulated (and has prognostic significance) in acute coronary syndromes.[44] RANTES is elevated in patients with advanced chronic HF and may have a role in disease progression via its effects on platelet-inflammatory cell interactions.[77] However, data on RANTES in chronic HF are sparse and further studies are needed.

IL-8

IL-8 is probably one of the best characterized neutrophil chemoattractants and degranulating agents. It is consistently found in macrophage-rich atherosclerotic plaques and it is thus implicated in early atherosclerotic progression.[79]

IL-8 is increased in patients with chronic HF with particularly high concentrations in those with the most both severe HF. Activated monocytes and platelets may contribute to increased levels of IL-8 in chronic HF.[72] IL-8 may be an important participant in both the systemic inflammatory response and the procoagulant activity in chronic HF. High IL-8 serum levels fall to near normal after haemodynamic recovery following ventricular assist device placement, suggesting that IL-8 may be marker of tissue damage.[80]

Adhesion molecules

Cell adhesion molecules (CAMs) are involved in the interactions between endothelial cells, leucocytes, and platelets. Thus, they have been implicated in a vast range of conditions including atherosclerosis, thrombosis, allograft rejection post-transplantation, and restenosis following coronary angioplasty.[54] Three families of proteins have been described so far. The intracellular cell adhesion molecule-1 (ICAM-1) and vascular cell adhesion molecule-1 (VCAM-1) belong to the immunoglobulin superfamily. Integrins form the second subfamily. The selectins cause a typical 'rolling' of leucocytes on the endothelial surface, which is mainly mediated by leucocyte (L)-selectin and platelet (P)-selectin.

The significance of CAMs in chronic HF is unclear. The failing myocardium, and in particular the microvascular endothelium, gives signals to assist in leucocyte infiltration, via the up-regulation and/or secretion of CAMs including P-selectin, e-selectin, L-selectin, ICAM-1 and VCAM-1. These molecules are important mediators of both endothelial–leucocyte adhesion and inflammatory responses.[81,82] Damage induced by oxygen free radicals and cytokine activation are stimulators of CAMs. The soluble forms of the adhesion molecules, generated by proteolytic cleavage of cell membrane-bound molecules, act as systemic activation signals for circulating cells.

There is increased endothelial production of adhesion molecules in chronic HF, increased expression of sICAM-1 and integrin CD11a/CD18 (lymphocyte function-associated antigen-1), and increased levels of soluble adhesion molecules. VCAM-1, E-selectin, and P-selectin are all also raised.[83,84] Soluble adhesion molecules (sVCAM-1 and sL-selectin) decrease after the implantation of mechanical circulatory support devices in patients with decompensated HF.

sICAM-1 increases with increasing severity of failure, which suggests that ICAM-1 may be associated with an adverse prognosis. High levels of sP-selectin or VCAM-1 are also independent predictors of outcome in patients with endstage HF.[84] However, data regarding the prognostic value of CAMs are inconsistent. The limited sample size and the different immunological actions of the studied CAMs are all possible explanations for the inconsistency. Furthermore, the different sCAMs vary differently with time, HF treatment, and heart transplantation.[83]

Downstream signalling pathways

NF-κB is a transcription factor mainly involved in stress-induced, immune, and inflammatory responses. Activation of NF-κB can be triggered by multiple stimuli, such as angiotensin II, TLR, IgG and reactive oxidant species (Fig. 16.4). Functional NF-κB requires formation of heterodimers of the p50 and p65 subunits.[85] Activation of NF-κB involves the degradation of its inhibitory proteins IκBs by specific kinases. The free NF-κB passes into the nucleus, where it binds to sites in the promoter regions of genes for inflammatory proteins such as TNFα, IL-1β, inducible NO synthase and adhesion molecules.[86] The activation of NF-κB leads to a coordinated increase in the expression of many genes, whose products are important mediators in the pathogenesis of chronic HF.

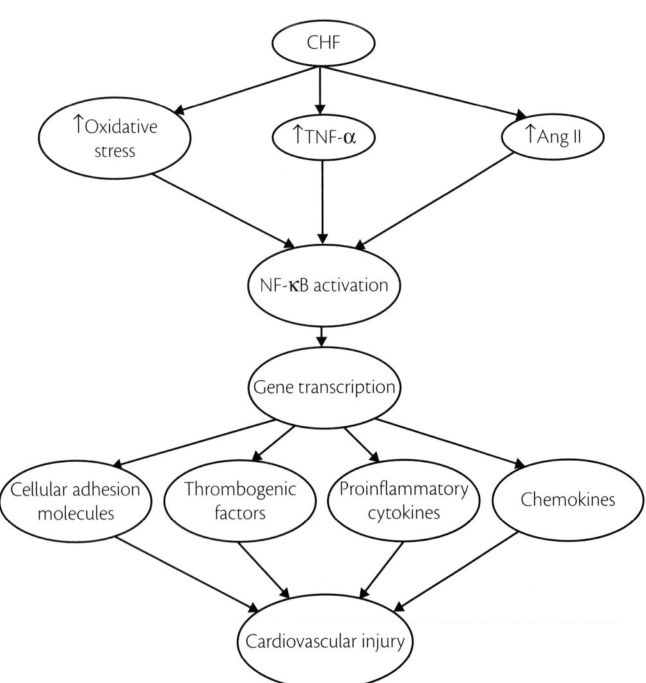

Fig. 16.4 Biological stimuli for the production and effects of NF-κB on the cardiovascular system in chronic heart failure.
From *Eur J Heart Fail* 2001;**3**:517–26, with permission.

NF-κB is activated in myocardial tissue of the failing human heart.[5] Activation of NF-κB ameliorates myocardial hypertrophy and is involved in pro and antiapoptic pathways in HF. Strategies targeting NF-κB improve the long-term prognosis in HF. In mice with targeted disruption of the NF-κB subunit p50, early survival after myocardial infarction is increased and ventricular dilatation is prevented, which is linked to decreased collagen production and deposition.[87]

Nitric oxide

The free-radical gas nitric oxide (NO) is enzymatically formed from L-arginine by three isoforms of NO synthase, which are all present in the heart:

- Endothelial NO synthase (eNOS) is expressed in endothelial cells of the coronary microvasculature and is also found in the subendocardial myocytes. eNOS is the source of vascular NO, acting as vasodilator.
- Neuronal NO synthase (nNOS) is found in the central and peripheral neuronal tissue as well as in cardiac myocytes.
- Inducible NO synthase (iNOS) can be expressed by many different cell types, including inflammatory cells, endothelial cells, and cardiac myocytes.[88]

NO inhibits platelet adherence and aggregation, induces vasodilatation, reduces the adherence of leucocytes to the endothelium, and suppresses the proliferation of vascular smooth muscle cells.[89]

iNOS expression is increased with increasing severity of HF. It is unclear whether wall stress or cytokine activation is the predominant stimulus for iNOS. TNFα is a potent inducer of iNOS expression in both endothelial and vascular smooth muscle cells resulting in enhanced NO production. NO can exert both negative inotropic and apoptotic effects on cardiac myocytes. Therapy with LVADs was found to normalize iNOS expression in association with diminished cardiomyocyte apoptosis in the failing heart.[89]

CRP

CRP is a simple downstream marker of inflammation. Il-6 is the primary stimulus for the hepatic production of CRP within 6 h of stimulus.[90] CRP can also be produced from vascular walls, particularly in the atherosclerotic intima of human coronary arteries. Left ventricular dysfunction, systemic underperfusion by low cardiac output, hypoxia, and venous congestion may all be sources of increased IL-6 and hence, CRP production.

CRP might worsen HF through multiple mechanisms (see Box 16.1). CRP is raised in chronic HF and higher plasma levels of CRP are associated with a worse haemodynamic and clinical profile; however, it is unclear whether the finding is related to active atherosclerosis.[91,92] Raised CRP is a predictor of future heart failure and adverse events in patients with vascular disease,[93] but its prognostic value in patients with established HF is less clear. There are no data in HF patients on the effects of treatment on CRP.

Box 16.1 Proinflammatory effects of CRP

- Activation of complement system
- Stimulation of cytokine production
  - Myocyte loss
  - Left ventricular remodelling and dysfunction[5,91]
- Attenuation of NO production
- Direct proinflammatory action on endothelial cells.

Novel inflammatory mediators

Leptin

Leptin is a major regulator of body mass and appetite.[94,95] In animal studies, it induces weight loss and anorexia and suppresses cardiac contractility through an NO-dependent pathway. Leptin is primarily produced by adipocytes, whereas its receptors are expressed in a variety of tissues, including the heart. Leptin is also related to fat mass in HF patients and therefore, it should be interpreted once corrected for fat mass.[96]. Leptin can modulate other cytokines including interference with NF-κB effects. Leptin is increased in noncachectic HF patients normal or even innapropriately low in cachectic patients—a paradox which may be related to sympathetic nervous activation.

Activin A

Activin A is a member of the TGFβ superfamily involved in growth, differentiation, and survival. Activin A is raised in patients with chronic HF. Activin A is involved in ventricular remodelling by enhancing MCP-1 production, the generation of $TGFβ_1$ and MMP, and specific gene expression associated with myocardial hypertrophy.[97]

TNF superfamily ligands

Fas and Fas ligand belong to the TNF receptor superfamily and might contribute to inflammation, apoptosis, and matrix degradation within the failing myocardium.[98]

The cross-linking of Fas with Fas ligand mediates apoptosis by triggering caspase activation. Soluble forms of Fas are raised in autoimmune diseases, myocarditis and severe chronic HF. Fas/Fas ligand are associated with left ventricular remodelling and may have prognostic value in chronic HF.

The osteoprotegerin receptor activator for NF-κB (RANK)/RANK ligand (RANKL) axis is another member of the TNF receptor superfamily, which is a mediator in both experimental and clinical HF.[99]

Anti-inflammatory targeting therapy

Immunomodulatory effects of traditional cardiovascular therapy

The beneficial effects of the traditional cardiovascular medications cannot be explained solely by their haemodynamic effects. Some drugs used in the treatment of chronic HF may also influence the persistent immune activation and inflammatory pathways.

Treatment with high doses of angiotensin converting enzyme (ACE) inhibitors reduces circulating levels of IL-6.[100] ACE inhibitors may affect TNFα and can reduce insulin-like growth factor-1 (IGF-1). Interestingly, ACE inhibitors may prevent NF-κB activation and MCP-1 expression, and reduce macrophage infiltration. Angiotensin II receptor antagonists down-regulate inflammation by reducing plasma levels of TNFα, IL-6, and brain natriuretic peptides in mild to moderate HF.[101]

Amlodipine reduces IL-6 levels, but with no effect on TNFα.[4] β-Adrenergic stimulation may modulate cytokine production from lymphocytes and monocytes. Carvedilol reduces IL-6.[102] On the other hand, long-term treatment with metoprolol has no significant effect on cytokine levels. The differential effects of α- and β-blockade on the cytokine network still need to be determined in more detail.

Statins may attenuate inflammatory responses and promote plaque stability independent of their cholesterol-lowering effects.[4,104] Statins reduce CRP levels and may be effective in preventing coronary events in patients with relatively low lipid levels but with elevated CRP.[103]

Apart from their short-term haemodynamic benefits, phosphodiesterase inhibitors can inhibit the production of TNFα and other cytokines in failing myocardium.[104] However, phosphodiesterase inhibitors are also related to an adverse outcome in chronic HF. Cardiac glycosides can also reduce levels of IL-6 and TNFα *in vivo*. Amiodarone causes a significant decrease in TNFα production by human mononuclear cells, suggesting a possible mechanism for its effect in HF.

However, some of the effects on the immune system may be secondary to improved left ventricular function and not a direct effect of the drugs. A nonpharmacological approach, physical training, induces beneficial changes in exercise capacity which are correlated with a reduction in inflammatory markers (Fig. 16.5).[105] Exercise training restores, at least partially, abnormal immuno-inflammatory responses by depressing systemic inflammation with reduced proinflammatory cytokine (TNFα and IL-6) expression at both circulation[106] and tissue[107] level. In consequence, there is a fall in oxidative stress as demonstrated by the reduced expression of iNOS and the increased activity of radical scavenger enzymes in skeletal muscle.[108] There is an inverse relation between iNOS expression and cytochrome *c* oxidase activity, suggesting that local anti-inflammatory effects may contribute to improved skeletal muscle oxidative metabolism with physical training.[109] The local anti-inflammatory effects of exercise may slow down or even reverse the catabolic wasting process associated with the progression of HF.

Anti-TNF studies: positive and negative results

Given the potential central role of TNFα, etanercept, a recombinant sTNFR type 2 protein, which functionally inactivates TNFα, has been tried as a treatment for chronic HF. An initial study showed beneficial effects on cardiac function and left ventricular remodelling in a small population with severe chronic HF. Subsequently, the long-term effects of etanercept were assessed by three large placebo-controlled trials: RENEWAL, RENAISSANCE, and RECOVER. The trials were terminated prematurely because of lack of evidence of beneficial effects.[110]

Inxiximab is a chimeric monoclonal antibody which directly binds to the transmembrane form of TNF. Its use was associated with time- and dose-related increase in death and HF hospitalization in patients with moderate/severe HF.[111] The xanthine derivative pentoxifylline, which exerts peripheral vasodilatory effects

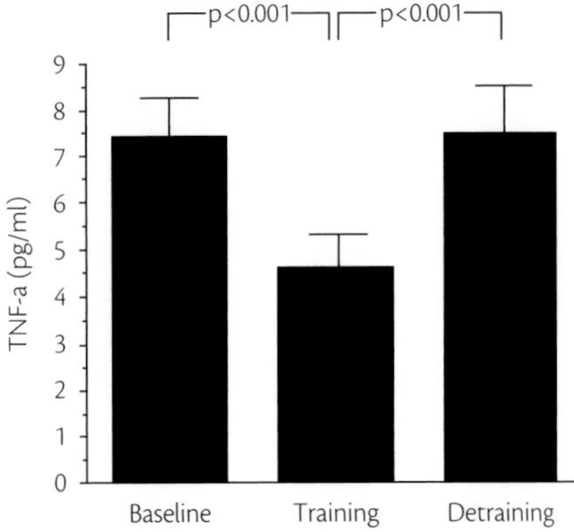

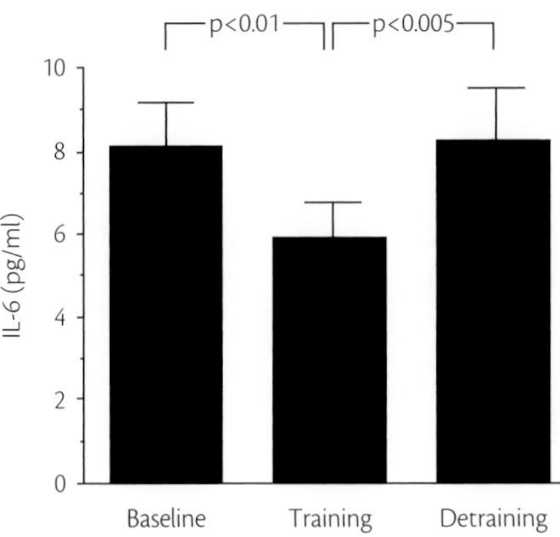

Fig. 16.5 The anti-inflammatory effect of physical training in patients with chronic heart failure. The effects of a training programme on TNFα and IL-6 are shown.
From *J Am Coll Cardiol* 2002;**39:**653–663, with permission.

and improves blood flow, also reduces TNFα. Treatment with pentoxifylline was associated with a significant improvement in functional class and LVEF, along with a decrease in circulating TNFα.[112] The observed changes did not correlate to each other, suggesting that the beneficial effects of pentoxifylline were independent of TNFα.

The failure of anti-TNFα therapy has led to much discussion. The intervention on a single cytokine may not be sufficient to have an impact on the progression of HF. TNFα is a pleiotropic cytokine, also implicated in cardioprotective pathways, at least early on in the disease process. It may be that immunomodulation is only or particularly valuable for those patients with strongly up-regulated inflammatory status. Etanercept and infliximab may even have increased the biological half-life of TNFα, or it may be that the dose used was not sufficient to inhibit TNFα function. The future of anti-TNF therapy is very uncertain. Other agents that modulate the production of TNFα, such as inhibitors of lysophosphatidic acid acyl transferase, p38 MAP kinases, NF-κB, and TNFα converting enzyme may be treatments of the future.

Intravenous immunoglobulin (IVIG) or interferon (INF)

IVIG administration improves LVEF, haemodynamics, and exercise capacity in patients with chronic HF, independent of aetiology.[113] Others have found no impact of IVIG on recent-onset idiopathic dilated cardiomyopathy.[104] To add to the controversory, long-term therapy results in improved LVEF, associated with a marked elevation of IL-10, IL-1 receptor antagonist, and sTNFR. IVIG also reduced chemokines and their receptors in peripheral blood mononuclear cells, suggesting that direct blockade of the chemokine network may be an approach for future intervention.

A pilot study of INF-1β for the treatment of virus-related dilated cardiomyopathy showed improvement in symptoms and quality of life but no change in objective variables.[104] It is being investigated in a large phase III trial.

Immunomodulation therapy: celacade

Celacade is an immunomodulation therapy designed to target chronic inflammation by activating the immune system's physiological anti-inflammatory response. A blood sample is rapidly exposed to a combination of physiochemical stressors *ex vivo* and then reinjected intramuscularly in an attempt to evoke beneficial immune responses. The physiological response of the immune system to the reinjected apoptotic cells is likely to increase inflammatory cytokine production, rather than impair it. Phase I and II clinical trials of celacade showed a low risk of side effects and improved quality of life in HF patients.[114,115] ACCLAIM, a phase III trial, did not show any significant reduction in mortality or cardiovascular hospitalization,[116] but there was a benefit in some subgroups, particularly those with NYHA II class HF and those without a history of previous myocardial infarction.

Promising immunomodulation therapeutic options

Immunoadsorption allows the removal of circulating autoantibodies, such as those against the β_1-adrenergic and muscarinergic receptors or troponin I. It improves cardiac structure and function and decreases oxidative stress and myocardial inflammation.[99,104] It may only be effective in patients with cardiodepressant autoantibodies or only in combination with IVIG acting additively or synergistically.

Thalidomide has both anti-inflammatory and antioncogenic properties and has recently been evaluated on a limited number of patients. Other immunomodulatory treatments have the potential to improve myocardial function. Pentraxins are cytokine-inducible genes, expressed in specific tissues, which reduce early myocardial damage after myocardial infarction. Drugs targeting the kinase activity of PI3Kγ—a major component of signal transduction controlling leucocyte migration—can reduce cardiac inflammation. The MMP system is involved in ventricular remodelling: its inhibition may have beneficial effects, particularly in acute HF where MMP expression is related to acute dilatation and failure. Gene therapy with MCP-1 blocker attenuates the development of cardiac remodelling after myocardial infarction. IL-10 and IL-1R antagonist exert cardioprotective effects in viral myocarditis and against ischaemia reperfusion injury in mice.

Activators of peroxisome proliferator-activated receptors reduce endotoxin-stimulated TNFα expression and cardiac hypertrophy by inhibiting NF-κB activation, thereby decreasing inflammatory response. Tranilast is a mast-cell stabilizing agent, which has been found to modulate compensated hypertrophy, ventricular remodelling, and the production of anti-inflammatory cytokines like IL-10.

Other emerging therapeutic targets including mannose-binding lectin, IL-18 and IL-6 antagonists, and T-cell and caspase inhibitors, which can tackle inflammation in the heart. More knowledge on inflammatory cytokines in HF and larger placebo-controlled randomized studies will allow the development of more effective therapeutic options. Finally, a promising immunomodulatory approach with respect to the efficacy of immunosuppressive therapy in patients with chronic inflammatory cardiomyopathy was examined in the randomized TIMIC Study, underlining the importance of endomyocardial biopsy in dilated cardiomyopathy. Eighty-five patients with biopsy-proven myocarditis and no evidence of myocardial viral genomes who received 6 months prednisone and azathioprine, in addition to conventional therapy for heart failure, showed a significant improvement of left-ventricular ejection fraction and a significant decrease in left-ventricular dimensions and volumes compared with baseline (anti-remodelling effect).[117]

References

1. Mann DL. Mechanisms, models in HF: A combinatorial approach. *Circulation* 1999;**100**:999–1008.
2. Mann DL, Young JB. Basic mechanisms in congestive heart failure: recognizing the role of proinflammatory cytokines. *Chest* 1994;**105**:897–904.
3. Rouleau JL. Treatment of congestive heart failure: present and future. *Can J Cardiol* 2005;**21**:1084–8.
4. Damas JK, Gullestad L, Aukrust P. Cytokines as new treatment targets in chronic heart failure. *Curr Control Trials Cardiovasc Med* 2001;**2**:271–7.
5. Anker SD, von Haehling S. Inflammatory mediators in chronic heart failure: an overview. *Heart* 2004;**90**:464–70.
6. Pearson TA, Mensah GA, Alexander RW, *et al.* Markers of inflammation and cardiovascular disease: application to clinical and public health practice: a statement for healthcare professionals from the Centers for Disease Control and Prevention and the American Heart Association. *Circulation* 2003;**107**:499–511.
7. Murray, DR, Dugan J. Overview of recent clinical trials in heart failure: what is the current standard of care?. *Cardiol Rev* 2000;**8**:340–347.
8. Mann DL, Deswal A, Bozkurt B, Torre-Amione G. New therapeutics for chronic heart failure. *Annu Rev Med* 2002;**53**:59–74.
9. Dibbs Z, Kurrelmeyer K, Kalra D, *et al.* Cytokines in heart failure: pathogenetic mechanisms and potential treatment. *Proc Assoc Am Physicians* 1999;**111**:423–8.
10. Anker SD, von Haehling S (2004). Inflammatory mediators in chronic heart failure: an overview. *Heart* 2004;**90**:464–70.
11. Anker SD, Egerer KR, Volk HD, Kox WJ, Poole-Wilson PA, Coats AJ. Elevated soluble CD14 receptors and altered cytokines in chronic heart failure. *Am J Cardiol* 1997;**79**:1426–30.
12. Genth-Zotz S, von Haehling S, Bolger AP, *et al.* Pathophysiologic quantities of endotoxin-induced tumor necrosis factor-alpha release in whole blood from patients with chronic heart failure. *Am J Cardiol* 2002;**90**:1226–30.
13. Niebauer J, Volk H-D, Kemp M, *et al.* Endotoxin and immune activation in chronic heart failure: a prospective cohort study. *Lancet* 1999;**353**:1838–42.
14. Paulus WJ. How are cytokines activated in heart failure?. *Eur J Heart Fail* 1999;**1**:309–12.
15. Charalambous BM, Stephens RC, Feavers IM, Montgomery HE. Role of bacterial endotoxin in chronic heart failure: the gut of the matter. *Shock* 2007;**28**:15–23.
16. Murray DR, Prabhu SD, Chandrasekar B (2000). Chronic beta-adrenergic stimulation induces myocardial proinflammatory cytokine expression. *Circulation* 2000;**101**:2338–41.
17. Schulze PC, Gielen S, Adams V, *et al.* Muscular levels of proinflammatory cytokines correlate with a reduced expression of insulinlike growth factor-I in chronic heart failure. *Basic Res Cardiol* 2003;**98**:267–74.
18. Hambrecht R, Schulze PC, Gielen S, *et al.* Reduction of insulin-like growth factor-I expression in the skeletal muscle of noncachectic patients with chronic heart failure. *J Am Coll Cardiol* 2002;**39**:1175–81.
19. Latres E, Amini AR, Amini AA, *et al.* Insulin-like growth factor-1 (IGF-1) inversely regulates atrophy-induced genes via the phosphatidylinositol 3-kinase/Akt/mammalian target of rapamycin (PI3K/Akt/mTOR) pathway. *J Biol Chem* 2005;**280**:2737–44.
20. Schulze PC, Fang J, Kassik KA, *et al.* Transgenic overexpression of locally acting IGF-1 inhibits ubiquitin-mediated muscle atrophy in chronic left ventricular dysfunction. *Circ Res* 2005;**97**:418–26.
21. Sandri M, Sandri C, Gilbert A, *et al.*. Foxo transcription factors induce the atrophy-related ubiquitin ligase atrogin-1 and cause skeletal muscle atrophy. *Cell* 2004;**117**:399–412.
22. Du J, Wang X, Miereles C, Bailey JL, *et al.* Activation of caspase-3 is an initial step triggering accelerated muscle proteolysis in catabolic conditions. *J Clin Invest* 2004;**113**:115–23.
23. Conraads VM, Hoymans VY, Vermeulen T, *et al.* Exercise capacity in chronic heart failure patients is related to active gene transcription in skeletal muscle and not apoptosis. *Eur J Cardiovasc Prev Rehabil* 2009;**16**:325–32.
24. Piepoli M, Clark AL, Volterrani M, Adamopoulos S, Sleight P, Coats AJS. Contribution of muscle afferents to the hemodynamic, autonomic, and ventilatory responses to exercise in patients with chronic heart failure: effects of physical training. *Circulation* 1996;**93**:940–52.
25. Levine B, Kalman J, Mayer L, Fillit HM, Packer M. Elevated circulating levels of tumor necrosis factor in severe chronic heart failure. *N Engl J Med* 1990;**323**:236–41.
26. Torre-Amione G, Kapadia S, Lee J, *et al.* Tumor necrosis factor-alpha and tumor necrosis factor receptors in the failing human heart. *Circulation* 1996;**93**:704–11.
27. Torre-Amione G, Stetson SJ, Youker KA, *et al.* Decreased expression of tumor necrosis factor-alpha in failing human myocardium after mechanical circulatory support : A potential mechanism for cardiac recovery. *Circulation* 1999;**100**:1189–93.
28. Birks EJ, Latif N, Owen V, *et al.* Quantitative myocardial cytokine expression and activation of the apoptotic pathway in patients who require left ventricular assist devices. *Circulation* 2001;**104**(12 Suppl 1):I233–40.
29. McMurray J, Abdullah I, Dargie HJ, Shapiro D. Increased concentrations of tumour necrosis factor in 'cachectic' patients with severe chronic heart failure. *Br Heart J* 1991;**66**:356–8.
30. Torre-Amione G, Kapadia S, Benedict C, Oral H, Young JB, Mann DL. Proinflammatory cytokine levels in patients with depressed left ventricular ejection fraction: a report from the studies of left ventricular dysfunction (SOLVD). *J Am Coll Cardiol* 1996;**27**:1201–6.
31. Deswal A, Petersen NJ, Feldman AM, Young JB, White BG, Mann DL. Cytokines and cytokine receptors in advanced heart failure: an analysis of the cytokine database from the Vesnarinone trial (VEST). *Circulation* 2001;**103**:2055–9.
32. Yokoyama T, Vaca L, Rossen RD, Durante W, Hazarika P, Mann DL. Cellular basis for the negative inotropic effects of tumor necrosis factor-α in the mammalian heart. *J Clin Invest* 1993;**92**:2303–12.
33. Wada H, Saito K, Kanda T, *et al.* Tumor necrosis factor-α (TNF-α) plays a protective role in acute viral myocarditis in mice: a study using mice lacking TNF-α. *Circulation* 2001;**103**:743–9.
34. Bolger AP, Anker SD. Tumour necrosis factor in chronic heart failure: a peripheral view on pathogenesis, clinical manifestations and therapeutic implications. *Drugs* 2000;**60**:1245–57.
35. Suematsu N, Tsutsui H, Wen J, *et al.* Oxidative stress mediates tumor necrosis factor-alpha-induced mitochondrial DNA damage and dysfunction in cardiac myocytes. *Circulation* 2003;**107**:1418–23.
36. Anker SD, Volterrani M, Egerer KR, *et al.* Tumour necrosis factor alpha as a predictor of impaired peak leg blood flow in patients with chronic heart failure. *Q J Med* 1998;**91**:199–203.
37. Ferrari R, Bachetti T, Confortini R, *et al.* Tumor necrosis factor soluble receptors in patients with various degrees of congestive failure. *Circulation* 1995;**92**:1479–86.
38. Valgimigli M, Ceconi C, Malagutti P, *et al.* Tumor necrosis factor-alpha receptor 1 is a major predictor of mortality and new-onset heart failure in patients with acute myocardial infarction: the Cytokine-Activation and Long-Term Prognosis in Myocardial Infarction (C-ALPHA) study. *Circulation* 2005;**111**:863–70.
39. Hamid T, Gu Y, Ortines RV, Bhattacharya C, Wang G, Xuan YT, Prabhu SD. Divergent tumor necrosis factor receptor-related remodeling responses in heart failure: role of nuclear factor-kappaB and inflammatory activation. *Circulation* 2009;**119**:1386–97.

40. MacGowan GA, Mann DL, Kormos RL, Feldman AM, Murali S. Circulating interleukin-6 in severe heart failure. *Am J Cardiol* 1997;**79**:1128–31.
41. Wollert KC, Drexler H. The role of interleukin-6 in the failing heart. *Heart Fail Rev* 2001;**6**:95–103.
42. Tsujinaka T, Fujita J, Ebisui C, *et al.* Interleukin 6 receptor antibody inhibits muscle atrophy and modulates proteolytic systems in interleukin 6 transgenic mice. *J Clin Invest* 1996;**97**:244–9.
43. Tsutamoto T, Hisanaga T, Wada A, *et al.* Interleukin-6 spillover in the peripheral circulation increases with the severity of heart failure, and the high plasma level of interleukin-6 is an important prognostic predictor in patients with congestive heart failure. *J Am Coll Cardiol* 1998;**31**:391–8.
44. Adamopoulos S, Parissis JT, Kremastinos DT. A glossary of circulating cytokines in chronic heart failure. *Eur J Heart Fail* 2001;**3**:517–26.
45. Vasan RS, Sullivan LM, Roubenoff R, *et al.* Inflammatory markers and risk of heart failure in elderly subjects without prior myocardial infarction: the Framingham Heart Study. *Circulation* 2003;**107**:1486–91.
46. Cesari M, Penninx BW, Newman AB, *et al.* Inflammatory markers and onset of cardiovascular events: results from the Health ABC study. *Circulation* 2003;**108**:2317–22.
47. Koukkunen H, Penttila K, Kemppainen A, *et al.* C-reactive protein, fibrinogen, interleukin-6 and tumor necrosis factor-alpha in the prognostic classification of unstable angina pectoris. *Ann Med* 2001;**33**:37–47.
48. Rauchhaus M, Doehner W, Francis DP, *et al.* Plasma cytokine parameters and mortality in patients with chronic heart failure. *Circulation* 2000;**102**:3060–7.
49. Dibbs Z, Thornby J, White BG, Mann DL. Natural variability of circulating levels of cytokines and cytokine receptors in patients with heart failure: implications for clinical trials. *J Am Coll Cardiol* 1999;**33**:1935–42.
50. Yamauchi-Takihara K. Gp130-mediated pathway and left ventricular remodeling. *J Card Fail* 2002;**8**(6 Suppl):S374–8.
51. Hirota H, Chen J, Betz UA, *et al.* Loss of a gp130 cardiac muscle cell survival pathway is a critical event in the onset of heart failure during biomechanical stress. *Cell* 1999;**97**:189–98.
52. Dinarello CA. Interleukin-1 and interleukin-1 antagonism. *Blood* 1991;**77**:1627–52.
53. Auron PE. The interleukin 1 receptor: ligand interactions and signal transduction. *Cytokine Growth Factor Rev* 1998;**9**:221–37.
54. Francis SE, Holden H, Holt CM, *et al.* Interleukin-1 in myocardium and coronary arteries of patients with dilated cardiomyopathy. *J Mol Cell Cardiol* 1998;**30**:215–23.
55. Cain BS, Meldrum DR, Dinarello CA, *et al.* Tumor necrosis factor-α and interleukin-1β synergistically depress human myocardial function. *Crit Care Med* 1999;**27**:1309–18.
56. Testa M, Yeh M, Lee P, *et al.* Circulating levels of cytokines and their endogenous modulators in patients with mild to severe congestive heart failure due to coronary artery disease or hypertension. *J Am Coll Cardiol* 1996;**28**:964–71.
57. Thiele RI, Daniel V, Opelz G, *et al.* Circulating interleukin-1 receptor antagonist (IL-1RA) serum levels in patients undergoing orthotopic heart transplantation. *Transpl Int* 1998;**11**:443–8.
58. Dinarello CA. Interleukin-18, a proinflammatory cytokine. *Eur Cytokine Netw* 2000;**11**:483–6.
59. Puren AJ, Fantuzzi G, Gu Y, Su MS, Dinarello CA. Interleukin-18 (IFNgamma-inducing factor) induces IL-8 and IL-1beta via TNFalpha production from non- CD14+ human blood mononuclear cells. *J Clin Invest* 1998;**101**:711–21.
60. Blankenberg S, Tiret L, Bickel C, *et al.* Interleukin-18 is a strong predictor of cardiovascular death in stable and unstable angina. *Circulation* 2002;**106**:24–30.
61. Yamaoka-Tojo M, Tojo T, Inomata T, Machida Y, Osada, K, Izumi T. Circulating levels of interleukin 18 reflect etiologies of heart failure: Th1/Th2 cytokine imbalance exaggerates the pathophysiology of advanced heart failure. *J Card Fail* 2002;**8**:21–7.
62. Seiler C, Pohl T, Wustmann K *et al.* Promotion of collateral growth by granulocyte-macrophage colony-stimulating factor in patients with coronary artery disease: a randomized, double blind, placebo-controlled study. *Circulation* 2001;**104**:2012–17.
63. Parissis JT, Adamopoulos S, Venetsanou KF, Mentzikof DG, Karas SM, Kremastinos DT. Clinical and neurohormonal correlates of circulating granulocyte-macrophage colonystimulating factor in severe heart failure secondary to ischemic or idiopathic dilated cardiomyopathy. *Am J Cardiol* 2000;**86**:707–10.
64. Heeschen C, Dimmeler S, Hamm CW, *et al.* Serum level of the antiinflammatory cytokine interleukin-10 is an important prognostic determinant in patients with acute coronary syndromes. *Circulation* 2003;**107**:2109–14.
65. Poe JC, Wagner DH Jr, Miller RW, Stout RD, Suttles J. IL-4 and IL-10 modulation of CD40-mediated signaling of monocyte IL-1beta synthesis and rescue from apoptosis. *J Immunol* 1997;**159**:846–52.
66. Silvestre JS, Mallat Z, Tamarat R, Duriez M, Tedgui A, Levy BI. Regulation of matrix metalloproteinase activity in ischemic tissue by interleukin-10: role in ischemia-induced angiogenesis. *Circ Res* 2001;**89**:259–264.
67. Stumpf C, Lehner C, Yilmaz A, Daniel WG, Garlichs CD. Decrease of serum levels of the anti-inflammatory cytokine interleukin-10 in patients with advanced chronic heart failure. *Clin Sci (Lond)* 2003;**105**:45–50.
68. Gullestad L, Aass H, Fjeld JG, *et al.* Immunomodulating therapy with intravenous immunoglobulin in patients with chronic heart failure. *Circulation* 2001;**103**:220–225.
69. Gamble JR, Khew-Goodall Y, Vadas MA. Transforming growth factor-beta inhibits E-selectin expression on human endothelial cells. *J Immunol* 1993;**150**:4494–503.
70. Tiedemann H, Asashima M, Grunz H, Knochel W. Pluripotent cells (stem cells) and their determination and differentiation in early vertebrate embryogenesis. *Dev Growth Differ* 2001;**43**:469–502.
71. Sanderson JE, Lai KB, Shum IO, Wei S, Chow LT. Transforming growth factor-beta expression in dilated cardiomyopathy. *Heart* 2001;**86**:701–8.
72. Damås JK, Gullestad L, Ueland T, *et al.* CXC-chemokines, a new group of cytokines in congestive heart failure—possible role of platelets and monocytes. *Cardiovasc Res* 2000;**45**:428–36.
73. Baggiolini M, Dewald B, Moser B. Interleukin-8 and related chemotactic cytokines: CXC and CC chemokines. *Adv Immunol* 1994;**55**:97–179.
74. Okada M, Matsumori A, Ono K, *et al.* Cyclic stretch upregulates production of interleukin-8 and monocyte chemotactic and activating factor/monocyte chemoattractant protein-1 in human endothelial cells. *Arterioscler Thromb Vasc Biol* 1998;**18**:894–901.
75. Shioi T, Matsumori A, Kihara Y, *et al.* Increased expression of interleukin-1 beta and monocyte chemotactic and activating factor/ monocyte chemoattractant protein-1 in the hypertrophied and failing heart with pressure overload. *Circ Res* 1997;**81**:664–71.
76. Zhou L, Azfer A, Niu J, *et al.* Monocyte chemoattractant protein-1 induces a novel transcription factor that causes cardiac myocyte apoptosis and ventricular dysfunction. *Circ Res* 2006;**98**:1177–85.
77. Aukrust P, Veland T, M¨uller F *et al.* Elevated circulating levels of C-C chemokines in patients with congestive heart failure. *Circulation* 1998;**97**:1136–43.
78. Pattison J, Nelson PJ, Huie P *et al.* RANTES chemokine expression in cell-mediated transplant rejection of the kidney. *Lancet* 1994;**343**:209–11.
79. Boisvert WA, Santiago R, Curtiss LK, Terkeltaub RA. A leukocyte homologue of the IL-8 receptor CXCR-2 mediates the accumulation of macrophages in atherosclerotic lesions of LDL receptor-deficient mice. *J Clin Invest* 1998;**101**:353–63.
80. Goldstein DJ, Moazami N, Seldomridge JA, *et al.* Circulatory resuscitation with left ventricular assist device support reduces interleukins 6 and 8 levels. *Ann Thorac Surg* 1997;**63**:971–4.

81. Devaux B, Scholz D, Hirche A, Klövekorn WP, Schaper J. Upregulation of cell adhesion molecules and the presence of low grade inflammation in human chronic heart failure. *Eur Heart J* 1997;**18**:470–9.
82. Noutsias M, Seeberg B, Schultheiss HP, Kuhl U. Expression of cell adhesion molecules in dilated cardiomyopathy. *Circulation* 1999;**99**:2124–31.
83. Andreassen AK, Nord y I, Simonsen S, *et al.* Levels of circulating adhesion molecules in congestive heart failure and after heart transplantation. *Am J Cardiol* 1998;**81**:604–8.
84. Yin WH, Chen JW, Jen HL, *et al.* The prognostic value of circulating soluble cell adhesion molecules in patients with chronic congestive heart failure. *Eur J Heart Fail* 2003;**5**:507–16.
85. Barnes PJ, Karin M. Nuclear factor-κB—a pivotal transcription factor in chronic inflammatory disease. *N Engl J Med* 1997;**336**:1066–71.
86. Satriano J, Schlondorff D. Activation and attenuation of transcription factor NF-κ B in the mouse glomerular mesangial cells in response to tumour necrosis factor-α, immunoglobulin G, and adenosine 3′:5′-cyclic monophosphate. Evidence for involvement of reactive oxygen species. *J Clin Invest* 1994;**94**:1629–36.
87. Frantz S, Hu K, Bayer B, *et al.* Absence of NF-kappaB subunit p50 improves heart failure after myocardial infarction. *FASEB J* 2006;**20**:1918–20.
88. Paulus WJ, Frantz S, Kelly R. Nitric oxide and cardiac contractility in human heart failure: time for reappraisal. *Circulation* 2001;**104**:2260–2.
89. Patten RD, DeNofrio D, El-Zaru M, *et al.* Ventricular assist device therapy normalizes inducible nitric oxide synthase expression and reduces cardiomyocyte apoptosis in the failing human heart. *J Am Coll Cardiol* 2005;**45**:1419–24.
90. Baumann H, Gauldie J. Regulation of hepatic acute phase plasma protein genes by hepatocyte stimulating factors and other mediators of inflammation. *Mol Biol Med* 1990;**7**:147–59.
91. Anand IS, Latini R, Florea VG, *et al.* C-reactive protein in heart failure: prognostic value and the effect of valsartan. *Circulation* 2005;**112**:1428–34.
92. Kardys I, Knetsch AM, Bleumink GS, *et al.* C-reactive protein and risk of heart failure. The Rotterdam Study. *Am Heart J* 2006;**152**:514–20.
93. Yin WH, Chen JW, Jen HL, *et al.* Independent prognostic value of elevated high-sensitivity C-reactive protein in chronic heart failure. *Am Heart J* 2004;**147**:931–938.
94. Berry C, Clark AL. Catabolism in chronic heart failure. *Eur Heart J* 2000;**21**:521–32.
95. Kennedy A, Gettys TW, Watson P, *et al.* The metabolic significance of leptin in humans: gender based differences in relation to adiposity, insulin sensitivity, and energy expenditure . *J Clin Endocrinol Metab* 1997;**82**:1293–300.
96. Leyva F, Anker SD, Egerer K, Stevenson JC, Knox WJ, Coats AJS. Hyperleptinaemia in chronic heart failure; relationships with insulin. *Eur Heart J* 1998;**19**:1547–51.
97. Yndestad A, Ueland T, Øie E, *et al.* Elevated levels of activin A in heart failure: potential role in myocardial remodeling. *Circulation* 2004;**109**:1379–85.
98. Yamaguchi S, Yamaoka M, Okuyama M, *et al.* Elevated circulating levels and cardiac secretion of soluble Fas ligand in patients with congestive heart failure. *Am J Cardiol* 1999;**83**:1500–3.
99. Aukrust P, Gullestad L, Ueland T, Damas JK, Yndestad A. Inflammatory and anti-inflammatory cytokines in chronic heart failure: Potential therapeutic implications. *Ann Med* 2005;**37**:74–85.
100. Gullestad L, Aukrust P, Ueland T, *et al.* Effect of high- versus low-dose angiotensin converting enzyme inhibition on cytokine levels in chronic heart failure. *J Am Coll Cardiol* 1999;**34**:2061–7.
101. Tsutamoto T, Wada A, Maeda K, *et al.* Angiotensin II Type I receptor antagonist decreases plasma levels of tumor necrosis factor-α, interleukin-6 and soluble adhesion molecules in patients with chronic heart failure. *J Am Col Cardiol* 2000;**35**:714–21.
102. Gullestad L, Ueland T, Brunsvig A, *et al.* Effect of metoprolol on cytokine levels in chronic heart failure-a substudy in the Metoprolol Controlled- Release Randomised Intervention Trial in Heart Failure (MERIT-HF). *Am Heart J* 2001;**141**:418–21.
103. von Haehling S, Anker SD. Statins for heart failure: at the crossroads between cholesterol reduction and pleiotropism?. *Heart* 2005;**91**:1–2.
104. Heymans S, Hirsch E, Anker SD, *et al.* Inflammation as a therapeutic target in heart failure? A scientific statement from the Translational Research Committee of the Heart Failure Association of the European Society of Cardiology. *Eur J Heart Fail* 2009;**11**:119–29.
105. Adamopoulos S, Parissis J. Immunomodulatory effects of physical training in chronic heart failure. *Hellenic J Cardiol* 2003;**44**:49–55.
106. Adamopoulos S, Parissis J, Karatzas D, *et al.* Physical training modulates proinflammatory cytokines and soluble Fas/soluble Fas ligand system in patients with chronic heart failure. *J Am Coll Cardiol* 2002;**39**:653–63.
107. Gielen S, Adams V, Möbius-Winkler S, Linke A, *et al.* Anti-inflammatory effects of exercise training in the skeletal muscle of patients with chronic heart failure. *J Am Coll Cardiol* 2003;**42**:861–8.
108. Linke A, Adams V, Schulze PC, *et al.* Antioxidative effects of exercise training in patients with chronic heart failure: increase in radical scavenger enzyme activity in skeletal muscle. *Circulation* 2005;**111**:1763–70.
109. Gielen S, Adams V, Linke A, *et al.* Exercise training in chronic heart failure: correlation between reduced local inflammation and improved oxidative capacity in the skeletal muscle. *Eur J Cardiovasc Prev Rehabil* 2005;**12**:393–400.
110. Mann DL, McMurray JJ, Packer M, *et al.* Targeted anticytokine therapy in patients with chronic heart failure: results of the Randomized Etanercept Worldwide Evaluation (RENEWAL). *Circulation* 2004;**109**:1594–602.
111. Chung ES, Packer M, Lo KH, Fasanmade AA, Willerson JT. Randomized, double-blind, placebo-controlled, pilot trial of infiximab, a chimeric monoclonal antibody to tumor necrosis factor-alpha, in patients with moderate-to-severe heart failure: results of the anti-TNF Therapy Against Congestive Heart failure (ATTACH) Trial. *Circulation* 2003;**107**:3133–40.
112. Bahrmann P, Hengst UM, Richartz BM, *et al.* Pentoxifylline in ischemic, hypertensive and idiopathic-dilated cardiomyopathy: effects on left-ventricular function, inflammatory cytokines and symptoms. *Eur J Heart Fail* 2004;**6**:195–201.
113. Gullestad L, Aass H, Fjeld JG, *et al.* Immunomodulating therapy with intravenous immunoglobulin in patients with chronic heart failure. *Circulation* 2001;**103**:220–5.
114. Torre-Amione G, Sestier F, Radovancevic B. Effects of a novel immune modulation therapy in patients with advanced chronic heart failure. results of a randomized, controlled, phase II trial. *J Am Coll Cardiol* 2004;**44**:1181–6.
115. Torre-Amione G, Sestier F, Radovancevic B, Young J. Broad modulation of tissue responses (immune activation) by Celacade may favorably influence pathologic processes associated with heart failure progression. *Am J Cardiol* 2005;**95**:30–40C.
116. Torre-Amione G, Anker SD, Bourge RC, *et al.* Results of a non-specific immunomodulation therapy in chronic heart failure (ACCLAIM trial): a placebo-controlled randomised trial. *Lancet* 2008;**371**:228–36.
117. Frustaci A, Russo MA, Chimenti C. Randomized study on the efficacy of immunosuppressive therapy in patients with virus-negative inflammatory cardiomyopathy: the TIMIC study. *Eur Heart J* 2009;**30**:1995–2002.

PART VI

The diagnosis of heart failure

17

Diagnosing heart failure

Henry J. Dargie and Theresa A. McDonagh

It is often said that heart failure (HF) is not a diagnosis *per se* but a clinical syndrome consisting of a constellation of symptoms and signs, which are ultimately due to cardiac dysfunction. Nevertheless it is important to diagnose the presence of HF accurately in order to facilitate the general and specific treatments that can modify its traditionally poor outlook.

The diagnosis of HF involves three distinct yet related phases. First there is the confirmation that the patient has HF, secondly the nature of the underlying cardiac dysfunction needs to be determined, and thirdly the actual aetiology of the cardiac dysfunction should be indentified.

Following confirmation of the diagnosis of HF some basic diagnostic tests must also be performed to determine the starting status of key parameters prior to initiation of therapy and to establish the presence of comorbidities.

Diagnosing possible heart failure

The first phase of an accurate diagnosis of HF is to suspect it. This is where the cardinal symptoms and signs of HF have their place in the diagnostic algorithm. Patients with chronic HF may complain of breathlessness, usually on effort, but with more severe disease they may describe orthopnea and paroxysmal nocturnal dyspnoea. The presence of fluid retention often prompts patients to complain of ankle swelling. Tiredness is also frequently a prominent symptom.

Many physical signs can be detected on examination. Traditionally more weight is given to diagnosing HF if the jugular venous pressure (JVP) is elevated or there are signs of peripheral oedema (Fig. 17.1). This usually presents first of all as ankle oedema but as the disease progresses sacral oedema, ascites, and pleural and pericardial effusions may develop

The pulse can be normal or there may be a tachycardia, most commonly atrial fibrillation (AF). The blood pressure may be low, normal, of high, depending on the stage of the disease and the underlying aetiology. Examination of the heart can also yield a number of abnormalities: a displaced apex beat, third and/or fourth heart sound, and potentially a number of murmurs—most notably the pansystolic murmurs of mitral and tricuspid regurgitation.

Unfortunately clinical symptoms and signs are not sufficiently accurate to diagnose HF. They are often insensitive, or where they are sensitive they lack specificity (see Table 17.1). Relying on clinical acumen alone leads to wrongly diagnosing HF in up to one-half of cases.[1,2] This is true in primary or secondary care. In the past clinical scoring systems such as the Framingham or Boston criteria were used to try to improve the accuracy of diagnosis.[3,4] However, these are not routinely used in clinical practice and are reserved for epidemiological studies, as other simpler and reproducible methods to infer the presence of HF have come into modern clinical practice.

Thus, symptoms and signs can be used to alert the clinician to the possible diagnosis of HF. The next stage is to improve the likelihood of cardiac dysfunction being detected. For this two tests should be done: the measurement of natriuretic peptides (NPs) and a 12-lead ECG.

Natriuretic peptides

Most work to date has been done with B-type natriuretic peptide (BNP/NT-proBNP; see Chapter 14). These circulating cardiac hormones are increased in terms of their circulating concentrations when patients have HF.[5–8] Numerous studies have shown that in both chronic and acute HF, elevated BNP concentrations have a high negative predictive accuracy (98–99%) for ruling out HF as a cause of the patient's symptoms. They are therefore very reliable, widely available diagnostic tests for HF and their use in encouraged in all international diagnostic cardiology guidelines.[9,10] Absolute cut-points for ruling out HF vary with the assay used; easily applicable ones are shown in Table 17.2.[11] In addition, they also provide important prognostic information as their concentrations rise in proportion to disease severity, with declining New York Heart Association (NHYA) class, and left ventricular ejection fraction (LVEF).[12,13] Values are high irrespective of the type of cardiac dysfunction underlying the diagnosis, i.e. in systolic dysfunction and in HF with normal ejection fraction (HeFNEF).[14] A raised BNP concentration does not equal a diagnosis of HF, as they are

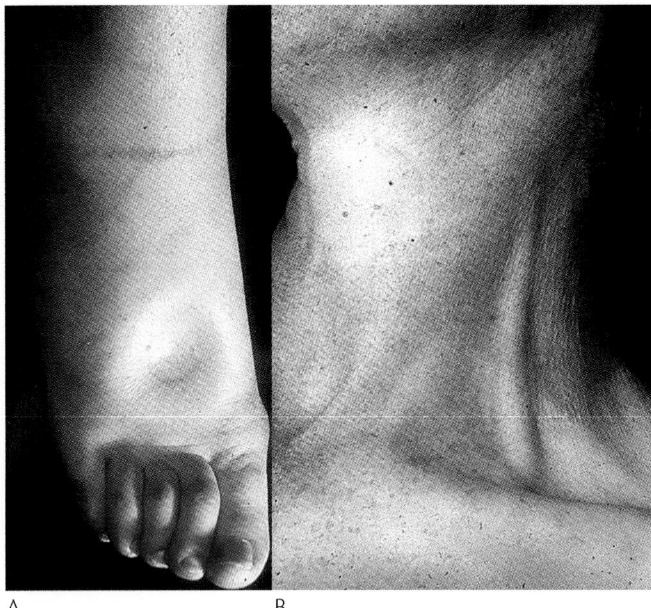

Fig. 17.1 Signs of congestion in heart failure: (A) peripheral oedema; (B) raised jugular venous pressure.

nonspecific markers of cardiac structural and functional disease as well as of renal impairment.[15] Their value is in flagging up that symptoms and signs may be due to cardiac dysfunction and should trigger referral for further cardiology assessment.

ECG

Patients suspected of HF should also have a 12-lead ECG. HF is very rarely present if the ECG is normal.[16,17] The negative predictive accuracy is not quite as high as with BNP but in most studies it is greater than 90%.[17] The ECG may also provide important information as to the underlying aetiology and give additional information that may help guide future therapy, e.g. the presence of a wide QRS complex.

If the BNP or the ECG is abnormal the patient should be referred for cardiology assessment to confirm or refute the presence of cardiac dysfunction (Fig. 17.2).[18]

Table 17.1 Sensitivity and specificity of clinical symptoms and signs in heart failure

Clinical features	Sensitivity (%)	Specificity (%)
Breathlessness	66	52
Orthopnoea	21	81
PND	33	76
History of oedema	23	80
Tachycardia	7	99
Pulmonary crackles	13	91
Oedema on examination	10	93
Third heart sound	31	95
Raised JVP	10	97

JVP, jugular venous pressure; PND, paroxysmal nocturnal dyspnoea.
From Sosin M, *A colour handbook of heart failure*, Mansion Publishing, London, 2006, with permission

Table 17.2 Suggested values of BNP and NT-proBNP for the diagnosis of heart failure

Setting	BNP	NT-proBNP
Acute	100 pg/mL	300 pg/mL
Chronic (primary care)	50 pg/mL	<60 years 50 pg/mL 60–75 years 100 pg/mL >75 years 250 pg/mL

BNP, B-type natriuretic peptide; GP, general practitioner; NT-proBNP, N-terminal pro-BNP.
Numbers have been rounded up for simplification.
Adapted from Cowie MR *et al. Br J Cardiol* 2010;**17**:76–80.

Before referral a chest radiograph should also be performed. This is less important diagnostically as about one-half of all patients with HF have a normal cardiothoracic ratio on the chest radiograph. However, it is useful for excluding other lung pathology, which may manifest as breathlessness.

Diagnosing heart failure: confirming cardiac dysfunction

The definition of HF mandates that cardiac dysfunction is present. There are many imaging modalities which can be used to determine this: echocardiography, radionuclide ventriculography, cardiac magnetic resonance (CMR), and invasive angiographic ventriculography (Fig. 17.3.

The most commonly used is echocardiography as it is noninvasive and widely available. This subject is covered in more detail in Chapter 19, however some important points are worthy of repetition here.

The first assessment which is made relates to the genre of cardiac dysfunction which underlies the HF, i.e. is there left ventricular systolic dysfunction (LVSD) or HeFNEF? LVSD is most accurately assessed echocardiographically by formally measuring the LVEF using the biplane Simpson's rule method.[19] Other parameters based on M-mode are less accurate, especially in the presence of coronary artery disease where there may be regional wall motion

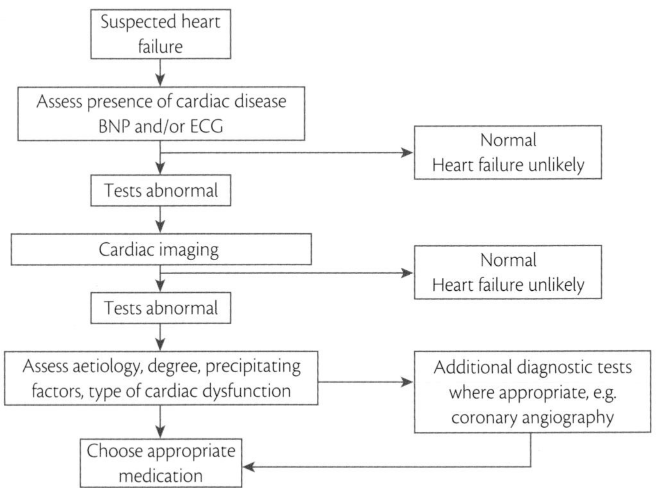

Fig. 17.2 Diagnostic algorithm for heart failure.
Adapted from the European Society of Cardiology guidelines: *Eur Heart J* 2005:**22**;1527.

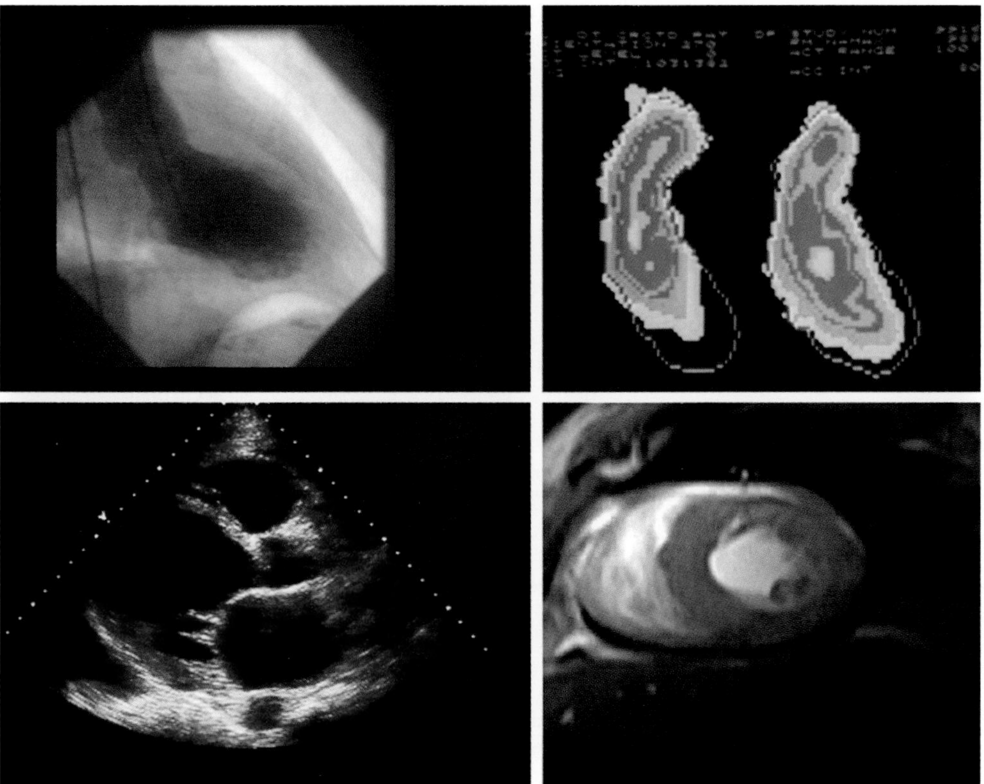

Fig. 17.3 Cardiac dysfunction—imaging modalities. Top left, angiographic ventriculography; top right, radionuclide ventriculography; bottom left, echocardiography; bottom right, cardiac magnetic resonance imaging.

abnormalities.[20] Methods such as wall motion score indices and 'eyeball' methods can be used to estimate ejection fraction when insufficient endocardium can be seen to formally calculate LVEF.[20] The confirmation of the presence of LVSD remains important: it is a measure of left ventricular function with both clinical and prognostic significance and was most often the criteria used for inclusion of patients into the landmark HF treatment trials, which have established role of renin–angiotensin–aldosterone system (RAAS) and sympathetic nervous system blockade.[21–23]

The diagnosis of HeFNEF by echocardiography is less clear-cut, with many abnormalities having been described in diagnostic algorithms.[24,25] However, criteria such as left ventricular hypertrophy and an increased left atrial volume are emerging as useful predictors of this syndrome (see Chapter 19).

Echocardiography can also provide useful information of the aetiology of the cardiac dysfunction regarding valve disease.

The other modalities tend to be used in more specific circumstances. Radionuclide ventriculography (RNVG) gives a more accurate and reproducible measure of LVEF than echocardiography (see Chapter 20). It is sometimes used when echocardiographic acoustic windows are suboptimal or when LVEF needs to be monitored, e.g. during anthracyline administration. It is important to stress that absolute values of LVEF vary with the technique used[25]—an LVEF of less 40% measured by RNVG is regarded as abnormal whereas the values for echocardiography (<50%) and CMR (<55%) are higher.

CMR is less widely available but provides a highly accurate assessment of cardiac structure and function, and it may become the standard of care in the future (see Chapter 21).

Angiographic assessment of left ventricular function tends only to be done when the patient is undergoing coronary angiography or during cardiac catheterization for another reason (see Chapter 24)

Diagnosing the aetiology of heart failure

Once the presence of cardiac dysfunction has been confirmed and its nature ascertained, the underlying cardiac pathology should be identified.

This usually involves further investigation, which in Western countries is often aimed at diagnosing the presence of significant coronary artery disease. However, as there are many potential aetiologies, tests may also focus on arrhythmias, valve disease, specific muscle diseased, genetics, metabolic, toxic, and infective causes, as described in other chapters of this book.

Baseline investigations

In addition baseline haematology is required, as anaemia can both cause and exacerbate HF and is potentially treatable. Assessing renal function and electrolytes is mandatory before starting therapy. Thyroid status should be measured—both hypo- and hyperthyroidism can cause HF and are commonly found in patients being treated with amiodarone. Liver function tests and serum sodium are also useful simple baseline prognostic markers. Ferritin should always be measured in the patient with diabetes and HF to exclude haemochromatosis. Creatinine kinase (CK) measurement can also alert clinicians to the presence of a muscular dystrophy and HF.

Summary

In conclusion, HF should be diagnosed by first having a high index of suspicion on clinical presentation. Secondly, the possibility of

Box 17.1 Future diagnostic criteria

- Symptoms and/or signs
  - Cardiac dysfunction
  - A raised biomarker, e.g. BNP

HF should be further refined by carrying out a NP measurement, and, if possible an ECG. If either of these is abnormal the patients needs to be referred for confirmation/exclusion of significant cardiac dysfunction as a cause of their symptoms. The nature of the cardiac dysfunction should be broadly categorized in to HF with systolic dysfunction or HeFNEF. The underlying aetiology of the heart disease should then be determined, if possible, and baseline assessments of renal function and parameters of common comorbidities should be determined.

This diagnostic process then sets the stage for the general pharmacotherapy of HF to begin, allows subgroups who will benefit from device therapy to be determined, defines the aetiology so that specific therapies aimed at targeting any potential reversal of the HF can be initiated, facilitates the treatment of comorbidity, and aids in risk stratification.

The diagnostic process is not yet perfect; HF remains difficult and complex to diagnose. In the future, the process will hopefully become more simple with the widespread use and utility of BNP. Ideally, we should strive for a more streamlined definition of HF which, like its relation myocardial infarction, will comprise not only appropriate symptoms and the presence of cardiac dysfunction but also a biomarker which has both diagnostic and prognostic accuracy, e.g. BNP (Box 17.1).

References

1. Clarke KW, Gray D, Hampton JR. Evidence of inadequate investigation and treatment of patients with heart failure. *Br Heart J* 1994;**71**(6):584–7.
2. Hillis GS, Al-Mohammad A, Wood M, Jennings KP. Changing patterns of investigation and treatment of cardiac failure in hospital. *Heart* 1996;**76**(5):427–9.
3. Eriksson H, Svardsudd K, Caidahl K, *et al.* Early heart failure in the population. The study of men born in 1913. *Acta Med Scand* 1988;**223**(3):197–209.
4. McKee PA, Castelli WP, McNamara PM, Kannel WB. The natural history of congestive heart failure: the Framingham study. *N Engl J Med* 1971;**285**(26):1441–6.
5. Davis M, Espiner E, Richards G, *et al.* Plasma brain natriuretic peptide in assessment of acute dyspnoea. *Lancet* 1994;**343**(8895):440–4.
6. Cowie MR, Struthers AD, Wood DA, *et al.* Value of natriuretic peptides in assessment of patients with possible new heart failure in primary care. *Lancet* 1997;**350**(9088):1349–53.
7. McDonagh TA, Robb SD, Murdoch DR, *et al.* Biochemical detection of left-ventricular systolic dysfunction. *Lancet* 1998;**351**(9095):9–13.
8. Maisel AS, Krishnaswamy P, Nowak RM, *et al.* Rapid measurement of B-type natriuretic peptide in the emergency diagnosis of heart failure. *N Engl J Med* 2002;**347**(3):161–7.
9. Dickstein K, Cohen-Solal A, Filippatos G, *et al.* ESC guidelines for the diagnosis and treatment of acute and chronic heart failure 2008: the Task Force for the diagnosis and treatment of acute and chronic heart failure 2008 of the European Society of Cardiology. Developed in collaboration with the Heart Failure Association of the ESC (HFA) and endorsed by the European Society of Intensive Care Medicine (ESICM). *Eur J Heart Fail* 2008 Oct;**10**(10):933–89.
10. Hunt SA, Abraham WT, Chin MH, *et al.* 2009 focused update incorporated into the ACC/AHA 2005 Guidelines for the Diagnosis and Management of Heart Failure in Adults: a report of the American College of Cardiology Foundation/American Heart Association Task Force on Practice Guidelines: developed in collaboration with the International Society for Heart and Lung Transplantation. *Circulation* 2009;**119**(14):e391–479.
11. Cowie M. Recommendations on the clinical ise of B-type natriuretic peptide testing (BNP or NTproBNP) in the UK and Ireland. *Br J Cardiol* 2010;**17**(2):76–80.
12. Gardner RS, Ozalp F, Murday AJ, Robb SD, McDonagh TA. N-terminal pro-brain natriuretic peptide. A new gold standard in predicting mortality in patients with advanced heart failure. *Eur Heart J* 2003;**24**(19):1735–43.
13. Anand IS, Fisher LD, Chiang YT, *et al.* Changes in brain natriuretic peptide and norepinephrine over time and mortality and morbidity in the Valsartan Heart Failure Trial (Val-HeFT). *Circulation* 2003;**107**(9):1278–83.
14. Parekh N, Maisel AS. Utility of B-natriuretic peptide in the evaluation of left ventricular diastolic function and diastolic heart failure. *Curr Opin Cardiol* 2009;**24**(2):155–60.
15. McDonagh TA, Holmer S, Raymond I, Luchner A, Hildebrant P, Dargie HJ. NT-proBNP and the diagnosis of heart failure: a pooled analysis of three European epidemiological studies. *Eur J Heart Fail* 2004;**6**(3):269–73.
16. Davie AP, Francis CM, Love MP, *et al.* Value of the electrocardiogram in identifying heart failure due to left ventricular systolic dysfunction. *BMJ* 1996;**312**(7025):222.
17. Zaphiriou A, Robb S, Murray-Thomas T, *et al.* The diagnostic accuracy of plasma BNP and NTproBNP in patients referred from primary care with suspected heart failure: results of the UK natriuretic peptide study. *Eur J Heart Fail* 2005;**7**(4):537–41.
18. Swedberg K, Cleland J, Dargie H, *et al.* Guidelines for the diagnosis and treatment of chronic heart failure: executive summary (update 2005): The Task Force for the Diagnosis and Treatment of Chronic Heart Failure of the European Society of Cardiology. *Eur Heart J* 2005;**26**(11):1115–40.
19. Schiller NB, Shah PM, Crawford M, *et al.* Recommendations for quantitation of the left ventricle by two-dimensional echocardiography. American Society of Echocardiography Committee on Standards, Subcommittee on Quantitation of Two-Dimensional Echocardiograms. *J Am Soc Echocardiogr* 1989;**2**(5):358–67.
20. McGowan JH, Martin W, Burgess MI, *et al.* Validation of an echocardiographic wall motion index in heart failure due to ischaemic heart disease. *Eur J Heart Fail* 2001;**3**(6):731–7.
21. Effect of enalapril on survival in patients with reduced left ventricular ejection fractions and congestive heart failure. The SOLVD Investigators. *N Engl J Med* 1991;**325**(5):293–302.
22. The Cardiac Insufficiency Bisoprolol Study II (CIBIS-II): a randomised trial. The CIBIS II Investigators. *Lancet* 1999;**353**(9146):9–13.
23. Pitt B, Zannad F, Remme WJ, *et al.* The effect of spironolactone on morbidity and mortality in patients with severe heart failure. Randomized Aldactone Evaluation Study Investigators. *N Engl J Med* 1999;**341**(10):709–17.
24. Paulus WJ, Tschope C, Sanderson JE, *et al.* How to diagnose diastolic heart failure: a consensus statement on the diagnosis of heart failure with normal left ventricular ejection fraction by the Heart Failure and Echocardiography Associations of the European Society of Cardiology. *Eur Heart J* 2007;**28**(20):2539–50.
25. Ray SG, Metcalfe MJ, Oldroyd KG, *et al.* Do radionuclide and echocardiographic techniques give a universal cut off value for left ventricular ejection fraction that can be used to select patients for treatment with ACE inhibitors after myocardial infarction?. *Br Heart J* 1995;**73**(5):466–9.

PART VII

Noninvasive investigation

18

Basic investigation of heart failure

Roy S. Gardner

Although the clinical history and examination may suggest a diagnosis of heart failure (HF), objective evidence of cardiac dysfunction is also required. A number of diagnostic tests can be reliably employed to identify patients with left ventricular systolic dysfunction (LVSD). However, HF with preserved systolic function is less reliably pinpointed, particularly as the syndrome is a mixed bag of conditions rather than a specific entity.

As well as investigating patients to identify the presence and severity of cardiac dysfunction and any relevant comorbidities, it is important to clarify the underlying aetiology. Some causes are potentially correctable with possible improvement in the degree of cardiac dysfunction. Appropriate investigations will also help to risk-stratify patients, identifying those suitable for advanced therapies such as device therapy (ICD, CRT, VAD) and cardiac transplantation.

Although echocardiography is currently the principal diagnostic test for patients with HF, cardiac magnetic resonance imaging (CMR) is now considered to be the 'gold standard' method of assessing cardiac function. The investigations that should be done, or at least considered, in the patient suspected of having HF are shown in Table 18.1. This chapter concentrates on the first-line investigations.

ECG

The ECG is a simple, inexpensive, reproducible, and readily available investigation that should be performed in every patient suspected of having HF. ECG changes are very common in patients with HF, and a normal ECG is associated with a high negative predictive value for HF (>90%): a patient with a completely normal ECG is most unlikely to have HF. The ECG can suggest the underlying aetiology (e.g. prior myocardial infarction—Fig. 18.1) and also help identify which patients might respond to particular therapies, such as cardiac resynchronization therapy (CRT—Fig. 18.2). There are a number of other ECG features or abnormalities that may be relevant in a patient with HF and these are shown in Table 18.2 and Table 18.3.

Bundle branch block

Left bundle branch block (LBBB; Fig. 18.2) is common in patients with HF. In the Italian Network chronic HF registry,[1] LBBB—diagnosed with a QRS duration greater than 140 ms rather than the widely accepted duration of over 120 ms—was found in 25.2% of individuals with chronic heart failure (CHF). LBBB was more prevalent in females and in patients with dilated cardiomyopathy, and found to be an independent predictor of all-cause death, as well as sudden death, in patients with CHF. LBBB was also shown to be an independent predictor of mortality in the CIBIS-2 study.[2] Further studies have since shown that accelerated QRS-interval widening is independently associated with deterioration of cardiac function,[3] and death or need for urgent cardiac transplantation.[4]

Right bundle branch block (RBBB) is also seen in patients with HF, and a broadened QRS (>120 ms)—whether secondary to LBBB or RBBB—can help to identify patients who may be suitable for cardiac resynchronization therapy (see Chapter 48).[5]

Laboratory tests

A number of laboratory tests should be considered mandatory in the assessment of the patient with suspected HF (see Table 18.1), and in the monitoring of patients commenced on HF therapy. Other tests can be performed depending on the clinical context. The most relevant laboratory tests are expanded on below.

Urea & electrolytes (U&Es)

The measurement of serum electrolytes and creatinine, and the estimation of glomerular filtration rate (eGFR) are important, both as a baseline and in the subsequent follow up of the patient with HF.

Serum sodium

Hyponatraemia (Na^+ <135 mmol/L) is frequently seen in patients with HF and its presence is a powerful adverse prognostic sign. It is commonly caused by haemodilution, diuretic therapy

Table 18.1 Basic investigations in conditions that may lead to heart failure

Aetiology	ECG	Bloods	Other investigation
Amyloid	P mitrale/pulmonale Low precordial QRS amplitude Abnormal axis Atrial arrhythmia (particularly AF)	Serum and urine electrophoresis ESR	CMR Cardiac catheterization Endomyocardial biopsy
Cardiac sarcoidosis	RBBB Conduction abnormalities Supraventricular and ventricular tachycardias	Serum ACE	Chest radiograph (bilateral hilar lymphadenopathy) Endomyocardial biopsy CMR
Haemochromatosis	Abnormalities are common	Ferritin Transferrin saturation	Genetic analysis (C282Y homozygosity) CMR (T2*) Endomyocardial biopsy
Dystrophinopathies (DMD and BMD)	Tall Rt precordial R waves ↑R/S ratio Deep Q waves in lateral leads	Markedly elevated CK (10–20×) Dystrophin (↓in DMD; abnormal molecular weight in BMD)	Genetic analysis
Myotonic dystrophy	Pathological Q waves (in the absence of CAD)	Mildly elevated CK	Genetic analysis Muscle biopsy EMG
Fabry's disease	Conduction abnormalities	↓α-Galactosidase A activity in males (may be normal in carriers)	Molecular studies
Pompe's disease		Elevated CK Acid α-glucosidase	Muscle biopsy Genetic analysis
Chagas' disease	Conduction abnormalities	Machado–Guerreiro complement fixation test	ELISA
Lyme disease	Conduction abnormalities Nonspecific ST/T wave abnormalities	Lyme serology (ELISA and western blot analysis)	
Löffler endocarditis	Atrial fibrillation Nonspecific T-wave abnormalities	Eosinophilia	
Myocarditis	Non-specifically abnormal ST/T abnormalities arrhythmias	Raised WCC and CRP	Cardiac MRI Endomyocardial biopsy Gallium scan

AF, atrial fibrillation; BMD, Becker muscular dystrophy; CAD, coronary artery disease; CK, creatine kinase; CMR, cardiac MRI; CRP, C-reactive protein; DMD, Duchenne muscular dystrophy; EMG, electromyography; ESR, erythrocyte sedimentation rate; RBBB, right bundle branch block; WCC, white cell count.

(particularly where a loop diuretic is used in combination with a thiazide), and release of arginine vasopressin (AVP). It can often be improved by fluid restriction or avoidance of diuretic combinations where possible. AVP receptor antagonists (e.g. tolvaptan) are being investigated as aquaretics,[6] and may be most valuable for the treatment of hyponatraemic HF patients. Hypernatraemia (Na^+ >150 mmol/L) is occasionally seen in patients who have become dehydrated from overdiuresis.

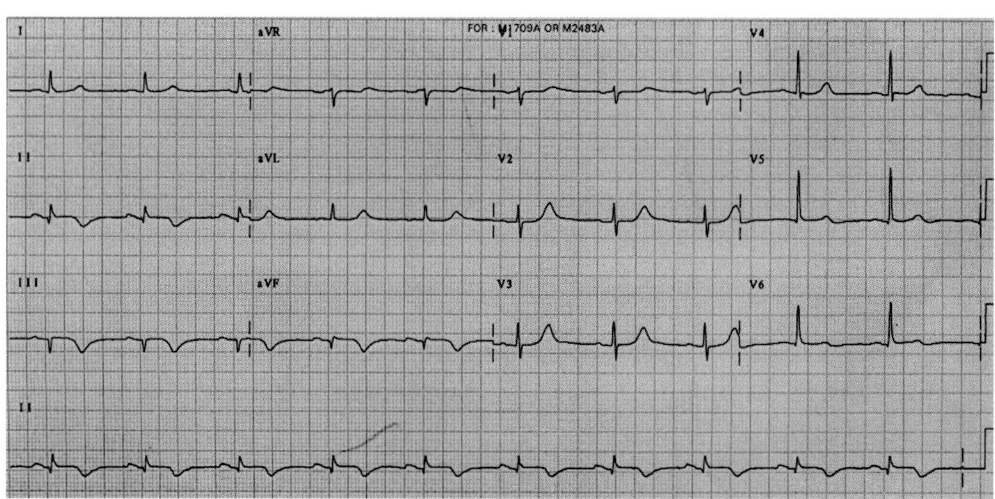

Fig. 18.1 ECG evidence of an old inferior myocardial infarction, with Q-waves and T-wave inversion in leads II, III, and aVf.

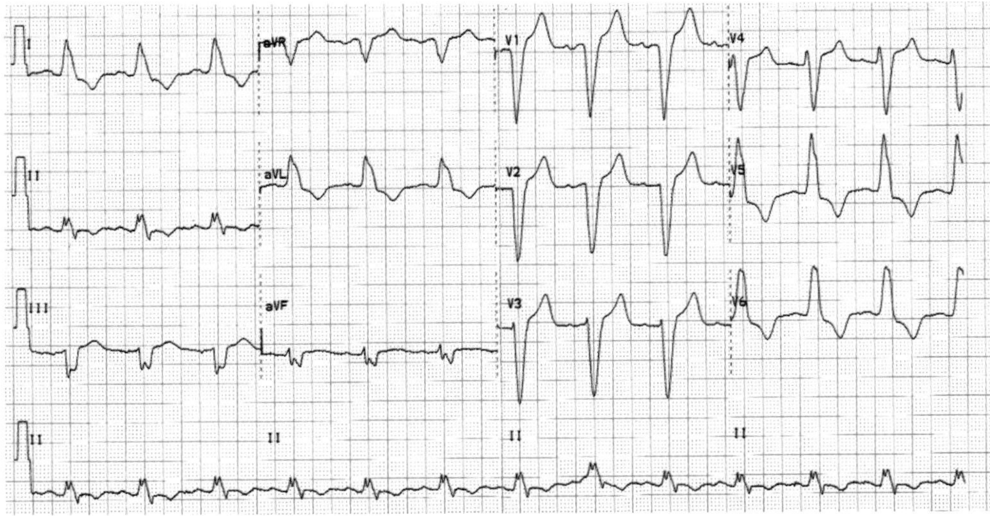

Fig. 18.2 ECG demonstrating left bundle branch block.

Table 18.2 ECG features and potential causes

ECG feature	Potential cause	Investigations/therapy to be considered
Sinus tachycardia	Decompensated HF Thyrotoxicosis Sepsis Anaemia	Echo FBC TFT Infection screen
Sinus bradycardia	Drug related (β-blocker, digoxin, amiodarone, etc.) Hypothyroidism Sick sinus syndrome	If necessary remove or modify cause TFT
P mitrale	Causes of left atrial dilation: Mitral valve disease LVH Restrictive cardiomyopathy	Echo
P pulmonale	Causes of right atrial dilatation: Chronic lung disease Tricuspid regurgitation	Echo PFT CXR
Atrial fibrillation/ flutter/ tachycardia	Decompensated HF Ischaemia/infarction Mitral valve disease Hyperthyroidism HCM Restrictive cardiomyopathy Sepsis Drugs (digoxin toxicity may precipitate tachycardia)	Echo TFT Digoxin level Infection screen Consider rate vs rhythm control; radiofrequency ablation
Ventricular arrhythmias	Decompensated HF Acute ischaemia/infarction Previous myocardial infarction (i.e. scar-related)	U&E Mg Tn Coronary angiography ICD
AV block	Drug toxicity (Beta-blocker, digoxin, amiodarone, etc) Ischaemia/infarction Sarcoidosis Myocarditis Lyme carditis Dystrophinopathies	Remove/treat cause CMR Lyme serology Pacemaker

Table 18.2 (cont'd.)

ECG feature	Potential cause	Investigations/therapy to be considered
Ischaemia/ infarction	Coronary heart disease	Tn Echo Coronary angiography CMR
LBBB	Myocardial infarction Dilated cardiomyopathy Hypertension	Echo Tn Coronary angiography Consider CRT
RBBB	Acute or chronic lung disease Myocardial infarction	CXR PFTs Echo CMR Consider CRT
LVH	Hypertension Aortic stenosis Hypertrophic cardiomyopathy Coarctation	Echo CMR
Small voltage complexes	Obesity Obstructive lung disease Cardiac amyloid Pericardial effusion	CXR PFT Echo CMR

CMR, cardiac MRI; CRT, cardiac resynchronization therapy; CXR, chest radiograph; FBC, full blood count; LVH, left ventricular hypertrophy; ICD, implantable cardioverted-defibrillator; LBBB, left bundle branch block; PFT, pulmonary function tests; RBBB, right bundle branch block; TFT, thyroid functions tests; Tn, troponin

Serum potassium

Hypokalaemia (K^+ <3.5 mmol/L) is commonly seen in patients on loop or thiazide diuretics, or those with secondary hyperaldosteronism. The hypokalaemic state increases the likelihood of arrhythmias, as well as the risk of side effects from digoxin therapy. Serum potassium levels can be increased with the use of potassium supplements, potassium-sparing diuretics, aldosterone antagonists, angiotension converting enzyme (ACE) inhibitors or angiotensin receptor blockers (ARBs). Conversely, hyperkalaemia (K^+>5.5 mol/L) is often caused by such therapy, and may require

Table 18.3 Common ECG features of heart failure conditions

Condition	ECG features
Ischaemia	ST depression
Acute MI	Regional ST elevation (STEMI) or ST depression (NSTEMI/posterior MI) or new LBBB
Established MI	Regional q waves and/or T-wave inversion
Dilated cardiomyopathy	Non-specific ST/T wave abnormalities
Restrictive cardiomyopathy	P mitrale/pulmonale; low precordial QRS amplitude; atrial arrhythmias
Hypertrophic cardiomyopathy	Usually abnormal (85%), with ST/T wave abnormalities and LVH particularly in the mid-precordial leads. Prominent inferior or precordial Q waves are also frequently seen (in up to 50%)
LV non-compaction	Usually abnormal with abnormalities that include LBBB or RBBB, fascicular block, atrial fibrillation, and ventricular tachycardia
Myocarditis	Nonspecifically abnormal: ST/T abnormalities, arrhythmias; may mimic STEMI (particularly with pericardial involvement)
Arrhythmogenic RV cardiomyopathy	Epsilon waves or localized prolongation (>110 ms) of the QRS complex in right precordial leads (V1–V3) VT (usually of RV origin—LBBB morphology)
Dystrophinopathies	Tall right precordial R waves with an increased R/S ratio; deep q waves in lateral leads; conduction disturbances
Cardiac sarcoid	Ventricular and supraventricular tachycardia; conduction disease
Cardiac amyloid	AF; small voltage QRS complexes
Lyme carditis	conduction disease

AF, atrial fibrillation; LBBB, left bundle branch block; LV, left ventricular; MI, myocardial infarction; RV, right ventricular.

either a reduction in dose or discontinuation of the offending drug. Hyperkalaemia increases the likelihood of bradycardia, and on occasions may require correction with dialysis or ultrafiltration.

Serum creatinine and eGFR

CHF, is not only a cardiac disorder, but rather a cardiorenal and neurohumoral syndrome, and a raised creatinine level is often a marker of coexisting renal dysfunction. Renal impairment is often associated with CHF as a result of renal hypoperfusion, diuretic treatment, disease-modifying HF therapy (ACE inhibitors, angiotensin II antagonists, aldosterone antagonists), as well as other concomitant medication and comorbidities such as diabetes. Serum creatinine concentration, which is often quoted as a barometer of renal impairment, is actually a poor indicator of renal function.[7] Therefore, estimation of the glomerular filtration rate (eGFR—Fig. 18.3) is preferred for the accurate assessment of renal function,[7] and the Modification of Diet in Renal Disease (MDRD) equations[8] have recently been validated in patients with severe chronic HF (Fig. 18.3).[9] A GFR below 60 mL/min/1.73 m^2 is associated with complications of renal disease.[7] Moreover, a GFR estimated by creatinine clearance (CrCl) is independently predictive of all-cause mortality in patients with asymptomatic[10] and symptomatic[10–13] LVSD.

(1) MDRD-1 equation:

$$\text{GFR} = 170 \times [\text{plasma creatinine}]^{-0.999} \times [\text{age}]^{-0.176} \times [0.762 \text{ if patient is female}] \times [1.180 \text{ if patient is black}] \times [\text{SUN}]^{-0.170} \times [\text{albumin}]^{+0.318}$$

(2) MDRD-2 (abbreviated) equation:

$$\text{GFR} = 186 \times [\text{Pcr}]^{-1.154}\ [\text{age}]^{-0.203} \times [0.742 \text{ if patient is female}] \times [1.212 \text{ if patient is black}]$$

(3) Cockcroft–Gault formula normalized to a body surface area of 1.73m^2, (creatinine clearance, expressed in mL/minute/1.73m^2):

$$\text{GFR (males)} = \frac{1.23 \times \text{weight (kg)} \times [140 - \text{age}]}{\text{plasma creatinine } (\mu\text{mol/L}) \times 1.73/\text{BSA}}$$

$$\text{GFR (females)} = \frac{1.03 \times \text{weight (kg)} \times [140 - \text{age}]}{\text{plasma creatinine } (\mu\text{mol/L}) \times 1.73/\text{BSA}},$$

$$\text{where BSA(m}^2) = \sqrt{[\text{weight (kg)} \times \text{height (cm)}/3600]}$$

Fig. 18.3 Equations used in the estimation of glomerular filtration rate (eGFR; expressed in mL/min/1.73 m^2).

Full blood count (FBC)

Haemoglobin

Anaemia (Hb <13 g/dL in men, <12 g/dL in women) is common in patients with chronic HF,[14] and the proportion of patients with anaemia increases with worsening NYHA functional class.[15] Anaemia is also associated with increased symptoms, more frequent hospitalizations and, in some studies, with an increased mortality rate.[15–17] The cause of anaemia in chronic HF is likely to be multifactorial. It has often been put down to an 'anaemia of chronic disease', but other potential causes include haemodilution and erythropoietin suppression due to coexisting renal dysfunction,[17] proinflammatory effects of cytokines activated in patients with chronic HF, and a response to ACE inhibitors.[18]

Liver function tests

Transaminases

Raised transaminases are frequently seen in HF patients with hepatic congestion. This can be associated with a rise in bilirubin and deranged clotting—a prolonged prothrombin time ('autoanticoagulation'). Deranged transaminases may also be a sign of drug toxicity (particularly from spironolactone or amiodarone).

Albumin

A low albumin (<30 g/L) is seen in patients with poor nutrition, those with a chronic illness, and those with renal loss. However, a raised albumin (>45 g/L) can be seen in dehydrated/overdiuresed patients or those with myeloma.

Thyroid function tests

Thyroid hormones have important effects on heart rate, cardiac contractility, the peripheral circulation, and the sympathetic nervous system. Concentrations of these hormones are frequently abnormal in patients with HF, particularly in those treated with amiodarone. Triiodothyronine (T_3) is low in patients with advanced HF, possibly due to a reduced conversion from thyroxine (T_4).

Both hypo- and hyperthyroidism can lead to the development of cardiac dysfunction. Hyperthyroidism initially induces a high

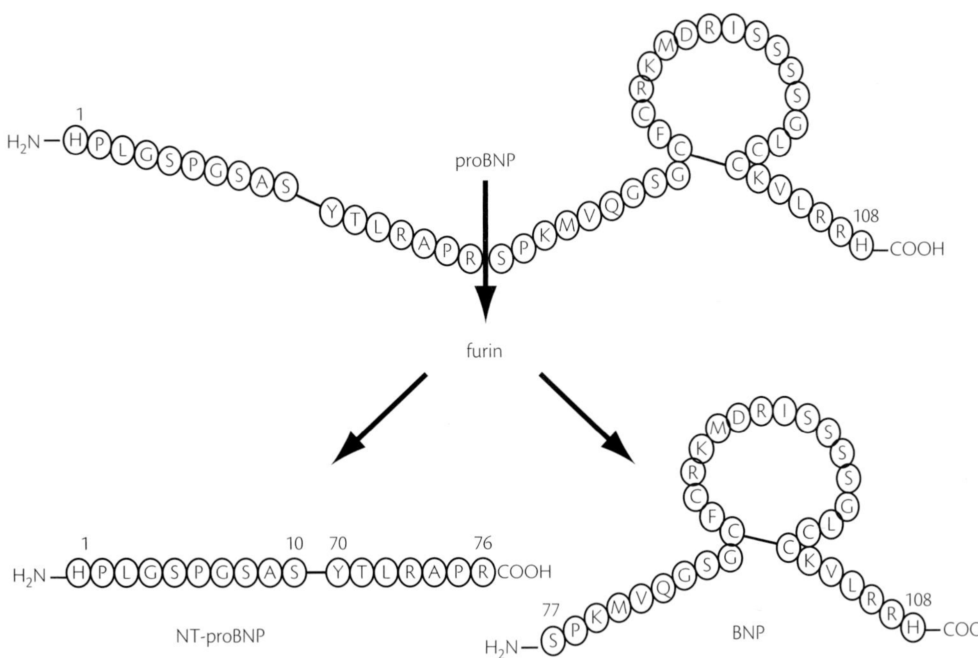

Fig. 18.4 The cleavage of proBNP by furin into B-type natriuretic peptide (BNP) and the inactive fragment, NT-proBNP

output state by an increase in heart rate and cardiac contractility, and the reduction in systemic vascular resistance. However, the incessant tachycardia and increased myocardial oxygen demand eventually may lead to left ventricular dilatation and a reduction in systolic function, resulting in a low output state. The situation may be further exacerbated by the increased risk of atrial fibrillation. Thyrotoxicosis-induced HF may be reversed by treatment (e.g. by propylthiouracil). In one study, 85% had resolution of left ventricular dysfunction on achieving euthyroidism.[19]

Hypothyroidism causes a low output state, mediated by reductions in heart rate and contractility. Cardiac function may worsen with coexisting HF and thyroxine replacement should be administered cautiously.

Natriuretic peptides

The B-type natriuretic peptides BNP and NT-proBNP (the inactive fragment of proBNP—Fig. 18.4), are well known to be increased in patients with both asymptomatic and symptomatic LVSD[20,21] increasing in proportion to the severity of chronic HF.[22] BNP is stable in whole blood for 3 days, can be measured by a rapid assay,[23] and increases only minimally following exercise.[24]

BNP can accurately detect LVSD in the general population,[25] but there is considerable debate about the potential role of BNP as a screening test for asymptomatic LVSD. The main role of BNP is currently as a 'rule-out' test to exclude HF due to its high negative predictive value (NPV) (up to 99%). One study has shown that BNP testing reduced the number of echocardiograms needed, and subsequent cost, in screening subjects for LVSD.[26]

Using a rapid point-of-care test for BNP, Dao *et al* first demonstrated that BNP was both a sensitive and specific test to diagnose HF in patients presenting to the Emergency Department with dyspnoea.[27] Indeed, the NPV was 98% for BNP less than 80 pg/mL, and the availability of BNP measurements could have potentially corrected 96.7% of the diagnoses missed by the Emergency Department physician. These findings were confirmed in a larger prospective study of 1586 patients.[28] Again, BNP was found to have a high NPV (96% at BNP <50 pg/mL) and in multiple logistic-regression analysis, BNP added significant predictive power to other clinical variables in identifying which patients had acute HF.

The European Society of Cardiology has recommended a diagnostic algorithm in for HF using natriuretic peptides in untreated

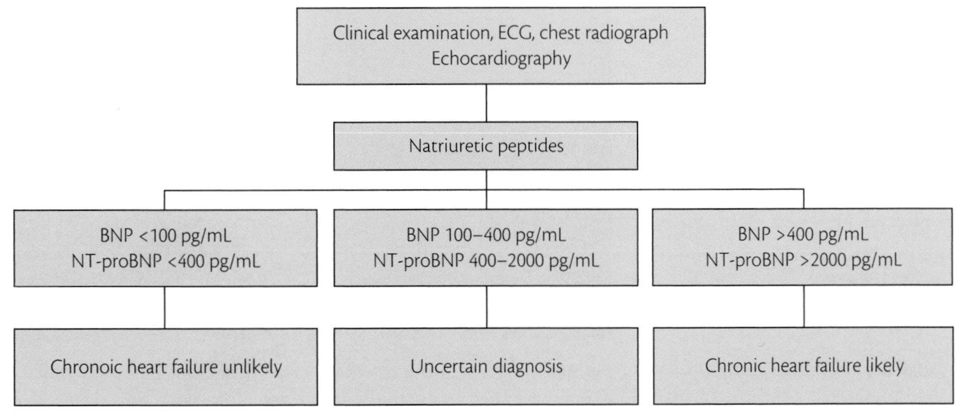

Fig. 18.5 Flowchart for the diagnosis of heart failure with natriuretic peptides in untreated patients with symptoms suggestive of heart failure. ESC Heart failure guidelines *Eur J Heart Fail.*

patients with symptoms of HF (Fig. 18.5). Although BNP/NT-proBNP concentrations increase with age, and are normally higher in men than in women, increased values indicate either a cardiac functional/structural abnormality or renal dysfunction, and require further investigation. They are discussed further in Chapter 14.

Other laboratory tests

Glucose

Diabetes mellitus is commonly associated with the presence of coronary heart disease, and thus HF (see chapter 32). Its presence is a strong independent predictor of mortality in patients with CHF.[29,30] The increased risk was later shown to be in patients with an ischaemic cardiomyopathy, rather than those with a dilated cardiomyopathy.[31]

Iron studies (ferritin ± C282Y genotyping)

Hereditary haemochromatosis (HH) is an autosomal recessive disorder in which a mutation of the *HFE* gene (most commonly a C282Y mutation) causes increased intestinal iron absorption. This, and other forms of iron overload, can lead to conduction system disease or dilated cardiomyopathy. The HH homozygous state has a prevalence of 0.45% in the United States,[17] with cardiac involvement being the presenting manifestation in 15% of individuals. Appropriate investigations include transferrin saturation, serum ferritin and, where appropriate, C282Y *HFE* mutation analysis.

Troponin

An elevated troponin I or T indicates myocyte necrosis and is seen both in acute coronary syndromes (ACS) and in acute myocarditis. Minor increases in cardiac troponin are frequently seen in advanced HF or during episodes of decompensation. Persistently elevated TnT concentrations have been shown to be associated with increasing left ventricular diastolic dimensions, decreasing left ventricular ejection fraction (LVEF), and increased risk of death.[32] An elevated troponin is an especially powerful adverse prognostic marker in HF patients who also have elevated natriuretic peptides.[33]

Caeruloplasmin

Wilson's disease is an autosomal recessive defect in cellular copper transport which usually leads to hepatic cirrhosis, but rarely can also lead to cardiomyopathy. As the incorporation of copper into caeruloplasmin is also impaired, there is a reduction in serum caeruloplasmin concentrations present in most patients with Wilson's disease.

Urate

Serum uric acid is often raised in patients on diuretics, and may be a precursor for the development of gout. Raised uric acid concentrations have been shown to be strongly related to circulating markers of inflammation in patients with HF,[34] and are independently predictive of an adverse prognosis.[35,36]

Genetic screen

Genetic testing and counselling are important in cases of suspected familial cardiomyopathy, usually where there is a family history. Serum creatine kinase (CK) should also be checked as it can be raised in myotonic dystrophy or the dystrophinopathies. Genetic causes of HF are further considered in Chapter 5.

Further tests

Other tests that may be considered include urinalysis, a myeloma screen, autoantibodies (including ANA) where systemic lupus erythematosus (SLE) is suspected, and urinary catecholamines for the investigation of phaeochromocytoma.

Table 18.4 Cardiothoracic ratio in large heart failure trials

Trial	Mean CTR (SD) or *(SEM)	Mean LVEF (%)
CIBIS(37)	0.55±0.07	25.4
DIG(38)	0.52±0.07	28.1
PRAISE	0.57±0.01*	21
PROVED	0.50±0.01*	–
RADIANCE	0.53±0.01	27
SOLVD-P	0.50±0.06	28
SOLVD-T	0.53±0.07	25
VHeFT	0.53±0.006	30
VHeFT II	0.53±0.006	29

CTR, cardiothoracic ratio; LVEF, left ventricular ejection fraction; SD, standard deviation; SEM; standard error of the mean.
Adapted from Petrie MC, *Eur J Heart Fail* 2003;**5**:117–19.

Chest radiograph

The chest radiograph is an important investigation in the diagnostic work-up of the breathless patient. However, a normal chest radiograph does not exclude a diagnosis of HF, as the cardiothoracic ratio (CTR) is normal (<0.5) in around 50% of cases. Indeed, there is a wealth of evidence from large HF trials showing that even patients with severe LVSD can have a normal heart size on chest radiograph (Table 18.4). Conversely, the chest radiograph may be suggestive of a cardiac abnormality when cardiomegaly (CTR >0.50) is present (Fig. 18.6) or if there evidence of pulmonary venous congestion, bilateral pleural effusions, or interstitial oedema.

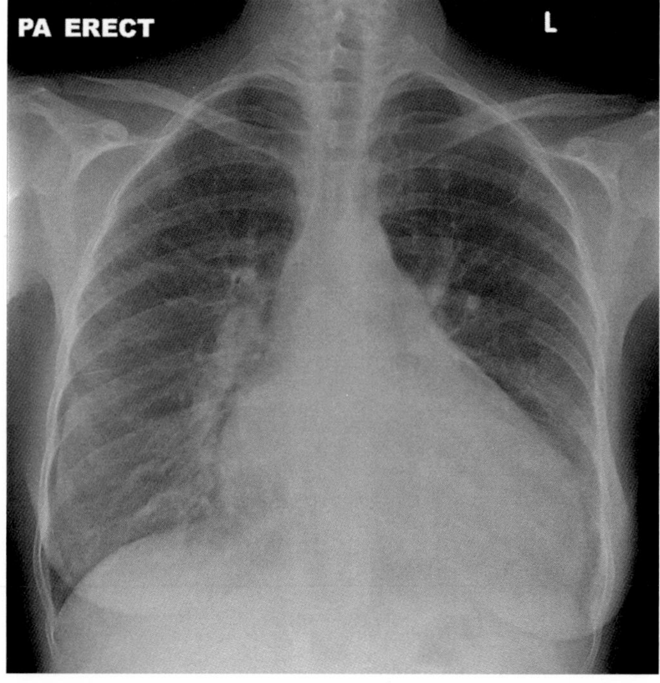

Fig. 18.6 PA chest radiograph of a 17-year old girl with gross cardiomegaly. There is also evidence of fluid in the horizontal fissure and upper lobe venous diversion.

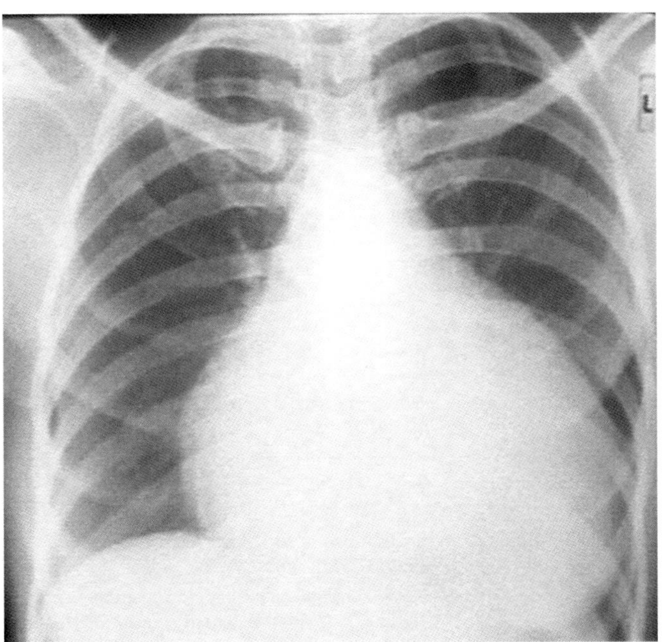

Fig. 18.7 PA chest radiograph of a patient with a pericardial effusion.

The chest radiograph can also help identify or exclude other causes of breathlessness, such as pericardial effusion (Fig. 18.7), bronchial carcinoma (Fig. 18.8), or emphysema.

Although an increased CTR may be supportive of a cardiac abnormality, it need not reflect a reduced LVEF. Indeed, in the registry population of the Coronary Artery Surgery Study,[39] two-thirds of patients with a CTR >0.50 had a normal LVEF. In the absence of LVSD, other causes of radiographic cardiomegaly include pericardial fat, left ventricular hypertrophy, pericardial effusion (Fig. 18.7), valvular dysfunction, and right heart dysfunction/dilatation.

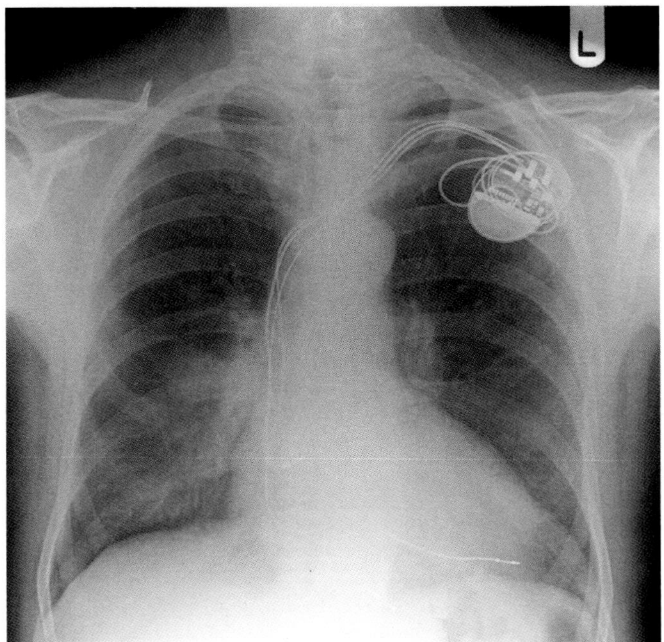

Fig. 18.8 Chest radiograph showing two causes for breathlessness: (1) a right hilar mass was identified post-CRT-P implantation for congestive heart failure, and (2) a subsequent biopsy revealed non-small-cell lung carcinoma.

Thus, a normal heart size does not exclude significant, or even severe, LVSD in a patient with suspected HF, and cardiomegaly is not necessarily specific for LVSD. This is in contrast to the normal 12-lead ECG which virtually rules out LVSD, and when abnormal can point to an underlying aetiology. Although the CTR adds little additional diagnostic information to that obtained from the 12-lead ECG, other findings on the chest radiograph, such as pulmonary congestion or oedema, may be supportive of a diagnosis of cardiac dysfunction.

However, the CTR is of considerable prognostic value in the patient with chronic HF and a low LVEF. A higher CTR is predictive of the risk of worsening symptoms, hospitalization and mortality. In addition, UK-HEART (United Kingdom HF evaluation and assessment of risk trial)—a multicenter prospective study designed to identify noninvasive markers of death and mode of death in patients with chronic HF—showed that a greater CTR was also predictive of sudden death (HR 1.43 (95% CI 1.20–1.71), $p < 0.04$ for a 10% increase in CTR).[40]

A higher CTR may also help predict response to therapy. In the DIG trial, the benefit of digoxin appeared to be greater among patients at high risk.[41] Those who were more symptomatic, had a lower ejection fraction, or greater CTR (>0.55) had a lower risk of experiencing death from, or hospitalization for, worsening chronic HF when randomized to digoxin compared to placebo.

Other investigations

Echocardiography is a key investigation in the assessment of the patient suspected of having HF. It allows a very accessible and non-invasive assessment of myocardial and valvular function. However, CMR is an emerging tool that allows an accurate and reproducible measurement of cardiac volumes and left ventricular mass, as well as characterizing cardiac tissue and identifying areas of infarction or infiltration. Invasive investigations include right and left heart catheterization and endomyocardial biopsy. These investigations are considered in more detail in subsequent chapters.

Summary

Each investigation highlighted above is a piece of a diagnostic jigsaw and no single test can confirm the clinical syndrome of HF without the presence of symptoms. However, a normal BNP/NT-proBNP and ECG argue strongly against the presence of HF. Conversely, a raised BNP/NT-proBNP can have causes other than HF, and cardiomegaly on the chest radiograph is not a prerequisite for the diagnosis either, as a significant proportion of patients with LVSD have a normal CTR. Thus, the accurate assessment of the patient suspected of having HF requires a detailed history and examination, as well as objective evidence of cardiac dysfunction from careful investigation using echocardiography or CMR.

References

1. Baldasseroni S, Opasich C, Gorini M, *et al.* Left bundle branch block is associated with increased 1-year sudden and total mortality rate in 5517 outpatients with congestive heart failure: A report from the Italian Network on Congestive Heart Failure. *Am Heart J* 2002;**143**:398–405.
2. Funck-Brentano C, Lancar R, Hansen S, *et al.* Predictors of medical events and of their competitive interactions in the Cardiac Insufficiency Bisoprolol Study 2 (CIBIS-2). *Am Heart J* 2001;**142**:989–97.

3. Shamim W, Yousufuddin M, Cicoria M, Gibson DG, Coats AJ, Henein MY. Incremental changes in QRS duration in serial ECGs over time identify high risk elderly patients with heart failure. *Heart* 2002;**88**:47–52.
4. Grigioni F, Carinci V, Boriani G, *et al.* Accelerated QRS widening as an independent predictor of cardiac death or the need for heart transplantation in patients with congestive heart failure. *J Heart Lung Transplant* 2002;**21**:899–901.
5. Cleland JG, Daubert JC, Erdmann E, *et al.* The effect of cardiac resynchronization on morbidity and mortality in heart failure. *N Engl J Med* 2005;**352**(15):1539–49.
6. Konstam MA, Gheorghiade M, Burnett JC Jr, *et al.* Effects of oral tolvaptan in patients hospitalized for worsening heart failure: the EVEREST Outcome Trial. JAMA 2007;**297**(12):1319–31.
7. Levey AS, Coresh J, Balk E. National Kidney Foundation practice guidelines for chronic kidney disease: evaluation, classification, and stratification. *Ann Intern Med* 2003;**139**:137–47.
8. Levey AS, Bosch JP, Lewis JB, Greene T, Rogers N, Roth D. A more accurate method to estimate glomerular filtration rate from serum creatinine: a new prediction equation. *Ann Intern Med* 1999;**130**: 461–70.
9. O'Meara E, Chong KS, Gardner RS, Jardine AG, Neilly JB, McDonagh TA. The Modification of Diet in Renal Disease (MDRD) equations provide valid estimations of glomerular filtration rates in patients with advanced heart failure. *Eur J Heart Fail* 2006;**8**(1):63–67.
10. Dries DL, Exner DV, Domanski MJ, Greenberg B, Stevenson LW. The prognostic implications of renal insufficiency in asymptomatic and symptomatic patients with left ventricular systolic dysfunction. *J Am Coll Cardiol* 2000;**35**(3):681–9.
11. Mahon N, Blackstone EH, Francis GS, Starling RC, Young JB, Lauer MS. The prognostic value of estimated creatinine clearance alongside functional capacity in ambulatory patients with chronic congestive heart failure. *J Am Coll Cardiol* 2002;**40**:1106–13.
12. Al-Ahmad A, Rand W, Manjunath G, *et al.* Reduced kidney function and anemia as risk factors for mortality in patients with left ventricular dysfunction. *J Am Coll Cardiol* 2001;**38**(4):955–62.
13. Hillege HL, Girbes ARJ, de Kam PJ, *et al.* Renal function, neurohormonal activation and survival in patients with chronic heart failure. *Circulation* 2000;**102**:203–10.
14. Ezekowitz JA, McAlister FA, Armstrong PW. Anemia is common in heart failure and is associated with a poor outcome. *Circulation* 2003;**107**:223–225.
15. Anand I, McMurray JJV, Whitmore J, Warren M, McCamish MA, Burton PB. Anemia and its relationship to clinical outcome in heart failure. *Circulation* 2004;**110**:149–54.
16. Horwich TB, Fonarow GC, Hamilton MA, MacLellan WR, Borer JS. Anemia is associated with worse symptoms, greater impairment in functional capacity and a significant increase in mortality in patients with advanced heart failure. *J Am Coll Cardiol* 2002;**39**:1780–6.
17. Al Ahmad A, Rand W, Manjunath G, *et al.* Reduced kidney function and anemia as risk factors for mortality in patients with left ventricular dysfunction. *J Am Coll Cardiol* 2001;**38**(4):955–62.
18. Plata R, Cornejo A, Arratia C, *et al.* Angiotensin-converting-enzyme inhibition therapy in altitude polycythaemia: a prospective randomised trial. *Lancet* 2002;**359**:663–6.
19. Wong F, Siu S, Liu P, Blendis LM. Brain natriuretic peptide: is it a predictor of cardiomyopathy in cirrhosis?. *Clin Sci (Lond)* 2001;**101**(6):621–8.
20. Lerman A, Gibbons RJ, Rodeheffer RJ, *et al.* Circulating N-terminal atrial natriuretic peptide as a marker for symptomless left-ventricular dysfunction. *Lancet* 1993;**341**:1105–9.
21. McDonagh TA, Cunningham AD, Morrison CE, *et al.* Left ventricular dysfunction, natriuretic peptides, and mortality in an urban population. *Heart* 2001;**86**:21–6.
22. Tsutamoto T, Wada A, Maeda K, *et al.* Attenuation of compensation of endogenous cardiac natriuretic peptide system in chronic heart failure -Prognostic role of brain natriuretic peptide concentration in patients with chronic symptomatic left ventricular dysfunction. *Circulation* 1997;**96**:509–16.
23. Murdoch DR, Byrne J, Morton JJ, *et al.* Brain natriuretic peptide is stable in whole blood and can be measured using a simple rapid assay: implications for clinical practice. *Heart* 1997;**78**:594–7.
24. McNairy M, Gardetto N, Clopton P, *et al.* Stability of B-type natriuretic peptide levels during exercise in patients with congestive heart failure. *Am Heart J* 2002;**143**:406–411.
25. McDonagh TA, Robb SD, Murdoch DR, Morton JJ, Ford I, Morrison CE *et al.* Biochemical detection of left-ventricular systolic dysfunction. *Lancet* 1998; **351**(9095):9–13.
26. Nielsen OW, McDonagh TA, Robb SD, Dargie HJ. Retrospective analysis of the cost-effectiveness of using plasma brain natriuretic peptide in screening for left ventricular systolic dysfunction in the general population. *J Am Coll Cardiol* 2003;**41**:113–120.
27. Dao Q, Krishnaswamy P, Kazanegra R, *et al.* Utility of B-type natriuretic peptide in the diagnosis of congestive heart failure in an urgent-care setting. *J Am Coll Cardiol* 2001; **37**(2):379–85.
28. Maisel AS, Krishnaswamy P, Nowak R, *et al.* Rapid measurement of B-type natriuretic peptide in the emergency diagnosis of heart failure. *N Engl J Med* 2002;**347**(3):161–7.
29. Shindler DM, Kostis JB, Yusuf S, *et al.* Diabetes mellitus: a predictor of morbidity and mortality in the Studies Of Left Ventricular Dysfunction (SOLVD) trials and registry. *Am J Cardiol* 1996;**77**:1017–20.
30. Prazak P, Pfisterer M, Osswald S, Buser P, Burkart F. Differences of disease progression in congestive heart failure due to alcoholic as compared to idiopathic dilated cardiomyopathy. *Eur Heart J* 1996;**17**(2):251–7.
31. Dries DL, Sweitzer NK, Drazner MH, *et al.* Prognostic impact of diabetes mellitus in patients with heart failure according to the etiology of left ventricular systolic function. *J Am Coll Cardiol* 2001;**38**:421–8.
32. Sato Y, Yamada T, Taniguchi R, *et al.* Persistently increased serum concentrations of cardiac troponin T in patients with idiopathic dilated cardiomyopathy are predicitve of adverse outcomes. *Circulation* 2001;**103**:369–74.
33. Metra M, Nodari S, Parrinello G, *et al.* The role of plasma biomarkers in acute heart failure. Serial changes and independent prognostic value of NT-proBNP and cardiac troponin-T. *Eur J Heart Fail* 2007;**9**(8):776–86.
34. Leyva F, Anker SD, Godsland IF, *et al.* Uric acid in chronic heart failure: a marker of chronic inflammation. *Eur Heart J* 1998;**19**(12):1814–22.
35. Anker SD, Leyva F, Poole-Wilson P, Coats AJ. Uric acid as independent predictor of impaired prognosis in patients with chronic heart failure [abstract]. *J Am Coll Cardiol* 1998;**31**:154–5A.
36. Batin P, Wickens M, McEntegart D, Fullwood L, Cowley AJ. The importance of abnormalities of liver function tests in predicting mortality in chronic heart failure. *Eur Heart J* 1995;**16**(11):1613–18.
37. CIBIS Investigators and Committees. A randomised trial of beta-blockade in heart failure: the Cardiac Insufficiency Bisoprolol Study (CIBIS). *Circulation* 1994;**90**:1765–1773.
38. Rathore SS, Curtis JP, Wang Y, Bristow MR, Krumholz HM. Association of serum digoxin concentration and outcomes in patients with heart failure. *JAMA* 2003;**289**(7):871–8.
39. Rihal CS, Davis KB, Kennedy JW, Gersh BJ. The utility of clinical, electrocardiographic, and roentgenographic variables in the prediction of left ventricular function. *Am J Cardiol* 1995;**75**(4):220–3.
40. Kearney MT, Fox KA, Lee AJ, *et al.* Predicting sudden death in patients with mild to moderate chronic heart failure. *Heart* 2004;**90**(10):1137–43.
41. The effect of digoxin on mortality and morbidity in patients with heart failure. The Digitalis Investigation Group. *N Engl J Med* 1997;**336**(8):525–33.

19

Echocardiography

Alison Duncan

Introduction

Heart failure (HF) is a complex syndrome that can result from any structural or functional cardiac disorder that impairs the ability of the heart to function as a pump to support a physiological circulation. The most common cause of HF in the United Kingdom is coronary artery disease (CAD); other aetiologies include hypertension, atrial fibrillation, cardiomyopathies, valvular heart disease, pericardial disease, and intracardiac shunts.[1] Transthoracic echocardiography has a decisive role in the diagnosis, treatment, and follow-up of patients with HF.[2] Indeed, its importance was underscored in the UK 2003 NICE Guidelines for Heart Failure,[3] and more recently in the American College of Cardiology/American Heart Association (ACC/AHA) guidelines for the diagnosis and management of HF, where echocardiography was endorsed as 'the single most useful diagnostic test in the evaluation of patients with heart failure. . .'.[4] Echocardiography utilizes ultrasound which has no known adverse biological effects, is noninvasive, and is a relatively low-cost imaging modality. The use of echocardiography in the diagnosis, therapeutic management, and serial follow-up of the increasing number of patients with HF has therefore potentially large health benefits with relatively low patient cost.

Echocardiographic assessment of left ventricular function

Abnormalities of left ventricular function may be apparent even before clinical signs of HF are evident. Comprehensive echocardiographic assessment of left ventricular function is therefore required. Table 19.1 outlines standard techniques for echo evaluation of left ventricular function. The minimal requirements are an assessment of (1) left ventricular size and shape, (2) global systolic function, (3) regional systolic function, (4) diastolic function, (5) intracardiac haemodynamics, and (6) left ventricular synchrony.

Assessment of left ventricular cavity size

Measurements of left ventricular cavity size (end-diastolic dimension, EDD and end-systolic dimension, ESD) are made from M-mode or two-dimensional cross-sectional imaging of the left ventricle at the level of the mitral valve tips at end diastole (q wave of the preceding cardiac cycle) and at end systole (aortic valve closure) (Fig. 19.1). Segmental wall thickness at end diastole (and thickening fraction from measurements at end systole) may also be determined using either method. Normal ranges for left ventricular cavity size are presented in Table 19.2.[4]

Assessment of global left ventricular systolic function

Fractional shortening and ejection fraction

Fractional shortening may be calculated using measures of left ventricular end-diastolic and end-systolic cavity size (as the percentage change in left ventricular cavity dimension in systole with respect to diastole):

$$\text{Fractional shortening (\%)} = [(\text{EDD} - \text{ESD})/\text{EDD}) \times 100]$$

Although fractional shortening accurately quantifies basal left ventricular function, it is reliable only in a symmetrically contracting heart without regional variability and thus is frequently inappropriate for the remodelled ventricles of many HF patients. Assessment of left ventricular systolic function thus depends more on values of left ventricular ejection fraction (LVEF). Calculation of LVEF is based on guidelines from the American Society of Echocardiography using the principle of slicing the left ventricle from mitral valve annulus to apex into a series of 20 discs.[5] The volume of each disc is calculated (using the diameter and thickness of the slice) and then all the discs are summated to provide left ventricular volumes at end diastole and end systole (Fig. 19.2). LVEF is calculated as:

$$[(\text{EDV-ESV})/\text{EDV}) \times 100]$$

Accuracy is improved by using diameters in two perpendicular planes (biplane apical four- and two-chamber). Normal ranges for left ventricular fractional shortening and LVEF are presented in Table 19.2. The ASE guidelines define an abnormal LVEF as less than 55%, with the cut-offs for moderately and severely reduced LVEF as 36–44% and under 35% respectively.

Table 19.1 Assessment of left ventricular function

Echo variable	Assessment
LV cavity size	M-mode/2D measurements
Global LV systolic function	Qualitative evaluation of size, shape, and LVEF
	Quantification of LV dimensions, volumes, fractional shortening, EF (Simpson's)
	Degree of LVH
	Doppler measurements (dP/dt in mitral regurgitation)
Regional systolic function	Qualitative evaluation (wall motion score index)
	Quantitative evaluation (M-mode or TDI)
	Newer techniques (strain, strain rate, tissue tracking)
Diastolic function	Transmitral flow velocities
	Annular tissue velocity (E:E′ ratio)
	Response to Valsalva manoeuvre
	Others (pulmonary vein flow, mitral flow propagation)
Synchrony	Doppler assessment of interventricular delay
	Intraventricular delay (M-mode, TDI, strain, 3D)
	Consequences of incoordination on global function

EF, ejection fraction; LV, left ventricular; LVH, left ventricular hypertrophy; TDI, tissue Doppler imaging.

The 'summation of discs' method assumes that the imaging planes are orthogonal and is absolutely dependent on detection of the endocardial border and therefore on image quality of the echocardiogram. Interobserver variability and beat-to-beat variability can be significant if image quality is suboptimal. Real-time three-dimensional echo imaging has the advantage of taking into account variation in ventricular shape in all directions rather than just the two biplane measurements (Fig. 19.3a), with good correlation with cardiac volumes obtained from cardiac magnetic resonance imaging (CMR). However, good-quality endocardial border definition is still required.[6]

Despite the historical use of LVEF as 'a measure of left ventricular systolic function', its use has distinct disadvantages. As an ejection-phase index, LVEF is highly load-dependent; thus, a change in LVEF over time may not necessarily be due to a change in the intrinsic contractility of the myocardium (a true measure of systolic function), but may merely reflect a change in the loading conditions. Nevertheless, LVEF and 'systolic function' continue to be used interchangeably in the literature. Moreover, since LVEF is affected by preload and afterload, it can give misleading information in several clinical situations; for example, the falsely high LVEF in severe mitral regurgitation when underlying left ventricular systolic function is abnormal, the low LVEF in severe aortic stenosis which can increase markedly after valve replacement, and the variable LVEF in atrial fibrillation. Furthermore, LVEF does not correlate with HF symptoms, exercise capacity, or myocardial oxygen consumption.[7] Despite these major limitations, echo measurement of LVEF continues to be standard practice, providing as it does not only the standard entry criterion for many HF clinical trials,[8–10] but guidance for therapeutic intervention such as defibrillator device therapy and timing of surgery for valve disease,[11,12] and affording prognostic information (predicting major adverse cardiac events, cardiovascular mortality, and sudden death) in the HF population.[13,14]

Left ventricular thickness and mass

The clinical importance of left ventricular mass relates to the identification of pathological left ventricular hypertrophy (LVH). In the echocardiographic substudy of the SOLVD trial, increased left ventricular mass was associated with high mortality and rate of cardiovascular hospital stays, independent of LVEF.[14] LVH may be secondary to other pathology (aortic valve disease or hypertension) or it may be a primary myocardial problem (hypertrophic cardiomyopathy, infiltrative cardiomyopathy). Physiological hypertrophy (in athletes or during pregnancy) is usually reversible. In elderly people, there is sometimes septal angulation and thickening that creates the impression of septal hypertrophy but the left ventricular mass is usually unchanged.

Left ventricular mass may be calculated using M-mode techniques and the formula:

$$\text{LV mass} = 1.04\,([\text{LVID} + \text{PWT} + \text{LVST}]^3 - \text{LVID}^3) - 14\,g$$

LV cavity dimensions by M-mode

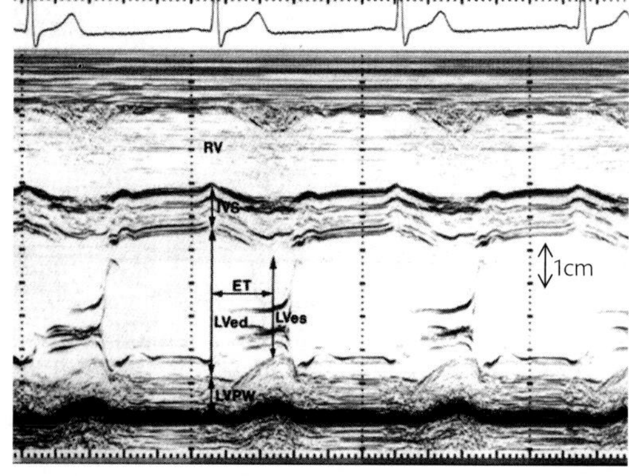

LV cavity dimensions by 2D

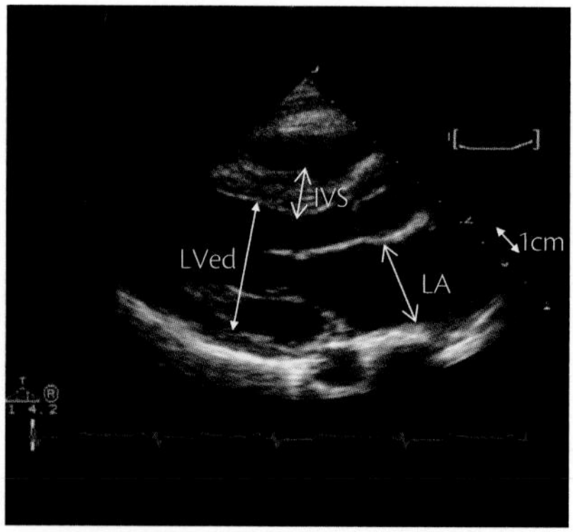

Fig. 19.1 Measurement of left ventricular cavity size. Left: left ventricular M-mode taken from a parasternal long-axis view at the level of the mitral valve tips. Right: still two-dimensional (2D) image from a parasternal long-axis view. In 2D imaging, left ventricular cavity size is measured endocardial border to endocardial border in a line at right angles to each wall passing through the mitral valve tips. ET, ejection time; IVS, interventricular septum; LA, left atrium; LVed, left ventricular cavity size at end diastole; LVes, left ventricular cavity size at end systole; LVPW, left ventricular posterior wall; RV, right ventricle.

Table 19.2 Left ventricular size, mass, and function

	Normal	Mild	Moderate	Severe
LV wall thickness				
IVSd/PW (cm)	0.6–1.2	1.3–1.5	1.6–1.9	≥2.0
LV dimension (women)				
LVIDd (cm)	3.9–5.3	5.4–5.7	5.8–6.1	≥6.2
LVIDd/BSA (cm/m^2)	2.4–3.2	3.3–3.4	3.5–3.7	≥3.8
LV dimension (men)				
LVIDd (cm)	4.2–5.9	6.0–6.3	6.4–6.8	≥6.9
LVIDd/BSA (cm/m^2)	2.2–3.1	3.2–3.4	3.5–3.6	≥3.7
LV volume (women)				
LV diastolic volume (mL)	56–104	105–117	118–130	≥131
LV systolic volume (mL)	19–49	50–59	60–69	≥70
LV volume (men)				
LV diastolic volume (mL)	67–155	156–178	179–201	≥202
LV systolic volume (mL)	22–58	59–70	71–82	≥83
LV volume index				
LV diastolic volume/BSA (mL/m^2)	35–75	76–86	87–96	≥97
LV systolic volume/BSA (mL/m^2)	12–30	31–36	37–42	≥43
LV function				
Fractional shortening (%)	25–43	20–24	15–19	<15
Ejection fraction (biplane Simpson's)	≥ 55	45–54	36–44	≤35
LV mass (women)				
LV mass (g)	66–150	151–171	172–182	≥182
LV mass/BSA (g/cm^2)	44–88	89–100	101–112	≥112
LV mass (men)				
LV mass (g)	96–200	201–227	228–254	≥254
LV mass /BSA (g/cm^2)	50–102	103–116	117–130	≥130

BSA, body surface area; LV, left ventricular.
Adapted from Lang RM, Bierig M, Devereaux RB, *et al.* Recommendations for chamber quantification. *J Am Soc Echocardiogr* 2005;**18**:1440–63.

where LVID is the left ventricular internal dimension during diastole, PWT is the posterior wall thickness, and IVST is the interventricular septal thickness.[15] Two-dimensional methods, including the truncated ellipsoid and the area–length formula, might be more appropriate for distorted ventricles with regional wall motion abnormalities. Both methods, however, rely heavily on geometric assumptions and are therefore subject to inaccuracies from foreshortening. These limitations may be partially overcome using three-dimensional echocardiographic techniques (Fig. 19.3b).

Normal ranges for left ventricular mass are presented in Table 19.2. LVH may be graded by reporting relative wall thickness (calculated as [2 × PWT]/LVEDD) and overall left ventricular mass, and reported as (1) normal; (2) concentric LVH (increased relative wall thickness with increased mass); (3) eccentric LVH (increased mass with normal relative wall thickness); (4) concentric remodelling (normal mass with increased relative wall thickness). Concentric changes suggest pressure overload (due to aortic stenosis or hypertension), while eccentric changes suggest volume overload (e.g. due to aortic regurgitation).

Doppler measures of left ventricular systolic function

Doppler echocardiography can evaluate indices of the isovolumic contraction phases of the cardiac cycle, which may be more representative of the left ventricular contractile state. The change in left ventricular pressure over time (dP/dt) is closely related to the mitral regurgitation trace obtained using echocardiography using continuous-wave Doppler across the mitral valve (Fig. 19.4). Assuming any change in left atrial pressure during systole has negligible effect on this pressure difference, a plot of left ventricular dP/dt can be generated from the first derivative of the pressure difference plot.[16] The faster the rise in ventricular pressure, the more coordinated the left ventricular systolic function.[17]

Alternatively, stroke distance can be calculated from the velocity time integral (VTI) of the left ventricular outflow tract using pulse-wave Doppler from an apical five-chamber view. The product of stroke distance (normally 18–22 cm) and left ventricular outflow tract area provides quantitative Doppler assessment of left ventricular stroke volume. Cardiac output may be subsequently calculated as the product of stroke volume and heart rate.

Assessment of regional left ventricular systolic function

Two-dimensional regional wall motion abnormalities

Regional wall motion abnormalities (RWMA) may occur in any dilated cardiomyopathy but are most commonly associated

End-diastolic volume

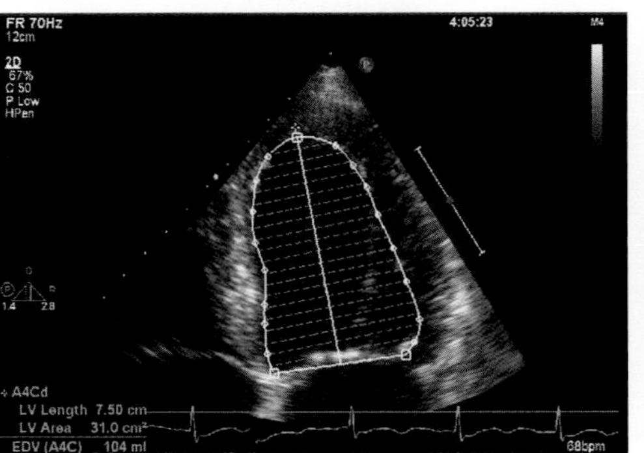

End-systolic volume

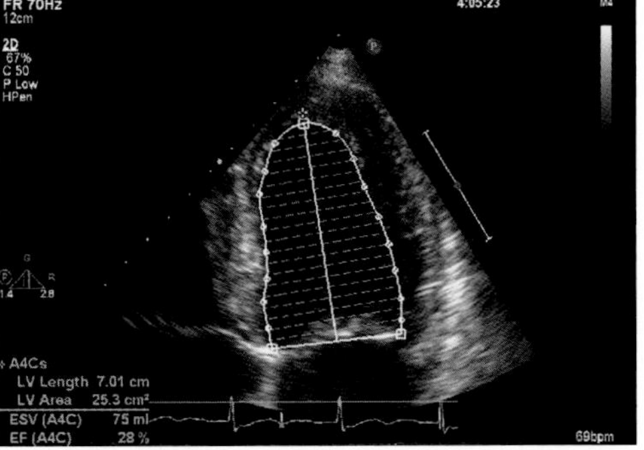

Fig. 19.2 Calculation of Simpson's biplane left ventricular ejection fraction. Left: still end-diastolic frame in apical four-chamber view calculating end-diastolic volume (EDV); right: still end-systolic frame in apical four-chamber view calculating end-systolic volume (ESV).

3D calculation of LV volumes and EF

3D calculation of LV Mass

A

B

Fig. 19.3 Calculation of left ventricular volumes using transthoracic three-dimensional (3D) echo. (A) Calculation of left ventricular volumes and ejection fraction. A 3D image set is acquired from the apex, the left ventricular border is traced in two planes, and the rest of the left ventricular border is tracked automatically to create a volume-rendered outline of the left ventricular throughout the cardiac cycle. From this, a mathematical model or 'cast' of the left ventricular is created using all 3D data points. Calculated left ventricular volume may be plotted against time during one cardiac cycle. End-diastolic and end-systolic volumes plus ejection fraction and sphericity index can be derived from these data. (B) Example of left ventricular mass calculation where apical four- and two-chamber sections have been created from a full volume dataset of the left ventricular, endocardial and epicardial borders of the left ventricular myocardium is identified and a biplane Simpson's rule calculation applied to derive both left ventricular and myocardial volumes. The latter is multiplied by the specific gravity of heart muscle to obtain the displayed mass.

with CAD. Echocardiography is an extremely useful tool for identifying left ventricular RWMA. Basic assessment of regional wall motion or thickening is usually assessed subjectively, and attributed to specific coronary territories. The right coronary artery usually supplies the right ventricle and left ventricular inferioseptal segments, the left anterior descending artery supplies the left ventricular anterior, anterioseptal, and apical segments, and the circumflex artery supplies the left ventricular lateral wall. However, there may be considerable variation and/or overlap between individual patients.

Qualitative assessment

A standard 16-segment model of the left ventricle (lateral, septal, inferior, anterior segments at the apex, midpapillary, and basal levels, and anteroseptal and posterior segments at the midpapillary and basal levels)[18] or more recently, a 17-segment model that includes a true apical segment,[19] is used to assess regional function. Each region is given a score where 1 is normal, 2 is hypokinetic (endocardial excursion <5 mm), 3 is akinetic (endocardial excursion <2 mm), and 4 is dyskinetic (endocardium moves outwards in systole). The overall wall motion score index, calculated by averaging the scores of all individual segments, is related to prognosis.[20] The technique is subjective, however, with variable reproducibility between centres, although its accuracy may be improved with the use of contrast agents that opacify the left ventricular cavity and enhance endocardial border delineation.

Quantitative assessment

Quantitation of regional function has been performed with a number of echocardiographic and Doppler modalities with increasingly reliable reproducibility (Table 19.3). Some techniques, such as M-mode and tissue Doppler imaging (TDI) are in routine clinical practice, while others are being investigated as possible measures of regional function that can detect subclinical disease in a similar fashion.

Longitudinal regional left ventricular systolic function

Assessment of annular longitudinal function by either measurement of amplitude (M-mode) or velocity (tissue Doppler) is a clinically useful tool for assessing systolic left ventricular function. Normal left ventricular contraction depends on the coordinate function of

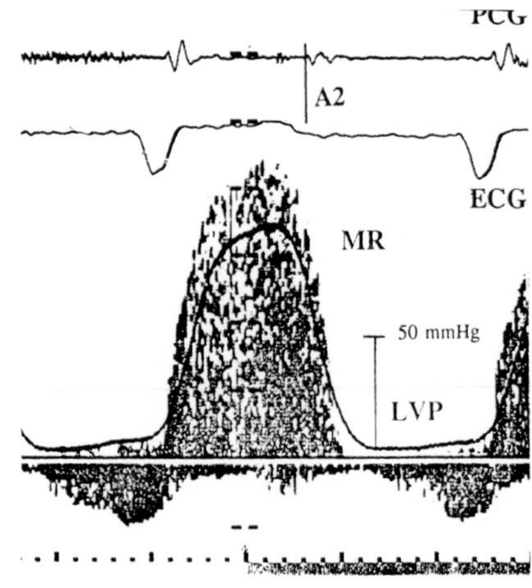

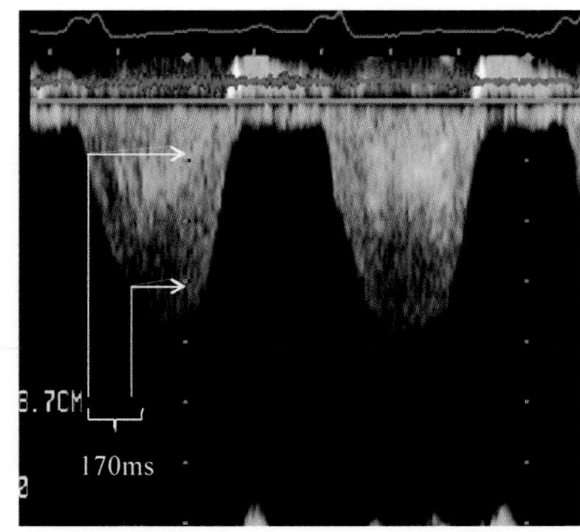

Fig. 19.4 Measurement of dP/dt. Left: change in left ventricular pressure (LVP, measured by tip manometer) is closely associated with mitral regurgitation (MR) trace obtained using transoesophageal echocardiography. Right: measurement of dP/dt: record MR at 100 mm/s and measure the time for the MR velocity jet to rise from 1 m/s to 4 m/s (i.e. from 4 mmHg to 36 mmHg). dP/dt >1200 mmHg/s (<27 ms between points) relates to normally timed left ventricular contraction whereas values <800 mmHg/s (>40 ms) suggests severely prolonged contractile state.

Table 19.3 Quantitative assessment of regional systolic function

	Radial	Longitudinal
Displacement and thickening	Colour kinesis	Annular M-mode
	Anatomical M-mode	Tissue tracking
Velocity	Speckle strain	TDI or speckle strain
Deformation	Speckle strain	TDI or speckle strain
Timing	TDI (time to peak systole or onset of diastole)	TDI (time to peak systole or onset of diastole)

TDI, tissue Doppler imaging.

longitudinally and circumferentially directed muscle fibres (twisting and untwisting with accompanying longitudinal shortening and lengthening), and loss of these interactions, evident early in left ventricular disease, are readily detected using echocardiography (Fig. 19.5). Abnormalities of the mitral annular motion have been described in a variety of conditions. Patients with acute myocardial infarction have reduced displacement more marked at the region of the annulus related to the site of infarct;[21] systolic long axis abnormalities may occur in 38–52% of HF patients with normal LVEF;[22,23] and reductions in long axis amplitude and velocity can be detected before reduction in LVEF or symptoms develop in hypertension, diabetes, 'diastolic HF', and hypertrophic cardiomyopathy among others.[24–26] Moreover, long axis amplitude is strongly related to LVEF,[27] and is a useful predictor of prognosis in a variety of clinical conditions.[28]

From digitally recorded tissue Doppler loops of one or more heart beats containing velocity data from the entire myocardium,

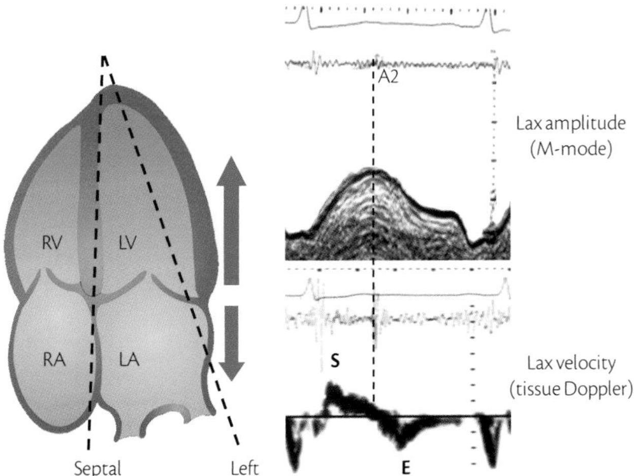

Fig. 19.5 Quantification of longitudinal cardiac motion. Left: schematic diagram of the motion of the lateral and septal long axis, which moves upwards towards the left ventricular apex during systole, returns to its original position in mid-diastole, and moves further away from away from the left ventricular apex during atrial contraction. Right top: corresponding M-mode of lateral M-mode long axis motion at the lateral wall. Note in a coordinate segment, the long axis motion peaks at aortic valve closure (A2), and amplitude is measured on the vertical scale. Right bottom: corresponding tissue Doppler velocity trace of the lateral wall (vertical scale). Note that the peak systolic velocity (S) corresponds with the peak rate of change of the systolic long axis amplitude, and the peak early diastolic velocity (E) corresponds to the peak rate of change of early backward motion of the lateral wall. LA, left atrium; LV left ventricle; RA, right atrium; RV, right ventricle.

two new tissue Doppler entities can be derived: (1) strain rate (the rate of deformation between two points a predefined distance apart)[29] and (2) speckle (tissue) tracking (echo software detects frame-to-frame migration of two-dimensional speckle signals from the myocardium from high-resolution two-dimensional imaging and then calculates myocardial strain independent of the angle of incidence) (Fig. 19.6).[30] From a 16-segment left ventricular model, the average motion amplitude toward the apex in systole for each segment can be measured and a 'global systolic contraction amplitude index' calculated.[31] Although reportedly useful in the early detection of subclinical heart disease, these newer techniques currently have the disadvantages of a large signal-to-noise ratio and wide inter- and intraobserver variability in measurements. Their specific advantages over M-mode or tissue velocity quantification of long axis function, that also detects subclinical disease therefore remain unclear. Their main use may be in the identification and measurement of left ventricular dyssynchrony.

Assessment of left ventricular diastolic function

A large proportion of patients who present with symptoms of HF have a LVEF within the normal range; these patients are frequently referred to as having 'diastolic HF.' The use of such a term is troublesome, not least because no simple definition of diastolic disease itself has emerged, but also because it presumes an understanding of the mechanisms leading to the disorder and therefore justification of the substitution of a mechanistic term for a descriptive phrase. 'Increased resistance to filling' has been suggested. However, whereas the resistance of a valve orifice or circulation can be readily identified in terms of pressure drop and flow, resistance to filling involves neither and so is poorly defined. This lack of gold standards by which discrete mechanisms can be assessed in individual patients is a major impediment to identifying and quantifying disturbances in disease. So is the reality that left ventricular filling is totally load-dependent. Nevertheless, a variety of echocardiographic techniques are frequently used to determine a series of abnormalities of diastolic function, the cornerstone of which is the measurement of transmitral flow (left ventricular filling) (Fig. 19.7). Pulmonary venous flow, left atrial size, and tissue doppler imaging (TDI) of the mitral annulus are also considered. These measurements have demonstrated considerable prognostic value in symptomatic and asymptomatic patients with either preserved or abnormal left ventricular systolic function.[32]

Diastole has traditionally been defined as the period in the cardiac cycle from the end of aortic ejection to the onset of ventricular tension development of the succeeding beat. It has four distinct phases:

- Isovolumic relaxation—between aortic valve closure and mitral valve opening.
- Early filling—accounting for 80% of ventricular filling in normal young subjects.
- Diastasis—as LA and left ventricular pressures equalize.
- Atrial systole—accounting for the remainder of ventricular filling.

Dominant A wave

Diastolic function is traditionally characterized in the literature according to severity. So-called 'mild diastolic dysfunction', usually present early in disease development (ischaemia, aortic stenosis,

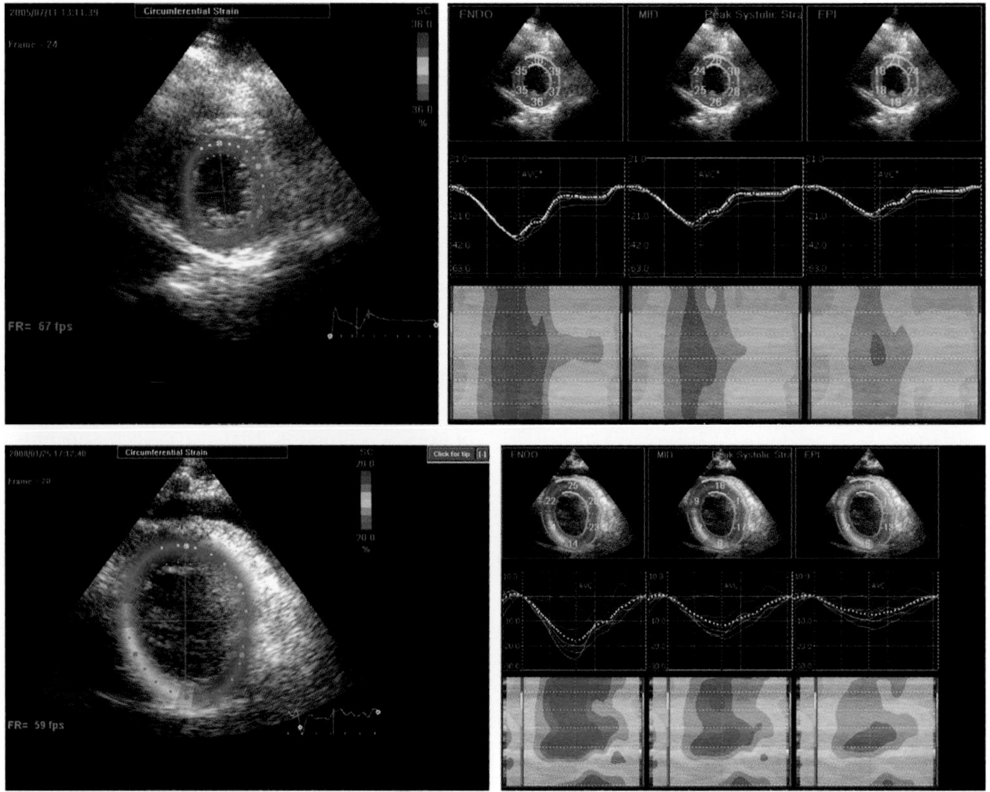

Fig. 19.6 Use of speckle tracking in assessment of left ventricular disease. Top: Short-axis end-systolic colour-coded radial strain image at the level of the papillary muscle of a subject with normal left ventricular function (left panel). The related strain curves for the endocardial, mid-myocardial, and epicardial layer of one cardiac cycle for the six segments within the short-axis view are given in the right panel. There is a gradual decline in circumferential strain from the endocardial to epicardial layers in all the segments. Bottom: Short-axis end-systolic colour-coded radial strain image at the level of the papillary muscle of a subject with prior posterior wall myocardial infarction (left panel). The related strain curves for the endocardial, mid-myocardial, and epicardial layers of one cardiac cycle of the six segments within the short-axis view are given in the right panel. There is considerable reduction of strain of each of the layers of the posterior segment.
From Adamu U, Schmitz F, Becker M, Kelm M, Hoffmann R. Advanced speckle tracking echocardiography allowing a three-myocardial layer-specific analysis of deformation parameters. *Eur J Echocardiogr* 2009;**10**:303–8, with permission.

hypertension, hypertrophy), is detected as prolongation of age-related isovolumic relaxation time (IVRT: time between aortic valve closure and mitral valve opening), decrease in early diastolic flow velocity (E-wave) and a greater reliance on atrial contraction (A-wave) to fill the left ventricle (E:A ratio <1). This pattern of left ventricular filling is usually attributed to 'impaired relaxation', although the exact meaning of the term is rarely specified in the literature (i.e. slow, delayed, or incomplete). In practice, it is nearly always associated with early diastolic incoordination (continued inward long axis shortening after the end of ejection, associated with outward motion elsewhere),[33] causing an abnormal shape change in early diastole which prevents the left ventricle from becoming spherical (Fig. 19.8). Such delayed contraction prolongs the fall in left ventricular pressure and profoundly affects early

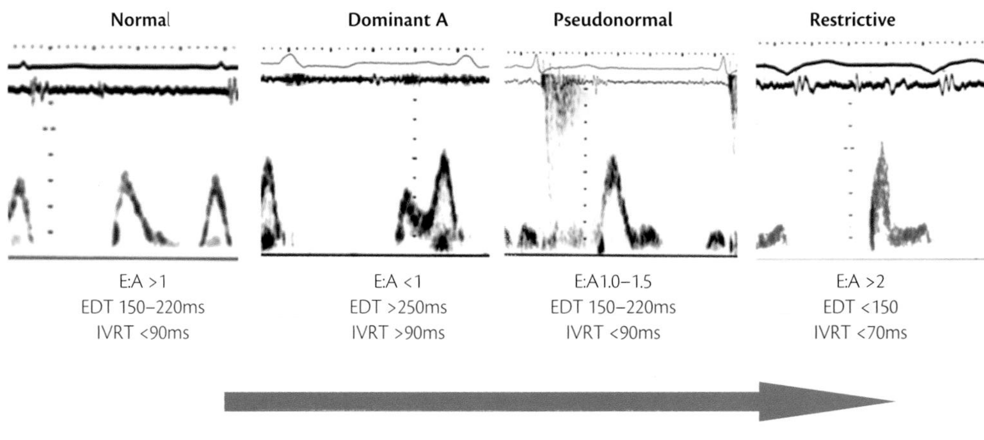

Fig. 19.7 A range of left ventricular filling patterns: normal, late diastolic (dominant A), pseudonormal, early diastolic (restrictive filling). EDT, E-wave deceleration time; IVRT, isovolumetric relaxation time/

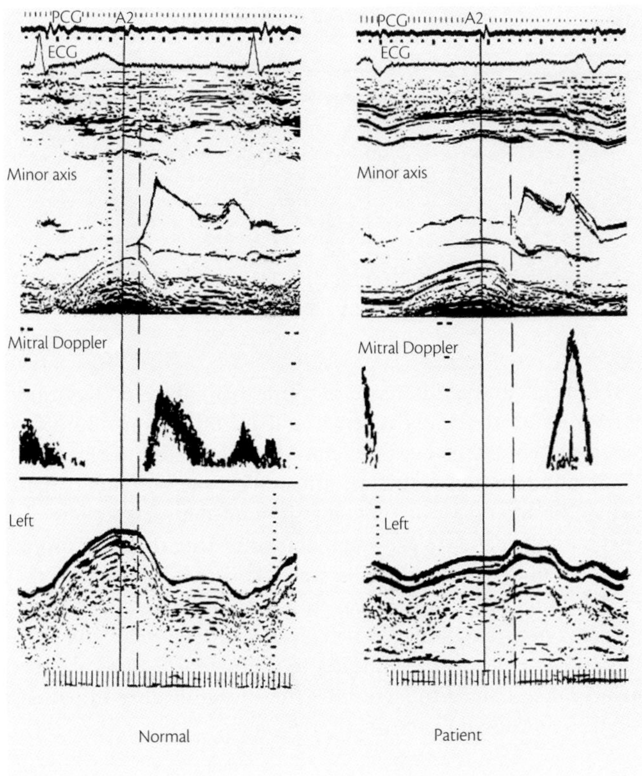

Fig. 19.8 Interaction between long axis incoordination and left ventricular filling. Long isovolumic relaxation time and isolated A wave would support a diagnosis of diastolic disease in the patient above. Prolonged isovolumic relaxation time is associated with increased tension in the left ventricle due to continued inward movement of the lateral long axis after the aortic valve has closed (A2), due in part to reduced long axis amplitude during systole and in part to delayed activation (patient has LBBB on ECG). LBBB results in a delay in the onset, and therefore a delay in the offset, of long axis amplitude.

From Henein MY, Gibson DG. Suppression of left ventricular early diastolic filling by long axis asynchrony. *Br Heart J* 1995;**73**(2): 151–7, with permission.

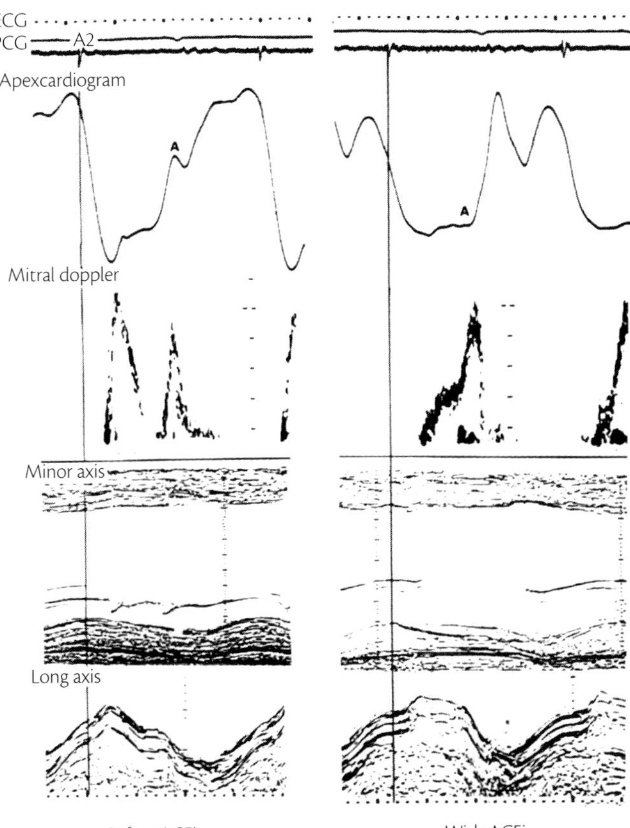

Fig. 19.9 Effect of ACE inhibition on left atrial pressure and left ventricular filling. Left ventricular filling and apexcardiogram from a patient with dilated cardiomyopathy and raised left atrial pressure (left) and response to ACE inhibition (right). Note the significant fall in end-diastolic pressure with treatment and reversal of left ventricular filling pattern, despite appearance of marked early diastolic long axis incoordination. ACEi, ACE inhibitor.

From Henein MY, Das SK, O'Sullivan C, Kakkar VV, Gillbe CE, Gibson DG. ACE inhibitors unmask incoordinate diastolic wall motion in restrictive left ventricular disease. *Heart* 1996;**75**:151–8, with permission.

diastolic filling, reducing its peak velocity or suppressing it altogether. Clinically, this pattern is associated with the combination of ventricular disease and a low or normal filling pressure. It may thus be unmasked by a Valsalva manoeuvre. It is also common in patients initially presenting with restrictive filling who have responded favourably to treatment with diuretic and angiotensin converting enzyme (ACE) inhibitor (Fig. 19.9).[34] This sequence of events illustrates how a patient may improve clinically at the same time that diastolic measurements become more abnormal. Moreover, filling with a dominant A is common in inducible ischaemia, during either angioplasty[35] or dobutamine stress.[36] It is even associated with activation abnormalities.[37] Thus echocardiographic disturbances occurring during diastole, which result in abnormalities of 'diastolic' function, may in fact have their origins much earlier in the cardiac cycle, during systole or even earlier, during activation.

Restrictive filling pattern

With disease progression, left ventricular fibrosis develops and chamber compliance reduces. Often referred to as 'severe diastolic dysfunction' in the literature, this form of left ventricular disease relates to the passive properties of the ventricle. It occurs when left atrial pressure is elevated such that early diastolic flow is extremely rapid, and left atrial and left ventricular pressures equalize quickly during early diastole. It is detected echocardiographically as a short (<40 ms) isovolumic relaxation time, an increased E:A ratio (>2) and a short E-wave deceleration time (<150 ms), which is often accompanied by a third heart sound (Fig. 19.10).

Acceleration and deceleration rates of the E-wave are both increased, implying high pressure gradients, both forward and reversed. Reduced A-wave amplitude is not usually caused by failure of left atrial contraction, since mechanical function can be demonstrated by direct measurement of left atrial pressure, by its indirect effect on the apex cardiogram, or by detecting retrograde blood flow into the pulmonary veins. The combination of an increased atrial pressure wave with no flow across the mitral valve demonstrates increased end-diastolic ventricular stiffness. Such 'restrictive filling' is good evidence of a raised left atrial pressure, which overrides any relaxation abnormality. It gives no direct information about the underlying diastolic disease. This may be specific, as occurs in amyloid or eosinophilic heart disease, or the high filling pressure may represent a complication of cavity dilation, hypertrophy, or diabetes, or even the simple result of fluid overload distending an otherwise normal ventricle. Whatever the underlying aetiology, a restrictive filling pattern should be regarded

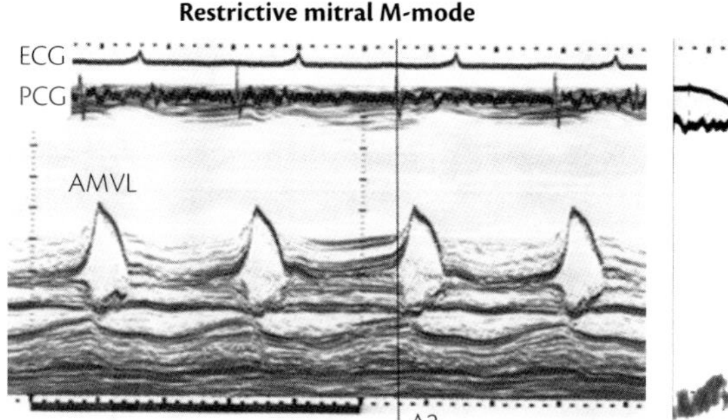

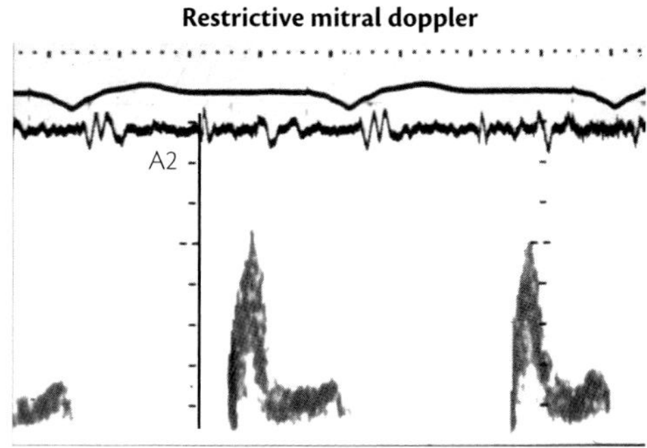

Fig. 19.10 Restrictive left ventricular filling. Left: Mitral valve leaflets open before the aortic valve has closed (A2) suggesting that left atrial pressure is significantly raised. Right: restrictive filling with associated third heart sound on a phonocardiogram.

as the result of a combination of diastolic disease and a high filling pressure, and identifies patients with a poor prognosis when detected at rest[38] or during stress.[39] Since a raised left atrial pressure is an important component of the clinical syndrome of HF, estimation of filling pressure should be an integral part of echocardiographic evaluation in these patients.

'Normal' filling pattern

Just as with isovolumic relaxation time, a raised left atrial pressure and diastolic disease have opposite effects on the E:A ratio, and so the combination of the two leads to a ratio between 1.0 and 2.0, often referred to by the unsatisfactory term 'pseudonormalization'.[40] The left ventricular filling pattern should not, however, be considered in isolation, so that recognizing pseudonormality is less of a problem than the literature might suggest. The majority of patients in whom the question arises are elderly people, in whom an E:A ratio greater than 1 would be unusual anyway. They also have clear evidence of structural left ventricular disease, either cavity dilatation or LVH. In a minority, pressure termination of forward atrial flow can be demonstrated, showing near restrictive filling. The ratio E:E′ (peak early diastolic velocity to peak ring velocity) may be useful in these circumstances. When this ratio is increased, then left atrial pressure is likely to be high. However, since a low value of E′ may be the result of reduced systolic amplitude, it may simply be a surrogate marker of left ventricular disease. A dominant E-wave in an elderly patient with ventricular disease should suggest a raised left ventricular filling pressure. Recognizing pseudonormality in young patients, in whom a dominant E-wave would in fact be normal, has received little attention in the literature.

Other measures of diastolic function include TDI, early left ventricular filling flow propagation slope (Vp), left atrial volumes, and pulmonary venous inflow. These measures are less dependent on loading conditions and heart rate and have been reported to be robust predictors of left ventricular filling pressures and cardiovascular mortality. For example, the ratio of peak early mitral inflow velocity to peak early diastolic myocardial velocity (E:E′ ratio) has been correlated with pulmonary capillary wedge pressure (an E:E′ ≤ 8 predicts a left ventricular end-diastolic pressure (LVEDP) of <15 mmHg while a ratio >15 predicts an LVEDP ≥15 mm Hg).[41] The reliability of the E:E′ ratio when it is in the 8–15 range in predicting LVEDP is, however, less convincing.[42] Moreover, with the extreme values (in which the relation is more certain), left atrial pressure is usually obvious from mitral filling pattern anyway. Alternative methods of estimating left atrial pressure include the ratio of peak early mitral inflow velocity to the slope of the propagation velocity (E:Vp ≥1.5 has been reported to predict a LVEDP >15 mmHg);[43] increased left atrial volume (>32 mL/m^2 predicts morbidity);[44] and a difference of more than 30 ms between pulmonary vein atrial flow reversal and mitral A-wave durations (reported to be a sensitive predictor of LVEDP >18 mmHg).[45]

Diastolic function is thus multifactorial; measurements made during diastole are not only highly load-dependent, but also depend on the patient's age and therapeutic drug regime. Absolute demarcation between isolated 'systolic' HF and 'diastolic' HF may be misleading, since many measures of diastolic function depend on events occurring much earlier in the cardiac cycle. The sensitivity of echo Doppler techniques to estimate left atrial pressure, however, has proved to have real clinical significance in patients with the clinical syndrome of HF.

Use of echo Doppler in assessment of intracardiac haemodynamics

Intracardiac pressure measurements have traditionally required invasive methods. This limitation, which also precludes serial measurements except in the intensive care context, can be circumvented with the use of echocardiographic techniques, which convert regurgitant velocity measurements into pressure drops using the Bernoulli equation modified to give the formula $4V^2$ (where V = velocity recorded across a regurgitant jet). Fig. 19.11 illustrates the use of echo Doppler in the estimation of right atrial pressure (from the properties of the inferior vena cava), right ventricular/pulmonary artery systolic pressure (from the tricuspid regurgitant trace), and pulmonary artery mean and diastolic pressures (from the pulmonary regurgitation trace).[46] As discussed earlier, a combination of long axis and echo Doppler can be used to estimate elevated left and right end-diastolic pressures.

Left ventricular synchrony

Maximal energy transfer from the myocardium to the circulation is dependent on the coordinate, though nonuniform, action of both circumferentially and longitudinally directed myocardial fibres. Loss of this interaction leads to ventricular dyssynchrony, usefully defined as 'incoordinate ventricular wall motion that reduces the extent of intrinsic energy transfer from myocardium to useful work on the circulation'. Its functional consequences are significant impairment of maximal cardiac function as a result of a reduction in the proportion of myocardial energy transmitted to the circulation (cycle efficiency).

Activation abnormalities are common in patients with HF and are a major contributor to left ventricular dyssynchrony. Patients with the combination of a long PR interval and left bundle branch block may have very early and prolonged left ventricular activation due to low action potentials that are not detected on a standard

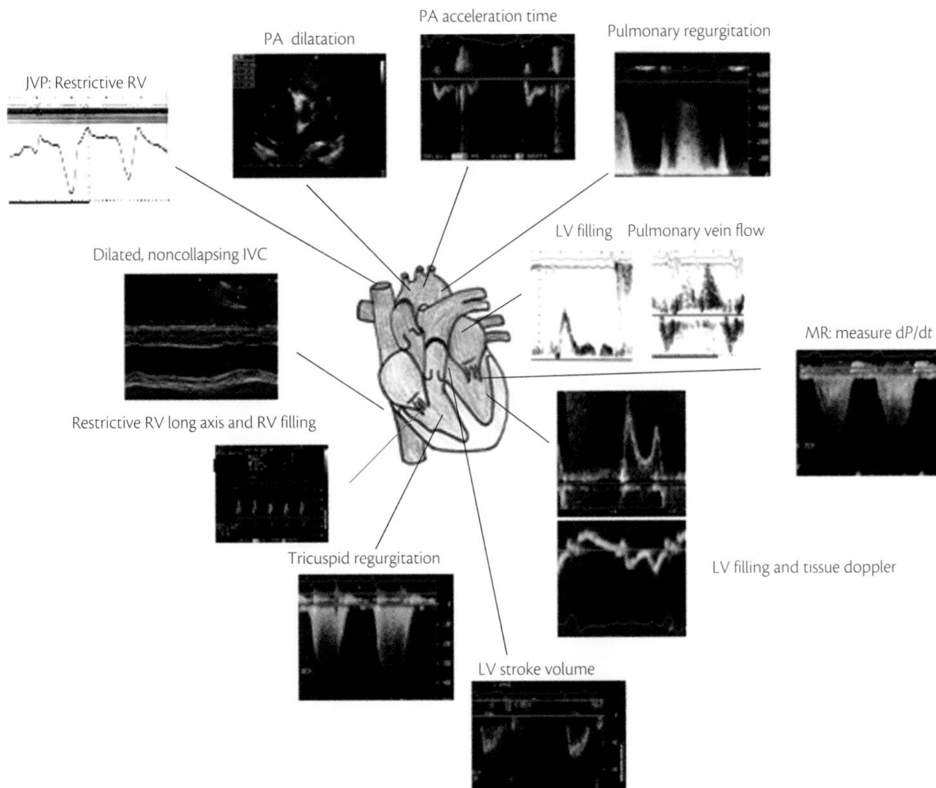

Fig. 19.11 Noninvasive haemodynamic assessment using echo. Right atrial pressure is estimated from inferior vena cava size and collapsibility, right ventricular systolic pressure from the peak tricuspid regurgitation velocity, right ventricular mean and end-diastolic pressure from pulmonary regurgitation velocity trace, and pulmonary vascular resistance from pulmonary acceleration time. Restrictive right ventricular function is determined from analysis of right ventricular long axis function, right ventricular filling pattern, hepatic vein flow, and jugular venous pressure trace. Restrictive left ventricular filling may be determined from analysis of left ventricular long axis function, left ventricular filling pattern, E:E′ ratio, and pulmonary venous flow. Mitral regurgitation (peak dP/dt) and stroke volume provide an estimate of left ventricular systolic function

12-lead ECG.[47] Such early left ventricular activation results in a 'presystolic' component of mitral regurgitation that lengthens the total duration of mitral regurgitation and significantly shortens available left ventricular filling time (Fig. 19.12, left).

Dyssynchrony is also major manifestation of CAD. Indeed, it has long been recognized that patients with chronic stable angina have asynchronous wall motion at rest, even in the absence of chest pain or ischaemic ECG changes. This is most obvious during the isovolumic periods, when the onset of long axis shortening may be so delayed during isovolumic contraction that it not only follows that of minor axis shortening, but results in long axis shortening during isovolumic relaxation.[35] Such continued inward movement is associated with 'postejection' mitral regurgitation and consequent shortening of left ventricular filling time at rest (Fig. 19.12, right).[33] This local mechanical dyssynchrony becomes even more exaggerated during pharmacological stress,[36] so that further shortening of left ventricular filling time at high heart rates (Fig. 19.13) may be enough to limit the normal increase in stroke volume during stress.

Measuring well-defined intervals in the cardiac cycle has long been established as a noninvasive means of assessing left ventricular function. The Tei index, described as 'a Doppler index of combined systolic and diastolic performance' is one such measure. It represents the sum of isovolumic contraction and relaxation times normalized to ejection time.[48] It thus depends on variables previously shown to be closely related to abnormal activation. Moreover the inclusion of ejection time introduces noise and limits its applicability. A more sensitive measure is total isovolumic time (t-IVT), which can be readily measured using simple echo Doppler techniques and derived as [60 – (total ejection time+total filling time)].

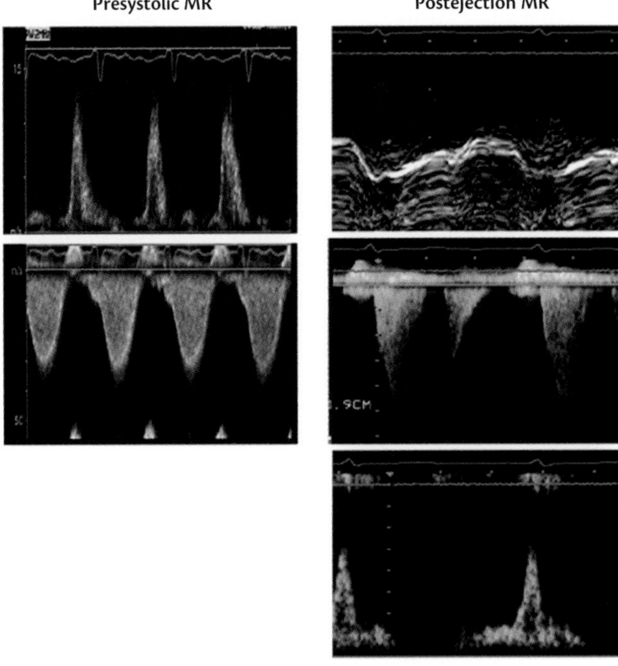

Fig. 19.12 Limitation of left ventricular filling time by long duration of mitral regurgitation. Left: long mitral regurgitation with a presystolic component that shortens available left ventricular filling time. Right: local incoordination in the left ventricular posterior wall in early diastole results in long postejection mitral regurgitation that limits left ventricular filling to late diastole.

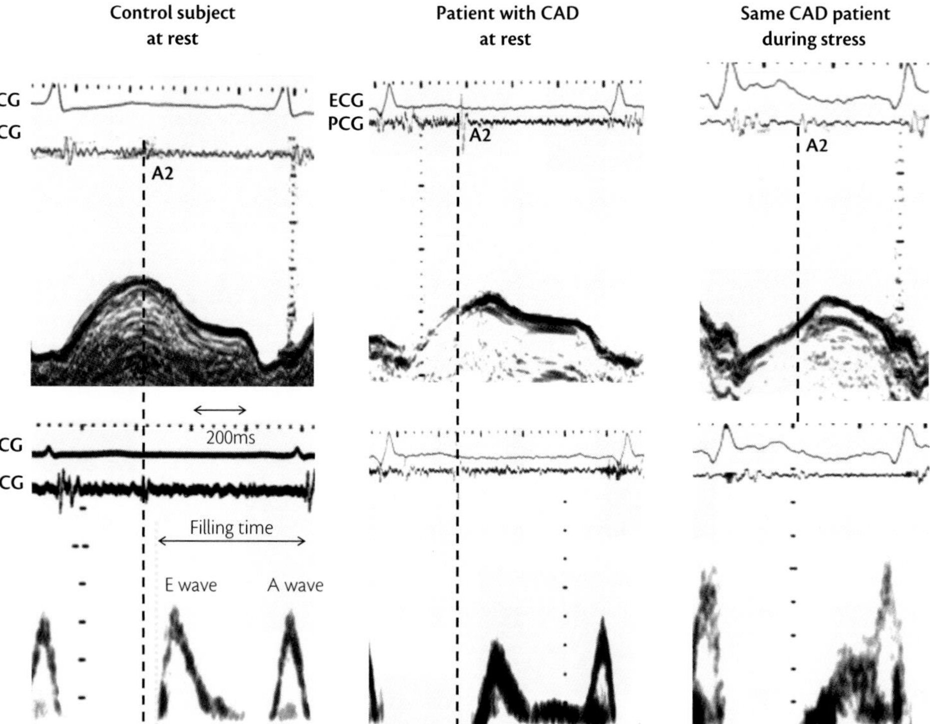

Fig. 19.13 Stress-induced regional dyssynchrony and shortening of left ventricular filling. Left: in a control subject, normal timing of retraction of the mitral annulus coincides with early diastolic filling (E wave). Middle: in a patient with coronary artery disease (CAD), continued inward movement of the long axis during early diastole at rest prolongs isovolumic relaxation time and delays early diastolic filling. Right: exaggerated early diastolic long axis incoordination during stress in the same patient with CAD significantly delays early diastolic filling, with overall limitation of filling time with respect to RR interval.

(Fig. 19.14).[49] The duration of left ventricular filling time combined with the duration of left ventricular ejection time provides an indication of the effectiveness of global cardiac synchrony. Its reciprocal, the time in the cardiac cycle when the ventricle is neither ejecting nor filling (the isovolumic time or 'wasted' time) provides a useful method of expressing the effects of regional dyssynchrony on global cardiac function.[50] When t-IVT is expressed in terms of seconds per minute, it is independent of heart rate, which is an advantage when comparing changes in global dyssynchrony with time (i.e. between rest and stress, or between baseline assessment and follow-up).

Unlike many echo measures including ejection fraction, total isovolumic time is related to the amount of ventricular dyssynchrony, peak stress cardiac output, and exercise capacity. Patients with the longest total isovolumic times are those with the most ventricular dyssynchrony,[50] the lowest cardiac output at peak stress (Fig. 19.15a)[52] and the lowest peak oxygen consumption during cardiopulmonary exercise testing (Fig. 19.15b).[53] Patients with the longest total isovolumic time (i.e. most global dyssynchrony) are potentially those most likely to benefit from cardiac resynchronization therapy (CRT).[54]

Thus, simple echo Doppler measures of global cardiac dyssynchrony may have benefit in the expanding field of predicting responders to CRT, quantifying the degree of response, and optimizing pacemaker settings.

Use of echo in therapeutic management of patients with heart failure

Echocardiography not only provides clinical measures and prognostic assessments in patients with HF but can also supply information to guide application of HF therapies.

Medical therapy

Echocardiographic LVEF is an entry criterion in many clinical trials designed to assess the therapeutic effect of various medical therapies in HF, including ACE inhibitors, β-blockers, and aldosterone antagonists.[8–10] A reduction in LVEF may highlight the detrimental effects on left ventricular function of cardiotoxic medications, including anthracycline chemotherapeutic agents.[55] A more detailed echocardiographic examination, assessing specifically left ventricular filling pattern and segmental incoordination, may demonstrate the beneficial effect of ACE inhibitors in off-loading the left ventricle, particularly in patients with raised left atrial pressure (restrictive filling pattern), reducing LVEDP, and unmasking segmental incoordination.[34]

Implantable cardioverter-defibrillators

Strategies for implantable cardioverter-defibrillators (ICDs) rely on LVEF for selecting patients for the devices.[11] Repeat LVEF assessment at 30–40 days after myocardial infarction and after initiation of optimal HF medical therapy is necessary to determine candidacy for ICD.

Cardiac resynchronization therapy

CRT reduces mortality, improves functional status, and increases LVEF in patients with severe left ventricle disease.[56–58] Current recommendations advocate that patients with LVEF 35% or less, moderate-to-severe HF symptoms, a widened QRS interval, and sinus rhythm should undergo CRT. Debate continues as to whether existing echo methods of assessing left ventricular dyssynchrony provide additional predictive value in determining those patients most likely to benefit from resynchronization.[59] The difficulty may lie in the type of echo measurement that is being used. In order for CRT to be successful, the baseline abnormality

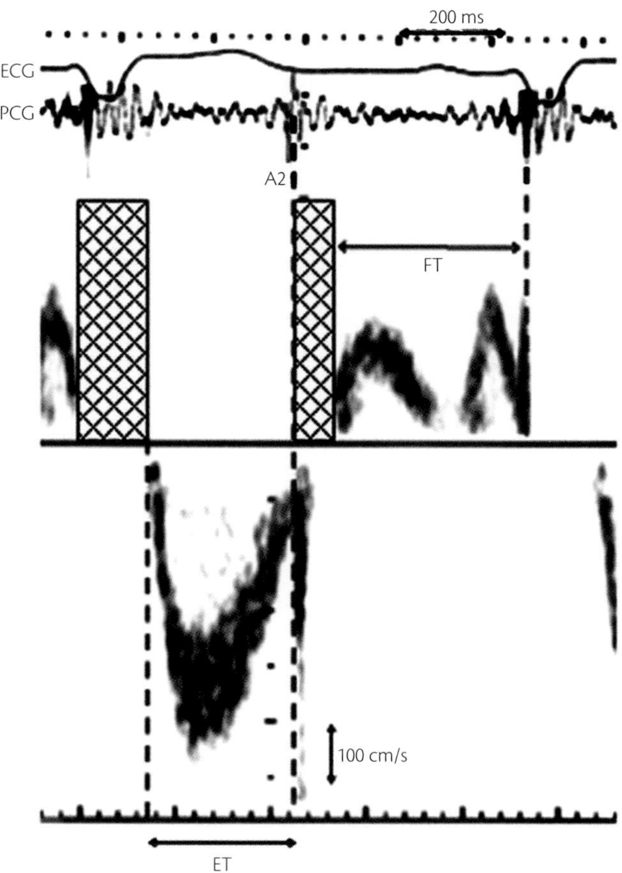

Fig. 19.14 Measurement of total isovolumic time. Left ventricular ejection and filling traces have been superimposed. The hatched areas represent the isovolumic periods, i.e. the time in the cardiac cycle when the left ventricular is neither ejecting nor filling. Total isovolumic time (t-IVT), the combination of isovolumic contraction and relaxation times expressed in s/min, is independent of heart rate. In this case the heart rate is 64 beats/min. The ejection time is 300 ms, so the total ejection time per minute is 0.30 × 64= 19.2 s/min. The filling time is 400 ms, so the total filling time per minute is 0.40 × 64 = 26.6 s/min. This gives t-IVT = 60 – (19.2 + 26.6) = 14.6 s/min.

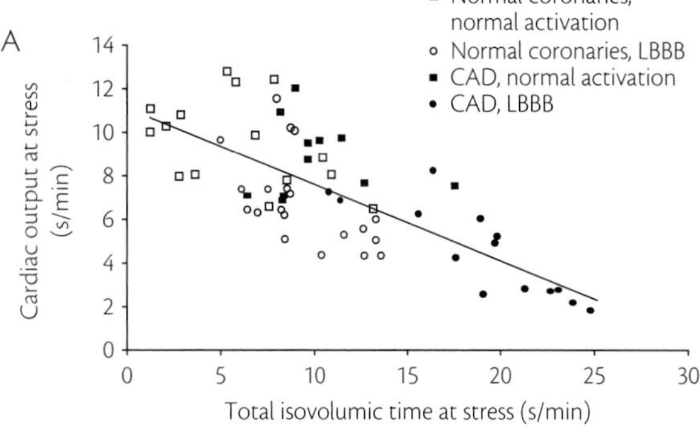

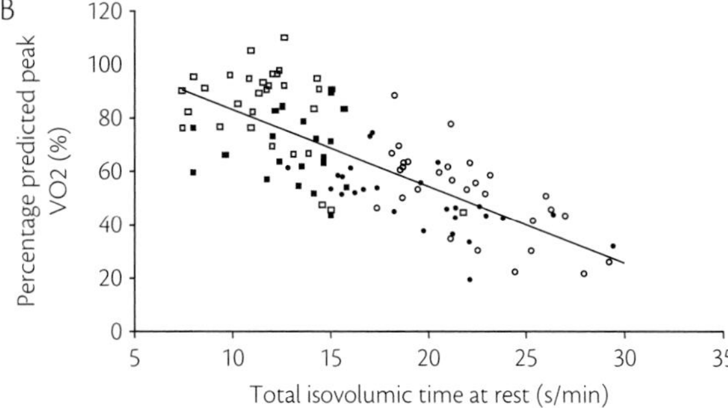

Fig. 19.15 Correlation between total isovolumic time, peak stress cardiac output, and exercise capacity. Top: Correlation between total isovolumic time and peak stress cardiac output. Patients with left bundle branch block (LBBB) and coronary artery disease (CAD) had the lowest cardiac output at peak stress. Bottom: Correlation between total isovolumic time and percentage predicted peak exercise capacity (Vo_2). Patients with (LBBB) had the longest total isovolumic time at rest and the lowest %predicted peak Vo_2, irrespective of whether CAD was present.

From Duncan AM, Francis DP, Henein MY, Gibson DG. Limitation of cardiac output by total isovolumic time during pharmacologic stress in patients with dilated cardiomyopathy: activation-mediated effects of left bundle branch block and coronary artery disease. *J Am Coll Cardiol* 2003;**41**:121–8, and Duncan A, Francis D, Gibson D, Henein M. Limitation of exercise tolerance in chronic heart failure: distinct effects of left bundle branch block and coronary artery disease. *J Am Coll Cardiol* 2004;**43**:1524–31, with permission

(regional dyssynchrony) not only needs to be present, but such regional dyssynchrony should also be haemodynamically limiting (i.e. result in global dyssynchrony). Indeed, patients with the most global dyssynchrony (long total isovolumic time >15 s/min and/or long interventricular delay >40 ms, as measured by the electromechanical delay between the right and left pre-ejection periods), have been shown to demonstrate significant clinical response to CRT.[54,58] Most studies, however, have concentrated on regional assessment of intraventricular dyssynchrony.

Echo markers of intraventricular dyssynchrony

Intraventricular dyssynchrony may be measured using a variety of echo techniques (M-mode, tissue Doppler, tissue tracking, and three-dimensional imaging). Although the assessment of regional dyssynchrony has gained great impetus in the literature in recent years, the relation between specific areas of regional dyssynchrony and their effect on global dyssynchrony, particularly during exercise, remains undefined. Moreover, since the publication of the PROSPECT trial, the reproducibility of various echo techniques for quantifying intraventricular dyssynchrony across different echo institutions has been seriously questioned.[60] Despite difficulties with reproducibility, multiple methods for assessing intraventricular dyssynchrony are quoted in the literature, including:

- septal–posterior delay >130 ms, as measured by M-mode[61]
- septal–posterior wall delay >65 ms, as measured by tissue Doppler (Fig. 19.16a)[62]
- systolic dyssynchrony index >33 ms, as measured by tissue Doppler (Fig. 19.16b)[63]
- anterior-septal to posterior wall peak strain >130 ms, as measured by tissue tracking[64]
- systolic dyssynchrony index >5%, as measured by three-dimensional endocardial border detection and segmental volume analysis.[65]

Assuming it is useful to use an echo-derived mechanical index to decide whether a patient should have CRT, and despite reported difficulties with the reproducibility of assessment of regional left ventricular dyssynchrony using techniques such as described above, determining the precise site of mechanical delay, especially if epicardial lead placement is being considered, should be useful in a patient being considered for CRT. It would also be helpful in

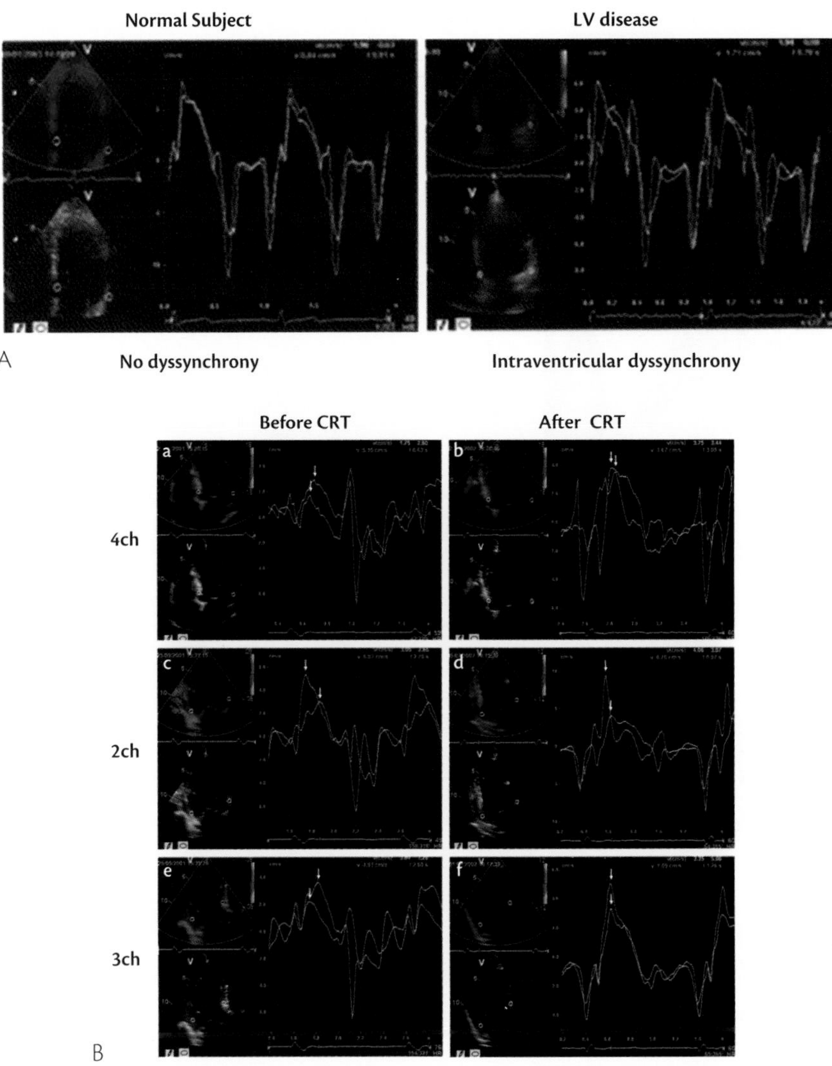

Fig. 19.16 Use of tissue Doppler in assessment of dyssynchrony. (A) Septal—lateral delay >65 ms. Left: Normal subject with no intraventricular dyssynchrony between septum (yellow curve) and lateral wall (green curve). Right: Severe intraventricular dyssynchrony between the septum and lateral wall. (B) Dyssynchrony Index from 12 segments >33 ms. A patient with left ventricular mechanical dyssynchrony in multiple segments before (panels a, c, e) and after (panels b, d, f) CRT. Before CRT, the apical four-chamber view (a) shows only mild delay of basal lateral segment over the basal septal segment of 30 ms. In the apical two-chamber view (c), there was severe delay in the basal inferior wall over the basal anterior wall of 130 ms which was significantly improved after CRT (d). In the apical long axis view (e), the basal posterior wall was delayed over the basal anteroseptal wall of 90 ms which was totally abolished after CRT (f). The peak systolic velocity during the ejection phase in each view is shown by the arrows.

(A) From Bax JJ, Ansalone G, Breithardt OA, *et al.* Echocardiographic evaluation of cardiac resynchronization therapy: ready for routine clinical use? A critical appraisal. *J Am Coll Cardiol* 2004;**44**:1–9, with permission; (B) Wth permission from Yu CM, Bax JJ, Monaghan M, Nihoyannopoulos P. Echocardiographic evaluation of cardiac dyssynchrony for predicting a favourable response to cardiac resynchronisation therapy. *Heart* 2004;**90**:17–22.

confirming that mechanical dyssynchrony is indeed the cause of a reduction in global left ventricular synchrony. Thus, when considering which echo index of dyssynchrony to use, a combination of both segmental and global measures is likely to produce the most useful information on both the degree and severity of mechanical dyssynchrony and its consequences on global left ventricular function. However, echo indices of dyssynchrony will only become credible and applicable after they have been shown to be predictive in large prospective randomized trials.

Pacing optimization

Continued presystolic mitral regurgitation in patients after implantation of a DDD or CRT pacing device(see Chapters 48 and 49) is associated with little or no clinical improvement. Echo Doppler techniques may be used to optimize the delay between pacing the right atrium and right ventricle (AV delay) in order to shorten or remove presystolic mitral regurgitation and thereby increase left ventricular filling time (Fig. 19.17).

The aim is to choose the shortest AV delay that still allows complete left ventricular filling by either the iterative method (whereby a long AV delay (e.g. 150 ms) is programmed on the pacemaker, the AV delay is then shortened in 20 ms stages until the A wave starts to be truncated, then the AV delay is gradually extended by 10-ms steps until the A wave is just complete) or the Ritter method (whereby a short AV delay (e.g. 50 ms) is programmed and the time from start QRS to end of A wave is measured (QAshort), then a long AV delay (e.g. 150 ms) is programmed and the time from start QRS to end of A wave (QAlong) is measured;

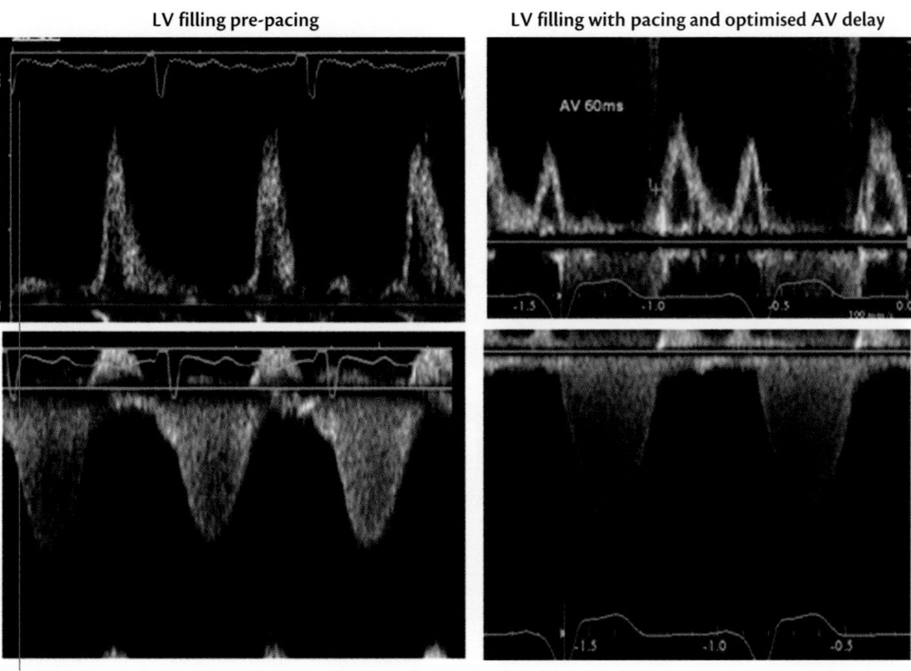

Fig. 19.17 Effect of pacing on left ventricular filling time when left ventricular filling limited by presystolic mitral regurgitation. Left: short left ventricular filling time before pacing due to pre-systolic mitral regurgitation. Right: after pacing and shortening the atrioventricular delay, the presystolic component of mitral regurgitation is removed, allowing significant increase in left ventricular filling time.

the optimal delay is then calculated as 'AVlong delay +QAlong – QAshort'). In theory, optimization of delay between pacing left and right ventricles (VV delay) with atriobiventricular pacemakers is possible, but no morbidity or mortality benefit has been documented for any of this. Moreover, optimization of pacemaker settings at rest takes no account of haemodynamic changes that occur during exercise or stress, which remains a major limitation of this technique.

Revascularization (viable myocardium)

Stunned or hibernating myocardium denotes viable but dysfunctional tissue. Increasing myocardial oxygen demand by stressing the heart with pharmacological agents (dobutamine or dipyridamole) can identify segments that are viable and potentially functional by inducing them to contract. Traditionally this requires qualitative assessment of wall motion score (whereby an akinetic segment becomes hypokinetic, or a hypokinetic segment thickens normally during low dose stress and then deteriorates again at high dose (biphasic response;[66] similar abnormalities may be quantitatively demonstrated using M-mode techniques, Fig. 19.18).[67]

Mitral valve surgery

'Functional' mitral regurgitation is multifactorial in patients with HF, and may be due to dilatation of the mitral annulus, malcoaptation of the mitral valve leaflets, and/or tethering of the mitral valve leaflets from remodelling-induced displacement of one or both papillary muscles. Physiological stress echo may be useful in planning mitral valve repair, particularly when combined with three-dimensional assessment during stress, since surgery has demonstrated efficacy even in advanced HF.[68]

Ventricular assist devices

Ventricular assist devices (a left ventricular assist device, LVAD or biventricular assist device, bi-VAD) are commonly used as bridges to heart transplantation or ventricular recovery. The pump sucks from the ventricle and ejects directly into the aorta, thus reducing wall stress and allowing the myocardium to recover. Echo can detect significant valvular disease, intracardiac shunts, significant right ventricular disease, or pulmonary hypertension preoperatively, and thrombus formation within the VAD or other causes of inflow cannula obstruction postoperatively.

Transplant

Many attempts have been made to assess the echocardiographic predictors of acute rejection, as the noninvasive diagnosis of episodes of rejection might obviate the need for repeated myocardial biopsy. Echocardiographic changes associated with rejection after cardiac transplantation include an increase in posterior wall thickness, an increase in left ventricular mass, and a decrease in diastolic compliance, with associated development of a restrictive mitral

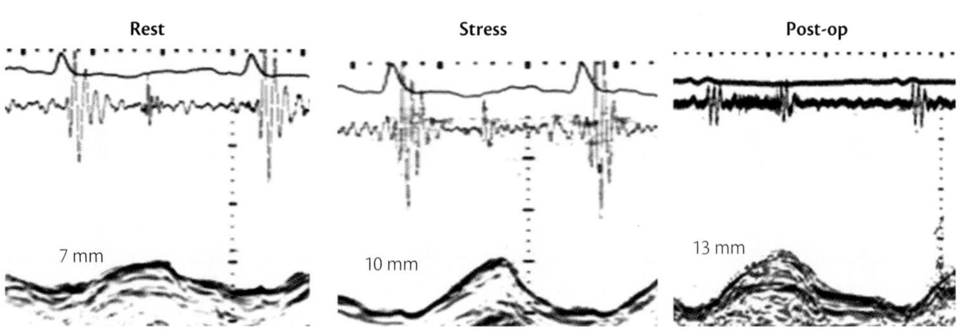

Fig. 19.18 Improved left ventricular long axis amplitude with stress predicts viable myocardium. Long axis M-mode recordings of lateral wall. There is a 30% increase in systolic amplitude with stress, suggesting the presence of viable myocardium, which was confirmed by significant increase in long axis amplitude at rest after revascularization.

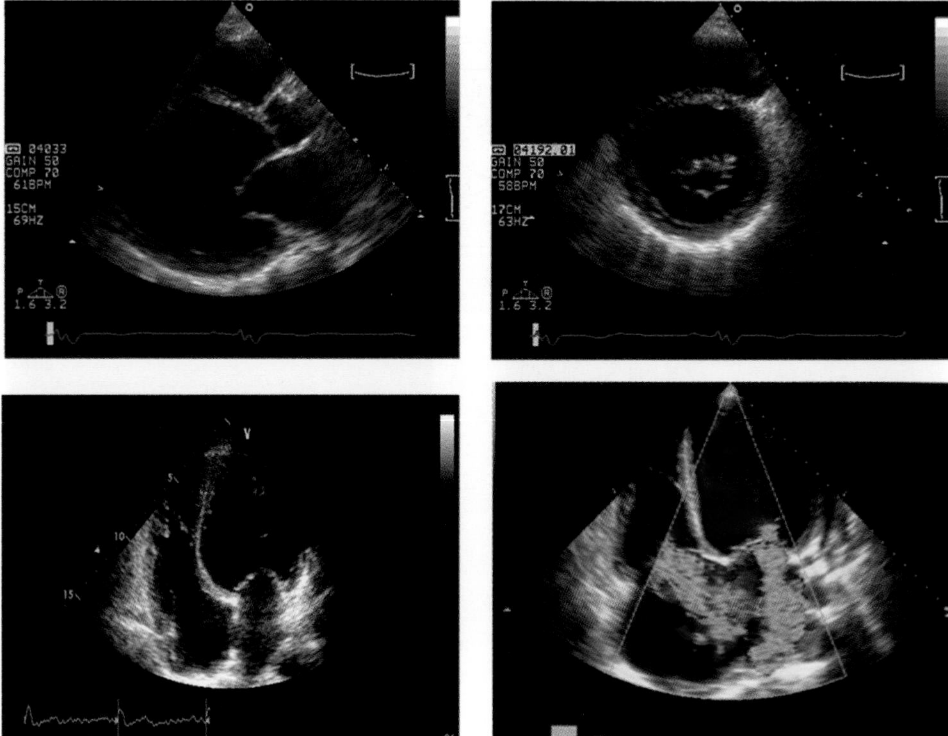

Fig. 19.19 Echo features of dilated cardiomyopathy. Top left: parasternal long axis view showing dilated left ventricular cavity size and tenting of mitral valve. Top right: parasternal short-axis view. Bottom left: spherical left ventricular with hypokinetic septum and dilated right ventricle. Bottom right: significant mitral and tricuspid regurgitation.

inflow pattern. Unfortunately, most of these changes indicate advanced rejection and therefore are of limited use as screening tools.

Specific echo findings in cardiomyopathies

Dilated cardiomyopathy

Echocardiographic findings in dilated cardiomyopathy include left ventricular dilatation, increased left ventricular end-diastolic volume, LVEF less than 40%, functional mitral regurgitation to varying degrees (Fig. 19.19), reduced left ventricular long axis amplitude, global and regional dyssynchrony, and pulmonary hypertension. There is no definite echocardiographic picture that differentiates different stages, but as the left ventricle becomes more dilated, wall stress increases (Laplace's law), resulting in both increased sphericity and myocardial oxygen consumption. RWMA are not specific to ischaemic cardiomyopathy and may be present in idiopathic cardiomypathy; dobutamine stress echo may be useful in differentiating between the two.[67]

The presence of right ventricular enlargement and dysfunction is variable but a poor prognostic sign if present. Tricuspid regurgitation is common and varies in severity.

The left ventricular filling pattern is highly variable in dilated cardiomyopathy, whether idiopathic or ischaemic. The early diastolic E wave is often dominant, and is associated with a short isovolumic relaxation time and a third heart sound which strongly suggests elevated LVEDP. Alternatively, ventricular filling may occur entirely during atrial systole, and be associated with a long isovolumic relaxation time and a fourth heart sound, which strongly suggests low or normal LVEDP. Finally, with sinus tachycardia, filling time at rest may be so short that only a single filling peak is recorded, consisting of superimposed E and A waves, and accompanied by a summation gallop. As discussed above, left ventricular filling time may be shortened even further during stress, and may become the rate-limiting step during exercise.

Hypertrophic cardiomyopathy

The echo pattern in hypertrophic cardiomyopathy is highly variable; there may be disproportionate septal hypertrophy in relation to the left ventricle posterior wall (ratio > 1.3:1.0), concentric LVH, in which the septal and posterior walls are equal in thickness, or hypertrophy confirmed to the apical segments. Significant left ventricular outflow tract obstruction is usual if asymmetric septal hypertrophy and systolic anterior motion of the mitral valve (SAM) are present (Fig. 19.20), but midcavity obstruction is also common, particularly when there is concentric LVH and the patient is hypovolaemic or on inotropes. Colour Doppler is useful for identifying the level of obstruction.

Left ventricular noncompaction

This is an inherited condition characterized by marked trabeculation, usually within the left ventricular apex. LVEF may be reduced, and areas of noncompaction may become substrates for left-sided thrombi and arrhythmias. To identify noncompaction, left-sided contrast agents are usually required. In apical views the trabeculation is usually seen as a partially contrast-filled layer. A ratio of >2:1 noncompacted (trabeculations) myocardium to compacted (normal) myocardium at end systole suggests left ventricular noncompaction.

Restrictive cardiomyopathy

Restrictive cardiomyopathy is a group of disorders characterized by limitation of left ventricular filling caused by increased left ventricular stiffness (decreased left ventricular compliance) during mid and late diastole. Amyloid infiltration is present in about half of these cases, and the aetiology is often undefined in the remainder.

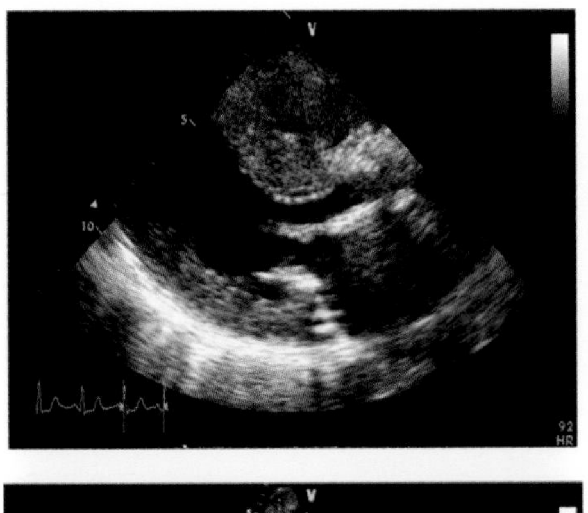

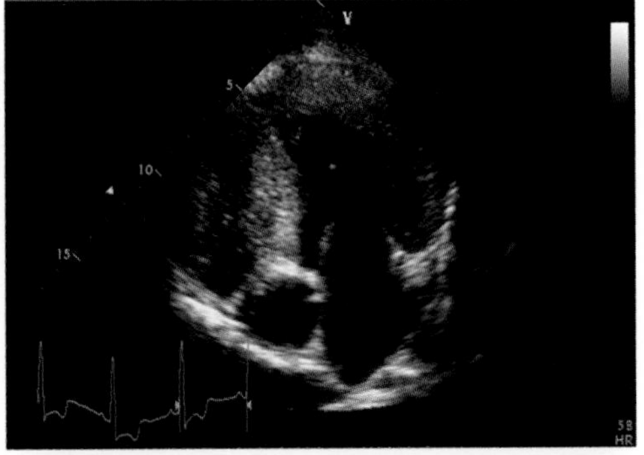

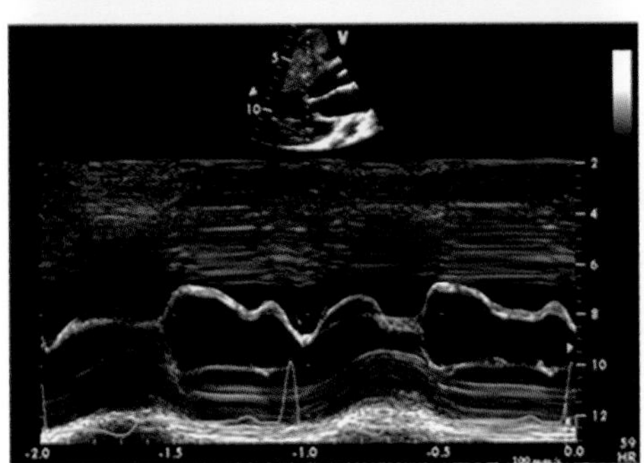

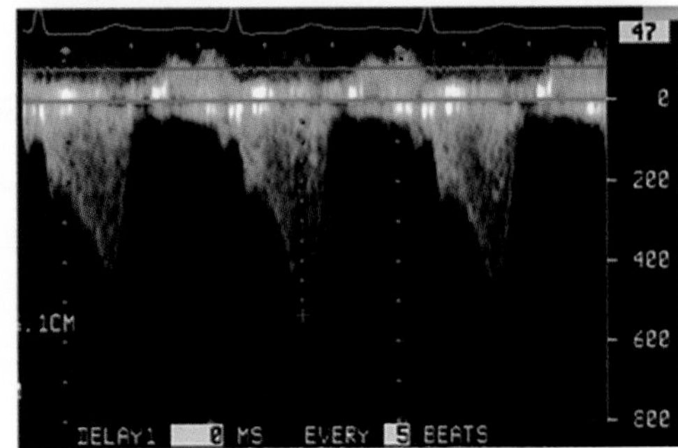

Fig. 19.20 Echo features of hypertrophic cardiomyopathy. Top left: Concentric left ventricular hypertrophy, with narrowing of left ventricular outflow tract. Top right: biventricular hypertrophy. Bottom left: systolic anterior motion of the mitral valve (SAM) detected readily by M-mode. Bottom right: significant left ventricular outflow tract obstruction, with velocity reaching 6 m/s. Symptoms of breathlessness may be due to dynamic left ventricular outflow tract obstruction or abnormal left ventricular diastolic function (usually prolonged isovolumic relation time, decrease in the rate of early diastolic filling, and increase in the atrial component of left ventricular filling).

Left ventricular cavity size is usually normal, although LVEF may be significantly reduced. Biatrial enlargement is usually present and peak inflow velocity during early diastole is often normal, but its duration is short, so acceleration and deceleration times are reduced, reflecting the combined effects of increased myocardial stiffness and a high left atrial pressure.[43] Restrictive filling does not represent a specific diagnosis, as patients with dilated cardiomyopathy or severe LVH may show restrictive physiology. Regardless of the underlying aetiology, these features regress when the left atrial pressure falls.

Right ventricular function

Right ventricular function has significant clinical relevance since it is highly related to prognosis[69] and has an important role in determining exercise capacity.[70] Assessing the size of the right ventricle may be difficult, because of its complex shape, but measuring end-diastolic length, the diameter at midcavity, and the diameter of the tricuspid annulus usually suffice (the latter should be <40 mm). Right ventricular function is assessed qualitatively and quantitatively, the latter by measuring tricuspid annular motion using M-mode (normal right ventricular amplitude is 15–20 mm in the absence of severe tricuspid regurgitation or pulmonary hypertension).

Identifying right ventricular pressure or volume overload can aid clinical assessment of right heart function. Although often considered together, they usually represent two different initial pathologies; right ventricular volume overload suggests right-sided valvular regurgitation or a right-to-left shunt. Pressure overload suggests pulmonary hypertension or pulmonary stenosis. Pressure overload can develop from volume overload, and occasionally vice versa, in which case features of both will be present. Assessing right ventricular size, free wall thickness, and septal motion are key since volume overload usually leads to increased cavity size and pressure overload usually leads to increased wall thickness (though the two findings may coexist), and volume overload is related to a flattened septum in diastole, whereas pressure overload is associated with a flattened septum in both systole and diastole.

Severe tricuspid regurgitation may be present in late left ventricular disease or if the primary pathology involves the right ventricle. In this case, the right atrium and right ventricle are usually both dilated, the right atrial pressure is increased, and the peak right AV pressure drop declines. The decline in pressure drop should not be taken as a sign of reduction in pulmonary artery pressure, particularly in patients who show clinical deterioration, but as a sign of increasing right atrial pressure. Restrictive right ventricular filling physiology is associated with poor prognosis in a fashion similar to left ventricular haemodynamics.

Chronic constrictive pericarditis

A rare, but clinically important, cause of HF is pericardial disease, and chronic constrictive pericarditis is an example of pure diastolic HF with a low cardiac output state. It is characterized by a thickened, adherent pericardium (Fig. 19.21) that restricts ventricular filling and limits chamber expansion and maximal diastolic volumes. Elevated filling pressures are required to maintain adequate cardiac output. End-diastolic pressures in all heart chambers are usually elevated and equalized. Compensatory mechanisms are activated but may ultimately fail, leading to elevated venous pressure, salt and water retention, and reduced cardiac output.

The clinical similarity between constrictive pericarditis and restrictive cardiomyopathy may make the differential diagnosis difficult in some cases, since both have stiff and incompliant left ventricle in late diastole and the left ventricle is unable to fill without a significant rise in LVEDP. However, constrictive pericarditis is an extracardiac constraint while restrictive cardiomyopathy is an intrinsic disease of the myocardium. Thus motion of the ventricular long axes and associated influence on vena caval flow help differentiate between the two conditions.

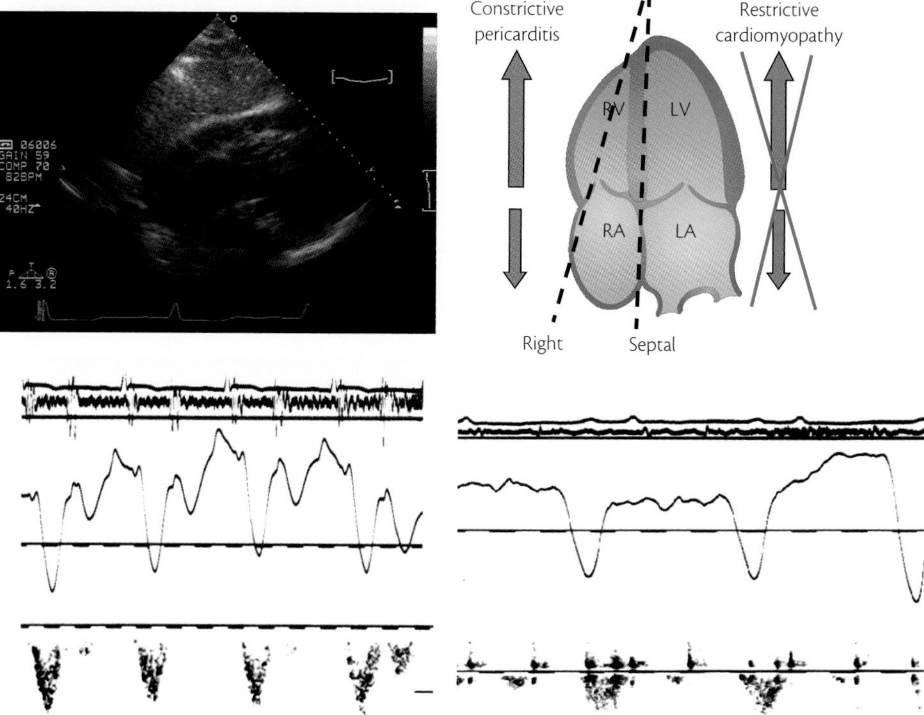

Fig. 19.21 Pathophysiology of pericardial constriction. Top left: subcostal view of pericardial adhesions between right ventricular/right atrial free wall and the visceral pericardium. Top right: in constrictive pericarditis, long axis function is maintained but is reduced in restrictive cardiomyopathy. Bottom left: apical systolic movement of right ventricular long axis corresponds to deep X descent in constrictive pericarditis (corresponding to systolic descent on superior vena cava flow). Bottom right: lack of apical systolic movement of right ventricular long axis reduces X descent on jugular venous pressure and produces dominant Y descent (corresponding to diastolic descent on superior vena cava flow).

Conclusion

Echocardiography is the single most useful noninvasive imaging tool in the HF population. It readily identifies patterns of disease, rapidly differentiating myocardial from structural or pericardial heart disease, and the dilated left ventricle from the hypertrophied left ventricle in a widely available clinical setting. More subtle echo techniques quantify the degree of left ventricular impairment, determine the presence of RWMA, differentiate restrictive left ventricular physiology from reduced early diastolic filling rates, quantify the degree of functional mitral regurgitation and pulmonary hypertension, identify occult right ventricular disease, and define the effects of abnormal activation on ventricular function. Echocardiography not only provides insights into the pathophysiological mechanisms underlying the various aetiologies of HF, but also identifies patients at high risk for cardiovascular morbidity and mortality and provides important data for therapeutic decision-making, including defining candidacy for medications, implantable cardiac devices, surgical procedures, and resynchronization. Thus, echocardiography continues to play a central role in the diagnosis and management of patients with HF.

References

1. Cowie MR, Wood DA, Coats AJ, *et al.* Incidence, aetiology of heart failure; a population-based study. *Eur Heart J* 1999;**20**:421–8.
2. Senni M, Rodeheffer RJ, Tribouilloy CM, *et al.* Use of echocardiography in the management of congestive heart failure in the community. *J Am Coll Cardiol* 1999;**33**:164–70.
3. National Institute for Clinical Excellence. *Management of chronic heart failure in adults in primary and secondary care. NICE Guideline No 5.* July 2003. Available at www.nice.org.uk
4. Hunt SA, Abraham WT, Chin MH, *et al.* ACC/AHA 2005 guideline update for the diagnosis and management of chronic heart failure in the adult: summary article: a report of the American College of Cardiology/American Heart Association Task Force on Practice Guidelines (Writing Committee to Update the 2001 Guidelines for the Evaluation and Management of Heart Failure). *J Am Coll Cardiol* 2005;**46**:e1–82.
5. Lang RM, Bierig M, Devereaux RB, *et al.* Recommendations for chamber quantification. *J Am Soc Echocardiogr* 2005;**18**:1440–63.
6. Jacobs LD, Salgo IS, Goonewardena S, *et al.* Rapid online quantification of left ventricular volume from real-time three-dimensional echocardiographic data. *Eur Heart J* 2006;**27**:460–8.
7. Franciosa JA, Park M, Levine TB. Lack of correlation between exercise capacity and indexes of resting left ventricular performance in heart failure. *Am J Cardiol* 1981;**47**:33–9.
8. Edner M, Bonarjee VV, Nilsen DW, Berning J, Carstensen S, Caidahl K. Effect of enalapril initiated early after acute myocardial infarction on heart failure parameters, with reference to clinical class and echocardiographic determinants. CONSENSUS II Multi-Echo Study Group. *Clin Cardiol* 1996;**19**:543–8.
9. The Cardiac Insufficiency Bisoprolol Study II (CIBIS-II): a randomised trial. *Lancet* 1999;**353**:9–13.
10. Pitt B, Zannad F, Remme WJ, Cody R, Castaigne A, Perez A, Palensky J, Wittes J. The effect of spironolactone on morbidity and mortality in patients with severe heart failure. Randomized Aldactone Evaluation Study Investigators. *N Engl J Med* 1999;**341**:709–17.
11. Moss AJ, Hall WJ, Cannom DS, *et al.* and MADIT Investigators. Improved survival with an implanted defibrillator in patients with coronary disease at high risk for ventricular arrhythmia. *N Engl J Med* 1996;**335:**1933–40.
12. Lee R, Marwick TH. Assessment of subclinical left ventricular dysfunction in asymptomatic mitral regurgitation. *Eur J Echocardiogr* 2007;**8**:175–84.
13. Sutton MSJ, Pfeffer MA, Plappert T, *et al.*, for the SAVE Investigators. Quantitative two-dimensional echocardiographic measurements are major predictors of adverse cardiovascular events after acute myocardial infarction. The protective effects of captopril. *Circulation* 1994;**89**:68–75.
14. Quinones MA, Breenberg BH, Kopelen HA, *et al.*, for the SOLVD Investigators. Echocardiogaphic predictors of clinical outcomes in

patients with left ventricular dysfunction enrolled in the SOLVD registry and trials: significance of left ventricular hypertrophy. *J Am Coll Cardiol* 2005;**35**:1237–44.

15. Devereux R, Reichek N. Echocardiographic determination of left ventricular mass in man. *Circulation* 1977;**55**:613–18.
16. Chen C, Rodriguez L, Lethor JP, *et al.* Continuous wave Doppler echocardiography for non-invasive assessment of left ventricular dP/dt and relaxation time constant from mitral regurgitant spectra in patients. *J Am Coll Cardiol* 1994;**23**:970–976.
17. Xiao HB, Brecker SJ, Gibson DG. Effects of abnormal activation on the time course of the left ventricular pressure pulse in dilated cardiomopathy. *Br Heart J* 1992;**68**:403–7.
18. Schiller NB, Shah PM, Crawford M, *et al.* Recommendations for quantitation of the left ventricle by two-dimensional echocardiography. *J Am Soc Echocardiogr* 1989;**2**:258–267.
19. Lang RM, Bierig M, Devereux RB, *et al.* American Society of Echocardiography's Nomenclature and Standards Committee; Task Force on Chamber Quantification; American College of Cardiology Echocardiography Committee; American Heart Association; European Association of Echocardiography, European Society of Cardiology. Recommendations for chamber quantification. *Eur J Echocardiogr* 2006;**7**:79–108.
20. Nishimura RA, Tajik AJ, Shub C, Miller FA Jr, Ilstrup DM, Harrison CE. Role of two-dimensional echocardiography in the prediction of in-hospital complications after acute myocardial infarction. *J Am Coll Cardiol* 1984;**4**:1080–7.
21. O'Sullivan CA, Ramzy IS, Li W, *et al.* The effect of the localization of Q wave myocardial infarction on ventricular electromechanics. *Int J Cardiol* 2002;**84**:241–7.
22. Yip G, Wang M, Zhang Y, Fung JW, Ho PY, Sanderson JE. Left ventricular long axis function in diastolic heart failure is reduced in both diastole and systole: time for a redefinition?. *Heart* 2002;**87**:121–5.
23. Yu CM, Lin H, Yang H, Kong SL, Zhang Q, Lee SW. Progression of systolic abnormalities in patients with 'isolated' diastolic heart failure and diastolic dysfunction. *Circulation* 2002;**105**:1195–201.
24. Tan YT, Wenzelburger F, Lee E, *et al.* The pathophysiology of heart failure with normal ejection fraction: exercise echocardiography reveals complex abnormalities of both systolic and diastolic ventricular function involving torsion, untwist, and longitudinal motion. *J Am Coll Cardiol* 2009;**54**:36–46.
25. Nishikage T, Nakai H, Lang RM, Takeuchi M. Subclinical left ventricular longitudinal systolic dysfunction in hypertension with no evidence of heart failure. *Circ J* 2008;**72**:189–94.
26. Ha JW, Lee HC, Kang ES, *et al.* Abnormal left ventricular longitudinal functional reserve in patients with diabetes mellitus: implication for detecting subclinical myocardial dysfunction using exercise tissue Doppler echocardiography. *Heart* 2007;**93**:1571–6.
27. Pai RG, Bodenheimer MM, Pai SM, Koss JH, Adamick RD. Usefulness of systolic excursion of the mitral anulus as an index of left ventricular systolic function. *Am J Cardiol.* 1991;**67**:222–4.
28. Sveälv BG, Olofsson EL, Andersson B. Ventricular long-axis function is of major importance for long-term survival in patients with heart failure. *Heart* 2008;**94**:284–9.
29. Artis NJ, Oxborough DL, Williams G, Pepper CB, Tan LB. Two-dimensional strain imaging: a new echocardiographic advance with research and clinical applications. *Int J Cardiol* 2008;**123**:240–8.
30. Adamu U, Schmitz F, Becker M, Kelm M, Hoffmann R. Advanced speckle tracking echocardiography allowing a three-myocardial layer-specific analysis of deformation parameters. *Eur J Echocardiogr* 2009;**10**:303–8.
31. S gaard P, Egeblad H, Kim WY, *et al.* Tissue Doppler imaging predicts improved systolic performance and reversed left ventricular remodeling during long-term cardiac resynchronization therapy. *J Am Coll Cardiol* 2002;**40**:723–30.
32. Franklin KM, Aurigemma GP. Prognosis in diastolic heart failure. *Prog Cardiovasc Dis* 2005;**47**:333–9.
33. Henein MY, Gibson DG. Suppression of left ventricular early diastolic filling by long axis asynchrony. *Br Heart J* 1995;**73**(2):151–7.
34. Henein MY, Das SK, O'Sullivan C, Kakkar VV, Gillbe CE, Gibson DG. ACE inhibitors unmask incoordinate diastolic wall motion in restrictive left ventricular disease. *Heart* 1996;**75**:151–8.
35. Henein MY, Priestley K, Davarashvili T, Buller N, Gibson DG. Early changes in left ventricular subendocardial function after successful coronary angioplasty. *Br Heart J* 1993;**69**:501–6.
36. Duncan AM, O'Sullivan CA, Carr-White GS, Gibson DG, Henein MY. Long axis electromechanics during dobutamine stress in patients with coronary artery disease and left ventricular dysfunction. *Heart* 2001;**86**:397–404.
37. Xiao HB, Lee CH, Gibson DG. Effect of left bundle branch block on diastolic function in dilated cardiomyopathy. *Br Heart J* 1991;**66**:443–7.
38. Pinamonti B, Zecchin M, Di Lenarda A, Gregori D, Sinagra G, Camerini F. Persistence of restrictive left ventricular filling pattern in dilated cardiomyopathy: an ominous prognostic sign. *J Am Coll Cardiol* 1997;**29**:604–12.
39. Duncan AM, Lim E, Gibson DG, Henein MY. Effect of dobutamine stress on left ventricular filling in ischemic dilated cardiomyopathy: pathophysiology and prognostic implications. *J Am Coll Cardiol* 2005;**46**:488–96.
40. Ommen SR, Nishimura RA, Appleton CP, *et al.* Clinical utility of Doppler echocardiography and tissue Doppler imaging in the estimation of left ventricular filling pressures: a comparative simultaneous Doppler catheterization study. *Circulation* 2000;**102**:1788–94.
41. Garcia MJ, Ares MA, Asher C, Rodriguez L, Vandervoort P, Thomas JD. An index of early left ventricular filling that combined with pulsed Doppler peak E velocity may estimate capillary wedge pressure. *J Am Coll Cardiol* 1997;**29**:448–54.
42. Mullens W, Borowski AG, Curtin RJ, Thomas JD, Tang WH. Tissue Doppler imaging in the estimation of intracardiac filling pressure in decompensated patients with advanced systolic heart failure. *Circulation* 2009;**119**:62–70.
43. Garcia MJ, Smedira NG, Greenberg NL, *et al.* Color M-mode Doppler flow propagation velocity is a preload insensitive index of left ventricular relaxation: animal and human validation. *J Am Coll Cardiol* 2000;**35**:201–8.
44. Takemoto Y, Barnes ME, Seward JB, *et al.* Usefulness of left atrial volume in predicting first congestive heart failure in patients ≥65 years of age with well-preserved left ventricular systolic function. *Am J Cardiol* 2005;**96**:832–6.
45. Rossi A, Loredana L, Cicoira M, *et al.* Additional value of pulmonary vein parameters in defining pseudonormalization of mitral inflow pattern. *Echocardiography* 2001;**18**:673–9.
46. Sorrell VL, Reeves WC. Noninvasive right and left heart catheterization. *Echocardiography* 2001;**18**:31–41.
47. Xiao HB, Brecker SJ, Gibson DG. Effects of abnormal activation on the time course of the left ventricular pressure pulse in dilated cardiomyopathy. *Br Heart J* 1992;**68**:403–7.
48. Tei C. New non-invasive index for combined systolic and diastolic ventricular function. *J Cardiol* 1995;**26**:135–6.
49. Duncan A, Francis D, Henein Y, Gibson D. Importance of left ventricular activation in determining myocardial performance (Tei) index: comparison with total isovolumic time. *Int J Cardiol* 2004;**95**:211–17.
50. Duncan A, O'Sullivan C, Gibson D, Henein M. Electromechanical interrelations during dobutamine stress in normal subjects and patients with coronary disease: comparison of changes in activation and inotropic state. *Heart* 2001;**85**:411–16.
51. Duncan A, Wait D, Gibson D, Daubert J. Left ventricular remodelling and haemodynamic effects of multisite biventricular pacing in patients

with congestive heart failure and activation disturbances. *Eur Heart J* 2003;**24**:430–41.

52. Duncan AM, Francis DP, Henein MY, Gibson DG. Limitation of cardiac output by total isovolumic time during pharmacologic stress in patients with dilated cardiomyopathy: activation-mediated effects of left bundle branch block and coronary artery disease. *J Am Coll Cardiol* 2003;**41**:121–8.
53. Duncan A, Francis D, Gibson D, Henein M. Limitation of exercise tolerance in chronic heart failure: distinct effects of left bundle branch block and coronary artery disease. *J Am Coll Cardiol* 2004;**43**:1524–31.
54. Duncan AM, Lim E, Clague J, Gibson D, Henein M. Predicting response to cardiac resynchronization therapy: comparison of segmental and global markers of dyssynchrony. *Eur Heart J* 2006;**27**:2426–32.
55. Youssef G, Links M. The prevention and management of cardiovascular complications of chemotherapy in patients with cancer. *Am J Cardiovasc Drugs* 2005;**5**:233–43.
56. Cazeau S, Leclercq M, Lavergne T, *et al.* for the MUltisite STimulation In Cardiomyopathies (MUSTIC) Study Investigators. Effects of multisite biventricular pacing in patients with heart failure and intraventricular conduction delay. *N Engl J Med* 2001;**344**:873–80.
57. Abraham WT, Fisher WG, Smith AL, *et al.* for the MIRACLE Study Group. Cardiac resynchronization in chronic heart failure. *N Engl J Med* 2002;**346**:1845–53.
58. Cleland JG, Daubert JC, Erdmann E, *et al.* Cardiac Resynchronization-Heart Failure (CARE-HF) Study Investigators. The effect of cardiac resynchronization on morbidity and mortality in heart failure. *N Engl J Med* 2005;**352**:1539–49.
59. Hawkins NM, Petrie MC, MacDonald MR, Hogg KJ, McMurray JV. Selecting patients for cardiac resynchronization therapy: electrical or mechanical dyssynchrony?. *Eur Heart J* 2006;**27**:1270–81.
60. Chung ES, Leon AR, Tavazzi L, *et al.* Results of the Predictors of Response to CRT (PROSPECT) trial. *Circulation* 2008;**117**:2608–16.
61. Pitzalis MV, Iacoviello M, Romito R, *et al.* Ventricular asynchrony predicts a better outcome in patients with chronic heart failure receiving cardiac resynchronization therapy. *J Am Coll Cardiol* 2005;**45**:65–9.
62. Bax JJ, Ansalone G, Breithardt OA, *et al.* Echocardiographic evaluation of cardiac resynchronization therapy: ready for routine clinical use? A critical appraisal. *J Am Coll Cardiol* 2004;**44**:1–9.
63. Yu CM, Bax JJ, Monaghan M, Nihoyannopoulos P. Echocardiographic evaluation of cardiac dyssynchrony for predicting a favourable response to cardiac resynchronisation therapy. *Heart* 2004;**90**:17–22.
64. Suffoletto MS, Dohi K, Cannesson M, Saba S, Gorcsan J 3rd. Novel speckle-tracking radial strain from routine black-and-white echocardiographic images to quantify dyssynchrony and predict response to cardiac resynchronization therapy. *Circulation* 2006;**113**:960–8.
65. Kapetanakis S, Kearney MT, Siva A, Gall N, Cooklin M, Monaghan MJ. Real-time three-dimensional echocardiography: a novel technique to quantify global left ventricular mechanical dyssynchrony. *Circulation* 2005;**112**:992–1000.
66. Picano E, Sicari R, Landi P, *et al.* Prognostic value of myocardial viability in medically treated patients with global left ventricular dysfunction early after an acute uncomplicated myocardial infarction: a dobutamine stress echocardiographic study. *Circulation* 1998;98:1078–84.
67. Duncan AM, Francis DP, Gibson DG, Henein MY. Differentiation of ischemic from nonischemic cardiomyopathy during dobutamine stress by left ventricular long-axis function: additional effect of left bundle-branch block. *Circulation* 2003;**108**:1214–20.
68. Bolling SF, Pagani FD, Deeb GM, Bach DS. Intermediate-term outcome of mitral reconstruction in cardiomyopathy. *J Thorac Cardiovasc Surg* 1998;**115**:381–6.
69. Ghio S, Gavazzi A, Campana C, *et al.* Independent and additive prognostic value of right ventricular systolic function and pulmonary artery pressure in patients with chronic heart failure. *J Am Coll Cardiol* 2001;37:183–8.
70. Webb-Peploe KM, Henein MY, Coats AJ, Gibson DG. Echo derived variables predicting exercise tolerance in patients with dilated and poorly functioning left ventricle. *Heart* 1998;**80**:565–9.

20

Nuclear medicine in heart failure

Pushan Bharadwaj and S. Richard Underwood

Introduction

Nuclear medicine, sometimes known as molecular imaging, involves the characterization and measurement of biological processes *in vivo* using small amounts of radiolabelled tracers. It is the most sensitive imaging technique in routine use, providing images of nano- or even picomolar concentrations of the tracer. In patients with heart failure (HF), biological processes such as myocardial perfusion, metabolism (both fatty acid and glucose), injury (including necrosis and apoptosis), and innervation are relevant and can be imaged.

The ideal tracer is a biological molecule labelled with an isotope of one of its constituent elements (carbon, oxygen, nitrogen, etc.), since the tracer will have biological properties identical to those of the natural compound. Such isotopes are positron emitters and are imaged by positron emission tomography (PET), which relies on detecting the synchronous 511-keV photons emitted in opposite directions when the positron annihilates with an electron in the surrounding tissue.

More common tracers use foreign elements such as iodine or technetium bound to a pharmaceutical that provides useful biological properties. These radiopharmaceuticals usually emit single gamma photons that are imaged by a gamma camera, often using single photon emission computed tomography (SPECT) to produce tomograms or three-dimensional images.

PET has some inherent advantages over SPECT, such as higher resolution and more reliable attenuation correction that simplifies quantification of the biological process being imaged. PET is however more expensive and, with the exception of fluorine-18, the very short-lived radionuclides have to be generated on site, requiring the additional expense of a cyclotron.

Nuclear imaging in an acute setting

Myocarditis

Indium-111 antimyosin antibody imaging is very sensitive for the detection of myocarditis.[1] Myocyte necrosis leads to loss of sarcolemmal integrity and exposes insoluble molecules such as the heavy chains of myosin to the radiopharmaceutical, leading to a positive image of necrotic cells. Indium antimyosin has been used to detect cell necrosis in other settings such as acute myocardial infarction and transplant rejection[2] but, regrettably, this agent is no longer commercially available.

Gallium-67 imaging is used to diagnose several chronic inflammatory conditions and fever of unknown origin although it provides a nonspecific signal. It is useful in Lyme myocarditis[3] and in the acute phase of Kawasaki's disease.[4] The incidence of histologically proven myocarditis is low (1.8%) in gallium-negative patients with dilated cardiomyopathy.[5]

Myocardial infarction

After cell death, the cardiac myocyte does not regenerate and contractile loss is permanent.[6] Noninvasive detection of myocardial injury is therefore important and imaging may be useful when ECG changes are absent or biomarkers cannot separate infarction from ischaemia.

Pyrophosphates

Technetium-99m chelates such as pyrophosphates and glucarates have been used in the detection of myocardial infarction. Pyrophosphates accumulate in areas of necrosis through their binding to exposed mitochondrial calcium.[7] A limitation, however, is that a positive signal is seen only after 24 h and up to several days and so the window of opportunity is relatively narrow.

Glucarates

Positively charged histones in the disintegrating nuclei of injured myocytes attract the negatively charged glucarate molecules and allow early imaging of infarction.[8] Animal studies have shown that glucarate is taken up by necrotic and not ischaemic tissue and images can be obtained as early as 1 h in nonreperfused zones.[9] Its rapid blood clearance and early uptake makes technetium-99m glucarate an attractive tool that is currently under investigation.[10]

Nuclear imaging in chronic heart failure

In contrast to acute HF, there are several areas in the management of chronic HF where radionuclide imaging is routine, including diagnosis of the underlying cause in newly presenting HF, assessment of myocardial viability and hibernation in ischaemic heart disease, and investigation before resynchronization pacing and defibrillator implantation.

Ischaemic heart disease

Myocardial perfusion scintigraphy (MPS) is an established and routine technique for the diagnosis of coronary artery disease.[11] There are fewer studies of its diagnostic accuracy in patients with left ventricular dysfunction but the sensitivity in this setting is extremely high.[12] Because nonischaemic myocardial scarring and inducible perfusion abnormalities also occur in primary and secondary muscle disorders, the specificity of the technique is not as high.[13,14] Features that suggest ischaemic heart disease are large areas of either transmural scarring or inducible ischaemia in a coronary distribution, impaired ventricular function in proportion to the loss of viable muscle, and predominant involvement of the left ventricle.

Viability and hibernation

It is important to distinguish between myocardial viability and hibernation. Although these terms are sometimes used interchangeably, they are different entities. Viable myocytes are alive, irrespective of their ability to function, and viable myocardium contains viable myocytes. Viability is not a dichotomy and there is a continuum from fully viable myocardium with no scarring, through partial thickness scarring to transmural scarring.

Hibernation is an ischaemic syndrome whereby viable myocardium loses its ability to contract but is able to recover contractile function once the ischaemia is abolished.[15] Hibernation was initially thought to be the result of reduced resting perfusion with contractile function being reduced in order to rematch oxygen supply and demand.[16] It is now thought to be the result of repetitive episodes of ischaemia and stunning that mimic chronic reduction of function.[17] It is likely that early hibernation is the same phenomenon as repetitive stunning but that changes in myocyte and myocardial structure later develop that may or may not be reversible. Hence, prolonged hibernating myocardium may lose its ability to recover and ultimately its viability through myocyte loss by apoptosis or necrosis.[18,19]

In order to detect hibernating myocardium, all imaging techniques rely upon detecting a triad of signs: viability, function, and ischaemia (Fig. 20.1). The imaging definition of hibernation is therefore muscle that is viable but akinetic and where inducible ischaemia can be demonstrated. Without all three of these markers, even an area of viable but akinetic myocardium is unlikely to be hibernating and it could for instance simply be an area of partial thickness scarring without hibernation where the scarring is sufficient to abolish function.

Several radionuclide techniques can be used to detect myocardial viability and hibernation.[20–22] They rely on the fact that all of the myocardial tracers are taken up only by viable cells, irrespective of the uptake mechanism. Hence, myocardial uptake reflects myocardial viability. In addition, tracers such as thallium-201, technetium-99m MIBI and tetrofosmin, nitrogen-13 ammonia, oxygen-15 water, and rubidium-82 have relatively high extraction and are fixed in the myocyte in proportion to delivery, hence they are dual tracers of viability and perfusion. When perfusion is less than 0.25mL min^{-1} g^{-1} or less than 30% of the blood flow in normal myocardium, recovery of function is unlikely after revascularization.[23] Preserved perfusion in areas of dysfunction indicates stunning.

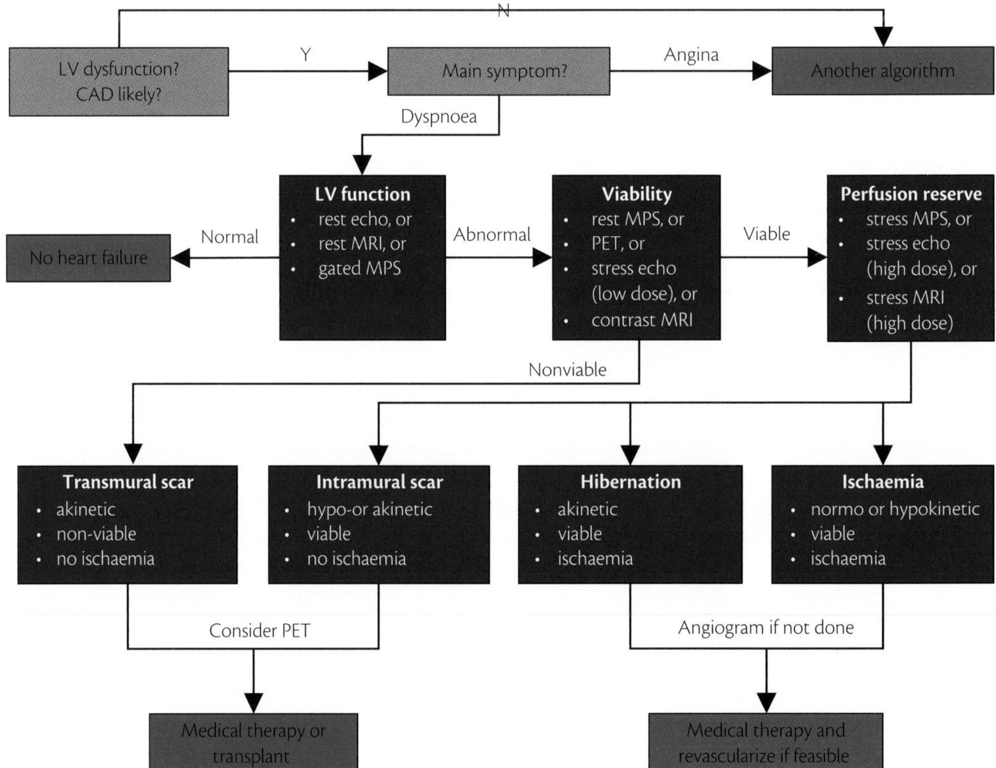

Fig. 20.1 Algorithm for the investigation of patients presenting with possible ischaemic heart disease and heart failure.
From Underwood SR, Bax JJ, vom Dahl J, *et al.* Imaging techniques for the assessment of myocardial hibernation. *Eur Heart J* 2004;**25**:815–36.

Perfusion imaging

Thallium-201

Thallium-201, injected as thallous chloride, is a potassium analogue and its retention is an energy-dependent process reflecting myocyte viability and perfusion.[24] Conventional imaging for the detection of myocardial ischaemia involves injection during stress (dynamic exercise or pharmacological). Imaging within 30 min of this stress injection reflects a combination of myocardial viability and perfusion. After this time, the thallium equilibrates between the intra- and extracellular spaces and takes up a distribution that reflects viability alone, irrespective of perfusion. Defects in the stress images that improve after redistribution, therefore, indicate hypoperfusion at the time of injection, or areas with inducible ischaemia. Redistribution imaging is normally performed 4 h after the stress injection, although imaging up to 24 h allows even better detection of viable myocardium at the expense of lower-quality images as the thallium is excreted.

Using conventional stress-redistribution imaging, areas of dysfunctional muscle with an inducible perfusion abnormality are likely to be hibernating.[25] However, redistribution can be slow and the simple stress-redistribution technique can underestimate myocardial viability.[26] More sensitive techniques involve a further injection of thallium at rest after stress-redistribution imaging (the reinjection technique)[27] or a separate day resting injection of thallium with early and delayed imaging (rest-redistribution) (Fig. 20.2).[28] Resting injections are best given under nitrate cover (e.g. after sublingual glyceryl trinitrate) in order to abolish resting hypoperfusion and to give the best chance of thallium reaching any viable myocyte.

Technetium-99m perfusion tracers

The technetium-based tracers MIBI and tetrofosmin have similar physiological properties to thallium although they have less avid extraction and are trapped within the myocyte and do not redistribute. Separate stress and rest injections are therefore required in order to detect inducible perfusion abnormalities. In contrast, technetium-99m has better imaging characteristics with a higher energy gamma emission (140 keV) and a shorter half-life (6 h). This leads to higher-resolution images, higher injected doses without excessive radiation exposure, and hence easier ECG gating for information on ventricular function.[29] The lack of redistribution means that viable but hypoperfused myocardium can be underestimated[30] and resting injections of MIBI and tetrofosmin should be injected under nitrate cover when assessing viability (Fig. 20.3).[31–34] Clinically relevant viability has been defined as resting MIBI or tetrofosmin uptake of more than 50–60% of maximum but attenuation in regions such as the inferior wall means that a lower threshold may be relevant.[35]

Metabolic imaging

The myocardium is very flexible in choice of substrates for energy production, but β-oxidation of fatty acids and glycolysis are the two main mechanisms of ATP production.[36] Under aerobic conditions, fatty acid oxidation is the pathway of choice but under hypoxic conditions, glucose metabolism predominates because of its greater efficiency.[37]

2-Fluorodeoxyglucose

Fluorine-18 is a positron-emitting radionuclide with a half-life of 110 min and it can therefore be imaged by PET without the need for on-site production. As 2-deoxy-2-(^{18}F)fluoro-D-glucose (FDG) it is widely used in oncology because of the affinity of rapidly dividing cells for the tracer. Uptake depends upon glucose transport, metabolism, and trapping within the cell and so FDG is a marker of glucose metabolism. Because normal myocardial metabolism uses fatty acids, if FDG is injected and imaged under fasting conditions there is no myocardial uptake but areas of glucose uptake indicate areas of current or recent ischaemia that have switched to glucose metabolism.[38] Alternatively, if FDG is injected after a glucose meal or during insulin and glucose infusion myocardial uptake is normal and defects indicate areas of scarring (Figs 20.4 and 20.5).

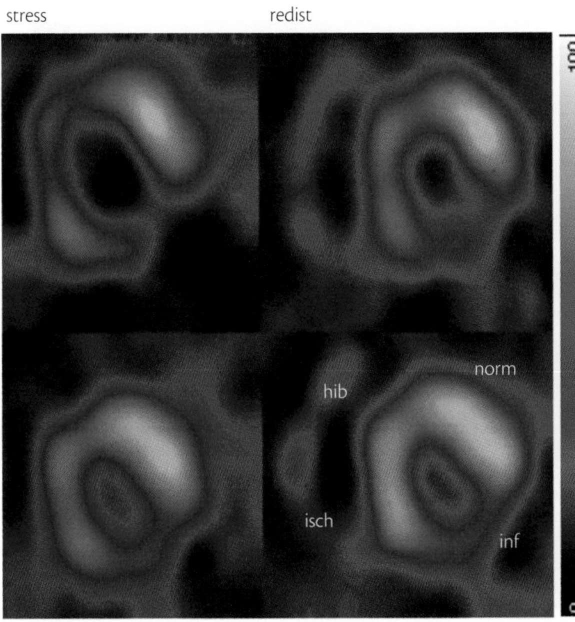

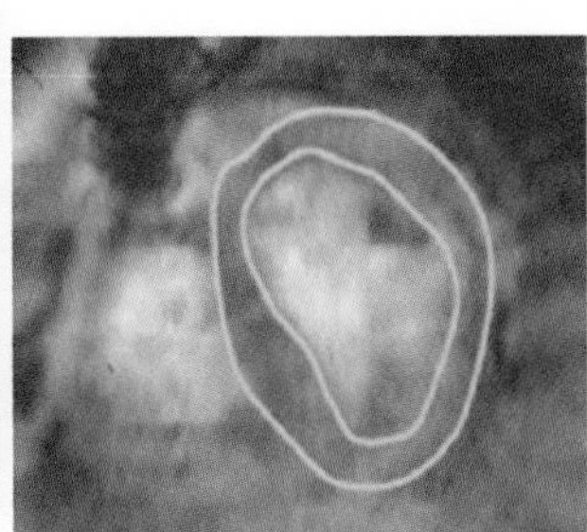

Fig. 20.2 Midventricular short-axis tomograms from a thallium-201 myocardial perfusion scan (MPS) (left) and end-systolic ciné gradient echo MRI with endo- and epicardial contours superimposed (right). The MPS images were acquired immediately after stress injection of thallium (stress), following redistribution of this injection (redist), and then on a separate day early (early rest) and late (late rest) after a resting injection of thallium. The combined images show: (1) Normal antero-lateral perfusion in viable and thickening muscle (norm); (2) partial-thickness inferolateral infarction with reduced thickening and some inducible ischaemia superimposed (inf); (3) inferoseptal ischaemia in fully viable and thickening myocardium (isch); (4) anteroseptal ischaemia in fully viable myocardium that does not thicken, in other words, hibernation (hib).

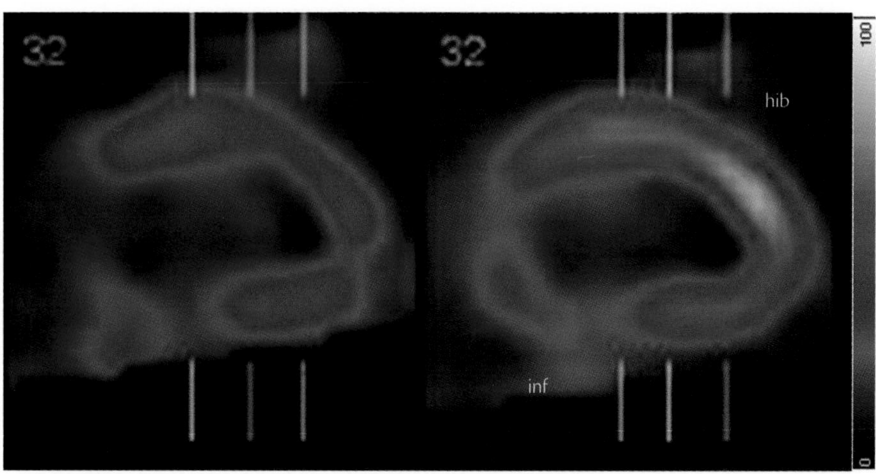

Fig. 20.3 Vertical long-axis tomograms after stress (left) and rest (right) injection of MIBI. The resting injection was given after sublingual glyceryl trinitrate. There is almost transmural infarction of the basal inferior wall (inf) and this area did not thicken on ECG-gated imaging, in keeping with the infarction. There is inducible ischaemia in fully viable myocardium in the apical anterior wall that also failed to thicken on ECG-gated imaging, indicating hibernation (hib).

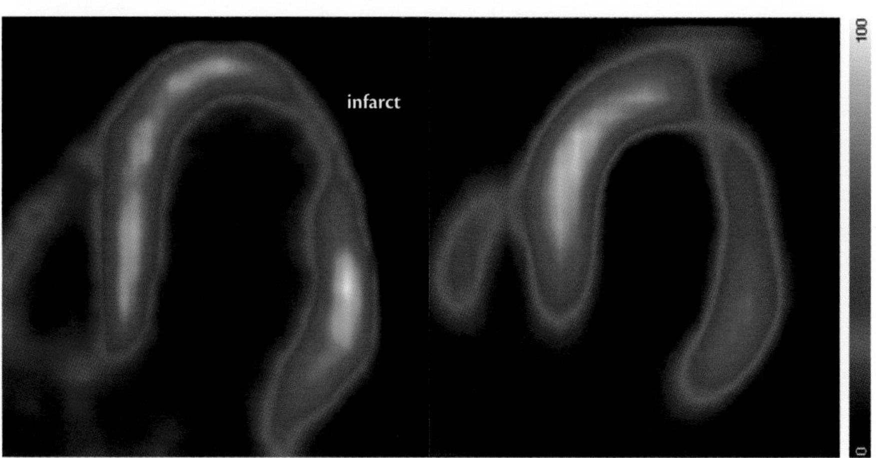

Fig. 20.4 Horizontal long-axis tomograms acquired using FDG PET (left) and tetrofosmin SPECT (right). The FDG was injected after a glucose load and acipimox. The tetrofosmin was injected after sublingual glyceryl trinitrate. There is partial thickness infarction of the apical lateral wall (infarct). The PET images have higher resolution but the pattern of tracer uptake is very similar indicating that both tracers can be used successfully to assess myocardial viability.

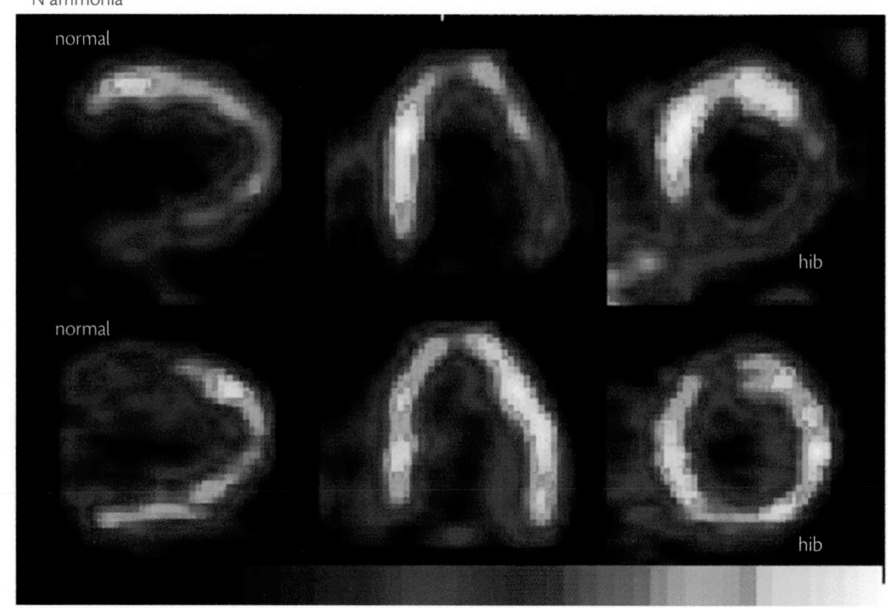

Fig. 20.5 Positron emission tomograms in vertical long-axis (left), horizontal long-axis (centre), and short-axis planes (right), acquired after resting injections of nitrogen-13 ammonia (top) and fluorine-18 2-fluorodeoxyglucose (FDG) with glucose loading (bottom).The inferolateral myocardium (hib) has normal viability (FDG uptake) but reduced resting perfusion (ammonia), which is the typical mismatched pattern of hibernation. The basal anterior wall (normal) has a reversed mismatch with normal resting perfusion (ammonia) and hence viability but reduced glucose metabolism (FDG). This emphasizes the importance of adequate glucose loading when FDG is used to assess viability.
Images courtesy of Professor Marcus Schwaiger, Munich.

Fatty acids

Straight-chain fatty acids can be labelled with radionuclides but their rapid metabolism complicates imaging. The β-methyl branched fatty acids are more suitable and the most widely used has been β-methyl-*p*-[^{123}I]-iodophenyl-pentadecanoic acid (BMIPP), although the tracer is currently only available commercially in Japan. When BMIPP is injected under fasting conditions it is extracted by the myocytes and converted into BMIPP-CoA, but it is not metabolized further. This results in high uptake and slow washout, making it very suitable for imaging.[39]

Images are usually compared with thallium or technetium images. Concordant defects are scar, whereas discordant defects with a larger metabolic defect are likely to be hibernating.[40,41] Discordant BMIPP defects have enhanced FDG uptake as a result of the metabolic shift[42] and have little fibrosis.[43] In a pooled study of 103 patients, 84% of segments with discordant BMIPP defects improved in function after revascularization but only 11% of those with concordant defects.[44]

Detection of hibernation

There are few large-scale studies of the accuracy of imaging techniques for predicting recovery of ventricular function after revascularization. Meta-analyses are confounded by different populations recruited, techniques used and imaging definitions of hibernation. For what it is worth, the weighted mean sensitivity and specificity for recovery of regional function after revascularization have been estimated as 92% and 63% for FDG PET, 87% and 54% for thallium MPS, 83% and 65% for technetium MPS, and 80% and 78% for dobutamine stress echocardiography. In general, all of the radionuclide techniques have similar accuracy and are said to be more sensitive but less specific than the dobutamine wall motion techniques.[45] In reality, though, the radionuclide techniques are more specific if the triad of signs referred to above is required before hibernation is diagnosed.

Fewer studies have looked at the improvement of global left ventricular function after revascularization but a similar trend is apparent in meta-analyses.[45] Fewer studies still have looked at more important measures such as symptoms and hard coronary events, but in nonrandomized observational studies patients with hibernation who are revascularized have better clinical outcome than those without hibernation, and the worst outcome is in patients with hibernation who are not revascularized. These observations can, however, only be hypothesis generating; randomized studies are needed to support the use of imaging in selecting patients with HF who will benefit from revascularization.

Cardiac innervation imaging

In the early stages of HF, increased sympathetic tone is helpful because it leads to increases in heart rate, contractility and venous return. As the syndrome progresses, this overactivity becomes unfavourable because of down-regulation and uncoupling of β-adrenoceptors, leading to progressive left ventricular dysfunction.[46] The sympathetic overactivity also increases the risk of arrhythmia mainly around focal areas of denervation.

Myocardial innervation can be imaged in a number of ways. [^{11}C]*meta*-hydroxyephedrine (HED) is an analogue of noradrenaline that concentrates in the presynaptic nerve terminal by the uptake-1 mechanism and provides high-quality PET images capable of quantification.[47] *Meta*-[^{123}I]iodobenzylguanidine (mIBG)is

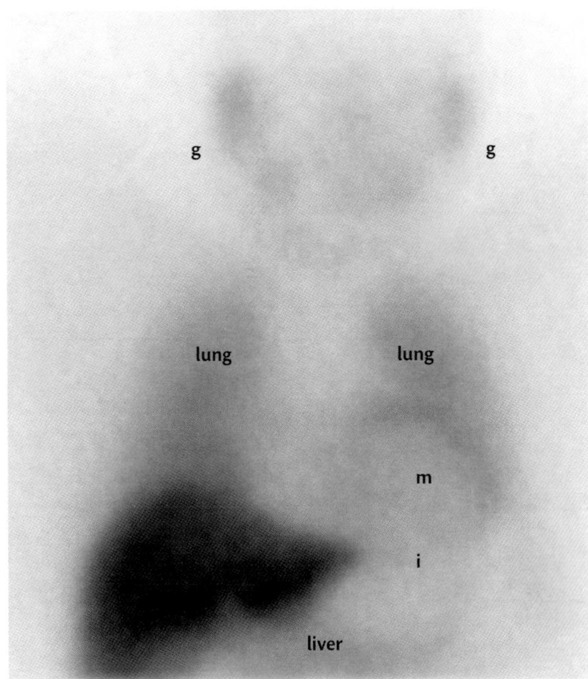

Fig. 20.6 Anterior projection image 4 h after injection of iodine-123 *meta*-iodobenzyl guanidine (mIBG). Myocardial uptake (m) is a measure of sympathetic innervation and tone. The patient had previous inferior infarction (i) with HF (NYHA 3). There is normal liver, lung and salivary gland (g) uptake. The heart to mediastinal ratio of mIBG uptake was 1.56, suggesting annual mortality in the region of 7% (see ADMIRE-HF study[58]).

a guanethedine analogue with a similar mechanism of uptake that is suitable for both planar and SPECT imaging. Initial mIBG uptake corresponds with the density of sympathetic innervation and washout rate, thereafter, with the frequency of nerve terminal firing and hence sympathetic activity. Uptake is quantified from the ratio of myocardial and mediastinal uptake and washout is measured from changes between 15-min and 4-h images (Fig. 20.6).[48]

Low myocardial uptake and rapid washout are associated with poor prognosis in both ischaemic HF and dilated cardiomyopathy[49,50] and myocardial uptake appears to be at least equal to left ventricular ejection fraction (LVEF) for predicting death and other major cardiac events.[51,52]

Other applications of mIBG imaging may be the prediction of life-threatening arrhythmias and hence the need for an implanted defibrillator, since ventricular arrhythmias may arise from the border of an area of scarring with viable muscle that is denervated (Fig. 20.7).[53] In a study, of 50 patients with previous myocardial infarction and left ventricular dysfunction, significant abnormality on semi-quantitative mIBG SPECT, was 77% sensitive and 75% specific for predicting ventricular arrhythmias on provocation testing.[54] Patients with appropriate defibrillator discharges have lower myocardial mIBG uptake than those without.[55,56]

The widest experience of the role of mIBG imaging for risk assessment in HF comes from the multicentre ADMIRE-HF study.[57,58] In this study, 964 patients with NYHA class II and III HF were studied with primary endpoints of HF progression, life-threatening arrhythmia, and cardiac death. There were 51 cardiac deaths in patients with heart to mediastinal ratio (HMR) of mIBG less than 1.6 compared with 2 in the high-uptake group, and 37% of patients with HMR less than 1.6 developed one of the endpoints

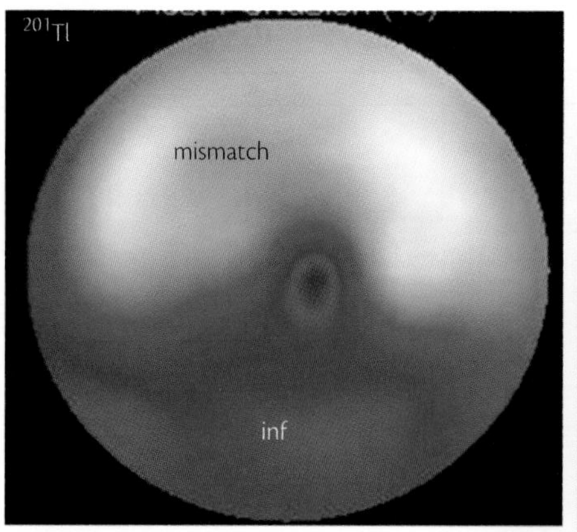

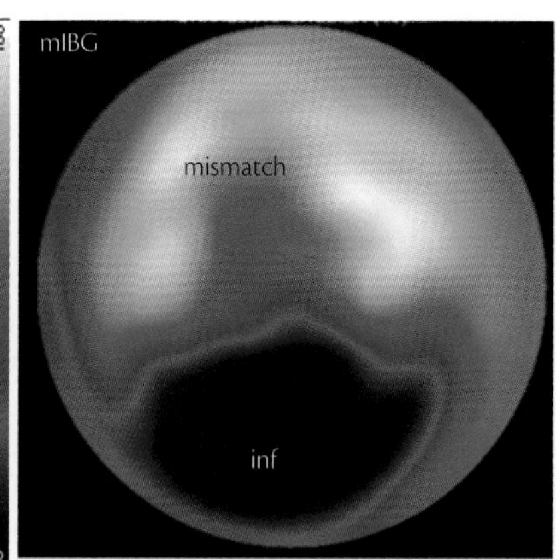

Fig. 20.7 Polar plots of thallium uptake (left) indicating myocardial viability, and mIBG uptake (right) indicating sympathetic innervation in the same patient as Fig. 20.6. There is almost transmural inferior infarction (inf), and a neighbouring area anteroapically of reduced innervation in viable myocardium (mismatch). The mismatch may be a substrate for arrhythmia.

compared with 15% with HMR greater than 1.6 ($p < 0.0001$). The negative predictive value of high HMR for cardiac death within 2 years was 98.8%. HF death was more common in the lowest group but arrhythmias were more common with intermediate HMR (1.2–1.6), suggesting that focal as opposed to global denervation is more likely to cause arrhythmias and sudden cardiac death.

Apoptosis imaging

Until the prospect of myocardial repair by stem cells becomes a reality, prevention of myocardial injury and cell death should be an important objective in the management of HF.[59] Apoptosis is a form of enzyme-mediated cell death that is responsible for loss of myocytes in a number of conditions such as ischaemia and reperfusion, with up to 30% of myocytes becoming apoptotic after reperfusion injury.[60,61] The process can be inhibited, and this is cardioprotective.[62,63]

Apoptosis is initiated by two pathways, intrinsic and extrinsic, with the final common step being activation of the caspase enzyme system.[64] Of the intracellular events that follow caspase activation, changes in phospholipid distribution in the cell membrane are central to apoptosis imaging. The maintenance of the lipid bilayer is energy dependent and one of the constituents, phosphatidyl serine (PS), is found in the inner layer. With caspase activation, the definition of the bilayer is lost and PS becomes externalized.[65] Annexin-V is an endogenous human protein with high affinity for PS that can be labelled with technetium-99m.[66]

Technetium-99m annexin imaging has been successfully demonstrated in patients with recent myocardial infarction who showed annexin uptake 2 h after revascularization, corresponding with MIBI defects at 6 weeks.[67] In the HF setting, however, the main problem for imaging is the small number of cells undergoing apoptosis. In healthy hearts the prevalence of apoptosis is 1–10 myocytes per 10^5 increasing to 80 to 250 per 10^5 in advanced HF.[68] In a study of 9 patients with dilated cardiomyopathy, annexin uptake was seen in patients with worsening left ventricular dysfunction raising the prospect of using annexin imaging for prognostication.[69] In another study, 5 of 18 patients with recent heart transplantation had myocardial annexin uptake associated with at least moderate transplant rejection, suggesting the potential for annexin imaging to detect rejection and reduce the need for endomyocardial biopsy (Fig. 20.8).[70]

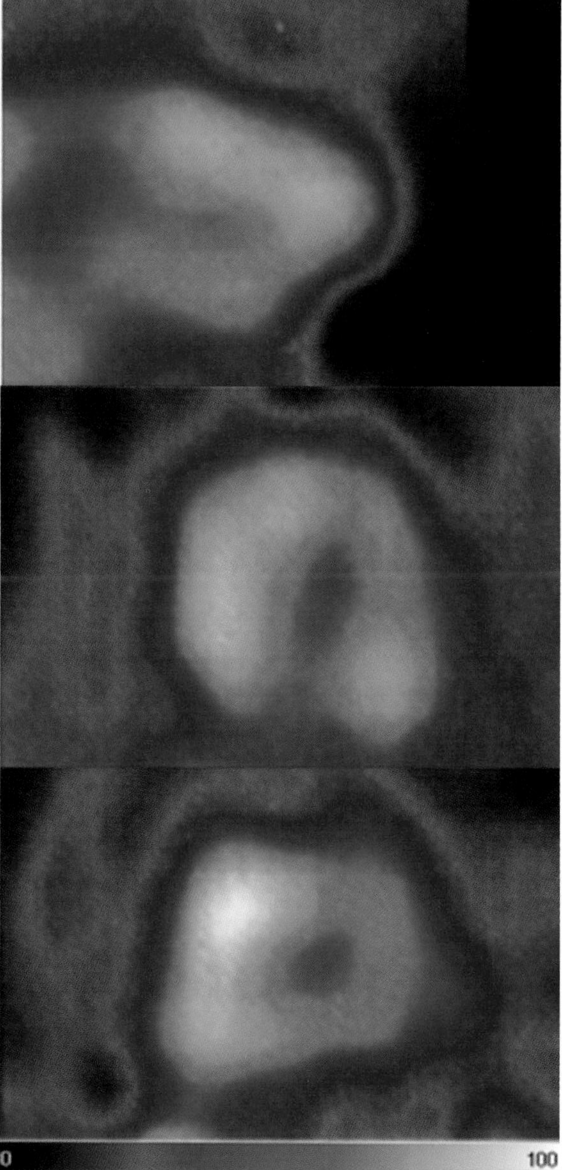

Fig. 20.8 Tomograms in vertical long-axis (top), horizontal long axis (centre), and short-axis planes (bottom) 9 months after orthotopic heart transplantation. The images show almost uniform myocardial uptake of ^{99m}Tc-annexin-V, most marked in the septum, indicating diffuse myocyte apoptosis and consistent with transplant rejection.

Adapted from Narula J, Acio ER, Narula N, *et al.* Annexin-V imaging for noninvasive detection of cardiac allograft rejection. *Nat Med* 2001;**7**:1347–52, with permission.

Radionuclide ventriculography

Radionuclide ventriculography (RNVG) is a mature technique that provides an accurate and reproducible method of assessing

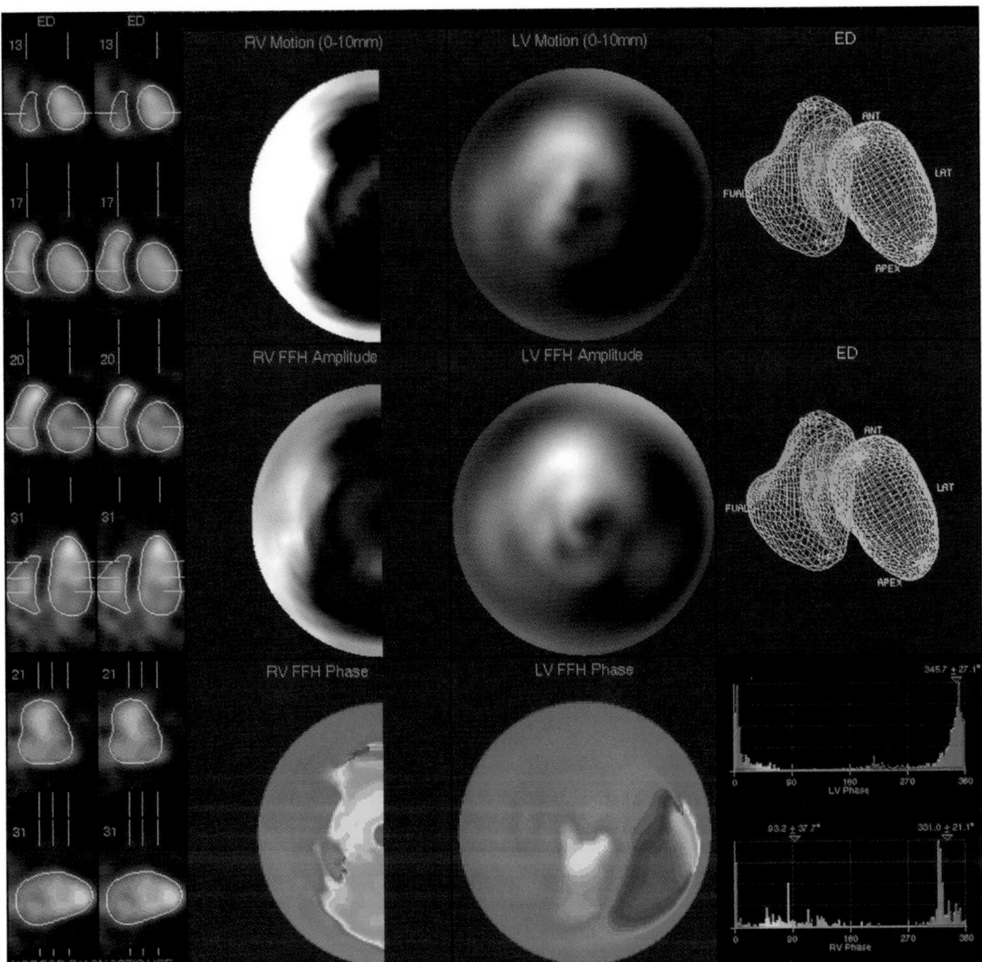

Fig. 20.9 ECG-gated blood pool SPECT for the assessment of ventricular function in a 76-year-old woman with alcoholic cardiomyopathy and heart failure. The polar plots of ventricular phase (bottom centre) show an area of almost paradoxical motion in the left ventricle inferolaterally (blue) and interventricular dyssynchrony (green in the right ventricle). After resynchronization pacing, NYHA class improved from III to I, left ventricular end-diastolic volume fell from 205 mL to 122 mL and left ventricular ejection fraction improved from 15% to 36%.

ventricular function. It is sometimes referred to as MUGA (multigated acquisition) but the acronym is not sufficiently descriptive and RNVG is preferred. The intracardiac blood pools are labelled with technetium-99m, usually by *in vivo* labelling in which sequential injections of a stannous agent and technetium-99m pertechnetate are given. The stannous ion reduces the pertechnetate once inside erythrocytes and it is fixed intracellularly by complexing.

Images are acquired after the tracer is in equilibrium with the blood pool (the equilibrium technique) and/or during its first pass through the central circulation (the first pass technique). The former mainly provides information on left ventricular function but the latter can also be used to assess right ventricular function and left-to-right shunting. Traditionally, image acquisition is planar in the left anterior oblique projection that best separates the left and right ventricles but emission tomographic imaging is used increasingly. Acquisition is gated to the ECG to provide 16–32 frames over the cardiac cycle, with each frame containing counts from an average cycle over what is typically a 10-min acquisition for planar imaging. Images can be acquired at rest and during dynamic exercise but stress tomographic imaging is not feasible because of motion during the longer acquisition.

In the planar equilibrium technique, left ventricular count changes over the cardiac cycle are used to calculate ejection fraction and other parameters of both global and regional function, including diastolic function. Ejection fraction measurements require the subtraction of counts from structures in front of and behind the left ventricle and these are usually estimated from a region of interest lateral to the left ventricle. The estimation of background is a source of inter- and intraobserver variability but the technique is otherwise accurate and reproducible because it makes no assumptions about ventricular geometry. In the tomographic technique, ventricular volumes can be measured either geometrically or by summing counts within the ventricles.[71,72]

Assessment of ventricular synchrony

Regional ventricular function is often assessed by Fourier analysis of count changes derived either from RNVG or from MPS, since myocardial count changes in MPS are related to myocardial thickening. Using either technique, Fourier analysis can also be applied to changes in geometry, for instance from the distance between the centre of the ventricle and the endocardium. Fourier analysis provides the parameters of phase and amplitude, which define the fundamental harmonic of contraction. Phase approximates to the time of end systole and can be expressed in milliseconds or more commonly as degrees or fraction of the cardiac cycle. Amplitude approximates to the magnitude of count changes through the cardiac cycle and hence to the extent of regional motion. Both parameters can be derived from whole ventricular counts, from regions or from individual image pixels. The histogram of phase values provides a simple method of displaying the mean and standard deviation of phase from any of these regions, and hence both inter- and intraventricular synchrony.

The combination of low LVEF and significant interventricular dyssynchrony measured by RNVG predicts improved systolic function 6 months after cardiac resynchronization therapy (CRT) (Fig. 20.9).[73] Similar analyses of MPS have shown a sensitivity and specificity of 70% and 74% respectively for predicting clinical improvement after CRT.[74,75]

Conclusion

- Radionuclide imaging is a simple and widely available method of obtaining information on the pathophysiology, extent, prognosis, and treatment options in patients with HF. It provides *in vivo* information noninvasively on myocardial perfusion, metabolism, innervation, or injury through necrosis and apoptosis.
- Perfusion imaging for the diagnosis of the cause of HF and imaging of myocardial viability and hibernation are routine techniques that should be available in all centres managing these patients.
- In the near future, cardiac adrenergic imaging will provide additional information on prognosis and selection criteria for implanted defibrillators.
- If imaging of injury through necrosis or apoptosis becomes a reality, tailor-made treatment directed at prevention of further injury and transplant rejection may become commonplace.
- Radionuclide ventriculography is a well-established and simple technique for assessing ventricular function that is both accurate and reproducible.
- Assessment of inter- and intraventricular synchrony by radionuclide techniques has the potential to assist selection of patients who will benefit from resynchronization pacing.

References

1. Yasuda T, Palacios IF, Dec GW, *et al.* Indium-111 monoclonal antimyosin antibody imaging in the diagnosis of acute myocarditis. Circulation 1987;**76**:306–11.
2. Narula J, Khaw BA, Dec GW, *et al.* Recognition of acute myocarditis masquerading as acute myocardial infarction. *New Engl J Med* 1993;**328**:100–4.
3. Jacobs JC, Rosen JM, Szer IS. Lyme myocarditis diagnosed by gallium scan. *J Pediatr* 1993;**105**:950–2.
4. Matsuura H, Ishikita T, Yamamoto S, *et al.* Gallium-67 myocardial imaging for the detection of myocarditis in the acute phase of Kawasaki disease (mucocutaneous lymph node syndrome): the usefulness of single photon emission computed tomography. *Br Heart J* 1987;**58**:385–92.
5. O'Connell JB, Henkin RE, Robinson JA, Subramanian R, Scanlon PJ, Gunnar RM. Gallium-67 imaging in patients with dilated cardiomyopathy and biopsy-proven myocarditis. *Circulation* 1984;**70**: 58–62.
6. Narula J, Zaret BL. Non-invasive detection of cell death: from tracking epitaphs to counting coffins. *J Nucl Cardiol* 2002;**9**:54–60.
7. Khaw BA. The current role of infarct avid imaging. *Semin Nucl Med* 1999;**29**:259–70.
8. Flotats A, Carrio I. Non-invasive in vivo imaging of myocardial apoptosis and necrosis. *Eur J Nucl Med Mol Imaging* 2003;**30**:259–70.
9. Orlandi C, Crane PD, Edwards DS *et al.* Early scintigraphic detection of experimental myocardial infarction in dogs with technetium-99m-glucaric acid. *J Nucl Med* 1991;**32**:263–8.
10. Morrison AR, Sinusas AJ. New molecular imaging targets to characterise myocardial biology. *Cardiol Clin* 2009;**27**:329–44.
11. Underwood SR, Anagnostopoulos C, Cerqueira M, *et al.* Myocardial perfusion scintigraphy: the evidence. *Eur J Nucl Med Mol Imaging* 2004;**31**:261–91.
12. Klocke FJ, Baird MG, Lorell BH, *et al.* ACC/AHA/ASNC guidelines for the clinical use of cardiac radionuclide imaging. *Circulation* 2003;**108**:1404–18.
13. Pasternac A, Noble J, Streulens Y, Elie R, Henschke C, Bourassa MG. Pathophysiology of chest pain in patients with cardiomyopathies and normal coronary arteries. *Circulation* 1982;**65**:778–89.
14. Miller WL, Hodge DO, Tointon SK, Rodeheffer RJ, Nelson SM, Gibbons RJ. Relationship of myocardial perfusion imaging findings to outcome of patients with heart failure and suspected ischemic heart disease. *Am Heart J* 2004;**147**:714–20.
15. Rahimtoola SH. The hibernating myocardium. *Am Heart J* 1982;**117**:211–21.
16. Schwarz ER, Speakman MT, vom Dahl J, Kloner RA. Hibernating myocardium: is there evidence for chronic flow reduction? *Heart Dis* 1999;**1**:155–62.
17. Braunwald E, Kloner RA. The stunned myocardium: prolonged, post-ischaemic ventricular dysfunction. *Circulation* 1982;**66**:1146–9.
18. Canty JM Jr, Fallavollita JA. Chronic hibernation and chronic stunning: a continuum. *J Nucl Cardiol* 2000;**7**:509–27.
19. Maes A, Flameng W, Nuyts J, *et al.* Histological alterations in chronically hypoperfused myocardium. Correlation with PET findings. *Circulation* 1994;**90**:735–45.
20. Bax JJ, Wijns W, Cornel JH, Visser FC, Boersma E, Fioretti PM. Accuracy of currently available techniques for prediction of functional recovery after revascularization in patients with left ventricular dysfunction due to chronic coronary artery disease: comparison of pooled data. *J Am Coll Cardiol* 1997;**30**:1451–60.
21. Allman KC, Shaw LJ, Hachamovitch R, Udelson JE. Myocardial viability testing and impact of revascularization on prognosis in patients with coronary artery disease and left ventricular dysfunction: a meta- analysis. *J Am Coll Cardiol* 2002;**39**:1151–8.
22. Underwood SR, Bax JJ, vom Dahl J, *et al.* Imaging techniques for the assessment of myocardial hibernation. *Eur Heart J* 2004;**25**: 815–36.
23. Gewirtz H, Fischman AJ, Abraham S, Gilson M, Strauss HW, Alpert NM. Positron emission tomographic measurements of absolute regional myocardial blood flow permits identification of nonviable myocardium in patients with chronic myocardial infarction. *J Am Coll Cardiol* 1994;**23**:851–9.
24. Bonow RO, Dilsizian V. Thallium-201 for assessment of myocardial viability. *Semin Nucl Med* 1991;**21**:230–41.
25. Rozanski A, Berman DS, Gray R, *et al.* Use of thallium-201 redistribution scintigraphy in the preoperative differentiation of reversible and nonreversible myocardial asynergy. *Circulation* 1981;**64**:936–44.
26. Liu P, Kiess MC, Okada RD, *et al.* The persistent defect on exercise thallium imaging and its fate after myocardial revascularisation: does it represent scar or ischaemia? *Am Heart J* 1985;**110**:996–1001.
27. Dilsizian V, Bonow RO. Current diagnostic techniques for assessing myocardial viability in patients with hibernating and stunned myocardium. *Circulation* 1993;**87**:1–20.
28. Sivaratnam DA, Bonow RO, Kalff V. Assessment of myocardial viability in dysfunctional myocardium. In: Ell PJ, Gambhir SS (eds.) *Nuclear medicine: clinical diagnosis and treatment*, pp. 1159–70. Churchill Livingstone, London, 1994.
29. Bonow RO, Dilsizian V. Thallium-201 and technetium-99m-sestamibi for assessing viable myocardium. *J Nucl Med* 1992;**33**:815–18.

30. Cuocolo A, Pace L, Ricciardelli B, Chiariello M, Trimarco B, Salvatore M. Identification of viable myocardium in patients with chronic coronary artery disease: comparison of thallium-201 scintigraphy with reinjection and technetium 99m-methoxyisobutylisonitrile. *J Nucl Med* 1992;**33**:505–11.
31. Bisi G, Sciagra R, Santoro GM, Rossi V, Fazzini PF. Technetium-99m-sestamibi imaging with nitrate infusion to detect viable hibernating myocardium and predict post revascularization recovery. *J Nucl Med* 1995;**36**:1994–2000.
32. Maurea S, Cuocolo A, Soricelli A, *et al.* Myocardial viability index in chronic coronary artery disease: technetium-99m-methoxy isobutyl isonitrile redistribution. *J Nucl Med* 1995;**36**:1953–60.
33. Udelson JE, Coleman PS, Metherall JA, *et al.* Predicting recovery of severe regional ventricular dysfunction: comparison of resting scintigraphy with ^{201}Tl and ^{99m}Tc-sestamibi. *Circulation* 1994;**89**: 2552–61.
34. Levine MG, McGill CC, Ahlberg AW, *et al.* Functional assessment with electrocardiographic gated single-photon emission computed tomography improves the ability of technetium-99 m sestamibi myocardial perfusion imaging to predict myocardial viability in patients undergoing revascularization. *Am J Cardiol* 1999;**83**:1–5.
35. Sciagra R, Pellegri M, Pupi A, *et al.* Prognostic implications of Tc-99 m sestamibi viability imaging and subsequent therapeutic strategy in patients with chronic coronary artery disease and left ventricular dysfunction. *J Am Coll Cardiol* 2000;**36**:739–45.
36. Neubauer S. The failing heart: an engine out of fuel. *N Engl J Med* 2007;**356**:1140–51.
37. Liedke AJ. Alterations of carbohydrate and lipid metabolism in the acutely ischemic heart. *Prog Cardiovasc Dis* 1981;**23**:321–36.
38. Schelbert HR. 18F-deoxyglucose and the assessment of myocardial viability. *Semin Nucl Med* 2002;**32**:60–9.
39. Knapp FF, Kropp J. Iodine-123-labelled fatty acids for myocardial single-photon emission tomography: current status and future perspectives. *Eur J Nucl Med* 1995;**22**:361–81.
40. Taki J, Nakajima K, Matsunari I, Banko H, Takada S, Tonami N. Impairment of regional fatty acid uptake in relation to wall motion and thallium-201 uptake in ischaemic but viable myocardium, assessment with iodine-123-labelled beta-methyl-branched fatty acid. *Eur J Nucl Med* 1995;**22**:1385–92.
41. Kawamoto M, Tamaki N, Yonekura Y, *et al.* Combined study with I-123 fatty acid and thallium-201 to assess ischemic myocardium. *Ann Nucl Med* 1994;**8**:47–54.
42. Tamaki N, Tadamura E, Kawamoto M, *et al.* Decreased uptake of iodinated branched fatty acid analog indicates metabolic alterations in ischemic myocardium. *J Nucl Med* 1995;**36**:1974–80.
43. Kudoh T, Tadamura E, Tamaki N, *et al.* Iodinated free fatty acid and ^{201}Tl uptake in chronically hypoperfused myocardium: histological correlation study. *J Nucl Med* 2000;**41**:293–6.
44. Tamaki N, Morita K, Kawai Y. The Japanese experience with metabolic imaging in the clinical setting. *J Nucl Cardiol* 2007;**14**(suppl 3):S145–52.
45. Schinkel AF, Bax JJ, Poldermans D, Elhendy A, Ferrari R, Rahimtoola SH. Hibernating myocardium: diagnosis and patient outcomes. *Curr Probl Cardiol* 2007;**32**:375–410.
46. Ungerer M, Böhm M, Elce JS, Erdmann E, Lohse MJ. Altered expression of beta-adrenergic receptor kinase and beta-adrenergic receptors in the failing human heart. *Circulation* 1993;**87**:454–63.
47. Bengel FM, Schwaiger M. Assessment of cardiac sympathetic neuronal function using PET imaging. *J Nucl Cardiol* 2004;**11**:603–16.
48. Carrio I. Cardiac neurotransmission imaging. *J Nucl Med* 2001;**42**:1062–76.
49. Merlet P, Benvenuti C, Moyse D, *et al.* Prognostic value of MIBG imaging in idiopathic dilated cardiomyopathy. *J Nucl Med* 1999;**40**:917–23.
50. Arimoto T, Takeishi Y, Niizeki T, *et al.* Cardiac sympathetic denervation and ongoing myocardial damage for prognosis in early stages of heart failure. *J Card Fail* 2007;**13**:34–41.
51. Merlet P, Valette H, Dubois-Rande J, *et al.* Prognostic value of cardiac metaiodo-benzylguanidine in patients with heart failure. *J Nucl Med* 1992;**33**:471–7.
52. Agostini D, Verberne HJ, Burchert W, *et al.* I-123-mIBG myocardial imaging for assessment of risk for a major cardiac event in heart failure patients: insights from a retrospective European multicenter study. *Eur J Nucl Med Mol Imaging* 2008;**35**:535–46.
53. Bax JJ, Boogers MM, Schuijf JD. Nuclear imaging in heart failure. *Cardiol Clin* 2009;**27**:265–76.
54. Bax JJ, Kraft O, Buxton AE, *et al.* 123-I-MIBG scintigraphy to predict inducibility of ventricular arrhythmias on cardiac electrophysiology testing. *Circ Cardiovasc Imaging* 2008;**1**:131–40.
55. Nagahara D, Nakata T, Hashimoto A, *et al.* Predicting the need for an implantable cardioverter defibrillator using cardiac metaiodobenzylguanidine activity together with plasma natriuretic peptide concentration or left ventricular function. *J Nucl Med* 2008;**49**:225–33.
56. Arora R, Ferrick KJ, Nakata T, *et al.* I-123 MIBG imaging and heart rate variability analysis to predict the need for an implantable cardioverter defibrillator. *J Nucl Cardiol* 2003;**10**:121–31.
57. Jacobson AF, Lombard J, Banerjee G, Camici P. ^{123}I-mIBG scintigraphy to predict risk for adverse cardiac outcomes in heart failure patients: design of two prospective multicenter international trials. *J Nucl Cardiol* 2009;**16**:113–21.
58. Jacobson AF, Senior R, Cerqueira M, *et al.* Myocardial iodine-123 meta-iodobenzylguanidine imaging and cardiac events in heart failure: results of the prospective ADMIRE-HF (AdreView Myocardial Imaging for Risk Evaluation in Heart Failure) study. *J Am Coll Cardiol* 2010;**55**:2212–21.
59. Orlic D, Kajstura J, Chimenti S, *et al.* Bone marrow cells regenerate infarcted myocardium. *Nature* 2001;**410**:701–5.
60. Brömme HJ, Holtz J. Apoptosis in the heart: when and why? *Mol Cell Biochem* 1996;**163–164**:261–75.
61. Fliss H, Gattinger D. Apoptosis in ischemic and reperfused rat myocardium. *Circ Res* 1996;**79**:949–56.
62. Strauss HW, Narula J, Blankenberg FD. Radioimaging to identify myocardial cell death and probably injury. *Lancet* 2000;**356**:180–1.
63. Yaoita H, Ogawa K, Maehara K, Maruyama Y. Attenuation of ischemia/reperfusion injury in rats by a caspase inhibitor. *Circulation* 1998;**97**:276–81.
64. Tait JF. Imaging of apoptosis. *J Nucl Med* 2008;**49**:1573–6.
65. Martin SJ, Reutelingsperger CP, McGahon AJ, *et al.* Early redistribution of plasma membrane phosphatidylserine is a general feature of apoptosis regardless of the initiating stimulus: inhibition by overexpression of Bcl-2 and Abl. *J Exp Med* 1995;**182**:1545–56.
66. Blankenberg FG, Katsikis PD, Tait JF, et al. In vivo detection and imaging of phosphatidylserine expression during programmed cell death. *Proc Natl Acad Sci U S A* 1998;95:6349–54.
67. Hofstra L, Liem IH, Dumont EA, *et al.* Visualisation of cell death in vivo in patients with acute myocardial infarction. *Lancet* 2000;**356**:209–12.
68. Wolters SL, Corsten MF, Reutelingsperger CPM, Narula J, Hofstra L. Cardiovascular molecular imaging of apoptosis. *Eur J Nucl Med Mol Imaging* 2007;**34**(suppl 1):S86–98.
69. Kietselaer BL, Reutelingsperger CP, Boersma HH, *et al.* Noninvasive detection of programmed cell loss with 99mTc-labeled annexin A5 in heart failure. *J Nucl Med* 2007;**48**:562–7.
70. Narula J, Acio ER, Narula N, *et al.* Annexin-V imaging for noninvasive detection of cardiac allograft rejection. *Nat Med* 2001;**7**:1347–52.
71. Botvinick EH, O'Connell JW, Kadkade PP, *et al.* Potential added value of three-dimensional reconstruction and display of single photon

emission computed tomographic gated blood pool images. *J Nucl Cardiol* 1998;5:245–55.

72. Harel F, Finnerty V, Gregoire J, *et al.* Comparison of left ventricular contraction homogeneity index using SPECT gated blood pool imaging and planar phase analysis. *J Nucl Cardiol* 2008;**15**: 80–5.
73. Toussaint JF, Lavergne T, Kerrou K, *et al.* Basal asynchrony and resynchronization with biventricular pacing predict long-term improvement of LV function in heart failure patients. *Pacing Clin Electrophysiol* 2003;**26**:1815–23.
74. Henneman MM, Chen J, Dibbets-Schneider P, *et al.* Can LV dyssynchrony as assessed with phase analysis on gated myocardial perfusion SPECT predicts response to CRT? *J Nucl Med* 2007;**48**:1104–11.
75. Adelstein EC, Saba S. Scar burden by myocardial perfusion imaging predicts echocardiographic response to cardiac resynchronization therapy in ischemic cardiomyopathy. *Am Heart J* 2007;**153**:105–12.

21

Heart failure imaged by cardiac magnetic resonance imaging

C. Parsai and S.K. Prasad

Introduction

Heart failure (HF) is a growing clinical condition resulting from a variety of primary or systemic disorders that impair the ability of the heart to meet systemic demands. Coronary artery disease (CAD), hypertension, and dilated cardiomyopathy (DCM) represent the most common aetiologies in the Western world, with a genetic background found in up to 30% of DCM.[1]

Although HF is largely a clinical diagnosis, imaging has become an essential part of patients' work-up complementing more invasive testing (e.g. coronary angiography, endomyocardial biopsy) and genetic testing. It is key to characterize myocardial and valvular structure and function; identify an underlying treatable substrate; risk-stratify patients; and guide decision-making for medical, surgical, or device therapies such as internal cardioverter-defibrillators (ICD) and cardiac resynchronization therapy (CRT). In addition, it provides measurements for assessing the effect of treatment, including percutaneous or surgical procedures.

As the prognosis of HF remains poor, particular emphasis has been placed on detection of early disease in patients at risk and in those with asymptomatic evidence of left ventricular damage as well as screening of relatives.

Although echocardiography remains the first imaging step,[1] cardiac magnetic resonance imaging (CMR) is now widely available and appears as an ideal complementary technique with the potential to address in a single 45–60 min scan an exhaustive evaluation of three-dimensional cardiac anatomy, function, tissue characterization, coronary and microvascular perfusion, valve disease, and coronary angiography.

The diagnostic and prognostic strengths of CMR as an integral part of the clinical workup of a HF patient are reviewed in a stepwise approach.

Technical aspects of CMR

Through a wide range of dedicated sequences, CMR can image in any selected plane, without interference from bones or lungs, regardless of patient's build, without ionizing radiation, and using relatively safe gadolinium contrast agents.

A standard protocol in a new-onset HF patient (Fig. 21.1) includes:

- Transaxial, coronal, and sagittal half-Fourier acquisition single-shot turbo spin-echo imaging (HASTE), offering a general overview of cardiac and extracardiac anatomy, detection of anomalous pulmonary venous drainage and large shunts.
- Steady-state free precession (SSFP): ciné imaging providing dynamic views of the heart during repeated breath-holds. Typically, three long-axis and a stack of short-axis planes are obtained from the atrioventricular (AV) groove to the apex of both ventricles. Reproducible and accurate assessments of biventricular volumes, mass, and ejection fraction (EF) are obtained by manual planimetry of endo- and epicardial borders or with semiautomated software.
- Tissue characterization without contrast agent:
  - T_1 and T_2-weighted turbo-spin echo sequences (TSE) are useful for assessing fat and the pericardium, helping the distinction between constrictive and restrictive cardiomyopathy
  - T_2-weighted short-tau inversion recovery (STIR) nulls myocardial fat and detects hyperintense areas of increased myocardial water content indicative of oedema or inflammation
  - $T_2{}^*$-weighted imaging, used in selected patients, allows myocardial iron quantification. By exploiting the dose-dependent loss of signal owing to greater field homogeneities, myocardial iron can be quantified.
- Perfusion imaging using gradient-echo imaging following intravenous gadolinium contrast injection:
  - Stress perfusion during pharmacological vasodilatation (commonly adenosine) identifies areas of inducible ischaemic-related subendocardial perfusion defects or perfusion defects at the microvascular level in nonischaemic cardiomyopathies.

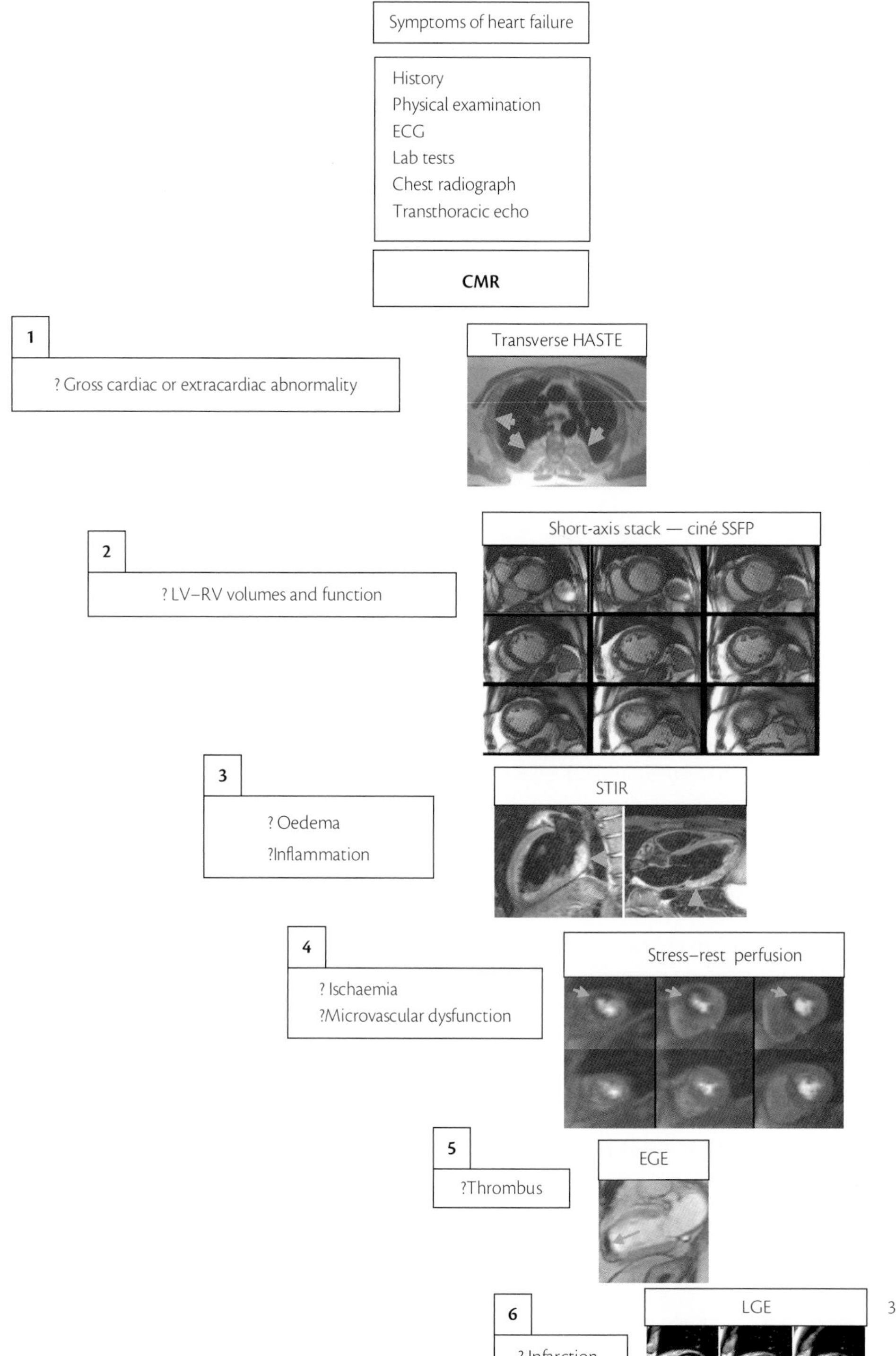

Fig. 21.1 CMR complements a classical clinical evaluation allowing in a stepwise approach the detection of gross cardiac or extracardiac pathologies (step1, extramedullary haematopoiesis in a thalassaemia patient, arrows), accurate and reproducible measurements of biventricular volume and function (step 2), detection of myocardial inflammation (step 3, STIR imaging showing localized oedema in myocarditis, arrows). Myocardial ischaemia or microvascular dysfunction can be identified by comparing rest and pharmacological stress perfusion (step 4, large area of inducible ischaemia in the left anterior descending artery territory, arrows). Thrombus can be detected immediately after gadolinium injection (step 5, apical thrombus, arrow) and fibrosis or myocardial infarction during late imaging (typical subendocardial LGE indicating previous infarction). EGE, early gadolinium imaging; HASTE, half-Fourier acquisition single-shot turbo spin-echo imaging; LGE, late gadolinium imaging; SSFP, steady-state free precession; STIR, short-tau inversion recovery.

- Rest perfusion performed at least 15 min after stress, to allow for clearance of gadolinium from blood, is compared to stress perfusion to identify inducible defects distinguishing them from artefacts.

- Early gadolinium imaging (EGE), typically 1–3 min after gadolinium administration, is a sensitive tool to detect dark, unenhanced intracardiac thrombi.
- Late gadolinium imaging (LGE) is performed 5–20 min after gadolinium administration using inversion recovery turbo-flash (IR GRE) or phase-sensitive inversion recovery sequences (PSIR). Gadolinium is an extracellular agent which accumulates in areas of increased interstitial space (secondary to fibrosis or infiltration) which appear as hyperintense. Thus, localization and extent of myocardial infarction, viability, stunning, and

hibernation can all be examined. In nonischaemic cardiomyopathies (NICM), the pattern of LGE provides diagnostic and prognostic clues.

Despite the use of a standardized approach to optimize performance and interpretation of CMR scans, available sequences are clinical instruments to achieve a diagnosis and are dynamically selected throughout the scan on the basis of the evolving picture.

Thus, CMR velocity mapping sequences can be added to the standard cardiomyopathy protocol for suspected valve disease or for quantification of intraventricular gradients with reproducible results.[2]

Limitations encountered in HF patients are mainly related to previous devices (mostly ICD and pacemakers). Imaging difficulties related to the patient's difficulty in performing breath-holds, or to atrial fibrillation, were previously considered to be major scanning limitations but can now be overcome by real-time imaging and fast single-shot LGE imaging acquiring one slice per heartbeat.

Clinical aspects

In HF, treatment and survival are directly related to the cause. While patients are generally rapidly classified as having normal (heart failure with normal ejection fraction, HeFNEF) or impaired left ventricular systolic function (heart failure with reduced ejection fraction, HeFREF) following a standard echocardiography, the next important diagnostic and prognostic step is to define whether patients have ischaemic or nonischaemic cardiomyopathy (NICM). This is usually based on the presence of epicardial CAD as imaged by invasive coronary angiography. However, this approach does not account for patients with NICM who also have concomitant coronary disease which may be incidental or partly contributing to myocardial dysfunction.

CMR offers the unique potential to assist the differential diagnosis step by step from delineation of EF to risk stratification (see Fig. 21.1).

Although many conditions causing HeFNEF in the early stages can progress to HeFREF, CMR diagnostic and prognostic features of the most frequent pathologies responsible for HF are discussed here according to their commonest presentation with a reduced or normal EF.

Heart failure with reduced ejection fraction

Aside from searching for a reversible condition responsible for HeFREF, CMR contributes to risk stratification and family screening. It can guide invasive therapy (e.g. percutaneous or surgical revascularization of viable myocardium, left ventricular lead positioning away from infarcted myocardium in CRT) and procedures such as endomyocardial biopsy and provide reproducible data for adequate follow-up under treatment.

Left ventricular dysfunction secondary to CAD (ischaemic cardiomyopathy)

CMR accurately assesses global and regional ventricular function, proximal coronary artery stenoses, and their repercussions. Following gadolinium contrast injection, first-pass perfusion can be quantified at rest and during stress. Microvascular obstruction and thrombus are visualized during early imaging, and infarction and residual viability are assessed during the late phase (Fig. 21.2).

Ischaemic cardiomyopathy (ICM) is characterized by a highly specific pattern of LGE validated by histopathology, typically affecting the subendocardium extending up to the epicardium in a pattern consistent with the wavefront phenomenon of ischaemic cell death (Fig. 21.2 C–D).[3] Recognition of this characteristic pattern coupled with assessment of perfusion has shed a new light on the diagnosis of ICM.

In presence of left ventricular dysfunction, LGE-CMR is more sensitive than coronary angiography at detecting CAD.[4] Interestingly, McCrohon *et al.* showed that among HF patients undergoing CMR, those with known CAD all had subendocardial or transmural enhancement, while DCM patients with unobstructed coronaries displayed three distinct patterns of LGE. The majority had no LGE (59%), but 13% exhibited an ischaemic pattern as a result of transient coronary occlusion and 28% had mid-wall LGE similar to the fibrosis found at autopsy. Similarly, LGE-CMR had a sensitivity of 86% and specificity of 93% for detection of CAD in new-onset HF patients with unobstructed coronaries.[5]

Transmurality of LGE predicts lack of postrevascularization functional improvement in ICM but also outperforms traditional markers of risk such as left ventricular ejection fraction (LVEF) by predicting the risk of inducible ventricular tachycardia, which increases the risk of death.[6] Similarly, silent infarction detected by LGE, even if small in size, carries a sevenfold increased risk of major cardiovascular events.[7]

To determine whether infarct size correlates with arrhythmias and risk of sudden death (SCD) in HF patients with left ventricular dysfunction, the large DETERMINE trial is still ongoing.

CMR contributes to predicting the success of CRT and to guiding patient selection. For example, the presence and transmurality of posterolateral scar has been linked to lack of response to CRT with a higher mortality when pacing occurred over the scarred area. CMR-derived dyssynchrony indices have also been used as predictors of CRT response.[8]

To ease left ventricular lead positioning, CMR has been used to image coronary venous anatomy prior to device implantation.[9]

Dilated cardiomyopathy

Dilated cardiomyopathy (DCM) is the third commonest cause of HF and the most frequent indication for heart transplantation. The aetiology of up to 50% of DCM remains unexplained following exclusion of significant CAD, active myocarditis, and a primary or secondary myocardial disease by coronary angiogram, echocardiography, and rarely endomyocardial biopsy.[10]

In addition to providing precise and reproducible quantification of LVEF and biventricular volumes, CMR offers the unique potential of searching noninvasively for an underlying aetiology by its ability to detect fibrosis, scarring, and infiltration.

Up to 28% of patients with systolic dysfunction of unknown aetiology have mid-wall LGE fibrosis, similar to autopsy findings (Fig. 21.3).[4] While the exact pathophysiology underlying this pattern of fibrosis remains uncertain, it is of strong prognostic significance. Assomull *et al.*,[11] who specifically studied the impact of mid-wall LGE in symptomatic DCM patients, showed that it was associated with increased mortality and cardiovascular events and was the best predictor of sudden cardiac death (SCD) and ventricular tachycardia. Similarly, Wu *et al.*[12] reported an eightfold increased prevalence of ventricular arrhythmias among ICD-eligible NICM patients with LGE, regardless of the segmental

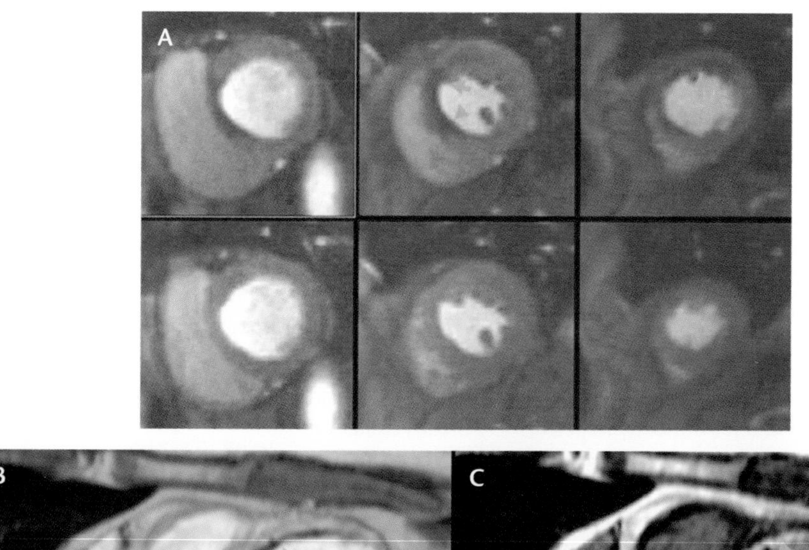

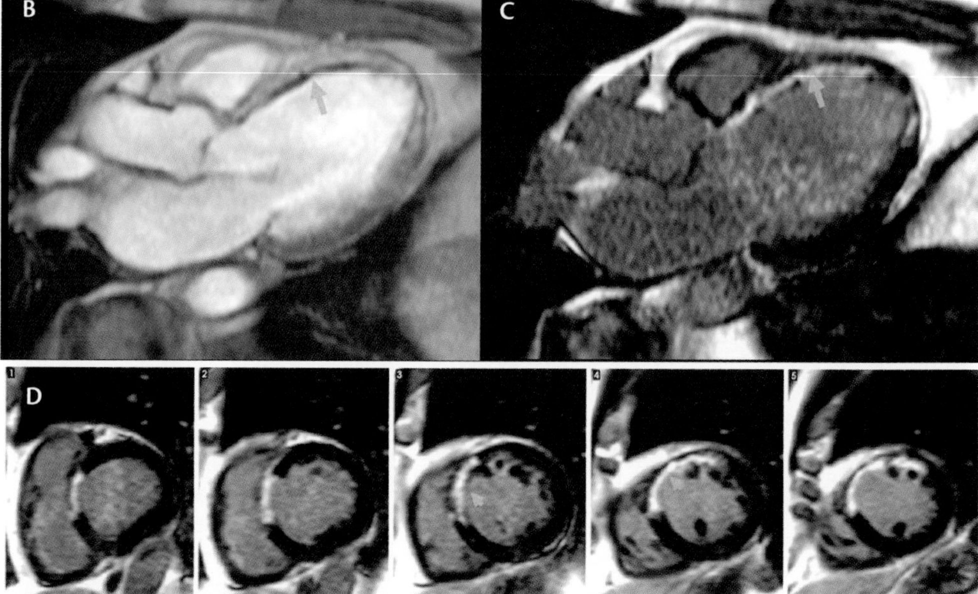

Fig. 21.2 CMR detects inducible ischaemia following pharmacological stress perfusion. A, top: inducible ischaemia during stress perfusion, arrows; A, bottom: rest perfusion showing normalization of myocardial perfusion. Microvascular obstruction is detected on early enhancement images (B, LVOT view with a dark rim of microvascular obstruction, arrow). LGE is typically subendocardial progressing to transmural (C–D, short-axis views displaying hyperintense areas consistent with infarction, arrowheads).

pattern of LGE (midwall, transmural or patchy) and persisting after adjustment for left ventricular volume index and functional class.

Of interest, a proportion of HF patients with unobstructed coronary arteries and systolic dysfunction classified as HF of unknown aetiology display an ischaemic pattern of LGE, highlighting the limitations of standard testing.[4,5] Valle *et al.*[5] reported a higher mortality rate and HF admissions among known ischaemic heart disease patients compared to DCM. In unrecognized ICM (normal angiogram but ischaemic pattern of LGE), the risk is similar to that of ischaemic patients, highlighting the role of LGE as a strong predictor of cardiac events beyond EF.

Myocarditis

Myocarditis, largely underdiagnosed clinically, is an important underlying cause of several myocardial diseases such as DCM and

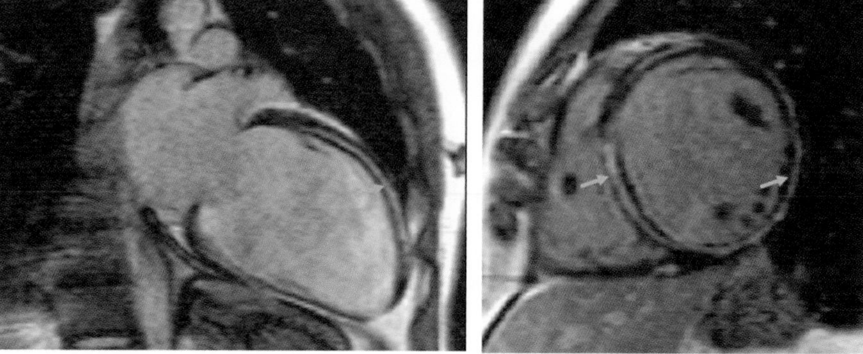

Fig. 21.3 Midwall distribution of LGE in DCM. Left panel, two-chamber view. Right panel, short-axis image with midwall enhancement (arrows).

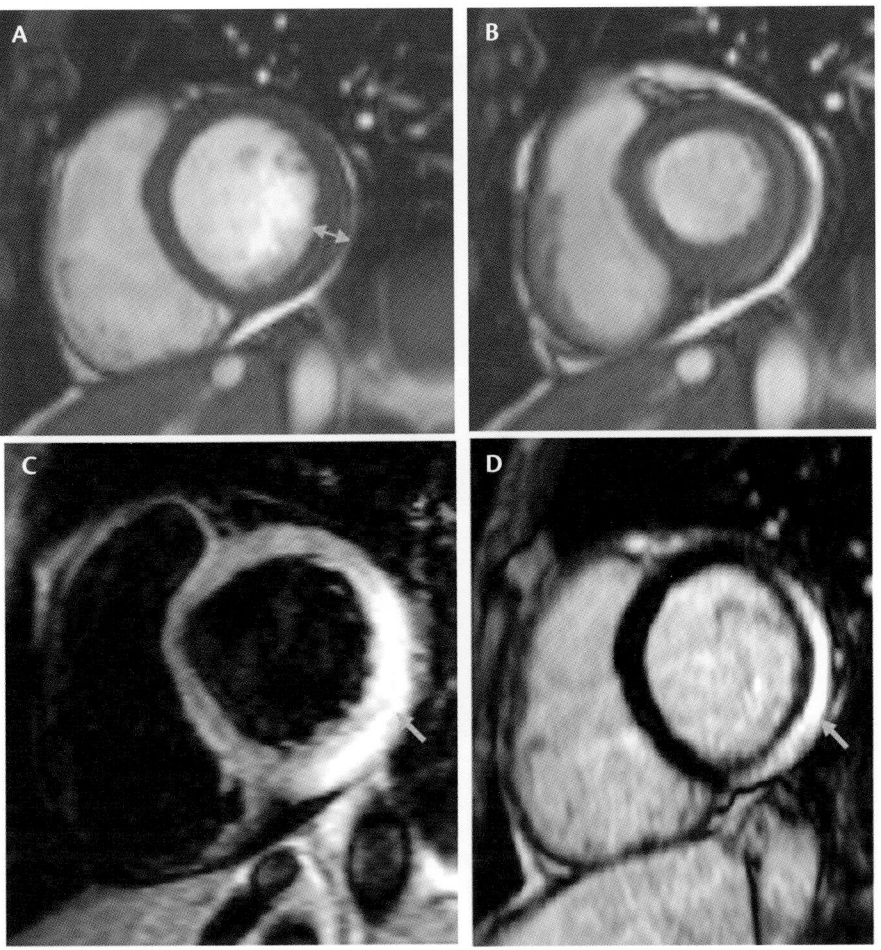

Fig. 21.4 Acute viral myocarditis resulting in thickened lateral wall with mild hypokinesia on ciné imaging. Short-axis ciné in diastole (A) and in systole (B). STIR images detect oedema (C: hyperintensity, arrow) and typical subepicardial LGE (D, arrow).

arrhythmogenic right ventricular cardiomyopathy (ARVC). Although endomyocardial biopsy has been the gold standard diagnostic tool, it is limited by insensitivity and its invasive nature. Among all imaging modalities, CMR appears to be the most powerful in diagnosing myocarditis, by detecting myocardial oedema in the early stages and irreversible fibrotic changes later in the disease process, distinguishing it from infarction and stress-induced cardiomyopathy.

Several aspects of the disease can be imaged by CMR:

- In the acute setting, aside from functional and morphological abnormalities, STIR sequences detect areas of hyperintense myocardial oedema and inflammation with good diagnostic accuracy (Fig. 21.4A–C).[13]
- Increased EGE matching areas of T_2-hyperintensity reflects myocardial hyperaemia and capillary leak.
- Associated pericarditis can be seen as pericardial T_2-hyperintensity and early gadolinium uptake.

As a consequence of myocardial necrosis, several LGE patterns can be seen:

- Typically, LGE is localized to the subepicardium of the inferolateral wall and less frequently to the anteroseptum (Fig. 21.4D). Usually focal, it can also be multifocal or diffuse but typically spares the subendocardium distinguishing it from ischaemia-mediated injury.[14]
- Localization of myocardial damage on CMR seems related to the type of virus and has been used to guide endomyocardial biopsy, enhancing the diagnostic accuracy.[13]
- Acutely, LGE extent has been inversely correlated with 3-year EF.[15]

Iron overload

Myocardial iron overload as a result of transfusion-dependant anaemia leads to diastolic and systolic HF, the leading cause of death in these patients despite iron-chelating therapy.

Intensive chelation therapy in the early stages of the disease appears essential to increase life expectancy. However, serum ferritin levels or liver iron are poorly correlated with myocardial iron load. CMR has made possible the noninvasive quantification of myocardial and liver iron as well as cardiac function in the same scan.

Anderson *et al.*[16] first described the utility of T_2^* relaxation time to measure iron levels from signal intensity decay. A single short-axis midventricular slice is acquired at nine different echo times to derive the T_2^* value arising from field inhomogeneities. The typical epicardial deposition of iron can be visualized *in vivo* (Fig. 21.5). Aside from monitoring accurately chelation therapy, T_2^* is also a predictive marker of HF and arrhythmias.[16] In a cross-sectional study, 89% of thalassaemia patients with new-onset HF had a T_2^* of less than 10 ms, defining severe cardiac iron overload.

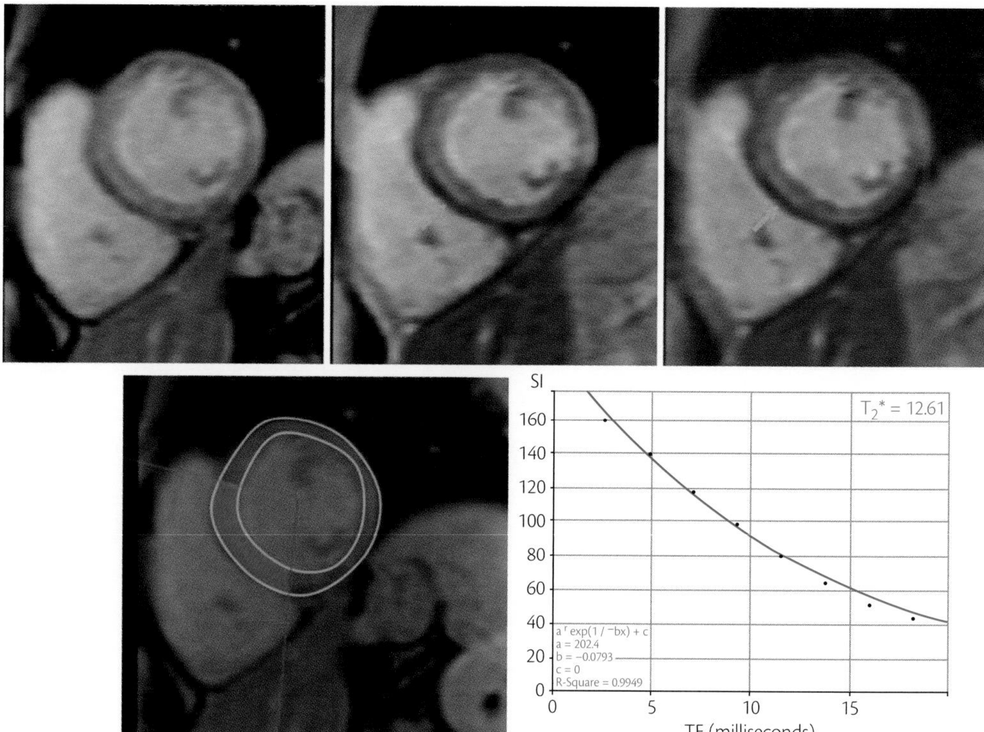

Fig. 21.5 Epicardial iron deposition (arrows) seen in iron-overload cardiomyopathy quantified from the time decay in signal intensity to derive a T_2^* value.

Modell *et al.*[17] studied the impact of T_2^* measurement in changing outcome among United Kingdom thalassaemia patients and noticed a dramatic reduction in mortality as a result of identification of severe myocardial iron overload and subsequent intensification of iron chelation.

Heart failure with normal ejection fraction

Many myocardial and nonmyocardial conditions can cause HeFNEF. Abnormal diastolic function is the main cause, easily diagnosed by Doppler echocardiography from evidence of abnormal relaxation, decreased compliance and increased filling pressures while left ventricular dimensions and LVEF are normal.[18] Alteration in left ventricular distensibility results from hypertension, CAD, restrictive, obstructive, and infiltrative cardiomyopathies.

While HeFNEF is diagnosed by two-dimensional and Doppler echocardiography, CMR is an ideal complementary tool to identify its underlying aetiology to target further management better.

Hypertensive heart disease

By providing precise and reproducible quantification of left ventricular volumes, LVEF, left ventricular mass, and wall thickness in any segment, CMR allows a precise detection of serial changes in an individual patient after initiation of treatment.[19]

In addition, secondary causes of hypertension, such as renal artery stenosis, coarctation, or adrenal adenomas can be sought during the same scan. The consequences of long-standing hypertension on aortic dimensions can also be assessed precisely.

LGE-CMR provides unique information to assist the differential diagnosis of hypertrophic cardiomyopathy or infiltrative diseases.

Interestingly, although up to 50% of patients may demonstrate patchy LGE, visibly enhanced myocardial regions are usually absent using LGE-CMR even in the presence of diffuse interstitial fibrosis, prompting the use of specific T_1-mapping techniques to quantify amount of collagen.[20]

Severity of diastolic dysfunction has been correlated to amount of CMR-detected fibrosis.[21]

Hypertrophic cardiomyopathy

Hypertrophic cardiomyopathy (HCM) is the most common cause of SCD in the young, including trained athletes, and an important substrate for HF disability at any age.[22]

Symptoms can be caused by a variety of mechanisms including left ventricular outflow tract obstruction, arrhythmias, impaired filling due to diastolic dysfunction or impaired systolic function.

Although ECG abnormalities can be the initial and sole clinical clue to HCM, the diagnosis is generally suspected by two-dimensional echocardiographic identification of an asymmetrically hypertrophied, nondilated left ventricle in the absence of another systemic or cardiac disease that is capable of producing the magnitude of wall thickening evident.

However, the distribution and magnitude of left ventricular hypertrophy (LVH) is highly heterogeneous among individuals harbouring the same HCM-causing mutant gene and a proportion of HCM patients are seemingly free from LVH during at least part of their clinical course.[23]

In addition, the detection of mild and localized increase in left ventricular wall thickness in trained athletes or long-term hypertensive patients adds to the diagnostic challenge, raising the differential diagnosis between HCM and physiological or secondary hypertrophy. This is further complicated by the presence of disease mimicking HCM such as amyloidosis or Fabry's disease and by the coexistence of hypertension and HCM in a proportion of patients.

By providing nonoblique images of high spatial resolution, with uniform contrast at the endocardial borders, encompassing all regions of the left ventricle, CMR has the potential to detect

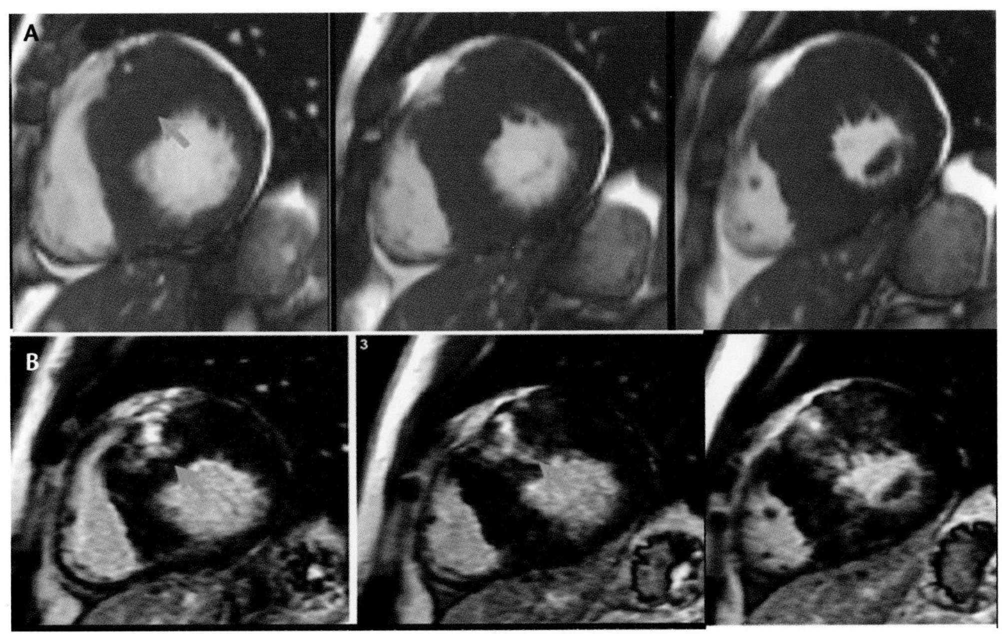

Fig. 21.6 HCM patient with marked asymmetrical septal hypertrophy on a stack of short-axis cinés (A, arrow) with patchy LGE in the area of hypertrophy (B, arrows)

segmental wall thickening in any area of the left ventricle (Fig. 21.6A).

Importantly, with the use of CMR, Maron *et al.*[24] identified a spectrum of distribution and pattern of left ventricular wall thickening in HCM patients. About 50% had regional hypertrophy, affecting mainly the basal anterior wall, with a normal left ventricular mass. A minority of HCM patients undetected with conventional imaging were characterized by areas of hypertrophy confined to the anterolateral wall, inferoseptum, and apex, more difficult to image by transthoracic echocardiography. CMR better delineated left ventricular apical aneurysms, affecting 2% of HCM patients, conferring increased risk of SCD, ventricular arrhythmias, thromboembolic strokes, and progressive HF.[25]

Microvascular dysfunction induced by coronary arteriole dysplasia or mismatch between increased left ventricular mass and coronary flow appears as circumferential stress perfusion defects on CMR and may contribute to the risk attributable to HCM.[26]

In vivo identification and quantification of fibrosis by LGE-CMR contributes to the diagnostic features found in up to 80% of HCM patients. Commonly, those segments with the greatest hypertrophy are those displaying more LGE, probably as the consequence of long-standing microvascular ischaemia, myocyte death, and fibrosis. Typical patterns include transseptal or RV septal fibrosis, confluent septal or multifocal LGE (Fig. 21.6B). The extent of LGE correlated with increased risk of SCD and HF and was predictive of nonsustained VT and atrial fibrillation.[27,28]

While HCM patients without LGE have an excellent prognosis (100% event-free survival at 6-year follow-up), LGE involving 5% or more of left ventricular mass, septal thickness 30 mm or more, and AF are independent predictors of death and ICD discharges.[28]

Among other prognostic markers, the extent of LVH with marked CMR-calculated left ventricular mass correlate both with the presence of a left ventricular outflow tract gradient and worse HF functional class.[24]

Amyloidosis

This infiltrative disease is characterized by the deposition of fibrillary amyloid proteins leading to thickened myocardial walls and diastolic dysfunction resulting in restrictive cardiomyopathy. The most common form, systemic AL amyloidosis, is derived from immunoglobulin light chains. Familial and age-related forms are also described. Cardiac involvement is frequent in the AL form and is associated with a poor prognosis, representing the main cause of death in 50%.

Although echocardiography can raise the suspicion of the diagnosis, endomyocardial biopsy provides the definitive diagnosis. Detection of early stage disease, which may respond to therapy, and exclusion of other disease mimicking amyloidosis, is crucial for patient management.

CMR offers unique diagnostic and prognostic information, helping the early detection of the disease. Typical findings include a small left ventricle with concentric left ventricular (and, inconsistently, right ventricular) wall thickening. Asymmetrical septal thickening mimicking HCM is found in up to 50% of patients. Other features include impaired long-axis function, thickened atrial walls and valve leaflets, dilated atria, and pericardial and pleural effusion. CMR excels by its unique ability to diagnose the macroscopic changes of myocardial tissue composition induced by amyloidosis, by the typical LGE-CMR pattern not seen in any other hypertrophic disease.[29]

Accumulation of amyloid in the myocardial interstitium results in peculiar gadolinium kinetics with faster washout of gadolinium from blood and myocardium. This often leads to a challenging LGE acquisition with inability to null the myocardium. Typically a predominant diffuse, global, and subendocardial LGE distribution (up to 69%) is found matching the distribution of amyloid on histology (Fig. 21.7).[29,30] The left ventricular midwall is often spared giving rise to a characteristic 'zebra striped' pattern of enhancement (Fig. 21.7B). LGE identified cardiac involvement in patients with AL amyloidosis with a sensitivity and specificity of 86% and correlated with severity of HF.[31]

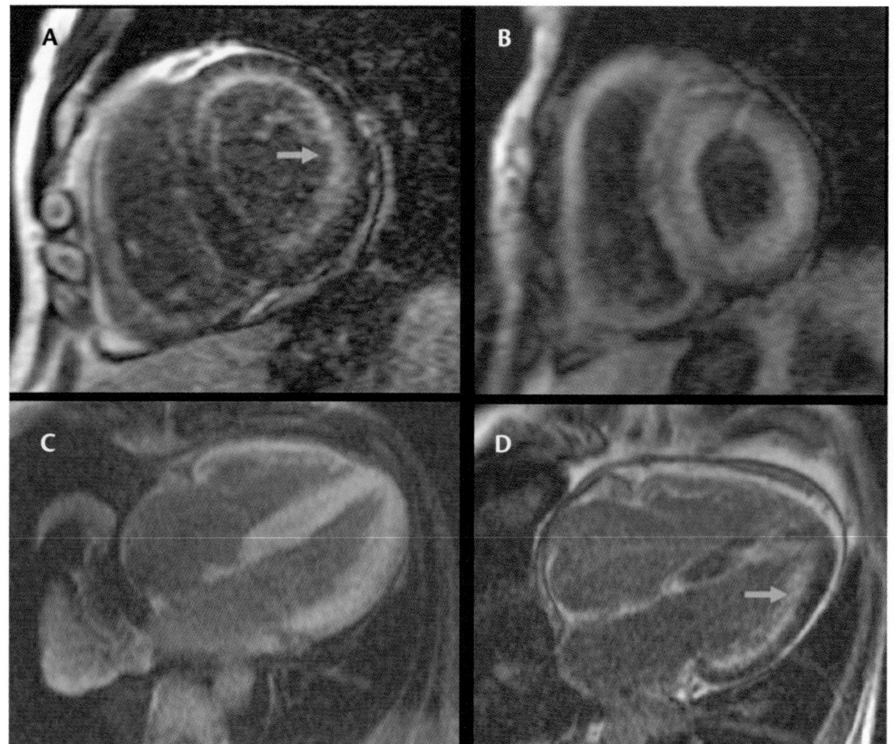

Fig. 21.7 Peculiar gadolinium kinetics in amyloidosis, leading to inability to null the myocardium, with circumferential subendocardial enhancement (A, D), sparing the midwall in a zebra pattern (B) or diffuse LGE (C).

Recently, Syed *et al.*[32] observed that LGE-CMR may detect early cardiac abnormalities in patients with amyloidosis and normal left ventricular wall thickness. Interestingly, while LGE helped the diagnosis, gadolinium kinetics, measured as intramyocardial T_1 gradient, reflecting cardiac amyloid burden, predicted survival. Thus, abnormal T_1 mapping may identify patients in whom early use of more intensive chemotherapy might be justified.[33]

Arrhythmogenic right ventricular cardiomyopathy

Arrhythmogenic right ventricular cardiomyopathy (ARVC) is an under-recognized clinical entity characterized by a fibrofatty replacement of the right ventricular myocardium, involving the left ventricle in up to 75% of cases.

Dilated right ventricle of unknown aetiology, arrhythmias originating from the right ventricular outflow tract, or SCD is often the initial presentation. Despite the fact that right ventricular enlargement and dysfunction are essential features of ARVC, signs of right ventricular failure were seen only in 6% of patients.[34] In spite of recent advances in genotyping, the clinical diagnosis remains challenging and relies on the ARVC Task Force criteria, poorly sensitive for detection of gene-carriers with limited disease expression and those with left-sided disease features.[35]

CMR, is the gold standard for assessing the right ventricle, and offers a complete morphological assessment of the right ventricle without restriction by acoustic windows, detecting global or regional right ventricular dysfunction, wall motion abnormalities, areas of thinning, or aneurysm formation (Fig. 21.8A, B). High temporal resolution transaxial ciné, done in dedicated centres by experienced observers, improves this assessment, reaching a sensitivity of 96% and specificity of 76%.[36]

T_1-weighted spin echo images were used initially with wide enthusiasm to detect fatty infiltration of the right ventricle free wall but proved of limited value due to difficulties in imaging the thin right ventricular wall and because some healthy individuals have right ventricular adipose infiltration.[37]

Initial reports focused on detection of right ventricular LGE as a marker of the disease. However, subsequent studies supported left ventricular LGE as the most discriminating diagnostic variable,[36] highlighting difficulties in distinguishing right ventricular LGE from myocardial fat, requiring substantially different inversion times compared to the left ventricle.

Left ventricular LGE commonly affects the subepicardium or the midwall (Fig. 21.8C, D) and predicts inducibility of sustained ventricular tachycardia (VT), fibrosis on endomyocardial biopsy, and right ventricular impairment even if its prognostic role still remains unclear.

While no single variable yet allows the detection of ARVC, CMR is an integral component of the diagnostic process in addition to ECG, echocardiography, and other standardized criteria.

Left ventricular noncompaction

Left ventricular noncompaction (LVNC) is an uncommon cardiac abnormality characterized by excessive and prominent trabeculations in the left ventricle (Fig. 21.9) associated with deep recesses. It results from failure of the trabecular regression which occurs during normal embryological development.

LVNC can be an isolated feature or associated with other congenital disorders or genetic syndromes, and may lead to progressive HF, ventricular arrhythmias, and thromboembolic manifestations.[38] It usually affects the left ventricle alone, but in fewer than 50% of cases, it can also involve the right ventricle. Features can overlap with DCM, HCM, and restrictive cardiomyopathy.

Although the diagnosis is generally made by echocardiography, CMR has the advantage of higher spatial resolution at the apex and the lateral wall. Hypertrabeculation, with a diastolic ratio of noncompacted over compacted myocardium of 2.3, distinguishes

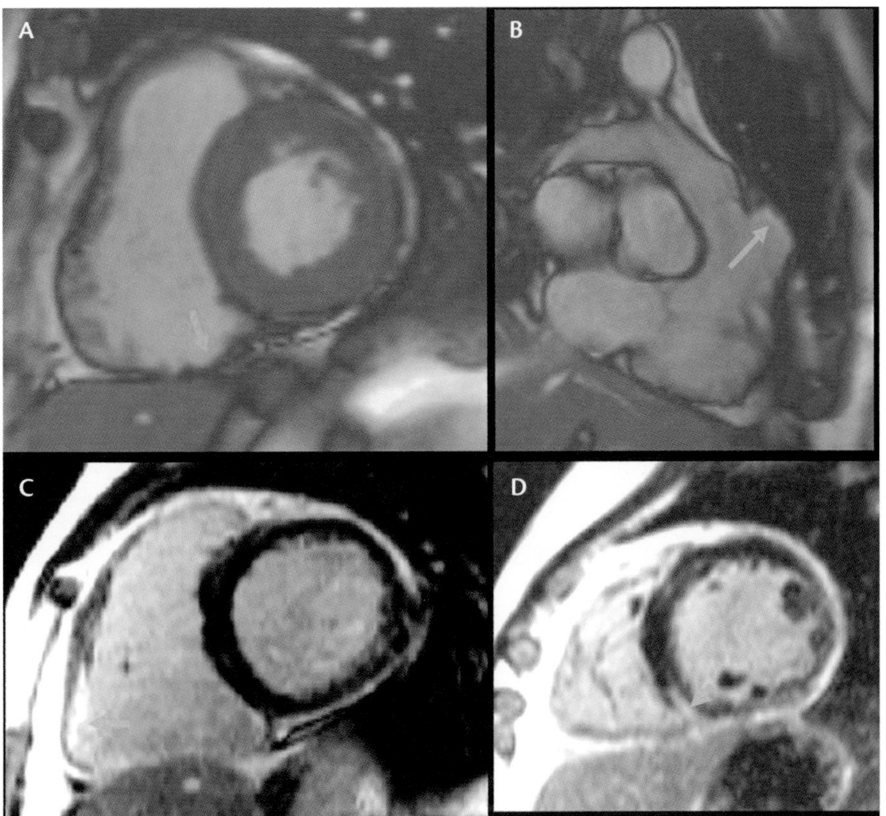

Fig. 21.8 Localized dyskinesia (A) or aneurysm formation (B, right ventricular outflow tract view with localized outflow tract aneurysm, arrow) suggestive of ARVC. LGE in the right ventricular free wall (C, arrow). In the left-sided form of the disease, areas of mid-wall LGE can be identified at right ventricle–left ventricle insertion points (D, arrow).

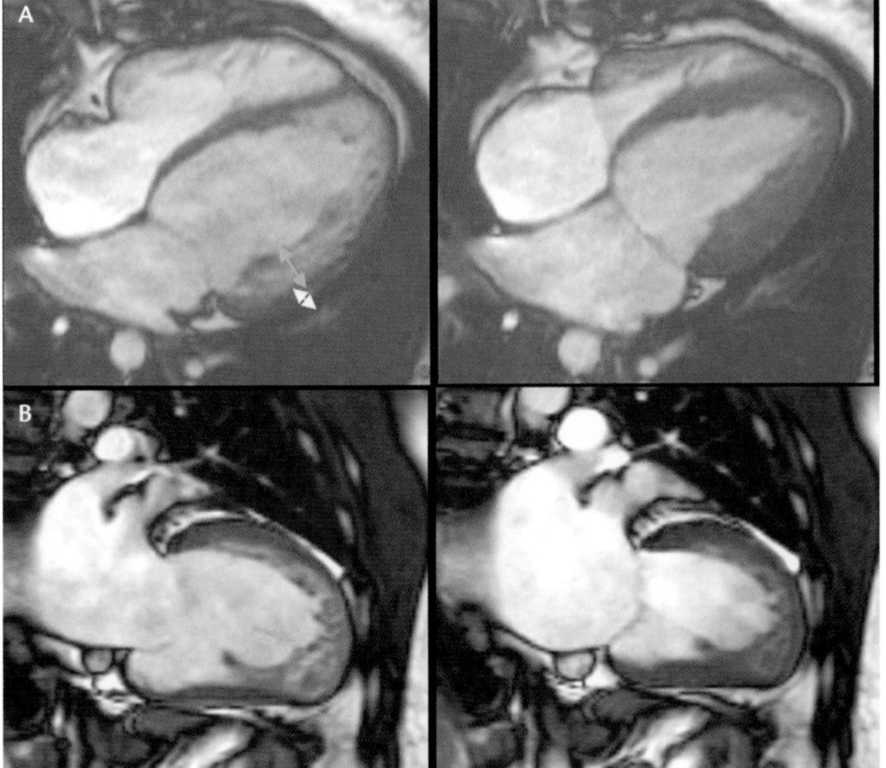

Fig. 21.9 Prominent trabeculations with deep recesses and a ratio of noncompacted over compacted myocardium of 2.3 identifies LVNC. (A) Four-chamber view in diastole and systole; orange arrow displays noncompacted, and white arrow compacted, myocardium. (B). Two-chamber view in diastole and systole.

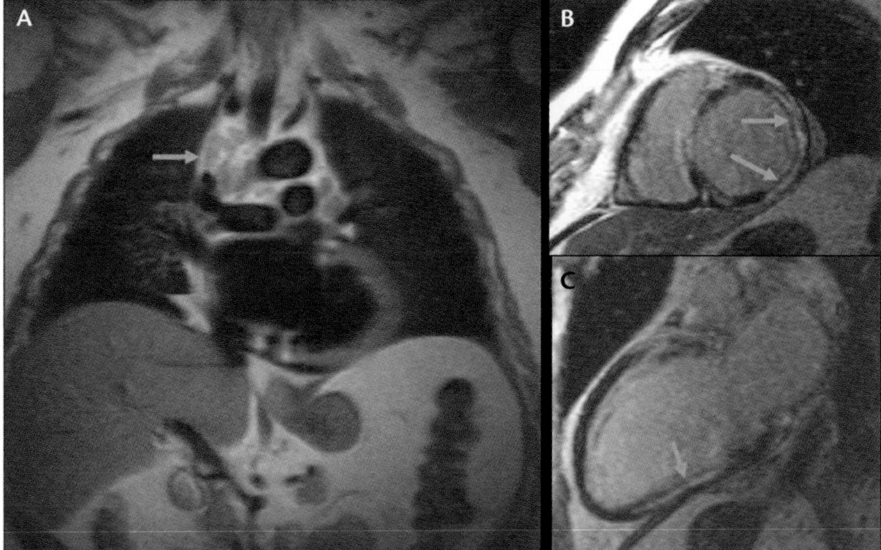

Fig. 21.10 Known extracardiac sarcoidosis patient displaying mediastinal lymphadenopathy on HASTE imaging (A, arrow) associated with diffuse midwall LGE. (B) Short-axis view, arrow. (C) Two-chamber view, arrows.

pathological from nonpathological conditions with a sensitivity of 86% and specificity of 99%.[39] Dursun *et al.*[40] reported three morphological findings: extensive spongy myocardium, prominent trabeculations with deep recesses, and thinned dysplastic myocardium with excessive trabeculations. The absence of well-formed papillary muscles also represents a clue to the diagnosis.

Interestingly, recent reports showed that trabecular LGE subendocardially, in the midwall or transmurally was a common finding, probably as a consequence of microvascular dysfunction.[40,41] The extent of LVNC and the amount and degree of trabecular LGE correlate with LVEF.[41]

Sarcoidosis

This multisystem granulomatous disease of unknown aetiology affects the myocardium in 50% of cases of fatal sarcoidosis, with cardiac dysfunction and SCD occurring in up to 67% of patients with evidence of cardiac sarcoidosis found at autopsy. Interestingly, only 23% of patients with cardiac involvement die from HF.[42] Clinical manifestations depend on the location and extent of granulomatous inflammation and vary from conduction defects and ventricular arrhythmias to diastolic and systolic HF.[43] As myocardial involvement alters the prognosis, an early diagnosis is crucial as current therapy may prevent death from cardiac failure and ventricular arrhythmias.

Endomyocardial biopsy and echocardiography are insensitive in identifying myocardial involvement: due to the patchy nature of the disease, relatively advanced stages of the disease tend to be detected. CMR detected myocardial involvement in patients with clinically diagnosed cardiac disease with a sensitivity of 100% compared with 50% for thallium SPECT and 20% for gallium SPECT.[44] Using T_2-weighted and STIR imaging, CMR identified areas of active inflammation which are reversible with treatment from areas of irreversible myocardial scarring detected by LGE.

In patients with biopsy-proven extracardiac sarcoidosis, LGE is twice as sensitive for cardiac involvement as the widely used clinical Japanese Ministry of Health and Welfare criteria.[45] Typical CMR findings include areas of focal signal hyperintensity on STIR imaging, corresponding to localized myocardial inflammation. Regional wall motion abnormalities and thinning inconsistent with anatomical coronary artery distribution can be identified on ciné imaging.

LGE as a consequence of granulomatous sarcoid infiltration includes midwall, subepicardial, or patchy patterns (Fig. 21.10).[46] In addition to providing diagnostic clues to the disease, LGE-CMR may be associated with adverse events, as even small regions of myocardial damage provide a substrate for ventricular arrhythmias and conduction disturbances.

Patel *et al.*[45] reported a 9-fold higher rate of adverse events and an 11-fold higher rate of cardiac death in sarcoidosis patients with myocardial damage detected by LGE-CMR. However, the negative predictive value of a negative CMR still remains unknown. Of interest, LGE can be used also to guide localization for endomyocardial biopsy and to monitor the efficacy of steroid therapy.[47]

Conclusions

Through a wide range of sequences, CMR is an ideal complementary tool, providing priceless information in the work-up of a cardiomyopathy patient. The ability of CMR to provide *in vivo* tissue characterization assists the diagnostic process and provides new measures for risk stratification. In addition, the absence of ionizing radiation offers the opportunity of family screening and regular follow-up.

References

1. Jessup M, Abraham WT, Casey DE, *et al.* 2009 focused update: ACCF/AHA Guidelines for the Diagnosis and Management of Heart Failure in Adults: a report of the American College of Cardiology Foundation/American Heart Association Task Force on Practice Guidelines: developed in collaboration with the International Society for Heart and Lung Transplantation. *Circulation* 2009;**119**(14):1977–2016.
2. Cawley PJ, Maki JH, Otto CM. Cardiovascular magnetic resonance imaging for valvular heart disease: technique and validation. *Circulation* 2009;**119**(3):468–78.
3. Kim RJ, Fieno DS, Parrish TB, *et al.* Relationship of MRI delayed contrast enhancement to irreversible injury, infarct age, and contractile function. *Circulation* 1999;**100**(19):1992–2002.
4. McCrohon JA, Moon JC, Prasad SK, *et al.* Differentiation of heart failure related to dilated cardiomyopathy and coronary artery disease using

gadolinium-enhanced cardiovascular magnetic resonance. *Circulation* 2003;**108**(1):54–9.

5. Valle-Munoz A, Estornell-Erill J, Soriano-Navarro CJ, *et al.* Late gadolinium enhancement-cardiovascular magnetic resonance identifies coronary artery disease as the aetiology of left ventricular dysfunction in acute new-onset congestive heart failure. *Eur J Echocardiogr* 2009;**10**(8):968–74.
6. Bello D, Fieno DS, Kim RJ, *et al.* Infarct morphology identifies patients with substrate for sustained ventricular tachycardia. *J Am Coll Cardiol* 2005;**45**(7):1104–8.
7. Kwong RY, Chan AK, Brown KA, *et al.* Impact of unrecognized myocardial scar detected by cardiac magnetic resonance imaging on event-free survival in patients presenting with signs or symptoms of coronary artery disease. *Circulation* 2006;**113**(23):2733–43.
8. Chalil S, Stegemann B, Muhyaldeen SA, *et al.* Effect of posterolateral left ventricular scar on mortality and morbidity following cardiac resynchronization therapy. *Pacing Clin Electrophysiol* 2007;**30**(10):1201–9.
9. Younger JF, Plein S, Crean A, Ball SG, Greenwood JP. Visualization of coronary venous anatomy by cardiovascular magnetic resonance. *J Cardiovasc Magn Reson* 2009;**11**(1):26.
10. Maron BJ, Towbin JA, Thiene G, *et al.* Contemporary definitions and classification of the cardiomyopathies: an American Heart Association Scientific Statement from the Council on Clinical Cardiology, Heart Failure and Transplantation Committee;Quality of Care and Outcomes Research and Functional Genomics and Translational Biology Interdisciplinary Working Groups;and Council on Epidemiology and Prevention. *Circulation* 2006;**113**(14):1807–16.
11. Assomull RG, Prasad SK, Lyne J, *et al.* Cardiovascular magnetic resonance, fibrosis, and prognosis in dilated cardiomyopathy. *J Am Coll Cardiol* 2006;**48**(10):1977–85.
12. Wu KC, Weiss RG, Thiemann DR, *et al.* Late gadolinium enhancement by cardiovascular magnetic resonance heralds an adverse prognosis in nonischemic cardiomyopathy. *J Am Coll Cardiol* 2008;**51**(25):2414–21.
13. Abdel-Aty H, Boye P, Zagrosek A, *et al.* Diagnostic performance of cardiovascular magnetic resonance in patients with suspected acute myocarditis: comparison of different approaches. *J Am Coll Cardiol* 2005;**45**(11):1815–22.
14. Friedrich MG, Sechtem U, Schulz-Menger J, *et al.* Cardiovascular magnetic resonance in myocarditis: A JACC White Paper. *J Am Coll Cardiol* 2009;**53**(17):1475–87.
15. Wagner A, Schulz-Menger J, Dietz R, Friedrich MG. Long-term follow-up of patients paragraph sign with acute myocarditis by magnetic paragraph sign resonance imaging. *MAGMA* 2003;**16**(1):17–20.
16. Anderson LJ, Holden S, Davis B, *et al.* Cardiovascular T2-star (T2*) magnetic resonance for the early diagnosis of myocardial iron overload. *Eur Heart J* 2001;**22**(23):2171–9.
17. Modell B, Khan M, Darlison M, Westwood MA, Ingram D, Pennell DJ. Improved survival of thalassaemia major in the UK and relation to T2* cardiovascular magnetic resonance. *J Cardiovasc Magn Reson* 2008;**10**(1):42.
18. Oh JK, Hatle L, Tajik AJ, Little WC. Diastolic heart failure can be diagnosed by comprehensive two-dimensional and Doppler echocardiography. *J Am Coll Cardiol* 2006;**47**(3):500–506.
19. Grothues F, Smith GC, Moon JC, *et al.* Comparison of interstudy reproducibility of cardiovascular magnetic resonance with two-dimensional echocardiography in normal subjects and in patients with heart failure or left ventricular hypertrophy. *Am J Cardiol* 2002;**90**(1):29–34.
20. Rudolph A, Abdel-Aty H, Bohl S, *et al.* Noninvasive detection of fibrosis applying contrast-enhanced cardiac magnetic resonance in different forms of left ventricular hypertrophy relation to remodeling. *J Am Coll Cardiol* 2009;**53**(3):284–91.
21. Moreo A, Ambrosio G, De Chiara B, *et al.* Influence of myocardial fibrosis on left ventricular diastolic function: noninvasive assessment by cardiac magnetic resonance and echo. *Circ Cardiovasc Imaging* 2009;**2**(6):437–43.
22. Maron BJ. Sudden death in young athletes. *N Engl J Med* 2003;**349**(11):1064–75.
23. Rickers C, Wilke NM, Jerosch-Herold M, *et al.* Utility of cardiac magnetic resonance imaging in the diagnosis of hypertrophic cardiomyopathy. *Circulation* 2005;**112**(6):855–61.
24. Maron MS, Maron BJ, Harrigan C, *et al.* Hypertrophic cardiomyopathy phenotype revisited after 50 years with cardiovascular magnetic resonance. *J Am Coll Cardiol* 2009;**54**(3):220–8.
25. Maron MS, Finley JJ, Bos JM, *et al.* Prevalence, clinical significance, and natural history of left ventricular apical aneurysms in hypertrophic cardiomyopathy. *Circulation* 2008;**118**(15):1541–9.
26. Petersen SE, Jerosch-Herold M, Hudsmith LE, *et al.* Evidence for microvascular dysfunction in hypertrophic cardiomyopathy: new insights from multiparametric magnetic resonance imaging. *Circulation* 2007;**115**(18):2418–25.
27. Adabag AS, Maron BJ, Appelbaum E, *et al.* Occurrence and frequency of arrhythmias in hypertrophic cardiomyopathy in relation to delayed enhancement on cardiovascular magnetic resonance. *J Am Coll Cardiol* 2008;**51**(14):1369–74.
28. Flett AS, Westwood MA, Davies LC, Mathur A, Moon JC. The prognostic implications of cardiovascular magnetic resonance. *Circ Cardiovasc Imaging* 2009;**2**(3):243–50.
29. Maceira AM, Joshi J, Prasad SK, *et al.* Cardiovascular magnetic resonance in cardiac amyloidosis. *Circulation* 2005;**111**(2):186–93.
30. Cheng AS, Banning AP, Mitchell AR, Neubauer S, Selvanayagam JB. Cardiac changes in systemic amyloidosis: visualisation by magnetic resonance imaging. *Int J Cardiol* 2006;**113**(1):E21–23.
31. Ruberg FL, Appelbaum E, Davidoff R, *et al.* Diagnostic and prognostic utility of cardiovascular magnetic resonance imaging in light-chain cardiac amyloidosis. *Am J Cardiol* 2009;**103**(4):544–9.
32. Syed IS, Glockner JF, Feng D, *et al.* Role of cardiac magnetic resonance imaging in the detection of cardiac amyloidosis. *JACC Cardiovasc Imaging*;**3**(2):155–64.
33. Maceira AM, Prasad SK, Hawkins PN, Roughton M, Pennell DJ. Cardiovascular magnetic resonance and prognosis in cardiac amyloidosis. *J Cardiovasc Magn Reson* 2008;**10**(1):54.
34. Hulot JS, Jouven X, Empana JP, Frank R, Fontaine G. Natural history and risk stratification of arrhythmogenic right ventricular dysplasia/cardiomyopathy. *Circulation* 2004;**110**(14):1879–1884.
35. Sen-Chowdhry S, McKenna WJ. The utility of magnetic resonance imaging in the evaluation of arrhythmogenic right ventricular cardiomyopathy. *Curr Opin Cardiol* 2008;**23**(1):38–45.
36. Sen-Chowdhry S, Prasad SK, Syrris P, *et al.* Cardiovascular magnetic resonance in arrhythmogenic right ventricular cardiomyopathy revisited: comparison with task force criteria and genotype. *J Am Coll Cardiol* 2006;**48**(10):2132–40.
37. Tandri H, Calkins H, Marcus FI. Controversial role of magnetic resonance imaging in the diagnosis of arrhythmogenic right ventricular dysplasia. *Am J Cardiol* 2003;**92**(5):649.
38. Oechslin EN, Attenhofer Jost CH, Rojas JR, Kaufmann PA, Jenni R. Long-term follow-up of 34 adults with isolated left ventricular noncompaction: a distinct cardiomyopathy with poor prognosis. *J Am Coll Cardiol* 2000;**36**(2):493–500.
39. Petersen SE, Selvanayagam JB, Wiesmann F, Robson MD, Francis JM, Anderson RH, Watkins H, Neubauer S. Left ventricular non-compaction: insights from cardiovascular magnetic resonance imaging. *J Am Coll Cardiol* 2005;**46**(1):101–5.
40. Dursun M, Agayev A, Nisli K, *et al.* MR imaging features of ventricular noncompaction: emphasis on distribution and pattern of fibrosis. *Eur J Radiol* 2010;**74**(1):147–51.
41. Dodd JD, Holmvang G, Hoffmann U, *et al.* Quantification of left ventricular noncompaction and trabecular delayed hyperenhancement with cardiac MRI: correlation with clinical severity. *AJR Am J Roentgenol* 2007;**189**(4):974–80.

42. Sharma S. Cardiac imaging in myocardial sarcoidosis and other cardiomyopathies. *Curr Opin Pulm Med* 2009;**15**(5): 507–512.
43. Ayyala US, Nair AP, Padilla ML. Cardiac sarcoidosis. *Clin Chest Med* 2008;**29**(3):493–508, ix.
44. Tadamura E, Yamamuro M, Kubo S, *et al.* Effectiveness of delayed enhanced MRI for identification of cardiac sarcoidosis: comparison with radionuclide imaging. *AJR Am J Roentgenol* 2005;**185**(1):110–15.
45. Patel MR, Cawley PJ, Heitner JF, *et al.* Detection of myocardial damage in patients with sarcoidosis. *Circulation* 2009;**120**(20):1969–77.
46. Ichinose A, Otani H, Oikawa M, *et al.* MRI of cardiac sarcoidosis: basal and subepicardial localization of myocardial lesions and their effect on left ventricular function. *AJR Am J Roentgenol* 2008;**191**(3):862–9.
47. Shimada T, Shimada K, Sakane T, *et al.* Diagnosis of cardiac sarcoidosis and evaluation of the effects of steroid therapy by gadolinium-DTPA-enhanced magnetic resonance imaging. *Am J Med* 2001;**110**(7):520–7.

22

CT imaging techniques

Joanne D. Schuijf, Laurens F. Tops, and Jeroen J. Bax

Introduction

In patients presenting with heart failure (HF), assessment of underlying aetiology is critical for optimal management. To differentiate between ischaemic and nonischaemic dilated cardiomyopathy, invasive coronary angiography is frequently performed. This technique is currently still considered the gold standard in the detection of coronary artery disease (CAD). In addition to accurate assessment of the presence, location, and severity of coronary artery lesions, the technique also provides the opportunity for direct intervention. On the other hand, the technique carries a small but not negligible risk of complications, while in many patients no clinically relevant abnormalities will be observed. Patients presenting with unexplained dilated cardiomyopathy and a low to intermediate likelihood of CAD may therefore benefit from a noninvasive imaging approach.

To this end, anatomical imaging with CT techniques has been proposed. With this technology, high-resolution images of the coronary arteries are obtained. In addition, detailed information on cardiac structures, and to some extent also function, can be derived. The aim of the current chapter is to provide an overview of the various applications of CT technology that may be relevant in the setting of HF.

CT techniques

Two CT-based modalities have been used for noninvasive anatomical cardiac imaging: electron beam CT (EBCT) and multidetector row CT (MDCT). Both techniques allow assessment of coronary calcifications and, during the administration of contrast, noninvasive coronary angiography. Developments have been particularly rapid for MDCT; in combination with its widespread availability this technique has become the most commonly CT technique in clinical practice.

During MDCT a gantry containing an X-ray tube and a detector system rotates around the patient to acquire multiple images during a single rotation. While initial systems allowed acquisition of 4 slices per rotation, current systems consist of up to 320 detector rows with submillimetre slice thickness. In addition, temporal resolution has been improved by faster rotation times as well as the introduction of dual-source CT systems. Nevertheless, most systems still require a low and stable heart rate to obtain good image quality, and β-blocking medication is frequently administered prior to MDCT imaging for this purpose.

During the administration of a bolus of iodinated contrast agent, a three-dimensional dataset of the entire heart is obtained within a single breath-hold of less than 10 s. Data acquisition is synchronized to the ECG to allow reconstruction of motion-free images. At present, several acquisition techniques are available, which are specified in Table 22.1. During ECG-gated spiral acquisition, the patient is moved continuously through the gantry at a slow speed while images are continuously acquired. This approach allows retrospective reconstruction of high-resolution datasets at any desired interval of the cardiac cycle. To reduce radiation exposure, dose modulation can be applied.[1] During dose modulation, the tube current is lowered during the phases that are expected not to be used for reconstruction of the coronary arteries. Although the images during these phases contain more noise and are of lower image quality, evaluation of noncoronary structures remains possible. More recently, prospective ECG-triggered, sequential scanning is increasingly applied.[1,2] Rather than continuous rotation of the X-ray tube, data acquisition is triggered by the ECG at a preselected phase. The patient is moved to the next position between successive acquisitions. Since imaging is performed during a small proportion of the cardiac cycle, considerable reduction has been achieved using this scanning mode. Heart rate needs to be stable and slow, however, as no other phases can be reconstructed retrospectively.

Diagnosis of coronary artery disease

Coronary calcium scoring

The presence of calcium in the coronary arteries is an accurate marker for CAD, as coronary calcifications occur exclusively in the presence of atherosclerosis. Moreover, coronary calcifications

Table 22.1 Acquisition protocols for noninvasive coronary angiography with MDCT

ECG		Table	LV function	Radiation dose
	Retrospective ECG gating	Continuous movement	Yes	High
	ECG-correlated tube modulation	Continuous movement	Yes	Moderate
	Prospective ECG, triggering	Sequential movement	No	Low

have high X-ray attenuation values, and are therefore easily recognized during CT imaging without contrast. Initially, data concerning coronary calcium have been obtained with EBCT. More recently, however, MDCT has become the most commonly applied technique for this purpose. An example of a patient with coronary calcium detected on MDCT is shown in Fig. 22.1. The traditional method to quantify coronary calcifications is the Agatston score.[3] Using this method, a score that can vary from 0 to over 1000 is obtained, thereby providing an estimate of the total atherosclerotic burden in the coronary arteries. Importantly, the absence of any calcium implies a very low likelihood of clinically relevant CAD. Extensive coronary calcifications on the other hand have been demonstrated to be strongly related with a higher likelihood of significant stenoses. Presumably, coronary calcium scoring may therefore allow rapid differentiation between ischaemic and nonischaemic aetiology in patients presenting with HF of unknown origin. This concept was investigated by Budoff *et al.*[4] in a cohort of 125 patients with reduced left ventricular ejection fraction (LVEF) and known coronary anatomy based on previous invasive coronary angiography. Coronary calcium scores as determined by EBCT were significantly higher in the 72 patients with ischaemic cardiomyopathy than in the 53 patients with nonischaemic cardiomyopathy (798 ± 899 vs 17 ± 51). Moreover, based on the presence of any calcium, 71 of 72 patients with ischaemic cardiomyopathy (sensitivity 99%) were correctly identified. However, the specificity of a calcium score of 0 was lower (83%) as a positive calcium score frequently occurred in the absence of significant stenosis. Indeed, despite the close correlation between the Agatston score and total atherosclerotic burden, a drawback remains the fact that the technique does not permit direct evaluation of the stenosis severity. High coronary calcium scores reflecting extensive calcifications can be observed in the absence of any luminal narrowing, whereas severe stenosis can be present at sites with minimal calcium. Accordingly, using a low calcium score to define a positive study will result in high sensitivity but low specificity for the presence of a significant stenosis. As illustrated in Table 22.2, specificity will improve when a higher threshold is used, but at the cost of sensitivity. Nonetheless, despite this limitation, coronary calcium scoring may represent a practical initial screening approach to determine whether an ischaemic origin is likely or not, thereby allowing more appropriate selection of further (invasive) evaluation. Interestingly, further research by the same investigators has suggested that coronary calcium scoring may be even a more accurate technique to distinguish ischaemic from nonischaemic cardiomyopathy than nuclear stress testing or resting echocardiography,[5,6] although evidently more data are needed.

Table 22.2 Diagnostic accuracy of different EBCT coronary calcium scores to differentiate ischaemic and nonischaemic cardiomyopathy

Threshold value	Sensitivity (%)	Specificity (%)	PPV (%)	NPV (%)	Accuracy (%)
>0	99	83	89	98	92
≥50	92	91	93	89	97
≥80	90	92	94	88	97
≥220	72	100	100	73	84

NPV: negative predictive value, PPV: positive predictive value.

From Budoff MJ, Shavelle DM, Lamont DH, *et al.* Usefulness of electron beam computed tomography scanning for distinguishing ischemic from nonischemic cardiomyopathy. *J Am Coll Cardiol* 1998;**32**(5):1173–8, with permission.

Noninvasive coronary angiography

As compared to coronary calcium scoring, contrast-enhanced noninvasive coronary angiography has several important advantages, including assessment of stenosis severity as well as the detection of noncalcified plaque in addition to calcified lesions. Accordingly, the technique may provide a more detailed assessment of the presence and severity of CAD, and thus facilitate rapid diagnosis. To evaluate the presence of significant (≥50% coronary lumen reduction) stenosis on MDCT, dedicated workstations are typically used. These workstations allow in addition to manual scrolling through the axial images, interactive manipulation of the dataset, including processing of three-dimensional reconstructions, curved multiplanar reformats, and maximum intensity projections. A clinical

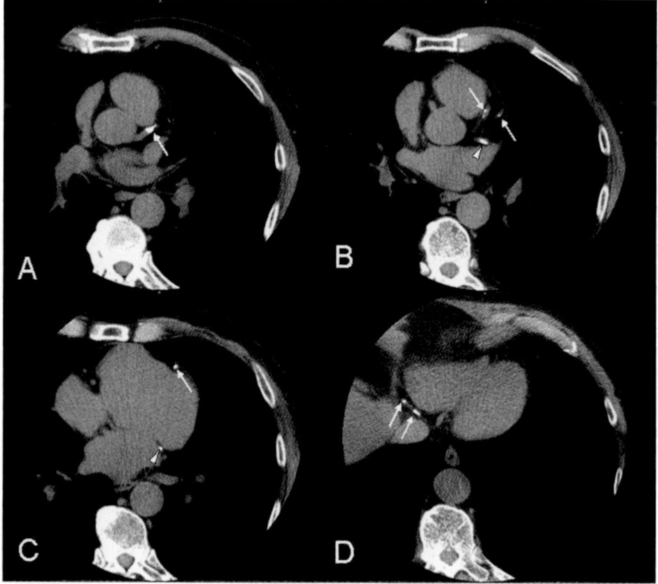

Fig. 22.1 Identification of coronary calcium as a marker for CAD with MDCT. Panels A, B, C, and D are representative 3.00 mm slices without contrast from the base towards the apex. In panel A, a dense calcification can be observed in the proximal left anterior descending coronary artery (LAD), as indicated by the arrow. As visible in panels B and C, the presence of calcifications continues in the mid and distal LAD (arrows) as well as in the left circumflex coronary artery (arrowheads). Finally, also in the distal right coronary artery the presence of calcium was identified (arrows in panel D). Accordingly, in this 65-year-old man, MDCT revealed substantial calcified plaque burden (total coronary calcium score 584), suggesting an increased likelihood of significant CAD.

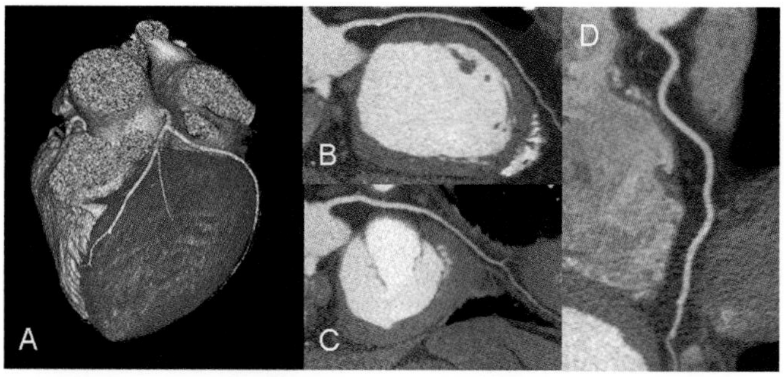

Fig. 22.2 Noninvasive coronary angiography with MDCT. In this 67-year-old patient presenting with left ventricular dilatation and reduced LVEF (34% on two-dimensional echocardiography), prospectively triggered 320-row MDCT was performed to rule out underlying CAD. Panel A is a three-dimensional volume-rendered reconstruction. Panels B, C, and D are curved multiplanar reconstructions of the left anterior descending coronary artery (LAD) (B), left circumflex coronary artery (C), and right coronary artery (D), providing an overview of the entire coronary artery in a single image. Only minor wall irregularities with minimal calcium in the LAD were observed, thereby excluding ischaemic origin of HF.

example of a patient presenting with HF and evaluated by MDCT coronary angiography is shown in Fig. 22.2.

In the general population, the diagnostic accuracy of MDCT to detect significant stenosis has been studied extensively against invasive coronary angiography. Using 64-slice MDCT, which is currently the most frequently used system, sensitivities and specificities exceeding 90% have been reported.[7] Moreover, negative predictive values are particularly high, indicating that the likelihood of CAD is very low for a normal MDCT angiogram. For this reason, MDCT may be an attractive tool to exclude significant CAD and thus avoid invasive coronary angiography in patients with a low to intermediate likelihood of having significant stenosis.[8]

However, particularly in the presence of extensive calcifications or motion artefacts, detected lesions are frequently overestimated on MDCT. As a result, somewhat lower positive predictive values have been reported. Although quantitative approaches that may improve accuracy are currently under development, these algorithms have not yet been fully validated. In addition, the information obtained by MDCT is restricted to anatomy and no information on the presence and extent of ischaemia is obtained. Indeed, the technique cannot differentiate between lesions that are haemodynamically relevant and those that are not. In many cases with abnormal findings on MDCT, additional evaluation is still needed to obtain a definite diagnosis and determine further management. As a result, the value of noninvasive coronary angiography with MDCT is limited in patients with a high clinical suspicion of having significant CAD. In these patients, direct evaluation with invasive coronary angiography remains preferable.

At present only limited studies have been performed dedicated to patients with HF. Andreini *et al.*[9] studied 61 consecutive patients admitted with HF of unknown aetiology using 16-slice MDCT. For comparative purposes, 139 patients undergoing invasive coronary angiography for other clinical indications were also investigated with MDCT. Overall, the technical success rate of the procedure was 97%. Importantly, MDCT allowed correct classification of ischaemic versus nonischaemic cardiomyopathy in all patients. Also on a segmental level, diagnostic accuracy in HF patients was high with a sensitivity and specificity of respectively 99% and 96%. Interestingly, sensitivity and negative predictive values were higher in the HF population than in the control population, probably because of the lower prevalence of CAD in this population (27.8% in the HF group vs 70.5% in the control group). In addition, it is likely that the reduced cardiac and coronary motion in HF may also have had a favourable effect on image quality and diagnostic accuracy.

Similar findings were recently reported using 64-slice MDCT.[10] In this study by Ghostine *et al.*,[10] all patients with significant stenoses (diameter reduction ≥50%) in two or more vessels were classified as having ischaemic cardiomyopathy. However, by definition, patients with single-vessel disease were only classified as having ischaemic cardiomyopathy in the presence of left main or proximal left anterior descending coronary artery stenosis. Using these criteria, MDCT correctly identified 60 of 62 (97%) patients without and 28 of 31 (90%) with ischaemic origin of HF. Although the impact on the patient-based analysis was minimal, the presence of extensive calcifications was identified as a major cause of reduced image quality and incorrect diagnosis on segmental level. In this regard, a stepwise approach incorporating coronary calcium scoring and noninvasive coronary angiography, as proposed by Cornily *et al.*,[11] may be particularly attractive. In their algorithm, coronary evaluation consisted of initial coronary calcium scoring followed by noninvasive coronary angiography in selected cases. Patients with a coronary calcium score of 1000 or higher were referred directly to invasive coronary angiography, based on the rationale not only that the performance of MDCT coronary angiography will be lower but also that many patients will have abnormal studies requiring further evaluation anyway. In the majority of patients, however, coronary calcium scores of less than 1000 were obtained. In these patients, MDCT was shown to accurately rule out CAD as the underlying cause of HF and thus avoid invasive coronary angiography in 21 of 27 (78%) patients. Although larger cohort studies are awaited, recently published guidelines for the diagnosis and treatment of patients with HF indicate that MDCT may indeed be considered to rule out underlying CAD noninvasively in patients with low to intermediate likelihood of significant CAD.[12]

Left ventricular dimensions and function

In addition to the coronary arteries, MDCT can also provide detailed information on chamber morphology and function. Importantly, datasets can be reformatted in any desired plane and, depending on the acquisition technique (see Table 22.1), reconstructed at multiple phases of the cardiac cycle. Typically, to assess left ventricular volumes and function, datasets are reformatted in the short- and long-axis orientation, as illustrated in Fig. 22.3. Subsequently, end-systolic and end-diastolic phases are determined by selecting the smallest and largest cross-sectional left ventricular cavity areas. The high contrast between the left ventricular cavity and the myocardium has facilitated the development of dedicated software algorithms that automatically detect endo- and epicardial borders. Consequently, end-diastolic and end-systolic volumes are derived to obtain LVEF.

Numerous studies have shown excellent correlations between MDCT and other imaging methods.[13–15] Overall, because its temporal resolution is inferior to that of two-dimensional echocardiography and MRI, a tendency of MDCT to overestimate end-systolic volume and thus slightly underestimate LVEF has been observed.

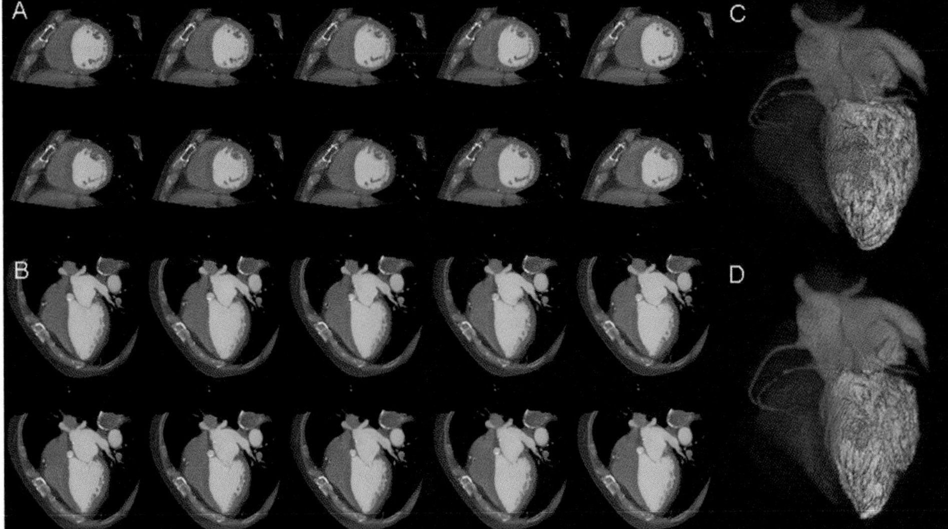

Fig. 22.3 Evaluation of left ventricular function with MDCT. In panels A and B, respectively, short-axis and long-axis views reconstructed throughout the cardiac cycle are provided, showing a dilated left ventricle with severely reduced wall motion. Using automated software (panels C and D) left ventricular volumes were calculated at 403 mL in end diastole and 327 mL in end systole, resulting in a LVEF of 19%.

Nevertheless, Yamamuro *et al.*[13] demonstrated that measurements between MDCT and MRI (the current gold standard for left ventricular function) were more closely related than measurements between two-dimensional echocardiography and MRI, suggesting that MDCT may be even more accurate than two-dimensional echocardiography in the evaluation of left ventricular function.

Displaying the images in ciné-loop format allows evaluation of segmental wall motion in addition to global function. Comparisons against two-dimensional echocardiography and MRI have revealed high accuracy of MDCT in identifying regional wall motion abnormalities. Amongst others, Mahnken *et al.*[16] observed an agreement of 86% between 16-slice MDCT and MRI. Moreover, using newer 64-slice MDCT technology, Henneman *et al.*[15] showed that 96% of segments were scored identically on 64-slice MDCT and two-dimensional echocardiography ($\kappa = 0.82$). Although patients with reduced left ventricular function were included in these investigations, only few studies have specifically focused on patients with HF. Butler *et al.*[17] studied 25 patients with an LVEF of less than 45% who underwent both two-dimensional echocardiography and MDCT. In this cohort with reduced LVEF (average 36 ± 8% on two-dimensional echocardiography), MDCT was shown to provide comparable results to two-dimensional echocardiography for both global and regional function.

Although MDCT may allow reliable assessment of left ventricular function, routine use of MDCT for the sole purpose of functional assessment is not recommended considering the radiation and contrast risks involved. Indeed, echocardiography and MRI remain the preferred techniques, and MDCT is considered only in patients with either suboptimal images during echocardiography or contraindications for MRI. In general, therefore, MDCT function analysis is usually only performed in conjunction with MDCT imaging for other purposes such as noninvasive coronary angiography.

Myocardial infarction

A growing body of literature indicates that MDCT may allow assessment of the presence and extent of myocardial infarction. End-diastolic wall thickness can easily be determined on MDCT, and the presence of end-diastolic wall thickness of less than 6 mm has been shown to correlate with the presence of larger, transmural myocardial infarctions.[18] Moreover, several investigations have confirmed that the observation of myocardial hypoenhancement reflects scar tissue. This concept, which dates back to experimental animal studies in the 1970s, is based on the kinetics of the contrast agent used for MDCT. As in MRI, MDCT imaging is performed during the administration of a bolus of contrast agent, reflecting first-pass perfusion. In both chronic and acute settings, the presence of hypoperfused areas on MDCT has been shown to correlate with triphenyltetrazolium chloride (TTC) staining as well as with the traditionally used imaging modalities. In a porcine model, Mahnken *et al.*[19] showed that hypoenhanced areas visualized by MDCT were strongly correlated to areas of myocardial necrosis on TTC staining and delayed enhancement MRI, although the mean size of infarction was slightly larger on MDCT (19.3 ± 4.5% of the left ventricle vs 18.7 ± 5.7% and 17.2 ± 4.0% of the left ventricle with TTC and MRI, respectively). Similar findings have been reported in humans comparing MDCT to either MRI or gated single-photon emission computed tomography (SPECT).[18,20,21] An example of early hypoenhancement on MDCT is shown in Fig. 22.4.

However, areas of decreased myocardial perfusion can represent either microvascular obstruction or areas of myocardial necrosis. Delayed enhancement imaging, which results in regional hyperenhancement of scar tissue similar to MRI, may possibly provide more accurate evaluation of myocardial infarction (see Fig. 22.4). Gerber *et al.*[22] showed that a combined MDCT protocol of early hypoenhancement and delayed enhancement imaging 10 min after contrast injection allowed characterization of myocardial infarction with contrast patterns highly similar to MRI. Between MDCT and MRI, areas of early hypoenhancement and late hyperenhancement showed good agreement on segmental basis (92% and 82%, respectively). Importantly, also absolute sizes of early hypoenhanced and late hyperenhanced myocardium were highly correlated without significant differences between the two techniques. Moreover, the presence and extent of early hypoenhanced and late hyperenhanced myocardium on MDCT has been shown to accurately predict functional recovery after 3 months.[23]

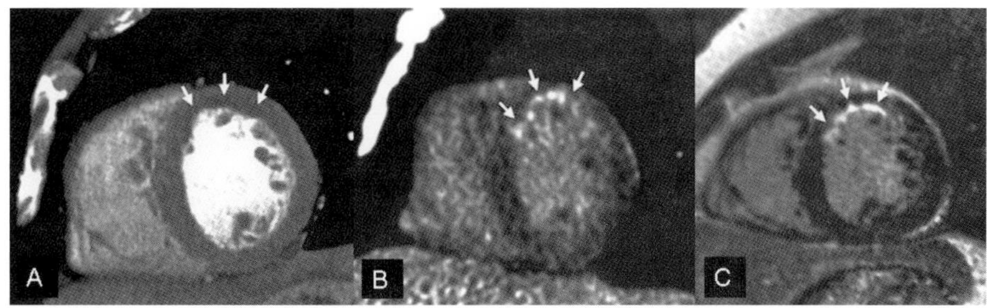

Fig. 22.4 Imaging of myocardial infarction with MDCT. Short-axis views obtained with MDCT (panels A and B) and MRI (panel C) in a patient with anterior myocardial infarction. In panels A and B, a region with respectively early hypoenhancement and late hyperenhancement is indicated by the arrows. Particularly for the late hyperenhancement, correlation with delayed enhancement MRI (panel C) was excellent.
From Mahnken AH, Koos R, Katoh M, *et al.* Assessment of myocardial viability in reperfused acute myocardial infarction using 16-slice computed tomography in comparison to magnetic resonance imaging. *J Am Coll Cardiol* 2005;**45**(12):2042–7, with permission.

Recently, le Polain de Waroux and colleagues[24] applied a combined coronary angiography and late enhancement protocol with MDCT to determine the underlying aetiology of HF. For this purpose, 71 patients presenting with left ventricular dysfunction of unknown origin underwent comprehensive evaluation with MDCT in addition to delayed enhancement MRI and invasive coronary angiography. MDCT coronary angiography correctly identified all patients with significant CAD on invasive coronary angiography. However, in two additional patients the severity of stenosis was overestimated on MDCT because of the presence of extensive calcifications. Using the delayed enhancement images, 28 of 29 (96%) patients with either subendocardial or transmural infarction on MRI were correctly identified on MDCT. In three patients, the observation of delayed enhancement on MDCT was not confirmed on MRI, resulting in a specificity of 92%. Importantly, combination of the information on coronary arteries and delayed enhancement was shown to allow accurate classification of patients with HF of definite or probable ischaemic origin. As compared to invasive coronary angiography in combination with MRI, sensitivity and specificity of 97% and 92%, respectively, were shown for MDCT. As suggested by the authors, MDCT may become an attractive modality for comprehensive assessment of aetiology in a single, rapid examination. Additional advantages include the more widespread availability and lower costs of MDCT as compared to MRI and the fact that patients with metallic implants can be safely studied. Disadvantages, however, remain the need for potentially nephrotoxic contrast agent, radiation dose, and the at present still somewhat variable image quality.

Cardiac vein anatomy

An application that is receiving increasing interest is visualization of the cardiac veins with MDCT. In highly symptomatic HF patients with wide QRS complex and depressed left ventricular function, cardiac resynchronization therapy (CRT) has emerged as an attractive treatment option that can provide substantial symptomatic benefit and reduce mortality. However, the presence of a suitable cardiac vein is mandatory for successful transvenous implantation of the left ventricular pacing lead. In this context, MDCT may become an attractive noninvasive technique to identify the presence of a suitable vein and guide lead implantation (Fig. 22.5). Indeed, several studies have demonstrated the feasibility of MDCT for the depiction of cardiac venous anatomy.[25,26] In addition, a good correlation with invasive venography has been demonstrated in patients referred for CRT implantation.[27] Interestingly, a possible association between the variation in cardiac venous anatomy and the history of a myocardial infarction was identified by van de Veire *et al.*[26] In 100 patients undergoing MDCT scanning, a left marginal vein was significantly less frequently observed in patients with a history of myocardial infarction, as compared with control patients and patients with CAD (27% vs 71% and 61%, respectively, $p < 0.001$).[26] Since the lack of a left marginal vein may hamper the positioning of the left ventricular pacing lead during CRT implantation,[28] preprocedural identification of patients in whom suitable branches are present is of critical importance. In this respect, MDCT may provide valuable information by noninvasively identifying patients who may be referred directly for an epicardial left ventricular lead placement using minimally invasive surgery.

Mitral valve geometry

HF patients with left ventricular systolic dysfunction (LVSD) frequently develop mitral regurgitation due to enlargement of the left ventricle leading to mitral valve annular dilatation and reduced leaflet coaptation. As the presence and severity of mitral

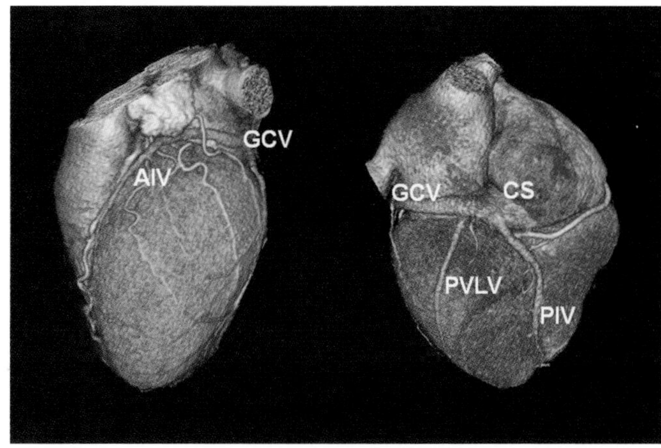

Fig. 22.5 Visualization of cardiac vein anatomy with MDCT. On the anterior view (left panel), the anterior interventricular vein (AIV) draining into the great cardiac vein (GCV) can be observed. The more posterior view (right panel) shows the posterior vein of the left ventricle (PVLV). Both the PVLV and the posterior interventricular vein (PIV) drain into the coronary sinus (CS), which eventually drains into the right atrium.

regurgitation negatively affect prognosis, additional mitral valve surgery during coronary bypass grafting should be considered in patients with ischaemic HF and mitral regurgitation. For optimal planning of the surgical procedure, detailed information of the shape of the left ventricle, the geometry of the valve, and the severity of mitral regurgitation is needed. Echocardiography remains the preferred technique, but some aspects may be evaluated by MDCT. As recently demonstrated by Delgado and colleagues, the high spatial resolution of MDCT allows for detailed evaluation of mitral valve geometry and its interaction with the left ventricle.[29] The authors showed that several variables that may be important in determining procedural strategy and success, including mitral valve annulus dimensions as well as mitral leaflet coaptation height and displacement of the papillary muscles, could be derived using this technique.

Moreover, the detailed visualization of cardiac anatomy may be of particular value in the setting of percutaneous mitral valve annuloplasty. During this procedure, the mitral annulus diameter is reduced by mean of a device inserted in the coronary sinus. The feasibility of this percutaneous procedure depends on the distance between the coronary sinus and the mitral annulus, and remodelling of the mitral annulus may be inefficient when the coronary sinus courses along the left atrial wall rather than along the mitral annulus. In addition, a course of the left circumflex coronary artery between the coronary sinus and the mitral valve annulus may be associated with risk of compression. In several investigations, MDCT has been applied to study the relation between the coronary sinus, mitral valve annulus and left circumflex, revealing a highly variable relation between these structures.[30,31] Accordingly, MDCT may provide valuable information for the selection of potential candidates for percutaneous mitral annuloplasty and could identify patients in whom percutaneous transvenous mitral annuloplasty may not be feasible.

Summary and conclusion

During the past decade, the rapid technological development of MDCT has allowed noninvasive coronary angiography. Owing to its high negative predictive value, the technique is particularly accurate in ruling out (significant) CAD. Accordingly, use of MDCT coronary angiography may be a reasonable approach to visualize coronary anatomy in patients presenting with HF of unknown origin and in whom extensive CAD is not expected. In addition, the technique can provide high-resolution images of cardiac structure and function. As a consequence, MDCT may allow a comprehensive cardiac evaluation in a single examination. However, this additional information is associated with increased radiation and contrast burden; use of MDCT for the sole purpose of assessing myocardial structure and function should therefore be restricted to patients in whom other imaging modalities are not feasible.

References

1. Hausleiter J, Meyer T. Tips to minimize radiation exposure. *J Cardiovasc Comput Tomogr* 2008;**2**(5):325–7.
2. Husmann L, Valenta I, Gaemperli O, *et al.* Feasibility of low-dose coronary CT angiography: first experience with prospective ECG-gating. *Eur Heart J* 2008;**29**(2):191–7.
3. Agatston AS, Janowitz WR, Hildner FJ, Zusmer NR, Viamonte M Jr, Detrano R. Quantification of coronary artery calcium using ultrafast computed tomography. *J Am Coll Cardiol* 1990;**15**(4):827–32.
4. Budoff MJ, Shavelle DM, Lamont DH, *et al.* Usefulness of electron beam computed tomography scanning for distinguishing ischemic from nonischemic cardiomyopathy. *J Am Coll Cardiol* 1998;**32**(5):1173–8.
5. Le T, Ko JY, Kim HT, Akinwale P, Budoff MJ. Comparison of echocardiography and electron beam tomography in differentiating the etiology of heart failure. *Clin Cardiol* 2000;**23**(6):417–20.
6. Budoff MJ, Jacob B, Rasouli ML, Yu D, Chang RS, Shavelle DM. Comparison of electron beam computed tomography and technetium stress testing in differentiating cause of dilated versus ischemic cardiomyopathy. *J Comput Assist Tomogr* 2005;**29**(5):699–703.
7. Meijer AB, YL O, Geleijns J, Kroft LJ. Meta-analysis of 40- and 64-MDCT angiography for assessing coronary artery stenosis. *AJR Am J Roentgenol* 2008;**191**(6):1667–75.
8. Schroeder S, Achenbach S, Bengel F, *et al.* Cardiac computed tomography: indications, applications, limitations, and training requirements: report of a Writing Group deployed by the Working Group Nuclear Cardiology and Cardiac CT of the European Society of Cardiology and the European Council of Nuclear Cardiology. *Eur Heart J* 2008;**29**(4):531–56.
9. Andreini D, Pontone G, Pepi M, *et al.* Diagnostic accuracy of multidetector computed tomography coronary angiography in patients with dilated cardiomyopathy. *J Am Coll Cardiol* 2007;**49**(20):2044–50.
10. Ghostine S, Caussin C, Habis M, *et al.* Non-invasive diagnosis of ischaemic heart failure using 64-slice computed tomography. *Eur Heart J* 2008;**29**(17):2133–40.
11. Cornily JC, Gilard M, Le Gal G, *et al.* Accuracy of 16-detector multislice spiral computed tomography in the initial evaluation of dilated cardiomyopathy. *Eur J Radiol* 2007;**61**(1):84–90.
12. Dickstein K, Cohen-Solal A, Filippatos G, *et al.* ESC Guidelines for the diagnosis and treatment of acute and chronic heart failure 2008: the Task Force for the Diagnosis and Treatment of Acute and Chronic Heart Failure 2008 of the European Society of Cardiology. Developed in collaboration with the Heart Failure Association of the ESC (HFA) and endorsed by the European Society of Intensive Care Medicine (ESICM). *Eur Heart J* 2008;**29**(19):2388–442.
13. Yamamuro M, Tadamura E, Kubo S, *et al.* Cardiac functional analysis with multi-detector row CT and segmental reconstruction algorithm: comparison with echocardiography, SPECT, and MR imaging. *Radiology* 2005;**234**(2):381–90.
14. Grude M, Juergens KU, Wichter T, *et al.* Evaluation of global left ventricular myocardial function with electrocardiogram-gated multidetector computed tomography: comparison with magnetic resonance imaging. *Invest Radiol* 2003;**38**(10):653–661.
15. Henneman MM, Schuijf JD, Jukema JW, *et al.* Assessment of global and regional left ventricular function and volumes with 64-slice MSCT: a comparison with 2D echocardiography. *J Nucl Cardiol* 2006;**13**(4):480–7.
16. Mahnken AH, Koos R, Katoh M, *et al.* Sixteen-slice spiral CT versus MR imaging for the assessment of left ventricular function in acute myocardial infarction. *Eur Radiol* 2005;**15**(4):714–20.
17. Butler J, Shapiro MD, Jassal DS, *et al.* Comparison of multidetector computed tomography and two-dimensional transthoracic echocardiography for left ventricular assessment in patients with heart failure. *Am J Cardiol* 2007;**99**(2):247–9.
18. Henneman MM, Schuijf JD, Dibbets-Schneider P, *et al.* Comparison of multislice computed tomography to gated single-photon emission computed tomography for imaging of healed myocardial infarcts. *Am J Cardiol* 2008;**101**(2):144–8.
19. Mahnken AH, Bruners P, Katoh M, Wildberger JE, Gunther RW, Buecker A. Dynamic multi-section CT imaging in acute myocardial infarction: preliminary animal experience. *Eur Radiol* 2006;**16**(3): 746–752.
20. Nikolaou K, Sanz J, Poon M, Wintersperger BJ, Ohnesorge B, Rius T *et al.* Assessment of myocardial perfusion and viability from routine contrast-enhanced 16-detector-row computed tomography of the heart: preliminary results. *Eur Radiol* 2005;**15**(5):864–871.

21. Mahnken AH, Koos R, Katoh M, *et al.* Assessment of myocardial viability in reperfused acute myocardial infarction using 16-slice computed tomography in comparison to magnetic resonance imaging. *J Am Coll Cardiol* 2005;**45**(12):2042–7.
22. Gerber BL, Belge B, Legros GJ, *et al.* Characterization of acute and chronic myocardial infarcts by multidetector computed tomography: comparison with contrast-enhanced magnetic resonance. *Circulation* 2006;**113**(6):823–33.
23. Lessick J, Dragu R, Mutlak D, *et al.* Is functional improvement after myocardial infarction predicted with myocardial enhancement patterns at multidetector CT? *Radiology* 2007;**244**(3):736–44.
24. le Polain de Waroux JB, Pouleur AC, Goffinet C, Pasquet A, Vanoverschelde JL, Gerber BL. Combined coronary and late-enhanced multidetector-computed tomography for delineation of the etiology of left ventricular dysfunction: comparison with coronary angiography and contrast-enhanced cardiac magnetic resonance imaging. *Eur Heart J* 2008;**29**(20):2544–51.
25. Jongbloed MR, Lamb HJ, Bax JJ, *et al.* Noninvasive visualization of the cardiac venous system using multislice computed tomography. *J Am Coll Cardiol* 2005;**45**(5):749–53.
26. Van de Veire NR, Schuijf JD, De Sutter J, *et al.* Non-invasive visualization of the cardiac venous system in coronary artery disease patients using 64-slice computed tomography. *J Am Coll Cardiol* 2006;**48**(9):1832–8.
27. Van de Veire NR, Marsan NA, Schuijf JD, *et al.* Noninvasive imaging of cardiac venous anatomy with 64-slice multi-slice computed tomography and noninvasive assessment of left ventricular dyssynchrony by 3-dimensional tissue synchronization imaging in patients with heart failure scheduled for cardiac resynchronization therapy. *Am J Cardiol* 2008;**101**(7):1023–9.
28. Bax JJ, Abraham T, Barold SS, *et al.* Cardiac resynchronization therapy: Part 1 issues before device implantation. *J Am Coll Cardiol* 2005;**46**(12):2153–67.
29. Delgado V, Tops LF, Schuijf JD, *et al.* Assessment of mitral valve anatomy and geometry with multislice computed tomography. *JACC Cardiovasc Imaging* 2009;**2**(5):556–65.
30. Choure AJ, Garcia MJ, Hesse B, *et al.* In vivo analysis of the anatomical relationship of coronary sinus to mitral annulus and left circumflex coronary artery using cardiac multidetector computed tomography: implications for percutaneous coronary sinus mitral annuloplasty. *J Am Coll Cardiol* 2006;**48**(10):1938–45.
31. Tops LF, van de Veire NR, Schuijf JD, *et al.* Noninvasive evaluation of coronary sinus anatomy and its relation to the mitral valve annulus: implications for percutaneous mitral annuloplasty. *Circulation* 2007;**115**(11):1426–32.

23

Metabolic exercise testing in chronic heart failure

Klaus K. Witte

Chronic heart failure (HF) is characterized by exercise intolerance usually due to breathlessness or fatigue in the presence of cardiac dysfunction. Hence when assessing a patient with such symptoms, in addition to appropriate cardiac imaging, some form of standardized exercise testing is important to measure objectively the degree and nature of the symptoms and confirm their aetiology. In addition, exercise capacity is a powerful predictor of mortality and is used as a marker of the need for cardiac transplantation. Although useful data can be gained from a standard treadmill-based exercise test,[1] or a corridor walk test, additional and independent information is available when the test is performed while measuring metabolic gas exchange.[2]

Definitions and variables

In patients with chronic HF, an exercise test with or without metabolic gas analysis gives important information about ischaemia, inducible arrhythmias, and prognosis.[3–6] Metabolic gas analysis during exercise is accurate and reproducible[7] and also a robust predictor of outcomes.[8,9]

During an incremental exercise test, patients exercise to exhaustion while wearing a tight-fitting mask or mouthpiece, and expired air is sampled to measure metabolic gas exchange. This can either be done by sampling from a large bag at intervals (Douglas bag method) or more commonly on a breath-by-breath basis. Oxygen uptake, minute ventilation (as a product of tidal volume and frequency of ventilation), and CO_2 production can be measured (Fig. 23.1). Exercise duration, heart rate, blood pressure changes, and peak heart rate are often quoted, but the variables most commonly used to describe the exercise response are peak O_2 consumption (pVo_2), anaerobic threshold (AT), and the derived variables of the relationship of ventilation to CO_2 production (VE/Vco$_2$ slope) and the ratio of CO_2 output to O_2 uptake (Vco_2/Vo_2; respiratory exchange ratio or RER).

Anaerobic and aerobic metabolism

Skeletal muscle cellular activity requires energy, which is stored in skeletal muscle myocytes in the form of creatine phosphate and glycogen. Creatine phosphate is rapidly accessible, but stores are sufficient for only a few seconds of work. The currency of energy transfer is in the breaking and reformation of the terminal phosphate bond of ATP. The energy released when this bond is broken is used for a cycle of linking and releasing of the two elements of the contractile structure, actin and myosin. The linking and subsequent release leads to conformational changes in the cell. If neighbouring cells perform this activity in a controlled and coordinated manner, contraction of the muscle can take place. Other cellular activities such as biosynthesis and active transport are also supported by the energy released from the hydrolysis of ATP.

Aerobic metabolism

The production of units of ATP, which must continuously be regenerated to allow cellular work to continue, depends largely upon the oxidation in the mitochondria of carbohydrates, fatty acids, and, in conditions of starvation, protein. Carbohydrate sources (such as glycogen) are converted initially to pyruvate, and then enter the tricarboxylic acid cycle (TCA or Krebs cycle), as acetyl-CoA, eventually forming CO_2, high-energy electrons, and hydrogen ions. On the other hand, fatty acids undergo β-oxidation but then also enter the TCA cycle as acetyl-CoA units. The release of the protons and the entry of the electrons into the electron transport chain is dependent on the consumption of O_2 and leads to the production of water and the regeneration of ATP (Fig. 23.2). An important part of the process is the reduction of nicotinamide adenine dinucleotide (NAD) to NADH. NADH is the route through which electrons enter the electron transport chain, in the process being oxidized again to NAD.

Anaerobic metabolism

In conditions where the supply of O_2 is not sufficient to keep up with demand, the impaired flow of electrons into the electron transfer chain would eventually inhibit energy production in the cell. In the absence of O_2, pyruvate cannot enter the TCA cycle, so, in order to allow the reoxidization of NADH to NAD, pyruvate is instead converted to lactate. This is termed anaerobic metabolism and leads to

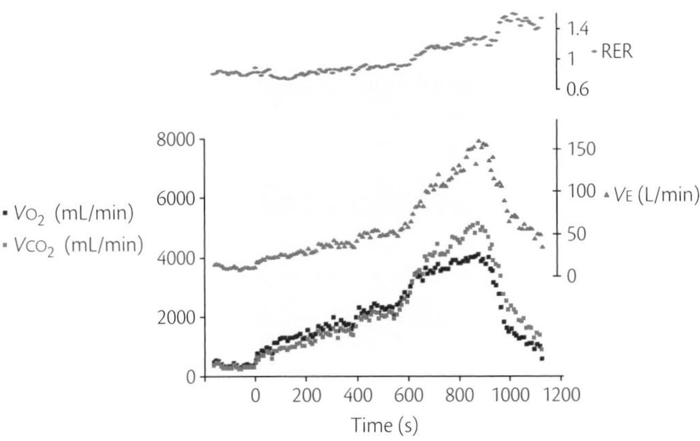

Fig. 23.1 Cardiopulmonary dataset from a control showing increases in O_2 uptake ($\dot{V}O_2$), CO_2 output ($\dot{V}CO_2$), ventilation ($\dot{V}E$), and respiratory exchange ratio (RER).

the production of fewer ATP molecules for each molecule of substrate than aerobic metabolism. When O_2 becomes available again, the lactate can be converted back to pyruvate and pass into the TCA cycle. Cellular metabolism can therefore continue in circumstances of relative O_2 deficiency, but is less efficient.

In most circumstances, both aerobic and anaerobic metabolism occur simultaneously in all cells, but in skeletal muscle cells, particularly at high workloads, anaerobic metabolism provides a greater proportion of the energy than at rest.

Energy substrates

The ratio of O_2 consumption to CO_2 production in the tissues is a function of the substrate used. When using glucose, each molecule of O_2 used leads to the formation of one molecule of CO_2:

$$C_6H_{12}O_6 + 6O_2 \rightarrow 6H_2O + 6CO_2$$

This leads to a respiratory quotient (RQ: Qco_2/Qo_2) of 1. Lipids are much more reduced than carbohydrate, and so when fatty acids are oxidized, the CO_2 production is lower than the rate of O_2 consumption with a correspondingly lower RQ of around 0.7:

$$C_{16}H_{32}O_2 + 23O_2 \rightarrow 16H_2O + 16CO_2 \text{ and } 16/23 = 0.7$$

where $C_{16}H_{32}O_2$ is palmitic acid, a commonly used fatty acid.

In humans at rest, there is a preponderance of fatty acid metabolism so the CO_2 production is lower than O_2 consumption and the RQ is around 0.7. The higher the proportion of carbohydrate used, the greater the required ventilatory response to eliminate the CO_2.

With metabolic gas exchange measurements, 'whole body' gas exchange is measured from the difference between inspired and expired O_2 and CO_2 at the mouth and is not a direct measure of cellular metabolism. As with RQ, O_2 consumption and CO_2 production measured at the mouth can be expressed as a ratio—the RER.

Oxygen consumption

During exercise there is a several-fold increase in O_2 consumption by skeletal muscle cells. The physiological adaptations to exercise include increased cardiac output from a resting level of 3.5 L/min to typically 20 L/min, with local arterial vasodilation to increase O_2 delivery to exercising muscles. There is a rightward shift of the oxyhaemoglobin dissociation curve encouraging unloading of O_2 in areas of acidosis, and there is increased ventilation up to 100 L/min.

The body's upper limit of O_2 utilization is determined by the maximal cardiac output,[10] arterial O_2 content, the fractional distribution of cardiac output to the exercising muscle,[11] and the ability of the muscle to extract O_2.[12] Ventilation is a limiting factor only when the ventilatory capacity is insufficient to eliminate the CO_2 produced by aerobic metabolism and the bicarbonate buffering of lactic acid,[13] or at the rarely achieved maximum voluntary ventilation (MVV).

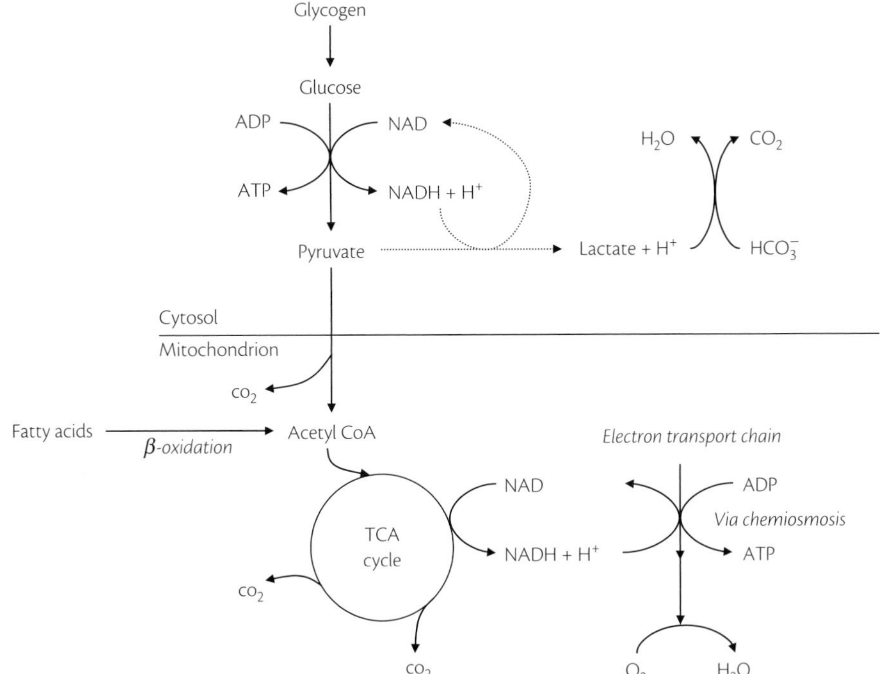

Fig. 23.2 Aerobic and anaerobic metabolism (dashed lines show the passage of protons into the electron transport chain).

The measurement of O_2 uptake at the mouth is traditionally recorded as O_2 consumption ($V\text{O}_2$). Strictly, O_2 is consumed at the cellular level, and only a small percentage of resting O_2 uptake is consumed by skeletal muscles. During exercise, most of the increase in O_2 uptake at the mouth reflects increased O_2 consumption in the skeletal muscles. Hence O_2 uptake at the mouth and O_2 consumption are assumed to be equivalent and the terms are used interchangeably. The value is presented either as an absolute (mL/min) or referenced to body weight (mL/kg per min).

Physiologists refer to the concept of maximal O_2 consumption ('$V\text{O}_{2\,max}$') as the O_2 consumption plateau reached where an increase in imposed workload no longer elicits an increase in $V\text{O}_2$. However, on most occasions, even normal individuals cannot tolerate the discomfort long enough to achieve a plateau in $V\text{O}_2$, and HF patients are almost never able to exercise to such plateau. A flattening of the $V\text{O}_2$–work rate relationship is therefore not seen. The term 'peak $V\text{O}_2$' should be used when a plateau is not reached, and is used as an index of peak exercise capacity.

Carbon dioxide output

Metabolic activity produces CO_2 and water as waste products. The amount of CO_2 produced for a given energy release, is determined by the substrate and how it is metabolized. As with O_2 consumption, the CO_2 production occurs in the metabolizing tissues but is measured at the mouth.

Ventilation

Ventilation (in L/min) is a product of frequency (f) and tidal volume (V_T) at the mouth. The relationship between O_2 consumption and workload during submaximal exercise is linear.[14] However, the ventilatory response is not related linearly to O_2 consumption ($V\text{O}_2$). Instead, there is a close relationship between the production of CO_2 ($V\text{CO}_2$) and minute ventilation ($V\text{E}$) (Fig. 23.3).[15–17] This relationship, termed the $V\text{E}/V\text{CO}_2$ slope, becomes steeper above the AT (see below).[16]

The relation between ventilation and CO_2 production is given by

$$V\text{E}/V\text{CO}_2 V\text{CO}_2 = 863/P\text{aO}_2 \times x\,(1 - V\text{D}/V\text{T}) \qquad \text{(Equation 23.1)}$$

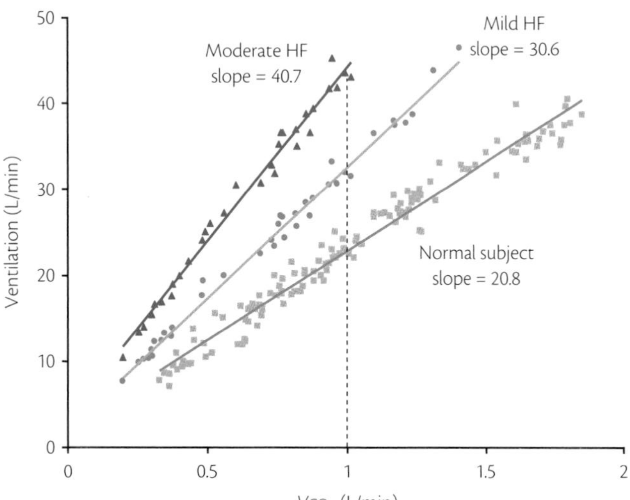

Fig. 23.3 The $V\text{E}/V\text{CO}_2$ slope in two patients with chronic heart failure and a control subject.

where 863 is a constant to standardize volume measurements, $P\text{aCO}_2$ is the arterial tension of CO_2 and $V\text{D}/V\text{T}$ is dead space as a fraction of tidal volume. A consequence is that, in the short term at least, $V\text{CO}_2$ is determined by ventilation: if an individual hyperventilates, $V\text{CO}_2$ increases as the CO_2 passing through the lungs is blown off.[18]

Equation 23.1 includes a calculation for dead space—lung tissue that is ventilated but not perfused, which includes bronchi, trachea, and underperfused alveoli. As a result of perfusion changes and the increased frequency of ventilation,[19] dead space ventilation as a fraction of tidal volume is greater in patients with chronic HF than in control subjects. This might contribute to exercise limitation and symptoms in patients with chronic HF; hence $V\text{D}/V\text{T}$ is frequently presented within a cardiopulmonary exercise report.

Derived variables

Several variables are commonly derived from the basic measurements. It must be borne in mind that derived variables especially suffer from a multiplication of errors when calculated from poorly performed tests.

Ventilatory equivalents

The ventilatory equivalents for O_2 ($V\text{eqO}_2$ or $V\text{E}/V\text{O}_2$) and CO_2 ($V\text{eqCO}_2$ or $V\text{E}/V\text{CO}_2$) give an impression of the instantaneous ventilation required at a particular time point for the metabolic gas in question and are usually plotted against work rate or time in a progressive test. Both decline slightly early during progressive exercise until the AT, at which point both increase. Both ventilatory equivalents for O_2 and CO_2 are higher in patients with chronic HF than in controls throughout exercise.

Respiratory exchange ratio

A problem with incremental testing in a population of individuals unused to maximal exercise tests is determining whether a maximum has been reached, or whether exercise is 'submaximal'. Where a genuine plateau in O_2 consumption is reached, then a maximum test can be inferred confidently. For most patients with HF, the RER ($V\text{CO}_2/V\text{O}_2$) is usually used.

When glucose is the metabolic substrate, the RER is 1.0 (1 mole of CO_2 is produced for each mole of O_2 consumed). The RER for lipid metabolism is around 0.7, as lipid is more highly reduced than glucose. At rest in patients and normal individuals alike, the ratio is around 0.7, representing the balance between fatty acid and glucose metabolism. However, as exercise progresses, ATP is generated increasingly from anaerobic metabolism. The shift away from aerobic metabolism leads to an increase in lactate production which is buffered in the blood by bicarbonate (HCO_3^-) ions. Carbonic acid dissociates to water and CO_2, which is then blown off at the mouth. As a consequence, CO_2 output increases relative to O_2 consumed, and the RER gradually rises above 1.0. A test is usually taken to be maximal when the RER exceeds 1.1 (although fit individuals may attain an RER of 1.4) and in practice in HF populations, an RER of 1.0 or more is often accepted. Higher RER levels improve the prognostic information of the data collected,[20] whereas those with low RER levels are much less informative.[21]

The anaerobic threshold

At low workload, aerobic metabolism is able to support energy production completely, and the need for anaerobic metabolism is low. During incremental exercise, there comes a point where the

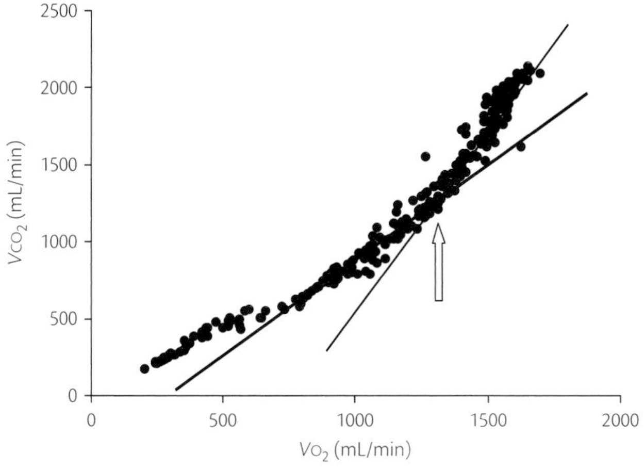

Fig. 23.4 The V-slope method to determine anaerobic threshold in a patient with chronic heart failure. The arrow demonstrates the estimated AT.

circulation can no longer deliver sufficient O_2 to the exercising muscle, and anaerobic metabolism supplies an increasing proportion of the ATP. At this point, lactate is generated, which is buffered by bicarbonate in the blood. Bicarbonate in turn is converted to water and CO_2, which is added to the metabolic CO_2 production and blown off at the lungs in order to maintain plasma pH at physiological levels. The result is a nonlinear increase in $\dot{V}CO_2$ relative to $\dot{V}O_2$, detectable from the metabolic gas exchange data.[22] The point at which this begins is termed the AT and can be identified by plotting $\dot{V}O_2$ against $\dot{V}CO_2$, known as the V-slope method (Fig. 23.4). AT is recorded as the O_2 consumption at this point.

The identification of a discrete AT point is arbitrary as the increase in CO_2 production is gradual,[23] but it can nevertheless be reasonably reliably estimated by expired air analysis.[24] There is a high correlation between the AT and $p\dot{V}O_2$,[25] making the anaerobic threshold a potentially useful submaximal measure of exercise capacity that is independent of patient motivation.[26]

There are other methods of identifying the AT; a second method depends upon the changing ventilatory response to CO_2 during exercise.[27] The relationship of $\dot{V}E$ to $\dot{V}CO_2$ (ventilatory equivalent for CO_2 or $Veqco_2$) can also be plotted against time, and the nadir gives another estimation of the AT (Fig. 23.5).

The relationship of ventilation to CO_2 is linear throughout early exercise, but after the AT, an increase in ventilation occurs out of proportion to the production of CO_2. This was initially thought to be a consequence of the acidosis due to lactic acid,[28] but plasma pH and CO_2 remain stable,[29] and the reason for the change in the ratio remains elusive. Nevertheless, some laboratories use the lowest point in the ratio before the rise as the AT. This method is highly reproducible. The 'crossing' method, using the point at which the ratio of CO_2 production and O_2 consumption passes 1.0, allows an estimation of the AT in more patients than the other methods but gives a higher value.[30]

$\dot{V}E/\dot{V}CO_2$ slope

During exercise, both CO_2 output and ventilation increase steadily. The relationship between the two is linear,[31] but in patients with HF, the slope of the relationship is increased (the slope is steeper), so that for a given CO_2 production, there is more ventilation (Fig. 23.4).[32] The $\dot{V}E/\dot{V}CO_2$ slope is directly related to both mortality and morbidity.[33] Peak $\dot{V}O_2$ and the $\dot{V}E/\dot{V}CO_2$ slope are inversely related to each other,[33,34] so that the more reduced the exercise capacity, the greater the ventilatory response to exercise (Fig. 23.6).

Other variables

Additional variables can contribute further information. Cyclic fluctuations in ventilation, known as early oscillatory breathing (EOV), are exacerbated in patients with chronic HF both at rest and during exercise.[35,36] There are at least two definitions of cyclical breathing, but patients with EOV by either definition have a worse prognosis.[37]

Although the relation between ventilation and O_2 uptake is not linear, the O_2 uptake efficiency slope (OUES) is derived by plotting $\dot{V}O_2$ as a function of $\log_{10}\dot{V}E$, which is an approximately linear relation.[38] The steeper the slope, the more O_2 is taken up for a given unit ventilation (Fig. 23.7). One advantage of the OUES is that it can be measured from submaximal data and does not depend upon reaching peak exertion. The OUES is predictive of prognosis even from submaximal tests.[39]

Combining peak variables occasionally offers greater prognostic power. For example, peak cardiac power output, the product of cardiac output and mean arterial blood pressure at peak exercise, relates to exercise capacity and outcome.[40] However, not all

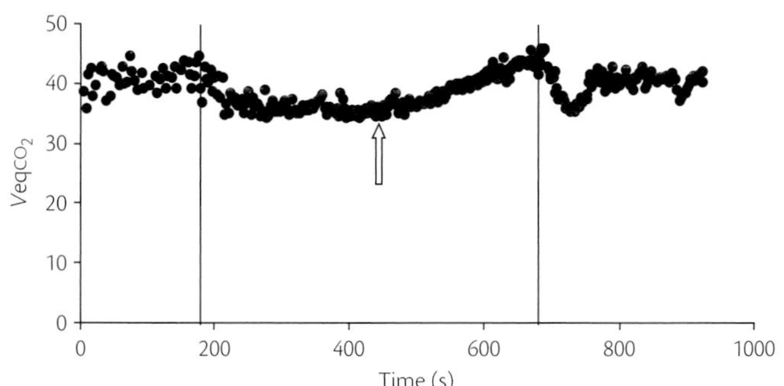

Fig. 23.5 The plot of ventilatory equivalent for CO_2 against ventilation for a patient with chronic heart failure. The markers show the onset and offset of treadmill exercise, and the arrow demonstrates the anaerobic threshold at the lowest point of the relationship during exercise.

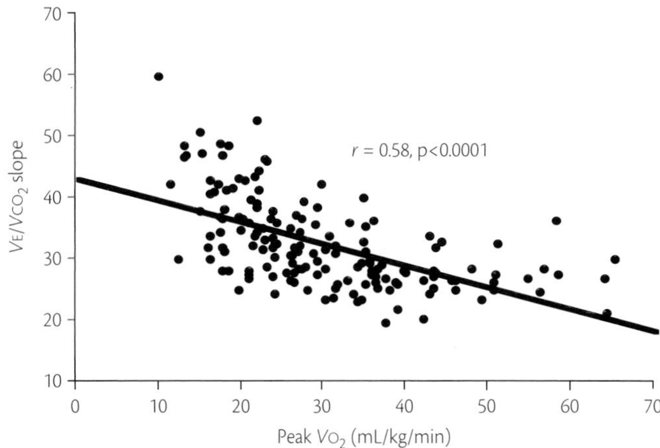

Fig. 23.6 The inverse relationship between $\dot{V}E/\dot{V}CO_2$ slope and $p\dot{V}O_2$.

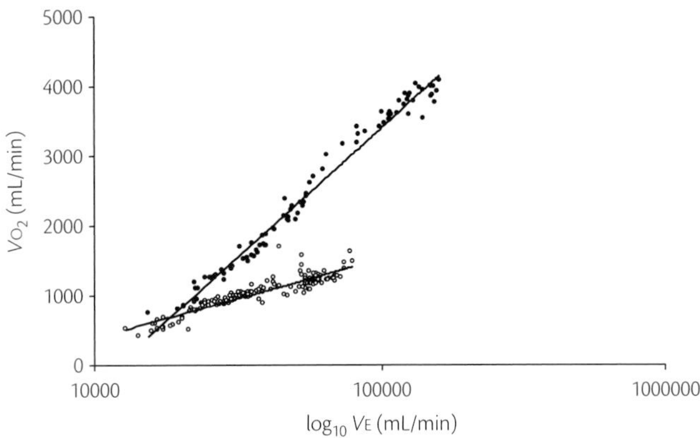

Fig. 23.7 The O_2 uptake efficiency slope in a patient (unfilled circles) and a control subject (filled circles). The slope is steeper in the control subject, implying greater O_2 uptake for a given ventilation.

combinations of peak variables are of greater predictive value than their constituent measurements.[41]

Can the cause of exercise intolerance in chronic HF be determined from peak variables?

The cause of exercise intolerance and the abnormal physiology during exercise in chronic HF (such as the increased *V*E/*V*CO_2 slope), and the relative contributions of central haemodynamics, peripheral vasculature, and skeletal muscle adaptations, are incompletely understood. Many variables, such as ventilation, cardiac power output, metabolic gas exchange kinetics,[42] heart rate and, of course, time, increase during an exercise test as a function of exercise load (and exercise duration in an incremental test). Thus, the exercise measures and derived variables will all correlate highly with each other, and all will correlate to some degree with prognosis.[43] Which is the most 'powerful' predictor will vary from dataset to dataset by random chance. There is a temptation to plot one variable as a function of another, and assume that the mathematically dependent variable plotted on the *y*-axis is somehow determined by the variable on the *x*-axis: this is certainly not the case. Correlation does not imply cause and effect. An absurd example is the observation that hair length (if measured accurately) will also increase as a function of duration of an exercise test, and would correlate closely with peak *V*O_2: however, increase in hair length is clearly not the determinant of peak *V*O_2. A more controversial example is the influence of chronotropic incompetence and whether it is a limitation of heart rate increase that determines exercise capacity. Chronotropic incompetence is more frequent and more severe in patients taking β-blockers than in those not taking them, yet they do not induce a reduction in peak O_2 consumption.[44,45] It cannot be assumed that any variable derived from an exercise test determines exercise capacity. It makes as much sense to state that exercise capacity, for example, determines peak cardiac power output or peak heart rate.

Methods of metabolic gas exchange measurement

The measurement of peak O_2 consumption (p*V*O_2) requires a form of exercise equipment, usually either a programmable treadmill or a stationary electromagnetically braked cycle, and a metabolic gas analyser. A 12-lead ECG monitor is used for safety and to determine heart rate. Ideally, the laboratory should be air-conditioned to achieve a stable temperature and humidity. Repeated exercise tests should take place at about the same time in the day, and not within 3 h of a main meal. Caffeine should be avoided for 6 h before a test. Subjects should be advised to wear comfortable shoes, and women should wear a loose shirt or vest under which the ECG electrodes can be applied to the skin.

All metabolic gas analysis systems must measure ventilation and analyse the concentrations of O_2 and CO_2 in expired air. In a typical system, subjects wear a mask or breathe through a mouthpiece (with a nose-clip) attached to a flow meter which allows the measurement of tidal volume (*V*T) and frequency of ventilation (*f*). These are used to derive total minute ventilation (*V*E). Connected to the flow meter is a sample tube which continuously aspirates a small volume of the expired and inspired air to measure the concentrations of O_2 and CO_2. By knowing *V*E and the concentrations of the metabolic gases, volumes of CO_2 produced and O_2 consumed can be derived.

Metabolic gas analysis

Mass spectrometry is the gold standard for gas analysis. It provides rapid and reliable online breath-by-breath assessment of O_2 and CO_2. Sampled gases are subjected to an electron beam and thereby converted to charged ions. These are then accelerated in an electric field and their direction altered by a magnetic field. Detectors produce an output according to the numbers of ions striking them. However, the equipment is expensive, and requires regular maintenance. Alternatives to mass spectrometry include paramagnetic analysers or gas chromatography linked to thermal conductivity detectors for O_2 analysis and infrared absorption detectors for CO_2.

Flow-sensing devices

The most common and maintenance-free devices for measuring flow are low-resistance turbines which are less affected by ambient temperature and humidity than alternative devices, but resistance and inertia of the vane can reduce sensitivity. Alternatives include pneumotachometers which measure a pressure drop across two capillary tubes, and anemometers which calculate air flow based upon the temperature change in a thin electrified wire stretched across the tube.

Although initial work was performed using intermittent bag collection of expired air, most equipment now measures ventilation and gas concentrations on a breath-by-breath basis. This requires a temporal adjustment of the gas analysis, which takes longer than the flow assessment, to maintain accuracy.[46]

Calibration

Small errors in sampling are magnified by the calculations performed during and after the test. The equipment should therefore be calibrated at least daily and preferably before each test. Mass spectrometry devices commonly use indicator dilution to give the flow signal, hence only one device needs to be calibrated to get all the signals of interest, whereas with the typical metabolic cart, there are three different devices—flow, O_2 and CO_2 meters. Exercise tests should be carried out and interpreted by experienced personnel, with appropriate support from equipment manufacturers. Equipment should be serviced regularly.

Preparation of the subject

The procedure must be explained in full to each subject. When a maximal test is being undertaken, it should be made clear before the test starts that the aim is to assess peak exercise capacity and that the subject will be encouraged to exercise to their limit. During the test, they should be asked to score their symptoms of breathlessness or fatigue according to a recognized rating of perceived exertion scale (such as the Borg score, Table 23.1),[47] and they should be discouraged from talking during the test. Simple signals should be agreed upon, such as raising of the left hand to stop the test. The subject should receive standardized encouragement at the midpoint of each stage, such as 'You're doing well', 'Keep it up'.

Subjects respond differently to the mask or the mouthpiece. The mouthpiece commonly causes distress and hypersalivation, but is associated with fewer gas leaks. In contrast, masks are more comfortable but have a higher incidence of leaks and a larger dead space volume. Both options should be available.

Haemodynamic assessment

Throughout the test, a 12-lead ECG should be monitored, and a hard copy is usually printed with each exercise stage or at appropriate intervals. Blood pressure and heart rate should also be recorded at these time points. Some devices allow intermittent determination of cardiac output by inert gas dilution. It is important to explain and demonstrate the procedure before the test.

Spirometry

Basic assessment of pulmonary status can be performed routinely on any subject undergoing an exercise test. Using the capnograph, and software within the metabolic cart, a maximal flow volume loop can recorded and forced expiratory volume in one second (FEV_1), forced vital capacity (FVC), and inspiratory volumes measured. The spirometry test should be judged to be satisfactory by the joining of the inspiratory and expiratory loops. The FEV_1 can be used to calculate MVV ($= FEV_1 \times 35$).[48]

Resting data

Before exercise begins, 3–5 min of resting data should be collected. This allows the subject to become familiar with the mouthpiece or mask, and the investigators to identify leaks and analyser problems. Baseline O_2 consumption should be between 3 and 5 mL/kg per min and the respiratory exchange ratio below 0.9. Baseline heart rate and blood pressure should be measured at the end of this phase.

Table 23.1 The Borg scale of perceived exertion

0	Nothing at all
0.5	Very, very slight
1	Very slight
2	Slight
3	Moderate
4	Somewhat severe
5	Severe
6	
7	Very severe
8	
9	Very, very severe
10	Maximal

Exercise protocols

Protocols for both stationary cycle and treadmill exercise are available and the choice of equipment is often dictated by the experience of the personnel and the space available in the laboratory. Treadmill-based exercise is more natural and often leads to a higher peak O_2 consumption since subjects also carry their own weight. In contrast, cycle exercise allows haemodynamic monitoring and more gradual increments in workload. Whatever form of exercise is used, whether it consists of steady and progressive increases in work, or more stepwise increases, the rate of increase of work must be slow enough to allow an adaptation of the slow metabolic gas kinetics seen in chronic HF. The protocol should aim for an exercise time of between 6 and 12 min, as this maximizes peak $\dot{V}O_2$.[49]

Treadmill exercise

The Bruce protocol[50] modified by the addition of a 'stage 0' at onset consisting of 3 min of exercise at 1.61 km/h (1 mile/h) with a 5% gradient is often used (Table 23.2). However, the steps between each stage are large, such that many subjects stop exercise immediately after a stage begins. Alternatives are the Balke protocol[51] which has a constant speed and gradual increase in incline (1% per minute), and the Naughton[52] protocol which has shorter stages with smaller increments in both speed and incline. Each of these has been criticized for excessive duration of exercise. More rapidly incremental protocols are more discriminatory between patients, but do not allow steady state metabolic gas exchange to be reached. During the test, the subject should be encouraged not to use the handrails except as a guide and balance. Dependence on handrails alters the work being performed and the reliability of the O_2 uptake data.[53]

Cycle exercise

Preparation of the subject for exercise on the stationary cycle proceeds as for treadmill exercise. The resistance (watts) against which the subject pedals is increased gradually until exhaustion. The ramp protocol is the most commonly employed and consists of continuous increments of workload aiming for 10 min of exercise.

Peak exercise and recovery

Exercise tests should be symptom-limited maximal tests. At peak exercise, heart rate and blood pressure should be measured and an ECG printed. The rating of perceived exertion and the reason for

Table 23.2 The Bruce protocol. An additional 'stage 0' is added to allow patients with severe exercise limitation to perform some exercise

Stage	Duration (s)	Speed (mile/h)	Grade (%)
0	180	1.0	5
1	180	1.7	10
2	180	2.5	12
3	180	3.4	14
4	180	4.2	16
5	180	5.0	18
6	180	5.5	20
7	180	6.0	22
8	180	6.5	22

stopping should be noted. Once the subject has signalled exhaustion, cycle resistance should be reduced to 0 or the treadmill should be slowed to minimum with no incline, and cycling or walking should continue for a further minute or so. Monitoring should continue until heart rate and gas exchange have returned to resting values.

What is peak exercise?

The point at which an increased load does not lead to an increase in O_2 consumption, is defined as '$Vo_{2\ max}$'. In most untrained subjects (and particularly HF patients), maximal O_2 consumption is rarely reached before exercise is discontinued due to fatigue or dyspnoea.[54] The O_2 consumption at termination of exercise is peak Vo_2 (pVo_2).The point from which pVo_2 is calculated is important. An RER of less than 1 is regarded as a submaximal test and the data must be interpreted in light of this.[54]

An RER consistently above 1.0 at the end of exercise suggests that close to peak exercise has been performed.[55] The prognostic value of peak O_2 consumption depends largely on the RER at peak.[21,56] The AT can be used to extrapolate the maximal O_2 consumption, but although useful, extrapolated $Vo_{2\ max}$ is less reliable than peak O_2 consumption.[57]

Analysis and interpretation

The data from the last 10 s of exercise are averaged to give peak ventilation (*V*E), O_2 consumption (Vo_2), and CO_2 production (Vco_2). The AT is also calculated (Box 23.1).

Safety of cardiopulmonary exercise testing and contraindications

Peak symptom-limited exercise testing using either a treadmill or a bicycle in a controlled setting is safe. In the largest published series of exercise testing in over 6000 men assessed for possible ischaemic heart disease, there were no deaths and the incidence of ventricular tachycardia, defined as three or more consecutive beats, was 1.1%.[58] In another series of 289 patients with severe left ventricular dysfunction (<35%), only one resuscitated cardiac arrest with ventricular fibrillation occurred, and nonsustained ventricular tachycardia occurred in 20%, with hypotension in 5%.[59] In a larger population of 607 patients enrolled in the Veterans Administration Cooperative Study-Vasodilator Heart Failure Trial (VHeFT), there was an incidence of arrhythmias necessitating termination of the test in only 1.6% of patients and no cardiac arrest or death.[60]

Box 23.1 Variables to be reported from an exercise test with metabolic gas exchange

- Indication
- Demographics: age, height, weight, BMI
- Baseline findings
- Exercise modality
- Exercise protocol
- Collection method—mask v mouthpiece
- Reasons for stopping exercise
- Complications
- Rating of perceived exertion (max score)
- Resting and peak heart rate and blood pressure
- Resting and peak Vo^2 and anaerobic threshold
- *V*E/*V*co² slope
- Electrocardiogram changes—ischaemia
- Possible aetiology of exercise impairment

Abnormalities of metabolic gas exchange in chronic heart failure patients

Patients with chronic HF typically have a reduced exercise time, lower than predicted peak O_2 consumption, and an elevated slope of the relationship between ventilation and CO_2 output (Fig. 23.3). The *V*E/*V*co$_2$ slope and pVo_2 are inversely related to each other and independently related to prognosis (Figs 23.6 and 23.8).

Reduced O_2 uptake—cardiac or peripheral

The aetiology of the impaired exercise capacity in patients with chronic HF remains incompletely understood. The haemodynamic hypothesis suggests that in particular individuals there is a single dominant pathology, either increased pulmonary fluid leading to breathlessness or poor skeletal muscle perfusion causing fatigue. However, regardless of the limiting symptom experienced during an exercise test, objective measures of exercise tolerance are similar in patient cohorts whichever symptom is dominant,[61] and the prognosis is related to the peak O_2 consumption achieved and not the nature of the symptoms experienced.[62] Furthermore, the type of exercise performed seems to influence whether individuals suffer breathlessness or fatigue. Slowly incrementing tests and cycle exercise are more likely to lead to fatigue;[63] in contrast, rapidly incremental exercise tests more frequently lead to breathlessness, even if the workload is standardized. Cycle exercise is more often stopped by fatigue than breathlessness compared with treadmill exercise, even when the same level of exercise is performed.[64,65] These findings suggest that there is a common underlying pathology resulting in symptoms; and that the symptoms are variably reported by patients depending upon context.

Central haemodynamics

Many studies have failed to show a significant link between exercise performance and left ventricular performance (Fig. 23.9).[66–72]

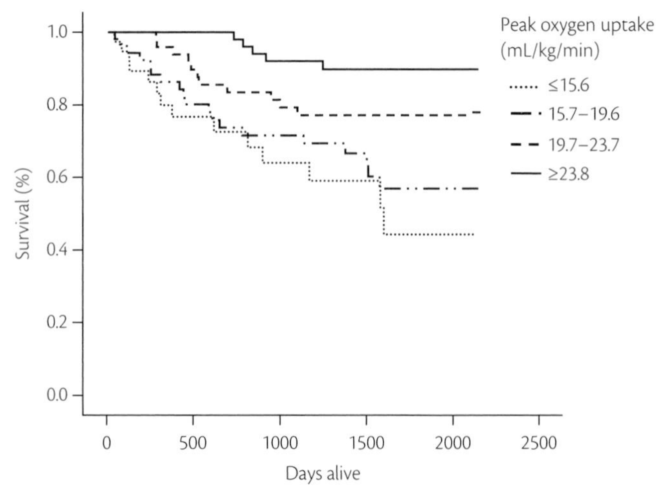

Fig. 23.8 The prognostic information from peak O_2 uptake by quartiles.

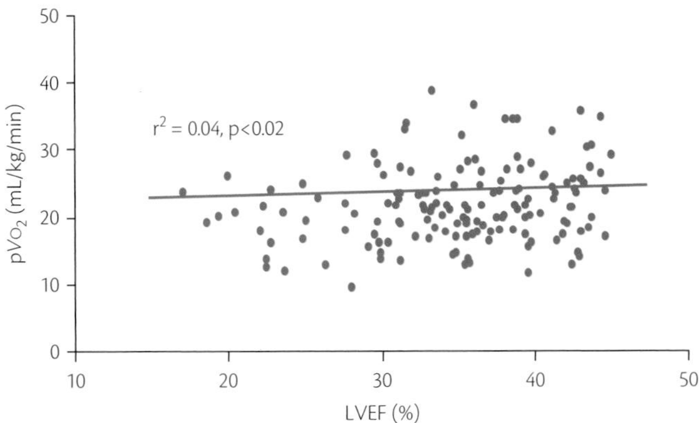

Fig. 23.9 The poor relationship between left ventricular function and peak O_2 consumption.

Furthermore, acute increases in resting cardiac contractility through inotropes[73,74] or cardiac transplantation,[75,76] increased cardiac output following mitral valvuloplasty,[77] and conversely, reductions in contractility and heart rate rise with β-blockers,[44] have no immediate impact on exercise capacity. In contrast, although exercise training can lead to impressive increases in exercise capacity which appears after a prolonged period of training, it has no effect on cardiac function.[78,79]

Chronotropic incompetence

Patients with chronic HF have a lower heart rate rise during exercise. This has been suggested as an aetiological factor in exercise intolerance in chronic HF. However, heart rate limitation seems not to reduce peak O_2 consumption in chronic HF patients,[44,45] and increasing heart rate during exercise has no beneficial effect.[80] It is therefore unlikely that chronotropic incompetence is a mediator, but rather a marker of impaired exercise capacity.[81,82] As such however, it is of course related to outcome in the same manner as other peak variables.

Lung function

Many investigators have described abnormalities of pulmonary function in patients with chronic HF. Spirometric variables are variously reported to be abnormal in heart failure,[83] although large numbers of patients have normal spirometry.[84,85] Nevertheless, some spirometric indices do correlate with exercise capacity,[86] particularly in patients with more modest symptoms.[87]

Large airways function is abnormal in some patients with chronic HF,[88] but although there is some reversibility of airways obstruction with nebulized β-agonists, this has no effect on exercise capacity.[89]

Bronchoconstriction is a major component of acute pulmonary oedema.[90,91] Cabanes *et al.*[92] suggested that there was an increase in bronchial reactivity in HF patients. This effect could be partially reversed with albuterol, a β-stimulant, and, paradoxically, with inhaled methoxamine, a bronchoconstrictor.[93] The hypothesis here was that if left atrial pressure increased as a result of exercise, the veins draining the distal bronchi into the left atrium might become congested, and methoxamine would improve exercise capacity by constricting these vessels. However, others have found no increase in bronchial hyperesponsiveness to stimulation with methacholine or sodium metabisulphite, no change in cough responsiveness to capsaicin, and no evidence for exercise-induced bronchospasm.[94]

Patients with chronic HF also have impaired transalveolar diffusion as measured by transcapillary carbon monoxide diffusion (DLco).[95] DLco is directly related to exercise capacity,[96] and the increased ventilatory response during exercise,[97] and hence is a prognostic marker.[98] It can be improved by ACE inhibitors (an effect countered by aspirin),[99], exercise training,[100] and sildenafil,[101] but not by ultrafiltration,[102] suggesting that the cause of the impaired diffusion is vascular, possibly endothelial, rather than being related to lung blood volume or haemodynamic status.

Diaphragmatic weakness has been implicated in the symptomatology of chronic HF. The histological abnormalities seen in the skeletal muscle of HF patients (see 'Skeletal muscle', below) are also seen in the diaphragm.[103] The ability to generate negative intrathoracic pressure is slightly reduced in heart failure patients when compared with controls.[104] This weakness, combined with reduced lung compliance leading to increased diaphragmatic work particularly in the supine position,[105] suggests that respiratory muscle could contribute to exercise limitation. However, overall diaphragmatic strength at rest appears to be well preserved,[106,107] and contractile diaphragmatic fatigue is uncommon in chronic HF patients during an exercise test.[108]

Finally, patients ventilate at the same proportion of their maximum ventilatory volume at peak exercise as control subjects, further refuting the suggestion that ventilatory capacity limits exercise in chronic HF.[109] However, as will be discussed in relation to skeletal muscle generally below, diaphragmatic fatigue causes sympathetic activation and a reduction in leg blood flow.[110,111] These changes could potentially contribute to the cycle of impaired muscle perfusion, worsening of the skeletal myopathy, and the abnormal ventilatory response to exercise.

Ventilation–perfusion mismatching

Ventilation–perfusion matching in the lung is commonly abnormal in patients with chronic HF. Ventilation, V, and perfusion, Q, are ideally equal, leading to a V/Q ratio of 1.0 in an idealized lung unit. Where perfusion is greater than ventilation ($V/Q < 1.0$), there is effective shunting of venous blood; where ventilation is greater than perfusion ($V/Q > 1.0$), there is 'wasted ventilation', or dead space. At rest in upright normal individuals, for example, there is a gradient of V/Q ratio from apex to base of the lung leading to dead space in the apices.

Increased dead space may be a cause of the elevated V_E/V_{CO_2} slope. Equation 23.1 suggests that when V_E/V_{CO_2} is increased, if Pa_{CO_2} is constant, then V_D/V_T must be increased. However, while this may be true, it does not imply that increased dead space ventilation is the cause of the increased V_E/V_{CO_2} slope. Several lines of evidence suggest that it may not be. Firstly, the exercise hyperventilation seen during exercise in chronic HF patients is present from the outset of exercise,[112,113] whereas any abnormalities in blood chemistry and increases in dead space ventilation would worsen as exercise progresses. Secondly, although during submaximal exercise V_D/V_T is higher in patients than controls, at peak exercise controls have a higher absolute dead space ventilation than patients.[85] Furthermore, some data suggest that apical lung perfusion is increased in heart failure patients at rest compared with controls[114] (which leads to better V/Q matching) and it does not deteriorate during exercise.[114] Thirdly, β-blockade with carvedilol reduces hyperventilation without changing V_D/V_T.[18] Finally, correcting for the increased dead space ventilation due to breathing frequency in chronic HF patients does not weaken the correlation between the increased ventilatory response to exercise and peak O_2 consumption,[32] and increasing anatomical dead space in normal individuals does not cause an increase in the V_E/V_{CO_2} slope.[115]

A conceptual problem with all hypotheses for the origin of the increased V_E/V_{CO_2} in HF that rely on pulmonary pathology is the absence of a physiological signal. Arterial blood gas tensions are normal or supranormal during exercise in patients with HF with a higher Pa_{O_2} and lower Pa_{CO_2} than in normal subjects.[116,117] Indeed, where blood gas tensions are abnormal, there is usually another explanation for the symptoms of breathlessness.[117] There is no dead space ventilation detector, and how increased dead space ventilation would be communicated to the respiratory centres in order to stimulate 'compensatory' hyperventilation is unclear. On the other hand, if there were a stimulus to excess ventilation arising outside the lungs, there would be a tendency to an excessive fall in arterial CO_2. Increasing dead space ventilation might thus be a physiological response to prevent even greater reductions in Pa_{CO_2}.

Peripheral haemodynamics

In chronic HF, despite impaired ventricular function, the blood pressure response to exercise is not usually abnormal (particularly at submaximal workloads),[118] as a consequence of increased peripheral resistance.[119,120] The increased peripheral vascular resistance is a result of chronically increased sympathetic tone and renin–angiotensin system activation. There is arterial smooth muscle hypertrophy and activation of fibroblasts with hyalinosis of the vascular wall.[121] These changes lead to reduced arterial compliance[122] and hence to poor vasodilatation in skeletal muscle arterioles during exercise.[123]

In addition, there is a reduced response to endogenous vasodilatory stimuli,[124,125] to infused hyperosmolar solutions,[126] and to pharmacological agents.[127] There are also increased in levels of endothelin, a powerful vasoconstrictor.[128]

Skeletal muscles

The skeletal muscles are abnormal in patients with chronic HF. There is general reduction in muscle bulk early in the course of heart failure,[138] and there is a shift from type I (slow twitch) to type IIb (fast twitch) fibres within skeletal muscles.[129] Type IIb fibres are more easily fatiguable and have less aerobic capacity than type I fibres. Capillary density is also reduced.[130] Hence there is an earlier need for anaerobic metabolism during exercise than normal. It is also becoming clear that perfusion within muscles and fibre recruitment may be impaired in chronic HF,[131] and muscle strength is also reduced,[132] as is endurance.[133] Exercise capacity in heart failure patients is related to both muscle strength and bulk,[134–136], and the reduction in endurance correlates with exercise performance.[137]

From a patient's point of view, the ability to perform repeated submaximal exercise (endurance) may be more important than peak force generation (strength), and early quadriceps fatiguability has been reported.[133,138] Fatigue is independent of acute changes in blood flow[163,139] and of central factors.[170] Fatiguability has been shown in a very small muscle group[167] in which blood flow is unlikely to be limited by cardiac reserve, suggesting that intrinsic muscle factors mediate fatiguability of muscle. It is not difficult to imagine how such abnormal muscles might lead to fatigue, but it is less clear how they might lead to breathlessness.

Ergoreceptors are muscle receptors sensitive to work. Stimulation of the receptors during exercise leads to ventilation and sympathetic activation—the ergoreflex. The degree of activation is in part related to the work performed per unit of muscle mass and to the metabolic state of the muscle. In normal subjects, for example, the ventilatory response to a given workload is much greater if the work is performed by arms rather than legs.[140] Furthermore, when normal subjects exercise with cuffs inflated to suprasystolic pressure, thus preventing the wash-out of the metabolic products of exercise, the ventilatory response to exercise is greater than in the control situation.[140]

The ergoreflex can be quantified by experiments involving cuff inflation around an exercising limb. During exercise in a normal subject, ventilation progressively increases with an increase in vascular resistance in the nonexercising limbs. There is a swift return to normal at the end of exercise. If a cuff is inflated at peak exercise proximal to the exercising muscle, the muscle is 'frozen' in its exercising state.[141] The consequent persisting increase in ventilation compared with the control response is the ergoreflex response.[142] In HF patients, presumably as a result of skeletal muscle abnormalities, the ergoreflex response generated by postexercise regional circulatory occlusion is much greater, both in terms of haemodynamic responses and in terms of the ventilatory response.[143,144] The reflex is sensitive to metabolic stimulation rather than movement.[145] The increased ventilatory response to exercise is proportional to the increased ergoreflex activity,[143] and a training programme can reduce the contribution of the ergoreflex to ventilation,[143] presumably by increasing the quality of the skeletal muscle.

The precise exercise product responsible for triggering the ergoreflex is not clear. Possibilities include potassium, particular as arterial potassium rises on exercise,[146,147] mirroring closely the increase in ventilation.[148] However, potassium rises during exercise do not demonstrate an inflection similar to that seen in the rise in ventilation during heavy exercise.[149] Furthermore, β-blockers lead to a greater rise in arterial potassium for a given workload, but do not increase minute ventilation.[150] Another possible contributor is prostaglandin production, as local prostaglandin levels in exercising muscle correlate with the ventilatory response.[151] However, patients taking regular aspirin, a powerful inhibitor of inflammatory prostaglandin production, do not demonstrate a clinically significant difference in ventilatory response to exercise compared with those not taking aspirin.[152]

In addition to a metabolic response to exercise, there are suggestions that nerve fibres sensitive to stretch might be involved in the response to ventilation. Muscle sympathetic nerve activity (MSNA) is related to the V_E/V_{CO_2} slope in chronic HF patients,[153] and passive limb movement leads to an increase in MSNA in chronic HF patients but not controls,[154] proportional to heart failure severity.[155] This suggests the existence of a mechanoreflex in addition to the metaboreflex.

The concept that peripheral muscle receptors sensitive to work, whether they be metabo- or mechanoreceptors, contribute to ventilation, and that this reflex is abnormal in patients with chronic HF, provides an elegant and unifying hypothesis explaining both breathlessness and fatigue in these patients.[156] On exercise, patients with heart failure have weak, structurally abnormal skeletal muscles, which are performing more work per unit muscle volume than normal muscle. In turn, this results in greater production of the metabolic products of exercise in the context of impaired perfusion. This leads to an increased stimulation of ergoreceptors sensitive to metabolic products, which stimulate increased ventilation relative to CO_2 production thus increasing the V_E/V_{CO_2} slope and reducing Pa_{CO_2}.

Sympathetic activation and ventilation

The increased sympathetic activation of chronic HF may also contribute to the ventilatory response to exercise. Acute and chronic β-blockade, although having little effect on maximal[157] or submaximal exercise capacity,[158,159] reduces submaximal and maximal ventilation during exercise, and also reduces the V_E/V_{CO_2} slope.[44,45] On the other hand, increasing presynaptic catecholamine levels leads to an increase in ventilation in normal subjects, perhaps by sensitizing the ergoreceptors.[160]

Use of data from metabolic gas exchange variables

Diagnosis, prognosis, and transplant assessment

In subjects referred for investigation of symptoms of breathlessness and fatigue, a carefully performed exercise test provides an objective measure of exercise capacity. Cardiopulmonary exercise testing gives an overall assessment of the severity of the pathophysiology of chronic HF, integrating skeletal muscle, lung, endothelial, and cardiac function.

Perhaps more than other single assessment, peak V_{O_2} is as a sensitive predictor of morbidity and mortality.[82,161] A peak V_{O_2} of less than 14 mL/kg per min has been used as a functional criterion for selecting patients for cardiac transplantation.[162] However, since the incorporation of β-blockers into routine management, patients have a better outlook for a given exercise capacity, and a pV_{O_2} of around 10–12 mL/kg per min is increasingly used as the cut-off identifying patients at especially high risk who might therefore benefit from transplantation.[163] Nevertheless, the value of pV_{O_2} as a risk assessment tool remains in the presence of optimal medical therapy,[164–166] and referral for transplant assessment can safely be deferred in patients with a pV_{O_2} greater than 18mL/kg per min.

More recently, it has become clear that an elevated V_E/V_{CO_2} slope provides additional and independent prognostic information.[167] Combining peak O_2 consumption and V_E/V_{CO_2} slope improves risk assessment in some [168] but not all studies.[41]

Differential diagnosis

Cardiopulmonary exercise testing can not only aid with prognostic assessment but can also assist in establishing the cause of symptoms of exercise intolerance in an individual. The most common differential diagnoses are chronic obstructive pulmonary disease (COPD), obesity, psychogenic hyperventilation, and poor effort. Data collected during a routine cardiopulmonary exercise test can add to clinical information and data from noninvasive imaging. Table 23.3 shows the cardiopulmonary exercise test variables seen with important differential diagnoses.

Response to therapy

With aggressive neurohormonal blockade, appropriate device therapy, and careful hospital and community-based management programmes, mortality rates of less than 10% and hospitalization rates of less than 20% per year can be achieved for many patients with chronic HF. Contemporary randomized, placebo-controlled studies exploring the effects of new therapies on mortality and morbidity therefore require ever-increasing numbers of subjects. As a noninvasive, reproducible, and repeatable surrogate for outcome and an objective measure of heart failure severity, exercise testing with or without metabolic gas exchange is increasingly used as an endpoint in studies in chronic HF. Improvements in exercise capacity in smaller studies can also help plan larger mortality studies. So, for example, early studies of cardiac resynchronization therapy showed improvements on in exercise capacity,[169–171] allowing better planning of the CARE-HF study using the earlier studies as a guide.[172]

Conclusions

In addition to helping with diagnosis in patients presenting with symptoms of exercise intolerance, cardiopulmonary metabolic exercise testing (CPET) provides reliable and objective information on prognosis in patients with chronic HF and can be used to stratify patients requiring transplant assessment. CPET is

Table 23.3 Results from cardiopulmonary exercise testing in patients with differential diagnoses

Variable	Chronic heart failure	Chronic obstructive airways disease	Obesity	Hyperventilation	Poor effort
pV_{O_2}	↓	↓	↓	↓	↓
AT	↓	↔/↓	↓	↔	Often impossible to determine or normal
RER at peak	↔	↔	↔	↓ at peak	↓
V_E/V_{CO_2}	↑	↑	↑/↔	↑/↔	↑/↔
Breathing reserve	↔/↑	↓	↑	↑	↓
Vital capacity	↓	↑	↓	↔	↑
$P_{ET}CO_2$	↑	↑	↔	↓	↔
Comments	Reduced $\Delta V_{O_2}/\Delta WR$, oscillatory breathing	Increased dead space, FEV_1 low	Physical examination confirms obesity	RER and ventilation ↑ prior to exercise, abrupt further increase in ventilation at onset of exercise	

pV_{O_2}; peak O_2 consumption, RER; respiratory exchange ratio, V_E/V_{CO_2}; relationship between ventilation and CO_2 production, $P_{ET}CO_2$; end-tidal CO_2, $\Delta V_{O_2}/\Delta WR$; ratio between change in O_2 consumption and change in work rate

noninvasive and low risk and can be easily repeated in order to monitor responses to therapy, in both daily clinical practice and research settings. However, the test must be carried out and interpreted in a controlled manner by experienced staff.

References

1. Myers J, Prakash M, Froelicher V, Do D, Partington S, Atwood JE. Exercise capacity and mortality among men referred for exercise testing. *N Engl J Med* 2002;**346**:793–801.
2. Clark AL, Coats AJS. Exercise endpoints in chronic heart failure. *Int J Cardiol* 2000;**73**:61–6.
3. Willens HJ, Blevins RD, Wrisley D, Antonishen D, Reinstein D, Rubenfire M. The prognostic value of functional capacity in patients with mild to moderate heart failure. *Am Heart J* 1987;**114**:377–82.
4. Cohn JN, Johnson GR, Shabetai R, *et al.* Ejection fraction, peak exercise oxygen consumption, cardiothoracic ratio, ventricular arrhythmias, and plasma norepinephrine as determinants of prognosis in heart failure. The V-HeFT VA Cooperative Studies Group. *Circulation* 1993;**87**(6 Suppl):VI5–16.
5. Francis GS, Goldsmith SR, Cohn JN. Relationship of exercise capacity to resting left ventricular performance and basal plasma norepinephrine levels in patients with congestive heart failure. *Am Heart J* 1982;**104**(4 Pt 1):725–31.
6. Hsich E, Gorodeski EZ, Starling RC, Blackstone EH, Ishwaran H, Lauer MS. Importance of treadmill exercise time as an initial prognostic screening tool in patients with systolic left ventricular dysfunction. *Circulation* 2009;**119**:3189–97.
7. Myers J. *Essential of cardiopulmonary exercise testing.* Human Kinetics, Champaign, IL, 1996.
8. Stelken AM, Younis LT, Jennison SH, *et al.* Prognostic value of cardiopulmonary exercise testing using percent achieved of predicted peak oxygen uptake for patients with ischemic and dilated cardiomyopathy. *J Am Coll Cardiol* 1996;**27**:345–52.
9. Myers J, Gullestad L, Vagelos R, Do D, Bellin D, Ross H, Fowler MB. Clinical, hemodynamic, and cardiopulmonary exercise test determinants of survival in patients referred for evaluation of heart failure. *Ann Intern Med* 1998;**129**(4):286–93.
10. Taylor HL, Buskirk E, Henschel A. Maximal oxygen intake as an objective measure of cardiorespiratory performance. *J Appl Physiol* 1955;**8**:73–80.
11. Andersen P, Saltin B. Maxial perfusion of skeletal muscle in man. *J Appl Physiol* 1985;**366**:233–49.
12. Vogel JA, Gleser MA. Effect of carbon monoxide on oxygen transport during exercise. *J Appl Physiol* 1972;**32**:234–9.
13. Whipp BJ, Ward SA. Coupling of ventilation to pulmonary gas axchange during exercise. In: Whipp BJ, Wasserman K (eds.) *Exercise: pulmonary physiology and pathophysiology*, p. 275. Marcel Dekker, New York, 1991.
14. Whipp BJ. Ventilatory control during exercise in humans. *Ann Rev Physiol* 1983;**45**:393–412.
15. Brown SE, Wiener S, Brown RA, Maratelli PA, Light RW. Exercise performance following a carbohydrate load in chronic airflow obstruction. *Am J Appl Physiol* 1985;**58**:1340–6.
16. Wasserman K, Van Kessel AL, Burton GB. Interaction of physiological mechanisms during exercise. *J Appl Physiol* 1967;**22**:71–85.
17. Cassaburi R, Whipp BJ, Wasserman K, Beaver WL, Koyal SN. Ventilatory and gas exchange dynamics in response to sinusoidal work. *J Appl Physiol Respirat Environ Exercise Physiol* 1977;**42**:300–11.
18. Agostoni P, Contini M, Magini A, *et al.* Carvedilol reduces exercise-induced hyperventilation: A benefit in normoxia and a problem with hypoxia. *Eur J Heart Fail* 2006;8:729–35.
19. Witte KK, Thackray SD, Nikitin NP, Cleland JG, Clark AL. Pattern of ventilation during exercise in chronic heart failure. *Heart* 2003;**89**:610–4.
20. Mezzani A, Corra U, Bosimini E, Giordano A, Giannuzzi P. Contribution of peak respiratory exchange ratio to peak VO2 prognostic reliability in patients with chronic heart failure and severely reduced exercise capacity. *Am Heart J* 2003;**145**:1102–7.
21. Ingle L, Witte KK, Cleland JG, Clark AL. The prognostic value of cardiopulmonary exercise testing with a peak respiratory exchange ratio of <1.0 in patients with chronic heart failure. *Int J Cardiol* 2008;**127**:88–92.
22. Stringer W, Wasserman K, Casaburi R. The VCO2/VO2 relationship during heavy, constant work rate exercise reflects the rate of lactic acid accumulation. *Eur J Appl Physiol Occup Physiol* 1995;**72**:25–31.
23. Hughson RH, Weisiger KW, Swanson GD. Blood lactate concentration increases as a continuous function in progressive exercise. *J Appl Physiol* 1987;**62**:1975–81.
24. Simonton CA, Higginbotham MB, Cobb FR. The ventilatory threshold: quantitative analysis of reproducibility and relation to arterial lactate concentration in normal subjects and in patients with chronic congestive heart failure. *Am J Cardiol* 1988;**62**:100–7.
25. Hoh H, Taniguchi K, Koike A, Doi M. Evaluation of severity of heart failure using ventilatory gas analysis. *Circulation* 1990;**81** (1 suppl 2):II31-II37.
26. Lipkin DP, Bayliss J, Poole-Wilson PA. The ability of a submaximal exercise test to predict maximal exercise capacity in patients with heart failure. *Eur Heart J* 1985;**6**:829–33.
27. Cohen-Solal A, Zannad F, Kayanakis JG, Gueret P, Aupetit JF, Kolsky H. Multicentre study of the determination of peak oxygen uptake and ventilatory threshold during bicycle exercise in chronic heart failure. Comparison of graphical methods, interobserver variability and influence of the exercise protocol. The VO2 French Study Group. *Eur Heart J* 1991;**12**:1055–63.
28. Wasserman K, Whipp BJ, Casaburi R. Respiratory control during exercise. In: Chrniak S, Widdicombe G (eds.) *Handbook of physiology*, vol 2, 515–619. American Physiological Society, Bethesda, MD, 1986.
29. Clark AL, Coats AJS. Usefulness of arterial blood gas estimations during exercise in patients with chronic heart failure. *Br Heart J* 1994;**71**:528–30.
30. Cohen-Solal A, Zannad F, Kayanakis JG, Gueret P, Aupetit JF, Kolsky H. Multicentre study of the determination of peak oxygen uptake and ventilatory threshold during bicycle exercise in chronic heart failure. Comparison of graphical methods, interobserver variability and influence of the exercise protocol. The VO2 French Study Group. *Eur Heart J* 1991;**12**:1055–63.
31. Witte KKA, Clark AL. Is the elevated slope relating ventilation to carbon dioxide production in chronic heart failure a consequence of slow metabolic gas kinetics? *Eur J Heart Fail* 2002;**4**:469–72.
32. Buller NP, Poole-Wilson PA. Mechanism of the increased ventilatory response to exercise in patients with chronic heart failure. *Br Heart J* 1990;**63**:281–3.
33. Francis DP, Shamim W, Davies LC, *et al.* Cardiopulmonary exercise testing for prognosis in chronic heart failure: continuous and independent prognostic value from VE/VCO2 slope and peak VO2. *Eur Heart J* 2000;**21**:154–61.
34. Davies SW, Emery TM, Watling MIL, Wannamethee G, Lipkin DP. A critical threshold of exercise capacity in the ventilatory response to exercise in heart failure. *Br Heart J* 1991;**65**:179–83.
35. Corrà U, Giordano A, Bosimini E, *et al.* Oscillatory ventilation during exercise in patients with chronic heart failure: clinical correlates and prognostic implications. *Chest* 2002;**121**(5):1572–80.
36. Leite JJ, Mansur AJ, de Freitas HF, *et al.* Periodic breathing during incremental exercise predicts mortality in patients with chronic heart failure evaluated for cardiac transplantation. *J Am Coll Cardiol* 2003;**41**(12):2175–81.
37. Ingle L, Isted A, Witte KK, Cleland JG, Clark AL. Impact of different diagnostic criteria on the prevalence and prognostic significance of

exertional oscillatory ventilation in patients with chronic heart failure. *Eur J Cardiovasc Prev Rehabil* 2009;**16**(4):451–6.

38. Baba R, Nagashima M, Goto M, *et al.* Oxygen uptake efficiency slope: a new index of cardiorespiratory functional reserve derived from the relation between oxygen uptake and minute ventilation during incremental exercise. *J Am Coll Cardiol* 1996;**28**(6):1567–72.
39. Davies LC, Wensel R, Georgiadou P, *et al.* Enhanced prognostic value from cardiopulmonary exercise testing in chronic heart failure by non-linear analysis: oxygen uptake efficiency slope. *Eur Heart J* 2006;**27**(6):684–90.
40. Williams SG, Cooke GA, Wright DJ, *et al.* Peak exercise cardiac power output; a direct indicator of cardiac function strongly predictive of prognosis in chronic heart failure. *Eur Heart J* 2001;**22**:1496–503.
41. Ingle L, Witte KK, Cleland JG, Clark AL. Combining the ventilatory response to exercise and peak oxygen consumption is no better than peak oxygen consumption alone in predicting mortality in chronic heart failure. *Eur J Heart Fail* 2008;**10**:85–8.
42. Witte KK, Thackray SD, Lindsay KA, Cleland JG, Clark AL. Metabolic gas kinetics depend upon the level of exercise performed. *Eur J Heart Fail* 2005;**7**:991–6.
43. Samejima H, Omiya K, Uno M, *et al.* Relationship between impaired chronotropic response, cardiac output during exercise, and exercise tolerance in patients with chronic heart failure. *Jpn Heart J* 2003;**44**:515–25.
44. Witte KKA, Thackray SDR, Nikitin NP, Cleland JGF, Clark AL. The effects of α- and β-blockade on ventilatory responses to exercise in chronic heart failure. *Heart* 2003;**89**:1169–73.
45. Witte KKA, Nikitin NP, Cleland JGF, Clark AL. The effects of long-term β-blockade on the ventilatory responses to exercise in chronic heart failure. *Eur J Heart Fail* 2005;4:612–617.
46. Proctor DN, Beck KC. Delay time adjustments to minimize errors in breath-by-breath measurement of Vo_2 during exercise. *J Appl Physiol* 1996;**81**(6):2495–9.
47. Borg G. Subjective effort and physical activities. *Scand J Rehab* 1978;**6**:108–13.
48. Jones RS, Buston MH, Wharton MJ. The effect of exercise on ventilatory function in the child with asthma. *Br J Dis Chest* 1962;**56**:78–86.
49. Buchfuhrer MJ, Hansen JE, Robinson TE, Sue DY, Wasserman K, Whipp BJ. Optimizing the exercise protocol for cardiopulmonary assessment. *J Appl Physiol* 1983;**55**:1558–64.
50. Bruce PA, McDonough IR. Stress testing in screening for cardiovascular disease. *Bull NY Acad Med* 1969;**45**:1288–305.
51. Balke B, Ware RW. An experimental study of physical fitness of Air Force personnel. *U S Armed Forces Med J* 1959;**10**:675–88.
52. Nagle FJ, Balke B, Naughton JP. Gradational step tests for assessing work capacity. *J Appl Physiol* 1965;**20**:745–8.
53. McConnell TR, Clark BA III. Prediction of maximal oxygen consumption during handrail-supported treadmill exercise. *J Cardiopulm Rehabil* 1987;**7**:324–31.
54. Ramos-Barbon D, Fitchett D, Gibbons WJ, Latter DA, Levy RD. Maximal exercise testing for the selection of heart transplantation candidates: limitation of peak oxygen consumption. *Chest* 1999;**115**:410–17.
55. Dickstein K, Aarsland T, Svanes H, Barvik S. A respiratory exchange ratio equal to 1 provides a reproducible index of submaximal cardiopulmonary exercise performance. *Am J Cardiol* 1993;**71**:1367–9.
56. Mezzani A, Corra U, Bosimini E, Giordano A, Giannuzzi P. Contribution of peak respiratory exchange ratio to peak VO2 prognostic reliability in patients with chronic heart failure and severely reduced exercise capacity. *Am Heart J* 2003;**145**:1102–7.
57. Butler NP, Poole-Wilson PA. Extrapolated maximal oxygen consumption. A new method for the objective analysis of respiratory gas exchange during exercise. *Br Heart J* 1988;**59**:212–17.
58. Myers J, Prakash M, Froelicher V, Do D, Partington S, Atwood JE. Exercise capacity and mortality among men referred for exercise testing. *N Engl J Med* 2002;**346**:793–801.
59. Squires RW, Allison TG, Johnson BD, Gau GT. Non-physician supervision of cardiopulmonary exercise testing in chronic heart failure: safety and results of a preliminary investigation. *J Cardiopulm Rehabil* 1999;**19**:249–53.
60. Tristani FE, Hughes CV, Archibald DG, Sheldahl LM, Cohn JN, Fletcher R. Safety of graded symptom-limited exercise testing in patients with congestive heart failure. *Circulation* 1987;**76** (6 Pt 2):VI54–8.
61. Clark AL, Sparrow JL, Coats AJ. Muscle fatigue and dyspnoea in chronic heart failure: two sides of the same coin? *Eur Heart J* 1995;**16**:49–52.
62. Witte KK, Clark AL. Dyspnoea versus fatigue: additional prognostic information from symptoms in chronic heart failure? *Eur J Heart Fail* 2008;**10**:1224–8.
63. Lipkin DP, Canepa-Anson R, Stephens MR, Poole-Wilson PA. Factors determining symptoms in heart failure: comparison of fast and slow exercise tests. *Br Heart J* 1986;**55**:439–45.
64. Fink LI, Wilson JR, Ferraro N. Exercise ventilation and pulmonary artery wedge pressure in chronic stable congestive heart failure. *Am J Cardiol* 1986;**57**:249–53.
65. Witte KKA, Clark AL. Cycle exercise causes a lower ventilatory response to exercise in chronic heart failure. *Heart* 2005;**91**:225–6.
66. Witte KK, Nikitin NP, De Silva R, Cleland JG, Clark AL. Exercise capacity and cardiac function assessed by tissue Doppler imaging in chronic heart failure. *Heart* 2004;**90**:1144–50.
67. Clark AL, Swan JW, Laney R, Connelly M, Somerville J, Coats AJ. The role of right and left ventricular function in the ventilatory response to exercise in chronic heart failure. *Circulation* 1994;**89**:2062–9.
68. Chandrashekhar Y, Anand IS. Relation between major indices of prognosis in patients with chronic congestive heart failure: studies of maximal exercise oxygen consumption, neurohormones and ventricular function. *Indian Heart J* 1992;**44**:213–16.
69. Carell ES, Murali S, Schulman DS, Estrada-Quintero T, Uretsky BF. Maximal exercise tolerance in chronic congestive heart failure. Relationship to resting left ventricular function. *Chest* 1994;**106**:1746–52.
70. Davies SW, Fussell AL, Jordan SL, Poole-Wilson PA, Lipkin DP. Abnormal diastolic filling patterns in chronic heart failure-relationship to exercise capacity. *Eur Heart J* 1992;**13**:749–57.
71. Higginbotham MB, Morris KG, Conn EH, Coleman RE, Cobb FR. Determinants of variable exercise performance among patients with severe left ventricular dysfunction. *Am J Cardiol* 1983;**51**:52–60.
72. Benge W, Litchfield RL, Marcus ML. Exercise capacity in patients with severe left ventricular dysfunction. *Circulation* 1980;**61**:955–9.
73. Ribeiro JP, White HD, Arnold JM, Hartley LH, Colucci WS. Exercise responses before and after long-term treatment with oral milrinone in patients with severe heart failure. *Am J Med* 1986;**81**: 759–64.
74. Petein M, Levine TB, Cohn JN. Persistent hemodynamic effects without long-term clinical benefits in response to oral piroximone (MDL 19,205) in patients with congestive heart failure. *Circulation* 1986;**73**(3 Pt 2):III230–6.
75. Leung TC, Ballman KV, Allison TG, *et al.* Clinical predictors of exercise capacity 1 year after cardiac transplantation. *J Heart Lung Transplant* 2003;**22**:16–27.
76. Douard H, Parrens E, Billes MA, Labbe L, Baudet E, Broustet JP. Predictive factors of maximal aerobic capacity after cardiac transplantation. *Eur Heart J* 1997;**18**:1823–8.
77. Marzo K, Herrmann HA, Rein A, Mancini D. Acute effect of balloon mitral valvuloplasty on exercise capacity ventilation and skeletal muscle oxygenation. *Circulation* 1991;**84**(Suppl II):11–72.

78. Smart N, Haluska B, Jeffriess L, Case C, Marwick TH. Cardiac contributions to exercise training responses in patients with chronic heart failure: a strain imaging study. *Echocardiography* 2006;**23**:376–82.
79. Jonsdottir S, Andersen KK, Sigurosson AF, Sigurosson SB. The effect of physical training in chronic heart failure. *Eur J Heart Fail* 2006;**8**:97–101.
80. Van Thielen G, Paelinck BP, Beckers P, Vrints CJ, Conraads VM. Rate response and cardiac resynchronisation therapy in chronic heart failure: higher cardiac output does not acutely improve exercise performance: a pilot trial. *Eur J Cardiovasc Prev Rehabil* 2008;**15**(2):197–202.
81. Witte KK, Clark AL. Chronotropic incompetence does not contribute to submaximal exercise limitation in patients with chronic heart failure. *Int J Cardiol* 2009;**134**:342–4.
82. Witte KK, Cleland JG, Clark AL. Chronic heart failure, chronotropic incompetence, and the effects of beta blockade. *Heart* 2006;**92**:481–6.
83. Moore DP, Weston AR, Hughes JMB, Oakley CM, Cleland JGF. Effects of increased inspired oxygen concentrations on exercise performance in chronic heart failure. *Lancet* 1992;**339**:850–3.
84. RS Wright, MS Levine, PE Bellamy, *et al.* Ventilatory and diffusion abnormalities in potential heart transplant recipients. *Chest* 1990;98:816–20.
85. Clark AL, Volterrani M, Swan JW, Coats AJS. Increased ventilatory response to exercise in chronic heart failure: relation to pulmonary pathology. *Heart* 1997;**77**:138–46.
86. Kraemer MD, Kubo SH, Rector TS, Brunsvold N, Bank AJ. Pulmonary and peripheral vascular factors are important determinants of peak exercise oxygen uptake in patients with heart failure. *J Am Coll Cardiol* 1993;**21**:641–8.
87. Ingle L, Shelton RJ, Cleland JG, Clark AL. Poor relationship between exercise capacity and spirometric measurements in patients with more symptomatic heart failure. *J Card Fail* 2005;**11**:619–23.
88. Witte KKA, Morice A, Clark AL, Cleland JGF. Airways resistance in chronic heart failure measured by impulse oscillometry. *J Cardiac Fail* 2002;**8**:225–31.
89. Witte KKA, Morice A, Clark AL, Cleland JGF. The reversibility of airways resistance in chronic heart failure. *J Cardiac Fail* 2004;**10**:149–154.
90. Light RM, George RB. Serial pulmonary function in patients with acute heart failure. *Arch Intern Med* 1983;**143**:429–433.
91. Peterman W, Barth J, Entzian P. Heart failure and airways obstruction. *Int J Cardiol* 1987;**17**:207–9.
92. Cabanes LR, Weber SN, Matran R, *et al.* Bronchial hyperresponsiveness to methacholine in patients with impaired left ventricular function. *N Engl J Med* 1989;**320**:1317–22.
93. Cabanes L, Costes F, Weber S, *et al.* Improvement in exercise performance by inhalation of methoxamine in patients with impaired left ventricular function. *N Engl J Med* 1992;**326**:1661–5.
94. Chua TP, Lalloo UG, Worsdell MY, Kharitonov S, Chung KF, Coats AJS. Airway and cough responsiveness and exhaled nitric oxide in non-smoking patients with stable chronic heart failure. *Heart* 1996;**76**:144–9.
95. Puri S, Baker BL, Oakley CM, Hughes JM, Cleland JG. Increased alveolar/capillary membrane resistance to gas transfer in patients with chronic heart failure. *Br Heart J* 1994;**72**:140–4.
96. Puri S, Baker BL, Dutka DP, Oakley CM, Hughes JM, Cleland JG. Reduced alveolar-capillary membrane diffusing capacity in chronic heart failure. Its pathophysiological relevance and relationship to exercise performance. *Circulation* 1995;**91**:2769–74.
97. Smith AA, Cowburn PJ, Parker ME, *et al.* Impaired pulmonary diffusion during exercise in patients with chronic heart failure. *Circulation* 1999;**100**:1406–10.
98. Guazzi M, Pontone G, Brambilla R, Agostoni P, Reina G. Alveolar-capillary membrane gas conductance: a novel prognostic indicator in chronic heart failure. *Eur Heart J* 2002;**23**:467–76.
99. Guazzi M, Marenzi G, Alimento M, Contini M, Agostoni P. Improvement of alveolar-capillary membrane diffusing capacity with enalapril in chronic heart failure and counteracting effect of aspirin. *Circulation* 1997;**95**:1930–6.
100. Guazzi M, Reina G, Tumminello G, Guazzi MD. Improvement of alveolar-capillary membrane diffusing capacity with exercise training in chronic heart failure. *J Appl Physiol* 2004;**97**:1866–73.
101. Guazzi M, Tumminello G, Di Marco F, Fiorentini C, Guazzi MD. The effects of phosphodiesterase-5 inhibition with sildenafil on pulmonary hemodynamics and diffusion capacity, exercise ventilatory efficiency, and oxygen uptake kinetics in chronic heart failure. *J Am Coll Cardiol* 2004;**44**:2339–48.
102. Agostoni PG, Guazzi M, Bussotti M, Grazi M, Palermo P, Marenzi G. Lack of improvement of lung diffusing capacity following fluid withdrawal by ultrafiltration in chronic heart failure. *J Am Coll Cardiol* 2000;**36**:1600–4.
103. Lindsay DC, Lovegrove CA, Dunn MJ, Bennett JG, Pepper JR, Yacoub MH, Poole-Wilson PA. Histological abnormalities of muscle from limb, thorax and diaphragm in chronic heart failure. *Eur Heart J* 1996;**17**:1239–50.
104. Carmo MM, Barbara C, Ferreira T, Branco J, Ferreira S, Rendas AB. Diaphragmatic function in patients with chronic left ventricular failure. *Pathophysiology* 2001;**8**:55–60.
105. Nava S, Larovere MT, Fanfulla F, Navalesi P, Delmastro M, Mortara A. Orthopnea and inspiratory effort in chronic heart failure patients. *Respir Med* 2003;**97**:647–53.
106. Hughes PD, Polkey MI, Harrus ML, Coats AJ, Moxham J, Green M. Diaphragm strength in chronic heart failure. *Am J Respir Crit Care Med* 1999;**160**:529–34.
107. Dayer MJ, Hopkinson NS, Ross ET, Jonville S, Sharshar T, K earney M, Moxham J, Polkey MI. Does symptom-limited cycle exercise cause low frequency diaphragm fatigue in patients with heart failure? *Eur J Heart Fail* 2006;**8**:68–73.
108. Kufel TJ, Pineda LA, Junega RG, Hathwar R, Mador MJ. Diaphragmatic function after intense exercise in congestive heart failure patients. *Eur Respir J* 2002;**20**:1399–405.
109. Clark AL, Davies LC, Francis DP, Coats AJ. Ventilatory capacity and exercise tolerance in patients with chronic stable heart failure. *Eur J Heart Fail* 2000;**2**:47–51.
110. St Croix CM, Morgan BJ, Wetter TJ, Dempsey JA. Reflex effects from a fatiguing diaphragm increase sympathetic efferent activity (MSNA) to limb muscle in humans. *J Physiol* 2000;**529**: 493–504.
111. Sheel AW, Derchak PA, Morgan BJ, Pegelow DF, Jacques AJ, Dempsey JA. Fatiguing inspiratory muscle work causes reflex reduction in resting leg blood flow in humans. *J Physiol* 2001;**537**(Pt 1):277–89.
112. Metra M, Dei Cas L, Panina G, Visioli O. Exercise hyperventilation chronic congestive heart failure, and its relation to functional capacity and hemodynamics. *Am J Cardiol* 1992;**70**:622–8.
113. Clark AL, Coats AJ. Relationship between ventilation and carbon dioxide production in normal subjects with induced changes in anatomical dead space. *Eur J Clin Invest* 1993;**23**:428–32.
114. Mohsenifar Z, Amin DK, Shah PK. Regional distribution of lung perfusion and ventilation in patients with chronic congestive heart failure and its relationship to cardiopulmonary hemodynamics. *Am Heart J* 1989;**117**:887–91.
115. Clark AL, Volterrani M, Piepoli M, Coats AJS. Factors which alter the relationship between ventilation and carbon dioxide production during exercise: implications for the understanding of the increased ventilatory response to exercise in chronic heart failure. *Eur J Appl Physiol* 1996;**73**:144–148.
116. Rubin SA, Brown HV. Ventilation and gas exchange during exercise in severe chronic heart failure. *Am Rev Respir Dis* 1984;**129** (2 Pt 2):S63–4.

117. Clark AL, Coats AJ. Usefulness of arterial blood gas estimations during exercise in patients with chronic heart failure. *Br Heart J* 1994;**71**:528–30.

118. Sullivan MJ, Knight JD, Higginbotham MB, Cobb FR. Relation between central and peripheral haemodynamics during exercise in patients with chronic heart failure. Muscle blood flow is reduced with maintenance of arterial perfusion pressure. *Circulation* 1989;**80**:769–81.

119. LeJemtal TH, Maskin CS, Chadwick B, Sinoway L. Near maximal oxygen extraction by exercising muscles in patients with severe heart failure: a limitation to the benefits of training. *J Am Coll Cardiol* 1983;**1**:662A.

120. LeJemtel TH, Maskin CS, Lucido D, Chadwick BJ. Failure to augment maximal limb blood flow in response to one-leg versus two-leg exercise in patients with severe heart failure. *Circulation* 1986;**74**:245–51.

121. Wroblewski H, Kastrup J, Norgaard T, Mortensen S-A, Haunso S. Evidence of increased microvascular resistance and arteriolar hyalinosis in skin in congestive heart failure secondary to idiopathic dilated cardiomyopathy. *Am J Cardiol* 1992;**69**:769–74.

122. Arnold JMO, Marchiori GE, Imrie JR, Burton GL, Pflugfelder PW, Kostuk WJ. Large artery function in patients with chronic heart failure. Studies of brachial artery diameter and haemodynamics. *Circulation* 1991;**84**:2418–25.

123. Zelis R, Nellis SH, Longhurst J, Lee G, Mason DT. Abnormalities in the regional circulations accompanying congestive heart failure. *Prog Cardiovasc Dis* 1975;**18**:181–99.

124. Kubo SH, Rector TS, Bank AJ, Williams RE, Heifetz SM. Endothelium-dependent vasodilation is attenuated in patients with heart failure. *Circulation* 1991;**84**:1589–96.

125. Katz SD, Biasucci L, Sabba C, *et al.* Impaired endothelium-mediated vasodilation in the peripheral vasculature of patients with congestive heart failure. *J Am Coll Cardiol* 1992;**19**:918–25.

126. Bank AJ, Rector TS, Burke MN, Tschumperlin LK, Kubo SH. Impaired forearm vasodilation to hyperosmolal stimuli in patients with congestive heart failure secondary to idiopathic dilated cardiomyopathy or to ischemic cardiomyopathy. *Am J Cardiol* 1992;**70**:1315–9.

127. Franciosa JA, Goldsmith SR, Cohn JN. Contrasting immediate and long-term effects of isosorbide dinitrate on exercise capacity in congestive heart failure. *Am J Med* 1980;**69**:559–66.

128. McMurray JJ, Ray SG, Abdullah I, Dargie HJ, Morton JJ. Plasma endothelin in chronic heart failure. *Circulation* 1992;**85**:1374–9.

129. Lipkin DP, Jones DA, Round JM, Poole-Wilson PA. Abnormalities of skeletal muscle in patients with chronic heart failure. *Int J Cardiol* 1988;**18**:187–95.

130. Schaufelberger M, Eriksson BO, Grimby G, Held P, Swedberg K. Skeletal muscle alterations in patients with chronic heart failure. *Eur Heart J* 1997;**18**:971–80.

131. Mancini DM, Walter G, Reichnek N, *et al.* Contribution of skeletal muscle atrophy to exercise intolerance and altered muscle metabolism in heart failure. *Circulation* 1992;**85**:1364–73.

132. Buller NP, Jones D, Poole-Wilson PA. Direct measurements of skeletal muscle fatigue in patients with chronic heart failure. *Br Heart J* 1991;**65**:20–24.

133. Minotti JR, Pillay P, Chang L, Wells L, Massie BM. Neurophysiological assessment of skeletal muscle fatigue in patients with congestive heart failure. *Circulation* 1992;**86**:903–8.

134. Volterrani M, Clark AL, Ludman PF, *et al.* Determinants of exercise capacity in chronic heart failure. *Eur Heart J* 1994;**15**:801–809.

135. Clark A, Coats A. Mechanisms of exercise intolerance in cardiac failure: abnormalities of skeletal muscle and pulmonary function. *Curr Opin Cardiol* 1994;**9**:305–14.

136. Minotti JR, Pillay P, Oka R, Wells L, Christoph I, Massie BM. Skeletal muscle size: relationship to muscle function in heart failure. *J Appl Physiol* 1993;**75**:373–81.

137. Wilson JR, Mancini DM, Simson M. Detection of skeletal muscle fatigue in patients with heart failure using electromyography. *Am J Cardiol* 1992;**70**:488–93.

138. Lipkin DP, Jones DA, Round JM, Poole-Wilson PA. Abnormalities of skeletal muscle in patients with chronic heart failure. *Int J Cardiol* 1988;**18**:187–95.

139. Minotti JR, Christoph I, Oka R, Weiner MW, Wells L, Massie BM. Impaired skeletal muscle function in patients with congestive heart failure. Relationship to systemic exercise performance. *J Clin Invest* 1991;**88**:2077–82.

140. Clark AL, Piepoli M, Coats AJ. Skeletal muscle and the control of ventilation on exercise: evidence for metabolic receptors. *Eur J Clin Invest* 1995;**25**:299–305.

141. Arnolda L, Conway M, Dolecki M, *et al.* Skeletal muscle metabolism in heart failure:a 31P nuclear magnetic resonance spectroscopy study of leg muscle. *Clin Sci* 1990;79:583–589.

142. Piepoli M, Clark AL, Coats AJS. Muscle metaboreceptors in the hemodynamic, autonomic and ventilatory responses to exercise in man. *Am J Physiol* 1995;**269**(*Heart Circ Physiol* **38**):H1428–36.

143. Piepoli M, Clark AL, Volterrani M, Adamopoulos S, Sleight P, Coats AJ. Contribution of muscle afferents to the hemodynamic, autonomic, and ventilatory responses to exercise in patients with chronic heart failure: effects of physical training. *Circulation* 1996;**93**:940–52.

144. Grieve DAA, Clark AL, McCann GP, Hillis WS. The Ergoreflex in patients with chronic stable heart failure. *Int J Cardiol* 1999;**68**:157–164.

145. Scott AC, Francis DP, Davies LC, Ponikowski P, Coats AJ, Piepoli MF. Contribution of skeletal muscle 'ergoreceptors' in the human leg to respiratory control in chronic heart failure. *J Physiol* 2000;**529** Pt 3:863–70.

146. Sjoggard G, Adams RA, Saltin B. Water and ion shifts in skeletal muscle of humans with intense dynamic knee extension. *Am J Physiol* 1985;**248**:R190–6.

147. Linton RAF, Band DM. The effects of potassium on carotid body chemoreceptor activity and ventilation in the cat. *Respir Physiol* 1985;**59**:65–70.

148. Paterson DJ, Robbins PA, Conway J. Changes in arterial plasma potassium and ventilation during exercise in man. *Respir Physiol* 1989;**78**:323–30.

149. McLoughlin P, Popham P, Bruce RCH, Linton RAF, Band DM. Plasma potassium and the ventilatory threshold in man. *J Physiol* 1990;**427**:44P.

150. Lim M, Linton RAF, Wolff CB, Band DM. Propranolol, exercise and arterial potassium. *Lancet* 1981;ii:591.

151. Scott AC, Wensel R, Davos CH, *et al.* Chemical mediators of the muscle ergoreflex in chronic heart failure: a putative role for prostaglandins in reflex ventilatory control. *Circulation* 2002;**106**:214–20.

152. Witte KK, Clark AL. The effect of aspirin on the ventilatory response to exercise in chronic heart failure. *Eur J Heart Fail* 2004;**6**:745–8.

153. Witte KK, Notarius CF, Ivanov J, Floras JS. Muscle sympathetic nerve activity and ventilation during exercise in subjects with and without chronic heart failure. *Can J Cardiol* 2008;**24**:275–8.

154. Middlekauff HR, Chiu J, Hamilton MA, *et al.* Muscle mechanoreceptor sensitivity in heart failure. *Am J Physiol Heart Circ Physiol* 2004;**287**:H1937–43.

155. Negrão CE, Rondon MU, Tinucci T, *et al.* Abnormal neurovascular control during exercise is linked to heart failure severity. *Am J Physiol Heart Circ Physiol* 2001;**280**:H1286–92.

156. Clark AL, Poole-Wilson PA, Coats AJ. Exercise limitation in chronic heart failure: central role of the periphery. *J Am Coll Cardiol* 1996;**28**:1092–102.

157. Australia/New Zealand Heart Failure Research Collaborative Group. Randomised, placebo-controlled trial of carvedilol in patients with

congestive heart failure due to ischaemic heart disease. *Lancet* 1997;**349**:375–80.

158. US Carvedilol Heart Failure Study Group. Carvedilol inhibits clinical progression in patients with mild symptoms of heart failure. *Circ* 1996;**94**:2800–6.
159. Cohn JN, Fowler MB, Bristow MR *et al*, for the US Carvedilol Heart failure Study Group. Safety and efficacy of carvedilol in severe heart failure. *J Cardiac Fail* 1997;**3**:173–9.
160. Clark AL, Galloway S, MacFarlane N, Henderson E, Aitchison T, McMurray JJ. Catecholamines contribute to exertional dyspnoea and to the ventilatory response to exercise in normal humans. *Eur Heart J* 1997;**18**:1829–33.
161. Francis DP, Shamim W, Davies LC, *et al.* Cardiopulmonary exercise testing for prognosis in chronic heart failure: continuous and independent prognostic value from VE/VCO(2)slope and peak VO(2). *Eur Heart J* 2000;**21**:154–61.
162. Mancini DM, Eisen H, Kussmaul W, Mull R, Edmunds LH Jr, Wilson JR. Value of peak exercise oxygen consumption for optimal timing of cardiac transplantation in ambulatory patients with heart failure. *Circulation* 1991;**83**:778–86.
163. Zugck C, Haunstetter A, Krüger C, *et al.* Impact of beta-blocker treatment on the prognostic value of currently used risk predictors in congestive heart failure. *J Am Coll Cardiol* 2002;**39**(10):1615–22.
164. Koelling TM, Joseph S, Aaronson KD. Heart failure survival score continues to predict clinical outcomes in patients with heart failure receiving beta-blockers. *J Heart Lung Transplant* 2004;**23**:1414–22.
165. Butler J, Khadim G, Paul KM, *et al.* Selection of patients for heart transplantation in the current era of heart failure therapy. *J Am Coll Cardiol* 2004;**43**:787–93.
166. Geisberg C, Goring J, Listerman J, Nading MA, Huang RL, Butler J. Impact of optimal heart failure medical therapy on heart transplant listing. *Transplant Proc* 2006;**38**:1493–5.
167. Chua TP, Ponikowski P, Harrington D, *et al.* Clinical correlates and prognostic significance of the ventilatory response to exercise in chronic heart failure. *J Am Coll Cardiol* 1997;**29**:1585–90.
168. Corrà U, Mezzani A, Bosimini E, Scapellato F, Imparato A, Giannuzzi P. Ventilatory response to exercise improves risk stratification in patients with chronic heart failure and intermediate functional capacity. *Am Heart J* 2002;**143**:418–26.
169. Cazeau S, Leclercq C, Lavergne T, *et al.*; Multisite Stimulation in Cardiomyopathies (MUSTIC) Study Investigators. Effects of multisite biventricular pacing in patients with heart failure and intraventricular conduction delay. *N Engl J Med* 2001; **344**:873–80.
170. Varma C, Sharma S, Firoozi S, McKenna WJ, Daubert JC; Multisite Stimulation in Cardiomyopathy (MUSTIC) Study Group. Atriobiventricular pacing improves exercise capacity in patients with heart failure and intraventricular conduction delay. *J Am Coll Cardiol* 2003;**41**:582–8.
171. Auricchio A, Stellbrink C, Sack S, *et al.*; Pacing Therapies in Congestive Heart Failure (PATH-CHF) Study Group. Long-term clinical effect of hemodynamically optimized cardiac resynchronization therapy in patients with heart failure and ventricular conduction delay. *J Am Coll Cardiol* 2002;**39**:2026–33.
172. Cleland JG, Daubert JC, Erdmann E, *et al.*; Cardiac Resynchronization-Heart Failure (CARE-HF) Study Investigators. The effect of cardiac resynchronization on morbidity and mortality in heart failure. *N Engl J Med* 2005;**352**:1539–49.

PART VIII

Invasive investigation

24

Invasive investigation

Roy S. Gardner

Catheter studies

The technique for human cardiac catheterization was first developed by Werner Forssmann. In 1929, he inserted a cannula into his own antecubital vein, through which he passed a catheter for 65 cm and then walked to the X-ray department, where a photograph was taken of the catheter lying in his right atrium. His approach was frowned upon and he was forced to give up cardiology for a career in urology. However, he was subsequently awarded the Nobel Prize in Physiology or Medicine in 1956, along with André Frédéric Cournand and Dickinson W. Richards who developed ways of applying his technique to heart disease diagnosis and research.

Despite advances in noninvasive imaging, there are frequent occasions when invasive investigation is required. This chapter aims to summarize these techniques and demonstrate how both right and left heart catheterization can offer valuable information about the patient.

Seldinger technique

The Seldinger technique (Fig. 24.1) was introduced by Dr Sven-Ivar Seldinger (1921–1998), a Swedish radiologist, in 1953.[1] Although originally described for percutaneous arteriography, the technique is now used to place catheters in a variety of locations including veins, arteries, or body cavities such as pleural or pericardial spaces.

Central venous cannulation

Obtaining central venous access is a key skill in the management of an ill patient, allowing invasive pressure monitoring, infusion of therapy, and access for procedures such as temporary pacing, pulmonary artery catheterization, and endomyocardial biopsy. The three routes commonly employed are the internal jugular vein, the subclavian vein, and the femoral vein.

The use of ultrasound to guide cannulation of the internal jugular vein significantly improves the success rate (100% compared to 88%, $p < 0.001$), decreases access time (mean of 9.8 s vs. 44.5 s, $p < 0.001$), and reduces the complication rate ($p < 0.001$) compared to cannulation using anatomical landmarks in over 600 patients.[2] In 2002, a technology appraisal from the UK National Institute for Health and Clinical Excellence (NICE) recommended that central venous cannulation (CVC) should be performed using direct vision where possible (e.g. Bard® Site-Rite® ultrasound system—Fig. 24.2).[3] However, NICE acknowledged that CVC using anatomical landmarks was a skill that should be maintained, particularly in emergency situations when direct vision equipment is not immediately available.

Internal jugular vein access

The internal jugular vein is most often used as it allows the catheter to be inserted under direct ultrasound guidance thus reducing the potential for complications such as carotid artery puncture or pneumothorax. Compared to a femoral approach, the site can be kept sterile. Indeed, a critical aspect in any invasive procedure is scrupulous attention to aseptic technique. The skin should be prepared and draped and local anaesthetic should be infiltrated into the skin and subcutaneous tissues. The catheter is flushed in preparation for insertion.

Place the patient supine in a head-down tilt. For a right internal jugular approach, rotate the head 30–45° to the left to open up the anterior triangle, which is formed by the sternal and clavicular heads of the sternomastoid muscle. The carotid artery can be palpated with the left hand, thus reducing the risk of an inadvertent arterial puncture. After making an incision in the skin, insert a 20 gauge needle at 45° to the skin lateral to the carotid artery, aiming for the right nipple in men and the right anterior superior iliac spine in women (Fig. 24.3). Once the vein is found, using the Seldinger technique, a J-tipped wire is advanced through the needle into the vein. It is important never to advance the wire against resistance and always to ensure that control and sight of the guide wire is maintained. The needle is then removed, leaving the wire in place over which is inserted a dilator. On removing the dilator, the catheter can then be gently twisted into position and the guide wire removed. The catheter is then sutured and the site covered with a sterile dressing. A check chest radiograph should be performed.

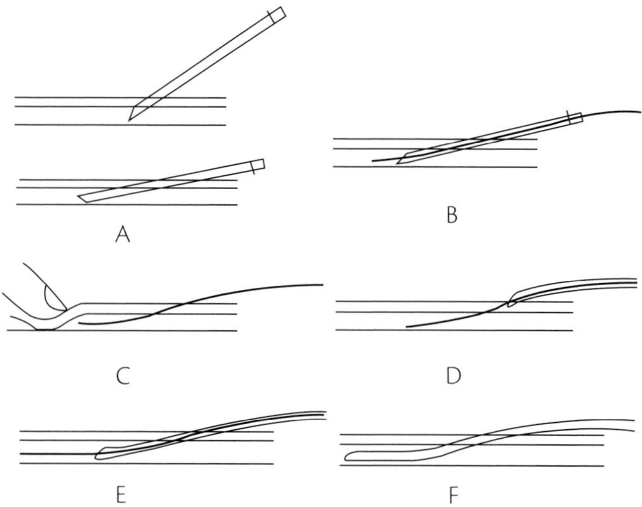

Fig. 24.1 The Seldinger technique: (A) The artery punctured. The needle pushed upwards. (B) The guidewire inserted. (C) The needle withdrawn and the artery compressed. (D) The catheter threaded onto the guide wire. (E) The catheter inserted into the artery. (F) the guide wire withdrawn.
From Seldinger SI. Catheter replacement of the needle in percutaneous arteriography; a new technique. *Acta Radiol* 1953;**39**:368–76.

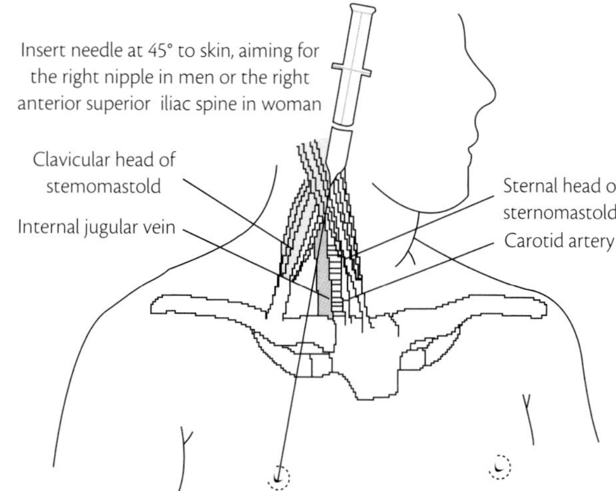

Fig. 24.3 Anatomy of right internal jugular vein.
Reproduced from Myerson SG, Choudhury RP, Mitchell A. *Emergencies in cardiology*, pp. 291–293, Oxford University Press, Oxford, 2005, with permission from Oxford University Press.

Subclavian vein access

The subclavian vein route can be more comfortable for patients, particularly if the catheter is expected to be *in situ* for a few days. However, this approach exposes the patient to a greater risk of pneumothorax and arterial puncture. The right subclavian vein is the preferred side for endomyocardial biopsy and temporary pacing (to avoid the side most commonly used for permanent systems). Again, the approach uses the Seldinger technique as described above using anatomical markings (Fig. 24.4).

Femoral vein access

The femoral approach is largely used for emergency access. Although it has a low rate of immediate complications, it is the site that is most prone to line infections. The vein lies medial to the femoral artery (Fig. 24.5). Again, this approach uses the Seldinger technique as described above.

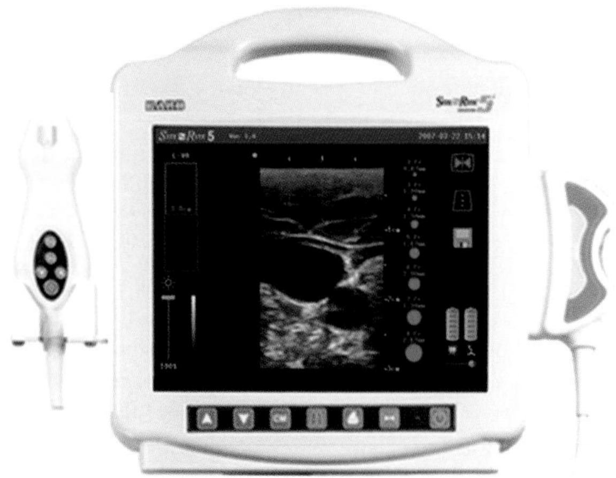

Fig. 24.2 An example of a portable ultrasound to facilitate central venous cannulation.

Complications of central venous cannulation

As with any invasive procedure, there are well-recognized complications that may result from CVC. These include bleeding, inadvertent arterial puncture, vascular damage including late vessel stenosis, pneumothorax (particularly with subclavian access), infection (especially femoral vein access), arrhythmia, and air embolism.

Central venous pressure

The central venous pressure (CVP) is usually measured from a catheter with its tip in the superior vena cava or from the proximal port of a pulmonary artery catheter lying in the right atrium.

The normal CVP waveform (Fig. 24.6) consists of three peaks (a, c, and v) and two descents (x and y). The a wave is the result of atrial contraction and immediately follows the p wave on the ECG, occurring at the end of diastole. As the atrium relaxes and pressure falls, there is a transient increase in atrial pressure (c wave) following the R wave on the surface ECG, produced by isovolumic right ventricular contraction causing closure of the tricuspid valve, displacing the valve into the right atrium.

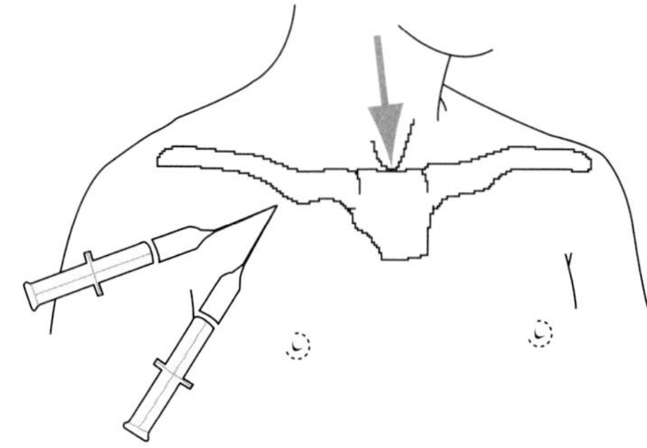

Fig. 24.4 Approach for cannulation of the right subclavian vein.
Reproduced from Myerson SG, Choudhury RP, Mitchell A. *Emergencies in cardiology*, pp. 291–293, Oxford University Press, Oxford, 2005, with permission from Oxford University Press.

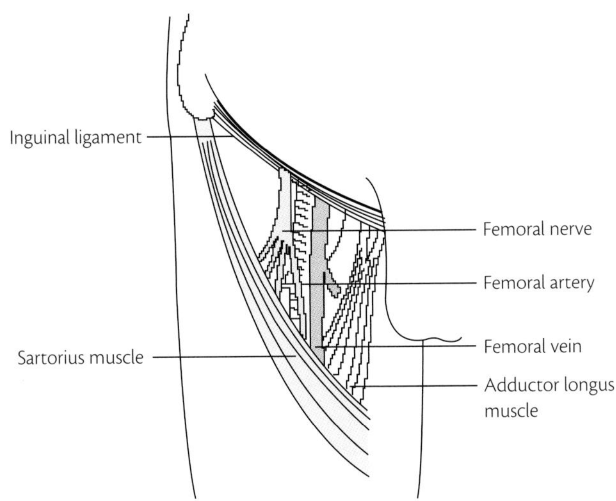

Fig. 24.5 The anatomy of the right femoral vein.
Reproduced from Myerson SG, Choudhury RP, Mitchell A. *Emergencies in cardiology*, pp. 291–293, Oxford University Press, Oxford, 2005, with permission from Oxford University Press.

The x descent represents the fall in atrial pressure during ventricular systole that occurs due to the effect of ventricular contraction on atrial geometry, and ongoing atrial relaxation. The v wave is caused by venous filling of the atrium during late ventricular systole (peaking just after the T wave on the ECG) when the tricuspid valve is still closed. When the valve opens, blood flows from the right atrium into the right ventricle, leading to a decrease in atrial pressure, represented by the y descent.

Following insertion of a central venous catheter into either the subclavian or internal jugular vein, central venous (i.e. right atrial) pressure can be measured by connecting the distal port of the catheter to pressure-monitoring equipment. The patient should be lying flat, and the pressure transducer placed and zeroed by opening to atmospheric pressure at the level of the patient's right atrium (fourth intercostal space in the midaxillary line). CVP should be measured at end expiration. A normal CVP is between 0 and 7 mmHg (10–15 cmH_2O). Causes of an elevated right atrial pressure include right ventricular infarction/failure, fluid overload, pulmonary hypertension, tricuspid stenosis or regurgitation, pulmonary stenosis, and left-to-right shunts (e.g. ventricular septal defect, VSD). There are also several classical abnormalities of the right atrial waveform, listed in Table 24.1.

Right heart catheterization

The pulmonary artery flotation catheter (PAC) was first invented by Jeremy Swan and William Ganz, from the Cedars-Sinai Medical Centre, Los Angeles, USA, the idea coming from the observation of sailing boats in the water.[4] A PAC can be used to measure pressures in the right heart (right atrium, right ventricle, pulmonary artery

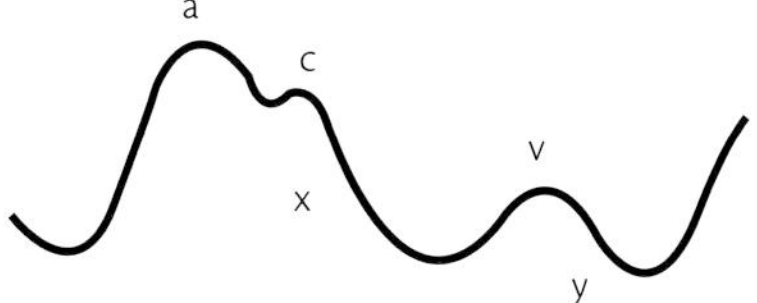

Fig. 24.6 The right atrial pressure wave form.

Table 24.1 Abnormalities of the right atrial waveform

Feature	Cause
Canon 'a' waves	AV dissociation (e.g. ventricular tachycardia, ventricular pacing, complete heart block)
Tall 'a' waves	Tricuspid stenosis
Tall 'v' waves	Tricuspid regurgitation
Brisk *x* descent	Pericardial tamponade
Brisk *y* (and *x*) descents	Pericardial constriction; myocardial restriction.

and pulmonary capillary wedge pressure), cardiac output (using thermodilution), and to assess pulmonary and systemic vascular resistance. It can also be used to detect intracardiac shunts (e.g. VSDs), as well as measure mixed venous oxygen saturation.

The Swan–Ganz catheter for the measurement of cardiac output has four ports: balloon tip, proximal port, distal port that sits in the pulmonary artery, and a thermistor located at the distal end of the catheter. The basic PAC has a balloon for flotation and a single lumen at the catheter tip. The catheters are ideally suited to be floated from the neck, rather than the femoral route.

Trials to study the benefits of PACs have been difficult to perform because of the extreme heterogeneity of the patient population. However, two recent multicentre prospective trials have been published that may radically reduce the use of PACs. The ESCAPE trial (Evaluation Study of Congestive Heart Failure and Pulmonary Artery Catheterization Effectiveness) looked specifically at the use of PACs in guiding the management of patients with decompensated chronic heart failure (HF) and concluded that there was no indication for the routine use of PACs.[5] In an intensive care population that included patients with acute myocardial infarction, the FACTT trial concluded that PACs did not improve survival or organ function but were associated with more catheter-related complications, mainly arrhythmias.[6] Furthermore, a meta-analysis of 13 randomized controlled studies involving over 5000 patients concluded that the use of the PAC neither increased overall mortality or days in hospital nor conferred benefit in critically ill patients.[7]

Thus PACs should be reserved for patients being assessed for cardiac transplantation, those in whom there is clinical uncertainty as to their haemodynamic status (e.g. right ventricular infarction), or those with established left ventricular dysfunction and acute change in fluid status, e.g. bleeding, sepsis, or renal failure. Normal values for PAC measurements are shown in Table 24.2.

Technique

The PAC is most easily manoeuvred via the superior vena cava from the internal jugular vein or the subclavian vein, but can be introduced through the inferior vena cava from the femoral vein. Because of the potential for ventricular arrhythmias—particularly on crossing the tricuspid valve and in the right ventricular outflow tract—the patient should be monitored and full resuscitation equipment should be available during manipulation of the PAC. In many centres, the PAC is manipulated according to pressure waveform (Fig. 24.7). However, it is good practice to use fluoroscopy in order to minimize complications.

Before use, all the lumens of the catheter should be flushed and the balloon inflated with 1.5 mL of air to test its integrity. The pressure line should then be connected to the distal port of the PAC and the transducer zeroed at the level of the right atrium. Insert the

Table 24.2 Cardiac conditions and findings on endomyocardial biopsy
(a) Normal values

Variable	Abbreviation	Normal range
Stroke volume	SV	70–100mL
Cardiac output	CO	4–6 L/min
Right atrial pressure	RAP	0–5 mmHg
Right ventricular pressure	RVP	20–25/0–5 mmHg
Pulmonary artery pressure	PAP	20–25/10–15 mmHg
Pulmonary capillary wedge pressure	PCWP	6–12 mmHg
Mixed venous oxygen saturation	SvO_2	70–75%

(b) Derived variables

Variable	Abbreviation	Calculation	Normal range
Cardiac index	CI	Cardiac output/BSA	2.5–3.5 L/min/m^3
Stroke index	SI	Stroke volume/ BSA	40–60 mL/m^2
Systemic vascular resistance	SVR	(MAP – RAP × 79.9)/CO	900–1100 dyne/s/cm^5
SVR index		(MAP – RAP × 79.9)/CI	1740–2400 dyne/s/m^2
Pulmonary vascular resistance	PVR	(PAP – PCWP × 79.9)/CO	25–125 dyne/s/cm^5

(c) Findings in cardiac conditions

Hypovolaemia	Sepsis	LV failure	RV failure	Tamponade	Acquired VSD
CVP	↓	↑	↑	↑	↑
PCWP	↓	↑	↓	↑	↑
CO	↓	↓	↓	↓	↓
SVR	↑	↑	↑	↑	↑
A-V SaO^2	↑	↑	↑	↑	↓

A-V SaO_2, difference in arterial and mixed venous oxygen saturations; LV, left ventricular; RV, right ventricular; VSD, ventricular septal defect.

From: p61 of Grubb & Newby. Need permission—previously obtained from Handbook

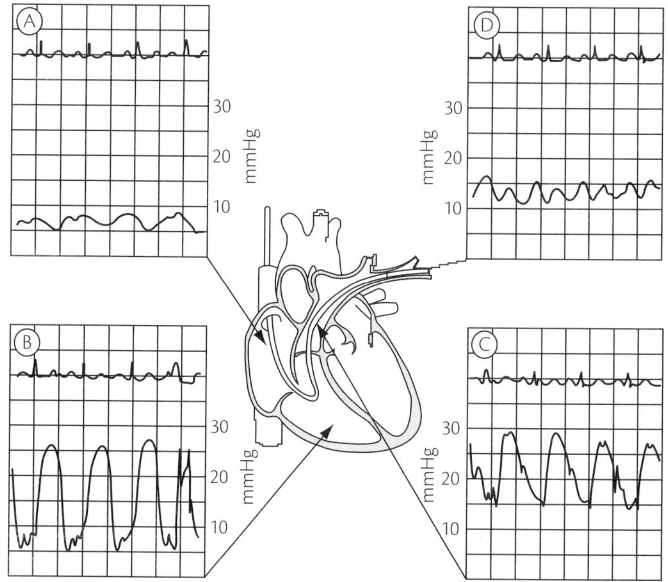

Fig. 24.7 Picture of waveforms in the right heart.
Reproduced from Myerson SG, Choudhury RP, Mitchell A. *Emergencies in cardiology*, pp. 295, Oxford University Press, Oxford, 2005, with permission from Oxford University Press.

catheter into the central venous cannula until its tip lies in the right atrium (15–20 cm from the right internal jugular or subclavian route). The characteristic right atrial tracing should be obtained (see 'Central venous pressure', above). To assist with transit through the right heart, the balloon is then inflated with 1.5 mL of air. On advancing the catheter, record the waveforms in the right ventricle (25–35 cm) and pulmonary artery (40–50 cm) in end expiration (Fig. 24.7). The right ventricular waveform is identified by an increase in systolic pressure and low diastolic pressure, which approximates right atrial pressure (RAP). The right ventricular end-diastolic pressure is measured at the R-wave of the ECG.

When the pulmonary capillary wedge pressure (PCWP) trace appears, the catheter should not be advanced further and the balloon should be deflated. If the pulmonary artery trace does not reappear, the catheter should be withdrawn by 2 cm and the balloon gently reinflated once the pulmonary artery trace does appear. A stable wedge position allows the catheter to be left in position with a pulmonary artery trace that then shows a PCWP trace on balloon inflation. It is important not to inflate the balloon if resistance is felt, or to leave the balloon inflated, because of the potential for trauma or pulmonary artery rupture. If the pressure trace continues to rise on balloon inflation, it suggests 'over-wedging' and the balloon should be deflated and the catheter withdrawn by 2 cm before reinflation. If the trace is damped, the catheter may be kinked or the lumen partially occluded with thrombus or affected by the presence of air bubbles.

Pulmonary capillary wedge pressure

The PCWP is a damped and delayed reflection of left atrial pressure. Although a good wedge trace has a left atrial waveform with a and v waves, the c wave is often difficult to discern. In a normal individual, the pulmonary artery diastolic pressure is similar to the mean PCWP (6–12 mmHg), because of low pulmonary vascular resistance. The mean PCWP cannot be higher than the mean pulmonary artery pressure. The optimal left atrial filling pressure (PCWP) in the presence of left ventricular systolic dysfunction is higher (*c.*14 mmHg).

There are several conditions where the PCWP does not give a fair representation of left atrial or left ventricular end-diastolic pressure. Where there is an elevation of pulmonary vascular resistance (e.g. with pulmonary hypertension, chronic obstructive airways disease, pulmonary embolism, hypoxaemia), the PCWP may exaggerate the actual left atrial pressure. Severe mitral regurgitation results in a prominent systolic (v) wave that may cause the PCWP trace to resemble the pulmonary artery trace (Fig. 24.8). In this situation, the a and v waves and mean PCWP pressures should all be recorded, with the left ventricular end-diastolic pressure (LVEDP) best approximated by measuring pressure prior to the regurgitant v wave. Another important example is mitral stenosis, where there is a pressure gradient caused by obstruction to blood flow between left atrium and left ventricle. As a result, left atrial pressure (estimated by PCWP) will exceed LVEDP.

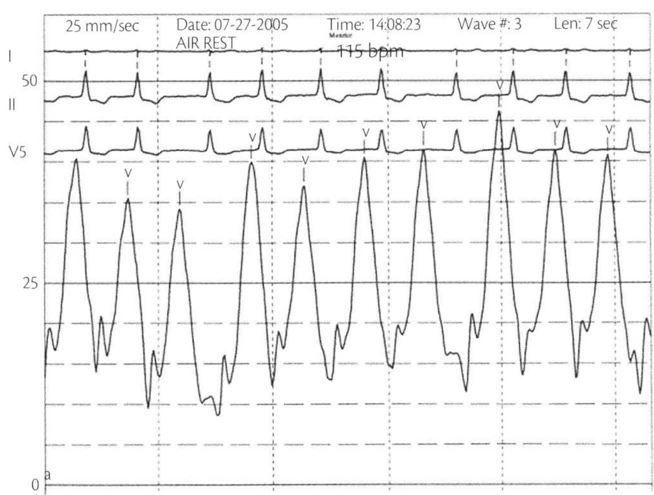

Fig. 24.8 Pulmonary capillary wedge pressure tracing from a patient with acute mitral regurgitation showing giant V waves. The rhythm is atrial fibrillation.

Cardiac output measurement—thermodilution technique

This technique uses a modification of the Fick principle. A fixed volume (such as 10 mL) of ice-cold saline is rapidly injected into the proximal port of the PAC. The rate of temperature change is detected by the thermistor at the catheter tip, 30 cm distal to the site of injection. The volume and temperature of injected saline are entered into a cardiac output computer which then derives the cardiac output from the change in temperature at the catheter tip. At least five measurements should be taken and averaged—more if the patient has atrial fibrillation or an unstable rhythm. The readings should fall within 10% of each other and those with irregular traces should be discarded. An important potential cause of error is significant tricuspid regurgitation, where some of the bolus falls back into the RA rendering the technique meaningless. Septal defects have a similar effect.

Vascular resistance

Vascular resistance (R) describes the resistance to flow offered by a circulation (primarily small arterioles—'resistance vessels'), and is calculated by the fraction of pressure gradient and mean flow (i.e. cardiac output). Although pulmonary vascular resistance (PVR) is commonly quoted in Wood units, systemic vascular resistance (SVR) is usually measured in absolute units (dyne s^{-1} cm^{-5}), by multiplying by a factor of 79.9. The normal ranges are shown in Table 24.2.

PVR is the resistance to flow offered by the pulmonary vasculature, and relies on the transpulmonary gradient (TPG—the pressure difference between the mean pulmonary artery pressure (PA_m) and mean left atrial pressure (LA_m)) and cardiac output (CO, in L/min), calculated using the following equations:

$$\text{TPG} = \text{PA}_m - \text{LA}_m \text{ (or PA}_m - \text{PCWP}_m\text{)}$$

$$\text{PVR} = \frac{TPG}{CO} \text{ (in Wood units) or}$$

$$\text{PVR} = \frac{79.9 \times TPG}{CO} \text{ (in dyne/sec/cm}^{-5}\text{)}$$

Mean PCWP is often used in lieu of LAP, accepting the limitations of PCWP in the estimation of LAP (see above).

The calculation of PVR is particularly important in the assessment of patients for cardiac transplantation, because an elevated PVR is a risk factor for premature death after transplantation.[8,9] An elevated PVR is commonly found in patients with chronic HF, particularly in the presence of valvular heart disease, and it may or may not be reversible. Irreversible pulmonary hypertension is an absolute contraindication to cardiac transplantation.[9] It is defined as:

- PVR >5 Wood units, or
- PVR index (PVRI) >6, or
- TPG >16 mmHg, or
- pulmonary artery systolic pressure >60 mmHg in addition to one of the three criteria above.

If the PVR is elevated (but<5), reversibility can be assessed with the use of oxygen and vasodilator therapy (such as with glyceryl trinitrate or sodium nitroprusside) while maintaining systolic blood pressure above 85 mmHg. If this is unsuccessful, or hypotension precludes the use of vasodilators, an infusion of dobutamine or insertion of an intra-aortic balloon pump (IABP) can be tried. If the PVR does fall, then the successful regime should be recorded in the notes and the PVR reassessed at least every 6 months. If the PVR can be reduced to less than 2.5 but at a cost of a fall in systolic blood pressure to less than 85 mmHg, the patient remains at high risk of right ventricular failure and death following cardiac transplantation.

SVR is the resistance offered by the peripheral circulation and is almost invariably raised in patients with chronic HF, due to the activation of the renin–angiotensin–aldosterone and sympathetic nervous systems, as well as the endogenous release of vasoconstrictors such as endothelin. SVR is calculated using the mean aortic and right atrial pressures, and CO in the following equation:

$$SVR = \frac{79.9\,\text{(mean aortic pressure} - \text{mean RA pressure)}}{Cardiac\ Output} \quad \text{(in dyne.sec.cm}^{-5}\text{)}$$

Mixed venous oxygen saturation

Assuming that there is no intracardiac shunt, mixed venous oxygen saturation can be measured from a pulmonary artery blood sample which should be taken slowly to avoid 'arterialization', i.e. pulmonary venous sampling. The normal mixed venous oxygen saturation is 70–75%. Low-output states result in increased tissue oxygen extraction, and so low mixed venous saturation. High mixed venous saturations occur in high-output states including septic shock or in low-output states where there is a left-to-right shunt, such as ventricular septal rupture.

Plasma lactate

In shock, tissue hypoxia prevents the aerobic metabolism of pyruvate into water and carbon dioxide. Instead, lactate is formed, which can be measured, offering useful data regarding tissue perfusion. A sample of either venous or arterial blood is collected into a heparin fluoride tube for analysis, although many arterial blood gas analysers now measure lactate as standard. A normal plasma lactate is 0.3–1.3 mmol/L. An initial rise in lactate may be seen after improving tissue perfusion, reflecting the washout from previously hypoperfused tissue.

Shunt calculation

Left-to-right shunts can be calculated by measuring oxygen saturations during cardiac catheterization ('a shunt run') with the chamber or vessel in which there is a step up in oxygen saturation indicating the level of the shunt. The ratio of pulmonary flow to systemic flow is given by:

$$\frac{Pulmonary\ flow}{Systemic\ flow} = \frac{Aortic\ SaO_2 - mean\ venous\ SaO_2}{98 - PA\ SaO_2}$$

where PF is pulmonary flow, SF is systemic flow, 98 is the assumed percentage oxygen saturation in the pulmonary veins, and mixed venous saturation is $\frac{3 \times SVC\ saturation + IVC\ saturation}{4}$.

Difficulty in placing the PAC

The commonest difficulty experienced with PACs is in steering the catheter into the pulmonary artery. There are several techniques that can aid successful positioning. With the balloon inflated, the catheter will float more readily through the tricuspid valve with the patient in the head-down position. Conversely, the head-up position can be used to aid flotation out of the right ventricle. Deep inspiration will increase right ventricular output transiently due to increased venous return, which may also help with catheter passage, particularly in patients with a low CO.

The catheter can also be stiffened or guided with the use of a long 0.25" (0.64mm) J-tipped wire introduced via the distal lumen to steer the wire up into the right ventricular outflow tract. A guide wire can be particularly useful from the femoral route when the catheter may point downward into the right ventricular apex. To avoid myocardial perforation in this situation, force should never be applied.

Complications of PACs

As well as the complications of CVC, there are several recognized adverse sequelae from the use of a PAC. These include:

- Arrhythmias—PACs can induce arrhythmias from their passage through the right heart. The arrhythmias are predominantly ventricular in origin, due to irritation of the right ventricular outflow tract. However, complete heart block can also occur secondary to stunning of the right bundle branch in patients who already have left bundle branch block. Atrial arrhythmias are less common.
- Pulmonary artery rupture—the risk of pulmonary artery trauma can be minimized by ensuring that the PAC is not pushed, nor the balloon inflated, against resistance.
- Pulmonary infarction—the risk of pulmonary infarction can be greatly reduced by avoiding the PAC balloon being inflated for prolonged periods of time.
- Valvular trauma—manipulation of the PAC can cause either tricuspid or pulmonary valve trauma. It is of particular importance to deflate the PAC balloon before withdrawing the catheter.
- Infection—potentially endocarditis.
- Catheter knotting—this is less likely with the use of fluoroscopy and the avoidance of excessive catheter loops. Where the catheter is seen to loop, it should not be pulled tight. Rather, advancing the catheter and manipulating it with a guide wire may untie the knot. Where this is not possible, the knot can often be snared from the femoral vein and should not be pulled through the internal jugular vein. However, rarely, vascular surgery may be required.

Left heart catheterization

Measurement of left ventricular end-diastolic pressure

The measurement of LVEDP (Fig. 24.9 and Fig. 24.10) contributes to the assessment of left ventricular filling pressures. The traces are recorded as part of a left heart catheterization study, where a catheter is placed directly into the left ventricle. The LVEDP is measured at the onset of isovolumic contraction (occasionally termed the C- or Z-point: see Fig. 24.9 and Fig. 24.10). This usually coincides with the R wave of the ECG, and is best recorded after the a wave in a LAP tracing. The normal LVEDP is less than 12 mmHg: it can be elevated in the presence of mitral or aortic incompetence, left ventricular systolic dysfunction, VSD, tamponade, or pericardial constriction. The LVEDP can also be elevated if there is myocardial hypertrophy (e.g. hypertensive heart disease) or myocardial infiltration (e.g. amyloid). Conversely, a low LVEDP is seen in hypovolaemia and mitral stenosis.

Pressure gradients

An assessment of aortic stenosis can be made during cardiac catheterization, by measuring the peak-to-peak (pullback) gradient, peak instantaneous gradient, mean gradient and, where the CO is known, the valve orifice area (Fig. 24.11). Indeed, until advances in echocardiography, pullback gradients were routinely performed in the assessment of patients with aortic stenosis.

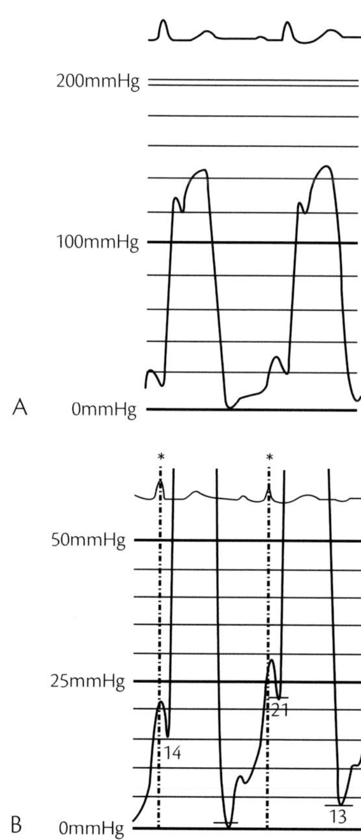

Fig. 24.9 (A) The left ventricular pressure trace is shown with a close-up view (B) of the left ventricular end-doastolic pressure (LVEDP). The point to assess the LVEDP equates to the peak of the R wave, indicated by (*). The mean of several traces should be taken (three if sinus rhythm, five if atrial fibrillation).
Adapted from our heart failure handbook.

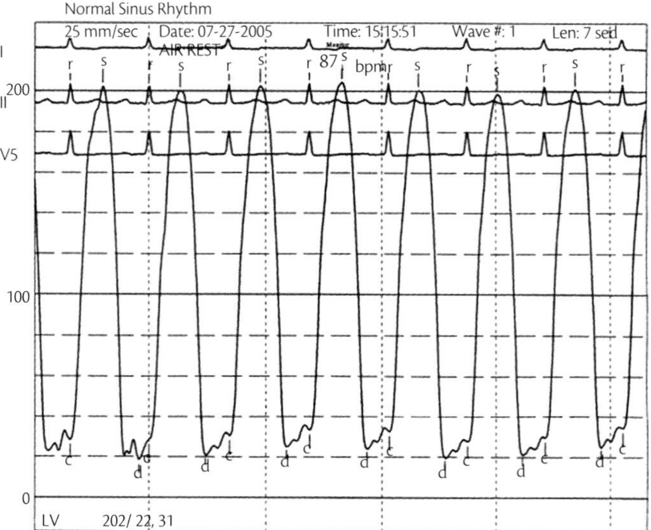

Fig. 24.10 Left ventricular pressure trace in patient with chronic heart failure and hypertension. The left ventricular systolic pressure reaches over 200 mmHg, with an end-diastolic pressure of 31 mmHg measured at the c-point.

In aortic stenosis, the peak-to-peak (pullback) gradient is obtained by the careful withdrawal of a catheter from the left ventricle into the aorta whilst constantly recording pressure. The gradient is generally lower, and a less accurate reflection of valve area, than the peak instantaneous gradient obtained by simultaneous recording of ventricular and ascending aortic pressure with either two catheters or a double lumen catheter (or, indeed, echocardiography) (Fig. 24.12). An alternative method of calculating an aortic gradient involves the simultaneous recording of ventricular and femoral arterial pressure, although this method has the potential for error due to the delay in pressure transmission and the alteration of the pressure waveform.

The Gorlin formula can be used to assess aortic valve area:
aortic valve area (cm2) =

$$\frac{Cardiac\ output\left(\frac{1}{min}\right)}{44.3 \times SEP \times HR \times \sqrt{Mean\ aortic\ gradient\ (mmHg)}}$$

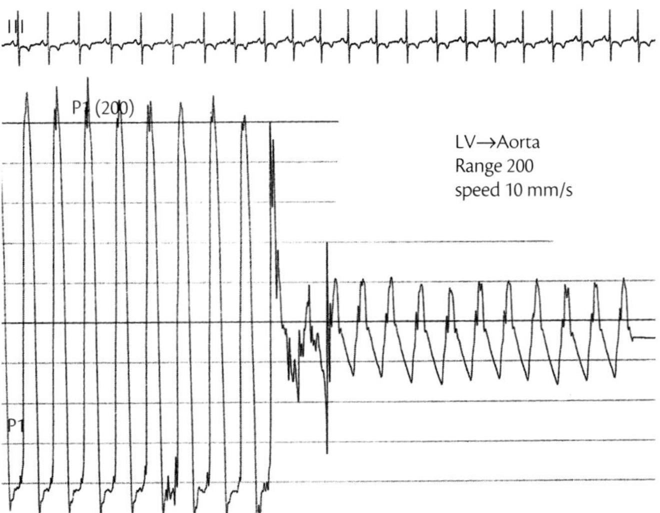

Fig. 24.11 Pressure trace from a pigtail catheter pulled back from the left ventricle into the ascending aorta illustrates an aortic valve gradient of 80 mmHg.

where SEP is systolic ejection period, i.e. the length of time where left ventricular pressure is greater than aortic pressure) and HR is the heart rate. In a similar way to simultaneous pressure recording in the assessment of aortic stenosis, mitral stenosis can be evaluated by simultaneous left ventricular pressure and PCWP (or left atrial pressure) measurement.

Constriction versus restriction

Despite very different underlying pathological processes, the clinical and haemodynamic findings in constriction and restriction are similar and may be difficult to differentiate. Both conditions present with enlarged atria, normal-sized ventricles, and normal systolic function. However, noncompliance of the ventricular myocardium (restriction) or pericardium (constriction) results in diastolic dysfunction.

The diagnosis of constriction may be suggested by thickening and/or calcification of the pericardium—best seen on cardiac CT. Pulsus paradoxus—the exaggeration of the normal reduction in blood pressure with inspiration—is often present in constriction, but rarely with restriction. There are some haemodynamic differences that may differentiate between the two conditions. The classical finding in constrictive pericarditis is the equalization of diastolic pressures (within 5 mmHg in the majority of cases) on simultaneous left and right heart catheterization. Furthermore, the right ventricular systolic pressure is nearly always below 60 mmHg (and usually <40 mmHg) in constriction, whereas it is frequently above 40 mmHg in restriction (Fig. 24.13). Table 8.7 on p. 84 highlights the main differences between the two conditions.

Coronary angiography

Although coronary angiography is often unnecessary for the routine management of a patient with HF, it can help to clarify the underlying aetiology and offer useful prognostic information (an ischaemic aetiology is associated with a higher risk of morbidity and mortality). Moreover, it should be considered in patients who have symptoms of ischaemia, in suspected ischaemic cardiomyopathy, or following cardiac arrest where revascularization may be appropriate.[10]

Although there is some support for revascularization in patients with ischaemic cardiomyopathy,[11] there are currently no trial data supporting the use of revascularization for the relief of HF symptoms. This is the subject of the first hypothesis of the forthcoming Surgical Treatment for Ischemic Heart Failure (STICH) trial which is due to report in 2011.[12] The second hypothesis of STICH compared surgical ventricular reconstruction in addition to CABG (coronary artery bypass grafting) with CABG alone:[13] although there was a reduction in left ventricle volume with ventricular reconstruction, the anatomical change was not associated with a greater improvement in symptoms or exercise tolerance or with a reduction in the rate of death or hospitalization for cardiac causes.

Revascularization should only be considered after balancing up the risks and potential benefits, and in the presence of viable myocardium (as detected by CMR, stress echo, or nuclear imaging).[14]

Contrast left ventriculography:

Contrast left ventriculography can provide important information regarding global and regional cardiac function and mitral regurgitation (Fig. 24.14), as well as the size and position of VSDs. It is an invasive procedure and is now infrequently performed in the

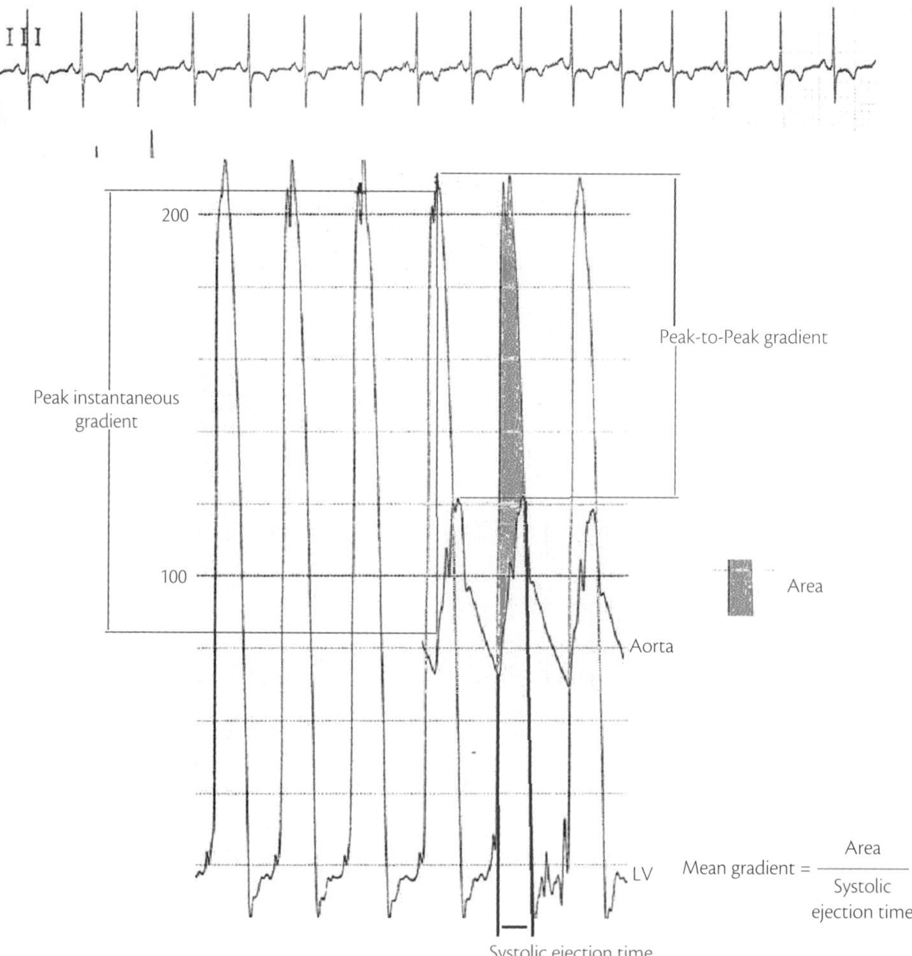

Fig. 24.12 Simultaneous left ventricular and aortic pressure tracing in a patient with aortic stenosis demonstrating three different measures of severity of stenosis. Mean gradient = area/systolic ejection time.

routine investigation of HF patients, as the quality of noninvasive imaging has greatly improved.

In order to achieve an adequate contrast injection, it is necessary to inject a relatively large volume of contrast over a short period of time. Typical settings are 30–45 mL of contrast at a rate of 10–15 mL/s, achieved by passing a catheter with multiple side holes into the mid left ventricular cavity and using a power injector to deliver contrast. An angled pigtail catheter is often used to minimize the catheter entanglement in the mitral valve apparatus, and hence reduce ectopy. It is of paramount importance that precautions are taken to prevent air embolism.

Images are best acquired in the 30° RAO projection (viewing the high lateral, anterior, apical, and inferior walls) and 45–60° LAO with 20° cranial tilt (viewing the lateral and septal walls: a useful view to assess for a VSD). Measurements can be obtained of ventricular volumes, and hence LVEF, and regional wall motion. LVEF can be calculated from the following equation:

$$\text{LVEF (\%)} = \frac{(\text{End diastolic volume} - \text{End systolic volume})}{\text{End diastolic volume} \times 100}$$

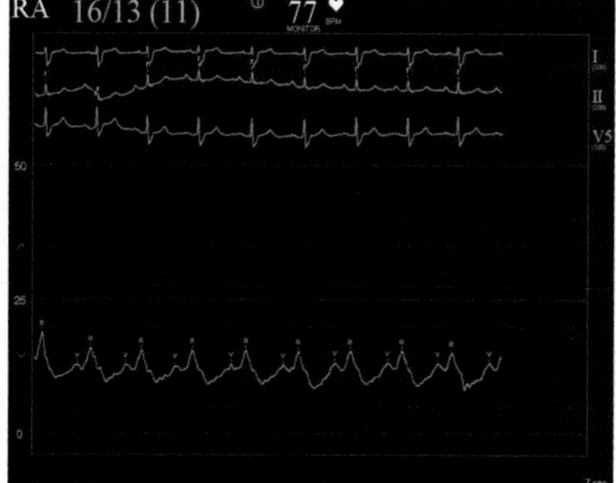

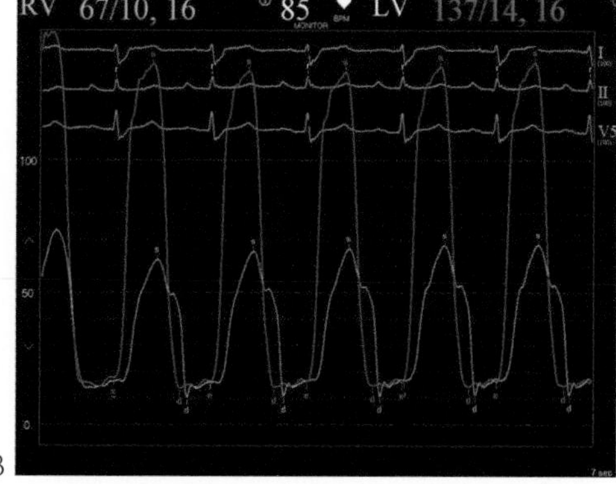

Fig. 24.13 (A) Right atrial pressure and (B) simultaneous right and left ventricular pressure tracings in a patient with restrictive cardiomyopathy.

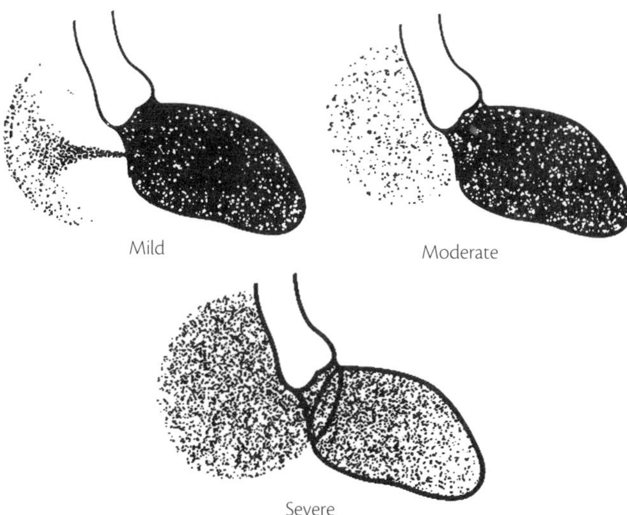

Fig. 24.14 Assessment of severity of mitral regurgitation from contrast left ventriculography.
From: figure 4–23: The Cardiac Catheterisation Handbook.

The severity of mitral regurgitation is assessed from the degree of opacification of the left atrium during contrast left ventriculography (Fig. 24.14).

Contraindications to contrast left ventriculography

When considering left ventricular contrast ventriculography, it is important to consider whether a noninvasive means of assessing ventricular or valvular function might be preferable. This is particularly true in patients with a significant left main coronary artery stenosis or aortic valve stenosis, mural thrombus, renal impairment, and in those with left ventricular systolic pressure 180 mmHg or more, or LVEDP 25 mmHg or more.

Complications of contrast left ventriculography

There are a number of complications of contrast left ventriculography:

- Cardiac arrhythmias—ventricular extrasystoles are common, and usually result from stimulation of the ventricular endocardium by the catheter or jet of contrast medium. They can be minimized by repositioning the catheter. Short runs of ventricular tachycardia can also occur, but usually resolve on removal of the catheter from the ventricle.
- Embolism—the embolization of air or thrombus during contrast injection can have catastrophic results. The risk of embolism should be minimized by meticulous technique in ensuring that the injector system is free of bubbles or thrombus. Contrast ventriculography should also be avoided in patients with known left ventricular thrombus.
- Intramyocardial staining—usually caused by improper positioning of the catheter so that it lies underneath a papillary muscle or one of the side holes abuts the endocardium. Small stains are of limited significance, but larger stains may be associated with refractory ventricular arrhythmias or even perforation and the development of cardiac tamponade.
- Contrast reactions—allergies to contrast media are reasonably common. However, it is more common to have powerful flushing sensations caused by vasodilatation.
- Fascicular block as the catheter is advanced into the left ventricle, transient left anterior fascicular block may occur as the anterior fascicle of the left bundle lies close to the left ventricular outflow tract. Patients who already have right bundle branch block and left posterior fascicular block may develop transient complete heart block.

Endomyocardial biopsy

In 1962, Sakakibara and Konno first reported their experience with transvascular cardiac biopsy. Eleven years later, Caves described transvenous endomyocardial biopsy to diagnose cardiac allograft rejection.

Right ventricular endomyocardial biopsies are commonly taken after heart transplantation to assess allograft rejection. Only in very rare instances is a left ventricular biopsy indicated (e.g. due to multiple previous right ventricular biopsies) because of the risk of systemic embolization. There are few occasions when an endomyocardial biopsy is necessary in patients with chronic HF, and there remains considerable controversy surrounding the use of this procedure to evaluate the cause of dilated cardiomyopathy. Current guidelines state that endomyocardial biopsy should not be performed in the routine evaluation of patients with HF.[15] Rare exceptions are where an infiltrative cardiac condition is suspected and the result would influence therapy, although diagnostic information can often be obtained by other methods (Table 24.3). In an acute presentation of new HF, endomyocardial biopsy is indicated if giant cell myocarditis is suspected, as the condition often progresses rapidly, and these patients should be considered for circulatory support and urgent listing for cardiac transplantation. Biopsies of intracardiac masses can also be undertaken, where the result is necessary prior to surgery (Fig. 24.15).[16] An example of normal histology is shown in Fig. 24.16.

Procedure

The patient should be adequately monitored by continuous ECG, pulse oximetry, and blood pressure. The following equipment should be immediately available in the event of a complication (see below): resuscitation trolley, temporary pacing line, pericardiocentesis tray, and chest drain kit.

Right ventricular endomyocardial biopsies are generally undertaken via the right internal jugular vein using a using an 8–9 F sheath with haemostasis valve, thorough which a 50-cm disposable bioptome is passed. Biopsies can also be taken from the femoral or subclavian veins, although the femoral route requires a long sheath and a 104-cm bioptome. The subclavian approach can be technically challenging, and for this reason is generally reserved for occasions when endomyocardial biopsy cannot be performed from other routes (e.g. jugular venous thrombosis), as the angle between the subclavian vein and superior vena cava angle is often too acute for the relatively stiff bioptome to negotiate easily. Often, by taking a more lateral approach, or by using a longer sheath, this difficulty can be overcome. In the unusual circumstance where left ventricular biopsy is necessary, this is invariably performed via the femoral artery.

Before use, the bioptome must first be checked to ensure that the jaws approximate tightly and that the 90° bend lines up with the bioptome handle. It is advisable to ask the patient to stop breathing when putting the bioptome into the sheath (and again when removing) in order to reduce the risk of air embolism.

Table 24.3 Interpretation of pulmonary artery flotation catheter data

Condition	Tissue biopsied	Stain(s)	Features
Amyloid (Fig. 24.17, Fig. 24.18)	Heart Buccal mucosa Rectum, kidney	Congo Red Sirius Red	Apple green birefringence. Myocytes are ringed by pink-staining extracellullar deposits of amyloid
Sarcoidosis (Fig. 8.3, p. 85)	Heart Hilar lymph nodes Lung, skin	H&E	Noncaseating granuloma with myocyte destruction and replacement fibrosis
Haemochromatosis (Fig. 8.4, p. 85)	Heart Liver	Perls stain (Prussian blue)	Granular intracellular cardiac myocyte deposits of haemosiderin are stained blue with both Perls stain
Endomyocardial fibrosis	Endomyocardium	H&E	
Viral myocarditis (Fig 8.1, p. 79)	Endomyocardium	H&E	Sensitivity as low as 35% due to transient and patchy myocardial involvement. Dallas histopathological criteria are on p. 78 in Chapter 8
Giant cell myocarditis (Fig. 8.2, p. 79)	Endomyocardium	H&E	widespread necrosis and inflammation with the presence of lymphocytes, histiocytes, eosinophils, as well as the characteristic multinucleated giant cells
Chagas' disease	Endomyocardium	H&E	Parasitization of myofibres by trypanosomes, accompanied by an inflammatory infiltrate
Heart transplant rejection (Fig. 24.19, Fig. 24.20)	Endomyocardium	H&E	Histological features include interstitial oedema, inflammatory infiltration and immunoglobulin deposition. More severe rejection is marked by myocyte death and occasionally interstitial haemorrhage.

H&E, haematoxylin and eosin.

Right ventricular biopsy

Using fluoroscopy, the bioptome is directed laterally along the superior vena cava into the mid-right atrium, at which point it is rotated anteriorly (anticlockwise) through the tricuspid valve, and advanced into the RV gradually rotating posteriorly to the interventricular septum. The position can be confirmed using 30° RAO and 60° LAO projections. At this point, the tip is withdrawn slightly when it abuts the endocardium (seen fluoroscopically and felt as slight resistance). The bioptome jaws are then opened and advanced on to the endocardial surface. The jaws are then closed and the bioptome withdrawn briskly but smoothly. Tissue is then gently removed from the jaws and placed in an appropriate preservative. In view of the various histopathological techniques, it is best to discuss preservative solutions with the pathologist prior to the procedure. Typically, 10% neutral buffered formalin is used. For the assessment of cardiac allograft rejection, 5–6 biopsy specimens are required because of the multifocal nature of rejection. In cases of suspected infiltrative disease, a cardiac MRI beforehand can reduce false-negative results by identifying areas of interest.

Histology specimens from a patient with cardiac amyloidosis are shown in Fig. 24.17 and Fig. 24.18. Illustrations of biopsy samples of patients with sarcoidosis, iron deposition, viral and giant cell myocarditis are shown in Figs 8.1–8.4 (pp. 79–85).

Heart transplant rejection

Despite much research in the pursuit of a surrogate marker of heart transplant rejection, nothing has been found to date that has successfully avoided the need for endomyocardial biopsy.

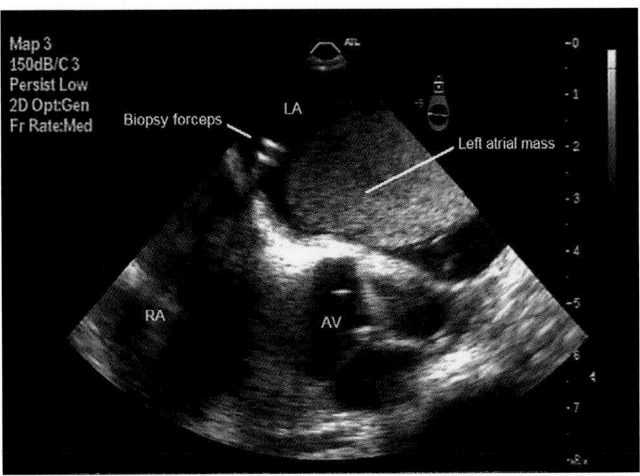

Fig. 24.15 Transoesophageal echocardiogram illustrating a trans-septal biopsy of a left atrial mass. RA, right atrium; LA, left atrium; AV, aortic valve.
From Jackson CE, Gardner RS, Connelly DT. A novel approach for a novel combination: a trans-septal biopsy of left atrial mass in recurrent phyllodes tumour. *Eur J Echocardiogr* 2009;**10**:171–2.

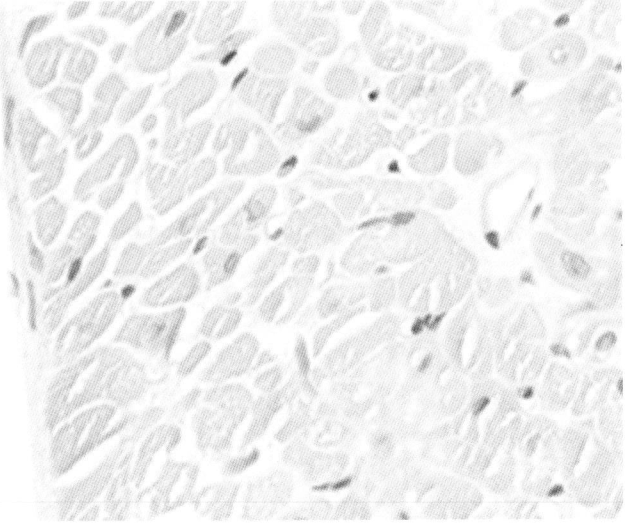

Fig. 24.16 Normal myocardium stained with haematoxylin and eosin (×400). The endocardium on the left is a thin uniform layer with underlying myocardium that comprises cardiac myocytes that are closely applied to one another with little intervening stroma that includes small blood vessels.
Courtesy of Dr Allan McPhaden, Glasgow Royal Infirmary

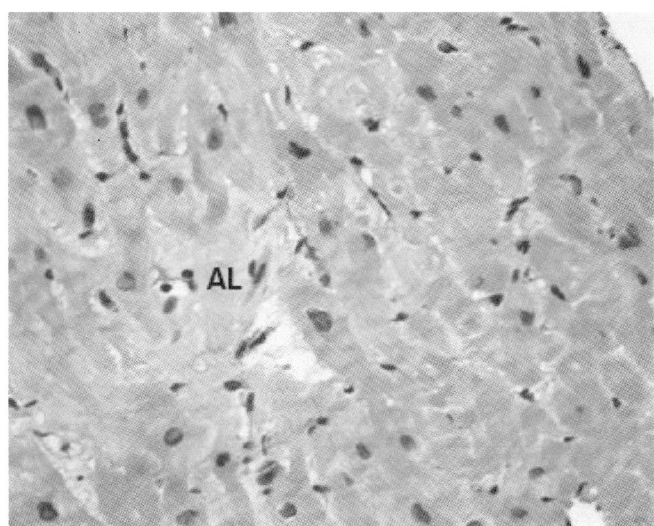

Fig. 24.17 Histopathology of cardiac amyloid, demonstrating apple green birefringence with polarized light. Congo Red ×200.
Courtesy of Dr Allan McPhaden, Glasgow Royal Infirmary.

Although rejection episodes are less frequent with advances in immunosuppressive regimes, endomyocardial biopsy remains the cornerstone investigation for the monitoring of rejection. Surveillance biopsies are generally performed weekly for the first 6 weeks, then fortnightly to 3 months, and then every 6 weeks for the remainder of the first postoperative year, because of the high incidence of rejection episodes during this time.

On light microscopy, histological features of rejection include interstitial oedema, inflammatory infiltration and immunoglobulin deposition (Box 24.1). More severe rejection is marked by myocyte death and occasionally interstitial haemorrhage.

Box 24.1 Grades of cellular rejection on endomyocardial biopsy (ISHLT scale)

0 No rejection

Ia Focal infiltrate without necrosis (Fig. 24.19)

Ib Diffuse but sparse infiltrate but without necrosis

II One focus only, with aggressive infiltration and/or focal myocyte damage

IIIa Multifocal aggressive infiltrates and/or myocyte damage

IIIb Diffuse inflammatory process with necrosis

IV Diffuse aggressive polymorphous infiltrate, and/or oedema, and/or haemorrhage, and/or vasculitis, with necrosis (Fig. 24.20).

Quilty

There is emerging evidence that Quilty—an endocardial infiltration of B-cell and T-cell lymphocytes found exclusively in endomyocardial biopsies from heart transplant recipients—may have a bearing on outcome following cardiac transplantation by representing subclinical rejection. Although the biopsy prevalence of Quilty is low (6–11%), the lifetime incidence of Quilty in cardiac transplant patients is high, with 50–74% of patients having at least one instance of Quilty during their posttransplant follow-up. Its significance is a matter of some debate.

Complications

In order to minimize the risk to patients, endomyocardial biopsies should be performed by expert operators in experienced centres. The risk of serious complication from endomyocardial biopsy is less than 1%. Even so, the procedure should still only be performed when there is a strong reason to believe that the results will have a significant impact on subsequent therapeutic decisions or prognosis.

Myocardial perforation

The most significant complication from endomyocardial biopsy is perforation—usually of the right ventricular free wall, which is

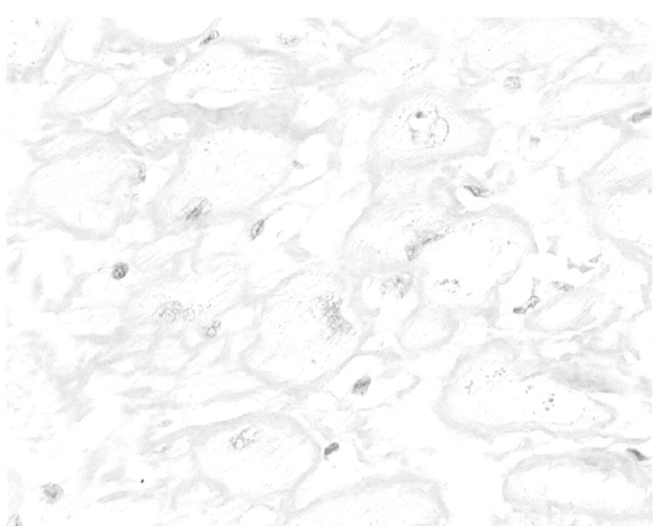

Fig. 24.18 Amyloidosis. Individual myocytes are ringed by pink-staining extracellullar deposits of amyloid in a case of primary amyloidosis. Sirius red ×400.
Courtesy of Dr Allan McPhaden, Glasgow Royal Infirmary.

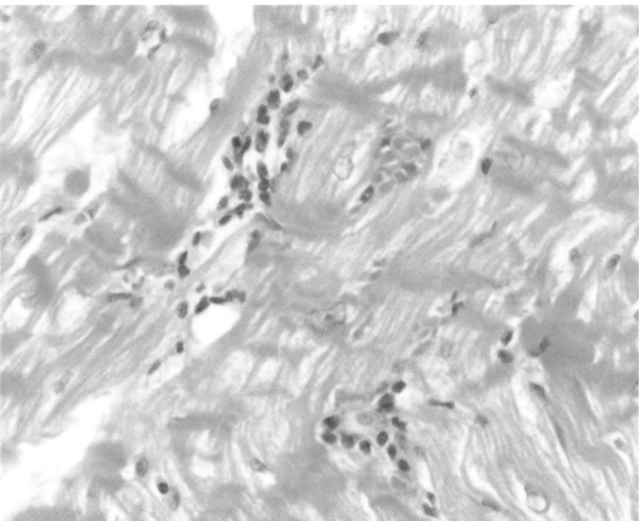

Fig. 24.19 Low grade cardiac allograft rejection. The myocardium contains small perivascular aggregates of mononuclear cells (ISHLT Grade 1a). Haematoxylin and eosin ×400.
Courtesy of Dr Allan McPhaden, Glasgow Royal Infirmary.

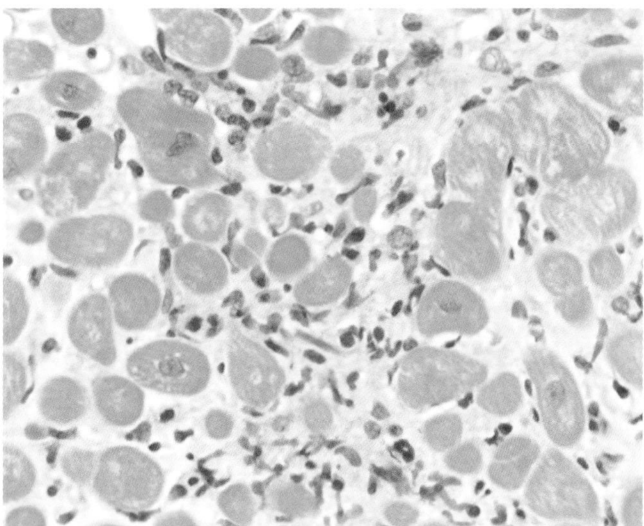

Fig. 24.20 High-grade cardiac allograft rejection. The myocardium contains perivascular aggregates of mononuclear cells with extension into the interstitium associated with mutiple foci of cardiac myocyte degeneration. Haematoxylin and eosin ×400.
Courtesy of Dr Allan McPhaden, Glasgow Royal Infirmary.

only 1–2 mm in thickness. Perforation can lead quickly to cardiac tamponade, and is often heralded by the patient experiencing sharp chest pain (less likely after cardiac transplantation), followed by an exaggerated vagal response (bradycardia and hypotension) that is frequently unresponsive to atropine administration. If a perforation is suspected, an echocardiogram should be performed without delay, before taking any further biopsies. Because of the risks of tamponade, a pericardiocentesis kit should always be immediately available in the biopsy room.

Arrhythmias

Although the presence of premature ventricular contractions is often an indication that the bioptome has crossed into the ventricle, and therefore to be expected, ventricular tachycardia can occur. This often responds to the bioptome (or sheath) being removed from the ventricular cavity. Sustained ventricular tachycardia may rarely result, requiring overdrive pacing, antiarrhythmic drugs, or electrical cardioversion.

Supraventricular arrhythmias can also occur as the bioptome, sheath, or guide wire stimulates the right atrium, particularly in cases where there are increased filling pressures. These are invariably transient.

Pneumothorax

A pneumothorax can be caused by puncture of the lung pleura, particularly when using a subclavian or a low internal jugular vein approach. The risk can be minimized by using direct vision (e.g. Site-Rite) and a mid-high internal jugular approach, or avoided altogether by using a femoral approach. If a pneumothorax is suspected, fluoroscopy of the lung edge or chest radiograph should be carried out without delay. A chest drain kit should always be available in the biopsy room.

Conduction disturbance

Pressure against the septum around the tricuspid valve apparatus from the bioptome or sheath can transiently induce right bundle branch block which is of particular concern in the third of HF patients who already have a left bundle branch block, when complete heart block or asystole can ensue. Removal of the insult usually resolves this problem, although occasionally a temporary pacing line may be required, and this should be immediately available.

Lead displacement

In the current era of advanced HF management, many patients have either an implanted cardioverter-defibrillator (ICD) or CRT-P/-D *in situ*. Where possible, right heart catheterization or right ventricular endomyocardial biopsy should be avoided until device leads have had the opportunity to bed down. This is especially true of passive fix leads, and in particular, coronary sinus left ventricle leads.

Other complications

Other complications that may result are air embolism or thromboembolism, nerve palsy, haematoma, inadvertent arterial puncture, arteriovenous fistula.

References

1. Seldinger SI. Catheter replacement of the needle in percutaneous arteriography; a new technique. *Acta Radiol* 1953;**39**:368–76.
2. Denys BG, Uretsky BF, Reddy PS. Ultrasound-assisted cannulation of the internal jugular vein. A prospective comparison to the external landmark-guided technique. *Circulation* 1993;**87**:1557–62.
3. *Guidance on the use of ultrasound locating devices for placing central venous catheters*. NICE, [2002]. http://www.nice.org.uk/nicemedia/pdf/Ultrasound_49_GUIDANCE.pdf.
4. Swan HJ, Ganz W, Forrester J, Marcus H, Diamond G, Chonette D. Catheterization of the heart in man with use of a flow-directed balloon-tipped catheter. *N Engl J Med* 1970;**283**:447–51.
5. Binanay C, Califf RM, Hasselblad V, *et al*. Evaluation study of congestive heart failure and pulmonary artery catheterization effectiveness: the ESCAPE trial. *JAMA* 2005;**294**:1625–33.
6. Wheeler AP, Bernard GR, Thompson BT, *et al*. Pulmonary-artery versus central venous catheter to guide treatment of acute lung injury. *N Engl J Med* 2006;**354**:2213–24.
7. Shah MR, Hasselblad V, Stevenson LW, *et al*. Impact of the pulmonary artery catheter in critically ill patients: meta-analysis of randomized clinical trials. *JAMA* 2005;**294**:1664–70.
8. Kirklin JK, Naftel DC, Kirklin JW. Pulmonary vascular resistance and the risk of heart transplantation. *J Heart Lung Transplant* 1988;**7**:331–6.
9. Mehra MR, Kobashigawa J, Starling R, *et al*. Listing criteria for heart transplantation: International Society for Heart and Lung Transplantation guidelines for the care of cardiac transplant candidates—2006. *J Heart Lung Transplant* 2006;**25**:1024–42.
10. Dickstein K, Cohen-Solal, A, Filippatos G, *et al*. ESC Guidelines for the diagnosis and treatment of acute and chronic heart failure. *Eur Heart J* 2008;**29**(19):2388–42.

11. Shanmugam G, Legare JF. Revascularization for ischaemic cardiomyopathy. *Curr Opin Cardiol* 2008;**23**:148–52.
12. Velazquez EJ, Lee KL, O'Connor CM, *et al.* The rationale and design of the Surgical Treatment for Ischemic Heart Failure (STICH) trial. *J Thorac Cardiovasc Surg* 2007;**134**:1540–7.
13. Jones RH, Velazquez EJ, Michler RE, *et al.* Coronary bypass surgery with or without surgical ventricular reconstruction. *N Engl J Med* 2009;**360**:1705–17.
14. Schinkel AF, Poldermans D, Elhendy A, Bax JJ. Assessment of myocardial viability in patients with heart failure. *J Nucl Med* 2007;**48**:1135–46.
15. Hunt SA, Abraham WT, Chin MH, *et al.* 2009 focused update incorporated into the ACC/AHA 2005 Guidelines for the Diagnosis and Management of Heart Failure in Adults: a report of the American College of Cardiology Foundation/American Heart Association Task Force on Practice Guidelines: developed in collaboration with the International Society for Heart and Lung Transplantation. *Circulation* 2009;**119**:e391–e479.
16. Jackson CE, Gardner RS, Connelly DT. A novel approach for a novel combination: a trans-septal biopsy of left atrial mass in recurrent phyllodes tumour. *Eur J Echocardiogr* 2009;**10**:171–2.

PART IX

Prognostication

25

Prognostication

Roy S. Gardner

Introduction

Recent advances in medical therapy, notably angiotensin converting enzyme (ACE) inhibitors, β-adrenoreceptor antagonists, and aldosterone antagonists, as well as device therapy have improved that prognosis such that even in patients with chronic heart failure (CHF) who are in New York Heart Association (NYHA) class IV, the annual mortality can be as low as 9.7%.[1] Nevertheless, many patients do not respond to medical therapy and remain symptomatically very limited with a poor prognosis. It is for such patients that cardiac transplantation and ventricular assist devices are options. However, identifying such patients is one of the great challenges of HF management.

The 1-year mortality following cardiac transplantation is approximately 19%.[2] The selection of candidates for cardiac transplantation is therefore heavily involved with identifying those patients whose annual mortality from HF exceeds this rate and who might therefore benefit prognostically from a transplant.

There are over 300 prognostic markers described in patients with HF, the most significant of which are shown in Table 25.1. Many studies have been carried out looking at clinical, haemodynamic, and neurohormonal variables to assist with risk stratification, although it is important to look at such data in the context of the latest disease-modifying therapy. The traditional markers, including left ventricular ejection fraction (LVEF) and the peak oxygen uptake (pVo_2), consistently offer useful prognostic information, although scoring systems involving a combination of markers have also been developed. More recently, neurohormones have been shown to demonstrate the greatest prognostic potential in identifying patients at the greatest risk of an adverse outcome.

Risk according to demographics

Age

The Framingham Heart Study showed that mortality increased with advancing age, with a 27% increase in mortality per decade in men and 61% increase per decade in women.[3] This is confirmed by other studies which have shown that increasing age is an independent risk factor for all-cause mortality and HF hospitalization.[4–9] However, despite the increased risk elderly HF patients currently face, their fate is substantially better than that it would have been 50 years ago. Further data from the Framingham study demonstrated a 5-year mortality of 54% in men and 40% in women in the period 1990–1999, compared to 65% and 66% in 1950–1969, in patients surviving at least 30 days after the onset of HF.[10]

Sex

Although there are occasional conflicting reports, women with HF are generally regarded to have a better outlook than men.[11,12] The Framingham study showed that between 1948 and 1988, women had a median survival time after diagnosis of 3.2 years compared to 1.7 years for men; after 5 years, 38% of women and 25% of men with CHF were alive.[11] In the period from 1990 to 1999, the 5-year survival had improved to 60% in women compared to 46% in men.[10]

A reduced risk in women has also been seen in modern therapeutic trials.[13–17] However, in the Italian Network on Congestive HF Registry,[18] no difference in outcome was found between men and women, and in the Studies of Left Ventricular Dysfunction (SOLVD) trial[19], where an ischaemic aetiology was more common, women were found to have a poorer prognosis than men.

In a study by Adams *et al.*,[20] women with nonischaemic HF had a significantly better outcome than men (male RR = 3.08). In contrast, ischaemic HF had a similar outcome in both men and women. A similar finding was also shown in a pooled analysis of over of 11,000 patients from five modern therapeutic randomized trials in patients with reduced LVEF (MERIT HF, PRAISE, PRAISE II, PROMISE, and VEST).[12] In multivariable analysis, male sex was associated with significantly worse prognosis, particularly for those with a nonischaemic aetiology of HF.

There were similar findings in a comparison of outcomes in 2400 women and 5199 men in the CHARM trial, which included patients with both reduced and normal LVEF.[15] Women had lower risks of most fatal and nonfatal outcomes; these differences were not explained by LVEF or the cause of HF.

Table 25.1 Powerful markers of an adverse outcome in patients with heart failure

Category	Prognostic marker	Relationship
Demographics	Age	Direct
Aetiology	Ischaemic heart disease	Direct
Comorbidity	Chronic renal failure	Direct
	Diabetes mellitus	Direct
	Body mass index	Inverse
Symptoms and signs	Pulse	Direct
	Blood pressure	Inverse
	NYHA class	Direct
	S3	Adverse
Therapy	ACE inhibitors/ARBs	Beneficial
	β-blocker	Beneficial
	Aldosterone antagonist	Beneficial
Laboratory tests	Sodium	Inverse
	Troponin	Direct
	Creatinine	Direct
	Haemoglobin	Inverse
ECG	QRS duration	Direct
	Heart rate variability	Inverse
	Nonsustained VT	Direct
Imaging	Left ventricular end-diastolic dimension	Direct
	Left atrial volume	Direct
	Left ventricular ejection fraction	Inverse
Haemodynamics	Peak Vo_2	Inverse
	6-minute walk	Inverse
	Pulmonary capillary wedge pressure	Direct
	Cardiac output	Inverse
Neurohormones	B-type natriuretic peptide/NT-proBNP	Direct
	Atrial natriuretic peptide	Direct
	Noradrenaline	Direct
	Adrenomedullin	Direct
	Endothelin-1	Direct
Scoring systems	Heart Failure Survival Score	Inverse
	Seattle Heart Failure Model	Direct

Race

In a prospective study of patients admitted with decompensated HF, African Americans had a similar mortality but greater functional decline and were around 8 years younger on presentation than white Americans.[21] In the SOLVD registry,[22] black patients with CHF were also at a greater risk of death and worsening HF, but had a higher prevalence of diabetes, prior stroke, and left ventricular dysfunction of a nonischaemic aetiology, making interpretation difficult. Physiological differences in the renin–angiotensin–aldosterone and neuroendocrine systems could account for any difference in outcome, with ACE inhibitors thought to be less effective at halting disease progression in black compared to white patients.

Climate

There is some evidence to suggest a significant seasonal variation in hospitalization and death from HF, with winter peaks most notable in the elderly population.[23,24] In one report at least a fifth of cases could be attributable to the associated seasonal increase in respiratory disease.[23]

Risk by aetiology

Chronic HF of ischaemic aetiology carries an greater risk of morbidity and mortality than that of a nonischaemic aetiology.[13] Exceptions to this rule are infiltrative causes of myocardial disease, such as amyloidosis and haemochromatosis.[25] Although an ischaemic aetiology is an independent predictor of mortality in patients with a reduced ejection fraction, patients with mild coronary artery disease appear to have a similar 5-year survival to those with a non–ischaemic cardiomyopathy.[8] There is some evidence that revascularization of ischaemic myocardium may improve prognosis,[26] although results from large prospective randomized trials are awaited.[27]

Risk according to coexisting disease

Chronic renal impairment

Renal impairment is often associated with HF due to renal hypoperfusion, and the use of diuretics, ACE inhibitors, angiotensin receptor antagonists, aldosterone antagonist, and other concomitant medication. Serum creatinine concentration, which is often quoted as a barometer of renal impairment, is actually a poor indicator of renal function.[28] An estimation of the glomerular filtration rate (GFR) is better for the accurate assessment of renal function,[28] and the Modification of Diet in Renal Disease (MDRD) equations[29] have recently been validated in patients with severe CHF (see Fig. 18.3, p. 180).[30] A GFR below 60 mL/min/1.73 m^2 is associated with complications of renal disease.[28] Moreover, a reduced GFR is independently predictive of all-cause mortality in asymptomatic[31] and symptomatic[31–34] left ventricular systolic dysfunction. In advanced HF, however, NT-proBNP appears to be a superior marker of prognosis.[35]

Diabetes mellitus

Diabetes mellitus is a strong independent predictor of mortality in patients with HF[36,37] and this increased risk was later shown to be in patients with an ischaemic cardiomyopathy, rather than those with a dilated cardiomyopathy.[38]

Alcohol abuse

Excessive intake of alcohol is also a strong independent predictor of mortality.[39] Importantly, with total abstinence from alcohol, patients with an alcoholic cardiomyopathy can demonstrate a significant improvement in LVEF and functional status.[40] However, the prognosis for those who continue to consume excess alcohol is poor.[41]

Psychosocial

HF patients with major depression are at an increased risk of death as well as hospitalization.[42] Social isolation is also a significant predictor of mortality.[43] Marital quality, as assessed by the marital satisfaction scale, predicts 4-year survival independent of NYHA class.[44]

Risk according to clinical variables

Symptoms

NYHA class

A higher NYHA class has frequently been shown to be an independent predictor of mortality.[8,17,18,45]

Quality of life

In a cohort of mild to moderate CHF, the Minnesota Living with Heart Failure Questionnaire (MLHFQ) was found to be an independent predictor of 1-year mortality or worsening HF.[46] However, there is no correlation between MLHFQ and traditional prognostic indicators, such as LVEF and p$\dot{V}O_2$.[47] Another health-related quality of life (HRQL) questionnaire has also been shown to predict mortality and CHF-related hospitalization.[48]

Syncope

Syncope in CHF, whether cardiac in origin or not, is independently predictive of sudden death.[49]

Signs

Cardiac signs

A heart rate above 86/min and systolic blood pressure below 119 mmHg are independently associated with a poorer outcome in CHF.[17,18,50] The prognostic importance of elevated jugular venous pressure and a third heart sound in patients with HF was evaluated in a retrospective analysis of the SOLVD treatment trial.[51] Both signs were associated with a significantly poorer NYHA class, but each was independently associated with an adverse outcome. A third heart sound was also an independent predictor of 1-year mortality in the Italian Network on Congestive HF Registry.[18]

Clinical profile

In a prospective analysis of 452 patients, subjects were classified by clinical assessment into four profiles: dry–warm, wet–warm, wet–cold, and dry–cold, on the basis of the absence/presence of signs of congestion, and evidence suggesting adequate or inadequate perfusion. Patients who were either wet–cold or wet–warm had an increased risk of death plus urgent transplantation on multivariate analysis.[52]

Body weight

Obesity, as defined by a body mass index (BMI) greater than 31, is not associated with increased mortality in patients with advanced CHF after 5 years of follow-up.[53] Paradoxically, an elevated BMI was shown to be an independent predictor of improved survival. This could be partly explained by higher blood pressure in the overweight and obese groups, allowing a significantly greater use of disease-modifying therapy. Low body weight and significant weight loss predict increased mortality, however, possibly reflecting a higher degree of cytokine activation.[54,55]

Exercise

Although a meta-analysis of small-scale trials of rehabilitation suggested that there may have been a survival benefit from exercise training,[56] the near-definitive HF-ACTION trial showed no effect of a formal training programme on survival. Training was associated with better quality of life.[57,58]

Risk according to drug therapy

There is compelling evidence that ACE inhibitors,[59–63], β-blockers[64–66] and aldosterone antagonists[67] are associated with better survival. The relation between some other drugs and survival is less clear-cut.

Diuretics

In a retrospective study, high doses of diuretic (>80 mg furosemide or equivalent per day) were independently associated with total mortality, sudden death, and pump failure death.[68] Another study corroborates this finding that diuretic dose relates to mortality.[69]

HMG CoA reductase inhibitors (statins)

Statin therapy is beneficial for the primary and secondary prevention of ischaemic heart disease[70,71]. However, two recent studies of rosuvastatin have shown that this statin does not alter prognosis in patients with HF, whether or not it is due to coronary heart disease.[72,73]

Amiodarone

Although it appears to be a relatively safe antiarrhythmic agent in CHF, there is conflicting information about the effect of amiodarone on mortality. In the GESICA study[74], there was a 28% relative risk reduction in mortality, but the mortality reduction was not verified in the larger, placebo-controlled CHF-STAT study.[75]

Digoxin

Although digoxin improves symptoms and reduces hospitalization in CHF, it has a neutral effect on mortality[76,77]. However, a post-hoc analysis of the DIG trial suggests that male subjects with higher serum digoxin concentrations(>1.2 ng/mL) have a higher mortality than patients receiving placebo.[78]

Hydralazine/isosorbide dinitrate

The combination of hydralazine and isosorbide dinitrate is associated with a lower mortality than placebo,[79] but is less effective than enalapril.[80] However, the A-HeFT study was stopped early because it showed that the addition of hydralazine and isosorbide dinitrate to standard care (including 69% on ACE inhibitors and 74% on β-blockers) in black patients was superior to placebo (43% RRR in all-cause mortality).[81]

Risk according to biochemistry and haematology

Electrolytes

Several studies have shown hyponatraemia to be an independent predictor of mortality[82–86] and hypokalaemia to be an independent predictor of sudden cardiac death[82]. Serum magnesium is not an independent risk factor for death in patients with moderate to severe CHF.[87]

Troponin

Over the past decade, an increasing number of studies has demonstrated that a significant proportion of patients with CHF (10–49%) have detectable troponin (Tn).[88] Persistently elevated Tn concentrations are associated with an adverse prognosis regardless of the aetiology of HF.[89] A raised Tn level is also associated with an adverse outcome in acute, and acute decompensated, HF.[88,90]

Urate

Serum uric acid is strongly related to circulating markers of inflammation in patients with HF.[91] Several studies have shown that a raised uric acid concentration is independently predictive of an impaired prognosis.[69,92] Interestingly, a retrospective study has suggested that long-term use of high-dose allopurinol could be associated with a reduced mortality, possibly by negating the adverse effect of an elevated urate concentration.[93]

Liver function tests

Abnormalities in liver function tests adversely affect prognosis in CHF, most notably AST and bilirubin.[69]

C-reactive protein

Inflammatory markers such as C-reactive protein (CRP), as well as the interleukins IL-4 and IL-6, increase during episodes of acute decompensation, returning to baseline once patients become compensated.[94] Patients admitted with decompensated HF who subsequently died or required readmission following discharge had a higher baseline CRP concentration than those who remained event free.[95] In the Val-HeFT trial, the cumulative likelihood of death or a first morbid event increased progressively with quartiles of serum CRP.[96]

Haemoglobin

Anaemia is an independent predictor of mortality in patients with new onset HF, [97] mild to moderate CHF[35] and advanced CHF.[105] Indeed, in the latter study, patients in the lowest haemoglobin (Hb) quartile were 86% more likely to die at 1 year than those in the highest Hb quartile. Hb is a significant predictor of progressive pump failure but not sudden death. Treatment of anaemia in CHF with subcutaneous erythropoietin and intravenous iron improves some aspects of the condition,[98] but large randomized controlled trials of erythropoietin in anaemic HF patients are awaited.

Red cell distribution width

Red cell distribution width is a readily available measure of the variation in erythrocyte volume. As well as offering prognostic information in CHF,[99] it is also a marker of adverse outcome in patients with acute HF, regardless of anaemia status.[100] It has prognostic value additional to that of B-type natriuretic peptide.[101]

White cell count

In a retrospective analysis of the SOLVD study, a white cell count (WCC) greater than 7000/mm^3 was an independent predictor of all-cause and cardiovascular mortality in patients with LVSD of ischaemic aetiology, but not in those with a dilated cardiomyopathy.[102]

Platelet function

Although platelet activity is increased in 22% of patients with stable CHF (vs 7% in normal controls), the degree of activation was similar in CHF of ischaemic and nonischaemic aetiologies and platelet activation was not related to either NYHA class or subsequent outcome.[103]

Erythrocyte sedimentation rate

An erythrocyte sedimentation rate (ESR) above the median value (14 mm/h) is associated with a poor survival, independent of age, NYHA class, LVEF, and peak Vo_2.[104,105]

Risk according to ECG

Atrial fibrillation

Atrial fibrillation (AF) is much more common in patients with CHF than in normal individuals, with prevalence ranging from 10% to 50%. Data assessing the outcome of AF in patients with CHF have been conflicting, with most showing no impact on survival.

In the V-HeFT study, atrial fibrillation did not increase major morbidity or mortality in mild to moderate HF.[106] A follow-up of patients in the SOLVD trials with asymptomatic left ventricular dysfunction or NYHA class II–III HF found that AF (present in only 6.4%) was a significant predictor of all-cause mortality,[107] primarily due to pump failure, as there was no increase in mortality from arrhythmia. Around 18% of patients in the CHARM series had AF at baseline which was independently linked to mortality, both in patients with either low or preserved LVEF.[108]

One study noted an improvement in the prognosis of AF in patients with CHF with the advent of ACE inhibitor therapy, amiodarone, and avoidance of class Ia antiarrhythmic drugs.[109]

Heart rate variability

In a prospective study, a standard deviation of R-R interval of less than 100 ms identified patients at increased risk of death due to progressive pump failure but not sudden cardiac death.[82] However, conversely, a retrospective analysis of data from the Veterans Affairs' Survival Trial of Anti-arrhythmic Therapy in Congestive Heart Failure, the lowest quartile of the standard deviation of R-R intervals was an independent predictor of sudden death, as well as total mortality.[110]

QRS duration

QRS prolongation (>120 ms) is an independent predictor of both total mortality and sudden death in patients with severe CHF (LVEF<30%).[111] In moderate CHF (LVEF 30–40%), however, QRS duration is associated only with increased mortality but not sudden death. Right bundle branch block is not associated with excess mortality.

In the Italian Network Network on Congestive registry,[112] left bundle breach block (LBBB)—diagnosed with a QRS duration in excess of 140 ms—was found in 25.2% of individuals with CHF. LBBB was more common in women and in patients with dilated cardiomyopathy, and was an independent predictor of all-cause death and sudden death in patients with CHF. LBBB was also an independent predictor of mortality in the CIBIS-2 study[17]. In two subsequent studies, accelerated QRS-interval widening was independently associated with deterioration of cardiac function,[113] and death or need for urgent cardiac transplantation.[114]

QT dispersion

In a substudy of Diamond-CHF,[115] QT dispersion was not a predictor of outcome and in another study QT dispersion and maximum QT interval were found to be univariate but not independent predictors of all-cause mortality and sudden death.[116]

Ventricular tachycardia

Patients with moderate to severe CHF who have evidence of non-sustained ventricular tachycardia (NSVT) on 24-h Holter monitoring have an increased risk of total mortality and sudden death.[82,117]

Risk according to imaging

Chest radiograph

A higher cardiothoracic ratio (CTR) is predictive of the risk of worsening symptoms, hospitalization, and mortality,[118] particularly in the patient with CHF and a low LVEF. In addition, UK-HEART (United Kingdom-Heart Failure Evaluation and Assessment of Risk Trial)—a multicentre prospective study designed to identify noninvasive markers of death and mode of death in patients with CHF—showed that a greater CTR was also predictive of sudden death.[119]

Echocardiography

Left ventricular dimensions (end-systolic and end-diastolic) independently predict all-cause mortality and sudden cardiac death.[82,120] Furthermore, HF patients with severe mitral or tricuspid regurgitation on echocardiography are also at increased risk of death.[121]

In a study using dobutamine echocardiography, patients with moderate to severe left ventricular dysfunction and viable or ischaemic myocardium had an adverse prognosis, independent of age and LVEF.[122]

Cardiac magnetic resonance imaging

There are few prognostic data from studies of cardiac magnetic resonance imaging (CMR) in patients with CHF. However, in a study of 279 patients with poor-quality echocardiograms, the presence of a reduced left ventricular function (<40%) on CMR stress testing was independently associated with all-cause mortality.[123]

Risk according to haemodynamics

Left ventricular ejection fraction

A lower ejection fraction is associated with a poorer outcome in patients with CHF.[17,118,124] A improvement in LVEF during exercise radionuclide ventriculography in mild CHF is a strong independent predictor of survival.[125]

Right ventricular ejection fraction

In a small study by Di Salvo *et al.*,[126] a right ventricular ejection fraction of 35% or more at exercise was an independent predictor of survival and more potent than peak Vo_2 or percentage of predicted Vo_2.

Peak Vo_2

Peak oxygen consumption (pVo_2) of less than 10 mL/kg/min is associated with a 1-year mortality of 77% compared with 21% for those patients who achieved a pVo_2 of 10–18 mL/kg per min.[127] pVo_2 has become widely accepted as a marker of prognosis,[7,118,128–131] as well as a marker for the timing of transplantation.[132] Initially, those patients with a pVo_2 of less than 14 mL/kg/min were identified as a high-risk cohort of patients, with a 1-year mortality of 30% compared with those with a value greater than 14 mL/kg/min who had a 1-year mortality of 6%. However, with widespread use of β-blockade, the cut-off has fallen to 12 mL/kg/min.[133]

Many studies have since attempted to 'fine-tune' the predictive power of pVo_2. As pVo_2 is affected by age, sex, body composition, and body conditioning, the percentage of predicted pVo_2 might be a better marker, but added minimal precision over pVo_2 alone.[134] As oxygen consumption is corrected for total body weight, and body fat consumes very little oxygen, body fat adjusted pVo_2 (pVo_2 lean) may provide greater prognostic precision, especially in female and obese subgroups.[135]

Six-minute walk test

The six-minute walk test is simple and noninvasive, and independently predicts morbidity and mortality in patients with mild–moderate[136] as well as advanced[137] CHF. However, in other studies, the six-minute walk test was only able to predict mortality in univariate analysis, and was not an independent predictor of survival.[138,139]

Invasive haemodynamic variables

There are inconsistent reports of the predictive power of right heart catheter data in CHF. No single variable consistently predicts outcome, although many studies have found the pulmonary capillary wedge pressure (PCWP) to be independently predictive of mortality.[140,141] Other studies have found other right heart pressure measurements to be similarly predictive of outcome.[142,143] Most studies were conducted prior to the routine use of modern disease-modifying therapy and so their relevance to today's practice is uncertain. There is a role for right heart catheterization in patient selection for cardiac transplantation, however, since an increased pulmonary vascular resistance has consistently been shown to increase the risk of early graft failure.[144,145]

Risk according to neurohormones

Adrenomedullin

This 52-amino-acid peptide is almost ubiquitously expressed throughout the human cardiovascular system. It has potent vasodilating and natriuretic effects, and is raised in HF in proportion to the severity of the disease.[146] Although adrenomedullin is an independent predictor of death or urgent cardiac transplantation in patients with mild–moderate CHF,[147] it is not as powerful a predictor of prognosis as endothelin-1 or NT-proBNP.[148,149] However, as plasma levels of adrenomedullin can be inaccurate because of its short half-life, an assay has been developed for the more stable midregional portion of the pro-peptide (MR-proADM) which may offer further prognostic information.[150]

Catecholamines

A high plasma noradrenaline (NA) level is an independent predictor of morbidity and mortality in LVSD patients with NYHA class I–II.[151] In a substudy of the Val-HeFT trial, a NA level above the median at baseline was an independent predictor of mortality, although not as powerful as B-type natriuretic peptide.[152] Interestingly, subjects with the greatest increase or greatest decrease in NE over the first 4 months of the study had the highest mortality risk, which complements preliminary data from the BEST study.[152]

Endothelin

Endothelin-1 is a 21-amino-acid structure with potent and long-lasting vasoconstricting properties that is elevated in patients with CHF. It independently predicts mortality, clinical deterioration, and the need for cardiac transplantation in patients with CHF.[153–157] However, one study showed that there was no difference in endothelin-1 concentrations between patients with mild CHF and healthy controls.[158] Endothelin also correlates positively with the degree of pulmonary hypertension in CHF,[159] which in itself has been shown to alter prognosis unfavourably.[160]

Natriuretic peptides

Atrial and B-type natriuretic peptides (ANP and BNP) are polypeptides that are produced in response to cardiac stretch. They stimulate natriuresis, induce vasodilatation, and are antiproliferative. They also inhibit the renin–angiotensin–aldosterone and sympathetic nervous systems.

Atrial natriuretic peptides

ANP and NT-proANP are raised in patients with CHF,[161,162] correlating closely with the severity of CHF, and are associated with increased mortality.[163] The midregional segment of the pro-atrial natriuretic peptide molecule (MR-proANP) is more stable in plasma than either proANP or mature ANP and is emerging as a promising biomarker. MR-proANP is an independent predictor of mortality in acutely decompensated HF,[164] and may be a better marker than BNP and its variants in patients with CHF.[165,166]

B-type natriuretic peptide

BNP and its N-terminal inactive fragment (NT-proBNP), are increased in both symptomatic and asymptomatic LVSD,[161] increasing in proportion to the severity of CHF.[167] Currently, they appear to be the most potent prognostic markers available in HF, and are predictive of morbidity and mortality in asymptomatic or minimally symptomatic LVSD,[151] in mild–moderate CHF,[138] and in patients with advanced HF referred for consideration of cardiac transplantation.[168]

Cytokines

Tumour necrosis factor

Tumour necrosis factor α (TNFα) is a proinflammatory cytokine and is increased in patients with severe CHF, particularly in those with cachexia.[169,170] Although TNF-α has not been shown to be an independent marker of prognosis, tumour necrosis factor soluble receptor-1 has.[171]

Interleukin-6

IL-6 is a proinflammatory and vasodepressor cytokine that mediates both inflammatory and immune responses: like TNFα, it is increased in patients with HF. In a study of NYHA class III patients, IL-6 was an independent predictor of mortality at 1 year, and was as least as predictive as LVEF.[172] In contrast, there were no significant differences in the plasma concentrations of IL-1, IL-10, IL-12, and TNFα between survivors and non-survivors. Plasma concentrations of IL-6 follow a circadian rhythm, peaking at midnight.[185]

Novel biomarkers

Several emerging biomarkers have shown promise as predictors in HF, and are currently being investigated (Table 25.2).[173] Many of them arise from our greater understanding of the pathophysiological processes in HF, in particular the components of novel neurohormonal pathways with possible roles—both protective and deleterious.

Table 25.2 Summary of novel biomarkers in acute and chronic heart failure

Biomarker	Plasma levels in ADHF	Independent prognostic information?	Levels altered with therapy?	Plasma levels in CHF	Independent prognostic information?	Levels altered with therapy?
MR-proANP	↑	Yes	U	↑	Yes	U
MR-proADM	U	U	U	↑	Yes	U
copeptin	↑	Yes	U	↑	Yes	U
Apelin	↔	No	No	↓	U	Yes
Urocortin	U	U	U	↑	U	U
CgA	↑	Yes	U	↑	Yes	No
CoQ_{10}	U	U	U	↓	Yes	U
Adiponectin	↑	Yes	U	↑	Yes	U
H-FABP	U	U	U	↑	Yes	Yes
MLC-1	U	U	U	↑	Yes	U
Osteopontin	U	U	U	↑	Yes	U
GDF-15	U	U	U	↑	Yes	U
Pentraxin-3	U	U	U	↑	Yes	U
Secretory sphingomyelinase	U	U	U	↑	Yes	U
CT-1	U	U	U	↑	Yes	U
Gal-3	↑	Yes	U	↑	U	No
ST2	↑	Yes	U	↑	Yes	U
Cystatin C	↑	Yes	U	↑	Yes	U
SP-B	↑	U	Yes	↑	U	Yes

↑: raised; ↓: reduced; ↔: no change; ADHF; acutely decompensated heart failure; CHF, congestive heart failure; U, unknown.

Adapted from Dalzel JR *et al. Biomark Med* 2009;**3**(5):483–93.

Risk according to composite scoring systems

Retrospective analyses have been used to develop composite scoring systems as predictive models that generate a more accurate and individual estimate of prognosis than single variables.[174–176] As with the single-variable studies, however, the scoring systems quickly become out of date with the development of new therapies, and the models are often derived and validated in different populations of patients.

EFFECT model

The EFFECT model was retrospectively derived and tested, and was intended for use in patients hospitalized for HF.[176] The derivation cohort included patients from the EFFECT study who presented with HF between 1999 and 2001. The model was then validated in a separate cohort presenting between 1997 and 1999. Multiple clinical characteristics (age, respiratory rate, systolic pressure, blood urea nitrogen, and serum sodium concentration) and comorbidities were included and the resultant scores correlated with 30-day and 1-year mortality. However, no information was given on background therapy, and the model was created prior to the routine use of natriuretic peptides. An online calculator is available at www.ccort.ca/CHFriskmodel.aspx.

Heart Failure Survival Score

One commonly used scoring system is the Heart Failure Survival Score (HFSS),[85] which was developed and validated in patients with advanced HF (NYHA III and IV). The score stratifies patients by risk—low, medium, and high (equating to a 1-year survival rate of 88%, 60%, and 35%, respectively)—of death or urgent transplantation and incorporates seven variables (heart rate, mean blood pressure, serum sodium, ejection fraction, pVo_2, presence of ischaemic heart disease, and conduction delay on electrocardiography; Fig 25.1). In an invasive version of the HFSS, PCWP was included as an eighth variable. Unfortunately, due to the timing of the original model, only a small percentage of patients involved in the initial HFSS study were established on current standards of medical or device therapy. In particular, the use of β-blockers and spironolactone was very low, and both can alter some of the variables used in the scoring system, as well as the prognosis of CHF. However, a later study validated the HFSS in patients on current therapy.[177] A conflicting study found that a simplified risk stratification model with only two variables—LVEF and Vo_2 or six-minute walk test—was superior to the HFSS.[178]

Coronary artery disease (yes = 1; no = 0)	(....... × 0.6931) =	+
Intraventricular conduction delay (y = 1; n = 0)	(....... × 0.6083) =	+
Left ventricular ejection fraction (%)	(....... × −0.0464) =	+
Heart rate (bpm)	(....... × 0.0216) =	+
Na^+ concentration (mmol/L)	(....... × −0.0470) =	+
Mean arterial pressure (mmHg)	(....... × −0.0255) =	+
Peak VO_2 (mL/minute/kg)	(....... × −0.0546) =	
	HFSS =	....

- High risk <7.19 35% 1-year survival.
- Mediun risk 7.20–8.09 60% 1-year survival.
- Low risk >8.10 88% 1-year survival.

Fig. 25.1 The Heart Failure Survival Score.

The Seattle Heart Failure Model

The Seattle Heart Failure Model (SHFM) was derived from the PRAISE-1 database of 1125 HF patients with the use of a multivariable Cox model. It was subsequently prospectively validated in five additional cohorts: ELITE-2, Val-HeFT, UW, RENAISSANCE, and INCHF involving 9942 HF patients and 17 307 person-years of follow-up.[174] Although no patients in the derivation cohort were on β-blockers, up to 72% of the validation population were. Importantly, the validation cohorts also included patients with a wide range of ages (14–100 years), ejection fractions (1–75%), and HF symptoms (NYHA class I–IV).

The SHFM accurately predicts survival of HF patients (Fig. 25.2) with the use of commonly obtained clinical characteristics (NYHA class, ischaemic aetiology, diuretic dose, LVEF, systolic BP, serum sodium, haemoglobin, percentage lymphocytes, uric acid, and serum cholesterol). It has a distinct advantage over the HFSS which relies on pVo_2 to calculate a score. The Seattle model also provides information about the likely mode of death. In an analysis of 10 538 ambulatory patients with predominantly systolic HF (NYHA class II–IV), the score was predictive of the risk of sudden death and of pump failure.[179]

Interestingly, renal function was not an independent predictor in the SHFM, and two extremely powerful prognostic markers—VO_2 and BNP/NT-proBNP—were not included in the development of the model, as the data were available in fewer that 1% of the patients in the six data sets. An online calculator is available at www.SeattleHeartFailureModel.org.

Summary

In clinical trials, the 1-year mortality of patients with severe CHF can be as low as 9.7%,[180] but perhaps the real challenge is identifying those patients at greatest risk of death, and therefore those who would benefit most from advanced therapies such as ventricular assist devices and cardiac transplantation.

Many variables have prognostic power in CHF but the markers vary in their success for predicting outcome because of the heterogeneous nature of HF and the populations in which the variables were studied. Many of the described variables are inter-related and although they may be strong univariate markers of prognosis, they can be competitively removed in any multivariate model.

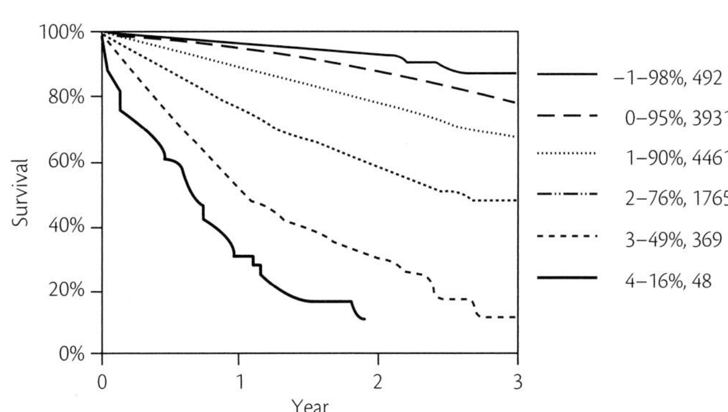

Fig. 25.2 The combined dataset of the derivation and five validation cohorts for a Seattle Heart Failure Score rounded to −1 to 4. The score. the predicted 1-year survival for the score, and the number of patients with that score are shown. From Levy WC *et al.* The Seattle Heart Failure Model: prediction of survival in heart failure. *Circulation* 2006; 113: 1424–33, with permission from Lippincott, Williams and Wilkins.

The ideal prognostic tool would be cost-effective, readily available, easy to measure, reproducible, minimally invasive, and both sensitive and specific. Until recently, the best single marker of prognosis was pVo_2, but many patients with CHF fail to achieve a true pVo_2, it is difficult to perform, and is not widely available. Many of the studies proposing the use of specific markers were carried out before the widespread use of β-blockers, ACE inhibitors, and spironolactone.

The HF survival score is currently used by many transplant centres to help identify patients who would benefit most from cardiac transplantation.[175] However, the score relies on seven variables being available for each patient, including pVo_2, and without one variable the score is useless.

The variables with perhaps the most promise as prognostic tools in CHF are the B-type natriuretic peptides. They are relatively cheap, are stable in whole blood for 3 days and can be measured on most modern autoanalysers.[181]

However, in view of the multifactorial nature of CHF, it seems likely that a combination of variables would be useful in the prediction of prognosis in HF. Large prospective studies are therefore required in order to further clarify the subject.

References

1. Cleland JG, Daubert JC, Erdmann E, *et al.* The effect of cardiac resynchronization on morbidity and mortality in heart failure. N Engl J Med 2005;352:1539–49.
2. Hosenpud JD, Bennet LE, Keck BM, Boucek MM, Novick RJ. ISHLT Registry Report: The Registry of the International Society for Heart and Lung Transplantation: Seventeenth Official Report—2000. J Heart Lung Transplant 2000;19:909–31.
3. Ho KK, Anderson KM, Kannel WB, et al. Survival after the onset of congestive heart failure in Framingham heart study subjects. Circulation 1993;88:107–15.
4. van Veldhuisen DJ, Boomsma F, de Kam PJ, et al. Influence of age on neurohormonal activation and prognosis in patients with chronic heart failure. Eur Heart J 1998;19:753–60.
5. Adams KF, Dunlap SH, Sueta CA, et al. Relation between gender, etiology and survival in patients with symptomatic heart failure. J Am Coll Cardiol 1996;28:1781–8.
6. Rich MW, Beckham V, Wittenberg C, Leven CL, Freedland KE, Carney RM. A multidisciplinary intervention to prevent the readmission of elderly patients with congestive heart failure. N Engl J Med 1995;333:1190–5.
7. Myers J, Gullestad L, Vagelos R, et al. Clinical, hemodynamic, and cardiopulmonary exercise test determinants of survival in patients referred for evaluation of heart failure. Ann Intern Med 1998;129:286–293.
8. Bart BA, Shaw LK, McCants CB, et al. Clinical determinants of mortality in patients with angiographically diagnosed ischemic or nonischemic cardiomyopathy. *J Am Coll Cardiol* 1997;**30**:1002–1008.
9. Rich MW, McSherry F, Williford WO, *et al.* Effect of age on mortality, hospitalizations and response to digoxin in patients with heart failure: The DIG study. *J Am Coll Cardiol* 2001;**38**:806–813.
10. Levy D, Kenchaiah S, Larson MG, *et al.* Long-term trends in the incidence of and survival with heart failure. *N Engl J Med* 2002;**347**:1397–402.
11. Ho KK, Anderson KM, Kannel WB, Grossman W, Levy D. Survival after the onset of congestive heart failure in Framingham Heart Study subjects. *Circulation* 1993;**88**:107–15.
12. Frazier CG, Alexander KP, Newby LK, *et al.* Associations of gender and etiology with outcomes in heart failure with systolic dysfunction: a pooled analysis of 5 randomized control trials. *J Am Coll Cardiol* 2007;**49**:1450–8.
13. Simon T, Mary-Krause M, Funck-Brentano C. Sex differences in the prognosis of congestive heart failure; Results from the cardiac insufficiency bisoprolol study (CIBIS II). *Circulation* 2001;**103**:375–80.
14. Ghali JK, Pina IL, Gottlieb SS, Deedwania PC, Wikstrand JC. Metoprolol CR/XL in female patients with heart failure: analysis of the experience in Metoprolol Extended-Release Randomized Intervention Trial in Heart Failure (MERIT-HF). *Circulation* 2002;**105**:1585–91.
15. O'Meara E, Clayton T, McEntegart MB, *et al.* Sex differences in clinical characteristics and prognosis in a broad spectrum of patients with heart failure: results of the Candesartan in Heart failure: Assessment of Reduction in Mortality and morbidity (CHARM) program. *Circulation* 2007;**115**:3111–20.
16. Adams KF Jr, Sueta CA, Gheorghiade M, *et al.* Gender differences in survival in advanced heart failure. Insights from the FIRST study. *Circulation* 1999;**99**:1816–21.
17. Funck-Brentano C, Lancar R, Hansen S, *et al.* Predictors of medical events and of their competitive interactions in the Cardiac Insufficiency Bisoprolol Study 2 (CIBIS-2). *Am Heart J* 2001;**142**:989–97.
18. Opasich C, Tavazzi L, Lucci D, *et al.* Comparison of one-year outcome in women versus men with chronic congestive heart failure. *Am J Cardiol* 2000;**86**:353–57.
19. Bourassa MG, Gurné O, Bangdiwala SI, *et al.* Natural history and patterns of current practice in heart failure. The Studies of Left Ventricular Dysfunction (SOLVD) investgators. *J Am Coll Cardiol* 1993;**22**:14–19A.
20. Adams KF, Dunlap SH, Sueta CA, *et al.* Relation between gender, etiology and survival in patients with symptomatic heart failure. *J Am Coll Cardiol* 1996;**28**:1781–8.
21. Vaccarino V, Gahbauer E, Kasl SV, *et al.* Differences between African Americans and whites in the outcome of heart failure: Evidence for a greater functional decline in African Americans. *Am Heart J* 2002;**143**:1058–67.
22. Dries DL, Exner DV, Gersh BJ, Cooper HA, Carson PE, Domanski MJ. Racial differences in the outcome of left ventricular dysfunction. *N Engl J Med* 1999;**340**:609–16.
23. Stewart S, McIntyre K, Capewell S, McMurray JJ. Heart failure in a cold climate: Seasonal variation in heart failure-related morbidity and mortality. *J Am Coll Cardiol* 2002;**39**:760–6.
24. Boulay F, Berthier F, Sisteron O, Gendreike Y, Gibelin P. Seasonal variation in chronic heart failure hospitalizations and mortality in France. *Circulation* 1999;**100**:280–6.
25. Felker GM, Thompson RE, Hare JM, Hruban RH, Clemetson DE, Howard DL *et al.* Underlying causes and long-term survival in patients with initially unexplained cardiomyopathy. *N Engl J Med* 2000;**342**:1077–84.
26. Di CM, Asgarzadie F, Schelbert HR, *et al.* Quantitative relation between myocardial viability and improvement in heart failure symptoms after revascularization in patients with ischemic cardiomyopathy. *Circulation* 1995;**92**:3436–44.
27. Velazquez EJ, Lee KL, O'Connor CM, *et al.* The rationale and design of the Surgical Treatment for Ischemic Heart Failure (STICH) trial. *J Thorac Cardiovasc Surg* 2007;**134**:1540–7.
28. Levey AS, Coresh J, Balk E. National Kidney Foundation practice guidelines for chronic kidney disease: evaluation, classification, and stratification. *Ann Intern Med* 2003;**139**:137–47.
29. Levey AS, Bosch JP, Lewis JB, Greene T, Rogers N, Roth D. A more accurate method to estimate glomerular filtration rate from serum creatinine: a new prediction equation. *Ann Intern Med* 1999;**130**:461–70.
30. O'Meara E, Chong KS, Gardner RS, Jardine AG, Neilly JB, McDonagh TA. The Modification of Diet in Renal Disease (MDRD) equations provide valid estimations of glomerular filtration rates in patients with advanced heart failure. *Eur J Heart Fail* 2006;**8**:63–7.

31. Dries DL, Exner DV, Domanski MJ, Greenberg B, Stevenson LW. The prognostic implications of renal insufficiency in asymptomatic and symptomatic patients with left ventricular systolic dysfunction. *J Am Coll Cardiol* 2000;**35**:681–9.
32. Mahon N, Blackstone EH, Francis GS, Starling RC, Young JB, Lauer MS. The prognostic value of estimated creatinine clearance alongside functional capacity in ambulatory patients with chronic congestive heart failure. *J Am Coll Cardiol* 2002;**40**: 1106–13.
33. Al-Ahmad A, Rand W, Manjunath G, *et al.* Reduced kidney function and anemia as risk factors for mortality in patients with left ventricular dysfunction. *J Am Coll Cardiol* 2001;**38**(4):955–62.
34. Hillege HL, Girbes ARJ, de Kam PJ, *et al.* Renal function, neurohormonal activation and survival in patients with chronic heart failure. *Circulation* 2000;**102**:203–10.
35. Gardner RS, Chong KS, O'Meara E, Jardine A, Ford I, McDonagh TA. Renal dysfunction, as measured by the modification of diet in renal disease equations, and outcome in patients with advanced heart failure. *Eur Heart J* 2007;**28**:3027–33.
36. Shindler DM, Kostis JB, Yusuf S, *et al.* Diabetes mellitus: a predictor of morbidity and mortality in the Studies Of Left Ventricular Dysfunction (SOLVD) trials and registry. *Am J Cardiol* 1996;**77**:1017–20.
37. Prazak P, Pfisterer M, Osswald S, Buser P, Burkart F. Differences of disease progression in congestive heart failure due to alcoholic as compared to idiopathic dilated cardiomyopathy. *Eur Heart J* 1996;**17**:251–7.
38. Dries DL, Sweitzer NK, Drazner MH, *et al.* Prognostic impact of diabetes mellitus in patients with heart failure according to the etiology of left ventricular systolic function. *J Am Coll Cardiol* 2001;**38**:421–8.
39. Prazak P, Pfisterer M, Osswald S, Buser P, Burkart F. Differences of disease progression in congestive heart failure due to alcoholic as compared to idiopathic dilated cardiomyopathy. *Eur Heart J* 1996;**17**:251–7.
40. Guillo P, Mansourati J, Maheu B, *et al.* Long-term prognosis in patients with alcoholic cardiomyopathy and severe heart failure after total abstinence. *Am J Cardiol* 1997;**79**:1276–8.
41. Lazarevic AM, Nakatani S, Neskovic AN, *et al.* Early changes in left ventricular function in chronic asymptomatic alcoholics: relation to the duration of heavy drinking. *J Am Coll Cardiol* 2000;**35**:1599–606.
42. Jiang W, Alexander J, Christopher E, *et al.* Relationship of depression to increased risk of mortality and rehospitalization in patients with congestive heart failure. *Arch Intern Med* 2001;**161**:1849–56.
43. Murberg TA, Bru E. Social relationships and mortality in patients with congestive heart failure. *J Psychosomatic Res* 2001;**151**:521–7.
44. Coyne JC, Rohrbaugh MJ, Shoham V, *et al.* Prognostic importance of marital quality for survival of congestive heart failure. *Am J Cardiol* 2001;**88**:526–9.
45. Pernenkil R, Vinson JM, Shah AS, Beckham V, Wittenberg C, Rich MW. Course and prognosis in patients > or = 70 years of age with congestive heart failure and normal versus abnormal left ventricular ejection fraction. *Am J Cardiol* 1997;**79**:216–19.
46. Hulsmann M, Berger R, Sturm B, *et al.* Prediction of outcome by neurohumoral activation, the six-minute walk test and the Minnesota Living with Heart Failure Questionnaire in an outpatient cohort with congestive heart failure. *Eur Heart J* 2002;**23**:886–91.
47. Ben-Gal T, Zafrir N, Berman M, *et al.* Self-assessed quality of life in patients evaluated for heart transplantation: correlation with prognostic indicators. *Transplant Proc* 2001;**33**:2904–5.
48. Konstam V, Salem D, Pouleur H, *et al.* Baseline quality of life as a predictor of mortality and hospitalization in 5,025 patients with congestive heart failure. SOLVD Investigations. Studies of Left Ventricular Dysfunction Investigators. *Am J Cardiol* 1996;**78**:890–5.
49. Middlekauff HR, Stevenson WG, Stevenson LW, Saxon LA. Syncope in advanced heart failure: high risk of sudden death regardless of origin of syncope. *J Am Coll Cardiol* 1993;**21**:110–16.
50. Pernenkil R, Vinson JM, Shah AS, Beckham V, Wittenberg C, Rich MW. Course and prognosis in patients > or = 70 years of age with congestive heart failure and normal versus abnormal left ventricular ejection fraction. *Am J Cardiol* 1997;**79**: 216–19.
51. Drazner MH, Rame JE, Stevenson LW, *et al.* Prognostic importance of elevated jugular venous pressure and a third heart sound in patients with heart failure. *N Engl J Med* **345**, 574–581. 2001.
52. Nohria A, Tsang SW, Fang JC, *et al.* Clinical assessment identifies hemodynamic profile that predict outcomes in patients admitted with heart failure. *J Am Coll Cardiol* 2003;**41**:1797–804.
53. Horwich TB, Fonarow GC, Hamilton MA, *et al.* The relationship between obesity and mortality in patients with heart failure. *J Am Coll Cardiol* 2001;**38**:789–95.
54. O'Connor, C. M., Anderson, SA, Meese, RB, *et al.* Clinical determinants of outcome in advanced heart failure: Insights from the PRAISE trial (abstr). *J Am Coll Cardiol* 1997;**129**, 246A.
55. Anker SD, Ponikowski P, Varney S, *et al.* Wasting as independent risk factor for mortality in chronic heart failure. *Lancet* 1997;**349**:1050–3 [erratum appears in *Lancet* 1997;**349**(9060):1258].
56. Piepoli MF, Davos C, Francis DP, Coats AJ. Exercise training meta-analysis of trials in patients with chronic heart failure (ExTraMATCH). *BMJ* 2004;**328**:189.
57. O'Connor CM, Whellan DJ, Lee KL, *et al.* Efficacy and safety of exercise training in patients with chronic heart failure: HF-ACTION randomized controlled trial. *JAMA* 2009;**301**:1439–50.
58. Flynn KE, Pina IL, Whellan DJ, *et al.* Effects of exercise training on health status in patients with chronic heart failure: HF-ACTION randomized controlled trial. *JAMA* 2009;**301**:1451–9.
59. The SOLVD Investigators. Effect of enalapril on survival in patients with reduced left ventricular ejection fractions and congestive heart failure. *N Engl J Med* 1991;**325**(5):293–302.
60. SOLVD Investigators. Effect of enalapril on mortality and the development of heart failure in asymptomatic patients with reduced left ventricular ejection fractions. *N Engl J Med* 1992;**327**(10):685–91.
61. Garg R, Yusuf S. Overview of randomized trials of angiotensin-converting enzyme inhibitors on mortality and morbidity in patients with heart failure. Collaborative Group on ACE Inhibitor Trials. [see comments]. *JAMA* 1995;**273**:1450–6. [erratum appears in *JAMA* 1995;**274**(6):462].
62. Pfeffer MA, Braunwald E, Moye LA, *et al.* Effect of captopril on mortality and morbidity in patients with left ventricular dysfunction after myocardial infarction. Results of the survival and ventricular enlargement trial. The SAVE Investigators. *N Engl J Med* 1992;**327**:669–77.
63. AIRE. Effect of ramipril on mortality and morbidity of survivors of acute myocardial infarction with clinical evidence of heart failure. The Acute Infarction Ramipril Efficacy (AIRE) Study Investigators. *Lancet* 1993;**342**:821–8.
64. Cleland PJ, McGowan J, Clark A. The evidence for beta-blockers in heart failure. *BMJ* 1999;**318**:824–5.
65. Packer M, Coats AJ, Fowler MB, *et al.* Effect of carvedilol on survival in severe chronic heart failure. *N Engl J Med* 2001;**344**:1651–8.
66. The CAPRICORN Investigators. Effect of carvedilol on outcome after myocardial infarction in patients with left ventricular dysfunction:the CAPRICORN randomised trial. *Lancet* 2001;**357**: 1385–90.
67. Pitt B, Zannad F, Remme WJ, *et al.* The effect of spironolactone on morbidity and mortality in patients with severe heart failure. Randomized Aldactone Evaluation Study Investigators. [see comments]. *N Engl J Med* 1999;**341**:709–17.

68. Neuberg GW, Miller AB, O'Connor CM, *et al.* Diuretic resistance predicts mortality in patients with advanced heart failure. *Am Heart J* 2002;**144**:31–8.
69. Batin, P, Wickens, M, McEntegart, D., Fullwood, L., and Cowley, A. J. The importance of abnormalities of liver function tests in predicting mortality in chronic heart failure. *Eur Heart J* 1995;**16**(11):1613–18.
70. Shepherd, J., Cobbe, S. M., Ford I, *et al.* Prevention of coronary heart disease with pravastatin in men with hypercholesterolaemia. *N Engl J Med* 1995;**333**:1301–7.
71. The Scandinavian Simvastatin Survival Study group. Randomised trial of cholesterol lowering in 4444 patients with coronary heart disease: The Scandinavian Simvastatin Survival Study. *Lancet* 1994;**344**:1383–9.
72. Kjekshus J, Apetrei E, Barrios V, *et al.* Rosuvastatin in older patients with systolic heart failure. *N Engl J Med* 2007;**357**:2248–61.
73. Tavazzi L, Maggioni AP, Marchioli R, *et al.* Effect of rosuvastatin in patients with chronic heart failure (the GISSI-HF trial): a randomised, double-blind, placebo-controlled trial. *Lancet* 2008;**372**:1231–9.
74. Doval HC, Nul DR, Grancelli HO, *et al.* Randomised trial of low-dose amiodarone in severe congestive heart failure. *Lancet* 1994;**344**:493–8.
75. Singh SN, Fletcher RD, Fisher SG, *et al.* Amiodarone in patients with congestive heart failure and asymptomatic ventricular arrhythmia. Survival Trial of Antiarrhythmic Therapy in Congestive Heart Failure. [see comments]. *N Engl J Med* 1995;**333**:77–82.
76. Anonymous. The effect of digoxin on mortality and morbidity in patients with heart failure. The Digitalis Investigation Group. [see comments]. *N Engl J Med* 1997;**336**:525–33.
77. Packer M, Gheorghiade M, Young JB, *et al.* Withdrawal of digoxin from patients with chronic heart failure treated with angiotensin-converting-enzyme inhibitors. RADIANCE Study. *N Engl J Med* 1993;**329**:1–7.
78. Rathore SS, Curtis JP, Wang Y, Bristow MR, Krumholz HM. Association of serum digoxin concentration and outcomes in patients with heart failure. *JAMA* 2003;**289**:871–8.
79. Cohn JN, Archibald DG, Ziesche S, *et al.* Effect of vasodilator therapy on mortality in chronic congestive heart failure: Results of a Veterans Administration Cooperative Study. *N Engl J Med* 1986;**314**:1547–52.
80. Cohn JN, Johnson G, Ziesche S, *et al.* A comparison of enalapril with hydralazine-isosorbide dinitrate in the treatment of patients with chronic congestive heart failure. *N Engl J Med* 1991;**325**(5):303–10.
81. Taylor AL, Ziesche S, Yancy C, *et al.* Combination of isosorbide dinitrate and hydralazine in blacks with heart failure. *N Engl J Med* 2004;**351**:2049–57.
82. Nolan J, Batin PD, Andrews R, *et al.* Prospective study of heart rate variability and mortality in Chronic Heart Failure. *Circulation* 1998;**98**:1510–16.
83. Lee WH, Packer M. Prognostic importance of serum sodium concentration and its modification by converting-enzyme inhibition in patients with severe chronic heart failure. *Circulation* 1986;**73**:257–67.
84. Parameshwar J, Keegan J, Sparrow J, Sutton GC, Poole Wilson PA. Predictors of prognosis in severe chronic heart failure. *Am Heart J* 1992;**123**:421–6.
85. Aaronson KD, Schwartz JS, Chen TM, Wong KL, Goin JE, Mancini DM. Development and prospective validation of a clinical index to predict survival in ambulatory patients referred for cardiac transplant evaluation. *Circulation* 1997;**95**:2660–7.
86. Cleland JGF, Dargie HJ, Ford I. Mortality in heart failure: Clinical variables of prognostic value. *Br Heart J* 1987;**58**:572–82.
87. Eichhorn EJ, Tandon PK, DiBianco R, *et al.* Clinical and prognostic significance of serum magnesium concentration in patients with severe chronic congestive heart failure: the PROMISE Study. *J Am Coll Cardiol* 1993;**21**(3):634–40.
88. Jackson CE, Dalzell JR, Gardner RS. Prognostic utility of cardiac troponin in heart failure: a novel role for an established biomarker. *Biomark Med* 2009;**3**(5):483–93.
89. Sato Y, Yamada T, Taniguchi R, *et al.* Persistently increased serum concentrations of cardiac troponin T in patients with idiopathic dilated cardiomyopathy are predicitve of adverse outcomes. *Circulation* 2001;**103**:369–74.
90. Fonarow GC, Peacock WF, Horwich TB, Phillips CO, Givertz MM, Lopatin M *et al.* Usefulness of B-type natriuretic peptide and cardiac troponin levels to predict in-hospital mortality from ADHERE. *Am J Cardiol* 2008;**101**:231–7.
91. Leyva F, Anker SD, Godsland IF, *et al.* Uric acid in chronic heart failure: a marker of chronic inflammation. [see comments]. *Eur Heart J* 1998;**19**:1814–22.
92. Anker SD, Leyva F, Poole-Wilson P, Coats AJ. Uric acid as independent predictor of impaired prognosis in patients with chronic heart failure [Abstract]. *J Am Coll Cardiol* 1998;**31**:154–55A.
93. Struthers AD, Donnan PT, Lindsay P, McNaughton D, Broomhall J, MacDonald TM. Effect of allopurinol on mortality and hospitalisations in chronic heart failure: a retrospective cohort study. *Heart* 2002;**87**:229–34.
94. Sato Y, Takatsu Y, Yamada T, *et al.* Serial circulating concentrations of C-reactive protein, interleukin (Il)-4 and Il-6 in patients with acute left heart decompensation. *Clin Cardiol* 1999;**22**(12):811–13.
95. Alonso-Martinez JL, Llorente-Diez B, Echegaray-Agara M, *et al.* C-reactive protein as a predictor of improvement and readmission in heart failure. *Eur J Heart Fail* 2002;**4**:331–6.
96. Anand IS, Latini R, Florea VG, *et al.* C-reactive protein in heart failure: prognostic value and the effect of valsartan. *Circulation* 2005;**112**:1428–34.
97. Ezekowitz JA, McAlister FA, Armstrong PW. Anemia is common in heart failure and is associated with poor outcomes: Insights from a cohort of 12065 patients with new-onset heart failure. *Circulation* 2003;**107**:223–5.
98. Silverberg DS, Wexler D, Blum M, *et al.* The use of subcutaneous erythropoietin and intravenous iron for the treatment of the anemia of severe, resistant congestive heart failure improves cardiac and renal function and functional cardiac class, and markedly reduces hospitalizations. *J Am Coll Cardiol* 2000;**35**:1737–44.
99. Al Najjar Y, Goode KM, Zhang J, Cleland JG, Clark AL. Red cell distribution width: an inexpensive and powerful prognostic marker in heart failure. *Eur J Heart Fail* 2009;**11**:1155–62.
100. Pascual-Figal DA, Bonaque JC, Redondo B, *et al.* Red blood cell distribution width predicts long-term outcome regardless of anaemia status in acute heart failure patients. *Eur J Heart Fail* 2009;**11**:840–6.
101. Jackson CE, Dalzell JR, Bezlyak V, *et al.* Red cell distribution width has incremental prognostic value to B-type natriuretic peptide in acute heart failure. *Eur J Heart Fail* 2009;**11**:1152–4.
102. Cooper HA, Exner DV, Waclawiw MA, Domanski MJ. White blood cell count and mortality in patients with ischemic and nonischemic left ventricular systolic dysfunction (an analysis of the Studies of Left Ventricular Dysfunction [SOLVD]). *Am J Cardiol* 1999;**84**:252–7.
103. Gurbel PA, Gattis WA, Fuzaylov SY, *et al.* Evaluation of platelets in heart failure: Is platelet activity related to etiology, functional class, or clinical outcomes? *Am Heart J* 2002;**143**:1068–75.
104. Sharma R, Rauchhaus M, Ponikowski PP, *et al.* The relationship of the erythrocyte sedimentation rate to inflammatory cytokines and survival in patients with chronic heart failure treated with angiotensin-converting enzyme inhibitors. *J Am Coll Cardiol* 2000;**36**:523–8.

105. Sharma R, Rauchhaus M, Ponikowski PP, *et al.* The relationship of the erythrocyte sedimentation rate to inflammatory cytokines and survival in patients with chronic heart failure treated with angiotensin-converting enzyme inhibitors. *J Am Coll Cardiol* 2000;**36**:523–8.
106. Carson PE, Johnson GR, Dunkman WB, Fletcher RD, Farrell L, Cohn JN. The influence of atrial fibrillation on prognosis in mild to moderate heart failure. The V-HeFT Studies. The V-HeFT VA Cooperative Studies Group. *Circulation* 1993;**87**:VI102–10.
107. Dries DL, Exner DV, Gersh BJ, Domanski MJ, Waclawiw MA, Stevenson LW. Atrial fibrillation is associated with an increased risk for mortality and heart failure progression in patients with asymptomatic and symptomatic left ventricular systolic dysfunction: A retrospective analysis of the SOLVD trials. *J Am Coll Cardiol* 1998;**32**:695–703.
108. Olsson LG, Swedberg K, Ducharme A, *et al.* Atrial fibrillation and risk of clinical events in chronic heart failure with and without left ventricular systolic dysfunction: results from the Candesartan in Heart failure-Assessment of Reduction in Mortality and morbidity (CHARM) program. *J Am Coll Cardiol* 2006;**47**:1997–2004.
109. Stevenson WG, Stevenson LW, Middlekauff HR, *et al.* Improving survival for patients with atrial fibrillation and advanced heart failure. *J Am Coll Cardiol* 1996;**28**:1458–63.
110. Bilchick KC, Fetics B, Djoukeng R, *et al.* Prognostic value of heart rate variability in chronic congestive heart failure (Veterans Affairs' Survival Trial of Antiarrhythmic Therapy in Congestive Heart Failure). *Am Heart J* 2002;**90**:24–8.
111. Iuliano S, Fisher SG, Karasik PE, *et al.* QRS duration and mortality in patients with congestive heart failure. *Am Heart J* 2002;**143**:1085–91.
112. Baldasseroni S, Opasich C, Gorini M, *et al.* Left bundle branch block is associated with increased 1-year sudden and total mortality rate in 5517 outpatients with congestive heart failure: A report from the Italian Network on Congestive Heart Failure. *Am Heart J* 2002;**143**:398–405.
113. Shamim W, Yousufuddin M, Cicoria M, Gibson DG, Coats AJ, Henein MY. Incremental changes in QRS duration in serial ECGs over time identify high risk elderly patients with heart failure. *Heart* 2002;**88**:47–52.
114. Grigioni F, Carinci V, Boriani G, *et al.* Accelerated QRS widening as an independent predictor of cardiac death or the need for heart transplantation in patients with congestive heart failure. *J Heart Lung Transplant* 2002;**21**:899–901.
115. Brendorp B, Elming H, Jun L, *et al.* QT Dispersion has no prognostic information for patients with advanced congestive heart failure and reduced left ventricular systolic function. *Circulation* 2001;**103**:831–5.
116. Brooksby P, Batin PD, Nolan J, *et al.* The relationship between QT intervals and mortality in ambulant patients with chronic heart failure. The united kingdom heart failure evaluation and assessment of risk trial (UK-HEART). *Eur Heart J* 1999;**20**:1335–41.
117. Doval HC, Nul DR, Grancelli HO, *et al.* Nonsustained ventricular tachycardia in severe heart failure. Independent marker of increased mortality due to sudden death. GESICA-GEMA Investigators. *Circulation* 1996;**94**:3198–203.
118. Cohn J, Johnson G, Shabetai R, *et al.* for the V-HEFT VA Cooperative studies group. Ejection fraction, peak exercise consumption, cardiothoracic ratio and plasma norepinephrine as determinates of prognosis in heart failure. *Circulation* 1993;**87**:V1-5–16.
119. Kearney MT, Fox KA, Lee AJ, *et al.* Predicting sudden death in patients with mild to moderate chronic heart failure. *Heart* 2004;**90**:1137–43.
120. Baker BJ, Leddy C, Galie N, *et al.* Predictive value of M-mode echocardiography in patients with congestive heart failure. *Am Heart J* 1986;**111**:697–702.
121. Koelling TM, Aaronson KD, Cody RJ, Bach DS, Armstrong WF. Prognostic significance of mitral regurgitation and tricuspid regurgitation in patients with left ventricular systolic dysfunction. *Am Heart J* 2002;**144**, 524–9.
122. Williams MJ, Odabashian J, Lauer MS, Thomas JD, Marwick TH. Prognostic value of dobutamine echocardiography in patients with left ventricular dysfunction. *J Am Coll Cardiol* 1996;**27**:132–9.
123. Hundley WG, Morgan TM, Neagle, CM, Hamilton CA, Rerkpattanapipat P, Link KM. Magnetic resonance imaging determination of cardiac prognosis. *Circulation* 2002;**106**:2328–33.
124. Cohn JN. Prognosis in congestive heart failure. [Review]. *J Cardiac Fail* 1996;**2**:S225–9.
125. Nagaoka H, Isobe N, Kubota S, *et al.* Myocardial contractile reserve as prognostic determinant in patients with idiopathic dilated cardiomyopathy without overt heart failure. *Chest* 1997;**111**:344–50.
126. Di ST, Mathier M, Semigran MJ, Dec GW. Preserved right ventricular ejection fraction predicts exercise capacity and survival in advanced heart failure. *J Am Coll Cardiol* 1995;**25**:1143–53.
127. Szlachcic J, Massie B, Kramer B, *et al.* Correlates and prognostic implication of exercise capacity in chronic congestive heart failure. *Am J Cardiol* 1985;**55**:1037–42.
128. Likoff MJ, Chandler SL, Kay HR. Clinical determinants of mortality in chronic congestive heart failure secondary to idiopathic or dilated cardiomyopathy. *Am J Cardiol* 1987;**59**:634–8.
129. Cicoira M, Davos C, Florea V, *et al.* Chronic heart failure in the very elderly: clinical status, survival, and prognostic factors in 188 patients more than 70 years old. *Am Heart J* 2001;**142**: 174–80.
130. Myers J, Gullestad L, Vagelos R, *et al.* Cardiopulmonary exercise testing and prognosis in severe heart failure: 14 mL/kg/min revisited. *Am Heart J* 2000;**139**:78–84.
131. Mejhert M, Linder-Klingsell E, Edner M, Kahan T, Persson H. Ventilatory variables are strong prognostic markers in elderly patients with heart failure. *Heart* 2002;**88**:239–43.
132. Mancini DM, Eisen H, Kussmaul W, *et al.* Value of peak exercise consumption for optimal timing of cardiac transplantation in ambulatory patients with heart failure. *Circulation* 1991;**83**:778–86.
133. O'Neill JO, Young JB, Pothier CE, Lauer MS. Peak oxygen consumption as a predictor of death in patients with heart failure receiving beta-blockers. *Circulation* 2005;**111**:2313–18.
134. Aaronson KD, Mancini DM. Is percentage of predicted maximal exercise oxygen consumption a better predictor of survival than peak exercise oxygen consumption for patients with severe heart failure? *J Heart Lung Transplant* 1995;**14**:981–9.
135. Osman AF, Mehra MR, Lavie CJ, *et al.* The incremental prognostic importance of body fat adjusted peak oxygen consumption in chronic heart failure. *J Am Coll Cardiol* 2000;**36**:2126–31.
136. Bittner V, Weiner DH, Yusuf S, *et al.* Prediction of mortality and morbidity with a six-minute walk test in patients with left ventricular dysfunction. *JAMA* 1993;**270**: 1702–7.
137. Shah MR, Hasselblad V, Gheorghiade M, *et al.* Prognostic usefullness of the six-minute walk in patients with advanced congestive heart failure secondary to ischemic or nonischaemic cardiomyopathy. *Am J Cardiol* 2001;**88**:987–93.
138. Hüllsmann M, Berger R, Sturm B, *et al.* Prediction of outcome by neurohumoral activation, the six-minute walk test and the Minnesota Living with Heart Failure Questionnaire in an outpatient cohort with congestive heart failure. *Eur Heart J* 2002;**23**:886–91.
139. Opasich C, Pinna GD, Mazza A, *et al.* Six-minute walking performance in patients with moderate-to-severe heart failure. *Eur Heart J* 2001;**22**:488–96.
140. Keogh AM, Baron DW, Hickie JB. Prognostic guides in patients with idiopathic or ischemic dilated cardiomyopathy assessed for cardiac transplantation. *Am J Cardiol* 1990;**65**:903–8.

141. Griffin BP, Shah PK, Ferguson J, Rubin SA. Incremental prognostic value of exercise hemodynamic variables in chronic congestive heart failure secondary to coronary artery disease or dilated cardiomyopathy. *Am J Cardiol* 1991;**67**:848–53.
142. Morley D, Brozena S. Assessing risk by hemodynamic profile in patients awaiting cardiac transplantation. *Am J Cardiol* 1994;**73**:379–83.
143. Komajda M, Jais P, Reeves F, Goldfarb B, Bouhour JB. Factors predicting mortality in idiopathic dilated cardiomyopathy. *Eur Heart J* 1990;**11**:824–31.
144. Kirklin JK, Naftel DC, Kirklin JW, *et al.* Pulmonary vascular resistance and the risk of heart transplantation. *J Heart Lung Transplant* 1988;**7**:331–6.
145. Erickson, KW, Constanzo-Nordin, MR, O'Sullivan, EJ, *et al.* Influence of preoperative transpulmonary gradient on late mortality after orthotopic heart transplantation. *J Heart Lung Transplant* 1990;**9**:526–37.
146. Jougasaki M, Wei C, McKinley LJ. Elevation of circulating and ventricular adrenomedullin in human congestive heart failure. *Circulation* 1995;**92**:286–9.
147. Pousset F, Masson F, Chavirovskaia O, *et al.* Plasma adrenomedullin, a new independant predictor of prognosis in patients with chronic heart failure. *Eur Heart J* 2000;**21**:1009–14.
148. Gardner RS, Chong V, Morton I, McDonagh TA. N-terminal brain natriuretic peptide is a more powerful predictor of mortality than endothelin-1, adrenomedullin and tumour necrosis factor-alpha in patients referred for consideration of cardiac transplantation. *Eur J Heart Fail* 2005;**7**:253–60.
149. Richards AM, Nicholls G, Yandle TG, *et al.* Plasma N-Terminal pro-brain natriuretic peptide and adrenomedullin: new neurohormonal predcitors of left ventricular function and prognosis after myocardial infarction. *Circulation* 1998;**97**:1921–9.
150. Adlbrecht C, Hulsmann M, Strunk G, *et al.* Prognostic value of plasma midregional pro-adrenomedullin and C-terminal-pro-endothelin-1 in chronic heart failure outpatients. *Eur J Heart Fail* 2009;**11**:361–6.
151. Tsutamoto T, Wada A, Maeda K, *et al.* Plasma brain natriuretic peptide level as a biochemical marker of morbidity and mortality in patients with asymptomatic or minimally symptomatic left ventricular dysfunction. *Eur Heart J* 1999;**20**:1799–807.
152. Anand IS, Fisher LD, Chiang YT, *et al.* Changes in brain natriuretic peptide and norepinephrine over time and mortality and morbidity in the valsartan heart failure trial (Val-HeFT). *Circulation* 2003;**107**:1278–83.
153. McMurray JJ, Ray SG, Abdullah I, Dargie HJ, Morton JJ. Plasma endothelin in chronic heart failure. *Circulation* 1992;**85**:1374–9.
154. Pousset F, Isnard R, Lechat P, *et al.* Prognostic value of plasma endothelin-1 in patients with chronic heart failure. *Eur Heart J* 1997;**18**:254–8.
155. Pacher R, Stanek B, Hülsmann M, *et al.* Prognostic impact of big endothelin-1 plasma concentrations compared with invasive haemodynamic evaluation in severe heart failure. *J Am Coll Cardiol* 1996;**27**:633–41.
156. Stanek B, Frey B, Hülsmann M, *et al.* Validation of big endothelin plasma levels compared with established neurohormonal markers in patients with severe chronic heart failure. *Transplantation proceedings* 1997; **29**, 595–596.
157. Hülsmann M, Stanek B, Frey B, Sturm B, *et al.* Value of cardiopulmonary exercise testing and big endothelin plasma levels to predict short-term prognosis os patients with chronic heart failure. *J Am Coll Cardiol* 1998;**32**:1695–700.
158. Daggubati S, Parks JR, and Overton RM. Adrenomedullin, endothelin, neuropeptide Y, atrial, brain, and C-natriuretic prohormone peptides compared as early heart failure indicators. *Cardiovasc Res* 1997;**36**:246–55.
159. Cody RJ, Haas GJ, Binkley PF, *et al.* Plasma endothelin correlates with the extent of pulmonary hypertension in patients with chronic congestive heart failure. *Circulation* 1992;**85**:504–9.
160. Rickenbacher PR, Trindade PT, Haywood GA, *et al.* Transplant candidates with severe left ventricular dysfunction managed with medical treatment: characteristic and survival. *J Am Coll Cardiol* 1996;**27**:1192–7.
161. Lerman A, Gibbons RJ, Rodeheffer RJ, *et al.* Circulating N-terminal atrial natriuretic peptide as a marker for symptomless left-ventricular dysfunction. *Lancet* 1993;**341**:1105–9.
162. Francis GS, Benedict C, Johnstone DE, *et al.* Comparison of neuroendocrine activation in patients with left ventricular dysfunction with and without congestive heart failure: a substudy of the Studies of Left Ventricular Dysfunction (SOLVD). *Circulation* 1990;**82**:1724–9.
163. McDonagh TA, Cunningham AD, Morrison CE, McMurray JJ, Ford I, Morton JJ, and Dargie HJ. Left ventricular dysfunction, natriuretic peptides, and mortality in an urban population. *Heart* 2001;**86**:21–26.
164. Gegenhuber A, Struck J, Dieplinger B, *et al.* Comparative evaluation of B-type natriuretic peptide, mid-regional pro-A-type natriuretic peptide, mid-regional pro-adrenomedullin, and Copeptin to predict 1-year mortality in patients with acute destabilized heart failure. *J Card Fail* 2007;**13**:42–9.
165. von Haehling S, Jankowska EA, Morgenthaler NG, *et al.* Comparison of midregional pro-atrial natriuretic peptide with N-terminal pro-B-type natriuretic peptide in predicting survival in patients with chronic heart failure. *J Am Coll Cardiol* 2007;**50**:1973–80.
166. Moertl D, Berger R, Struck J, *et al.* Comparison of midregional pro-atrial and B-type natriuretic peptides in chronic heart failure: influencing factors, detection of left ventricular systolic dysfunction, and prediction of death. *J Am Coll Cardiol* 2009;**53**:1783–90.
167. Tsutamoto T, Wada A, Maeda K, *et al.* Attenuation of compensation of endogenous cardiac natriuretic peptide system in chronic heart failure: prognostic role of plasma brain natriuretic peptide concentration in patients with chronic symptomatic left ventricular dysfunction. *Circulation* 1997;**96**:509–16.
168. Gardner RS, Ozalp F, Murday AJ, Robb SD, McDonagh TA. N-terminal pro-brain natriuretic peptide. A new gold standard in predicting mortality in patients with advanced heart failure. *Eur Heart J* 2003;**24**:1735–43.
169. Levine B, Kalman J, Mayer L, *et al.* Elevated circulating levels of tumour necrosis factor in severe chronic heart failure. *N Engl J Med* 1990;**323**:236–41.
170. McMurray JJ, Abdullah I, Dargie HJ, *et al.* Increased concentrations of tumour necrosis factor in 'cachectic' patients with severe chronic heart failure. *Br Heart J* 1991;**66**:356–8.
171. Rauchhaus M, Doehner W, Francis DP. Plasma cytokine parameters and mortality in patients with chronic heart failure. *Circulation* 2000;**102**:3060–7.
172. Kell R, Haunstetter A, Dengler TJ. Do cytokines enable risk stratification to be improved in NYHA functional class III patients? *Eur Heart J* 2002;**23**:70–8.
173. Dalzell JR, Jackson CE, McDonagh TA, Gardner RS. Novel biomarkers in heart failure: an overview. *Biomark Med* 2009;**3**(5):483–93.
174. Levy WC, Mozaffarian D, Linker DT, *et al.* The Seattle Heart Failure Model: prediction of survival in heart failure. *Circulation* 2006;**113**:1424–33.
175. Aaronson KD, Schwartz JS, Chen TM, Wong KL, Goin JE, Mancini DM. Development and prospective validation of a clinical

index to predict survival in ambulatory patients referred for cardiac transplant evaluation. *Circulation* 1997;**95**:2660–7.

176. Lee DS, Austin PC, Rouleau JL, Liu PP, Naimark D, Tu JV. Predicting mortality among patients hospitalized for heart failure: derivation and validation of a clinical model. *JAMA* 2003;**290**:2581–7.

177. Koelling TM, Joseph S, Aaronson KD. Heart failure survival score continues to predict clinical outcomes in patients with heart failure receiving beta-blockers. *J Heart Lung Transplant* 2004;**23**:1414–22.

178. Zugck C, Kruger C, Kell R, *et al.* Risk stratification in middle-aged patients with congestive heart failure: prospective comparison with the heart failure survival score (HFSS) and a simplified two-variable model. *Eur J Heart Fail* 2001;**3**:577–85.

179. Mozaffarian D, Anker SD, Anand I, *et al.* Prediction of mode of death in heart failure: the Seattle Heart Failure Model. *Circulation* 2007;**116**:392–8.

180. Cleland JG, Daubert JC, Erdmann E, *et al.*, and Cardiac Resynchronization-Heart Failure (CARE-HF) Study Investigators. The effect of cardiac resynchronization on morbidity and mortality in heart failure. *N Engl J Med* 2005;**352**(15): 1539–49.

181. Murdoch DR, Byrne J, Morton JJ, *et al.* Brain natriuretic peptide is stable in whole blood and can be measured using a simple rapid assay: implications for clinical practice. *Heart* 1997;**78**: 594–7.

PART X

Comorbidities: the patients with heart failure and . . .

26

Diastolic heart failure

Andrew L. Clark

The vast majority of clinical trials in patients with chronic heart failure (CHF) have been conducted in patients with left ventricular systolic dysfunction (LVSD). Although defining CHF can be difficult, its pragmatic definition requiring symptoms compatible with the syndrome in the presence of cardiac dysfunction makes LVSD relatively easy to identify. This is the appeal of the left ventricular ejection fraction (LVEF) as a measurement—a normal range can be established, and those people who are breathless on exertion and whose ejection fraction falls below the normal range are labelled as having heart failure (HF).

This pragmatic approach to identifying patients who should be treated leaves a large group of people who have undoubted symptoms compatible with a diagnosis of CHF, but who have normal (or at most mildly impaired) left ventricular systolic function. There are many reports suggesting that perhaps half of all patients with HF fall into this category, and various labels are used.

- Diastolic HF implies that there is some objective abnormality of diastolic function to explain the symptoms: in turn, there is the implication that 'normal' diastolic function is well described, allowing diastolic dysfunction to be well defined.[1]
- HF with preserved systolic function (or variants thereof) implies that systolic function is normal and that any abnormality must be restricted to diastole.
- HF with normal ejection fraction (HeFNEF) is a more pragmatic description, but does imply that there is some way of being certain that the symptoms are due to the heart, even if the heart appears normal on imaging.

There is a range of difficulties in discussing 'diastolic HF'. Despite the apparent commonness of the condition in epidemiological studies,[2,3] many clinicians, even HF specialists, are sceptical about the diagnosis and its frequency.[4–6] Unlike the situation with clinical trials of patients with systolic left ventricular dysfunction, it has proved difficult to recruit patients to diastolic HF trials, and the more stringent the requirements for objective evidence of diastolic dysfunction, the more difficult it has been to recruit. A further surprise, perhaps, is that no clinical trial has yet demonstrated robust survival evidence for any specific HF therapy in patients with diastolic HF, suggesting that diastolic HF may be pathophysiologically distinct.

Pathophysiology

Patients with systolic left ventricular dysfunction have impaired diastolic function, too, often due to increased fibrous tissue. In those with HF and normal systolic function, the defect lies with predominant impairment of left ventricular filling. This will usually happen with a ventricle that is 'stiff' and has decreased compliance—that is, the relation between pressure and volume is shifted so that it requires a greater pressure than normal to increase the volume of the left ventricle prior to the next contraction. Ventricular filling (and subsequent stroke volume) is preserved, but at a cost of an increase in left ventricular diastolic pressure.

The increased left ventricular diastolic pressure is necessarily accompanied by an increase in left atrial pressure, and, in turn, pulmonary venous pressure. The pulmonary venous hypertension causes the lungs to stiffen, and can result in pulmonary oedema formation if it becomes very severe. Breathlessness is an obvious consequence.

A variety of changes might be seen in the heart. Left ventricular hypertrophy is very common, and might be considered a defining feature of 'diastolic dysfunction'. Similarly, left atrial dilatation is an almost inevitable consequence, and in its absence, an alternative for breathlessness should be sought.

End-diastolic pressure–volume relation

If this description of diastolic HF is correct, then there should be an upward shift in the end-diastolic pressure–volume relation of the left ventricle (Fig. 26.1A). An increase in end-diastolic pressure would not constitute 'diastolic dysfunction', but could simply represent increased preload. Measuring the pressure–volume relation is difficult, and has to be performed over a wide range as the relation between the two variables is nonlinear (Fig. 26.1B): stiffness,

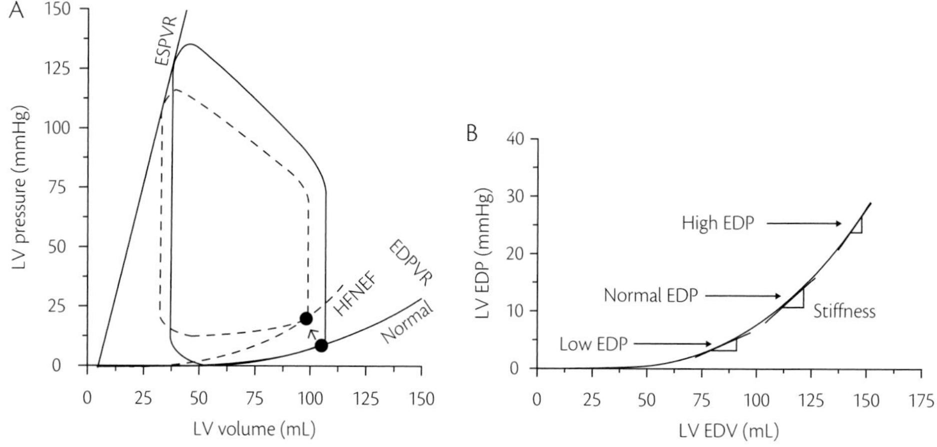

Fig. 26.1 (A) Pressure–volume relations within the left ventricle. For HeFNEF to be due to diastolic dysfunction, the end - diastolic pressure–volume relation (EDPVR) should be shifted upwards and to the left so that to reach a given left ventricular volume, the pressure required is greater. (B) The EDPVR is nonlinear: at higher volumes, the stiffness (measured as a tangent to the line) increases so that for a given increase in volume, the pressure change is greater than at smaller left ventricular volumes. Thus, simply demonstrating increased stiffness of the heart does not establish the presence of diastolic dysfunction.

represented by the slope of the relation between pressure and volume, increases with volume and pressure.

However, where the end-diastolic pressure–volume relation has been specifically measured, there is little evidence of a consistent alteration in the relation: in fact, quite the reverse. In individual subjects with apparent HF and normal ejection fraction, the relation might be normal, increased, or decreased (Fig. 26.2).[4,7,8]

Transmitral flow

A major feature of diastolic dysfunction is an alteration in transmitral diastolic blood flow. In the normal (young) adult, most ventricular filling occurs early in diastole and is largely passive (although there is some evidence that there may be an active component from left ventricular suction). The contribution of left atrial contraction to left ventricular filling is small. The transmitral filling pattern seen on Doppler echocardiography is thus typically a large E or 'early' wave and a small A or 'atrial' wave.

As diastolic HF develops and left ventricle compliance decreases, the transmitral blood flow pattern changes. The E wave becomes relatively smaller and the A wave larger as atrial contraction becomes an important determinant of left ventricular filling. The A wave becomes larger than the E wave—so called 'E:A reversal'. At the same time, the rate of decline of flow from the peak of the E wave, usually brisk, decreases, thus prolonging the E wave deceleration time and abbreviating the mid-diastolic diastasis.

Ultimately, a pattern of 'pseudonormalization' may develop in which the left ventricular diastolic pressure has risen sufficiently high that atrial contraction is no longer able adequately to compensate for the decline in early filling and left atrial pressure rises further. Most left ventricular filling now reverts to being early and passive with a smaller contribution from atrial contraction: this time, however, at a cost of very high left atrial pressure and a very brisk E wave deceleration time.

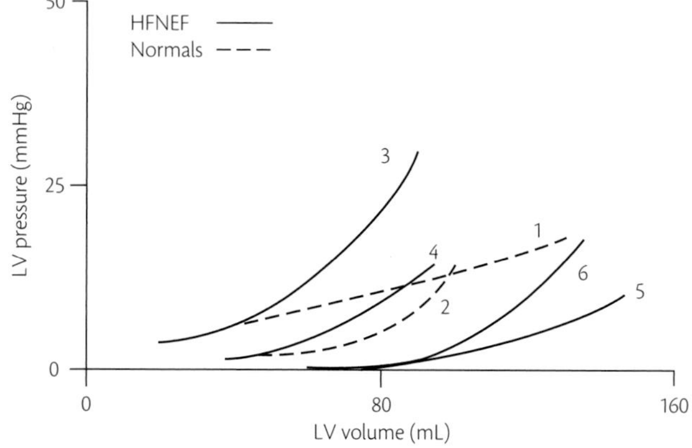

Fig. 26.2 Left ventricular end-diastolic pressure–volume relations from individual patients. Not that for patients with HeFNEF, the relation might be the same as normal or shifted to left or right.

Diagnosis of diastolic dysfunction

The definitive diagnosis of diastolic dysfunction rests with analysis of pressure–volume loops recorded from the left ventricle during diastole. This is impractical for routine clinical practice, meaning that cardiac imaging, and in particular echocardiography with Doppler analysis of transmitral blood flow, has become the diagnostic method most widely used. However, transmitral blood flow is highly dependent on filling conditions,[9] and so the analysis of diastolic function has to be broader. The key components of echocardiographic analysis are the assessment of transmitral flow, the assessment of motion of the mitral valve annulus, and assessment of pulmonary venous blood flow. In addition, evidence of cardiac structural changes (particularly left atrial dilation and left ventricular hypertrophy) is important.

Tissue Doppler interrogation of the mitral annulus particularly targets long-axis function of the left ventricle and is achieved by setting the filters and gains of the echo machine to record information of the relatively slow-moving tissues (over ranges of centimetres per second) as opposed to blood (moving over ranges of metres per second). In health, there is a movement of the base towards the apex recorded as the S wave, and during diastole E and A motion corresponding to the transmitral E and A waves. The tissue movements are known as E′ and A′ (or E_m and A_m, or E_a and A_a, 'm' meaning mitral and 'a' annular).

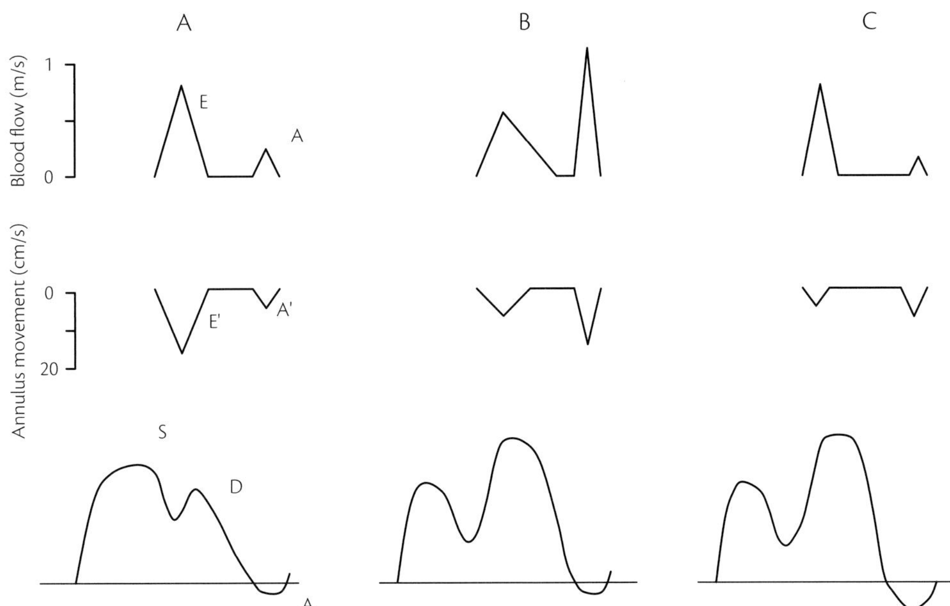

Fig. 26.3 Schematic of echocardiographic changes in diastolic dysfunction. The top row is transmitral blood flow; the middle row is movement of the mitral valve annulus with tissue Doppler, and the bottom row is pulmonary venous blood flow. A is the normal state: The mitral E wave is much greater than the A wave; most pulmonary blood flow is in systole. With increasing diastolic dysfunction (B), the mitral A wave becomes larger than the E ('E:A reversal'); the mitral annular is similarly affected and most pulmonary vein flow is in diastole. Finally, with severe diastolic dysfunction, the E:A ratio reverses again ('pseudonormalization'), but with a very short E wave; mitral annular motion is much reduced, with the ratio of E to E′ reduced. Pulmonary venous blood flow is further dominated by diastolic flow, with an increasing retrograde A wave.

There are two distinct pulses of blood flow into the left atrium from the pulmonary veins: one during systole (the larger in health) and one during diastole. There is some reversal of flow back into the pulmonary veins during atrial systole—the A wave.

Integrating these three movements is the major method for assessing diastolic function (Fig. 26.3). As left ventricular compliance falls and left atrial pressure rises, there is first a phase of abnormal relaxation during which there is reversal of the E:A ratio accompanied by reduction in E′ and reversal of the E′:A′ ratio. The diastolic component of pulmonary venous flow increases. Then, as diastolic function worsens, 'pseudonormalization' of transmitral flow is accompanied by more and more marked reduction in mitral annular diastolic motion, greater increases in diastolic pulmonary venous flow, and more marked reversal of pulmonary venous flow during atrial contraction.

A variety of methods for estimating diastolic pressures from echocardiographic data has been described, but the one in most widespread use is the ratio between transmitral E and mitral annular E′ motion. There is a linear relation between the E:E′ ratio and left ventricular filling pressure.[10] In health, the ratio is usually below 10, and a ratio above 20 strongly suggests that left atrial pressure is above 20 mmHg. A particular advantage of using the ratio is that it remains helpful in patients who have atrial fibrillation.

Epidemiology and clinical pattern

Perhaps as many as 60% of patients with CHF have HeFNEF (Fig. 26.4).[2,11] The cause of the HF is much more likely to be related to uncontrolled hypertension than in patients with systolic dysfunction.[12] Epidemiological data regularly suggest that patients with diastolic HF compared with systolic HF are: older by about 10 years or so; have a lower haemoglobin; are more likely to be overweight; are more likely to have atrial fibrillation (AF); are more likely to have diabetes; and are far more likely to be female.[2,13,14] The proportion of patients with 'preserved systolic function' has increased with time.[2]

It is difficult to be certain whether diastolic HF exists in a chronic state: the strong association with AF, particularly incident AF,[11] and hypertension, lead to the suggestion that apparent HeFNEF might be an acute condition, more likely to present as acute pulmonary oedema and rapidly resolving with treatment.[15] In this scenario, an acute event precipitates an episode of HF and an admission to hospital, but the resolution of symptoms means that such patients are likely to be under-represented in outpatient populations in

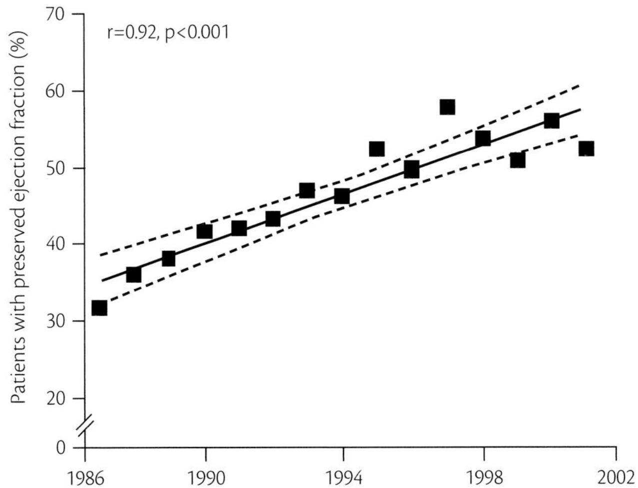

Fig. 26.4 The proportion of patients with heart failure who have a normal ejection fraction increased between 1986 and 2002.

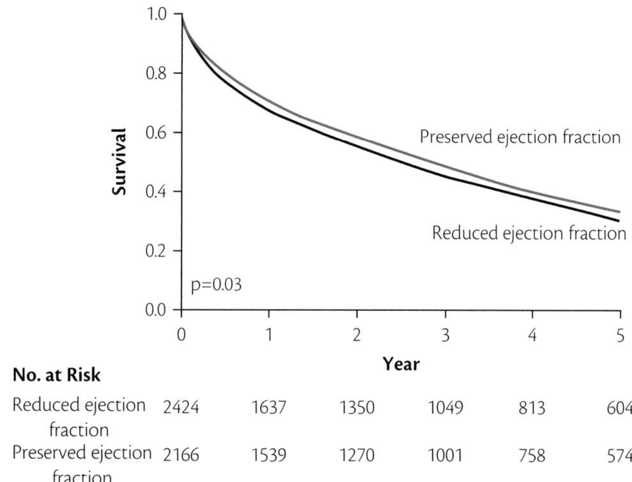

Fig. 26.5 The prognosis of patients with heart failure appears to be similar regardless of whether left ventricular ejection fraction is reduced.

CHF clinics. In some patients, then, it might be that there has been transient systolic dysfunction that has resolved before any left ventricular imaging has taken place.

The prognosis of patients with HF and normal ejection fraction remains controversial. Some studies suggest that the prognosis is just the same as for patients with impaired left ventricular function,[3] slightly better,[2] or much better.[16] The general consensus is that the prognosis is similar regardless of ejection fraction (Fig. 26.5).

Diagnostic difficulties

Abnormal diastolic function estimated from echocardiography is extremely common in patients with LVSD. Very grossly abnormal diastolic function in the absence of systolic dysfunction is much less common, and most patients diagnosed as having 'diastolic HF' have much less marked abnormalities of diastolic function. A difficulty then arises as the changes of diastolic dysfunction are in many cases indistinguishable from the effects of ageing on the heart.

Reliable echocardiographic criteria for the diagnosis of diastolic dysfunction have proved elusive.[17] There may be up to a 16-fold difference in the prevalence of diastolic dysfunction depending upon which measure is chosen. Various complex methodologies for accounting for the effects of age on diastolic function have been proposed, but these do not all reliably correlate with each other. There is a very marked degree of overlap for many of the proposed measured of diastolic function between breathless patients (labelled as diastolic HF) and an age-matched reference population.[18] A further complicating issue is that very many patients with apparent diastolic HF are in AF, making assessment of transmitral flow fraught.

Some authors have even suggested that detailed assessment of diastolic dysfunction may not be necessary.[19] Such a radical approach glosses over the usual effects of ageing where there is selective impairment of the longitudinal component of systolic contraction and consequent reduction in mitral annular velocities,[20] as compared with preservation of normal global indices of left ventricular systolic function.[21,22]

The final position might then seem to be that what distinguishes a patient with diastolic HF from an older person without HF is simply the presence of symptoms of breathlessness—in both, similar changes in the diastolic properties of the heart have happened.

An obvious problem with such an approach is that there is a long list of potential causes of breathlessness. This has led some to suggest that in many patients with supposed diastolic HF there may be another cause for breathlessness; for example, Caruana and colleagues suggest that more than 95% of such patients had an alternative explanation for symptoms of breathlessness.[23]

One cause of breathlessness in elderly people that is often overlooked is that of muscle wasting and lack of skeletal muscle fitness. Exercise capacity and breathlessness is strongly related to skeletal muscle bulk, and loss of bulk and muscle quality is extremely common with age (for review, see reference 24). The relation between muscle bulk and quality and exercise capacity is a recurrent theme in studies of patients with CHF due to LVSD,[25,26] but the issue has not been studied in patients with diastolic HF.

A further point to consider is that the definition of a 'normal' ejection fraction has larger arisen from the criteria used to define patients for inclusion into trials of systolic HF. The lower end of the normal range, conventionally taken as 45% or 50% when measured by echo, is almost certainly too low and does not take into account change in ejection fraction: a breathless patient whose ejection fraction has fallen from 75% to 50% may be labelled as having 'diastolic HF' when their systolic function is clearly markedly impaired compared with their normal. In recognition, US guidelines now state that the lower end of the normal range should be 55%,[27] but such a definition immediately presents a new problem: perhaps as many as a quarter of apparently normal people might be labelled as having impaired LV systolic function.[28]

It may be, too, that patients with 'diastolic HF' actually have more subtle abnormalities of systolic function than can simply be accounted for by measuring LVEF. We and others have shown that many patients have abnormal long-axis systolic function with normal LVEF,[29,30] and a key study actually studying patients as they develop symptoms (that is, during exercise) demonstrates that most patients with HeFNEF have widespread abnormalities of both systolic and diastolic function that become much more obvious on exercise.[31]

Lessons from clinical trials

Clinical trials into the effectiveness of treatment for HF due to diastolic dysfunction have now been conducted. None has shown benefit for a specific treatment, but the data accumulated do shed some light on the problem. The trials have had different definitions of the HF syndrome, and a generally trend is that the more rigorous the definition of HF, the more difficult it was to recruit patients to the trial (Table 26.1).

An ancillary study of the DIG trial of digoxin in HF[32] specifically focused on those with HF and normal LVEF. The majority had NYHA class II symptoms. Digoxin had no effect on outcome. The definition of HF was not very robust: a past history of limitation of activity coupled with basal crackles and some oedema is a very common collection of symptoms and signs, even in the absence of cardiac pathology.

In the CHARM-Preserved limb of the CHARM programme,[33] candesartan had no effect on outcome. The definition of HF was again very inclusive. It is very striking that small numbers of

Table 26.1 Summary of heart failure clinical trials

Trial	N	Age	% male	% AF	LVEF (%)	On loop (%)	NT - proBNP	Definition of heart failure
DIG (digoxin)	988	67	60	0	55	76[a]		Current or past symptoms (fatigue, dyspnoea, orthopnoea, limitation of activity) Signs: rales, ↑JVP, oedema, S3 Pulmonary congestion on CXR
CHARM-Preserved (candesartan)	3 023	67.2	60	20	54	75[a]	376 (mild DD) 1419 (more severe DD)[b]	NYHA II/III >4 weeks Hospital admission for cardiac cause Oedema 30%; orthopnoea 20%; crackles 15%; high JVP 7%; S3 5%; upper-zone redistribution 3%
I-Preserve (irbesartan)	4 128	72	40	17 (29% with history)	60	52	c.340 pg/mL	Heart failure symptoms; AND LVEF ≥45% AND HF hospitalization within 6 months (II–III) (44%) Or No hospitalization (III–V) AND corroborative evidence (congestion on CXR; LA dilation or LVH on echo; LBBB)
PEP-CHF (perindopril)	850	75	43	20	65	45	c.400 pg/mL	Treated with diuretics for CHF AND cardiovascular hospitalization within 6 months AND ≥3 clinical criteria Exertional breathlessness, orthopnoea or PND; ankle swelling; improved breathlessness with diuretic therapy; increased JVP; previous clinical pulmonary oedema; previous MI; cardiothoracic ratio >0.55; previous radiological pulmonary oedema. AND ≥ 2 echo criteria LV WMI 1.4–1.6 (LVEF 40—50) LA >.25 mm/m2 body surface area or .40 mm IVS posterior wall ≥ 12 mm impaired LV filling (ESC criteria)
Seniors (nebivolol)	2 128	76	63	20	36 (35% >35%)	86a	n/a	Admission with heart failure in previous 6 months OR LVEF ≤ 35% in previous 6 months

[a] Loop not differentiated from thiazide diuretic in report.

[b] Data from echocardiographic substudy (N = 181), Grewal J, McKelvie RS, Persson H, *et al.* Usefulness of N-terminal pro-brain natriuretic peptide and brain natriuretic peptide to predict cardiovascular outcomes in patients with heart failure and preserved LVEF. *Am J Cardiol* 2008;**102:**733–7.)

To convert pg/mL to pmol/L, divide by 8.457.

CXR, chest radiograph; JVP, jugular venous pressure; LA, left atrium; LBBB, left bundle branch block; LVEF, left ventricular ejection fraction; LVH, left ventricular hypertrophy; n/a, not available; PND, paroxysmal nocturnal dyspnoea.

patients had 'hard' signs of HF at randomization, and the harder the sign, the lower the number of patients.

There was a similar finding in I-Preserve which tested the possible role of irbesartan.[34] The definition of HF was tighter than in previous trials. In PEP-CHF,[35] the angiotensin converting enzyme (ACE) inhibitor perindopril was tested, again showing no beneficial effect on outcome. The HF definition was much the strictest of the trials under discussion, and of note, it was much harder to recruit patients to this trial.

In a much smaller trial, the Hong Kong Diastolic Heart Failure study,[36] whilst diuretics relieved symptoms, there was no effect of either irbesartan or ramipril used in addition. There was a similar decline in NT-proBNP in all three groups.

Finally, the SENIORS study of nebivolol in older patients with HF[37] did not have an ejection fraction inclusion criterion: around one-third had an ejection fraction over 35%. Although nebivolol use was associated with a reduction in event rate, there was no effect on all-cause mortality. There was no difference in the effect of nebivolol between those with a low or a 'high' ejection fraction. However, as the results are only reported above and below a cut-off of 35%, it is impossible really to assess how many patients might have had true diastolic HF.

Other points to note are that, where values are given, the NT-proBNP was not high, and, indeed, many of the patients not only had results in the normal range,[38] but would have had a result that puts them below the diagnostic threshold recommended by the European Society of Cardiology (ESC).[39] Another striking feature is that (where the data are given) the proportion of patients actually being treated with a loop diuretic is low for a population with CHF. Event rates were also low. Such a thing is common in HF trials, but conspicuous in diastolic HF trials. In PEP-CHF,[40] for example, the sample size calculation was based on data suggesting that older patients with HF and a recent hospital admission had an annual mortality of 10–20%, a readmission rate for HF of 30%, and a risk of death or readmission of about 50%, but in the trial, only around 25% reached a primary endpoint.

A further remarkable feature of the results from clinical trials of HF generally is that there is an extremely strong relation between LVEF and survival.[41,42] The relation between increasing LVEF and increasing survival is very potent and seen in most databases examined. The finding simply does not sit happily with the suggestion that the outcome for patients with CHF is the same regardless of left ventricular systolic function. A possible explanation is that there may be two groups of patients: those with 'systolic HF' in whom an increasing ejection fraction is beneficial; and a second, pathophysiologically distinct, group with 'diastolic HF' in whom ejection fraction is irrelevant. Such a division does not seem very likely.

Unresolved issues

Do patients with 'diastolic heart failure' have heart disease at all?

Underlying many discussions of HF is the position that while many patients have symptoms of breathlessness and fatigue, there is no certainty that the symptoms come from the heart. The approach of comparing indices of diastolic function between elderly breathless women and young healthy men is not satisfactory, and where an appropriate comparator population is used, there is often no echocardiographic difference between patients and normal subjects.

Many of the patients included in clinical trials and epidemiological studies almost certainly did not have HF. That is not to say that they did not have symptoms of breathlessness, and nor is it to say that they did not have a poor prognosis: indeed, we may just be seeing that the presence of breathlessness is a poor prognostic feature in elderly people regardless of the underlying cause.

As outlined above, the diagnosis of diastolic HF, despite the extensive research into potential echocardiographic variables to define it, remains a diagnosis of exclusion. For many patients, the diagnosis of diastolic HF will miss true underlying pathology and potentially prevent appropriate therapy.

What is needed is some objective measure that defines HF as present that is independent of echocardiographic variables. Such a method may be natriuretic peptide measurement. The N-terminal pro-B-type natriuretic peptide (NT-proBNP) has been most widely studied. It is released from the heart in response to myocardial stretch, and its increase is related to the severity of HF symptoms and to left ventricular size (and ejection fraction).[43]

The ESC has recently revised its guidelines for the diagnosis of HF to suggest that below a threshold value for NT-proBNP of 400 pg/mL, HF is unlikely. Such a threshold suggests that many patients in the diastolic HF trials did not have HF at all, so it is perhaps not surprising that therapies directed at CHF did reduce mortality.

Some have suggested that it might be unreasonable to expect NT-proBNP to rise in diastolic dysfunction as no stretch is involved: there is, however, an increase in wall stress which will cause NT-proBNP to rise. Data from a subgroup of 375 patients in the PEP-CHF study show that the threshold suggested by the ESC does indeed select out those patients with a worse prognosis;[44] below the threshold value, death rates are not appreciably greater than in an age-matched population.

In line with these ideas, we have found that patients with a diagnosis of diastolic HF had greater awareness of breathlessness for a given level of ventilation during exercise than control subjects, and, indeed, control subjects with the same echocardiographic markers of diastolic dysfunction but no symptoms.[45] In a similar group of patients diagnosed as having diastolic HF, we have found that the patients were every bit as symptom limited as patients with confirmed HF due to LVSD, but had values for NT-proBNP in the normal range.[46]

If they do have heart disease, is it 'heart failure'?

Even if an individual with symptoms of HF can definitely be labelled as having some cardiac pathology as the cause, the old mantra that HF is a syndrome, not a diagnosis, remains vitally important. It can be very easy to diagnose HeFNEF in someone presenting, say, with acute pulmonary oedema, and to assume that this represents a definitive statement. Such an approach will lead to patients with underlying acute ischaemia, mitral regurgitation, paroxysmal arrhythmia, or hypertension being mismanaged.

In practice, before a final diagnosis of HeFNEF is reached, these alternatives must be treated as appropriate or excluded.

If they do have heart failure, is it 'diastolic'?

Some patients do have HF with a normal ejection fraction, but the distinction between 'diastolic' and 'systolic' HF based on a single variable—left ventricular ejection fraction—is to oversimplify the complex relations between all parts of the cardiac cycle. Detailed research into myocardial contraction has repeatedly demonstrated that the majority of patients with diastolic HF have systolic abnormalities as well.

Concluding remarks

'Diastolic HF' has entered the common parlance of cardiology and some HF specialists. Some specialists remain sceptical, however. The diagnosis in fact covers many different groups of patients and it is a mistake to try and treat them as all being the same. 'Diastolic HF' as a diagnostic umbrella includes many patients with no cardiac explanation for their symptoms; it includes some with other cardiac pathology; and it includes some with HF and systolic dysfunction.

The most likely way forward for unravelling some of the complexities discussed is the use of NT-proBNP to define in the first instance patients who actually have cardiac pathology. Only once such an apparently independent index of cardiac function is used can investigators be certain that they are truly dealing with cardiac illness and not the echocardiographic changes of age.

References

1. Zile MR, Brutsaert DL. New concepts in diastolic dysfunction, diastolic heart failure: part I: diagnosis, prognosis, measurements of diastolic function. *Circulation* 2002;**105**:1387–1393.
2. Owan TE, Hodge DO, Herges RM, Jacobsen SJ, Roger VL, Redfield MM. Trends in prevalence and outcome of heart failure with preserved ejection fraction. *N Engl J Med* 2006;**355**:251–9.
3. Bhatia RS, Tu JV, Lee DS, *et al*. Outcome of heart failure with preserved ejection fraction in a population-based study. *N Engl J Med* 2006;**355**:260–9.
4. Burkhoff D, Maurer MS, Packer M. Heart failure with a normal ejection fraction: is it really a disorder of diastolic function?. *Circulation* 2003;**107**:656–8.
5. Maurer MS, King DL, El-Khoury Rumbarger L, Packer M, Burkhoff D. Left heart failure with a normal ejection fraction: identification of different pathophysiologic mechanisms. *J Card Fail* 2005;**11**:177–87.
6. Brutsaert DL, De Keulenaer GW. Diastolic heart failure: a myth. *Curr Opin Cardiol* 2006;**21**:240–8.
7. Liu CP, Ting CT, Lawrence W, Maughan WL, Chang MS, Kass DA. Diminished contractile response to increased heart rate in intact human left ventricular hypertrophy: systolic versus diastolic determinants. *Circulation* 1993;**88**:1893–906.
8. Kawaguchi M, Hay I, Fetics B, Kass DA. Combined ventricular and arterial stiffening in patients with heart failure and preserved ejection fraction: implications for systolic and diastolic reserve limitations. *Circulation* 2003;**107**: 714–720.
9. Stoddard MF, Pearson AC, Kern MJ, Ratcliff J, Mrosek DG, Labovitz AJ. Influence of alteration in preload on the pattern of left ventricular diastolic filling as assessed by Doppler echocardiography in humans. *Circulation* 1989;**79**:1226–36.
10. Nagueh SF, Mikati I, Kopelen HA, Middleton KJ, Quiñones MA, Zoghbi WA. Doppler estimation of left ventricular filling pressure in sinus tachycardia. A new application of tissue Doppler imaging. *Circulation* 1998;**98**:1644–50.
11. Hogg K, Swedberg K, McMurray J. Heart failure with preserved left ventricular systolic function: epidemiology, clinical characteristics, and prognosis. *J Am Coll Cardiol* 2004;**43**:317–27.
12. Yip GWK, Ho PPY, Woo KS, *et al*. Comparison of frequencies of left ventricular systolic and diastolic heart failure in Chinese living in Hong Kong. *Am J Cardiol* 1999;**84**:563–7.
13. Hogg K, Swedberg K, McMurray J. Heart failure with preserved left ventricular systolic function; epidemiology, clinical characteristics, and prognosis. *J Am Coll Cardiol* 2004;**43**:317–27.
14. Owan T, Redfield M. Epidemiology of diastolic heart failure. *Prog Cardiovasc Dis* 2005;**47**:320–32.
15. Banerjee P, Clark AL, Nikitin N, Cleland JG. Diastolic heart failure. Paroxysmal or chronic? *Eur J Heart Fail* 2004;**6**:427–31.
16. Philbin EF, Rocco TA Jr, Lindenmuth NW, Ulrich K, Jenkins PL. Systolic versus diastolic heart failure in community practice: clinical features, outcomes, and the use of angiotensin-converting enzyme inhibitors. *Am J Med* 2000;**109**:605–13.
17. Petrie MC, Hogg K, Caruana L, McMurray JJ. Poor concordance of commonly used echocardiographic measures of left ventricular diastolic function in patients with suspected heart failure but preserved systolic function: is there a reliable echocardiographic measure of diastolic dysfunction? *Heart* 2004;**90**:511–17.
18. Sim MF, Ho SF, O'Mahony MS, Steward JA, Buchalter M, Burr M. European reference values for Doppler indices of left ventricular diastolic filling. *Eur J Heart Fail* 2004;**6**:433–8.
19. Zile MR, Gaasch WH, Carroll JD, *et al.*Heart failure with a normal ejection fraction: is measurement of diastolic function necessary to make the diagnosis of diastolic heart failure?. *Circulation* 2001;**104**:779–82.
20. Nikitin NP, Witte KK, Ingle L, Clark AL, Farnsworth TA, Cleland JG. Longitudinal myocardial dysfunction in healthy older subjects as a manifestation of cardiac ageing. *Age Ageing* 2005;**34**:343–9.
21. Klein AL, Leung DY, Murray RD, Urban LH, Bailey KR, Tajik AJ. Effects of age and physiologic variables on right ventricular filling dynamics in normal subjects. *Am J Cardiol* 1999;**84**:440–8.
22. Pfisterer ME, Battler A, Zaret BL. Range of normal values for left and right ventricular ejection fraction at rest and during exercise assessed by radionuclide angiocardiography. *Eur Heart J* 1985;**6**:647–55.
23. Caruana L, Petrie MC, Davie AP, McMurray JJ. Do patients with suspected heart failure and preserved left ventricular systolic function suffer from 'diastolic heart failure' or from misdiagnosis? A prospective descriptive study. *BMJ* 2000;**321**:215–18.
24. Thompson LV. Age-related muscle dysfunction. *Exp Gerontol* 2009;**44**:106–11.
25. Anker SD, Swan JW, Volterrani M, *et al*. The influence of muscle mass, strength, fatigability and blood flow on exercise capacity in cachectic and non-cachectic patients with chronic heart failure. *Eur Heart J* 1997;**18**:259–69.
26. Harrington D, Clark AL, Chua TP, Anker SD, Poole-Wilson PA, Coats AJ. Effect of reduced muscle bulk on the ventilatory response to exercise in chronic congestive heart failure secondary to idiopathic dilated and ischemic cardiomyopathy. *Am J Cardiol* 1997;80:90–3.
27. Lang RM, Bierig M, Devereux RB *et al.*; Chamber Quantification Writing Group; American Society of Echocardiography's Guidelines and Standards Committee; European Association of Echocardiography. Recommendations for chamber quantification: a report from the American Society of Echocardiography's Guidelines and Standards Committee and the Chamber Quantification Writing Group, developed in conjunction with the European Association of Echocardiography, a branch of the European Society of Cardiology. *J Am Soc Echocardiogr* 2005;**18**:1440–63.
28. Mahadevan G, Davis RC, Frenneaux MP, *et al*. Left ventricular ejection fraction: are the revised cut-off points for defining systolic dysfunction sufficiently evidence based?. *Heart* 2008;**94**:426–8.
29. Nikitin NP, Witte KK, Clark AL, Cleland JG. Color tissue Doppler-derived long-axis left ventricular function in heart failure with preserved global systolic function. *Am J Cardiol* 2002;**90**:1174–7.
30. Petrie MC, Caruana L, Berry C, McMurray JJ. 'Diastolic heart failure' or heart failure caused by subtle left ventricular systolic dysfunction?. *Heart* 2002;**87**:29–31.
31. Tan YT, Wenzelburger F, Lee E, *et al*. The pathophysiology of heart failure with normal ejection fraction: exercise echocardiography reveals complex abnormalities of both systolic and diastolic ventricular function involving torsion, untwist, and longitudinal motion. *J Am Coll Cardiol* 2009;**54**:36–46.
32. Ahmed A, Rich MW, Fleg JL, *et al*. Effects of digoxin on morbidity and mortality in diastolic heart failure: the ancillary digitalis investigation group trial. *Circulation* 2006;**114**:397–403.
33. Yusuf S, Pfeffer MA, Swedberg K, *et al.*; CHARM Investigators and Committees. Effects of candesartan in patients with chronic heart failure and preserved left-ventricular ejection fraction: the CHARM-Preserved Trial. *Lancet* 2003;**362**:777–81.
34. Massie BM, Carson PE, McMurray JJ, *et al.*; I-PRESERVE Investigators. Irbesartan in patients with heart failure and preserved ejection fraction. *N Engl J Med* 2008;**359**:2456–67.
35. Cleland JG, Tendera M, Adamus J, Freemantle N, Polonski L, Taylor J; PEP-CHF Investigators. The perindopril in elderly people with chronic heart failure (PEP-CHF) study. *Eur Heart J* 2006;**27**:2338–45.
36. Yip GW, Wang M, Wang T, *et al*. The Hong Kong diastolic heart failure study: a randomised controlled trial of diuretics, irbesartan and ramipril on quality of life, exercise capacity, left ventricular global and regional function in heart failure with a normal ejection fraction. *Heart* 2008;**94**:573–80.
37. Flather MD, Shibata MC, Coats AJ, *et al.*; SENIORS Investigators. Randomized trial to determine the effect of nebivolol on mortality and cardiovascular hospital admission in elderly patients with heart failure (SENIORS). *Eur Heart J* 2005;**26**:215–25.

38. Raymond I, Groenning BA, Hildebrandt PR, *et al.* The influence of age, sex and other variables on the plasma level of N-terminal pro brain natriuretic peptide in a large sample of the general population. *Heart* 2003;**89**:745–751.
39. ESC Guidelines for the diagnosis and treatment of acute and chronic heart failure 2008: the Task Force for the Diagnosis and Treatment of Acute and Chronic Heart Failure 2008 of the European Society of Cardiology. *Eur Heart J* 2008;**29**:2388–2442.
40. Cleland JG, Tendera M, Adamus J, *et al.* Perindopril for elderly people with chronic heart failure: the PEP-CHF study. The PEP investigators. *Eur J Heart Fail* 1999;**1**:211–7.
41. Curtis JP, Sokol SI, Wang Y, *et al.* The association of left ventricular ejection fraction, mortality, and cause of death in stable outpatients with heart failure. *J Am Coll Cardiol* 2003;**42**:736–42.
42. Pocock SJ, Wang D, Pfeffer MA, *et al.* Predictors of mortality and morbidity in patients with chronic heart failure. *Eur Heart J* 2006;**27**:65–75.
43. Richards AM, Nicholls MG, Yandle TG, *et al.* Neuroendocrine prediction of left ventricular function and heart failure after acute myocardial infarction. The Christchurch Cardioendocrine Research Group. *Heart* 1999;**81**:114–20.
44. Cleland JG, Taylor J, Tendera M. Prognosis in heart failure with a normal ejection fraction. *N Engl J Med* 2007;**357**:829–30.
45. Witte KK, Nikitin NP, Cleland JG, Clark AL. Excessive breathlessness in patients with diastolic heart failure. *Heart* 2006;**92**:1425–9.
46. Ingle L, Cleland JG, Clark AL. Perception of symptoms is out of proportion to cardiac pathology in patients with 'diastolic heart failure'. *Heart* 2008;**94**:748–53.

27

Right heart failure

Andrew L. Clark

Most discussions of heart failure (HF) focus on the left ventricle and its dysfunction. The right heart is, of course, commonly affected in HF, both by the same disease processes as affect the left heart, and as a consequence of left heart disease. The right heart itself is much less commonly affected in isolation, but patients with heart disease do commonly present with 'right HF'.

Anatomy and physiology

The right heart is the low pressure segment of the circulation responsible for pumping blood to the lungs. In contrast to the left ventricle, the right ventricle is more coarsely trabeculated, and usually has a prominent moderator band. There is a papillary muscle arising from the interventricular septum attached to the tricuspid valve, but no septal papillary muscle in the left heart. The aortic and mitral valves are in continuity with each other, but the pulmonary valve is a separate structure arising from the infundibulum of the right ventricle. The inflow and outflow portion of the right ventricle are thus separated.

The arrangement of muscle fibres is different between the ventricles: there is no middle layer of circumferential fibres in the right ventricle, unlike the left, with the result that the right ventricle is more reliant on longitudinally aligned fibres.[1] A key difference between right and left ventricles is that the right is working against a very much lower impedance,[2] and the right heart is very sensitive to changes in afterload.[3] A final physiological consideration is that the left ventricle contributes very importantly to right ventricular function:[4] in a dog model, even if the right ventricular free wall was removed altogether, the right ventricle still generated near normal pressure.[5] The right ventricle is subject to the same haemodynamic mechanisms as the left: as the right heart fails, so a higher filling pressure is required to maintain right heart output. Typically, in health, the central venous pressure is around zero.

The filling pressure required is, of course, the haemostatic pressure tending to drive fluid out of the vasculature. With worsening of right heart function, the haemostatic pressure will ultimately exceed the forces tending to retain fluid in the vasculature (principally the colloid osmotic pressure and the resistance provided by the basement membrane) or to drain that fluid away (the lymphatic drainage). As this point is reached, oedema fluid starts to form in the tissues.

Although abrupt damage to the right ventricle in adult life can be catastrophic, normal exercise capacity in the absence of the right heart from the circulation is possible, and in some studies there is little direct relation between right ventricular function and exercise capacity.[6]

Assessment of right ventricular function

The complex shape of the right ventricle has historically made it difficult to assess its size, shape, and function.

Echocardiography

The echocardiogram is, of course, much more readily available than other techniques for assessing right heart function. Although the right ventricle is the part of the heart lying closest to the transthoracic echo probe, its function can be difficult to assess. It is not possible to measure the right ventricular ejection fraction accurately because of the shape of the ventricle. Various indices have been derived;[7] perhaps the most useful is the tricuspid annular plane systolic excursion (TAPSE) which is easy to measure and reproducible: an M-mode cursor is placed across the lateral tricuspid valve annulus from the apical four-chamber view and used to measure the movement of the tricuspid valve plane during right ventricular systole (Fig. 27.1). Fractional area change, again measured from the apical view, is also used but is less reproducible.

Doppler echocarcardiography is very commonly used to estimate the pulmonary artery pressure as some degree of tricuspid regurgitation (TR) is very common. It is important to remember that the velocity of TR recorded gives an estimate of the pressure drop between right ventricle and right atrium: an estimate of right atrial pressure has to be added to give the pulmonary artery pressure, and the assumption is made that there is no significant pulmonary stenosis.

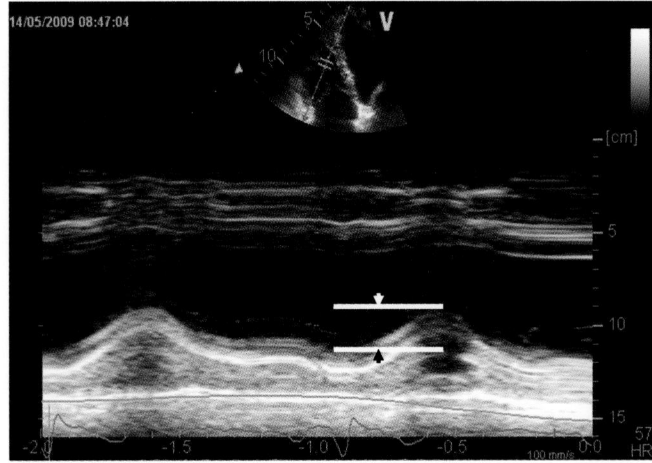

Fig. 27.1 Tricuspid annular plane systolic excursion (TAPSE) measured in a normal heart.

Nuclear techniques can be used to determine right ventricular ejection fraction without the complex geometry of the right ventricle mattering too much, but the best measures of right ventricular function come from CT and cardiac magnetic resonance (CMR) imaging. Both techniques give comparable data including right (and left) ventricular volumes and ejection fractions, myocardial mass measurements and morphological information. CMR is now the standard technique, and much more accurate than echocardiographic measurements.[8]

Syndrome of right heart failure

Older textbooks of cardiology often referred to HF in terms of pairings: forward versus backward failure; acute versus chronic; right versus left, and so on. The syndrome of right HF is characterized by fluid retention and manifests most commonly as ankle oedema.

The fluid excess has to be in the order of 5 L before it is clinically noticeable; individuals may tolerate volumes in excess of 20 L before seeking help. As the fluid collects under the influence of gravity, the ankles are usually first affected, extending up to the thighs and abdominal walls. The sacrum is a common collection site in bed-bound patient. Oedema affecting the external genitalia is common in men. Ultimately, pleural and pericardial effusions form, as does ascites. The old-fashioned terms anasarca (Gk: ανα-, throughout; σάρξ, flesh) and dropsy are sometimes applied to the clinical syndrome.

Fluid retention as a manifestation of right HF is usually accompanied by raised neck veins, but occasionally right HF may be suspected in the presence of raised neck veins alone. Superior vena cava obstruction or more localized venous obstruction (such as subclavian vein obstruction) will not result in ankle swelling.

Differential diagnosis and investigations

Peripheral oedema is not diagnostic of right HF. The most common cause is dependent oedema, followed by impaired venous drainage (Table 27.1). It is vital to consider the differential diagnosis before starting treatment with loop diuretic: the cycle of elderly patient with hypertension—calcium antagonist—ankle oedema—loop diuretic—gout is all too common. Obesity is increasingly common, and fat legs are treated with diuretic to little effect!

Table 27.1 Differential diagnosis of ankle oedema; common causes are listed

Cause	Comments
Dependent oedema	Sedentary lifestyle
Venous insufficiency	Past history of DVTs; iron staining; varicose veins
Drugs	Dihydropyridine calcium antagonists
Hypoalbuminaemia	Nephrotic syndrome
Lymphoedema	High protein fluid; woody swelling
Fat	Generalized obesity
Venous obstruction	IVC obstruction; retroperitoneal fibrosis
Fluid overload	Pregnancy; iatrogenic
Arthritis	Pain and stiffness common
Cardiac	

DVT, deep venous thrombosis; IVC, inferior vena cava.

An outline of the differential diagnosis of right HF is shown in Table 27.2. Any patient presenting with ankle oedema should have a urine dipstick test, and a biochemical profile to assess renal and hepatic synthetic function.

A 12-lead ECG gives invaluable clues as to the cause of right HF (Figs 27.2 and 27.3). Simple spirometry is helpful in suggesting whether cor pulmonale is likely, and a chest radiograph is vital (Fig. 27.4). The first step in imaging the heart is echocardiography, and a transoesophageal echocardiogram (TOE) can be very helpful where the patient has unexplained pulmonary hypertension or suspected congenital heart disease.

CT and CMR scanning may be necessary, and CMR in particular is helpful in cases where right ventricular cardiomyopathy is suspected.

Cardiac catheterization is vital in giving direct haemodynamic information: in particular, it is the only way to measure the pulmonary artery pressure with certainty, and the pressure changes of constrictive pericarditis can only be obtained this way.

Specific syndromes of right heart failure

Acute ischaemic heart disease

Patients with acute myocardial infarction frequently have right ventricular involvement. In patients with anterior infarction, there is a

Table 27.2 Outline of differential diagnosis of right heart failure

Cause	Examples
Left-sided heart failure	Left ventricular failure Mitral valve disease
Congenital heart disease	Atrial septal defect Right ventricle as systemic ventricle
Pulmonary hypertension	Primary Cor pulmonale Thromboembolic
Pericardial disease	Constrictive pericarditis
Primary right heart disease	Ischaemia Valvular disease (e.g. carcinoid) Specific cardiomyopathy

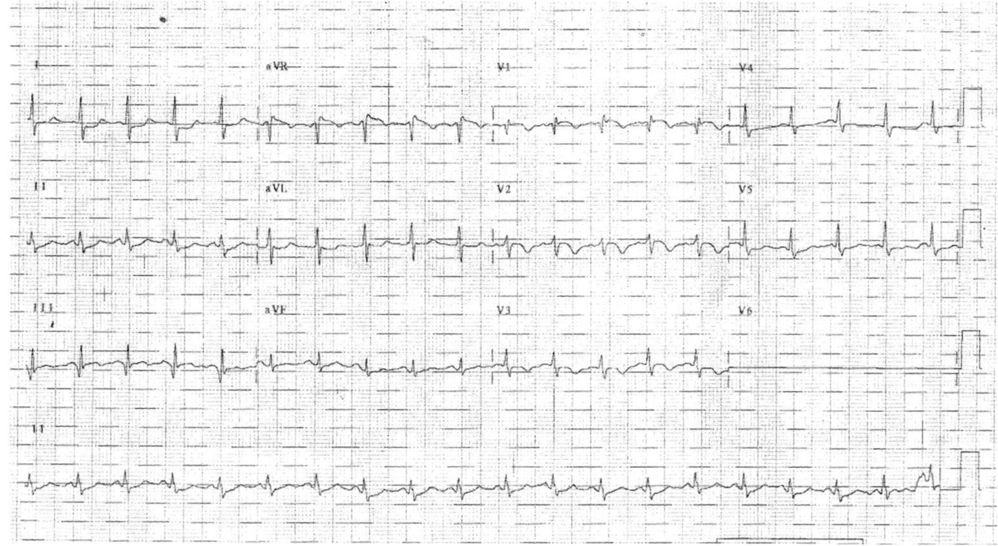

Fig. 27.2 12-lead ECG from a 39-year-old man with acute right heart failure 72 h after weight reduction surgery. Points to note are the sinus tachycardia, the S1Q3T3 pattern and changes in the right sided chest leads (lead V6 not recorded). The diagnosis was acute pulmonary embolism.

relation between the degrees of left and right ventricular dysfunction reflecting damage to the shared interventricular septum.[9] The clinical picture is usually dominated by the left ventricular damage.

After inferior myocardial infarction, usually caused by obstruction to the right coronary artery, there is little relation between right and left ventricular dysfunction. Predominant damage of the right ventricular free wall can lead to a picture of cardiogenic shock (hypotension and oliguria) in the presence of a clear chest radiograph and normal or near normal left ventricular function on echocardiography. The echo will often demonstrate impaired right ventricular function, although bedside images in coronary care units are often of indifferent quality and the right ventricle can be difficult to assess. ST segment elevation in lead V4R is sensitive and specific for right ventricular infarction.[10]

Other useful bedside investigations include pulmonary artery catheterization. The pulmonary artery catheter has fallen into disrepute as a general guide to the management of patients in intensive care,[11,12] but it remains extremely helpful in guiding treatment in specific situations. Where right ventricular infarction is the cause of acute HF, the central venous pressure will be high and pulmonary capillary wedge pressure (PCWP) will be low.

The diagnosis is important to make: orthodox treatment of acute HF aimed at reducing filling pressure with diuretic and vasodilators will make the situation worse. Diuretics and vasodilators should be stopped; and large volumes of fluid may be necessary to keep the right ventricular filling pressure high enough to maintain cardiac output. Percutaneous transluminal coronary angioplasty (PTCA) may be helpful in restoring some right ventricular function.

Primary pulmonary hypertension

Primary pulmonary hypertension (see Chapter 31) should be suspected in a young woman presenting with apparent right HF. As pulmonary hypertension advances, cardiac output becomes fixed as the right ventricle is generating its maximal amount of work at rest. Any exertion leads to breathlessness as the extra oxygen demand of the exercising muscles can only be met by increasing oxygen extraction. The mixed venous oxygen saturation can fall to extremely low levels and reflects right heart function.

Pulmonary thromboembolic disease

Acute large pulmonary emboli can be confused with HF on occasion, and can certainly result in acute right HF. The acute pulmonary

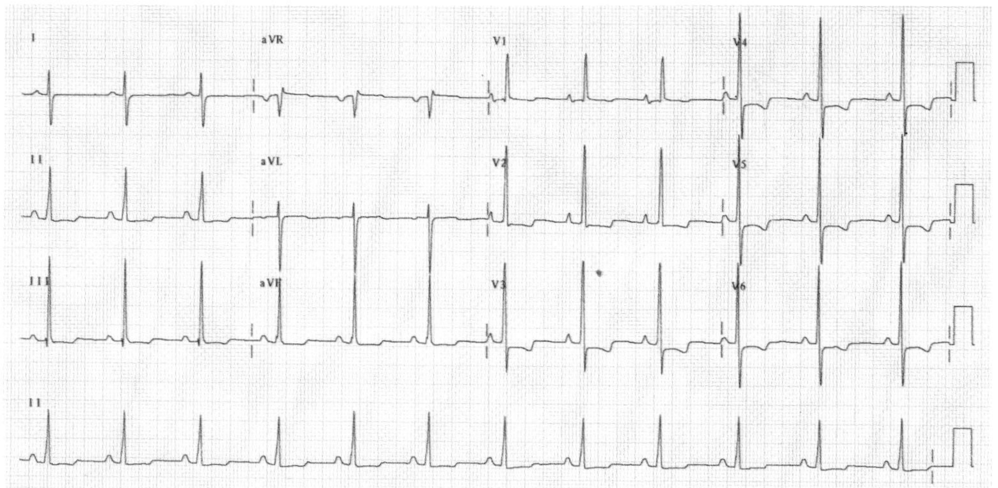

Fig. 27.3 12-lead ECG from a 17-year-old woman with chronic ankle oedema and breathlessness on exertion, diagnosed as asthma. There is right axis deviation and changes in the chest leads consistent with right ventricular hypertrophy. The diagnosis was primary pulmonary hypertension.

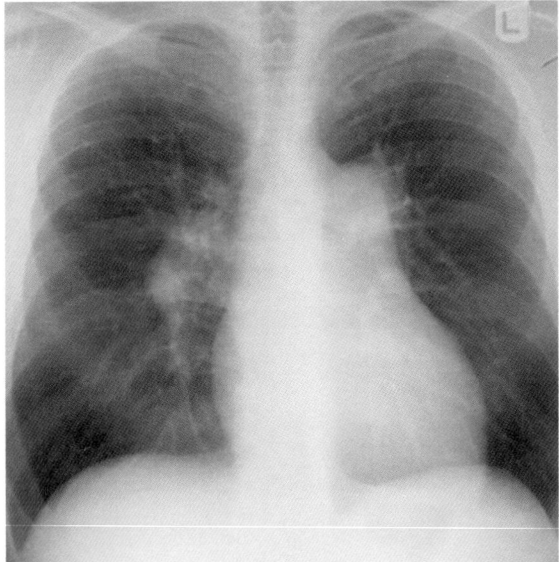

Fig. 27.4 Plain chest radiograph of the same patient as in Figure 27.3, showing a dilated pulmonary artery with peripheral pruning suggestive of pulmonary hypertension.

obstruction results in an abrupt increase in right ventricular afterload, to which the right ventricle is very sensitive. The right ventricle dilates and pulmonary artery pressure rises rapidly.

Left ventricular function becomes compromised as it becomes underfilled, and hypoxia develops due to ventilation–perfusion mismatching. At first sight, hypoxia seems an odd development as vascular obstruction should simply lead to an increase in dead space, but generalized ventilation–perfusion mismatching occurs leading to right-to-left shunting.[13]

The most important part of the management of pulmonary emboli is to think of the diagnosis in the first place. Various scoring schemes are reported that help estimate the risk that a pulmonary embolus is present,[14] but these can only be used once the diagnosis is considered.

Repeated pulmonary emboli may rarely lead to chronic pulmonary hypertension (Chapter 31). Chronic embolic occlusion of the pulmonary circulation appears to result from incomplete resorption and removal of initial emboli. Contrast CT scanning is helpful in establishing the diagnosis. It is a very important diagnosis to reach in a patient presenting with right HF and pulmonary hypertension because the surgical treatment, pulmonary thrombendarterectomy, although dangerous, is potentially curative.[15]

Cor pulmonale

Chronic cor pulmonale is the long-term consequence of lung disease in patients with chronic airways disease. The most potent stimulus to generating pulmonary hypertension in such patients is hypoxia: chronic hypoxia results in pulmonary vascular remodelling following hypoxic vasoconstriction.[16] The increased pulmonary vascular resistance in turn leads to pulmonary hypertension, right ventricular hypertrophy, and right ventricular failure.

The clinical features are of right HF: marked fluid retention with dependent oedema and raised jugular venous pressure in a patient with chronic productive cough and breathlessness. Patients are frequently cyanosed. Examination of the heart is usually limited by chest hyperinflation. The key investigation is spirometry: most patients have marked reductions in FEV_1 and FVC.

The echocardiogram is often unhelpful because of the overinflated lungs: it will, however, usually show good left ventricular function, and may show evidence of right ventricular hypertrophy and pulmonary arterial hypertension.

Patients with cor pulmonale should be assed for long-term oxygen therapy, the only intervention to have a marked impact on survival.[17] It should be considered for patients with an arterial oxygen tension less than 55 mmHg or saturation less than 88%.

Oxygen therapy has to be given for at least 19 h/day to be effective.[18]

Chronic rheumatic heart disease

The right-sided heart valves are almost never affected by rheumatic disease on their own,[19] but some involvement of the tricuspid valve is common in patients who have other valves affected.[20,21] Tricuspid stenosis causes right HF with predominant fluid retention and anasarca. Giant A waves in the jugular venous pulse and very slow y descent are important clinical clues. Tricuspid stenosis will protect the patient with mitral stenosis from pulmonary oedema by reducing right heart output.

Although TR can be caused by the rheumatic process itself, secondary regurgitation due to dilation of the right ventricle and tricuspid valve ring is more common. Prominent clinical features of TR are abdominal bloating and discomfort from the swollen liver and fullness in the neck due to the giant cV waves of TR in the jugular veins. Tricuspid valve surgery is often necessary at the time of valve surgery for rheumatic mitral valve disease, often in the form of a tricuspid valve ring.

An increasingly common clinical problem is that of chronic right HF and TR some time after surgery for left-sided valvular disease. Up to two-thirds of patients undergoing isolated mitral valve replacement will have significant TR after 10 years.[22] Significant TR is associated with a worse long-term prognosis.[23] There is some evidence to suggest that an aggressive approach to the tricuspid valve at the time of initial mitral valve surgery reduces the risk of long-term TR,[24] but selection of patients for repeat surgery many years after an initial valve replacement is difficult.

Other valvular heart disease

The tricuspid valve can be affected by other pathologies. In particular, endocarditis affecting the tricuspid valve, particularly associated with intravenous drug use, can result in severe TR due either to destruction or to surgical removal of the valve. Although in the short term most individuals can tolerate tricuspid valve removal, a proportion of patients develop intractable right HF later. The decision to replace the valve is difficult: it is vital to be certain the patient no longer uses intravenous drugs. Long-term anticoagulation is often needed.

Carcinoid tumours are rare gastrointestinal tumours that produce 5-hydroxytryptamine (5-HT, serotonin). If a carcinoid tumour should metastatize to the liver, then the serotonin is no longer cleared by the liver from the circulation and it will reach the heart. Serotonin causes fibrosis of the tricuspid valve with involvement of the pulmonary valve.

The diagnosis of carcinoid tumour has usually been made by the time the patient presents to a cardiologist, but should be suspected in a patient with unexplained TR, particularly if there are systemic symptoms such as flushing, diarrhoea, and bronchospasm. TR is the dominant cardiac lesion. Although the outcome is bleak once carcinoid heart disease has developed,[25] patients often die from the consequences of TR rather than carcinomatosis, and so surgery should be offered to selected patients.[26]

Atrial septal defect

Unoperated atrial septal defects (ASDs) commonly present late in life, and commonly present as right HF with apparently normal left ventricular function. It used to be said that approximately half of patients with unoperated ASDs died by the age of 50, but this observation is based on ASDs large enough to have been detected on chest radiographs. Smaller defects are compatible with normal life expectancy.

Obvious clues to the diagnosis are the physical signs of a right ventricular heave and pulmonary flow murmur. The fixed splitting of the second heart sound may not be very clear. The ECG will show evidence of right ventricular hypertrophy or right bundle branch block, and may show right axis deviation in a secundum defect or left if the defect is a primum one.

The echocardiogram will very often confirm the diagnosis, although the interatrial septum is often poorly seen. Some flow across the interatrial septum will usually be detectable, and the right heart appears dilated and overloaded. TOE usually allows a definitive diagnosis and allows assessment of the defect for percutaneous closure.

Coronary angiography will determine closure technique: if the patient has normal coronary arteries, percutaneous closure is usually possible for all but very large defects. Surgical closure may be needed for those with nonsecundum defects, very large defects, and those needing revascularization.

A particular mention should be made of sinus venosus ASDs. These are malalignment defects higher in the atrial septum than secundum defects (Fig. 27.5). The superior vena cava enters the right atrium over-riding the defect, usually at the same point as the right upper pulmonary vein. The defect is easily missed on echocardiography, and even on TOE if it is not specifically sought. Any patient thought to have primary pulmonary hypertension should have a TOE performed by an experienced operator to exclude this possible treatable lesion.

Congenital heart disease

An unusual problem discussed in more detail in Chapter 7 is that of failure of a systemic right ventricle. Older patients born with transposition of the great vessels who have been palliated with a Mustard or Senning procedure have a right ventricle supporting the systemic circulation. Patients with congenitally corrected transposition have similar physiology. The systemic right ventricle is likely to fail in early middle age.

Pericardial constriction

Constrictive pericarditis can be a difficult diagnosis to make clinically, and it is common for a patient to wait several years with recurring symptoms before being diagnosed.

Pathology

Constriction can develop as the consequence of any inflammatory process affecting the pericardium. Tuberculosis was once the commonest cause in industrialized societies, but has become rare. Trauma (particularly post-cardiac surgery), previous acute pericarditis, uraemia and connective tissue diseases are causes, although many patients have no known specific cause.

The pericardium gradually thickens with the two layer becoming adherent and densely fibrosed. Calcification is common, and may extend into the myocardium making eventual surgical therapy difficult.

Clinical picture

Constrictive pericarditis may take years to develop. The clinical picture is dominated by right HF with apparently normal or near normal left ventricular function. Peripheral oedema develops together with symptoms of liver congestion and ascites. The ascites can be very striking and may be confused with endstage liver disease, particularly as 'cardiac cirrhosis' may develop.

Fatigue, muscle wasting, and frank cachexia are common as the disease progresses, together with atrial fibrillation.

Pathophysiology

The pericardium in constrictive pericarditis acts to restrain filling of the heart, with the maximum volumes of the different chambers essentially individually fixed. In consequence of impaired ventricular filling in diastole, atrial pressure rises, and thus the moment the atrioventricular valves open in diastole, there is a sudden rush of blood from atria to ventricles that is abruptly halted as soon as the maximum volume of the ventricles is reached. These phenomena result in a raised jugular venous pressure, abrupt y descent (the x descent is preserved, giving a prominent M- or W-shaped wave form to the JVP) and loud third heart sound; and a 'dip-and-plateau' pressure trace recorded from the ventricles. As the constriction usually affects all cardiac chambers, there is equalization of the diastolic pressure in all cardiac chambers (Fig. 27.6).

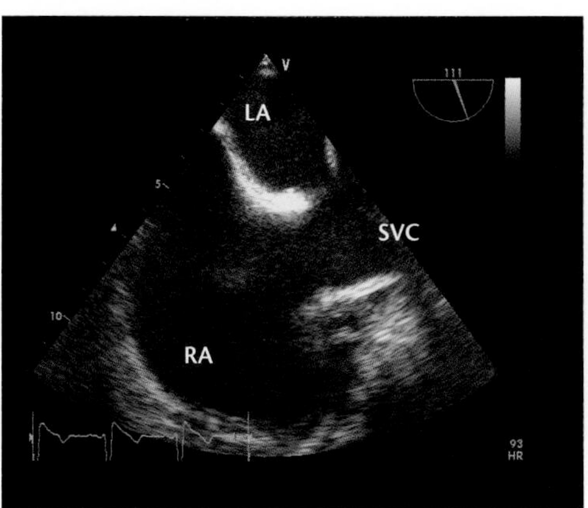

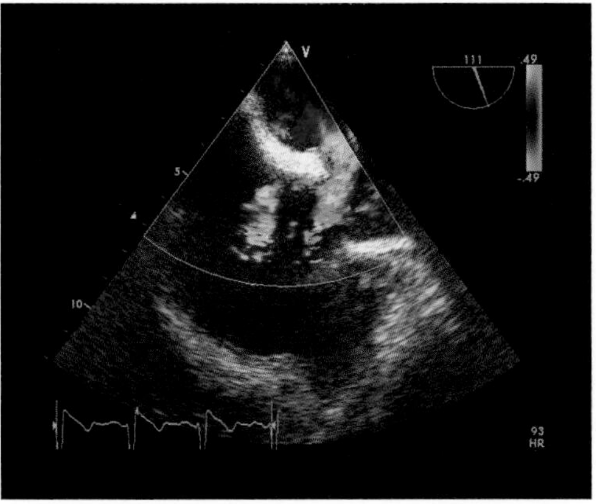

Fig. 27.5 Two frames from a transoesophageal echocardiogram. The interatrial septum is shown with a defect high in the septum highlighted by the colour flow image. LA, left atrium; RA, right atrium; SVC, superior vena cava.

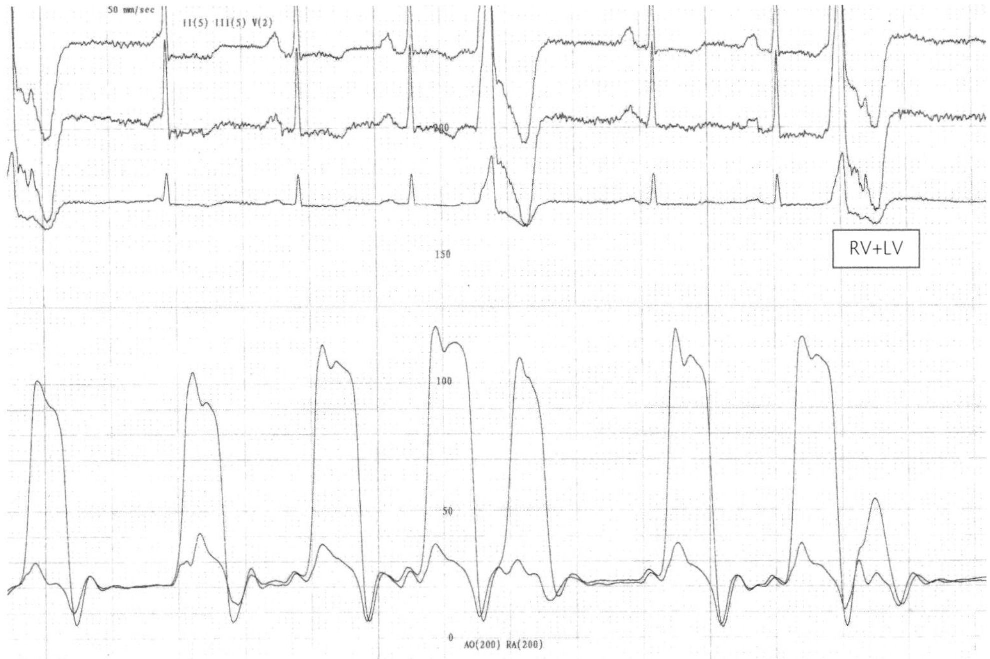

Fig. 27.6 Simultaneous recordings of pressures from left and right ventricles. The patient is in sinus rhythm with ectopics. The diastolic pressures are identical with a 'dip-and-plateau' wave form strongly suggestive of constrictive pericarditis.

Diagnosis

The key to diagnosing constrictive pericarditis is actually to suspect it. The chest radiograph may demonstrate pericardial constriction, and CT or CMR imaging of the heart may demonstrate the thickened pericardium.

The echocardiogram may sometimes show pericardial thickening, but the key echocardiographic feature is abnormal transmitral and tricuspid diastolic blood flow with respiration. There is a great exaggeration of the normal pattern: during inspiration, there is an increase in transtricuspid flow and marked reduction in transmitral flow, which is reversed in expiration.[27] The interventricular septum is often seen to bounce early in diastole as a consequence of the rapid filling, and may be seen to move markedly from side to side during the respiratory cycle.

Cardiac catheterization with careful simultaneous measurement of pressures in the different cardiac chambers (particularly right and left ventricles; and right atrium and left ventricle) will confirm the haemodynamics of constriction. Occasionally the signs may be missed in a patient who has been treated with high doses of diuretic. If there is a strong clinical suspicion of constriction, an acute fluid load of 500 mL saline can bring out the haemodynamic features.

The major differential diagnosis is restrictive cardiomyopathy. The two conditions can be similar clinically and distinguishing between the two is vital. Restriction is usually caused by some infiltrative process such as amyloidosis; the result is a small-voltage ECG and thickened myocardium on echocardiography. The septal bounce is not seen in restriction, nor is pericardial calcification.

The haemodynamics of restriction are also subtly different: the left-sided filling pressures are typically higher than the right (whereas they are identical in constriction), and pulmonary hypertension is frequent (whereas pulmonary artery pressure is rarely significantly raised in constrictive pericarditis).

Treatment

Although constrictive pericarditis is a potentially 'curable' cause of right HF, pericardectomy is a difficult and dangerous operation with a mortality rate of up to 15%.[28] The difficulty lies with the visceral pericardium's dense adherence to the myocardium and difficulty identifying a tissue plane between peri- and myocardium. In many patients, the pericardium is incompletely excised and recurrence of constriction is common. Fewer than one-half of patients are free of symptoms at 10 years postoperatively.[29] Perhaps the most important prognostic indicator is the extent of left ventricular damage preoperatively;[30] the left ventricle can be damaged by the combination of extension of fibrosis from the pericardium and atrophy. It is important to make the diagnosis of constrictive pericarditis and operate as quickly as possible to maximize the chances of recovery.

Arrhythmogenic right ventricular cardiomyopathy

Arrhythmogenic right ventricular cardiomyopathy (ARVC) is a rare cardiomyopathy specifically affecting the right ventricle. There is gradual loss of right ventricular myocytes, probably by apoptosis, and their replacement by fibrous and fatty tissue. Involvement of the right ventricle is often patchy, but the inflow area, apex, and infundibulum are most commonly affected and form the so-called 'triangle of dysplasia'.[31] Late in the course of the disease, the left ventricle can be involved as well.

ARVD is genetically determined and inherited as an autosomal dominant with variable penetrance. In some patients, the abnormality is in the cardiac ryanodine receptor, but many other variants have been described.[32]

The dominant clinical feature is ventricular tachycardia of right ventricular origin (so the 12-lead ECG shows a left bundle branch block pattern). In some patients, symptoms of right HF can dominate. The diagnosis can be difficult to reach: echocardiographic imaging is often normal early in the course of the disease.

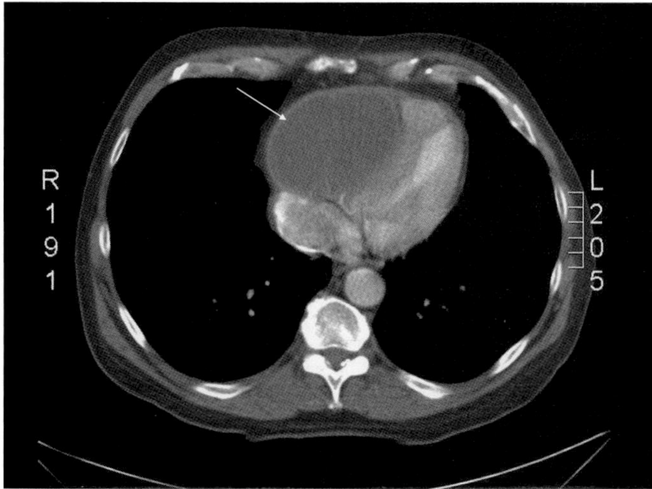

Fig. 27.7 CT scan from a 57-year-old man presenting with right heart failure. A large pericardial cyst (arrowed) was causing compression of the right heart.

Myocardial biopsy may miss patches of involvement. CMR is particularly helpful in detecting areas of fatty replacement of right ventricular myocardium.

Management is usually dominated by the need to control arrhythmias, with β-blockers being helpful and many patients needing an implantable defibrillator. Heart transplantation may be needed for uncontrollable HF or arrhythmia.

Uhl's anomaly has some similarity to ARVD, but is characterized by failure of right ventricular myocardium to develop in fetal life.[33,34] Uhl's anomaly presents with severe right HF in early life.

Miscellaneous

Other rare pathologies can cause right HF, such as right atrial tumours and traumatic damage to the tricuspid valve. Pacemaker leads can cause thrombosis, infection or tricuspid valve damage leading to right HF. External compression of the heart can cause right HF (Fig. 27.7). An occasional patient with an acquired intracardiac shunt can present with right HF (Fig. 27.8).

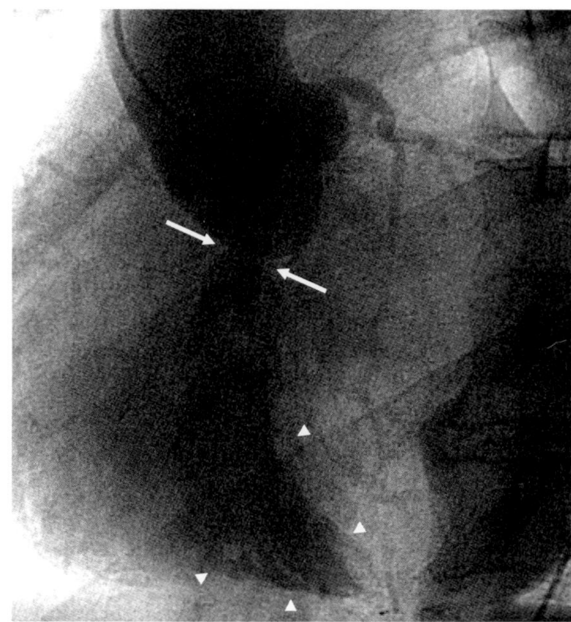

Fig. 27.8 Aortogram from a 27-year-old woman who presented with right heart failure. She had a continuous murmur, and the aortogram shows a ruptured sinus of Valsalva aneurysm (arrows) with the right ventricular cavity outlined (arrow heads).

References

1. Sanchez-Guintana D, Anderson RH, Ho SY. Ventricular myoarchitecture in tetralogy of Fallot. *Heart* 1996;**76**:280–6.
2. Redington AN, Rigby ML, Shinebourne EA, *et al.* Changes in the pressure-volume relation of the right ventricle when its loading conditions are modified. *Br Heart J* 1990;**63**:45–9.
3. Shekerdemian LS, Bush A, Lincoln C, Shore DF, Petros AJ, Redington AN. Cardiopulmonary interactions in healthy children and children after simple cardiac surgery: the effects of positive and negative pressure ventilation. *Heart* 1997;**78**:587–93.
4. Damiano RJ Jr, La Follette P Jr, Cox JL, Lowe JE, Santamore WP. Significant left ventricular contribution to right ventricular systolic function. *Am J Physiol* 1991;261(5 Pt 2):H1514–24.
5. Hoffman D, Sisto D, Frater RW, Nikolic SD. Left-to-right ventricular interaction with a noncontracting right ventricle. *J Thorac Cardiovasc Surg* 1994;**107**:1496–502.
6. Clark AL, Swan JW, Laney R, Connelly M, Somerville J, Coats AJ. The role of right and left ventricular function in the ventilatory response to exercise in chronic heart failure. *Circulation* 1994;**89**:2062–9.
7. Lee KS, Abbas AE, Khandheria BK, Lester SJ. Echocardiographic assessment of right heart hemodynamic parameters. *J Am Soc Echocardiogr* 2007;**20**:773–82.
8. Helbing WA, Bosch HG, Maliepaard C, *et al.* Comparison of echocardiographic methods with magnetic resonance imaging for assessment of right ventricular function in children. *Am J Cardiol* 1995;**76**:589–94.
9. Caplin JL, Dymond DS, Flatman WD, Spurrell RA. Global and regional right ventricular function after acute myocardial infarction: dependence upon site of left ventricular infarction. *Br Heart J* 1987;**58**:101–9.
10. Lopez-Sendon J, Coma-Canella I, Alcasena S, Seoane J, Gamello C. Electrocardiographic findings in acute right ventricular infarction: sensitivity and specificity of electrocardiographic alterations in right precordial leads V4R, V3R, VI, V2 and V3. *J Am Coll Cardiol* 1985;**6**:1273–9.
11. Harvey S, Harrison DA, Singer M, *et al.*; PAC-Man study collaboration. Assessment of the clinical effectiveness of pulmonary artery catheters in management of patients in intensive care (PAC-Man): a randomised controlled trial. *Lancet* 2005;**366**:472–7.
12. Binanay C, Califf RM, Hasselblad V, *et al.*; ESCAPE Investigators and ESCAPE Study Coordinators. Evaluation study of congestive heart failure and pulmonary artery catheterization effectiveness: the ESCAPE trial. *JAMA* 2005;**294**:1625–33.
13. Altemeier WA, Robertson HT, McKinney S, Glenny RW. Pulmonary embolization causes hypoxemia by redistributing regional blood flow without changing ventilation. *J Appl Physiol* 1998;**85**:2337–2343.
14. Wells PS, Anderson DR, Rodger M, *et al.* Derivation of a simple clinical model to categorize patients probability of pulmonary embolism: increasing the models utility with the SimpliRED D-dimer. *Thromb Haemost* 2000;**83**:416–20.
15. Thistlethwaite PA, Kaneko K, Madani MM, Jamieson SW. Technique and outcomes of pulmonary endarterectomy surgery. *Ann Thorac Cardiovasc Surg* 2008;**14**:274–82.
16. Burger CD. Pulmonary hypertension in COPD: a review and consideration of the role of arterial vasodilators. *COPD* 2009;**6**: 137–44.
17. Long term domiciliary oxygen therapy in chronic hypoxic cor pulmonale complicating chronic bronchitis and emphysema. Report of the Medical Research Council Working Party. *Lancet* 1981;**1**:681–6.

18. Nocturnal Oxygen Therapy Trial Group. Continuous or nocturnal oxygen therapy in hypoxemic chronic obstructive lung disease: a clinical trial. *Ann Intern Med* 1980;**93**:391–8.
19. Finnegan P, Abrams LD. Isolated tricuspid stenosis. *Heart* 1973;**35**:1207–10.
20. Yousof AM, Shafei MZ, Endrys G, Khan N, Simo M, Cherian G. Tricuspid stenosis and regurgitation in rheumatic heart disease: a prospective cardiac catheterization study in 525 patients. *Am Heart J* 1985;**110**:60–4.
21. Henein MY, O'Sullivan CA, Li W, *et al.* Evidence for rheumatic valve disease in patients with severe tricuspid regurgitation long after mitral valve surgery: the role of 3D echo reconstruction. *J Heart Valve Dis* 2003;**12**:566–72.
22. Porter A, Shapira Y, Wurzel M, *et al.* Tricuspid regurgitation late after mitral valve replacement: clinical and echocardiographic evaluation. *J Heart Valve Dis* 1999;**8**:57–62.
23. Song H, Kim MJ, Chung CH, *et al.* Factors associated with development of late significant tricuspid regurgitation after successful left-sided valve surgery. *Heart* 2009;**95**:931–6.
24. Dreyfus GD, Corbi PJ, Chan KM, Bahrami T. Secondary tricuspid regurgitation or dilatation: which should be the criteria for surgical repair?. *Ann Thorac Surg* 2005;**79**:127–32.
25. Pellikka PA, Tajik AJ, Khandheria BK, *et al.* Carcinoid heart disease. Clinical and echocardiographic spectrum in 74 patients. *Circulation* 1993;**87**:1188–96.
26. Connolly HM, Nishimura RA, Smith HC, Pellikka PA, Mullany CJ, Kvols LK. Outcome of cardiac surgery for carcinoid heart disease. *J Am Coll Cardiol* 1995;**25**:410–6.
27. Oh JK, Hatle LK, Seward JB, *et al.* Diagnostic role of Doppler echocardiography in constrictive pericarditis. *J Am Coll Cardiol* 1994;**23**:154–62.
28. Trotter MC, Chung KC, Ochsner JL, McFadden PM. Pericardiectomy for pericardial constriction. *Am Surg* 1996;**62**:304–7.
29. Ling LH, Oh JK, Schaff HV, *et al.* Constrictive pericarditis in the modern era: evolving clinical spectrum and impact on outcome after pericardiectomy. *Circulation* 1999;**100**:1380–6.
30. Ha JW, Oh JK, Schaff HV, *et al.* Impact of left ventricular function on immediate and long-term outcomes after pericardiectomy in constrictive pericarditis. *J Thorac Cardiovasc Surg* 2008;**136**:1136–41.
31. McKenna WJ, Thiene G, Nava A, *et al.* Diagnosis of arrhythmogenic right ventricular dysplasia/cardiomyopathy. Task Force of the Working Group Myocardial and Pericardial Disease of the European Society of Cardiology and of the Scientific Council on Cardiomyopathies of the International Society and Federation of Cardiology. *Br Heart J* 1994;**71**:215–8.
32. Basso C, Corrado D, Marcus FI, Nava A, Thiene G. Arrhythmogenic right ventricular cardiomyopathy. *Lancet* 2009;**373**:1289–300.
33. Uhl HS. A previously undescribed congenital malformation of the heart: almost total absence of the myocardium of the right ventricle. *Bull Johns Hopkins Hosp* 1952;**91**:197–209.
34. Gerlis LM, Schmidt-Ott SC, Ho SY, Anderson RH. Dysplastic conditions of the right ventricular myocardium: Uhl's anomaly vs arrhythmogenic right ventricular dysplasia. *Br Heart J* 1993;**69**: 142–50.

28

Anaemia

Peter van der Meer and Dirk J. van Veldhuisen

Prevalence and incidence of anaemia in heart failure patients

In patients with chronic heart failure (HF), anaemia is frequently diagnosed. The prevalence of anaemia depends on the severity of heart failure and the diagnostic criteria used to define it. The criteria of the World Health Organization (haemoglobin <12 g/dL (7.5 mmol/L) in women, haemoglobin <13 g/dL (8.1 mmol/L) in men) are most commonly used in the majority of studies appearing on the topic. Recently a study was performed in 2653 patients randomized in the CHARM Program.[1] This substudy revealed that anaemia was equally common in patients with CHF and preserved (27%) or reduced (25%) left ventricular ejection fraction (LVEF). The presence of anaemia was associated with diabetes, low body mass index, higher systolic and lower diastolic blood pressure, and recent heart failure (HF) hospitalization. In the study, more than one-half of the anaemic patients had impaired renal function (glomerular filtration rate <60 mL/min), compared with less than 30% of the nonanaemic chronic HF patients. In 2008, a meta-analysis was conducted to address the relationship between anaemia and mortality in patients with chronic HF. In this analysis, examining more than 150 000 patients, anaemia was frequently observed, being found in over one-third of the chronic HF patients. The presence of anaemia was associated with a doubled mortality risk in patients with systolic as well as diastolic HF (Fig. 28.1). When assessing the mortality risk by using multivariate analyses, anaemia remained an independent risk factor for mortality in chronic HF patients.[2]

The incidence of anaemia is much more difficult to determine than the prevalence. Data from the OPTIMAAL trial suggest, though, that in a population without anaemia at baseline who had a heart attack complicated by the development of HF, the incidence of anaemia was 10% in the first year.[3]

Aetiology of anaemia in patients with heart failure

Renal dysfunction

Chronic HF and renal failure are two entities that are often seen together, with prevalences ranging from 20% to 40%.[4] Renal failure plays an important role in the aetiology of anaemia in chronic HF patients (Table 28.1).[5,6] Renal function has been shown to be a useful predictor of morbidity and mortality in patients with HF, both in those with impaired and in those with preserved ejection fraction.[7] The interaction between mortality, renal failure, chronic HF, and anaemia was analysed by using a registry on more than 1 million patients. The study showed that renal failure, chronic HF, and anaemia are additive in their effects on increasing mortality.[8,9] The annual mortality rate increased from 4% in patients without anaemia, HF, and renal failure to 23% in patients with the combination of renal failure, CHF, and anaemia (Fig. 28.2).

The relationship between anaemia and HF is complex. Anaemia may lead to increased cardiac workload, resulting from an increased heart rate and stroke volume. As a response to the increased workload, the heart may undergo remodelling, marked by left ventricular hypertrophy and dilation, eventually leading to chronic HF. Renal failure itself may cause HF through hypertension and accelerated coronary atheroma. In established chronic HF, anaemia will worsen cardiac function with an increased mortality risk. On the other hand, chronic HF can also cause renal failure due to decreased cardiac output and blood pressure, and to a lesser extent, to venous congestion which subsequently reduces renal perfusion. This impaired renal perfusion may lead to chronic renal ischaemia, resulting in lower erythropoietin (EPO) levels and ultimately inducing anaemia, leading to an increased cardiac workload completing the vicious circle. Recently the cycle has been called 'cardio-renal anaemia syndrome'.[10]

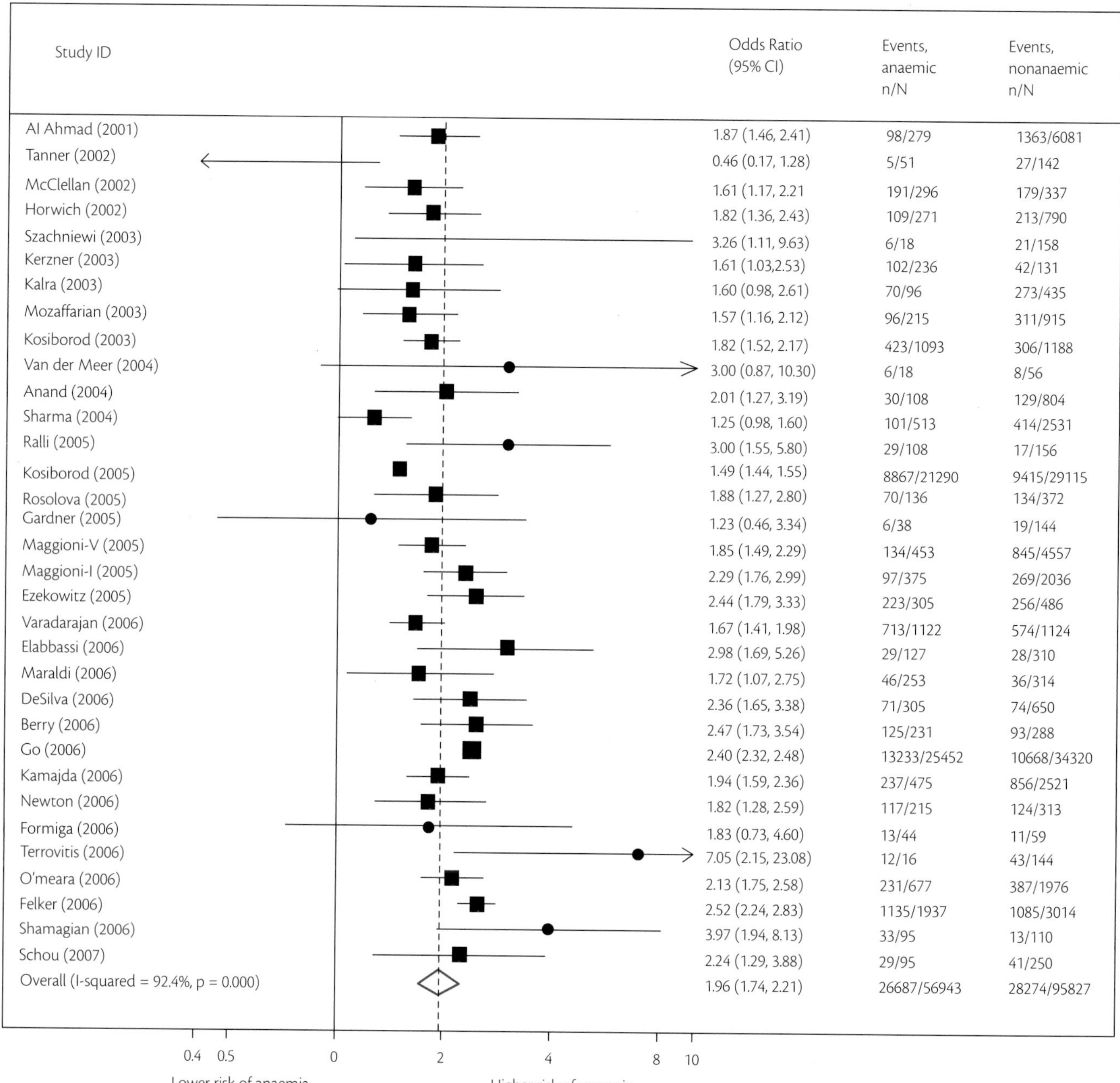

Fig. 28.1 Meta-analysis: the effect of anaemia on mortality in patients with chronic heart failure.
From Groenveld HF, Januzzi JL, Damman K, *et al.* Anemia and mortality in heart failure patients a systematic review and meta-analysis. *J Am Coll Cardiol* 2008;**52**:818–27, with permission.

A novel observation has been the relation between red cell distribution width (RDW) and outcome in patients with CHF.[11] RDW is a measure of variation in red blood cell size. In a single centre study, increasing RDW was an independent predictor of adverse outcome, even in models containing natriuretic peptide levels and haemoglobin.[12] Why RDW should predict outcome is unclear. It is independent of anaemia as a marker and it may reflect processes including inflammation and nutritional deficiencies.

Deficiencies in iron, folate, and vitamin B_{12}

Since only a minority of chronic HF patients have severe renal failure, other factors play a role in the aetiology of anaemia. Several studies showed that iron, folic acid, or vitamin B_{12} deficiencies are commonly observed in chronic HF patients.[13] In a study of 173 ambulatory patients with chronic HF, just fewer than 20% of patients were anaemic: 6% were vitamin B_{12} deficient, 13% iron deficient, and 8% folate deficient.[14] The cause of these deficiencies may be related to a reduced uptake of iron and vitamins, and related to poor nutrition, malabsorption, and cardiac cachexia.[15] Furthermore, the use of aspirin and oral anticoagulation can lead to microscopic amounts of gastrointestinal blood loss, contributing to the iron-deficiency anaemia. However, measuring iron status in chronic HF patients is difficult. Several markers including ferritin and transferrin are acute-phase proteins and they may be elevated in inflammatory conditions such as HF. The difficulty of identifying patients with iron deficiency by serum markers was

Table 28.1 Possible causes of anaemia in patients with chronic heart failure

Possible cause	Mechanism
Haemodilution	Fluid retention—'pseudoanaemia'
Renal dysfunction	Intrinsic renal disease Renal artery stenosis Raised venous pressure/low arterial pressure
Haematinic deficiency	Poor intake Poor absorption Increased blood loss
Chronic disease	Chronic inflammation EPO resistance
Iatrogenic	ACE inhibitors, β-blockers

ACE, angiotensin converting enzyme; EPO, erythropoietin.

emphasized by a Greek study. In this small study, 39 anaemic patients with severe chronic HF were included. Bone marrow biopsies were performed in all patients and the authors measured iron content in the bone marrow. They found that as many as 73% of the patients were iron deficient, despite normal serum iron and ferritin levels.[16] However, it is unrealistic to routinely perform bone marrow biopsies to detect iron deficiency in anaemic chronic HF patients, therefore newer markers including hepcidin and soluble transferrin receptor may be of value since they are less influenced by inflammation.

Hepcidin is a hormone released by the liver that prevents iron leaving the plasma pool. It is reduced in anaemia and hypoxia (encouraging iron uptake and hence haemoglobin synthesis) and increased in iron overload. Crucially, it is induced by inflammation, and appears important in the generation of the anaemic of chronic inflammation. Its role in chronic HF has only recently started to be explored, and its importance is not yet clear.[17]

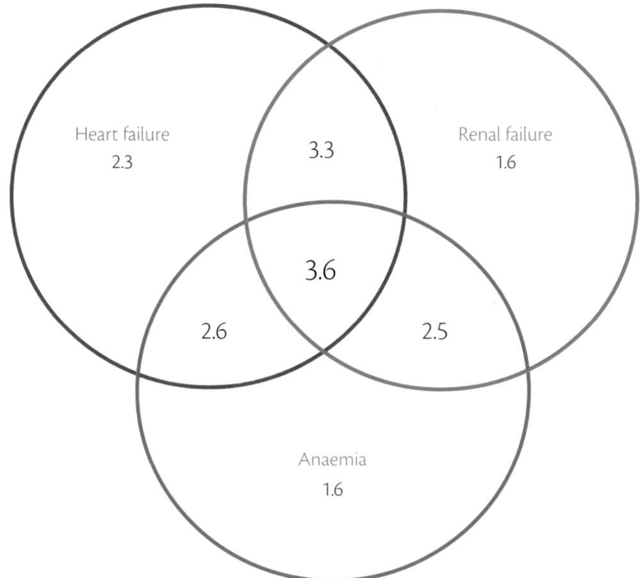

Fig. 28.2 The interactive effects of anaemia, heart failure, and renal failure on all-cause mortality risk. The risk from no anaemia, heart failure, or renal failure is taken as the reference value, 1.0.

From Herzog CA , Muster HA , Li S , Collins AJ. Impact of congestive heart failure, chronic kidney disease, and anemia on survival in the Medicare population. *J Card Fail* 2004; ;**10**:467–72.

Anaemia due to haemodilution

In chronic HF, the presence of haemodilution has been investigated in several small mechanistic studies. Impaired renal perfusion in chronic HF causes activation of the renin–angiotensin system (RAS), resulting in salt and fluid retention, and consequently increases extracellular volume (ECV). Anaemic HF patients have an elevated ECV, which is significantly correlated to lower haemoglobin levels.[17,18] The increased ECV in chronic HF causes haemodilution, which may result in pseudoanaemia. In these small studies, the anaemic HF patients received higher doses of diuretics but nevertheless had an elevated ECV. Importantly, although fluid retention was related to anaemia, signs of fluid retention with physical examination were absent which may indicate that haemodilution is present before clinical manifestation of fluid retention can be observed.

Anaemia of chronic disease

EPO regulates erythroid-cell proliferation in the bone marrow. EPO expression is inversely related to tissue oxygenation and haemoglobin levels, and there is a semilogarithmic relation between the EPO response (log) and the degree of anaemia (linear). EPO responses in the anaemia of chronic disease are inadequate for the degree of anaemia. Such a response has been seen in some studies of patients with chronic HF, but others have found that endogenous EPO levels are elevated in HF, proportional to the severity of symptoms, and are independent predictors of survival.[19] A significant proportion (one-third) of anaemic HF patients had higher EPO levels than one would expect based on the severity of anaemia.[20] These relatively high endogenous EPO levels suggest resistance of the bone marrow to the hormone in a proportion of anaemic HF patients. In contrast, most patients with kidney disease show relatively low EPO levels, and although endogenous EPO levels are still elevated in such patients, they are inappropriately low for the degree of anaemia. It has been observed that patients with chronic HF express elevated levels of TNFα,[21] which in turn may reduce the hematopoietic proliferation. Experimental data support this hypothesis and the proliferative capacity of the bone marrow progenitor cells in mice with HF was shown to be reduced to approximately 50% of control mice.[22]

Pharmacological treatment and anaemia

The use of angiotensin converting enzyme (ACE) inhibitors and β-blockers may also lead to anaemia. It has been shown that intervention in the RAS results in reduced haematopoietic activity. A substudy of SOLVD showed that patients randomized to enalapril significantly had a 56% higher risk of developing anaemia.[23] In order to elucidate the mechanism involved, it has been shown that serum of anaemic chronic HF patients inhibited *in vitro* the proliferation of bone marrow derived erythropoietic progenitor cells of healthy donors by almost one-fifth.[24] The hormone responsible for the inhibition of haematopoiesis is *N*-acetyl-seryl-aspartyl-lysyl-proline (Ac-SDKP). Levels of this haematopoiesis inhibitor, which is almost exclusively degraded by ACE, were significantly higher in anaemic chronic HF patients. There was a clear correlation between Ac-SDKP levels and proliferation of erythroid progenitor cells, thereby linking haematopoiesis to the RAS. However, it must be emphasized that there is no question about the importance of ACE inhibitors in chronic HF and the potential side effects on haematopoiesis are no contraindication to prescribe this drug in anaemic chronic HF patients. The relation between β-blockade and hematopoiesis is less well known. In a large β-blocker trial in chronic HF, there has been the suggestion that the use of β-blockers is associated with occurrence of anaemia.[25]

Treatment of anaemia

Considering the increased mortality risk associated with anaemia, trials have been designed to increase haemoglobin levels. Because the pathophysiology underlying anaemia is complex, different approaches have been used to increase haemoglobin levels. Of these, treatment with EPO, intravenous iron, or the combination of both has been studied extensively.

Iron therapy

The use of iron has been investigated in several small trials with chronic HF patients. Three recent trials showed beneficial effects in anaemic and nonanaemic HF patients.[26–28] Intravenous iron therapy without EPO resulted in a clear increase in haemoglobin levels. In addition, iron therapy reduced NT-proBNP levels in anaemic patients with chronic HF and moderate renal failure.[26] This effect was accompanied by an improved quality of life, exercise capacity, and cardiac function. In another study almost one-half of the patients were considered iron deficient, and they showed, as expected, the highest haemoglobin response to iron therapy. Remarkably, even in the non-iron-deficient group, iron therapy resulted in a modest increase in haemoglobin levels.[27]

In the largest trial of intravenous iron, FAIR-HF, 459 patients with CHF defined as having iron deficiency on the basis of a ferritin level less than 100 μg/L, or between 100 and 299 μg/L if the transferrin saturation was less than 20%, were randomized to receive intravenous iron to achieve repletion or placebo.[29] Although there were no differences in mortality between the groups, iron therapy was associated with marked improvement in symptoms and in six-minute walk test distance (Fig. 28.3). The benefits were seen regardless of whether the patients were actually anaemic at baseline or not.

Erythropoeitin treatment

For decades, EPO has been used to treat anaemia in patients with end stage renal disease. More recently, EPO has also been used in the treatment of anaemia in other conditions, such as malignancies and chronic HF. The first studies in chronic HF patients were published almost 10 years ago and showed a beneficial effect on surrogate cardiovascular endpoints, including cardiac performance, exercise time, and renal function.[30,31] Recently, the effects of darbepoetin alfa (a longer-acting erythropoietin analogue) have been investigated in several larger trials in patients with chronic HF.[32–34] These studies showed that treatment with darbepoetin alfa was safe and effectively raised haemoglobin levels, and that exercise capacity and quality of life improved. To investigate the role of EPO in anaemic chronic HF patients further, a meta-analysis was performed[35] which included a total of 650 patients from 7 studies. EPO treatment was associated with a highly significant 41% lower risk of HF hospitalization (Fig. 28.4). No significant

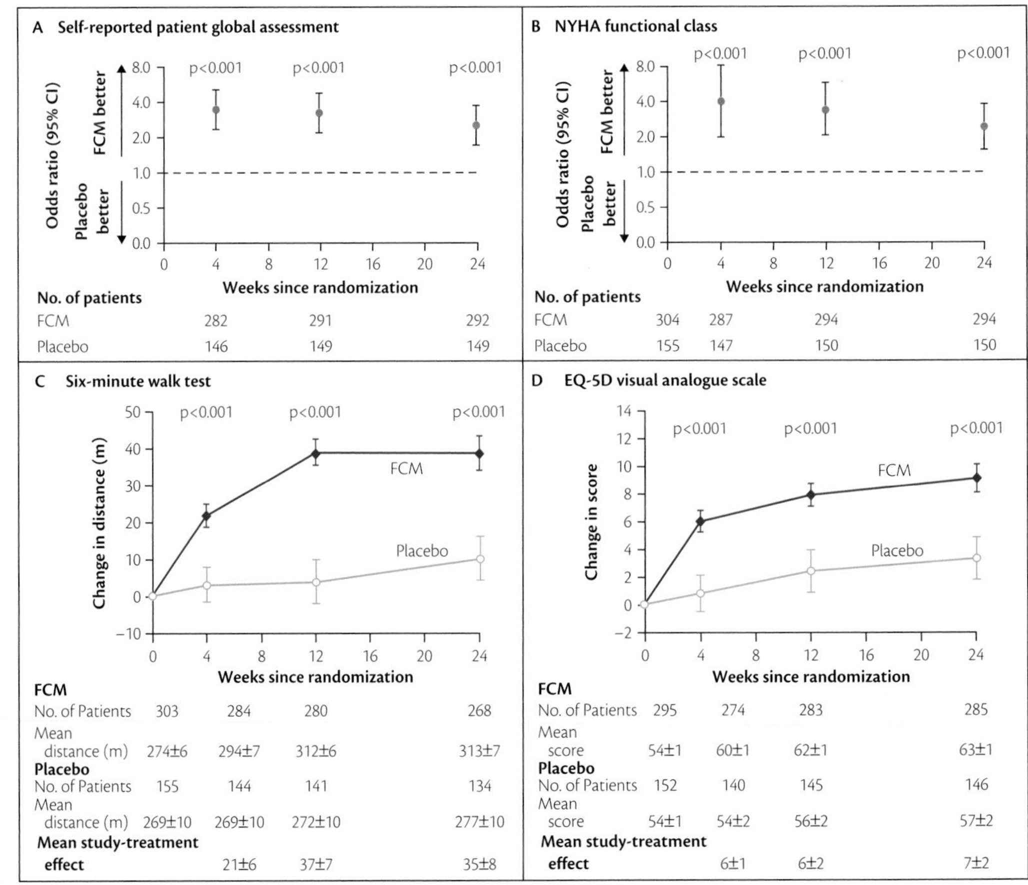

Fig. 28.3 Results from the FAIR-HF study of intravenous iron in patients with chronic heart failure and iron deficiency. EQ-5D, European Quality of Life—5 Dimensions (EQ-5D) visual analogue scale; FCM, ferric carboxymaltose.[47]
From Anker SD, Comin Colet J, Filippatos G, *et al.* Ferric carboxymaltose in patients with heart failure and iron deficiency. *N Engl J Med* 2009;**361**(25):2436–48, with permission.

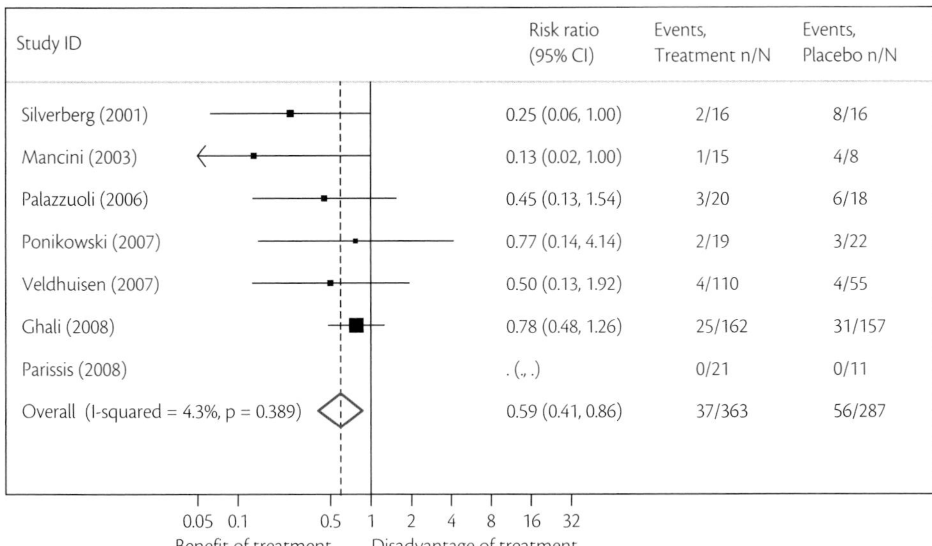

Fig. 28.4 Meta-analysis: the effect of erythropoietin on hospitalization for heart failure.
From van der Meer P, Groenveld HF, Januzzi JL Jr, van Veldhuisen DJ. Erythropoietin treatment in patients with chronic heart failure: a meta-analysis. *Heart* 2009;**95**:1309–14, with permission.

difference in the mortality risk between the two groups was observed. In addition, the prevalence of hypertension or venous thrombosis was similar in both groups. Taking all the data from these small clinical trials together, it seems that in chronic HF, treatment with EPO is not associated with a higher mortality rate or more adverse events, whereas a possible beneficial effect on HF hospitalization is seen. However, these findings need to be confirmed in a large clinical trial. Currently, a phase III morbidity and mortality trial, the RED-HF (Reduction of Events with Darbepoetin alfa in Heart Failure) trial is being conducted and will provide important data on safety and efficacy.[36]

How safe is erythropoietin treatment?

Recently, concerns about the cardiovascular safety of erythropoietin have been raised. Two separate studies, Correction of Hemoglobin and Outcomes in Renal Insufficiency (CHOIR)[37] and Cardiovascular Risk reduction by Early Anemia Treatment with Epoetin beta (CREATE),[38] both studied two different erythropoietin regimens, to examine the optimal target level of haemoglobin in patients with chronic kidney disease. Both studies revealed that higher haemoglobin levels were associated with a worse outcome in anaemic patients with severe renal failure. The two trials formed also the backbone of a meta-analysis examining the effect of EPO on raising haemoglobin to different targets in patients with kidney disease.[39] This analysis revealed a 17% higher mortality rate in patients randomized to a higher haemoglobin target. In addition, the latter patients also had a higher rate of poorly controlled blood pressure and arteriovenous access thrombosis. On the basis of these studies, the current guidelines recommend target haemoglobin levels of 10–12 g/dL (6.3–7.5 mmol/L).

However, it is important to notice that in all these studies, no placebo group was included. The first placebo-controlled trial was performed by Pfeffer and colleagues. They included in TREAT (Trial to Reduce Cardiovascular Events with Aranesp Therapy) more than 4000 patients with type II diabetes and renal failure not requiring dialysis.[40] The median achieved haemoglobin concentrations were 12.5 g/dL (7.8 mmol/L) in the patients who received darbepoetin alfa and 10.6 g/dL (6.6 mmol/L) in the patients in the placebo group. The authors report no differences between the two groups in the overall rates of death or combined cardiovascular endpoints. Importantly, of the patients assigned to darbepoetin alfa, 101 patients experienced a stroke, compared to 53 patients randomized to placebo (hazard ratio 1.92), which is statistically significantly different. There was only a marginal difference in quality of life. Therefore, in patients with chronic renal failure who do not require dialysis, the benefit of darbepoetin alfa to correct anaemia do not outweigh the risk of stroke for most patients.

These findings in renal disease are remarkable, and seem to be in contrast with the data in patients with chronic HF.[5] It needs to be emphasized that in these studies in chronic kidney disease, only a minority of patients suffered from HF and the aetiology of anaemia in both conditions is different. Furthermore, renal function, although impaired, was on average considerably less impaired in the chronic HF studies than in the kidney trials. Taking these factors into consideration, one must conclude that more data on the treatment of anaemia in chronic HF is needed before recommendations can be made as discussed above.

Pleiotropic effects of erythropoeitin in the heart

Besides haematopoietic effects, EPO is also involved the protection against ischaemic injury and stimulation of angiogenesis. In recent years, a functional EPO–EPO-receptor system has been demonstrated in nonhaematopoietic cells including the brain and the heart. This suggests that besides stimulating haematopoiesis, EPO also plays a role as a pleiotropic survival and growth factor.

In animal models, EPO administration during cardiac ischaemia/reperfusion injury reduced infarct size and improved haemodynamics.[41] The acute effect of EPO on infarct size are at least partly related to an antiapoptotic effects.[42,43] The beneficial findings of EPO were not only demonstrated in mice and rats, but also in rabbits and canines. Therefore, as a next step, a small safety study in patients with acute myocardial infarction undergoing percutaneous intervention was performed. Intravenous single high-dose darbepoetin alfa in acute myocardial infarction was both safe and well tolerated.[44] Furthermore, darbepoetin treatment stimulated the mobilization of endothelial progenitor cells (EPCs). Currently, several trials are recruiting patients to investigate the effect of EPO on infarct size and left ventricular function in patients presenting with acute myocardial infarction.

Besides acute cardioprotection, through inhibition of apoptosis, EPO has also shown to induce the formation of new capillaries in the heart after ischaemic injury. In a rat model of chronic HF, EPO administration 3 weeks after myocardial infarction improved cardiac performance which was associated with a significant increase in capillary density.[45] The mechanism of neovascularization is related to both stimulation of endothelial cell proliferation and mobilization of EPCs from the bone marrow.[46] Being aware of the pleiotropic effects of EPO, it is tempting to speculate that the beneficial effects of EPO in anaemic patients with chronic HF might be related to neovascularization. However, further studies are needed to investigate whether nonhematopoietic effects of EPO play a role in patients with chronic HF.

Conclusions

Anaemia has been identified as a common comorbidity in patients with HF; approximately one-third of all chronic HF patients have anaemia, according to a recent meta-analysis. It has become clear that morbidity and mortality is significantly higher in patients suffering from anaemia. The aetiology of anaemia in chronic HF is diverse including renal failure, haematinic deficiencies, pharmacological intervention, haemodilution, and anaemia of chronic disease with EPO resistance of the bone marrow. Several small clinical trials have shown a beneficial effect of EPO on exercise capacity and quality of life in anaemic patients with chronic HF. Currently, a large morbidity and mortality trial evaluating the effects of correction of anaemia with darbepoietin is being conducted. Until the results of this trial are available, the treatment of anaemic chronic HF patients should only be assessed in clinical trials, particularly in light of recent developments in patients with chronic renal failure.

References

1. O'Meara E, Clayton T, McEntegart MB, *et al.* Clinical correlates and consequences of anemia in a broad spectrum of patients with heart failure: results of the Candesartan in Heart Failure: Assessment of Reduction in Mortality and Morbidity (CHARM) Program. *Circulation* 2006;**113**:986–94.
2. Groenveld HF, Januzzi JL, Damman K, *et al.* Anemia and mortality in heart failure patients a systematic review and meta-analysis. *J Am Coll Cardiol* 2008;**52**:818–27.
3. Anker SD, Voors A, Okonko D, *et al.* Prevalence, incidence, and prognostic value of anaemia in patients after an acute myocardial infarction: data from the OPTIMAAL trial. *Eur Heart J* 2009;**30**: 1331–9.
4. Hillege HL, Girbes AR, de Kam PJ, *et al.* Renal function, neurohormonal activation, and survival in patients with chronic heart failure. *Circulation* 2000;**102**:203–10.
5. Kazory A, Ross EA: Anemia: the point of convergence or divergence for kidney disease and heart failure? *J Am Coll Cardiol* 2009;**53**:639–47.
6. van der Meer P, van Veldhuisen DJ. Anaemia and renal dysfunction in chronic heart failure. *Heart* 2009;**95**:1808–12.
7. Hillege HL, Nitsch D, Pfeffer MA, *et al.* Renal function as a predictor of outcome in a broad spectrum of patients with heart failure. *Circulation* 2006;**113**:671–8.
8. Herzog CA, Muster HA, Li S, Collins AJ. Impact of congestive heart failure, chronic kidney disease, and anemia on survival in the Medicare population. *J Card Fail* 2004;**10**:467–72.
9. de Silva R, Rigby AS, Witte KK, *et al.* Anemia, renal dysfunction, and their interaction in patients with chronic heart failure. *Am J Cardiol* 2006;**98**:391–8.
10. Silverberg DS, Wexler D, Iaina A, Steinbruch S, Wollman Y, Schwartz D: Anemia, chronic renal disease and congestive heart failure—the cardio renal anemia syndrome: the need for cooperation between cardiologists and nephrologists. *Int Urol Nephrol* 2006;**38**:295–310.
11. Felker GM, Allen LA, Pocock SJ, *et al.* Red cell distribution width as a novel prognostic marker in heart failure: data from the CHARM Program and the Duke Databank. *J Am Coll Cardiol* 2007;**50**:40–7.
12. Al-Najjar Y, Goode KM, Zhang J, Cleland JGF, Clark AL. Red cell distribution width: an inexpensive and powerful prognostic marker in heart failure. *Eur J Heart Failure* 2009;**11**:1155–62.
13. Cromie N, Lee C, Struthers AD. Anaemia in chronic heart failure: what is its frequency in the UK and its underlying causes? *Heart* 2002;**87**:377–8.
14. Witte KK, Desilva R, Chattopadhyay S, Ghosh J, Cleland JG, Clark AL. Are hematinic deficiencies the cause of anemia in chronic heart failure? *Am Heart J* 2004;**147**:924–30.
15. Anker SD, Sharma R: The syndrome of cardiac cachexia. *Int J Cardiol* 2002;**85**:51–66.
16. Nanas JN, Matsouka C, Karageorgopoulos D, *et al.* Etiology of anemia in patients with advanced heart failure. *J Am Coll Cardiol* 2006;**48**:2485–9.
17. Adlbrecht C, Kommata S, Hulsmann M, *et al.* Chronic heart failure leads to an expanded plasma volume and pseudoanaemia, but does not lead to a reduction in the body's red cell volume. *Eur Heart J* 2008;**29**:2343–50.
18. Westenbrink BD, Visser FW, Voors AA, *et al.* Anaemia in chronic heart failure is not only related to impaired renal perfusion and blunted erythropoietin production, but to fluid retention as well. *Eur Heart J* 2007;**28**:166–71.
19. van der Meer P, Voors AA, Lipsic E, *et al.* Prognostic value of plasma erythropoietin on mortality in patients with chronic heart failure. *J Am Coll Cardiol* 2004;**44**:63–7.
20. van der Meer P, Lok DJ, Januzzi JL, *et al.* Adequacy of endogenous erythropoietin levels and mortality in anaemic heart failure patients. *Eur Heart J* 2008;**29**:1510–15.
21. Rauchhaus M, Doehner W, Francis DP, *et al.* Plasma cytokine parameters and mortality in patients with chronic heart failure. *Circulation* 2000;**102**:3060–7.
22. Iversen PO, Woldbaek PR, Tonnessen T, Christensen G. Decreased hematopoiesis in bone marrow of mice with congestive heart failure. *Am J Physiol Regul Integr Comp Physiol* 2002;**282**:R166–72.
23. Ishani A, Weinhandl E, Zhao Z, *et al.* Angiotensin-converting enzyme inhibitor as a risk factor for the development of anemia, and the impact of incident anemia on mortality in patients with left ventricular dysfunction. *J Am Coll Cardiol* 2005;**45**:391–9.
24. van der Meer P, Lipsic E, Westenbrink BD, *et al.* Levels of hematopoiesis inhibitor N-acetyl-seryl-aspartyl-lysyl-proline partially explain the occurrence of anemia in heart failure. *Circulation* 2005;**112**:1743–7.
25. Komajda M, Anker SD, Charlesworth A, *et al.* The impact of new onset anaemia on morbidity and mortality in chronic heart failure: results from COMET. *Eur Heart J* 2006;**27**:1440–6.
26. Toblli JE, Lombrana A, Duarte P, Di Gennaro F. Intravenous iron reduces NT-pro-brain natriuretic peptide in anemic patients with chronic heart failure and renal insufficiency. *J Am Coll Cardiol* 2007;**50**:1657–65.
27. Bolger AP, Bartlett FR, Penston HS, *et al.* Intravenous iron alone for the treatment of anemia in patients with chronic heart failure. *J Am Coll Cardiol* 2006;**48**:1225–7.
28. Okonko DO, Grzeslo A, Witkowski T, *et al.* Effect of intravenous iron sucrose on exercise tolerance in anemic and nonanemic patients with symptomatic chronic heart failure and iron deficiency

FERRIC-HF: a randomized, controlled, observer-blinded trial. *J Am Coll Cardiol* 2008;**51**:103–12.

29. Anker SD, Comin CJ, Filippatos G, *et al.* Ferric carboxymaltose in patients with heart failure and iron deficiency. *N Engl J Med* 2009;**361**(25):2436–48.
30. Silverberg DS, Wexler D, Sheps D, *et al.* The effect of correction of mild anemia in severe, resistant congestive heart failure using subcutaneous erythropoietin and intravenous iron: a randomized controlled study. *J Am Coll Cardiol* 2001;**37**:1775–80.
31. Silverberg DS, Wexler D, Blum M, *et al.* The use of subcutaneous erythropoietin and intravenous iron for the treatment of the anemia of severe, resistant congestive heart failure improves cardiac and renal function and functional cardiac class, and markedly reduces hospitalizations. *J Am Coll Cardiol* 2000;**35**:1737–44.
32. van Veldhuisen DJ, Dickstein K, Cohen-Solal A, *et al.* Randomized, double-blind, placebo-controlled study to evaluate the effect of two dosing regimens of darbepoetin alfa in patients with heart failure and anaemia. *Eur Heart J* 2007;**28**:2208–16.
33. Klapholz M, Abraham WT, Ghali JK, *et al.* The safety and tolerability of darbepoetin alfa in patients with anaemia and symptomatic heart failure. *Eur J Heart Fail* 2009;**11**:1071–7.
34. Ghali JK, Anand IS, Abraham WT, *et al.* Randomized double-blind trial of darbepoetin alfa in patients with symptomatic heart failure and anemia. *Circulation* 2008;**117**:526–35.
35. Van der Meer P, Groenveld HF, Januzzi JL Jr, van Veldhuisen DJ. Erythropoietin treatment in patients with chronic heart failure: a meta-analysis. *Heart* 2009;**95**:1309–14.
36. McMurray JJ, Anand IS, Diaz R, *et al.* Design of the Reduction of Events with Darbepoetin alfa in Heart Failure (RED-HF): a Phase III, anaemia correction, morbidity-mortality trial. *Eur J Heart Fail* 2009;**11**:795–801.
37. Singh AK, Szczech L, Tang KL, *et al.* Correction of anemia with epoetin alfa in chronic kidney disease. *N Engl J Med* 2006;**355**:2085–98.
38. Drueke TB, Locatelli F, Clyne N, *et al.* Normalization of hemoglobin level in patients with chronic kidney disease and anemia. *N Engl J Med* 2006;**355**:2071–84.
39. Phrommintikul A, Haas SJ, Elsik M, Krum H. Mortality and target haemoglobin concentrations in anaemic patients with chronic kidney disease treated with erythropoietin: a meta-analysis. *Lancet* 2007;**369**:381–8.
40. Pfeffer MA, Burdmann EA, Chen CY, *et al.* A trial of darbepoetin alfa in type 2 diabetes and chronic kidney disease. *N Engl J Med* 2009;**361**(21):2019–32.
41. Lipsic E, Schoemaker RG, van der Meer P, Voors AA, van Veldhuisen DJ, van Gilst WH. Protective effects of erythropoietin in cardiac ischemia: from bench to bedside. *J Am Coll Cardiol* 2006;**48**:2161–7.
42. van der Meer P, Lipsic E, Henning RH, *et al.*: Erythropoietin improves left ventricular function and coronary flow in an experimental model of ischemia-reperfusion injury. *Eur J Heart Fail* 2004;**6**:853–9.
43. Parsa CJ, Matsumoto A, Kim J, *et al.* A novel protective effect of erythropoietin in the infarcted heart. *J Clin Invest* 2003;**112**: 999–1007.
44. Lipsic E, van der Meer P, Voors AA, *et al.* A single bolus of a long-acting erythropoietin analogue darbepoetin alfa in patients with acute myocardial infarction: a randomized feasibility and safety study. *Cardiovasc Drugs Ther* 2006;**20**:135–41.
45. Lipsic E, Westenbrink BD, van der Meer P, *et al.* Low-dose erythropoietin improves cardiac function in experimental heart failure without increasing haematocrit. *Eur J Heart Fail* 2008;**10**:22–9.
46. Westenbrink BD, Lipsic E, van der Meer P, *et al.* Erythropoietin improves cardiac function through endothelial progenitor cell and vascular endothelial growth factor mediated neovascularization. *Eur Heart J* 2007;**28**:2018–27.
47. Rabin R, de Charro, F. EQ-5D: a measure of health status from the EuroQol Group. *Ann Med* 2001;**33**:337–43.

29

Renal dysfunction

Darren Green and Philip A. Kalra

Introduction

Up to 55% of patients with heart failure (HF) have evidence of chronic kidney disease (CKD) stages 3–5 (estimated glomerular filtration rate (eGFR) of 15–59 mL/min, see Fig. 29.1), and mortality rises in proportion to fall in GFR (see Fig. 29.2).[1] In such patients, advanced CKD is as prognostically important as left ventricular ejection fraction (LVEF).[2] HF and its treatment may also play an important role in the pathophysiology of acute kidney injury (AKI), with a further associated risk of adverse outcome. Cardiovascular disease is the leading cause of death in patients with CKD, and structural cardiac abnormalities are highly prevalent in dialysis patients.

Epidemiology

Mortality in patients who have both renal and cardiovascular disease is very much higher than in the general population. The difficulty in defining a precise epidemiological association between HF and CKD is that much of the available data are derived from clinical trials and studies that have strict inclusion/exclusion criteria. These selection criteria limit the understanding of how renal disease impacts on other medical conditions, not just HF, as patients with advanced CKD in particular are typically excluded from clinical trials. However, the majority of elderly patients with HF will have some degree of CKD, as may many younger patients. A prospective cohort study of all comers to a HF clinic found that less than 17% of patients had a normal creatinine clearance (which was the previously used surrogate for eGFR).[2] The presence of renal impairment in patients with HF confers a major detrimental impact upon survival. For patients with advanced CKD, mortality increases by 1% for each 1 mL/min fall in creatinine clearance.[2]

HF is prone to develop and progress in patients of all ages with endstage renal disease (ESRD). Many factors contribute, including hypertension (found in >90% of patients with ESRD), anaemia, and fluid overload. 74% of patients have echocardiographic evidence of left ventricular hypertrophy (LVH) when starting renal replacement therapy (RRT), 36% left ventricular dilatation, 15% severe left ventricular dysfunction; and 4.5% of the patients having dialysis fulfil ACC/ASA/ESC criteria for ICD implantation based on primary and secondary prevention studies of patients with HF.[3–5] Foley *et al.*[6] followed a cohort of 259 patients from the time of starting dialysis for a mean of 41 months, and assessed baseline and follow-up echocardiography. In this study 70% of patients had an increase in left ventricular mass index (LVMI) and 50% an increase in left ventricular cavity volume at the end of the study compared to baseline values; 33% of patients developed HF, one-half of which were *de novo* episodes. Furthermore, each 10-mmHg rise in mean arterial pressure was associated with a relative risk of *de novo* HF of 1.44.

Table 29.2 shows the relative annual mortality figures for patients with anaemia, CKD and HF, or with combinations of these conditions[7] in a study of a random cohort of 5% of Medicare database patients (1 321 156 subjects). The patients were subdivided according to the presence or absence of anaemia, CKD (excluding ESRD) and HF, identified as comorbidities on Medicare claims. The relative risk of death in the presence of these diseases, matched for age and other comorbidities against the remainder of the cohort, is shown. The annual mortality was 4% for patients with no history of anaemia, CKD, or HF; 8% for patients with CKD; and 23% for patients with all three comorbidities.

As a general rule, all-cause mortality rises significantly as GFR falls. The excess mortality includes a disproportionate number of deaths due to left ventricular pump failure[8] and the mortality risk is equally high in patients with both systolic and diastolic dysfunction.[9] Data from the United States Renal Data System shows that cardiomyopathy, congestive HF, or pulmonary oedema is the primary cause of mortality in dialysis patients with a rate of 11.4 events per 1000 patient years.[10]

Definition of the cardiorenal syndrome

The term 'cardiorenal syndrome' has been used to describe the common finding of AKI in patients admitted to hospital with decompensated HF. The term has also been used to describe a worsening of renal function in response to HF treatment, and the

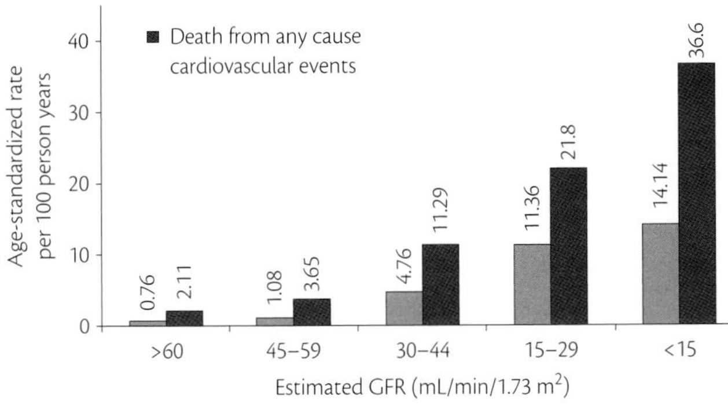

Fig. 29.1 Rates of death and cardiovascular events by eGFR.
Modified from Go AS, Chertow GM, Fan D, McCulloch CE, Hsu C. Chronic kidney disease and the risks of death, cardiovascular events, and hospitalization. *New Engl J Med* 2004;**351**:1296–305.

barrier to management that it may cause. Ronco *et al.*[11] classify the interaction of chronic as well as acute cardiorenal disease into five types of cardiorenal syndrome (Table 29.3). Decompensated HF as a cause or effect of AKI is type 1 or 3 respectively, CHF as a cause and effect of CKD is type 2 or 4 respectively. Type 5 is classed as cardiovascular and renal end-organ damage from a common underlying pathology, most often diabetes mellitus, atherosclerosis, and/or hypertension. Though categorized as separate clinical entities, each of these types of cardiorenal syndrome is more likely in the context of another. For example, AKI is more likely in a patient with decompensated HF if the patient has underlying diabetes, associated CKD, and coronary artery disease (CAD) than if the patient does not have such a history. What is more, because dysfunction of one organ system may cause or exacerbate dysfunction of the other, a 'snowball' effect can occur. This in part explains the poor outcome in patients with both heart and kidney failure.

Pathophysiology of the cardiorenal syndrome

Cardiovascular and renal disease may be due to the same underlying disease. Furthermore, CKD is an independent risk factor for developing cardiovascular disease, particularly CAD and LVH. CAD is responsible for more than one-half of incident cases of HF,[12] and arterial disease is a major cause of renal disease.

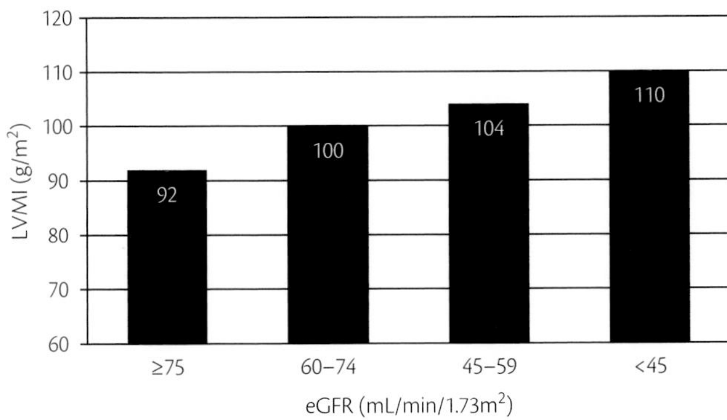

Fig. 29.2 The correlation of left ventricular mass index (LVMI) and eGFR.
Modified from Levin A, Singer J, Thompson C, Ross H, Lewis M. Prevalent left ventricular hypertrophy in the predialysis population: identifying opportunities for intervention. *Am J Kidney Dis* 1996;**27**:347–54.

Table 29.1 Stages of chronic kidney disease based on eGFR

Stage	eGFR (mL/min/1.73 m²)
1	≥90
2	60–89
3a	45–59
3b	30–44
4	15–29
5	<15 or RRT

Modified from Levey AS, Coresh J, Balk E, *et al.* National Kidney Foundation Practice Guidelines for Chronic Kidney Disease: Evaluation, Classification and Stratification. *Ann Intern Med* 2003;**139**:137–47.

Common underlying disease

Hypertension and LVH

Hypertension is extremely common in patients with CKD and it is associated with a high rate of *de novo* cardiac failure and ischaemic heart disease, especially in those on dialysis. Even modestly elevated blood pressure is associated with LVH and cardiomyopathy. However, in the study of dialysis patients by Foley *et al.*[6] discussed above, only a mean arterial pressure of 106 mmHg or more was independently associated with *de novo* HF—tight control of hypertension is fundamental to the renal physician's practice. However, in ESRD mortality is most strongly associated with a low blood pressure[6] and pump failure will lead to a low blood pressure irrespective of renal function. Hence, if a dialysis patient develops significant HF, their requirement for antihypertensive therapy may need to be re-evaluated.

Three-quarters of all dialysis patients have echocardiographic evidence of LVH. The presence of LVH in ESRD is associated with an adjusted relative risk of cardiac death of 2.7 (95% CI 0.9–8.2).[13] LVH develops early in CKD; in a study of 175 consecutive patients attending a predialysis clinic, LVMI increased as creatinine clearance fell and LVH was independently associated with age and systolic hypertension.[14] Aggressive management of hypertension in such patients can cause LVH to regress to the level seen in their nonhypertensive counterparts,[15] thereby potentially improving outcome. Figure 29.2 demonstrates that there is a link between LVMI and eGFR even in the early stages of CKD.[16]

Table 29.2 Relative annual mortality figures for patients who have had in patient hospital visits relating to anaemia, CKD and HF. The baseline annual mortality for patients with no history of anaemia, CKD or HF is 4%

Risk factor	Hazard ratio
No anaemia, CHF, or CKD	1.00
Anaemia only	1.60
CKD only	1.64
CHF only	2.25
CHF and CKD	3.30
Anaemia, CHF, and CKD	3.63

CHF, congestive heart failure; CKD, chronic kidney disease.

Adapted from Herzog C, Muster H, Li S, Collins A. Impact of congestive heart failure, chronic kidney disease, and anemia on survival in the Medicare population. *J Card Fail* 2004;**10**:467–72.

Table 29.3 Classification of the cardiorenal syndrome

Type 1	Acute cardiorenal syndrome	AKI secondary to acute HF
Type 2	Chronic cardiorenal syndrome	CHF causing progressive CKD
Type 3	Acute renocardiac syndrome	AKI or glomerulonephritis with cardiac complications
Type 4	Chronic renocardiac syndrome	CKD as a cause of cardiovascular morbidity
Type 5	Secondary cardiorenal syndrome	Heart failure and CKD with a common cause

AKI, acute kidney injury; CHF, congestive heart failure; CKD, chronic kidney disease
Adapted from Ronco C, Haapio M, House AA, Anavekar N, Bellomo R. Cardiorenal syndrome. *J Am Coll Cardiol* 2008;**52**:1527–39.

Table 29.4 Relative risk of hospitalization due to heart failure according to degree of albuminuria, measured by albumin/creatinine ratio, listed by quartiles

Albumin/Creatinine ratio (mg/mmol)	<0.22	0.22—0.57	0.58—1.62	>1.62
All patients	1	1.19	1.95	3.79
Diabetic patients	1	0.72	1.83	3.65
Nondiabetic patients	1	1.45	1.86	2.93

Adapted from Gerstein HC, Mann J, Yi Q, *et al.* Albuminuria and risk of cardiovascular events, death, and heart failure in diabetic and non-diabetic individuals. *JAMA* 2001;**286**(4):421–6.

Atherosclerosis

Atherosclerosis is a multisystem disease. CAD is the most common cause of HF, and 40% of patients with CKD have evidence of CAD.[17] CKD is a proatherosclerotic condition and, in turn, atherosclerosis can lead to and exacerbate CKD. Vascular damage occurs at a microvascular level in the kidney and is very often independent of renal artery stenosis (RAS). The intrarenal arterial disease will lead to chronic glomerular damage. Smoking is independently associated with the development, and risk of progression, of CKD and the pathway is likely to involve the same atheromatous processes that contribute to CAD. The mechanisms by which CKD can exacerbate coronary artery atherosclerosis are discussed below.

Diabetes mellitus and the metabolic syndrome

Diabetic nephropathy is responsible for 20% of all new dialysis cases in the UK.[18] Worldwide, this rises to as much as 40% in the United States and 55% in parts of the Indian subcontinent.[19] In addition, up to 7.5% of the prevalent dialysis population have type 2 diabetes that developed after RRT was started.[20] Insulin resistance and chronic hyperglycaemia both lead to endothelial dysfunction, in which the usual antiatheromatous properties of vascular endothelium are disrupted. Subsequent macrovascular disease manifests most often as CAD and CKD. Microvascular disease is responsible for diabetic cardiac autonomic neuropathy and early endothelial disruption in the kidneys produces proteinuria which is a reliable marker of progressive CKD.[21] Patients with a urine albumin-to-creatinine ratio of 30–299 mg/g, a range termed 'microalbuminuria', have a 9.2-fold risk of progression to established diabetic nephropathy compared to a control group of patients with no microalbuminuria.[22]

Microalbuminuria is independently associated with a relative risk of cardiovascular mortality of 1.87 in diabetic patients (compared to those without albuminuria) and in a 10-year follow-up of diabetic patients with microalbuminuria, 9% of all-cause mortality was attributed to HF.[23] In the Heart Outcomes Prevention Evaluation (HOPE) trial, microalbuminuria was associated with an adjusted relative risk of 3.23 for hospitalization for HF. Importantly, this was similar for diabetic and nondiabetic patients, indicating a significant risk of HF for patients with other proteinuric illnesses (Table 29.4).[24]

Diabetes mellitus is often part of the metabolic syndrome, in which there is coexistent obesity, hypertension, high triglycerides, and LDL cholesterol, and high circulating levels of prothrombotic/proinflammatory markers. These are all risk factors for cardiovascular and renal vascular damage, which emphasizes why diabetes is associated with such a high cardiorenal morbidity and mortality.

Renin–angiotensin pathway

CKD can contribute to overactivation of the renin–angiotensin–aldosterone system (RAAS) which in turn both contributes to the development of cardiovascular disease and further exacerbates CKD, thereby initiating a pathway of progressive cardiorenal disease.

One of the primary purposes of the RAAS is to adapt to a drop in blood pressure in order to maintain vital organ blood flow. Angiotensin II causes sodium retention, expansion of the extracellular compartment, vasoconstriction, and restoration of organ perfusion. CKD causes chronic overactivation of the RAAS, and this appears to play a prominent pathophysiological role in the subsequent progression and exacerbation of intrarenal (and cardiac) damage.

Angiotensin II causes postglomerular arteriolar vasoconstriction, leading to intrarenal hypertension and glomerular damage. Its systemic vasoconstrictive activity also leads to LVH. Angiotensin II and aldosterone up-regulate activity of proinflammatory cytokines such as fibroblast growth factor (FGF), platelet-derived growth factor (PDGF) and transforming growth factor β_1 (TGFβ_1). These cytokines contribute to endothelial dysfunction, thereby promoting CAD and renal vascular disease, and are associated with intrarenal and myocyte fibrosis. Progression of CKD and HF can follow, ultimately resulting in an ever worsening cycle of progressive cardiorenal organ damage (Fig. 29.3).

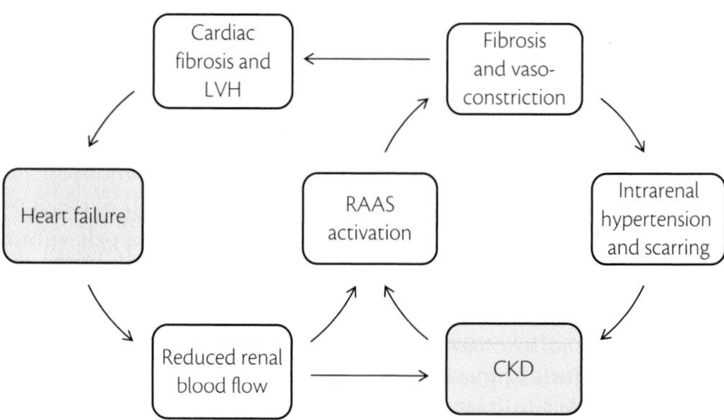

Fig. 29.3 Simplified schematic diagram showing the central role of RAAS activation in the pathogenesis of the cardiorenal syndrome in patients with heart failure and chronic kidney disease (CKD). LVH, left ventricular hypertrophy.

Renal disease as a cause of cardiovascular disease

Vascular stiffness

The excess of vascular disease in patients with CKD is largely due to underlying risk factors. One particular problem relates to vascular calcification and associated arterial stiffness. There is a fivefold increase in vascular calcification of the coronary arteries in dialysis patients compared to other patients with coronary atheroma,[25] and there is evidence of more widespread 'medial' calcification within the arterial tree. This is again associated with an excess of mortality.[26] The calcification starts developing in the early stages of CKD and is present in over 50% of patients at the time of starting dialysis.[27] Once calcification is present, it continues to progress, though some medications have been shown to slow this progression. In some patients, renal transplantation will halt progression.[28]

The pathophysiology of calcification is complex and involves an interplay between many predisposing factors including hyperphosphataemia, hypercalcaemia, and hyperparathyroidism, all of which can stimulate calcification of vascular smooth muscle cells and within the vascular matrix; CKD also leads to a reduction in endogenous inhibitors of calcification, such as fetuin A. Vascular calcification and renal bone abnormalities are now both encompassed by the term 'chronic kidney disease–mineral bone disorder' (CKD-MBD).

The clinical manifestation of calcification within the larger 'conduit' arteries is an increase in vascular stiffness which can be measured noninvasively with pulse wave velocity (PWV). An increase in PWV is associated with LVH and increased LVMI (and with reduced coronary filling), all of which may eventually predispose to HF.[29] Indeed, in some small studies, increased PWV, and thus vascular stiffness, has been shown to be more important than hypertension in the development of LVH.

That CKD-MBD represents a major cardiovascular risk highlights the importance of strict adherence to a 'renal' diet and appropriate use of phosphate binders at an early stage of CKD. However, there are possible risks of calcification associated with long-term use of high doses of oral calcium, as used in phosphate binders, although there is currently no proof of the association.

Endothelial dysfunction and Inflammation

Endothelial dysfunction plays an important role in HF. It leads to a loss of the usual endothelium-mediated vasodilatory response to nitric oxide (NO) which is in turn an independent predictor of cardiovascular mortality in patients with HF. RAAS activation, mediated by CKD, exacerbates endothelial dysfunction by increased the production of reactive oxygen species (ROS).[30] Patients are less able to reduce afterload (which is increased by the vascular stiffness discussed above). Endothelial dysfunction has also been linked with abnormal myocardial remodelling and CAD.

CKD is a major contributor to endothelial dysfunction. Although an elevated serum creatinine, and its mathematical transformation into eGFR, is used to signify CKD, there is a host of other metabolites that are not routinely measured in CKD, many of which contribute to oxidative stress that in turn leads to end organ damage. Further, some circulating pro-inflammatory cytokines, such as interleukin-6 (IL-6), are normally excreted via the kidneys but cannot be removed by dialysis. These accumulate in advanced CKD and contribute further to the endothelial dysfunction.[31] C-reactive protein (CRP) is a surrogate marker of the *in vivo* inflammation and is often raised in CKD, particularly in patients with tunnelled venous catheters as access for haemodialysis.[32] Chronically elevated CRP in dialysis patients is associated with increased cardiovascular mortality, although not specifically from HF.[33]

Salt and water retention

AKI as a primary event may lead to acute decompensated HF, even in patients with previously normal cardiac function. Retention of sodium and fluid occur as a result of renal injury and also as a result of attempts to resuscitate the unwell patient with intravenous fluid. When AKI supervenes, patients with underlying cardiovascular disease may also find that their medication, particularly diuretics and angiotensin converting enzyme (ACE) inhibitors, are stopped on admission to hospital, which increases the likelihood of a secondary episode of HF. Furthermore, electrolyte and metabolite disorders may develop which can further exacerbate decline in cardiac function. Specifically, renal acidosis is associated with pulmonary hypertension and right HF, and electrolyte disturbances leave patients at risk of arrhythmia and loss of effective atrial activity.

Patients with AKI and HF are difficult to manage. If oliguric AKI occurs and does not respond to early resuscitation, patients are at particular risk if acute pulmonary oedema or significant hyperkalaemia occur. They are unlikely to respond to diuretics, and so haemodialysis or haemofiltration are often necessary and should be considered early in the clinical course.

Chronic salt and water retention in advanced CKD can contribute to hypertension and ventricular dilation. In one study, Kayikcioglu *et al.*[34] managed hypertension in haemodialysis patients using dietary salt restriction and modification of dialysis target weight to control blood pressure, with no antihypertensive drugs. They achieved a target blood pressure of less than 140/90 mmHg in 90% of patients. Symptomatic hypotension was common but reduced to 7% of cases at 12 months. There was a reduction in LVMI from 164±64 to 112±36 g/m^2 during follow-up.[35]

Anaemia

Anaemia is a risk factor for both the development of HF, and its poor outcome, independent of concurrent or causative CKD. Given the high incidence of anaemia associated with CKD, the contributory importance and treatment of anaemia has to be considered when managing the patient with CKD and HF. Figure 29.1 outlines the additive effect on mortality of coexistent anaemia, CKD, and HF.

Arteriovenous fistula formation

An arteriovenous (AV) fistula is the preferred access for haemodialysis. It carries a three times lower risk of infection than tunnelled dialysis lines and there is a lower all-cause mortality in patients who dialyse via a fistula.[36] However, the creation of a shunt from the high-pressure arterial circulation into the lower-pressure venous system leads to circulatory changes and, ultimately, cardiac remodelling, which may cause high-output cardiac failure in a few individuals.

As little as 1 week after fistula formation, cardiac output may increase by up to 15%. There is an increased venous return and sympathetic activation with resultant resting tachycardia, and an increase in left ventricular end-diastolic volume, indicative of a greater circulating volume. The changes are thought in part to be a consequence of neurohormonal responses to the reduced vascular resistance that follows AV fistula formation, and patients with high-flow fistulae have higher circulating levels of natriuretic peptides because of the high volume state. There is also eccentric hypertrophy of the left ventricle in response to dilatation.[37] Although the majority of haemodialysis patients tolerate their fistula without any noticeable circulatory problems, a few patients are at risk of high-output cardiac failure. In such cases, ligation of the fistula must be considered as a therapeutic option. Male sex and use of proximal vessels for fistula formation are independent risk factors for the need for fistula ligation.

Renal artery stenosis

Atherosclerotic renovascular disease (ARVD) is common, and it is frequently seen in association with other cardiovascular diseases such as CAD, peripheral vascular disease, and stroke.[38] As would be expected, HF is also common in patients with ARVD. We found that ARVD was detectable in approximately one-third of elderly patients presenting acutely to hospital with HF.[39] In addition, 54% of a UK outpatient cardiac failure population had atherosclerotic renal artery stenosis (RAS) greater than 50%.[40] Conversely, HF is present in 38% of elderly US patients with ARVD[41] and HF leads to an almost threefold increase in mortality risk compared to patients with ARVD but without HF.[42] In many patients with ARVD and HF, there is normal LVEF, but patients with HF have higher filling pressures, higher LVMI, and greater prevalence of diastolic dysfunction than patients without HF.[42] Systematic echocardiographic studies of cardiac structure and function in ARVD have shown that only 5% of patients had normal hearts, that the prevalence of LVH was twice as great as in CKD patients without ARVD, and that changes progress over time.[43,44]

Heart failure as a cause of kidney disease

Patients admitted with decompensated HF have a worse outcome if there is associated AKI. A rise in serum creatinine of as little as 9 μmol/L is associated with both a prolonged inpatient stay and increased mortality.[45] The amount of change in creatinine is of more prognostic significance than the baseline creatinine.[46] In one study of 1004 patients admitted to hospital with decompensated HF, 25% had a rise in serum creatinine of more than 26.5 μmol/L (0.3 mg/dL). The presence of diabetes mellitus, hypertension, or CKD were independent predictors of postadmission AKI.[47] Anaemia, age, and the use of drugs blocking the RAAS and diuretics are predictors of AKI in the setting of acute hospitalization for HF. However, the precise pattern of risk is difficult to define because the definition of AKI varies from study to study. A 0.3 mg/dL rise in creatinine was defined as 'worsening renal function' (WRF) in the POSH study (the Prospective Outcomes Study in Heart failure). WRF was independently associated with higher serum creatinine levels on admission (odds ratio (OR) 3.02), pulmonary oedema (OR 3.35), but previous history of atrial fibrillation appeared to confer protection against WRF (OR 0.35). WRF was associated with an increase in average length of inpatient stay of 2 days but readmission rates and, importantly, mortality, were not affected.[48]

The fact that AKI usually occurs very soon after hospital admission for HF suggests that low-output cardiac failure is important in its pathogenesis. Drugs blocking the RAAS lead to reduced renal perfusion and have a deleterious effect on renal function, due to actions on glomerular haemodynamics (that are beneficial when perfusion is better). However, hypotension and a low cardiac output state are not present in all patients who develop renal dysfunction. Other factors are important and there is an association between higher right atrial pressures and lower GFR.[49] Thus venous congestion and volume overload appear to contribute to AKI, a pathogenetic theory supported by experimental models in which temporary occlusion of renal veins leads to a temporary decline in GFR.[49] Similar pathological mechanisms may also account for the evolution of CKD in chronic HF given that lower ejection fraction does not correlate closely with the likelihood of progression of CKD, and CKD may occur in cases where there is normal LVEF.

Heart failure therapy in patients with CKD

Improving heart failure prognosis in CKD

Drugs that act on the renin–angiotensin–aldosterone pathway

The landmark trials of ACE inhibitors in patients with chronic HF excluded patients with significant renal impairment, and evidence for the use of blockers of the RAAS in patients with CKD and HF often comes from nonrandomized trials. For example, in a study of 1704 patients with systolic HF and CKD (mean eGFR 43 mL/min), ACE inhibitor was associated with an all-cause survival benefit of 4% compared to a propensity-score matched 'control' group not on ACE inhibitor. There was a similar reduction in all hospital admissions.[50] A rise in serum creatinine after starting an ACE inhibitor is not associated with a poor renal outcome, provided that the rise is not inexorable. In patients with HF, a rise in creatinine of up to 30% followed by stable renal function should be accepted and should not lead to stopping the drug or further investigation, whereas a greater rise raises the possibility of ARVD: renal imaging may be indicated in selected cases.

The benefit of ACE inhibitors in patients with ESRD but no HF is less clear. A theoretical benefit is the potential for reduction in left ventricular mass given that LVH is associated with the risk of progression to cardiac dilation and HF, and of course, mortality.[3] However, ACE inhibitors have been shown to improve survival as a secondary endpoint in observational studies of dialysis patients.[51] As ACE inhibitors may cause hyperkalaemia, electrolyte changes should be very closely monitored in dialysis patients

Angiotensin II receptor blockers (ARBs) have a similar beneficial profile in CKD to ACE inhibitors. They also have a similar profile of adverse effects, so that converting from ACE inhibitor to ARB in cases of hyperkalaemia is unlikely to improve matters; however, a change may be indicated in cases of cough related to the use of an ACE inhibitor . Aliskiren, the first commercially available drug to inhibit renin directly, can improve neurohumoral markers of HF,[52] but its effects on clinical outcomes have not been fully evaluated.

Spironolactone, an aldosterone receptor antagonist, improves survival in HF[53] but at the expense of increasing risk of hyperkalaemia, and its use in patients with CKD is thus limited. The RALES trial excluded patients with significant renal impairment.[53] Dual blockade of the RAAS using a combination of two classes of drugs is commonplace in nephrology and is generally considered safe for treatment of HF.[54] An important exception is dual blockade including spironolactone in patients with CKD stages 4 and 5, in whom the risk of hyperkalaemia is considerable.

β-Blockers

β-Blockade confers significant survival benefit in patients with stage 3 CKD, CAD, and HF (OR 0.75 vs matched patients not on β-blockade).[55] Dialysis patients with HF also benefit, (2-year all-cause mortality, carvedilol vs placebo 51.7% vs 73.2%, $p < 0.001$)[56] and are less likely to develop *de novo* HF if pre-emptively prescribed a β-blocker (OR 0.69 vs matched patients not on β-blocker).[57] However, β-blockers appear to be underused in patients with CKD compared to matched patients without renal impairment,[55] despite poor renal function having little adverse effect on the efficacy of β-blockade in treatment of HF. In elderly patients with a low GFR there is a modest tendency to bradyarrhythmias leading to drug discontinuation (2.3% vs 0.8% in placebo).[58]

Digoxin

As is the case with β-blockers, the efficacy of digoxin is not affected by CKD and it does not correlate with GFR.[59] However, digoxin toxicity is more common in patients with CKD as the drug is partially eliminated by the kidney; for those patients with ESRD, the drug is not removed by dialysis. Digoxin can also contribute to hyperkalaemia and drugs such as calcium gluconate, used in the management of hyperkalaemia, can exacerbate the arrhythmic risk of digoxin toxicity. As digoxin does not confer the same survival benefit as β-blockers in HF, it should not be considered a first-line therapy for HF in patients with CKD.

Peritoneal dialysis

The principal of removing ascites to treat HF was first demonstrated 60 years ago. The possibility of using peritoneal dialysis as a management strategy for chronic HF in patients with and without CKD is now also gaining support. In one small study ($n = 17$, mean age 64±9 years), patients with refractory HF who were started on peritoneal dialysis had a significant survival benefit (82% 12-month survival) and fewer hospital admissions (reduction from 62±16 to 11±5 days per patient per year).[60] In refractory HF, the ability of the kidneys to generate a diuresis is blunted, as is their response to large-dose diuretics. Offloading fluid from the circulation by removal during peritoneal dialysis will improve haemodynamics—for example, by reducing right atrial pressure—so improving cardiac function and renal perfusion. There is a trend towards offering peritoneal dialysis rather than haemodialysis to patients with CKD stage 5 and coexistent HF. The theory is that patients with markedly impaired ventricular function will benefit from gradual fluid removal and so be less likely to suffer collapse relating to hypotension, and/or serious arrhythmias that might result from haemodialysis. However, the evidence to support this practice is conflicting and derived from small, nonrandomized studies.

One drawback that may prevent more widespread application of peritoneal dialysis (PD) in patients with HF and earlier stages of CKD is that patients need to be mobile and quite physically able to manage the technique; even where assisted PD programmes are available, the patient will be expected to manage all or some of their therapy. A 5-L bag of dialysis fluid weighs 5 kg and carrying two or more of these to a PD machine is an effort for any dialysis patient.

Anaemia management

Treatment of anaemia with erythropoiesis-stimulating agents (ESAs) and intravenous iron is associated with an improvement in cardiac function, and symptom and diuretic burden in HF. The effect is less marked in such patients who also have CKD.[61] The symptom benefit may not equate to survival benefit. TREAT (Trial to Reduce Cardiovascular Endpoints with Aranesp Therapy) aimed to show a benefit in using ESAs to achieve a higher than usual target haemoglobin (13 g/dL) in diabetic predialysis CKD patients. However, there was an excess of thromboembolic events and cerebrovascular events in the ESA arm compared to placebo.[62] The FAIR-HF trial[63] compared intravenous iron therapy with placebo in patients with NYHA class II or III HF and biochemical evidence of iron deficiency, but excluded patients with renal impairment (mean eGFR 64 mL/min). It showed a functional and symptomatic benefit without the adverse event profile of TREAT—there was a small but statistically significant improvement in haemoglobin in the treatment arm (13.0 ± 1 g/dL vs 12.5 ± 1 g/dL in placebo, $p < 0.001$).

Management of the acute admission with heart failure

Diuretics

The nephrotoxicity and decline in renal function with diuretic therapy may cause a therapeutic dilemma. Patients with decompensated HF with either associated AKI or underlying CKD are more likely to suffer further AKI due to diuretic drugs, and the adverse effect is even more pronounced in patients receiving blockers of the RAAS. ACE inhibitors (or ARBs) may have to be stopped during an acute admission due to AKI or hyperkalaemia, but they should be reintroduced when the acute risk has passed.

Patients with AKI or CKD are less responsive to diuretics than patients without renal impairment. The use of high doses of diuretics is correlated with poor outcome in HF, and the association is most likely due to the diuretic resistance seen in patients with the more severe forms of the cardiorenal syndrome, and in those with very poor haemodynamic status, in turn a marker of the most severe HF. It is important to note that using diuretics to improve urine output in acutely unwell patients will not improve renal function (in fact it may worsen it in those with hypovolaemia), and so diuretics should only be used when the removal of excesses of fluid is clinically required. Therapeutic B-type natriuretic peptide (BNP, nesiritide) does not reduce the need for diuretic, nor increase urine output in patients admitted acutely with HF.[64] Nitrates, and also hydralazine, are useful alternatives to blockade of the RAAS when HF exacerbations are complicated by AKI. However, hypotension may preclude their use.

In the acute setting, if nitrates are unable to stabilize a patient with severe HF coupled with AKI and diuretic resistance, the treatment options become quite limited, at which point haemofiltration may need to be considered (see below).

Inotropes

Positive inotropic agents were once regularly used for treating acute admissions with decompensated HF, but this practice has now fallen from favour. Low doses of dopamine interact with specific receptors in the kidney resulting in an increase in renal blood flow without apparent significant inotropic effect, and hence dopamine continues to be used by some at a 'renal dose', with the aim of improving the response to diuretics, and reducing the incidence and progression of AKI.[65] Unfortunately any data which has shown benefits of low dose dopamine regimes have derived from small-scale selected nonrandomized studies.

Haemofiltration

Haemofiltration is the ultrafiltration of fluid from the body via an extracorporeal machine. It uses the same principle as that used to offload fluid from haemodialysis patients, and it can now be achieved with portable machines designed specifically for haemofiltration only. Ultrafiltration has the advantage over diuretic therapy in that more rapid fluid and sodium removal is possible during the early phase of an admission with decompensated HF, minimizing the tendency to deterioration of renal function or hypotension that might accompany high dose diuretic therapy. The controlled nature of the haemofiltration process may thus benefit patients with labile blood pressure response during treatment. Studies have shown a short-term improvement in outcome when using haemofiltration instead of intravenous diuresis as first-line therapy for acute admissions with HF,[66] but longer-term outcome results are still awaited.

There is little evidence to support the use of PD in the management of acute HF. The logistics and safety of inserting a PD catheter in an acutely unwell patient, followed by its immediate use, are likely to preclude its becoming a standard therapy.

Diagnostic and therapeutic use of B-type natriuretic peptide

The evidence behind the use of BNP as a diagnostic tool has come from studies that either excluded patients with significant CKD, or studies that showed reduced clinical efficacy of BNP in the context of coexistent CKD. Given the prevalence of kidney disease in the HF population and vice versa, it is vital to have better understanding of BNP in such scenarios. Ventricular hypertrophy, dilatation, and abnormalities of function, as well as extracellular fluid accumulation, are commonplace in CKD patients, making the diagnosis of HF difficult. BNP is a potentially useful clinical tool in these circumstances.

Difficulties in interpretation arise because BNP levels may be elevated in CKD in the absence of HF. BNP correlates strongly with LVH, commonplace in CKD. BNP is partly metabolized in the renal parenchyma, so levels will also tend to be elevated in patients with reduced renal function. It is not removed by dialysis, but posthaemodialysis BNP levels show a fall that correlates with ultrafiltration volume. An elevated BNP is less likely to occur in patients using PD. BNP is probably still useful in diagnosing HF in ESRD, but only if higher diagnostic cut-offs (e.g. 200 pg/mL) are used, which reduces the sensitivity of the test. Its use should not replace clinical judgment.[64,67,68]

Although BNP increases renal perfusion, its therapeutic use does not reduce the occurrence of AKI in decompensated HF in patients with pre-existent CKD.[69] BNP reduces distal tubular reabsorption of sodium, leading to effective diuresis, an effect which is lost in CKD where glomerular or tubular disease predominate. The blunting of this effect may contribute to the high occurrence of HF in CKD patients, as such patients are less able to mount an effective response to fluid overload.

Acute pulmonary oedema and renal artery stenosis

A small number of patients with bilateral significant renal artery stenosis (RAS) present with sudden onset 'flash' pulmonary oedema, which can be life threatening.[70] These patients can be recognized by the absence of overt CAD, and the presence of severe, often accelerated, hypertension, AKI, and evidence of widespread atheroma (particularly arterial bruits). The Angioplasty and Stenting for Renal Artery Lesions (ASTRAL) trial has shown that endovascular intervention (angioplasty and stenting) with medical therapy does not reduce cardiovascular events and mortality in over 800 patients with significant RAS, when compared to medical therapy alone.[71] However, the study did not examine the effect of revascularization on HF, and nor has any previous trial. Despite the absence of conclusive benefit, the clinical consensus is that patients with 'flash' pulmonary oedema and RAS should be urgently treated with endovascular renal revascularization and there are many reports of subsequent successful clinical outcomes.[72]

Conclusion

Heart failure in CKD carries an excess mortality through a heterogeneous series of pathophysiological interactions. Prevention of LVH through blood pressure management and volume control, and early modification of risk factors for CAD is vital. A change in eGFR and proteinuria are early indicators of adverse cardiovascular outcome and, thus also indicate the need for early therapeutic intervention. Simple medical therapy, such as β-blockers and drugs that act on the RAAS, are effective but underused in patients with HF and renal impairment. These agents are safe provided that patients are appropriately monitored. Management of HF in the setting of acute or chronic kidney disease is complicated by the potentially nephrotoxic effect of many current therapies. PD and haemofiltration are measures that may yet improve the outcome of cardiorenal disease.

References

1. Go AS, Chertow GM, Fan D, McCulloch CE, Hsu C. Chronic kidney disease and the risks of death, cardiovascular events, and hospitalization. *New Engl J Med* 2004;**351**:1296–305.
2. McAlister FA, Ezekowitz J, Tonelli M, Armstrong PW. Renal insufficiency and heart failure: prognostic and therapeutic implications from a prospective cohort study. *Circulation* 2004;**109**:1004–9.
3. Foley RN, Parfrey PS, Harnett JD, Kent GM. The prognostic importance of left ventricular geometry in uremic cardiomyopathy. *J Am Coll Cardiol* 1995;**5**:2024–31.
4. Parfrey PS, Foley RN. The clinical epidemiology of cardiac disease in chronic renal failure. *J Am Soc Nephrol* 1999;**10**:1606–15.
5. Saravanan P, Freeman G, Davidson NC. Risk assessment for sudden cardiac death in dialysis patients: How relevant are conventional cardiac risk factors? *Int J Cardiol* 2009;doi:10.1016/j.ijcard.2009.03.048.
6. Foley RN, Parfrey PS, Harnett JD, Kent GM, Murray DC, Barrett PE. Impact of hypertension on cardiomyopathy, morbidity and mortality in end-stage renal disease. *Kidney Int* 1996;**49**:1379–85.
7. Herzog C, Muster H, Li S, Collins A. Impact of congestive heart failure, chronic kidney disease, and anemia on survival in the Medicare population. *J Card Fail* 2004;**10**:467–72.
8. Dries DL, Exner DV, Domanski MJ, Greenberg B, Stevenson LW. The prognostic implications of renal insufficiency in asymptomatic and symptomatic patients with left ventricular systolic dysfunction. *J Am Coll Cardiol* 2000;**35**:681–9.
9. Campbell RC, Sui X, Filippatos G, *et al.* Association of chronic kidney disease with outcomes in chronic heart failure: a propensity-matched study. *Nephrol Dial Transplant* 2009;**24**:186–93.
10. Section H—Mortality and causes of death. In: *USRDS 2008 Annual Data Report* 2008, pp. 619–70.
11. Ronco C, Haapio M, House AA, Anavekar N, Bellomo R. Cardiorenal syndrome. *J Am Coll Cardiol* 2008;**52**:1527–39.
12. Fox KF, Cowie MR, Wood DA, *et al.* Coronary artery disease as the cause of incident heart failure in the population. *Heart* 2001;**22**: 228–236.
13. Silberberg JS, Barre PE, Prichard SS, Sniderman AD. Impact of left ventricular hypertrophy on survival in end-stage renal disease. *Kidney Int* 1989;**36**:286–90.

14. Levin A, Singer J, Thompson C, Ross H, Lewis M. Prevalent left ventricular hypertrophy in the predialysis population: identifying opportunities for intervention. *Am J Kidney Dis* 1996;**27**:347–54.
15. Cannella G, Paoletti E, Delfino R, Peloso G, Molinari S, Traverso GB. Regression of left ventricular hypertrophy in hypertensive dialyzed uremic patients on long-term antihypertensive therapy. *Kidney Int* 1993;**44**:881–6.
16. Verma A, Anavekar NS, Meris A, *et al.* The relationship between renal function and cardiac structure, function, and prognosis after myocardial infarction: the VALIANT *Echo Study. J Am Coll Cardiol* 2007;**50**:1238–45.
17. Stack AG, Bloembergen WE. Prevalence and clinical correlates of coronary artery disease among new dialysis patients in the United States: a cross-sectional study. *J Am Soc Nephrol* 2001;**12**:1516–23.
18. Farrington K, Hodsman A, Casula A, Ansell D, Feehally J. Chapter 4: ESRD prevalent rates in 2007 in the UK: national and centre-specific analyses. In: *UK Renal Registry 11th Annual Report* 2007, pp. 43–68.
19. Ritz E, Rychlík I, Locatelli F, Halimi S. End-stage renal failure in type 2 diabetes: A medical catastrophe of worldwide dimensions. *Am J Kidney Dis* 1999;**34**:795–808.
20. Catalano C. De novo diabetes in dialysis patients: when diabetes is not diabetic nephropathy. *Nephrol Dial Transplant* 1996;**11**:938–41.
21. Hadi HA, Suwaidi JA. Endothelial dysfunction in diabetes mellitus. *Vasc Health Risk Manag* 2007;**3**:853–76.
22. Nelson RG, Knowler WC, Pettitt DJ, Saad MF, Charles MA, Bennett PH. Assessment of risk of overt nephropathy in diabetic patients from albumin excretion in untimed urine specimen. *Arch Intern Med* 1991;**151**:1761–5.
23. Rossing P, Hougaard P, Borch-Johnsen K, Parving H. Predictors of mortality in insulin dependent diabetes: 10 year observational follow up study. *BMJ* 1996;**31**:779–84.
24. Gerstein HC, Mann J, Yi Q, *et al.* Albuminuria and risk of cardiovascular events, death, and heart failure in diabetic and nondiabetic individuals. *JAMA* 2001;**286**:421–6.
25. Braun J, Oldendor FM, Moshage W, Heidler R, Zeitler E, Luft F. Electron beam computed tomography in the evaluation of cardiac calcification in chronic dialysis patients. *Am J Kidney Dis* 1996;**27**: 394–401.
26. London GM. Arterial media calcification in end-stage renal disease: impact on all-cause and cardiovascular mortality. *Nephrol Dial Transplant* 2003;**18**:1731–40.
27. Hujairi NM, Afzali B, Goldsmith DJ. Cardiac calcification in renal patients: what we do and don't know. *Am J Kidney Dis* 2003;**43**:234–43.
28. Moe SM, O'Neill KD, Reslerova M, *et al.* Natural history of vascular calcification in dialysis and transplant patients. *Nephrol Dial Transplant* 2004;**19**:2387–93.
29. Wang M, Tsai W, Chen J, Cheng M, Huang J. Arterial stiffness correlated with cardiac remodelling in patients with chronic kidney disease. *Nephrology* 2007;**12**:591–7.
30. Bongartz LG, Cramer MJ, Doevendans PA, Joles JA, Braam B. The severe cardiorenal syndrome: 'Guyton revisited'. *Eur Heart J* 2005;**26**:11–17.
31. Tripepi G, Mallamaci F, Zoccali C. Inflammation markers, adhesion molecules, and all-cause and cardiovascular mortality in patients with ESRD: searching for the best risk marker by multivariate modeling. *J Am Soc Nephrol* 2005;**16**:s83–8.
32. Hung AM, Ikizler TA. Hemodialysis central venous catheters as a source of inflammation and its implications. *Sem Dial* 2008;**21**:401–4.
33. Apple FS, Murakami MM, Pearce LA, Herzog CA. multi-biomarker risk stratification of N-terminal pro-B-type natriuretic peptide, high-sensitivity C-reactive protein, and cardiac troponin T and I in end-stage renal disease for all-cause death. *Clin Chem* 2004;**50**:2279–85.
34. Kayikcioglu M, Tumuklu M, Ozkahya M, *et al.* The benefit of salt restriction in the treatment of end-stage renal disease by haemodialysis. *Nephrol Dial Transplant* 2009;**24**:956–62.
35. Ozkahya M, Toz H, Qzerkan F, *et al.* Impact of volume control on left ventricular hypertrophy in dialysis patients. *J Nephrol* 2002;**15**: 655–60.
36. Fluck R, Rao R, van Schalkwyk D, Ansell D, Feest T. The UK Vascular Access Survey—follow-up data and repeat survey (chapter 5). *Nephrol Dial Transplant* 2007;**22**(Suppl 7):vii51–7.
37. MacRae JM. Vascular access and cardiac disease: is there a relationship? *Curr Opin Nephrol Hyperten* 2006;**15**:577–82.
38. Shurrab A, MacDowall P, Wright J, Mamtora H, Kalra P. The importance of associated extra-renal vascular disease on the outcome of patients with atherosclerotic renovascular disease. *Nephron Clin Prac* 2003;**93**:51–7.
39. MacDowall P, Kalra Pa, O'Donoghue DJ, Waldek S, Mamtora H, Brown K. Risk of morbidity from renovascular disease in elderly patients with congestive cardiac failure. *Lancet* 1998;**352**:13–16.
40. de Silva R, Loh H, Rigby AS, *et al.* Epidemiology, associated factors, and prognostic outcomes of renal artery stenosis in chronic heart failure assessed by magnetic resonance angiography. *Am J Cardiol* 2007;**100**:273–9.
41. Kalra PA, Guo H, Kausz AT, *et al.* Atherosclerotic renovascular disease in United States patients aged 67 years or older: risk factors, revascularization, and prognosis. *Kidney Int* 2005;**68**:293–301.
42. Kane GC, Xu N, Mistrik E, Roubicek T, Stanson AW, Garovic VD. Renal artery revascularization improves heart failure control in patients with atherosclerotic renal artery stenosis. *Nephrol Dial Transplant* 2009;1–7.
43. Wright JR, Shurrab AE, Cooper A, Kalra PR, Foley RN, Kalra PA. Progression of cardiac dysfunction in patients with atherosclerotic renovascular disease. *QJM* 2009;**102**:695–704.
44. Wright JR, Shurrab AE, Cooper A, Kalra PR, Foley RN, Kalra PA. Left ventricular morphology and function in patients with atherosclerotic renovascular disease. *J Am Soc Nephrol* 2005;**16**:2746–53.
45. Gottlieb S. The prognostic importance of different definitions of worsening renal function in congestive heart failure. *J Card Fail* 2002;**8**:136–41.
46. Smith GL, Vaccarino V, Kosiborod M, *et al.* Worsening renal function: what is a clinically meaningful change in creatinine during hospitalization with heart failure? *J Card Fail* 2003;**9**:13–25.
47. Forman DE, Butler J, Wang Y, *et al.* Incidence, predictors at admission, and impact of worsening renal function among patients hospitalized with heart failure. *J Am Coll Cardiol* 2004;**43**:61–7.
48. Cowie MR, Komajda M, Murray-Thomas T, Underwood J, Ticho B. Prevalence and impact of worsening renal function in patients hospitalized with decompensated heart failure: results of the prospective outcomes study in heart failure (POSH). *Eur Heart J* 2006;**27**:1216–22.
49. Ljungman S, Laragh J, Cody R. Role of the kidney in congestive heart failure. Relationship of cardiac index to kidney function. *Drugs* 1990;**39**(Suppl 4):10–21.
50. Ahmed A, Love T, Sui X, Rich M. Effects of ACE inhibitors in systolic heart failure patients with chronic kidney disease: a propensity score analysis. *J Card Fail* 2009;**12**:499–506.
51. Yancy CW, Lopatin M, Stevenson LW, De Marco T, Fonarow GC. Clinical presentation, management, and in-hospital outcomes of patients admitted with acute decompensated heart failure with preserved systolic function: a report from the Acute Decompensated Heart Failure National Registry (ADHERE) Database. *J Am Coll Cardiol* 2006;**47**:76–84.
52. McMurray JJ, Pitt B, Latini R, *et al.* Effects of the oral direct renin inhibitor aliskiren in patients with symptomatic heart failure. *Circ Heart Fail* 2008;**1**:17–24.
53. Rales investigators. Effectiveness of spironolactone added to an angiotensin-converting enzyme inhibitor and a loop diuretic for severe chronic congestive heart failure (the Randomized Aldactone Evaluation Study [RALES]. *Am J Cardiol* 1996;**78**:902–7.

54. Young JB, Dunlap ME, Pfeffer MA, *et al.* Mortality and morbidity reduction with Candesartan in patients with chronic heart failure and left ventricular systolic dysfunction: results of the CHARM low-left ventricular ejection fraction trials. *Circulation* 2004;**110**:2618–26.
55. Ezekowitz J, McAlister FA, Humphries KH, *et al.* The association among renal insufficiency, pharmacotherapy, and outcomes in 6,427 patients with heart failure and coronary artery disease. . *J Am Coll Cardiol* 2004;**44**:1587–92.
56. Cice G, Ferrara L, D'Andrea A, D'Isa S. Carvedilol increases two-year survival in dialysis patients with dilated cardiomyopathy—a prospective, placebo-controlled trial. *J Am Coll Cardiol* 2003;**43**:1438–44.
57. Abbott K, Trespalacios F, Agodoa L, Taylor A, Bakris G. Beta-blocker use in long-term dialysis patients. *Arch Intern Med* 2004;**164**:2465–71.
58. Cohen-Solal A, Kotecha D, van Veldhuisen DJ, *et al.* Efficacy and safety of nebivolol in elderly heart failure patients with impaired renal function: insights from the SENIORS trial. *Eur J Heart Fail* 2009;**11**:872–80.
59. Shlipak MG, Smith GL, Rathore SS, Massie BM, Krumholz HM. Renal function, digoxin therapy, and heart failure outcomes: evidence from the digoxin intervention group trial. *J Am Soc Nephrol* 2004;**15**:2195–203.
60. Sánchez J, Ortega T, Rodríguez C, *et al.* Efficacy of peritoneal ultrafiltration in the treatment of refractory congestive heart failure. *Nephrol Dial Transplant* 2010;**25**:605–61.
61. Silverberg D, Wexler D, Blum B, Iaina A. Anemia in chronic kidney disease and congestive heart failure. *Blood Purif* 2003;**21**:124–30.
62. Pfeffer M, Burdmann E, Chen C, *et al.* A trial of darbepoetin alfa in type 2 diabetes and chronic kidney disease. *N Engl J Med* 2009;**361**:2019–32.
63. Anker SD, Comin Colet J, Filippatos G, *et al.* Ferric carboxymaltose in patients with heart failure and iron deficiency. *N Engl J Med* 2009;**361**:2436–48.
64. Dhar S, Pressman GS, Subramanian S, *et al.* Natriuretic peptides and heart failure in the patient with chronic kidney disease: a review of current evidence. *Postgrad Med J* 2009;**85**:299–302.
65. Elkayam U, Ng TM, Hatamizadeh P, Janmohamed M, Mehra A. Renal vasodilatory action of dopamine in patients with heart failure: magnitude of effect and site of action. *Circulation* 2008;**117**:200–5.
66. Bart BA, Boyle A, Bank AJ, *et al.* Ultrafiltration versus usual care for hospitalized patients with heart failure: the Relief for Acutely Fluid-Overloaded Patients With Decompensated Congestive Heart Failure (RAPID-CHF) trial. *J Am Coll Cardiol* 2005;**46**:2043–6.
67. McCullough PA, Sandberg KR. B-type natriuretic peptide and renal disease. *Heart Fail Rev* 2003;**8**:355–8.
68. Cataliott A, Malatino L, Jougasak IM, *et al.* Circulating natriuretic peptide concentrations in patients with end-stage renal disease: role of brain natriuretic peptide as a biomarker for ventricular remodeling. *Mayo Clin Proc* 2001;**76**:1111–19.
69. Witteles RM, Kao D, Christopherson D, *et al.* Impact of nesiritide on renal function in patients with acute decompensated heart failure and pre-existing renal dysfunction a randomized, double-blind, placebo-controlled clinical trial. *J Am Coll Cardiol* 2007;**50**:1835–40.
70. Pickering T, Herman L, Devereux R, *et al.* Recurrent pulmonary oedema in hypertension due to bilateral renal artery stenosis: treatment by angioplasty or surgical revascularisation. *Lancet* 1988;**8610**:551–2.
71. Wheatley K, Ives N, Gray R, *et al.* The ASTRAL investigators. Revascularization versus medical therapy for renal artery stenosis. *N Engl J Med* 2009;**361**:1953–62.
72. Levey AS, Coresh J, Balk E, *et al.* National Kidney Foundation Practice Guidelines for Chronic Kidney Disease: Evaluation, Classification and Stratification. *Ann Intern Med* 2003;**139**:137–47.

30

Chronic lung disease

Michael Greenstone, Simon P. Hart, and Nathaniel M. Hawkins

Chronic obstructive pulmonary disease (COPD) and heart failure (HF) commonly occur in the same patient and the presence of one will affect the prognosis from the other. There is a growing body of evidence linking COPD and vascular events. When the National Health and Nutrition Examination Survey population was stratified by forced expiratory volume in 1 s (FEV_1) and examined for cause of death, then the risk of death from cardiovascular disease was as much as fivefold greater in those with the lowest FEV_1 compared to the highest.[1] Studies in Malmo and Baltimore showed that those with the most rapidly declining FEV_1 were most likely to die of cardiovascular disease. Low baseline FEV_1 also predicts stroke mortality, all-cause cancer mortality, and death from nonrespiratory, noncardiac causes.[2] Thus cardiac disease and respiratory function are strongly correlated: although smoking is the obvious common risk factor, the relationship still stands in nonsmokers. It is possible that FEV_1 is a marker for an ill-defined environmental factor such as poor nutrition but it could also be a marker of a systemic process of chronic tissue damage and abnormal repair.

The mechanisms behind the association remain conjectural but inflammation, hypoxia, oxidative stress, and sympathetic nervous system malfunction may all be important.[3] In experimental models, inflammation can drive both the genesis and progression of atherosclerotic plaques. Decline in FEV_1 correlates with raised inflammatory markers such as C-reactive protein (CRP) and fibrinogen, and the inflammatory component of COPD may explain many of the 'systemic' features of the condition such as muscle weakness and weight loss. Patients with COPD seem to have increased arterial stiffness compared with appropriately matched normal subjects, although abnormalities of endothelial dysfunction are inconsistently found.[4] As yet, there is no convincing evidence that treating airway inflammation in COPD with steroids affects cardiovascular mortality, but there is growing interest in the possibility that statins reduce airway inflammation[5] and the combination of statin and inhaled steroids might be associated with decreased mortality in COPD.[6]

Although COPD is set to become the third leading cause of death worldwide, cardiovascular disease is the most important cause of both morbidity and mortality in patients with mild or moderate COPD and the leading cause of hospitalization. Until recently, it was thought that patients with severe COPD died from respiratory failure rather than myocardial infarction. The attribution was usually made from review of the notes rather than autopsy, however, and recent unselected data based on autopsy suggested the leading causes of death in patients dying within 24 h of admission with an 'acute exacerbation of COPD' was cardiac failure followed by pneumonia and thromboembolic events: all were more common than respiratory failure.[7] In one of the largest drug trials examining mortality in COPD, cardiovascular causes and malignancy were as common as acute exacerbations as a cause of death.[8] Recent reviews have emphasized the high incidence of coronary disease in contributing to mortality in cohorts of patients with COPD.[3,9]

The prevalence of COPD in the HF population is not well described, but a recent review[10] noted widely variable prevalence rates (9–52%) with a trend towards higher rates in more recent studies. The rise may reflect the comorbidities of an ageing population or a growing awareness of COPD and the wider availability of spirometry to make the diagnosis. In large studies of patients hospitalized with HF, the reported prevalence of COPD varied from 9% to 41% (median 26%). However, in many cohorts the diagnosis of COPD was based on self-report rather than spirometry and therefore likely to be subject to considerable inaccuracy. Most studies found a higher prevalence of COPD in those HF populations with normal left ventricular ejection fraction (LVEF), suggesting that COPD is more likely to be diagnosed if left ventricular systolic dysfunction (LVSD) is excluded. Using the Scottish Continuous Morbidity recording database, which looks at disease trends in primary care, the prevalence of COPD in the HF population was approximately sevenfold higher than in the general population and seemed to be steadily increasing.[11]

There is less information about the prevalence of HF in a COPD population, but in unselected groups the prevalence of LVSD ranged from 10% to 46% of reviewed studies.[12]

The diagnosis of COPD

The Global Initiative against Chronic Obstructive Lung Disease (GOLD) defines COPD[13] as 'a disease characterized by airflow limitation that is not fully reversible. The airflow limitation is usually both progressive and associated with an abnormal inflammatory response of the lungs to noxious particles or gases' (see Box 30.1). The definition is important because it emphasizes that the diagnosis requires an objective demonstration of limitation of flow in the airways (ideally by spirometry) and that this narrowing is relatively fixed, in contrast to asthma where the narrowing is largely reversible with treatment or the passage of time. The definition emphasizes the progressive nature of the condition and the recognition of the inflammatory component dictates some of the treatment choices.

Spirometry is a simple technique which is increasingly available in primary care and almost universally in secondary care. It measures FEV_1 and compares it with the total amount that can be forcibly exhaled (forced vital capacity or FVC) after a full inspiration. If the ratio of the two measurements is less than 70%, then airflow obstruction is present. Reversibility studies may be required to distinguish COPD from asthma. Once airflow obstruction is confirmed, then the absolute value of FEV_1 compared to the value predicted from a matched normal population is useful for stratification (Table 30.1).

The requirement to demonstrate airflow obstruction ensures the individuals with recurrent cough and sputum (a pragmatic epidemiological definition used by the Medical Research Council to define 'chronic bronchitis' and equivalent to GOLD stage 0) are not diagnosed as having COPD in the face of essentially normal lung function. Hypersecretory bronchitis is almost universal amongst chronic smokers, has a much better prognosis than COPD, and is unlikely to cause breathlessness. COPD affects only 1 in 6 long-term smokers, so not all breathless smokers can be assumed to have COPD even if they have a productive cough. Although most COPD patients have a 20 pack-year smoking history, the condition is increasingly recognized in nonsmokers, particularly in the developing world where environmental smoke and other toxins may be important.[14]

Table 30.1 Classification of COPD by severity

Stage	Characteristics
0: At risk	Normal spirometry. Chronic symptoms (cough, sputum production)
I: Mild COPD	FEV_1/FVC <70% and FEV_1 ≥80% predicted, with or without chronic symptoms (cough, sputum production)
II: Moderate COPD	FEV_1/FVC <70%; 30% ≤ FEV_1 < 80% predicted (IIA: 50% ≤ FEV_1 < 80% predicted) (IIB: 30% ≤ FEV_1 < 50% predicted), with or without chronic symptoms (cough, sputum production, dyspnoea)
III: Severe COPD	FEV_1/FVC < 70% and FEV_1 < 30% predicted, or the presence of respiratory failure,a or clinical signs of right HF

[a] Respiratory failure: Pa_{O_2} <8.0 kPa (60 mmHg) with or without Pa_{CO_2} >6.7 kPa (50 mmHg) while breathing air at sea level.

Box 30.1 The diagnosis of COPD

COPD is characterized by airflow obstruction. The airflow obstruction is usually progressive, not fully reversible and does not change markedly over several months. Airflow obstruction is defined by a reduced FEV_1 and a reduced FEV_1/FVC ratio such that FEV_1 is less than 80% predicted and FEV_1/FVC is less than 0.7. Making a diagnosis relies on clinical judgement based on a combination of history, physical examination, and confirmation of the presence of airflow obstruction using spirometry.[a]

The diagnosis of asthma

There is no universally agreed definition.[b] A history of atopy, cough, wheeze, chest tightness, and variable breathlessness is usual. Symptoms are often worse at night or early morning and may be precipitated by cold air, exercise, or allergen exposure. A good history and response to inhaled treatment makes the diagnosis more likely. A normal spirogram when the individual is not symptomatic does not exclude the diagnosis. In patients with obstructive spirometry, a change in FEV_1 >12% and greater than 400 mL in response to inhaled bronchodilators is useful evidence in favour of asthma.

[a] National Institute for Clinical Excellence. *Chronic obstructive pulmonary disease. Management of chronic obstructive pulmonary disease in adults in primary and secondary care.* February 2004.
[b] British Thoracic Society/Scottish Intercollegiate Network. *British guidelines on the management of asthma. A national clinical guideline.* May 2008.

Clinical assessment of the patient with chronic lung disease

It is important that cardiologists recognize isolated chronic lung disease in patients under their care because the diagnosis may obviate the need for cardiac investigation and treatment. In patients with both cardiac and respiratory disease, it is axiomatic that treatment of both conditions and the recognition of the predominant one may allow better treatment and more informed prognostication.

The clinical history and examination may allow a relatively confident identification of the patient whose predominating problem is chronic lung disease. Patients with COPD usually have a long history of productive cough and consultations for 'chest infections' which are usually mild exacerbations of their COPD. At this point, wheeze usually predominates but early inspiratory crackles at the lung bases are sometimes heard and may be misinterpreted as indicating pulmonary oedema if the patient has a cardiac history. Careful examination after the exacerbation has settled will usually show diminished chest expansion with quiet breath sounds even if no wheeze is audible.

The pattern of breathlessness is not very helpful in distinguishing respiratory from cardiac disease, but prominent wheeze is more suggestive of COPD. Orthopnoea is seen with advanced COPD and is also a prominent symptom in patients with diaphragmatic weakness due to neuromuscular disease. Paroxysmal nocturnal dyspnoea is thought of as a feature of HF, but may occur in patients with asthma and less commonly in patients with very advanced COPD. Chest pain is an under-reported symptom in COPD but is usually fairly clearly associated with new infective symptoms or linked to bouts of prolonged coughing. The distinction from ischaemic cardiac pain can usually be made on the basis of its lack of severity and its localized nature.

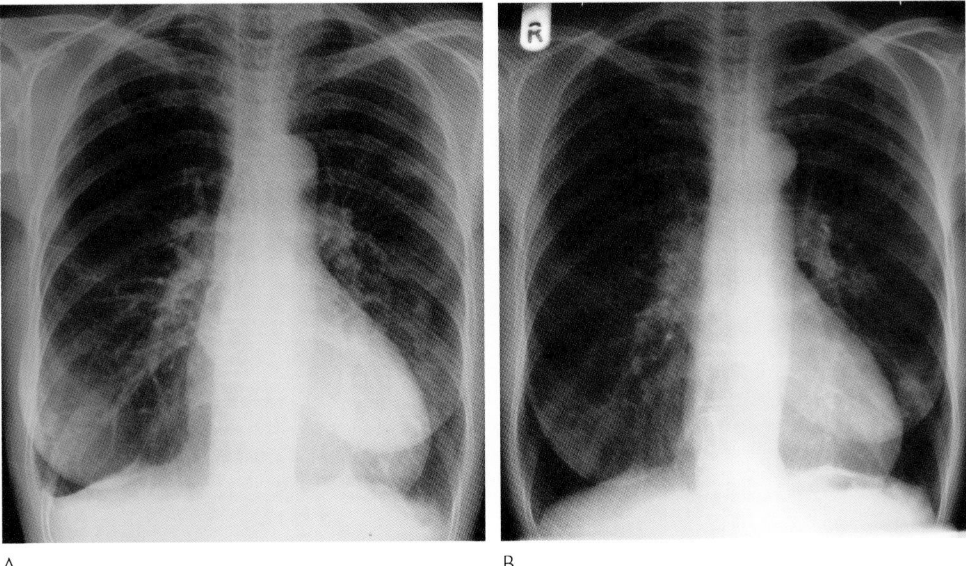

Fig. 30.1 A 60-year-old woman with severe COPD and cardiac failure secondary to mitral valve disease and impaired left ventricular systolic function. (A) There are small bilateral pleural effusions, Kerley B lines at the right base, and pulmonary venous distension in the left upper lobe. There is no venous diversion to the right upper lobe because of her severe emphysema. (B) Following treatment the costophrenic angles are preserved and the subtle changes in the left upper lobe have resolved.

Central cyanosis (observed on the tongue rather than the lips) is hard to detect with confidence if oxygen saturations are much above 88%, but its presence almost invariably indicates respiratory failure due to advanced lung disease. Signs of hyperinflation (a barrel chest, pursed lip breathing, and the use of accessory muscles of respiration) point to severe COPD. The development of peripheral oedema is a milestone in the natural history of COPD and usually indicates that the patient should be considered for long-term oxygen therapy (LTOT) when other causes have been considered. It is when patients present acutely with peripheral oedema that the difficulty distinguishing cardiac from respiratory disease is greatest. In most COPD patients cardiac auscultation is unremarkable, in part because overinflated lungs make the heart sounds hard to hear, and venous pressure may not be raised. The mechanism of peripheral oedema in COPD is complex (see 'The heart in COPD', below).

In the presence of COPD, the radiological appearances of HF may be atypical. Most commonly, the characteristic pulmonary venous distension is attenuated because of underperfusion of an emphysematous upper lobe (Fig. 30.1). Another trap for the unwary is the patient with 'refractory HF' who is eventually found to have interstitial lung disease, usually idiopathic pulmonary fibrosis (IPF). The clinical picture is of increasingly intrusive dyspnoea and perhaps dry cough in the presence of basal and axillary 'Velcro-like' late inspiratory crackles which are persistent and best heard with the patient supine. The chest radiograph appearances are sometimes normal or may show small lung fields with diffuse lower-zone reticulation (Fig. 30.2). The diagnosis, once suspected, is easily confirmed with high-resolution CT scanning which shows subpleural basal changes with honeycombing, interlobular septal thickening and traction bronchiectasis most marked in the lower zones (Fig. 30.3). The appearances are usually sufficiently specific to obviate the need for thoracoscopic lung biopsy.

The heart in COPD

As COPD progresses, worsening ventilation–perfusion relationships in the lung cause chronic hypoxia, leading in turn to vasoconstriction of pulmonary arterioles and remodelling of the pulmonary

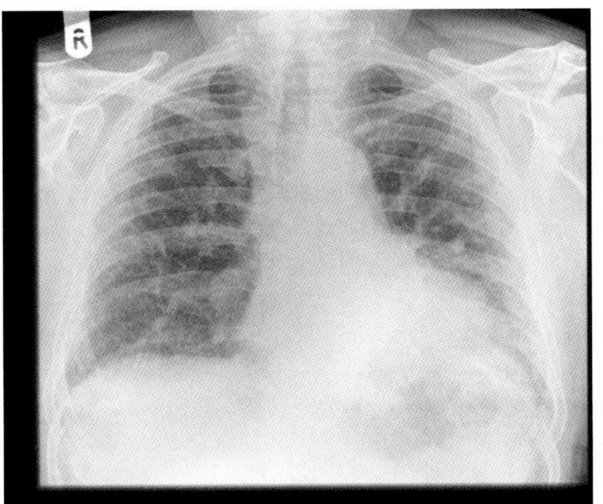

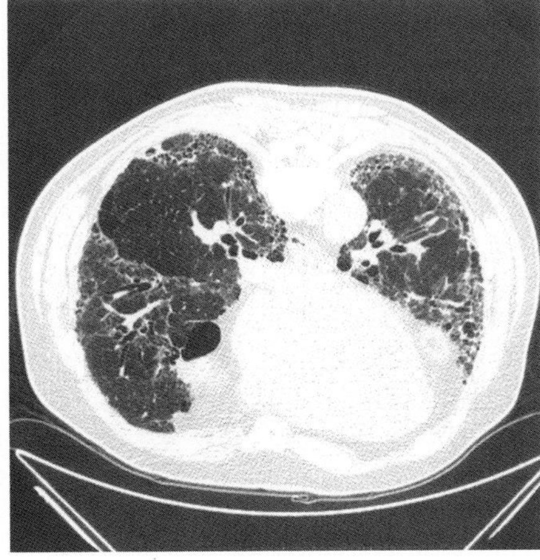

Fig. 30.2 A 74-year-old man with previous coronary artery surgery and hypertension with a 3-month history of progressive dyspnoea. (A) Plain chest radiograph shows borderline cardiomegaly and 'congested' lung fields with interstitial shadowing. (B) Prone high-resolution CT shows bilateral lower lobe fibrosis with predominantly subpleural reticulation and honeycombing suggestive of IPF.

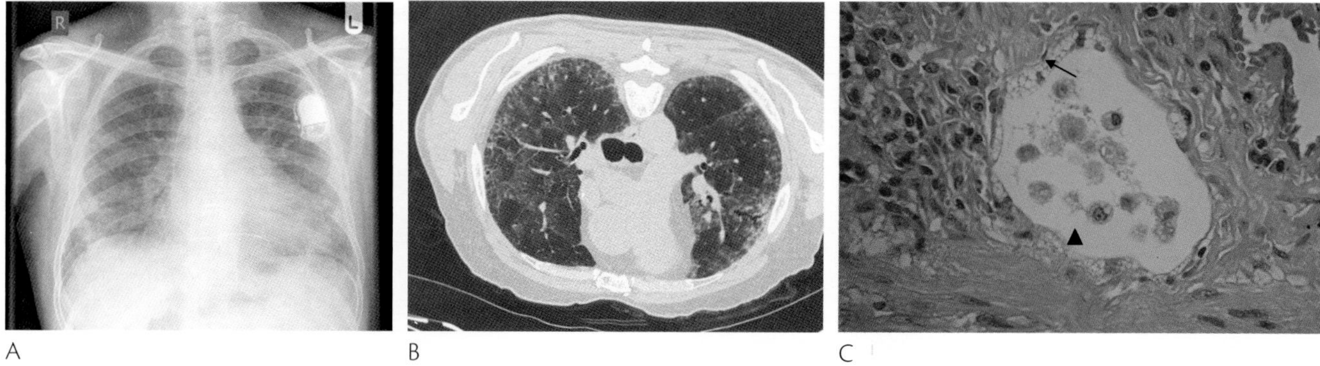

Fig. 30.3 Amiodarone pulmonary toxicity. (A) Chest radiograph demonstrating bilateral interstitial shadowing. The patient has a ventricular pacemaker and has had previous coronary artery bypass surgery. (B) High-resolution CT scan, performed with the patient lying prone, showing bilateral fibrosis and ground-glass change. (C) Histology of a video-assisted thoracoscopic lung biopsy demonstrating foamy type II alveolar epithelial cells (arrow) and alveolar spaces filled with macrophages (arrowhead). Other areas of the biopsy showed interstitial chronic inflammation and fibrosis, and scattered areas of organizing pneumonia.

vasculature. All three layers of the pulmonary arteriolar walls are involved and the mechanism is probably more complicated that pure hypoxic vasoconstriction,[15] which may explain the disappointing response of the raised pulmonary artery pressures to LTOT. Pulmonary hypertension in COPD carries a poor prognosis, but the pressure is rarely markedly elevated at rest. Pulmonary artery pressure may become quite abnormal on exercise, during sleep, or at the time of an exacerbation, and contribute to disability over and beyond that due to the airflow obstruction alone.

Echocardiography is often unsatisfactory in patients with COPD because of the poor acoustic window, but in many oedematous COPD patients the right atrial pressure is normal with a right ventricle which may be enlarged but apparently contracting well. Measurements of right ventricular ejection fraction are usually unremarkable. Oedematous patients with acute exacerbations of their COPD usually have an increase in their pulmonary artery pressure which returns to the (elevated) baseline as hypoxia improves. Some of these patients will have haemodynamic evidence of right HF as judged by an acute elevation in right ventricular end diastolic pressure (RVEDP) measured invasively at the time of an exacerbation.[16] It is now thought that an increase in RVEDP on exercise stretches the right atrium thereby increasing sympathetic activation and activating the renin–angiotensin–aldosterone system causing salt and water retention. A further potential contributor to fluid retention is that an increase in RVEDP may lead to abnormal interventricular septal motion, thereby impairing left ventricular function.[17]

Patients with pulmonary fibrosis are often very hypoxic but rarely become as polycythaemic or oedematous as patients with COPD. The difference perhaps reflects the more rapid downhill trajectory of IPF and the fact that COPD patients may be hypoxic for years before they are identified and treated with LTOT. A more significant difference is the presence of hypercapnia in the COPD group. Carbon dioxide decreases renal blood flow, glomerular filtration rate. and sodium and water excretion as hydrogen ions are exchanged for sodium and the renal tubules retain bicarbonate ions (HCO_3^-) to buffer the acidosis.

The absence of recent type 2 respiratory failure in an oedematous COPD patient should prompt further investigation for an alternative cause for the oedema.

Lung function testing for the diagnosis of COPD

Spirometry is necessary to allow a firm diagnosis of COPD. Peak expiratory flow (PEF) meters are useful for recognizing changes in airway calibre in patients monitoring their own asthma or documenting recovery in an individual with an exacerbation of airflow obstruction, but are inadequate for making a definitive new diagnosis of COPD. The PEF manoeuvre is effort-dependent and poor technique (if not identified) can lead to an incorrect diagnosis. Conversely, some patients with established COPD may have relatively well-preserved flow rates because of the timing of airway collapse in relation to the lung volume. The reason is that PEF is a measurement recorded during the early part of expiration whereas in emphysema the problem is at the alveolar level where the loss of radial traction allows small airways to close prematurely at lower lung volumes. There is also a wide normal range of values so it is usually deviations from a patient's 'normal' reading that are most helpful, except in the acute setting when a very low reading may be diagnostic.

The diagnosis of COPD requires the demonstration of an obstructive ventilatory defect defined by an abnormal ratio of FEV_1 to FVC (<70%). The ratio is not particularly helpful in stratifying the severity of the COPD. Comparison of observed against predicted FEV_1 then allows the severity of the disease to be assigned.

As an example, consider a 60-year-old man 1.72 m tall with predicted values for FEV_1 of 3.1 L and FVC of 4.0 L. He undergoes spirometry because of breathlessness. His values are 0.9 L for FEV_1 and 1.5 L for FVC. The FEV_1/FVC ratio is 60%, which confirms the diagnosis of airflow obstruction. Assuming reversibility to inhaled bronchodilators is minimal, the diagnosis of COPD is established but might be considered mild on the basis that the ratio of 60% is not far below the threshold (>70%) above which COPD is not diagnosed. However, when the observed FEV_1 is compared to the predicted value (allowing for age, sex, and height) he is diagnosed as having very severe disease (<30%) and which may result in recurrent hospital admissions with exacerbations, or preclude potentially curative surgery were he to develop lung cancer.

Sometimes more detailed lung function tests are required, particularly if the mildness of the airflow obstruction seems at variance with the clinical picture. The measurement of lung volumes and gas transfer are carried out routinely in lung function laboratories and are sometimes useful in the identification of a restrictive or mixed defect. In a pure restrictive lung disease, such as IPF, there is usually a symmetrical reduction in lung volumes (FEV_1, FVC, RV (residual volume), and TLC (total lung capacity)) together with a reduction in gas transfer of carbon monoxide (CO) expressed as reductions in TLco (transfer factor) and Kco (the gas transfer coefficient, the transfer factor corrected for alveolar volume). Patients with mixed defects, such as the concurrence of COPD and pulmonary fibrosis, or COPD and obesity, show obstructive spirometry but have small lung volumes as measured by TLC. The Kco, if low, may help identify patients with emphysema or fibrosis, both of which may be associated with relatively normal spirometry. When fibrosis and emphysema coexist the measurement is often markedly reduced and disability may be very severe.

A raised Kco is seen with so-called extrapulmonary restriction where the lungs themselves are functioning well but there is a problem with chest wall mechanics such as spinal deformity, weak respiratory muscles, or (most commonly) morbid obesity. With the possible exception of the notoriously difficult diagnosis of chronic thromboembolic disease, the combination of normal spirometry and transfer factor in a symptomatic patient virtually excludes the lungs as a cause for breathlessness. When cardiac and respiratory disease are both present, then a cardiopulmonary exercise test can be useful for apportionment as well as the identification of confounders such as hyperventilation or poor effort.

Lung function testing in cardiac disease

Even with an apparently uncomplicated myocardial infarct, there is abnormal pulmonary gas exchange as judged by an increase in the alveolar–arterial (A-a) gradient. Postulated mechanisms include basal airway closure, low cardiac output with greater desaturation of mixed venous blood, and ventilation–perfusion mismatch.[18]

In mild acute HF, there is a measurable reduction in vital capacity (VC) which takes several weeks to return to normal even though the radiological appearances have resolved. Wheeze may be a prominent auscultatory finding in acute pulmonary oedema (so-called cardiac asthma) and is traditionally attributed to peribronchial oedema. A more likely mechanism is mucosal swelling and reflex bronchoconstriction secondary to raised pulmonary vascular resistance.[19]

In the acute setting, there is often diagnostic uncertainty as to whether acute breathlessness is cardiac or respiratory in origin. If the PEF is in excess of 200 L/min, then cardiac disease is probably the explanation; if it is less than 100 L/min, then a respiratory cause is more likely.[20] Where there is still diagnostic uncertainty, natriuretic peptides may be useful. Pulmonary hypertension, cor pulmonale, and COPD are associated with intermediate elevations of this marker, but a level above 500 pg/mL is highly suggestive of primary cardiac disease. A level below 100 pg/mL has a high negative predictive value.

The situation in chronic HF is different because of respiratory muscle fatigue and wasting which contributes to loss of lung volume: nevertheless, patients with endstage HF show little if any evidence of airflow obstruction.[21,22]

Effect of comorbidity on outcome

Acute exacerbations of COPD are usually caused by viral or bacterial infection but rarely if ever by HF. Conversely, worsening HF is potentially multifactorial, and poor drug compliance, inappropriate prescribing, worsening ischaemia, arrhythmias, and infection are often implicated. A review of recent studies attributed respiratory infection as a frequent cause with an incidence of as much as 20% of HF exacerbations.[23] Patients hospitalized with HF have worse outcomes if they also have a COPD diagnosis.[24]

β-Blockers in patients with HF and COPD

β-Adrenoceptor blockade

The β-adrenoreceptors are G-protein-linked cell-surface receptors that mediate different effects in different tissues in response to catecholamines, particularly adrenaline (epinephrine) and noradrenaline (norepinephrine). β_1 receptors in the heart mediate increased heart rate and contractility, and β_1 antagonists have beneficial effects in patients with myocardial ischaemia or HF, and in the postoperative period. Relaxation of bronchial smooth muscle leading to bronchodilatation is mediated by activation of β_2 receptors. Concerns regarding the use of β-antagonists (β-blockers) initially arose following reports of acute bronchospasm in asthmatic patients given nonselective β-blockers, which block both β_1 and β_2 receptors.[25–27] The question is whether these observations can be extrapolated to patients with COPD, a disease of older people caused by long-term exposure to tobacco smoke in whom heart disease often coexists.

Underuse of β-blockers in patients with heart failure and COPD

In contrast to asthma, the airflow obstruction that characterizes COPD is largely (but not completely) irreversible following administration of bronchodilators, including β_2 agonists. Although the benefits of β-blockade in patients with HF due to LVSD are compelling and include a substantial improvement in survival,[28] almost all trials excluded patients with significant pulmonary disease, documented COPD, or bronchodilator therapy. Evidence from several studies suggests that β-blockers are underused in patients with both HF and COPD. For example, in a large primary care survey in Scotland, only 18% of patients with HF and COPD were prescribed β-blockers compared with 41% for those without COPD.[29] In the Euro Heart Failure Survey, 'pulmonary disease' was the most powerful independent predictor of β-blocker underuse (odds ratio 0.35),[30] and an Australian analysis revealed similar underuse of β-blockers at hospital discharge in patients with HF and airways disease.[31]

Do β-blockers make lung function worse in patients with COPD?

Although the definition of cardioselectivity varies, cardioselective β-blockers such as bisoprolol and nebivolol exhibit much greater affinity for β_1 receptors than for β_2 receptors. Carvedilol is the only noncardioselective β-blocker approved for treating HF. Theoretically, worsening of airflow obstruction should be less of an issue with cardioselective β-blockers compared with nonselective antagonists, which in patients with airways disease (asthma and COPD) undoubtedly reduce FEV_1, antagonize β-agonists, increase breathlessness, and necessitate withdrawal of patients from studies.[32] The long-term impact of β-blockade on COPD exacerbations is unknown, but is particularly important in patients with HF. Should an acute exacerbation of COPD necessitate abrupt β-blocker withdrawal, rebound ischaemia, ventricular arrhythmias, and death may follow.[33]

A Cochrane Library meta-analysis concluded that long-term cardioselective β-blockade is safe and well tolerated in COPD.[34] However, the quality of the reviewed evidence was poor—all of the studies were of short duration, included small numbers of patients, and focused mainly on lung function rather than clinically important outcomes such as exercise capacity, exacerbation rates, and quality of life. Furthermore, no study included any patients with HF. The β-blocker doses used were those employed for treating hypertension or angina, whereas in HF initial low doses are gradually titrated upwards. Information is particularly limited for β-blockers known to confer benefit in HF: many trials used metoprolol, whereas only two single-dose studies used bisoprolol and none used carvedilol or nebivolol. The same caveats apply to the evidence for β-blockade in patients with severe COPD. The few existing studies are small, of limited duration, predominantly used metoprolol, had no dose titration, and excluded patients with HF. However, bisoprolol caused a small but significant reduction in FEV_1 (−70 mL vs +120 mL with placebo) after 4 months' treatment in a recent randomized trial in 27 patients with coexisting HF and moderate or severe COPD.[35] Reversibility following inhaled a β_2-agonist and static lung volumes were not impaired by bisoprolol, and measures of health status showed a small, but nonsignificant, improvement with bisoprolol.

Because of a lack of large adequately powered trials, the true effects of long-term cardioselective β-blockade on airways disease in COPD are unknown. Serial home measurements of PEF are not helpful for disease monitoring in COPD. However, there is some evidence that a β-blocker confers benefit on patients with HF and coexisting COPD. In the Valsartan Heart Failure Trial, 140 (22%) of the 628 participants with physician-recorded COPD received β-blockers. Mortality over a mean of 23 months was approximately 17% in patients with HF and COPD who received a β-blocker, compared with 31% in those with not prescribed β-blockers, although there was no statistical adjustment for baseline differences.[36] A retrospective Canadian study of 11 942 elderly patients hospitalized for HF undoubtedly more accurately represents a 'real life' population of patients with HF.[37] The proportion with LVSD was unknown, and only 242 (6%) of the 3834 patients with concurrent COPD received β-blockers. Mortality during median follow-up of 21 months was lower in those prescribed β-blockers, after comprehensive adjustment for age, sex, comorbidity, and propensity scores (HR 0.78 [95% CI 0.63–0.95]). A more recent study of 2230 patients with COPD confirmed the association between β-blocker use and improved survival.[38]

On the basis of the available evidence, cardioselective β-blockers should be tried in patients with both HF and COPD, but gradual titration of dosage is especially important and extra vigilance is recommended to detect any deterioration in airways symptoms. Whether the noncardioselective carvedilol is as safe is simply not clear, but it has been successfully used in many patients with coexistent HF and airways disease.[39]

Amiodarone pulmonary toxicity

Epidemiology of amiodarone pulmonary toxicity

Amiodarone was developed as an antianginal drug in 1961, but its antiarrhythmic properties soon became apparent and by 1980 it was widely prescribed in the UK and continental Europe for the treatment of a variety of cardiac arrhythmias. However, lung disease in patients treated with amiodarone was first described only when it was used as an investigational drug in the US in the early 1980s. At the time fewer than 500 American patients had been treated,[40,41] yet an association between amiodarone and pulmonary toxicity had never been reported in Europe despite over 500 000 patient–years of experience (although it may have been missed). In six cases (incidence 1.4%) of amiodarone pulmonary toxicity (APT) reported in 1982, the daily maintenance dose of amiodarone ranged between 600 and 800 mg/day, with treatment durations of between 4 weeks and 8 months.[40] Subsequent reports over the next 10 years bore out that the risk of APT was dose-related (generally 400 mg/day or higher) and that clinical manifestations usually appeared within a few weeks or months of initiating treatment.[42]

The clinical features of APT are a gradual onset of breathlessness, fever, and sometimes chest pain, with crackles on auscultation of the lungs, a high erythrocyte sedimentation rate (ESR), and new pulmonary shadowing on the chest radiograph. Sometimes a pleural effusion develops. APT may be asymptomatic. A high-resolution CT scan of the chest usual reveals a mixture of alveolar and interstitial shadowing which may be symmetrical or asymmetrical. Of course, none of these clinical or radiological features is specific, so other diagnoses need to be considered and excluded, including pneumonia, HF, eosinophilic pneumonia, bronchoalveolar cell carcinoma, and idiopathic interstitial pneumonias (such as IPF and cryptogenic organizing pneumonia). A baseline chest radiograph before commencing amiodarone therapy is very helpful in excluding some of the latter diagnoses. It is possible that some reported cases of APT, particularly those occurring with lower amiodarone doses (e.g. 200 mg/day), longer durations of therapy, and with mainly fibrotic patterns on CT in fact represent coincidental cases of idiopathic interstitial pneumonias rather than amiodarone toxicity. The histological picture is one of oedema, inflammation, and fibrosis occurring in a nonspecific pattern. There may be areas of organizing pneumonia and type II pneumocyte hyperplasia, which is a general response to alveolar epithelial injury. However, a characteristic feature of APT is the presence of foamy macrophages, which are found in the alveoli in the lung biopsy or in the bronchoalveolar lavage fluid if bronchoscopy is performed.[43]

Mechanism of amiodarone pulmonary toxicity

The mechanism of APT seems to be directly related to the peculiar pharmacokinetics of amiodarone. Following absorption from the gastrointestinal tract, lipid-soluble amiodarone is distributed to fat and many other tissues and little remains in the blood, which accounts for its enormous apparent volume of distribution (5000 L/70 kg). Its half-life is long (>30 days) and after slow release from the tissues, amiodarone is metabolized by the liver and eliminated in the bile.

Amiodarone and its metabolite desethylamiodarone, both cationic amphiphilics, are preferentially distributed in fat, lung, thyroid, kidney, and liver.[44,45] Macrophages in various tissues show lipidosis and a characteristic foamy appearance on light microscopy with multilamellar lysosomal inclusions on electron microscopy.[46] Each 200-mg tablet of amiodarone contains about 75 mg of iodine, which may be detected radiologically by increased attenuation of the liver, spleen, and pulmonary infiltrates on CT scanning.[47,48]

However, the CT findings, and the presence of foamy macrophages in the alveoli and in the skin, reflect exposure to amiodarone, and as such they are necessary but not sufficient to invoke a diagnosis of APT. The tissue accumulation mirrors sites of toxic effects of amiodarone, so drug sequestration is probably the main determinant of toxicity. However, the precise mechanisms of amiodarone-induced tissue injury remain unknown.[49]

Treatment of amiodarone pulmonary toxicity

Amiodarone and desethylamiodarone can be detected in the lung 1 year after discontinuation of therapy,[50] which is reflected in clinical observations that improvement may take many months after stopping the drug. Corticosteroids are commonly administered systemically, although there is a lack of good-quality evidence to support their use. Furthermore, the histological pattern is not one that naturally associates itself with steroid responsiveness. If a response to steroids is demonstrated by clinical, radiological, and lung function improvement, then a prolonged course may be needed to cover the period of amiodarone clearance from the lung. Although improvement is common once the diagnosis had been made with complete clearing of radiological opacities in a majority of patients, mortality is high (21–33% of hospitalized patients). Retreatment with amiodarone following a period of drug withdrawal has been reported to lead to recurrent APT.[51]

References

1. Sin DD, Wu L, Man SFP. The relationship between reduced lung function and cardiovascular mortality. *Chest* 2005;**127**:1952–59.
2. Hole DJ, Watt GC, Davey-Smith G, Hart Cl, Gillis CR, Hawthorne VM. Impaired lung function and mortality risk in men and women: findings from the Renfrew and Paisley Prospective Population Study. *BMJ* 1996;**313**:711–15.
3. MacNee W, Maclay J, McAllister D. Cardiovascular injury and repair in chronic obstructive pulmonary disease. *Prc Am Thorac Soc* 2008;**5**:824–33.
4. Burghuber OC, Valipour A. Knowing chronic obstructive pulmonary disease by heart. Cumulating evidence of systemic vascular dysfunction. *Am J Respir Crit Care Med* 2009;**180**:487–90.
5. Young RP, Hopkins R, Eaton TE. Potential benefits of statins on morbidity and mortality in chronic obstructive pulmonary disease: a review of the evidence. *Postgrad Med J* 2009;**85**:414–21.
6. Soyseth V, Brekke PH, Smith P, Omland T. Statin use is associated with reduced mortality in chronic obstructive pulmonary disease. *Eur Resp J* 2007;**29**:279–83.
7. Zvezdin B, Milutinov S, Kojicic M, *et al.* A post-mortem analysis of major causes of early death in patients hospitalised with chronic obstructive pulmonary disease. *Chest* 2009;**136**:376–80.
8. McGarvey LP, John M, Anderson JA, Zvarich M, Wise RA; TORCH Clinical Endpoint Committee. Ascertainment of cause-specific mortality in COPD: operations of the TORCH Clinical Endpoint Committee. *Thorax* 2007;**62**:411–15.
9. Sin DD, Anthonisen NR, Soriano JB, Agusti AG. Mortality in COPD: role of comorbidities. *Eur Resp J* 2006;**28**:1245–57.
10. Hawkins NM, Petrie MC, Jhund PS, Chalmers GW, Dunn FG, McMurray JJ. Heart failure and chronic obstructive pulmonary disease: diagnostic pitfalls and epidemiology. *Eur J Heart Fail* 2009;**11**:130–9.
11. Hawkins NM, Jhund PS, Simpson CR, *et al.* Primary care burden and treatment of patients with heart failure and chronic obstructive pulmonary disease in Scotland. *Eur J Heart Fail* 2010;**12**:17–24.
12. Rutten FH, Cramer M-JM, Lammers J-WJ, Grobbee DE, Hoes AW. Heart failure and chronic obstructive pulmonary disease: an ignored combination? *Eur J Heart Fail* 2006;**8**:706–11.
13. update: global strategy for the diagnosis, management, and prevention of COPD. Available at: www.goldcopd.com. Accessed 31 December 2009.
14. Salvi SS, Barnes PJ. Chronic obstructive pulmonary disease in non-smokers. *Lancet* 2009;**374**:733–43.
15. Naeije R. Pulmonary hypertension and right heart failure in chronic obstructive pulmonary disease. *Proc Am Thorac Soc* 2005;**2**:20–2.
16. Weitzenblum E, Apprill M, Oswald M, Chaouat A, Imbs JL. Pulmonary haemodynamics in patients with chronic obstructive pulmonary disease before and during an episode of peripheral edema. *Chest* 1994;**105**:1377–82.
17. O'Donnell DE, Parker CM. COPD exacerbations. 3:Pathophysiology. *Thorax* 2006;**61**:354–61.
18. Gibson JG. *Clinical tests of respiratory function*. Chapman & Hall, London, 1996.
19. Snashall PD, Chung KF. Airway obstruction and bronchial hyperresponsiveness in left ventricular failure and mitral stenosis. *Am Rev Respir Dis* 1991;**144**:945–56.
20. McNamara RM, Cionni DJ. Utility of the peak expiratory flow rate in the differentiation of acute dyspnoea :cardiac vs pulmonary origin. *Chest* 1992;**101**:129–32.
21. Wright RS, Levine MS, Bellamy PE, *et al.*Ventilatory and diffusion abnormalities in potential heart transplant recipients. *Chest* 1990;**98**:816–20.
22. Clark AL, Volterrani M, Swan JW, Coats AJS. Increased ventilatory response to exercise in chronic heart failure: relation to pulmonary pathology. *Heart* 1997;**77**:138–46.
23. Mosterd A,Hoes AW. Reducing hospitalisation for heart failure. *Eur Heart J* 2002;**23**:842–5.
24. Macchia A, Monte S, Romero M, D'Ettore A, Tognoni G. The prognostic influence of chronic obstructive pulmonary disease in patients hospitalised for chronic heart failure. *Eur J Heart Fail* 2007;**9**:942–8.
25. McNeill RS. Effect of a beta-adrenergic-blocking agent, propranolol, on asthmatics. *Lancet* 1964;**2**:1101–2.
26. Zaid G, Beall GN. Bronchial response to beta-adrenergic blockade. *N Engl J Med* 1966;**275**:580–4.
27. Raine JM, Palazzo MG, Kerr JH, Sleight P. Near-fatal bronchospasm after oral nadolol in a young asthmatic and response to ventilation with halothane. *Br Med J (Clin Res Ed)* 1981;**282**:548–9.
28. Cleland JG, McGowan J, Clark A, Freemantle N. The evidence for beta blockers in heart failure. *BMJ* 1999;**318**:824–5.
29. Hawkins NM, Jhund PS, Simpson CR, *et al.* Primary care burden and treatment of patients with heart failure and chronic obstructive pulmonary disease in Scotland. *Eur J Heart Fail* 2010;**12**:17–24.
30. Komajda M, Follath F, Swedberg K, *et al.* The EuroHeart Failure Survey programme a survey on the quality of care among patients with heart failure in Europe. Part 2: treatment. *Eur Heart J* 2003;**24**:464–74.
31. Wlodarczyk JH, Keogh A, Smith K, McCosker C. CHART: congestive cardiac failure in hospitals, an Australian review of treatment. *Heart Lung Circ* 2003;**12**:94–102.
32. Wunderlich J, Macha HN, Wudicke H, Huckauf H. Beta-adrenoceptor blockers and terbutaline in patients with chronic obstructive lung disease. Effects and interaction after oral administration. *Chest* 1980;**78**:714–20.
33. Eichhorn EJ. Beta-blocker withdrawal: the song of Orpheus. *Am Heart J* 1999;**138**(3 Pt 1):387–9.
34. Salpeter S, Ormiston T, Salpeter E. Cardioselective beta-blockers for chronic obstructive pulmonary disease. *Cochrane Database Syst Rev* 2005:CD003566.
35. Hawkins NM, MacDonald MR, Petrie MC, *et al.* Bisoprolol in patients with heart failure and moderate to severe chronic obstructive pulmonary disease: a randomized controlled trial. *Eur J Heart Fail* 2009;**11**:684–90.

36. Staszewsky L, Wong M, Masson S, *et al.* Clinical, neurohormonal, and inflammatory markers and overall prognostic role of chronic obstructive pulmonary disease in patients with heart failure: data from the Val-HeFT heart failure trial. *J Card Fail* 2007;**13**: 797–804.
37. Sin DD, McAlister FA. The effects of beta-blockers on morbidity and mortality in a population-based cohort of 11,942 elderly patients with heart failure. *Am J Med* 2002;**113**:650–6.
38. Rutten FH, Zuithoff NP, Hak E, Grobbee DE, Hoes AW. Beta-blockers may reduce mortality and risk of exacerbations in patients with chronic obstructive pulmonary disease. *Arch Intern Med* 2010; **170**:880–7.
39. Shelton RJ, Rigby AS, Cleland JG, Clark AL. Effect of a community heart failure clinic on uptake of beta blockers by patients with obstructive airways disease and heart failure. *Heart* 2006;**92**:331–6.
40. Rotmensch HH, Liron M, Tupilski M, Laniado S. Possible association of pneumonitis with amiodarone therapy. *Am Heart J* 1980;**100**: 412–3.
41. Sobol SM, Rakita L. Pneumonitis and pulmonary fibrosis associated with amiodarone treatment: a possible complication of a new antiarrhythmic drug. *Circulation* 1982;**65**:819–24.
42. Sunderji R, Kanji Z, Gin K. Pulmonary effects of low dose amiodarone: a review of the risks and recommendations for surveillance. *Can J Cardiol* 2000;**16**:1435–40.
43. Martin WJ 2nd, Osborn MJ, Douglas WW. Amiodarone pulmonary toxicity. Assessment by bronchoalveolar lavage. *Chest* 1985;**88**: 630–1.
44. Darmanata JI, van Zandwijk N, Duren DR, *et al.* Amiodarone pneumonitis: three further cases with a review of published reports. *Thorax* 1984;**39**:57–64.
45. Plomp TA, Wiersinga WM, Maes RA. Tissue distribution of amiodarone and desethylamiodarone in rats after repeated oral administration of various amiodarone dosages. *Arzneimittelforschung* 1985;**35**:1805–10.
46. Adams PC, Holt DW, Storey GC, Morley AR, Callaghan J, Campbell RW. Amiodarone and its desethyl metabolite: tissue distribution and morphologic changes during long-term therapy. *Circulation* 1985;**72**:1064–75.
47. Ren H, Kuhlman JE, Hruban RH, Fishman EK, Wheeler PS, Hutchins GM. CT-pathology correlation of amiodarone lung. *J Comput Assist Tomogr* 1990;**14**:760–5.
48. Kuhlman JE, Teigen C, Ren H, Hruban RH, Hutchins GM, Fishman EK. Amiodarone pulmonary toxicity: CT findings in symptomatic patients. *Radiology* 1990;**177**:121–5.
49. Reasor MJ, Kacew S. An evaluation of possible mechanisms underlying amiodarone-induced pulmonary toxicity. *Proc Soc Exp Biol Med* 1996;**212**:297–304.
50. Esinger W, Schleiffer T, Leinberger H, *et al.* [Steroid-refractory amiodarone-induced pulmonary fibrosis. Clinical features and morphology after an amiodarone-free interval of 3 months]. *Dtsch Med Wochenschr* 1988;**113**:1638–41.
51. Veltri EP, Reid PR. Amiodarone pulmonary toxicity: early changes in pulmonary function tests during amiodarone rechallenge. *J Am Coll Cardiol* 1985;**6**:802–5.

31

Pulmonary hypertension

T.J. Corte and S.J. Wort

Introduction and classification

Pulmonary hypertension (PH) is defined haemodynamically as an increase in mean pulmonary arterial pressure (mPAP) of at least 25 mmHg at rest, as assessed by right heart catheterization (RHC). At the 2008 World Symposium on Pulmonary Hypertension in Dana Point, mPAP of 20–25 mmHg was considered abnormal, and the term 'pre-PH' was proposed to signify this.[1] Previously, the definition of PH included exercise-induced PH (mPAP ≥30 mmHg on exercise).[2] However, the data for exercise-induced PH is limited, and the recent reclassification of PH does not include exercise-induced PH in its definition.

PH is a severe, progressive disorder, which may be idiopathic, or related to a spectrum of medical disorders. The clinical classification of PH was revised at the Dana Point symposium (Table 31.1).[1] PH is classified into five groups with specific pathological, pathophysiological, and therapeutic characteristics. PH associated with left heart disease was identified as a distinct subgroup, with subcategories including PH related to systolic and diastolic dysfunction and valvular heart disease

PH may be considered pre- or postcapillary (Table 31.2).[3] Precapillary PH is defined as mPAP 25 mmHg or more, with pulmonary capillary wedge pressure (PCWP) 15 mmHg or less and a normal or reduced cardiac output (CO). PH associated with left heart disease is considered postcapillary, and defined on haemodynamic terms as having mPAP 25 mmHg or more, PCWP greater than 15 mmHg, and a normal or reduced CO. Furthermore, postcapillary PH can be considered in two subgroups: passive PH (in which the transpulmonary gradient, TPG ≤12 mmHg) and reactive or disproportionate PH (in which the TPG >12 mmHg).

The transpulmonary gradient is the drop from mPAP to left atrial (or pulmonary capillary wedge) pressure, and is measured at right heart catheterization. A low TPG in the face of PH implies that the pulmonary circulation is likely to be structurally normal and that the PH is purely secondary to the back pressure effect of raised left heart filling pressure; whereas a high TPG implies that secondary changes have occurred to the pulmonary vasculature.

Prevalence and prognostic implications of pulmonary hypertension in left heart disease

The prevalence of PH in left heart disease increases with the severity of functional impairment. Forty to seventy per cent of patients with isolated diastolic dysfunction, and up to 60% of those with left ventricular systolic dysfunction (LVSD) have PH at presentation.[3,4] In patients with valvular heart disease, the prevalence of PH increases with the severity of the valvular defect, and is reported in up to 100% of cases with severe left heart valvular disease.[5]

In general when PH develops in association with left heart disease, patients have a worse prognosis. In a chronic heart failure (HF) study, the mortality rate was higher in patients with PH (28%) than in those without PH (17%) at 28 months.[6] PH (pulmonary vascular resistance >6–8 Wood's units; TPG >16 mmHg) is also associated with an increased postoperative risk of right HF after cardiac transplantation.[7]

Histopathology of pulmonary hypertension associated with left heart disease

The histopathology of PH associated with left heart disease is characterized by pulmonary venous distension and thickening and pulmonary capillary and lymphatic dilatation, as well as interstitial oedema and alveolar haemorrhage. Over time, pulmonary vascular remodelling may lead to the classic changes of the distal pulmonary vasculature seen in pulmonary arterial hypertension (PAH) including medial hypertrophy, intimal proliferation and fibrosis, and adventitial changes (Fig. 31.1).[8,9]

Table 31.1 Dana Point classification of pulmonary arterial hypertension

1	PAH
1.1	Idiopathic PAH
1.2	Heritable
1.2.1	BMPR2
1.2.2	ALK1, endoglin (with or without hereditary haemorrhagic telangectasia)
1.2.3	Unknown
1.3	Drug and toxin induced
1.4	Associated with:
1.4.1	Collagen tissue diseases
1.4.2	HIV infection
1.4.3	Portal hypertension
1.4.4	Congenital heart diseases
1.4.5	Schistosomiasis
1.4.6	Chronic haemolytic aneamia
1.5	Associated with significant venous or capillary involvement
1.5.1	Pulmonary veno-occlusive disease
1.5.2	Pulmonary capillary haemangiomatosis
1.6	Persistent PH of the newborn
2	PH with left heart disease
2.1	Left-sided atrial or ventricular heart disease
2.2	Left-sided valvular heart disease
3	PH associated with lung diseases and/or hypoxaemia
3.1	COPD
3.2	Interstitial lung disease
3.3	Other pulmonary diseases with mixed restrictive and obstructive pattern
3.4	Sleep-disordered breathing
3.5	Alveolar hypoventilation disorders
3.6	Chronic exposure to high altitude
3.7	Developmental abnormalities
4	CTEPH
5	PH with unclear multifactorial mechanisms
5.1	Haematologic disorders: myeloproliferative disorders, splenectomy
5.2	Systemic disorders: sarcoidosis, pulmonary Langerhans cell histiocytosis, lymphangioleiomyomatosis, neurofibromatosis, vasculitis
5.3	Metabolic disorders: glycogen storage disease, Gaucher's disease, thyroid disorders
5.4	Others: tumoral obstruction, fibrosing mediastinitis, chronic renal failure on dialysis

COPD, chronic obstructive pulmonary disease; CTEPH, chronic thromboembolic pulmonary hypertension; PAH, pulmonary arterial hypertension; PH, pulmonary hypertension.

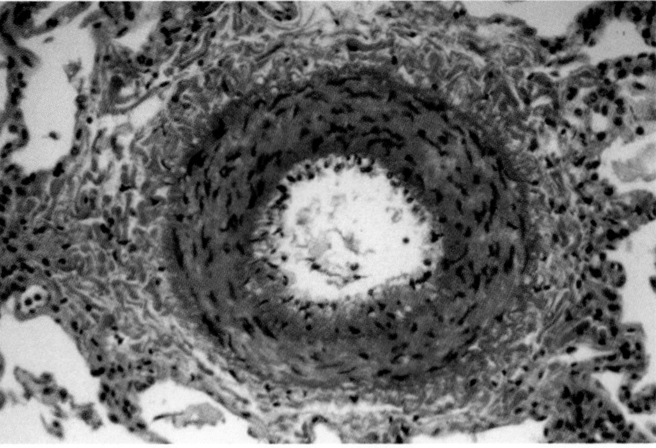

Fig. 31.1 Histopathology of pulmonary artery in pulmonary hypertension (expansion of all three layers of the pulmonary artery is present in PH).
Image courtesy of Peter Dorfmuller.

Pathophysiology of pulmonary hypertension associated with left heart disease

The pathophysiology of PH related to left heart disease is complex, and may be best considered as a combination of passive and active mechanisms. Passive pulmonary venous stretch resulting from backward transmission of elevated left heart filling pressures is important (Table 31.2). Purely passive PH is usually reversible with acute vasodilator testing, and may be more responsive to chronic HF treatment.[10]

However, in some cases there is an additional active component, leading to PH 'out of proportion' to the underlying left heart disease. In such patients, mPAP is disproportionately elevated above left heart filling pressures, leading to an elevation in TPG

Table 31.2 Haemodynamic definitions of pulmonary hypertension

Definition	Characteristics[a]	Clinical groups
PH	Mean PAP ≥25 mmHg	All
Precapillary PH	Mean PAP ≥25 mmHg PCWP ≤15 mmHg CO normal or reduced	PAH PH due to lung diseases CTEPH Miscellaneous PH
Postcapillary PH	Mean PAP ≥25 mmHg PCWP >15 mmHg CO normal or reduced	PH due to left heart disease
Passive	TPG ≤12 mmHg	
Reactive (out of proportion)	TPG >12 mmHg	

[a] All values measured at rest.
CO, cardiac output; CTEPH, chronic thromboembolic pulmonary hypertension; PAH, pulmonary arterial hypertension; PAP, pulmonary arterial pressure; PCWP, pulmonary capillary wedge pressure; PH, pulmonary hypertension; TPG, transpulmonary gradient.
Adapted from the European Cardiology Society (ECS)/European Respiratory Society (ERS) PH guidelines.

and a consequent increase in pulmonary vascular resistance (PVR). This elevation in PVR is attributed to an increase in the vasomotor tone of the distal pulmonary vasculature from pulmonary vasoconstriction and pulmonary vascular remodelling.[11]

Pulmonary vascular remodelling results from increase in cell number in all components of the vessel wall. This leads to a narrowed lumen and increase in vascular resistance proportional to radius[4]. Although the formation of plexiform lesions, characteristic of severe PAH, are not generally seen in PH associated with left heart disease, true remodelling of resistance vessels has been reported. These fixed, obstructive lesions lead to PH that is generally unresponsive to acute vasodilator testing.

It is not clear why pulmonary vascular remodelling and disproportionate PH develop in only some chronic HF patients. It is possible that pulmonary vascular remodelling develops in response to chronic activation of stretch receptors located in the left atrium and pulmonary veins. Patients with congestive cardiac failure also have endothelial dysfunction, and raised serum endothelin-1 (ET-1) levels, a pathological mediator known to be important in vascular remodelling in PAH.[12 13]

Other potential pathophysiological mechanisms include hypoxic pulmonary vasoconstriction and *in situ* thrombosis.

Diagnosis of pulmonary hypertension in left heart disease

Recognition of PH may be delayed, as it is often masked by the clinical picture of the underlying left heart disease. Symptoms including dyspnoea and fatigue are common to both PH and left heart disease. Physical signs reflective of PH (such as a loud pulmonary component of the second heart sound) are often difficult to hear. Signs of right HF (including peripheral oedema) are generally late findings.

It may be difficult to distinguish between PH associated with diastolic dysfunction and true PAH. Left ventricular diastolic dysfunction should be suspected (rather than PAH) in the presence of one or more of a number of clinical or echocardiographic risk factors (Box 31.1).[3,14] However, a definite diagnosis of PH associated with left heart disease is only possible following RHC.

Box 31.1 Factors favouring diagnosis of LVSD in the presence of PH as assessed by Doppler echocardiography

Clinical features

- Age >65 years
- Elevated systolic blood pressure
- Elevated pulse pressure
- Obesity, metabolic syndrome
- Hypertension
- Coronary artery disease
- Diabetes mellitus
- Atrial fibrillation

Echocardiography

- Left atrial enlargement
- Concentric remodelling of the left ventricle (relative wall thickness >0.45)
- Left ventricular hypertrophy
- Presence of echocardiographic indicators of elevated left ventricular filling pressure

Interim evaluation (after echocardiography)

- Symptomatic response to diuretics
- Exaggerated increase in systolic blood pressure with exercise
- Re-evaluation of chest radiograph consistent with heart failure

Adapted from the European Cardiology Society (ECS)/European Respiratory Society (ERS) pulmonary hypertension guidelines, and Hoeper MM, Barbera JA, Channick RN, *et al.* Diagnosis, assessment, and treatment of non-pulmonary arterial hypertension pulmonary hypertension. *J Am Coll Cardiol* 2009;**54**:S85–96

Right heart catheter

RHC remains the gold standard for the diagnosis of PH. It allows the measurement of mPAP, PCWP, and CO, and subsequent calculation of TPG and PVR. These data are important for the diagnosis of PH associated with left heart disease, and its subdivision into passive and active categories (Table 31.2).

The role of acute vasodilator testing is not clear in PH due to left heart disease. In general, patients with passive PH will have acute vasodilator reversibility, whereas patients with disproportionate PH will have fixed disease, unresponsive to vasodilator testing.[10] At present, vasoreactivity testing is recommended for patients referred for cardiac transplantation.[15] In these patients, lack of response to vasodilator testing is associated with increased risk of post-transplantation right ventricular failure and early mortality.[16]

A variety of agents are used for vasoreactivity testing, including nitrous oxide, phosphodiesterase-5 (PDE-5) inhbitors, prostanoids, and other vasodilators.

In the diagnosis of left ventricular diastolic dysfunction, the role of exercise testing, or volume challenge, remains unclear (Fig. 31.2). However, in some patients with apparently 'normal' left ventricular filling pressures (often following diuretic therapy and fluid restriction prior to RHC), an increase in pressure following exercise or fluid challenge may unveil occult left ventricular dysfunction.[14]

RHC is a moderately invasive procedure, and so a number of noninvasive investigations are often used in the assessment for PH.

Echocardiography

Continuous Doppler flow echocardiography is the best noninvasive tool for the assessment of PH associated with left heart disease. Echocardiography allows estimation of the systolic PAP from the maximal velocity of the tricuspid regurgitation jet (in the presence

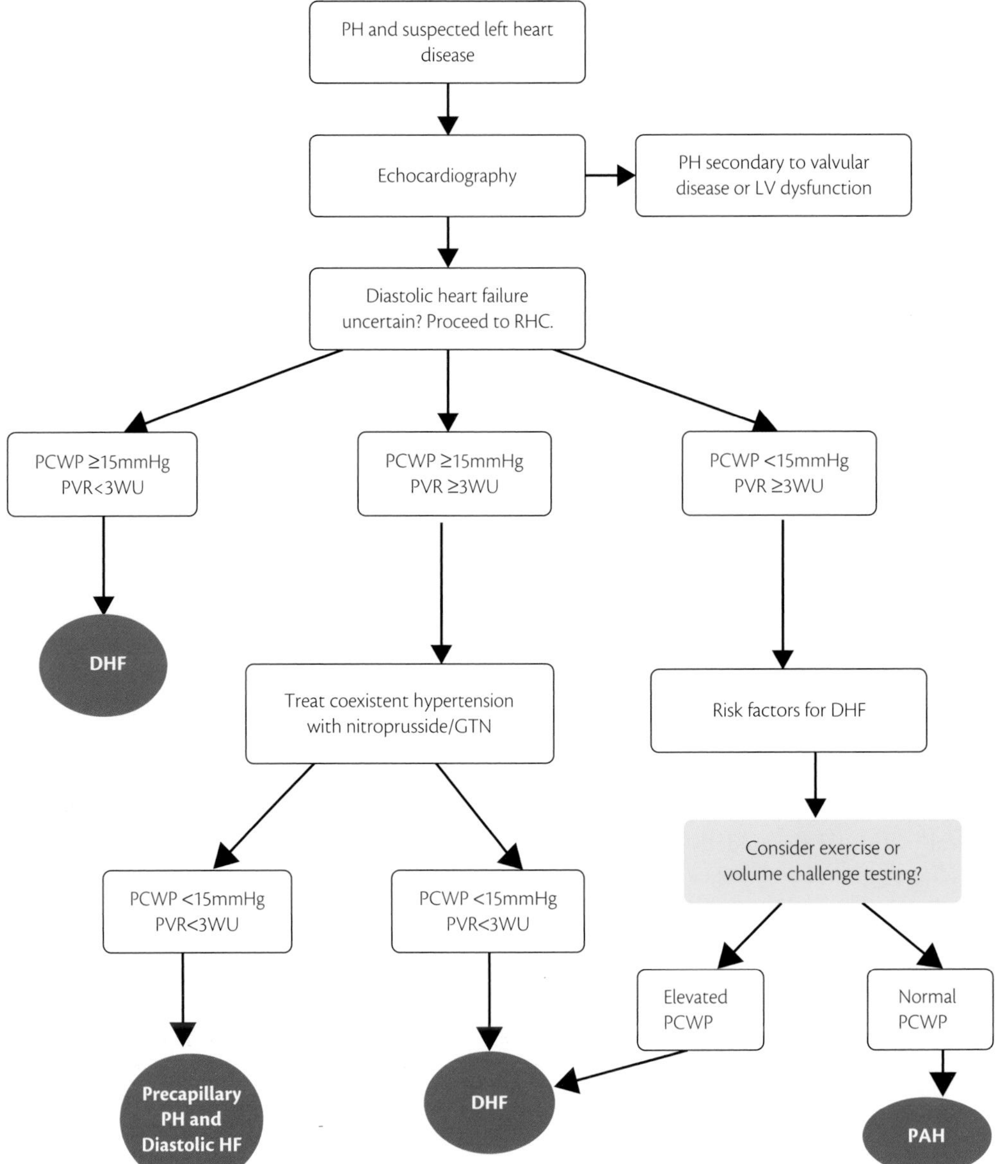

Fig. 31.2 Diagnostic algorithm for pulmonary hypertension associated with left ventricular diastolic dysfunction. DHF, diastolic heart failure; GTN, glyceryl trinitrate; PCWP, pulmonary capillary wedge pressure; PVR, pulmonary vascular resistance; RHC, right heart catheterization; WU, Wood units.

of tricuspid regurgitation). However, echocardiography also complements RHC as it provides other, structural and functional cardiac information.

Left ventricular systolic function is assessed by the left ventricular ejection fraction (LVEF). In contrast, left ventricular diastolic dysfunction is more difficult to assess, although there are several echocardiographic findings that should arouse suspicion for diastolic dysfunction (Table 31.3).[3,14] Left ventricular filling pressures may be estimated by the ratio of mitral valve flow velocity (E) divided by early diastolic lengthening velocities (E′). However, accurate evaluation of left ventricular filling pressures requires RHC.

Other noninvasive investigations

B-type natriuretic peptide (BNP) is released in response to atrial and ventricular wall stretch. Plasma BNP concentrations are elevated in PAH, and are associated with poorer outcomes.[17] However, in BNP concentrations are also elevated in left heart disease. Therefore, it is not clear whether increased BNP levels are useful in identification or prognostic evaluation of PH in left heart disease.

Cardiopulmonary exercise tests (CPET) may be useful to identify early, or exercise-induced, PH as a cause of exercise-limitation in patients with underlying left heart disease. However, patients are often unable to perform a CPET, and six-minute walk testing is used instead. In patients with PAH, lower six-minute walk test distance portends a poorer prognosis.[18,19]

Cardiac MRI (CMR) provides the most accurate measurement of right ventricular mass and ejection fraction. Its role in the diagnosis of PH in this patient group is promising, but needs further study.

The main and segmental pulmonary artery size may be measured on CT scanning. There are few data to support the use of CT scanning in the diagnosis of PH in patients with left heart disease.

Table 31.3 Summary of long-term treatment trials with endothelin receptor antagonists in heart failure

Study name	Endothelin receptor antagonist	Subjects	Outcome
RITZ 1–5	Intravenous tezosentan (25–100 mg/h)	Acute heart failure	No difference in all endpoints
VERITAS 1 and 2	Intravenous tezosentan	Acute heart failure	No difference in dyspnoea at 24 h or survival at 7days Mild haemodynamic benefit No survival difference at 6 months
REACH 1	High dose bosentan (250 mg twice a day)	Chronic heart failure (WHO class IIIb–IV)	Early hepatotoxicity (10% versus 2% receiving placebo) Trial terminated early Trend towards clinical improvement in those receiving 6 months bosentan
ENABLE 1 and 2	Bosentan (125 mg twice a day)	Chronic heart failure (WHO class IIIb– IV)	No improvement in endpoints Early toxicity with clinical worsening of heart failure with bosentan
ENCOR	Enrasentan	Chronic heart failure (WHO class II–III)	Increased adverse events, heart failure hospitalizations and trend towards increased mortality with enrasentan
EARTH	Darusentan	Chronic heart failure (WHO class II–IV)	Increased adverse events, and worsening of cardiac failure in darusentan groups No benefit with darusentan

RITZ, Randomized Intravenous TeZosentan Study; VERITAS, Value of Endothelin Receptor Inhibition with Tezosentan in Acute Heart Failure Studies.

Management of pulmonary hypertension related to left heart disease

General principles

Management of PH related to left heart disease centres on the treatment of the underlying disorder with medications such as diuretics, angiotensin converting enzyme (ACE) inhibitors, β-adrenoreceptor blockers, or other interventions.[10] In patients with valvular heart disease, corrective valve surgery is recommended, and is usually associated with clinical improvement, and resolution of the PH.[5,20] The improvement may take several weeks to months, and may be incomplete, due to the fixed obstructive changes of pulmonary vascular remodelling.

Supplemental oxygen is recommended to reverse resting hypoxaemia in appropriate patients. Full assessment and treatment of comorbidities (including pulmonary emboli and obstructive sleep apnoea) is important. Early referral for cardiac transplantation is essential for selected cases. Patients with endstage cardiac failure and PH may be candidates for cardiac transplantation (in milder, largely reversible forms of PH), or heart–lung transplantation when PH is severe and/or fixed.

Specific therapy for pulmonary hypertension

Specific PH therapy is not routinely recommended for patients with PH secondary to heart disease, as there have been no successful placebo-controlled trials of disease-targeted PH therapies in this patient group.[3,21] There is a potential risk of increasing intrapulmonary shunting and ventilation–perfusion mismatch, particularly with pulmonary vasodilators. However, the risk may be ameliorated by treatment to reduce left ventricular filling pressures. A number of pharmceutical trials have been performed, and the results are summarized below.

Nitric oxide and prostacyclin therapy

Nitric oxide (NO) and prostacyclin are potent pulmonary vasodilators. Both NO and prostacyclin have been shown to improve pulmonary haemodynamics acutely, with decreased PVR, and pulmonary arterial pressures.[22–24] In patients with left heart disease, inhaled NO leads to a decrease in PVR, with an increase in left ventricular filling pressures. However, an international trial using intravenous epoprostenol in patients with severe left ventricular failure (FIRST trial) was terminated prematurely because of a trend towards increased mortality in patients receiving epoprostenol.[25]

Endothelin-1 receptor antagonists

The endothelin system is activated in chronic HF, and elevated plasma ET-1 (and its precursor big-ET1) levels are associated with increased morbidity and mortality in patients with left heart disease.[26,27] Plasma ET-1 levels correlate with the symptomatic and haemodynamic severity of the HF.[28,29] Intravenous infusions of ET-1 lead to increased systemic vascular resistance, and decreased cardiac index.[30] ET-1 acts via two receptor subtypes (ET_A and ET_B receptors). Both receptor subtypes lead to pulmonary vasoconstriction, and vascular smooth muscle proliferation. Activation of ET_B receptors also leads to vasodilation (via NO and prostacyclin), antiproliferative and antithrombotic effects, and clearance of ET-1. It is unclear whether selective ETA blockade is advantageous in chronic HF.

In preliminary small studies using the endothelin-1 receptor antagonists (ETRAs) bosentan, darusentan, and BQ-123, there was an acute improvement in mPAP, right atrial pressure, PCWP, and CO.[31–33] Intravenous bosentan led to acute improvement in pulmonary haemodynamics in 24 patients with chronic HF.[29] Acute treatment with the ETA receptor antagonist sitaxentan led to significant decreases in pulmonary arterial pressures and PVR.[34] In a large placebo-controlled study of patients with acute decompensated HF, intravenous tezosentan led to an acute reduction in left ventricular filling pressures, and increased cardiac index.[35]

Longer-term studies have not confirmed a benefit for the use of ETRAs in patients with PH associated with left heart disease.

The Research on Endothelin Antagonists in Chronic Heart Failure (REACH-1) study, a placebo-controlled study using bosentan, was terminated early because of elevated hepatic transaminase levels.[36] However, there was a trend towards reduced HF mortality and morbidity with bosentan. The Endothelin Antagonist Bosentan or Lowering Cardiac Events in Heart Failure (ENABLE 1 and 2) studies did not show any benefit of bosentan over placebo with regard to morbidity or mortality.[37] In a further study with enrasentan (Enrasentan Cooperative Randomized Evaluation, ENCOR study), no benefit was shown.[38] The Endothelin A Receptor Antagonist Trial in Heart Failure (EARTH) study also showed no difference of left ventricular end-systolic volume on CMR imaging in patients treated with darusentan or placebo.[39] The results of the ETRA trials in cardiac failure patients are summarized in Table 31.3.

It is somewhat difficult to reconcile the negative results in the trials described above with the positive findings in acute studies. One explanation for the disparity is that patients who have PH disproportionate to their underlying left heart disease are more likely to benefit from specific PH therapy, and many of the trials discussed included all patients with congestive HF, not only patients specifically with PH who might be expected to benefit. Alternatively, it is possible that the acute haemodynamic response to ETRAs does not lead to a sustained clinical benefit, or that any benefit is masked by the use of other HF therapies.[40,41] Currently, the use of ETRAs is not recommended for the treatment of PH associated with left heart disease.

Phosphodiesterase-5 inhibitors

In PAH, NO mediates pulmonary vasodilation via cyclic guanosine monophosphate (cGMP), which is degraded by phosphodiesterases (particularly PDE-5). In PH, PDE-5 is up-regulated. PDE-5 inhibitors, such as sildenafil, cause pulmonary vasodilation, anti-proliferative actions on pulmonary vascular smooth muscle cells, and protection from ischaemic reperfusion injury. In PAH, sildenfil is associated with increased six-minute walk test distance, and improved pulmonary haemodynamics at 12 weeks, with a sustained clinical benefit at 12 months.[42]

In chronic HF, sildenafil acutely lowers PVR and pulmonary arterial pressures, and improves endothelium-dependent flow-mediated pulmonary vasodilation.[43–45] Longer-term studies have shown that sildenafil is associated with improvement in exercise capacity, and CO and skeletal muscle blood flow during exercise.[46,47] A study of 34 patients with symptomatic HF and PH, showed an improvement in six-minute walk test distance, quality of life, exercise capacity, and fewer hospitalizations for HF, with sildenafil compared to placebo at 12 weeks. Despite these promising results, the routine use of sildenafil in patients with PH associated with left heart disease cannot be recommended. There is an urgent need for further longer-term trials, particularly in patients with PH disproportionate to the underlying heart disease.

To date, there have been no trials specifically addressing patients with left ventricular diastolic HF, in which PH is common. The PhosphodiesteRasE-5 Inhibition to Improve Quality of Life And EXercise Capacity in Diastolic Heart Failure (RELAX) study, a double-blind, placebo-controlled clinical trial using sildenafil, is currently under way. The primary endpoint of the study is the change in exercise capacity as assessed by peak VO_2 after 24 weeks of treatment with sildenafil or placebo.

Summary

PH is common in patients with left heart disease, and is associated with increased morbidity and mortality. The underlying pathophysiological mechanisms are complex, including both passive and active components. PH disproportionate to the underlying left heart disease may be attributable to reactive pulmonary vascular remodelling. Left ventricular diastolic dysfunction may be difficult to diagnose, but is best assessed with echocardiography and RHC. Management of PH is focused on treatment of the underlying left heart disease, and reversal of hypoxaemia. There is no supporting evidence for the routine use of specific PH therapies at present. However, there is some suggestion that PDE-5 inhibitors may be useful, and their safety and efficacy needs to be formally evaluated in controlled trials before further recommendations are made.

Further reading

Galie N, Ghofrani HA, Torbicki A, Barst RJ, Rubin LJ, Badesch D, *et al.* Sildenafil citrate therapy for pulmonary arterial hypertension. *New Engl J Med* 2005;**353**(20):2148–57.

Galie N, Hoeper MM, Humbert M, *et al.* Guidelines for the diagnosis and treatment of pulmonary hypertension: The Task Force for the Diagnosis and Treatment of Pulmonary Hypertension of the European Society of Cardiology (ESC) and the European Respiratory Society (ERS), endorsed by the International Society of Heart and Lung Transplantation (ISHLT). *Eur Heart J* 2009;**30**(20):2493–537.

Gibbs S. Consensus statement on the management of pulmonary hypertension in clinical practice in the UK and Ireland. *Thorax* 2008;**63**(S2):ii1–41.

Guazzi M, Samaja M, Arena R, Vicenzi M, Guazzi MD. Long-term use of sildenafil in the therapeutic management of heart failure. *Journal of the American College of Cardiology* 2007;50(22):2136–44.

Hoeper MM, Barbera JA, Channick RN, *et al.* Diagnosis, assessment, and treatment of non-pulmonary arterial hypertension pulmonary hypertension. *J Am Coll Cardiol* 2009;**54**(1 Suppl):S85–96.

Kelland NF, Webb DJ. Clinical trials of endothelin antagonists in heart failure: publication is good for the public health. *Heart* 2007;**93**(1):2–4.

Kelland NF, Webb DJ. Clinical trials of endothelin antagonists in heart failure: a question of dose? *Exp Biol Med (Maywood)* 2006;**231**(6):696–9.

Kirkby NS, Hadoke PW, Bagnall AJ, Webb DJ. The endothelin system as a therapeutic target in cardiovascular disease: great expectations or bleak house? *Br J Pharmacol* 2008;**153**(6):1105–19.

Lewis GD, Shah R, Shahzad K, *et al.* Sildenafil improves exercise capacity and quality of life in patients with systolic heart failure and secondary pulmonary hypertension. *Circulation* 2007;**116**(14):1555–62.

Melenovsky V, Borlaug BA, Rosen B, *et al.* Cardiovascular features of heart failure with preserved ejection fraction versus nonfailing hypertensive left ventricular hypertrophy in the urban Baltimore community: the role of atrial remodeling/dysfunction. *J Am Coll Cardiol* 2007;**49**(2):198–207.

Simonneau G, Robbins IM, Beghetti M, Channick RN, *et al.* Updated clinical classification of pulmonary hypertension. *J Am Coll Cardiol* 2009;**54**(1 Suppl S):S43–54.

Simonneau G. Proceedings of the 3rd World Symposium on Pulmonary Arterial Hypertension. Venice, Italy, June 23–25, 2003. *J. Am. Coll. Cardiol* 2004;**43**(12 Suppl S): S1–90.

References

1. Simonneau G, Robbins IM, Beghetti M, *et al.* Updated clinical classification of pulmonary hypertension. *J Am Coll Cardiol* 2009;**54** (1 Suppl):S43–54.
2. Simonneau G, Galie N, Rubin LJ, *et al.* Clinical classification of pulmonary hypertension. *J Am Coll Cardiol* 2004;**43**:5–12S.

3. Galie N, Hoeper MM, Humbert M, *et al.* Guidelines for the diagnosis and treatment of pulmonary hypertension: The Task Force for the Diagnosis and Treatment of Pulmonary Hypertension of the European Society of Cardiology (ESC) and the European Respiratory Society (ERS), endorsed by the International Society of Heart and Lung Transplantation (ISHLT). *Eur Heart J* 2009;**30**: 2493–537.
4. Ghio S, Gavazzi A, Campana C, *et al.* Independent and additive prognostic value of right ventricular systolic function and pulmonary artery pressure in patients with chronic heart failure. *J Am Coll Cardiol* 2001;**37**:183–8.
5. Vahanian A, Baumgartner H, Bax J, *et al.* Guidelines on the management of valvular heart disease: The Task Force on the Management of Valvular Heart Disease of the European Society of Cardiology. *Eur Heart J* 2007;**28**:230–68.
6. Abramson SV, Burke JF, Kelly JJ Jr, *et al.* Pulmonary hypertension predicts mortality and morbidity in patients with dilated cardiomyopathy. *Ann Intern Med* 1992;**116**:888–95.
7. Addonizio LJ, Gersony WM, Robbins RC, *et al.* Elevated pulmonary vascular resistance and cardiac transplantation. *Circulation* 1987;**76**:V52–5.
8. Pietra GG, Capron F, Stewart S, *et al.* Pathologic assessment of vasculopathies in pulmonary hypertension. *J Am Coll Cardiol* 2004;**43**:25–32S.
9. Tuder RM, Abman SH, Braun T, *et al.* Development and pathology of pulmonary hypertension. *J Am Coll Cardiol* 2009;**54**:S3–9.
10. Oudiz RJ. Pulmonary hypertension associated with left-sided heart disease. *Clin Chest Med* 2007;**28**:233–41, x.
11. Delgado JF, Conde E, Sanchez V, *et al.* Pulmonary vascular remodeling in pulmonary hypertension due to chronic heart failure. *Eur J Heart Fail* 2005;**7**:1011–16.
12. Love MP, McMurray JJ. Endothelin in chronic heart failure: current position and future prospects. *Cardiovasc Res* 1996;**31**:665–74.
13. Cowburn PJ, Cleland JG, McArthur JD, *et al.* Endothelin-1 has haemodynamic effects at pathophysiological concentrations in patients with left ventricular dysfunction. *Cardiovasc Res* 1998;**39**: 563–70.
14. Hoeper MM, Barbera JA, Channick RN, *et al.* Diagnosis, assessment, and treatment of non-pulmonary arterial hypertension pulmonary hypertension. *J Am Coll Cardiol* 2009;**54**:S85–96.
15. Costanzo MR, Augustine S, Bourge R, *et al.* Selection and treatment of candidates for heart transplantation. A statement for health professionals from the Committee on Heart Failure and Cardiac Transplantation of the Council on Clinical Cardiology, American Heart Association. *Circulation* 1995;**92**:3593–612.
16. Costard-Jackle A, Fowler MB. Influence of preoperative pulmonary artery pressure on mortality after heart transplantation: testing of potential reversibility of pulmonary hypertension with nitroprusside is useful in defining a high risk group. *J Am Coll Cardiol* 1992;**19**:48–54.
17. Nagaya N, Nishikimi T, Uematsu M, *et al.* Plasma brain natriuretic peptide as a prognostic indicator in patients with primary pulmonary hypertension. *Circulation* 2000;**102**:865–70.
18. Miyamoto S, Nagaya N, Satoh T, *et al.* Clinical correlates and prognostic significance of six-minute walk test in patients with primary pulmonary hypertension. Comparison with cardiopulmonary exercise testing. *Am J Resp Crit Care Med* 2000;**161**:487–92.
19. Sitbon O, Humbert M, Nunes H, *et al.* Long-term intravenous epoprostenol infusion in primary pulmonary hypertension: prognostic factors and survival. *J Am Coll Cardiol* 2002;**40**:780–8.
20. Roques F, Nashef SA, Michel P, *et al.* Risk factors and outcome in European cardiac surgery: analysis of the EuroSCORE multinational database of 19030 patients. *Eur J Cardiothorac Surg* 1999;**15**:816–22; discussion 22–3.
21. Gibbs S. Consensus statement on the management of pulmonary hypertension in clinical practice in the UK and Ireland. *Thorax* 2008;**63**:ii1–41.
22. Fojon S, Fernandez-Gonzalez C, Sanchez-Andrade J, *et al.* Inhaled nitric oxide through a noninvasive ventilation device to assess reversibility of pulmonary hypertension in selecting recipients for heart transplant. *Transplant Proc* 2005;**37**:4028–30.
23. Loh E, Stamler JS, Hare JM, Loscalzo J, Colucci WS. Cardiovascular effects of inhaled nitric oxide in patients with left ventricular dysfunction. *Circulation* 1994;**90**:2780–5.
24. Haraldsson A, Kieler-Jensen N, Nathorst-Westfelt U, Bergh CH, Ricksten SE. Comparison of inhaled nitric oxide and inhaled aerosolized prostacyclin in the evaluation of heart transplant candidates with elevated pulmonary vascular resistance. *Chest* 1998;**114**:780–6.
25. Califf RM, Adams KF, McKenna WJ, *et al.* A randomized controlled trial of epoprostenol therapy for severe congestive heart failure: The Flolan International Randomized Survival Trial (FIRST). *Am Heart J* 1997;**134**:44–54.
26. McMurray JJ, Ray SG, Abdullah I, Dargie HJ, Morton JJ. Plasma endothelin in chronic heart failure. *Circulation* 1992;**85**:1374–9.
27. Kirkby NS, Hadoke PW, Bagnall AJ, Webb DJ. The endothelin system as a therapeutic target in cardiovascular disease: great expectations or bleak house? *Br J Pharmacol* 2008;**153**:1105–19.
28. Cody RJ, Haas GJ, Binkley PF, Capers Q, Kelley R. Plasma endothelin correlates with the extent of pulmonary hypertension in patients with chronic congestive heart failure. *Circulation* 1992;**85**:504–9.
29. Kiowski W, Sutsch G, Hunziker P, *et al.* Evidence for endothelin-1-mediated vasoconstriction in severe chronic heart failure. *Lancet* 1995;**346**:732–6.
30. Cowburn PJ, Cleland JG, McArthur JD, MacLean MR, McMurray JJ, Dargie HJ. Pulmonary and systemic responses to exogenous endothelin-1 in patients with left ventricular dysfunction. *J Cardiovasc Pharmacol* 1998;**31**(Suppl 1):S290–3.
31. Sutsch G, Kiowski W, Yan XW, *et al.* Short-term oral endothelin-receptor antagonist therapy in conventionally treated patients with symptomatic severe chronic heart failure. *Circulation* 1998;**98**:2262–8.
32. Spieker LE, Mitrovic V, Noll G, *et al.* Acute hemodynamic and neurohumoral effects of selective ET(A) receptor blockade in patients with congestive heart failure. ET 003 Investigators. *J Am Coll Cardiol* 2000;**35**:1745–52.
33. Cowburn PJ, Cleland JG, McArthur JD, MacLean MR, McMurray JJ, Dargie HJ. Short-term haemodynamic effects of BQ-123, a selective endothelin ET(A)-receptor antagonist, in chronic heart failure. *Lancet* 1998;**352**:201–2.
34. Givertz MM, Colucci WS, LeJemtel TH, *et al.* Acute endothelin A receptor blockade causes selective pulmonary vasodilation in patients with chronic heart failure. *Circulation* 2000;**101**:2922–7.
35. Torre-Amione G, Young JB, Colucci WS, *et al.* Hemodynamic and clinical effects of tezosentan, an intravenous dual endothelin receptor antagonist, in patients hospitalized for acute decompensated heart failure. *J Am Coll Cardiol* 2003;**42**:140–7.
36. Mylona P, Cleland JG. Update of REACH-1 and MERIT-HF clinical trials in heart failure. Cardio.net Editorial Team. *Eur J Heart Fail* 1999;**1**:197–200.
37. Teerlink JR. Recent heart failure trials of neurohormonal modulation (OVERTURE and ENABLE): approaching the asymptote of efficacy? *J Card Fail* 2002;**8**:124–7.
38. Abrahams W. Progress in clinical trials: ENCOR. *Clin Cardiol* 2001;**24**:481–3.
39. Anand I, McMurray J, Cohn JN, *et al.* Long-term effects of darusentan on left-ventricular remodelling and clinical outcomes in the EndothelinA Receptor Antagonist Trial in Heart Failure (EARTH): randomised, double-blind, placebo-controlled trial. *Lancet* 2004;**364**:347–54.
40. Kelland NF, Webb DJ. Clinical trials of endothelin antagonists in heart failure: publication is good for the public health. *Heart* 2007;**93**:2–4.
41. Kelland NF, Webb DJ. Clinical trials of endothelin antagonists in heart failure: a question of dose? *Exp Biol Med (Maywood)* 2006;**231**:696–9.

42. Galie N, Ghofrani HA, Torbicki A, *et al.* Sildenafil citrate therapy for pulmonary arterial hypertension. *N Engl J Med* 2005;**353**:2148–57.
43. Lepore JJ, Maroo A, Bigatello LM, *et al.* Hemodynamic effects of sildenafil in patients with congestive heart failure and pulmonary hypertension: combined administration with inhaled nitric oxide. *Chest* 2005;**127**:1647–53.
44. Guazzi M, Tumminello G, Di Marco F, Fiorentini C, Guazzi MD. The effects of phosphodiesterase-5 inhibition with sildenafil on pulmonary hemodynamics and diffusion capacity, exercise ventilatory efficiency, and oxygen uptake kinetics in chronic heart failure. *J Am Coll Cardiol* 2004;**44**:2339–48.
45. Katz SD, Balidemaj K, Homma S, Wu H, Wang J, Maybaum S. Acute type 5 phosphodiesterase inhibition with sildenafil enhances flow-mediated vasodilation in patients with chronic heart failure. *J Am Coll Cardiol* 2000;**36**:845–51.
46. Guazzi M, Samaja M, Arena R, Vicenzi M, Guazzi MD. Long-term use of sildenafil in the therapeutic management of heart failure. *J Am Coll Cardiol* 2007;**50**:2136–44.
47. Lewis GD, Shah R, Shahzad K, *et al.* Sildenafil improves exercise capacity and quality of life in patients with systolic heart failure and secondary pulmonary hypertension. *Circulation* 2007;**116**:1555–62.

32

Diabetes mellitus

Andrew Jamieson

Introduction

Heart failure (HF) and diabetes mellitus (DM) are both increasing in prevalence worldwide, and HF is a serious and increasingly common comorbid factor in the patient with DM. The patient with HF and DM may present particular problems in relation to a number of management areas. As a consequence, it is increasingly important that practitioners dealing with patients with HF have some knowledge of the interplay between DM and HF and the potential pitfalls encountered when treating the diabetic patient with HF, and vice versa.

Epidemiology

The initial observations from the Framingham Heart Study population demonstrated that HF was twice as common in men with DM and five times as common in women with DM aged 45–74 as compared to their age-matched controls, and the risk of HF was independent of age, the presence of hypertension, obesity, coronary artery disease (CAD), or dyslipidaemia.[1] Furthermore, in patients with DM aged 65 or less, the prevalence of HF was even greater—four times higher in men with DM and eight times higher in women with DM. The increased risk of developing HF conferred by DM in women was confirmed in the HERS population where DM was the strongest predictor of HF, more so than the presence of CAD.[2]

The presence of DM itself is also an independent predictor of developing HF following myocardial infarction,[3] and if developed predicts a poorer outcome than in nondiabetic patients—greater even than the presence of CAD.[4,5] Furthermore, patients hospitalized with HF have a poorer outcome if they have DM, with a blood glucose level of more than 10 mmol/L being associated with a poor outcome.[6,7]

Prevalence and incidence of heart failure in patients with diabetes mellitus

Prevalence of heart failure in patients with diabetes mellitus

Population-based studies have estimated that 0.3–0.5% of the population have both DM and HF,[8,9] whereas the prevalence of HF in patients with DM is between 12–22%, becoming more prevalent with age (Table 32.1).[8,10]

Prevalence of diabetes mellitus in patients with heart failure

The prevalence of DM in patients with left ventricular systolic dysfunction (LVSD) varies significantly dependent upon the population studied. The background prevalence of DM is 4–7% in northern hemisphere populations,[8,11] but varies from 6% to 44% in patients with varying degrees of severity of HF (Table 32.2). Studies of treatment of HF due to LVSD have consistently demonstrated that 20–30% of patients with HF have DM,[12–16] although a similar prevalence was observed in patients with HF and preserved left ventricular function.[17]

By contrast, hospital-based studies have demonstrated consistently higher prevalence of DM in patients with HF ranging from 34% to 44%.[18,19] Although it appears that intervention studies underestimate the true prevalence of DM in patients with HF, it is still abundantly clear that the prevalence of DM in patients with HF is significantly higher than the background prevalence of DM in the non-HF-affected population.

Incidence of heart failure in diabetes mellitus

The Framingham study identified DM as an important independent risk factor for developing HF.[1] This has been confirmed by a number

Table 32.1 Prevalence and incidence of heart failure and diabetes mellitus in related circumstances

	Prevalence			Incidence	
	General population	**HF in DM**	**DM in HF**	**HF in DM**	**DM in HF**
Population-based studies[a]	DM 4–15% (population and age dependent) HF 1–4% (age dependent)[8,9,11]	12% 22% aged >64 years [10]	6–44%[18,19]	Hazard ratio 1.74–8 (age dependent) Odds ratio 2.0–2.8[1,8,10]	28.8% with DM vs. 18.3% without DM (3 years)[26]
Clinical trials	N/A	N/A	11–41% [12–16]	2.3—11.9 per 1000 person-years (HbA_{1c} related)[20] 13.3% in placebo group of MICRO-HOPE (4.2 years)[23]	5.9–7.4% (3 years) 13–20% (7.7 years, NYHA class dependent)[27–29]

DM, diabetes mellitus; HF, heart failure.
[a] Includes epidemiological, registry and population-based studies with endpoints including hospitalization.

of population-based studies in the US and Europe, which all confirm with some consistency an age-adjusted odds ratio for developing HF of around 2 compared with nondiabetic subjects.[1,8,10] The annual incidence of HF in patients with DM has been assessed in five studies.[20–24] The UKPDS reported HF incidence rates of 2.3–11.9 per 1000 patient-years over a 10-year follow-up period. The DIABHYCAR study determined the annual incidence rate of HF requiring hospitalization in subjects with DM and estimated it to be 1% (10 per 1000 patient-years). A large diabetic population (48 000 subjects with a mean age of 58 years) was studied and demonstrated an incidence rate of 4.5–9.2 per 1000 patient-years. This study only recorded those who were hospitalized with the principal diagnosis of HF, thus excluding less severe cases and underestimating the true incidence of HF. The MICRO-HOPE substudy placebo group of patients with DM had an incidence of HF of 13.3% over 4.5 years.

A retrospective cohort study of over 16 000 patients with and without type 2 DM followed for 6 years confirmed that patients with DM were much more likely to develop HF than those without (incidence rate 30.9 vs. 12.4 cases per 1000 person-years, giving a rate ratio of 2.5), and in particular the rate of developing HF was greatest in younger age groups (age 45–54 with DM vs. no DM odds ratio 8.6; age 75–84, odds ratio 1.2). In addition to the effect of age, the authors also concluded that poor glycaemic control and obesity were also important factors affecting the development of HF in patients with type 2 DM.

Thus, the incidence of HF in DM is significantly greater than the nondiabetic population, and whilst the size of the diabetic population increases, the potential burden of HF comorbidity is increasing too, perhaps at a rate greater than expected based on the rise in diabetes cases.[25]

Incidence of diabetes mellitus in heart failure

In one population-based study in elderly Italians, the odds ratio for developing DM in patients with HF was 1.6 versus patients without HF, with the absolute incidence of DM in the HF group 28% over 3 years.[26] Within the context of clinical trials, the incidence of DM in patients with HF is 5.9–7.4% over 3 years,[27,28] while the BIPS demonstrated an incidence of DM in patients without HF of 13% over a mean of 7:7 years versus 15% in patients with NYHA class II and 20% in patients with NYHA class III HF.[29] Clearly, DM is an independent risk factor for developing HF, but it is apparent that HF is an independent risk factor for developing DM. However, the mechanism behind this increased risk is unclear.

Background information: rising prevalence of diabetes mellitus

The worldwide prevalence of DM is alarmingly high. Current estimates suggest that over 200 million people have diabetes worldwide, with the total number projected to be 300 million by 2025.[33] In developed countries over 25% of people aged 65 or older will have diabetes.

Patients with diabetes have an excess burden of vascular complications, both macrovascular (i.e. coronary artery disease, cerebrovascular disease, peripheral arterial disease and HF) and microvascular (i.e. diabetic retinopathy, nephropathy and neuropathy), and three out of four deaths in patients with DM are attributed to cardiovascular causes.[20] In addition to hyperglycaemia, the diabetic patient

Table 32.2 Prevalence of diabetes mellitus in populations with and without LVSD based on a measure of LVEF

	Study type	Mean age (range)	LVEF measure	Prevalence of LVSD (%)	Symptomatic/ asymptomatic (%)	Prevalence of DM with LVSD (%)	Prevalence of DM without LVSD (%)
Glasgow[30]	Epidemiological	50 (25–74)	<30% <35%	2.9 7.7	77% asymptomatic	12.4	2.5
ECHOES, England[9]	Epidemiological—primary care	61 (>45)	<40%	1.8	1.0/0.8	30	3.8
Olmstead, USA[31]	Epidemiological	63 (>45)	≤50% ≤40%	6.5 1.8	N/A	17 15	6.8
Copenhagen[33]	Prospective—hospital	69 (N/A)	<45%	All included	All included were symptomatic	25.5	N/A

DM, diabetes mellitus; LVEF, left ventricular ejection fraction; LVSD, left ventricular systolic dysfunction

has an increased prevalence of other key cardiovascular risk factors, namely hypertension, obesity, dyslipidaemia, and chronic kidney disease (CKD). It is likely that the interaction of hyperglycaemia with these cardiovascular risk factors leads to the development of structural and functional changes in the vasculature and myocardium which contribute to the excess prevalence of HF in patients with DM.

The rise in the prevalence of obesity together with the reclassification of the diagnostic criteria for DM has led to an increased awareness of diabetes. This has led to the implementation of screening of individuals at risk for developing DM, e.g. those with obesity or positive family history of DM. Similarly, improved patient access to diagnostic testing, the application of evidence-based cardiovascular prevention strategies for patients with DM, improved detection and treatment of renal disease, and increasing use of revascularization strategies for coronary and peripheral vascular disease have all contributed to the increase in size of the patient population with DM, and in particular those surviving with HF or the substrates to develop HF.

Diagnosis and aetiology of diabetes mellitus

Diagnosis

In 1997, the diagnostic criteria and aetiological classification of DM were updated.[34] The critical changes made were firstly, the lowering of the level of fasting blood glucose required to diagnose DM to 7 mmol/L or greater; to propose the routine use of fasting blood glucose rather than the standard 75-g oral glucose tolerance test; and the introduction of a new category of abnormal glucose regulation—impaired fasting glucose (Table 32.3).

Most recently, the use of a single measure of HbA_{1c} (the glycosylated fraction of haemoglobin typically used to monitor glycaemic control) to diagnose DM (random $HbA_{1c} \geq 6.5\%$) has been advocated, although this is still a matter of considerable debate.[35,36]

Table 32.3 Diagnostic criteria and classification of aetiology of diabetes mellitus[34]

Diagnostic criteria	Classification
Fasting blood glucose ≥7 mmol/L[a]	Type 1 DM Autoimmunity: islet cell antibodies present in the majority of individuals, e.g anti-GAD65 antibodies
2-hour post 75-g OGTT Blood glucose ≥ 11.1 mmol/L	Type 2 DM Insulin resistance and centripetal obesity
Random blood glucose ≥ 11.1 mmol/L[a]	Others: Pancreatic disease, e.g. cystic fibrosis, acute or chronic pancreatitis, pancreatectomy Endocrine disease, e.g. acromegaly, thyrotoxicosis, Cushing's syndrome, primary hyperaldosteronism, hereditary haemochromatosis
Impaired FBG ≥6 mmol/ and <7 mmol/L	

FBG, fasting blood glucose, OGTT, oral glucose tolerance test.

[a] In the presence of symptoms compatible with DM, e.g. polydipsia, polyuria. A further fasting sample is required 4–6 weeks later if there are no symptoms present to confirm the diagnosis.

Aetiology

Type 1 DM accounts for 5–10% of cases of DM and is characterized by an absolute deficiency of insulin, most commonly in the context of associated cellular autoimmunity directed towards the pancreatic beta cells. Between 80% and 90% of those affected have evidence of autoimmunity against pancreatic beta cells, e.g. the presence of anti-islet cell antibodies, or anti-GAD_{65} antibodies. As a consequence, individuals with type 1 DM require insulin therapy lifelong from diagnosis and are prone to developing ketoacidosis. Such individuals are also at high risk of developing the classic manifestations of DM such as diabetic retinopathy and nephropathy in young adulthood, and have a reduced life expectancy principally due to cardiovascular deaths.

Type 2 DM is characterized by the presence of peripheral tissue insulin resistance and elevated insulin concentrations and is typically found in individuals who are centrally obese. As time progresses, the continuum from normal glucose tolerance to the development of DM in susceptible individuals with insulin resistance is associated with a gradual rise in fasting and meal-stimulated insulin concentrations associated with rising levels of fasting and postprandial blood glucose. The precise mechanism of insulin resistance is still unclear, although peripheral tissue resistance (principally adipose tissue and skeletal muscle) to the transmembrane and intracellular effects of insulin associated with fasting and postprandial hyperinsulinaemia, the presence of centripetal obesity and abnormal regulation of hepatic glucose production and fatty acid metabolism are contributory features. At some point, the progressive rise in insulin concentration will plateau for a variable period of time, and subsequently begin to fall leading to an eventual state of relative or absolute insulin deficiency. This fall in insulin production is related to the presence of impaired beta cell function, which is virtually always present when type 2 DM is diagnosed. The rate of decline in beta cell function in cases of type 2 DM varies between individuals but clearly contributes to the progressive hyperglycaemia seen in type 2 DM, the progressive failure of glycaemic response to agents such as sulphonylureas, and the increasing requirement for exogenous insulin to maintain levels of glycaemic control as the duration of type 2 DM continues.

Based on the key aetiological observations regarding the development of type 2 DM, interventions to control blood glucose levels in patients with type 2 DM are directed at reducing insulin resistance, directly stimulating remaining beta cell insulin release, and modifying meal-related insulin release. Insulin therapy in type 2 DM is usually initiated once one or a combination of these approaches has been tried and deemed to have failed by the treating clinician.

Risk factors for developing heart failure in diabetic patients

The two most common risk factors for the development of HF are the presence of CAD and arterial hypertension. Both of these are more prevalent in patients with DM than nondiabetic subjects and clearly this impacts upon the increased prevalence and incidence of HF in diabetic patients.

In addition to these two major risk factors, a number of features associated with DM have been identified as independent risk factors for developing HF. Poor glycaemic control, increasing BMI, increasing age, the use of insulin,[24] the presence of any measurable renal insult from microalbuminuria to endstage renal failure (ESRF),[10,24] and duration of DM are all independent risk factors for the development of HF in patients with DM. For instance, a 1% reduction in HbA_{1c} in UKPDS reduced the risk of HF by 16%,[20] and a 2.5-unit increase in BMI increases the risk of HF by 12%.[24]

Diabetic cardiomyopathy

Although most registry-based studies and intervention trials for the treatment of chronic HF suggest that the principal cause of LVSD in patients with DM is ischaemic in origin, a sizeable proportion appear to arise from the entity sometimes referred to as 'diabetic cardiomyopathy'.[37] The existence of a specific diabetic cardiomyopathy has long been debated and attempts made to characterize specific pathological and diagnostic features. The initial description was based on a small number of individuals noted to have a clinical diagnosis of HF but with no evidence of prior CAD or hypertension.[38] Using this simple clinical approach suggested that diabetic cardiomyopathy was a rare entity. However, further investigation has revealed a range of abnormalities in the diabetic heart which suggests not only that diabetic cardiomyopathy is a real entity, but also that it is extremely prevalent in patients with DM. These abnormalities are summarized in Table 32.4.[37,39]

The initial feature of diabetic cardiomyopathy appears to be the development of features of diastolic dysfunction, and this early feature correlates closely with HbA_{1c} in diabetic patients.[40] Although it is suggested that diastolic dysfunction may account for approximately one-half of all HF cases,[31] studies of patients with both type 1 and type 2 DM have suggested that diastolic dysfunction is much more common than previously reported in subjects who are free of clinically detectable heart disease.[41–43]

Once present, diastolic dysfunction has a prognosis similar to systolic dysfunction and the combination of either left ventricular hypertrophy, CAD, or both has a profound deleterious effect on the diabetic heart.[3–7] Thus, in addition to optimizing glycaemic control, rigorous attention to blood pressure and cardiovascular risk modification is essential in the patient with DM.

Table 32.4 Clinical, pathological, and molecular features of diabetic cardiomyopathy

Clinical features	**Absence of arterial hypertension**
	Absence of coronary artery disease
	Symptoms and/or signs of HF
Echocardiographic features	LV diastolic dysfunction evidenced by:
	reduced early and increased late diastolic transmitral flow (reversed E:A ratio)
	restrictive LV filling pattern
	Tissue Doppler measurements at mitral valve annulus to quantify longitudinal myocardial lengthening/shortening
	Left atrial volume index >40 mL/min^2
CMR	Greater morphological and functional parameter assessment
	Comparable measures of LV filling to echocardiography
	Allows other assessments, e.g. myocardial fat measurement
Pathological features	Myocardial fibrosis
	Cardiomyocyte hypertrophy
	Increased myocardial fat
Molecular mechanisms	Conventional coronary risk factors
	Hyperglycaemia
	Reactive oxygen species
	Nitric oxide
	Poly(ADP-ribose) polymerase
	PKC
	Altered intracellular calcium homeostasis
	Dysfunctional RAAS
	Hypoxia-inducible factor-1
	VEGF

Treating hyperglycaemia in diabetes mellitus

Fasting and postprandial hyperglycaemia are the key diagnostic features of DM and this is clearly responsible for the development of the microvascular complications of DM, and is an important factor in the genesis of the excess burden of cardiovascular complications seen in patients with DM; however, the management of the patient with DM should not be simply glucocentric.

The management of cardiovascular risk, with the purpose of reducing end-organ damage, specifically HF, is complex and requires meticulous attention to the control of blood pressure, aggressive modification of dyslipidaemia, appropriate use of antiplatelet therapy, and constant attention to lifestyle modification (Table 32.5).

Crucially, treating hypertension in diabetics reduces both microvascular and macrovascular complications. In particular, tight blood pressure control in UKPDS reduced new cases of HF by 44%.[44] However, this benefit did not persist after relaxation of blood pressure control, suggesting that aggressive blood pressure control should be instituted when first detected and maintained lifelong.[45,46]

Treating hyperglycaemia to reduce the vascular complications of DM seems intuitively straightforward. However, the first study that attempted to address this question suggested that pharmacological measures to lower blood glucose levels in patients with type 2 DM with the sulphonylurea drug tolbutamide actually resulted in an excess of cardiovascular deaths.[47] This study has been the centre of much controversy and more recently a number of well-conducted, informative studies have assessed the benefit, if any, of blood glucose lowering via pharmacological intervention in patients with type 1 and type 2 DM.

Principal amongst these studies has been the UKPDS.[48] This UK-based study assessed the value of 'tight' glycaemic control requiring escalating doses of oral hypoglycaemic agents, insulin or both (i.e. treatment based on achieving near normal fasting or postprandial blood glucose levels), versus 'conventional' glycaemic control (i.e. treatment based on symptom control). Overall, the application of the tight control approach resulted in an absolute reduction in HbA_{1c} of approximately 1% compared to the conventional treatment group,[48] which translated into a number of clear

Table 32.5 'Four corners' approach to modifying risk of cardiovascular disease in patients with diabetes mellitus

Hypertension	**Hyperglycaemia**
Aggressive treatment of hypertension to minimize risk of development of LVH and subsequent LVSD Target based blood pressure: ≤130/75 mmHg Lower blood pressure target in presence of end-organ damage, e.g. microalbuminuria: ≤120/70 mmHg Promote use of RAS blockade: ACEI/ARB/DRI/AA Do not avoid use of BB therapy due to presence of DM or fear of hypoglycaemic unawareness. Use evidence-based therapies, e.g. carvedilol, bisoprolol. Patients with DM are at increased risk of hyperkalaemia during treatment with AA/ACE-I/ARB therapy, and monitoring of eGFR and serum K^+ is recommended.	Optimal long-term control of hyperglycaemia. A target HbA_{1c} of 6.0–7.5% is likely to minimize the microvascular and macrovascular adverse effects of hyperglycaemia Complex combinations of oral agents, GLP-1 analogues and insulin may be required to reach this target Complex regimens to lower HbA_{1c} are associated with greater risks of significant hypoglycaemia, weight gain and possibly cardiovascular adverse effects Patients with HF should not receive TZD therapy. Metformin is safe in stable CHF but monitoring of renal function and temporary cessation during intercurrent illness is required
Hyperlipidaemia	Antiplatelet therapy/smoking cessation
Patients with known vascular disease should receive lipid-lowering therapy with an HMGCoA reductase inhibitor in line with local/national guidance, e.g. NICE, JBS2 Diabetes is recognized as a 'CHD-equivalent' in a number of national guidelines, and lowering of Total and LDL-Cholesterol with an HMGCoA reductase inhibitor is recommended even in the absence of clinical vascular disease. Addition of other therapies, including fibrates, should be considered Patients with early diabetic cardiomyopathy may benefit from treatment with HMGCoA reductase inhibitor therapy more than those with advanced HF.	Antiplatelet therapy with aspirin or clopidogrel should be used when there is evidence of existing vascular disease, (i.e. in line with guidance on secondary prevention of CHD). Use of aspirin in patients with DM but without clinically apparent vascular disease is not routinely recommended due to concerns regarding risk-benefits of this approach (i.e. risk of bleeding vs. reduction in vascular events). There are no data to support the use of aspirin in the absence of vascular disease in patients with diabetes Smoking cessation will limit the risk of further vascular events, including progressive retinopathy in diabetic patients.

benefits in terms of vascular risk modification. Although there was no clear significant benefit of tight glycaemic control on the overall risk of myocardial infarction, treatment with metformin in obese patients with type 2 DM did result in a significant reduction in the risk of myocardial infarction. Overall, the risk of developing HF increased by 8% for every 1% absolute rise in HbA_{1c} in keeping with the intuitive notion of good glycaemic control reducing the risk of HF.[20]

Although prolonged follow-up of the UKPDS demonstrated that HbA_{1c} measures in the tight control group and the conventional control group gravitated towards each other after study completion, a legacy effect was demonstrable in the tight control group beyond the period of strict tight control.[49] This translated to 10 years of clear benefits in terms of a reduction in myocardial infarction of 15% ($p = 0.01$) in the sulphonylurea-treated group, and a reduction in myocardial infarction of 33% ($p < 0.005$) and death from any cause of 27% ($p = 0.002$) in those overweight patients treated with metformin.[49]

The cornerstone of the management of all patients with DM is lifestyle modification aimed at maximizing daily activity, stopping tobacco exposure, attaining as near an ideal weight and BMI as practical, and encouraging healthy eating habits to minimize salt, saturated fat, refined carbohydrate, and excess calorie intake.[50] However, in the case of type 1 DM and the vast majority of cases of type 2 DM, adjunctive therapy with either oral agents, insulin, or both is necessary, not just to relieve the symptoms of hyperglycaemia, but to achieve as near normal blood glucose control as possible with the hope of minimizing DM-related complications including HF.

Oral hypoglycaemic agents

Until the mid 1990s, the only oral agents available for treating hyperglycaemia in DM were old drugs, or their mildly altered derivatives. Since the late 1990s, however, two new classes of agents have become widely available for treating hyperglycaemia in DM, with other novel agents in development (Table 32.6).

Metformin

Metformin is a biguanide drug which has been available for treating type 2 DM for over 40 years. Its precise mode of action is unclear, but it does reduce hepatic gluconeogenesis and peripheral insulin resistance leading to a reduction in both fasting and postprandial hyperglycaemia. Metformin is widely used for the treatment of type 2 DM worldwide, with most national guidelines suggesting it as the first-line oral agent for type 2 DM once lifestyle modification has been implemented and is no longer sufficient to maintain the set glycaemic target.[51] Metformin is frequently used in combination with other oral agents, insulin, and other injectable agents in type 2 DM, and is used in patients with type 1 DM when there is clinical evidence of insulin resistance.

Metformin's popularity stems from its positive association with reducing cardiovascular events in obese patients with type 2 DM in the UKPDS.[52] Within the UKPDS, metformin treatment was associated with a reduction myocardial infarction which was sustained at 10 years of follow-up.[49]

The major limitation to treatment with metformin is its propensity to cause gastrointestinal upset, particularly nausea and diarrhoea, which necessitates discontinuation of the drug in up to 20% of cases. Much less common is the potential for megaloblastic anaemia due to interference with vitamin B_{12} absorption. Metformin is renally excreted, and can accumulate in the presence of renal impairment. Current guidance in the UK suggests that withdrawal of metformin be considered when serum creatinine reaches 150 μmol/L or eGFR falls below 30 mL/min.[53]

Of greater concern is the association between metformin and lactic acidosis. This association, although well documented, is extremely rare and spontaneous isolated cases of metformin-induced lacticacidosis are extremely uncommon (less than 1 case per 100 000 treated patients).[54,55] In clinical practice, it is wise to

Table 32.6 Drug classes used to lower blood glucose in patients with diabetes mellitus

Class of agent	Example	Mode of action	Typical use	Side effects
Biguanide	Metformin	Reduce hepatic gluconeogenesis; increase peripheral tissue insulin sensitivity	First line after lifestyle modification. Combined with all other classes.	Gastrointestinal upset Vitamin B_{12} deficiency (rare) Lactic acidosis (rare, associated with intercurrent hypoxia-associated illness)
Sulphonylurea	Glipizide Gliclazide Glimepiride	Bind to ATP-dependent K^+ channel on beta cell membrane Promote release of preformed insulin	Second-line agent. Especially if symptomatic hypoglycaemia or BMI near normal	Hypoglycaemia Weight gain Relatively rapid loss of efficacy
Thiazolidinedione (glitazone)	Pioglitazone Rosiglitazone	Agonist of PPARγ; increases insulin sensitivity	Second-line agent. Especially if insulin resistance an issue and no cardiovascular risk factors.	Weight gain, oedema, HF, dilutional anaemia
α-Glucosidase inhibitor	Acarbose	Inhibits intestinal α-glucosidase and limits glucose absorption after meals	Can be used instead of metformin if not tolerated. Add on to all drug classes	Gastrointestinal upset, especially flatulence Hypoglycaemia rare, and does not respond to nonmonosaccharide sugars
Meglitinide	Repaglinide Nateglinide	Bind to ATP-dependent K+ channel on beta cell membrane (distinct from SU). Promote release of preformed insulin	Similar to Sulphonylureas, but pre-prandial use limits acceptability	Hypoglycaemia Weight gain
DPP-IV inhibitor	Sitagliptin Vildagliptin Saxagliptin	Inhibit degradation of GLP-1, enhance glucose-dependent insulin stimulation and suppress glucagon release to lower blood glucose	Second-line agent. Use in combination with metformin, sulphonylurea or thiazolidinedione	Nausea, skin rashes Weight gain and hypoglycaemia uncommon
Incretin mimetics	Exenatide Liraglutide	Mimic effect of endogenous GLP-1, to enhance glucose-dependent insulin stimulation and suppress glucagon release to lower blood glucose after meals. Reduced gastric emptying and possible central effect on satiety.	Second-line agent. Especially if obese with features of insulin resistance	Nausea, gastrointestinal upset Acute pancreatitis (exenatide)
Insulin	Rapid acting Long acting Human/ analogue/ porcine		All cases of type 1 DM. Type 2 DM after metformin monotherapy has failed or after trials of multiple oral agents.	Hypoglycaemia Weight gain

PPARγ peroxisome proliferator agonist receptor gamma; SU, sulphonylurea.

withdraw metformin temporarily in patients undergoing diagnostic procedures with the use of contrast, and those patients with HF who experience intercurrent illness which might be associated with tissue hypoxia, e.g. acute decompensated HF, myocardial infarction, or pneumonia. Similarly, patients with HF treated with metformin should have regular monitoring of renal function to ensure that metformin can be withdrawn in the event of a rapid decline in renal function, or in the context of a slow decline to a level where concern about accumulation outweighs potential benefits on glycaemic control and cardiovascular event reduction.

Sulphonylurea drugs

Initial experience with sulphonylureas was tempered by the UGDP experience[47] and some observational and retrospective studies suggest that these drugs are associated with increased cardiovascular mortality.[56,57] Subsequent investigations using newer agents with different properties have established the class as a popular choice for treating hyperglycaemia in patients who are no longer satisfactorily controlled on metformin alone.

However, neither the UKPDS nor ADVANCE studies demonstrated any adverse cardiovascular mortality effects associated with the use of sulphonylureas.[49,58] Their rapid onset of action and low cost is particularly attractive when treating symptomatic patients, but on the downside, use of sulphonylureas to achieve tight glycaemic control is associated with weight gain and significant potential for symptomatic hypoglycaemia.[58,59] Furthermore, sulphonylureas appear to exhibit a rather more rapid decline in efficacy over time than either metformin or thiazolidinediones,[60] making their use as first-line agents less attractive.

Thiazolidinediones

Thiazolidinediones (TZDs, glitazones) are modulators of the peroxisome proliferator-activated receptor γ (PPAR-γ), and increase the sensitivity of skeletal muscle, adipose tissue and liver to insulin.[61] As single agents, thiazolidinediones have a similar magnitude and duration of effect on glycaemic control to metformin,[60] with lower risks of hypoglycaemia than sulphonylureas. However, they have two adverse effects that have limited their use in the treatment of patients with DM, especially those with or at risk of developing HF—weight gain and fluid retention.

Weight gain with thiazolidinediones is similar or greater than that seen with sulphonylureas, although it is often associated with some modest benefits on lipid profiles.[60] Fluid retention is mediated via the kidney, and peripheral oedema and HF are both increased in users of thiazolidinediones. Although it appears that thiazolidinediones do not directly affect left ventricular function,[62] there is no question that they do cause HF, even in the presence of normal left ventricular function.[63,64]

Perhaps the greatest controversy surrounding thiazolidinediones is the suggestion that they may increase the risk of myocardial infarction or death. Initial evidence suggested that pioglitazone may have a modest beneficial effect on cardiovascular outcomes in patients with type 2 DM.[65] However, a controversial meta-analysis of data pertaining to rosiglitazone suggested that it was associated with a 43% increased risk of myocardial infarction.[66] This result was followed by a raft of publications which have confirmed that both thiazolidinediones increase rates of peripheral oedema, HF, and hospitalization due to HF.[54,63]

A retrospective cohort study of adverse cardiovascular events associated with thiazolidinedione use demonstrated no difference in the incidence of myocardial infarction in those treated with either pioglitazone or rosiglitazone, although the risk of death or HF was higher in those treated with rosiglitazone. This translated into a numbers needed to harm (NNH) of 120 for HF and 293 for death, for users of rosiglitazone rather than pioglitazone.[63] However, it should be borne in mind that the absolute event rates quoted (risk of myocardial infarction plus HF plus death, pioglitazone 5.3% vs rosiglitazone 6.9% over 6 years) equate to a 10-year risk of cardiovascular disease that barely reaches 10%.

Thiazolidinediones are available for use in the treatment of type 2 DM worldwide, either in combination with oral agents, or insulin in selected cases. They are not recommended for use in patients with known HF, and should be used with caution in patients at risk of developing HF.[64]

Table 32.7 Treatment of diabetic patients with or without heart failure; results of selected intervention studies.

Study name	Total study population (n)	Diabetes (n)	No diabetes (n)	RR of mortality (95% CI) Diabetes	RR of mortality (95% CI) No diabetes	Ratio of RR of mortality (95% CI) Diabetes vs. no diabetes
β-Blockers						
MERIT-HF [12]	3991	985	3006	0.81 (0.57–1.15)	0.62 (0.48–0.79)	
CIBIS-II [72]	2647	312	2335	0.81 (0.52–1.27)	0.66 (0.54–0.81)	
COPERNICUS [73]	2287	586	1701	0.68 (0.47–1.00)	0.67 (0.52–0.85)	
Pooled data		1883	7042	0.77 (0.61–0.96)	0.65 (0.57–0.74)	1.19 (0.91–1.55)
ACE inhibitors: HF						
CONSENSUS [14]	253	56	197	1.06 (0.65–1.74)	0.64 (0.46–0.88)2231	
SAVE [74]	2231	492	1739	0.89 (0.68–1.16)	0.82 (0.68–0.99)	
SMILE [75]	1556	303	1253	0.44 (0.22–0.87)	0.79 (0.5–1.15)	
SOLVD—prevention [76]	4228	647	3581	0.75 (0.55–1.02)	0.97 (0.83–1.15)	
SOLVD—treatment [76]	2569	663	1906	1.01 (0.85–1.21)	0.84 (0.74–0.95)	
TRACE [5]	1749	237	1512	0.73(0.57–0.94)	0.85 (0.74–0.97)	
Pooled data		2398	10188	0.84 (0.70–1.00)	0.85 (0.78–0.92)	1.00(0.80–1.25)
DM without HF	Placebo rate of HF	ACEI treated rate of HF				
HOPE [77]	11–15%	9%				
EUROPA [78]	No difference with respect to DM status					
Aldosterone antagonists						
RALES [79]	No difference shown or outcomes not stratified with respect to with diabetes					
EPHESUS [80]						
Angiotensin receptor blockers						
Val-HeFT [81]	Valsartan therapy did not prevent the primary endpoint in patients with HF and DM					
CHARM overall [82,83]	Trend to lesser effect of candesartan on preventing HF in patients with DM					
CHARM preserved [17]	Nonsignificant trend in reduction in HF in patients with DM					
I-PRESERVED [84]	No effect of Irbesartan on reducing onset of HF, and no benefit with respect to DM diagnosis					
Others (not specifically targeting patient with DM or HF)						
IDNT [85]	Irbesartan more effective than amlodipine in preventing new HF in patients with DM					
VALUE [86]	Valsartan more effective than amlodipine in preventing new HF in patients with DM					
RENAAL [87]	Losartan reduces HF incidence in patients with DM and preserved LV function by 32%					
LIFE [88]	Losartan reduced the risk of developing HF in patients with DM more than atenolol, RR = 0.41.					

DM, diabetes mellitus; HF, heart failure; LV, left ventricular.

Insulin

Insulin is the longest-serving therapeutic option for the treatment of DM. Multiple formulations exist and several means of insulin administration are used in an attempt to mimic physiological insulin profiles and restore normal blood glucose profiles in patients with DM. The use of insulin in the treatment of patients with type 2 DM is increasingly common, principally due to the increasing use of glycaemic targets promoted by national and international expert committees.[67]

Patients with HF exhibit increased resistance to insulin, mediated via a variety of different mechanisms. As a consequence, insulin doses required to achieve adequate glycaemic control in type 2 patients with HF are substantially higher than in patients with type 1 DM or type 2 DM without HF.

UKPDS did not show that insulin treatment increased the incidence of HF or mortality.[48] However, some studies have found that the use of insulin in patients with DM is an independent predictor for the development of HF, as well as being associated with increased mortality.[24,68–70] Diabetics without HF commenced on insulin may also have a higher rate of hospitalization due to HF than those commenced on sulphonylureas.[70] The CHARM study also demonstrated a greater risk of mortality than for non-insulin-treated patients.[71] A further retrospective analysis of patients with advanced HF suggested that insulin treatment was an independent predictor of mortality.[69] Therefore, at present there are no prospective evaluations of insulin therapy in patients with DM with or without HF to advise on the precise role of insulin treatment.

Other drugs

A number of other drugs are available for patient use to lower blood glucose in patients with DM. At present there are no data to determine their efficacy or otherwise in the management of the patient with DM and HF.

Heart failure treatments in patients with diabetes mellitus

Data on treatment efficacy for HF patients with DM are largely derived from subgroup analyses from the major HF treatment trials (Table 32.7).

ACE inhibitors

ACE inhibitors are widely used to treat hypertension, microalbuminuria, and proteinuria in patients with DM. Their benefits in the treatment of HF are well established, although in patients with DM the benefits are less apparent (Table 32.7).[90]

β-Blockers

β-Blockers are effective treatments for HF. In patients with HF and DM the benefits of β-blocker therapy are similar to those seen in nondiabetic subjects in reducing mortality and hospitalization due to HF (Table 32.7).[90]

A major concern regarding the application of β-blocker therapy is the potential for this class of drugs to alter insulin sensitivity and alter hypoglycaemia awareness. Hypoglycaemia results in a pronounced activation of the sympathetic nervous system, and release of cortisol and glucagon. These responses aim to increase hepatic glucose output, and increase blood supply to the brain and other glucose sensitive tissues. The UKPDS assessed the rates of hypoglycaemia in patients with hypertension and DM and did not discern any difference in the rate of hypoglycaemia in patients treated with atenolol or captopril,[44] whereas one study of elderly diabetic patients suggested that insulin-treated patients were more likely to experience severe hypoglycaemia than those treated with sulphonylureas.[91]

In general, there are few or no data to suggest that β-blockers used to treat HF in patients with DM specifically affect hypoglycaemic awareness or recovery from symptomatic hypoglycaemia, or adversely alter lipid metabolism to the detriment of patients. Furthermore, the benefits of treatment with β-blockers in terms of reduction in critical endpoints far outweighs any potential effects on other measures.

Other drugs

There are no specific data in relation to the effect of digoxin in patients with HF and DM. However, DM did not affect the benefit of hydralazine plus isosorbide dinitrate in A-HeFT.[89] Thiazide diuretics have the potential to increase fasting blood glucose levels although their effect on reducing blood pressure, preventing HF and reducing strokes far outweigh any minor effect on glycaemic control.[90]

Practice points

Table 32.8 lists a number of key practice points that are worth paying attention to in day-to-day practice when dealing with the patient with HF and DM.

Summary

DM and HF are increasingly common conditions, and may therefore frequently coexist. Diabetes imparts a greater risk of morbidity

Table 32.8 Practice points for daily management of patients with heart failure and diabetes

Practice point	Risks	Action
Hyperkalaemia	Long standing DM Type 4 renal tubular acidosis ACEI/ARB/AA use NSAID use	Monitor serum potassium regularly and during intercurrent illness Withdraw or modify doses of offending drugs
Hypoglycaemia	Sulphonylurea use Insulin use Injection site lipohypertrophy Unexpected exercise/ missed meals Worsening renal function	Measure renal function Examine injection sites Modify dose/timing of SU or insulin Correct any reversible causes of renal impairment
Renal impairment	DM duration Hypertension Cigarette smoking ACEI/ARB/renin inhibitors Peripheral vascular disease Dehydration/ excessive diuretic use NSAID use	Correct any intercurrent precipitant Withhold metformin and ACEI/ARB/renin inhibitors until condition improved Consider withdrawal or dose modification of metformin and ACEI/ARB/renin inhibitors

ACEI, angiotensin converting enzyme inhibitor; ARB, angiotensin receptor blocker; DM, diabetes mellitus; NSAID, nonsteroidal anti-inflammatory drug.

and mortality on the patient with HF and complicates the management of HF, and vice versa. Optimizing cardiovascular risk factors is essential for limiting adverse outcomes for both conditions, and patients with diabetes mellitus are, at present, still less likely to receive optimal care whether as a result of fear of application of some evidence-based strategies, or the inability to tolerate a number of therapeutic agents. Glycaemic control is an important factor in the management of the patient with DM and HF, and optimized patient-specific approaches are most likely to minimize adverse events while maximizing the opportunity for reducing long-term complications.

References

1. Kannel WB, Hjortland M, Castelli WP. Role of diabetes in congestive heart failure: the Framinhgam study. *Am J Cardiol* 1974;**34**:29–34.
2. Bibbins-Domingo K, Lin F, Vittinghoff E. Predictors of heart failure among women with coronary disease. *Circulation* 2004;**110**:1424–30.
3. Carrabba N, Valenti R, Parodi G, Santoro GM, Antoniucci D. Left ventricular remodelling and heart failure in diabetic patients treated with primary angioplasty for acute myocardial infarction. *Circulation* 2004;**110**:1974–9.
4. Mukamal, KJ, Nesto RW, Cohen MC, *et al.* Impact of diabetes on long-term survival after acute myocardial infarction: comparability of risk with prior myocardial infarction. *Diabetes Care* 2001;**24**:1422–7.
5. Melchior T, Kober L, Madsen CR, *et al.* Accelerating impact of diabetes mellitus on mortality in the years following an acute myocardial infarction: TRACE Study Group Trandolapril Cardiac Evaluation. *Eur Heart J* 1999;**20**:973–8.
6. Newton JD, Squire IB. Glucose and haemoglobin in the assessment of prognosis after first hospitalisation for heart failure. *Heart* 2006;**92**:1441–6.
7. Berry C, Brett M, Stevenson K, McMurray JJV, Norrie J. Nature and prognostic importance of abnormal glucose tolerance and diabetes in acute heart failure. *Heart* 2008;**94**:296–304.
8. Thrainsdottir IS, Aspelund T, Thorgeirsson G, *et al.* The association between glucose abnormalities and heart failure in the population-based Reykjavik study. *Diabetes Care* 2005;**28**:612–16.
9. Davies M, Hobbs F, Davis R, *et al.* Prevalence of left-ventricular systolic dysfunction and heart failure in the Echocardiographic Heart of England Screening study: a population based study. *Lancet* 2001;**358**:439–44.
10. Bertoni AG, Hundley WG, Massing MW, Bonds DE, Burke GL, Goff DC Jr. Heart failure prevalence, incidence, and mortality in the elderly with diabetes. *Diabetes Care* 2004;**27**:699–703.
11. Harris MI, Flegal KM, Cowie CC, *et al.* Prevalence of diabetes, impaired fasting glucose, and impaired glucose tolerance in U.S. Adults. The Third National Health and Nutrition Examination Survey 1988–1994. *Diabetes Care* 1998;**21**:518–24.
12. MERIT-HF Investigators. Effect of metoprolol CR/XL in chronic heart failure. Metoprolol CR/XL Randomised Intervention Trial in Congestive Heart Failure (MERIT-HF). *Lancet* 1999;**353**:2001–7.
13. Poole-Wilson PA, Swedberg K, Cleland JG, *et al.* Comparison of carvedilol and metoprolol on outcomes in patients with chronic heart failure in the Carvedilol or Metoprolol European Trial (COMET): randomised controlled trial. *Lancet* 2003;**362**:7–13.
14. CONSENSUS Trial Study Group. Effects of enalapril on mortality in severe congestive heart failure. Results of the Cooperative North Scandinavian Enalapril Survival Study (CONSENSUS). *N Engl J Med* 1987;**316**:1429–35.
15. Cohn JN, Tognoni G. A randomised trial of the angiotensin-receptor blocker valsartan in chronic heart failure. *N Engl J Med* 2001;**345**:1667–75.
16. Pitt B, Poole-Wilson PA, Segal R, *et al.* Effect of losartan compared with captopril on mortality in patients with symptomatic heart failure: randomised trial—the Losartan Heart Failure Survival Study Elite II. *Lancet* 2000;**355**:1582–7.
17. Yusuf S, Pfeffer MA, Swedberg K, *et al.* Effects of candesartan in patients with chronic heart failure and preserved left ventricular ejection fraction: the CHARM-preserved Trial. *Lancet* 2003;**362**:777–81.
18. Adams KF Jr, Fonarow GC, Emerman CL, *et al.* ADHERE Scientific Advisory Committee and Investigators. Characteristics and outcomes of patients hospitalised for heart failure in the United States: rationale, design, and preliminary observations from the first 100,000 cases in the Acute Decompensated Heart Failure National Registry (ADHERE). *Am Heart J* 2005;**149**:209–16.
19. Greenberg BH, Abraham WT, Albert NM, *et al.* Influence of diabetes on characteristics and outcomes in patients hospitalised with heart failure: A report from the Organized Program to Initiate Lifesaving Treatment in Hospitalized Patients with Heart Failure (OPTIMIZE-HF). *Am J Heart* 2007;**154**:27.e1–277.e8.
20. Stratton IM, Adler AI, Neil HAW, Matthews DR, Manley SR, Cull CA, Hadden D, Turner RC, Holman RR. Association of glycaemia with macrovascular and microvascular complications of type 2 diabetes (UKPDS 35): prospective observational study. *BMJ* 2000;**321**:405–12.
21. Vaur I, Gueret P, Lievre M, Chabaud S, Passa P. Development of congestive heart failure in type 2 diabetic patients with microalbuminuria or proteinuria: observations from the DIABHYCAR (Type 2 DIABetes, Hypertension, Cardiovascular, Events and Ramipril) study. *Diabetes Care* 2003;**26**:855–60.
22. Iribarren C, Karter AJ, Go AS, Ferrara A, Liu JY, Sidney S, Selby JV. Glycemic control and heart failure among adult patients with diabetes. *Circulation* 2001;**103**:2668–73.
23. Heart Outcome Prevention Evaluation (HOPE) Study Investigators. Effects of ramipril on cardiovascular and microvascular outcomes in people with diabetes mellitus: results of the HOPE study and MICRO-HOPE substudy. *Lancet* 2000;**355**:253–9.
24. Nichols GA, Gullion CM, Koro CE, Ephross SE, Brown JB. The incidence of congestive heart failure in type 2 diabetes. *Diabetes Care* 2004;**27**:1879–84.
25. Kamalesh M, Nair G. Increasing prevalence of diabetes among patients with congestive heart failure. *Int J Cardiol* 2005;**104**:77–80.
26. Amato L, Paolisso G, Cacciatore F, *et al.* Congestive heart failure predicts the development of non-insulin-dependent diabetes mellitus in the elderly. The Osservatorio Geriatrico Regione Campania Group. *Diabetes Metab* 1997;**23**:213–18.
27. Yusuf S, Ostergren JB, Gerstein HC, *et al.* Effects of candesartan on the development of a new diagnosis of diabetes mellitus in patients with heart failure. *Circulation* 2005;**112**:48–53.
28. Vermes E, Ducharme A, Bourassa MG, Lessard M, White M, Tardif JC. Enalapril reduces the incidence of diabetes in patients with chronic heart failure: insight from the studies of left ventricular dysfunction (SOLVD). *Circulation* 2003;**107**:1291–6.
29. Tenenbaum A, Motro M, Fisman EZ, *et al.* Functional class in patients with heart failure is associated with the development of diabetes. *Am J Med* 2003;**114**:271–5.
30. McDonagh TA, Morrison CE, Lawrence A, *et al.* Symptomatic and asymptomatic left-ventricular systolic dysfunction in an urban population. *Lancet* 1997;**350**:829–833.
31. Redfield MM, Jacobsen SJ, Burnett JC Jr, Mahoney DW, Bailey KR, Rodeheffer RJ. Burden of systolic and diastolic ventricular dysfunction in the community: appreciating the scope of the heart failure epidemic. *JAMA* 2003;**289**:194–202.
32. Kistorp C, Galatius S, Gustafsson F, Faber J, Corell P, Hildebrandt P. Prevalence and characteristics of diabetic patients in a chronic heart failure population. *Int J Cardiol* 2005;**100**:281–287.
33. King H, Aubert RE, Herman WH. Global burden of diabetes, 1995–2025: prevalence, numerical estimates, and projections. *Diabetes Care* 1998;**21**:1414–31.

34. The Expert Committee on the Diagnosis and Classification of Diabetes Mellitus. Report of the Expert Committee on the Diagnosis and Classification of Diabetes Mellitus. *Diabetes Care* 1997;**20**:1183–97.
35. International Expert Committee. International expert committee report on the role of the A1c assay in the diagnosis of diabetes. *Diabetes Care* 2009;**32**:1327–34.
36. Kilpatrick ES, Bloomgarden ZT, Zimmet PZ. Is haemoglobin A1c a step forward for diagnosing diabetes? *BMJ* 2009;**339**:b4432.
37. Boudina S, Abel ED. Diabetic cardiomyopathy revisited. *Circulation* 2007;**115**:3213–23.
38. Rubler S, Dlugash J, Yuceoglu YZ, Kumral T, Branwood AW, Grishman A. New type of cardiomyopathy associated with diabetic glomerulosclerosis. *Am J Cardiol* 1972;**30**:595–602.
39. Khhavandi K, Khavandi A, Asghar O, *et al.* Dilated cardiomyopathy—a distinct disease? *Baillieres Best Pract Res Clin Endocrinol Metab* 2009;**23**:347–60.
40. Shishehbor MH, Hoogwerf BJ, Schoeenhagen P, *et al.* Relation of hemoglobin A1c to left ventricular relaxation in patients with type 1 diabetes mellitus and without overt heart failure. *Am J Cardiol* 2003;**91**:115114–17.
41. Poirier P, Bogaty P, Garneau C, Marois L, Dumesnil JG. Diastolic dysfunction in normotensive men with well-controlled type 2 diabetes: importance of maneuvers in echocardiographic screening for preclinical diabetic cardiomyopathy. *Diabetes Care* 2001;**24**:5–10.
42. Shivalkar B, Dhondt D, Goovaerts I, *et al.* Flow mediated dilatation and cardiac function in type 1 diabetes mellitus. *Am J Cardiol* 2006;**97**:77–82.
43. Di Bonito P, Moio N, Cavuto L, *et al.* Early detection of diabetic cardiomyopathy: usefulness of tissue Doppler imaging. *Diabet Med* 2005;**22**:1720–5.
44. UKPDS Group. Tight blood pressure control and risk of macrovascular and microvascular complications in type 2 diabetes. *BMJ* 1998;**317**:703–13.
45. Holman RR, Paul SK, Bethel MA, Neil HAW, Matthews DR. Long-term follow-up after tight control of blood pressure in type 2 diabetes. *N Engl J Med*, 2008;**359**:1565–76.
46. Perreault S, Dragomir A, White M, Lalonde L, Blais L, Berard A. Better adherence to antihypertensive agents and risk reduction of chronic heart failure. *J Intern Med* 2009;**266**:207–18.
47. Meinert CL, Knatterud GL, Prout TE, *et al.* A study of the effects of hypoglycemic agents on vascular complications in patients with adult-onset diabetes. *Diabetes* 1970;**19**:789–830.
48. UKPDS Group. UKPDS 33: intensive blood-glucose control with sulphonylureas or insulin compared with conventional treatment and risk of complications in patients with type 2 diabetes. *Lancet* 1998;**352**:837–51.
49. Holman RR, Paul SK, Bethel MA, Matthews DR, Neil HAW.10-year follow-up of intensive glucose control in type 2 diabetes. *N Engl J Med* 2008;**359**:1577–89.
50. SIGN Guideline Committee. *SIGN 55—management of diabetes.* Scottish Intercollegiate Guideline Network, 2001.
51. Nathan DM, Buse JB, Davidson MB, *et al.* Medical management of hyperglycaemia in type 2 diabetes: a consensus algorithm for the initiation and adjustment of therapy. *Diabetes Care* 2009;**32**:193–203.
52. UKPDS study group. Effect of intensive blood-glucose control with metformin on complications in overweight patients with type 2 diabetes (UKPDS 34). *Lancet* 1998;**352**:854–65.
53. Shaw JS, Wilmot RL, Kilpatrick ES. Establishing pragmatic estimated GFR thresholds to guide metformin prescribing. *Diabetic Med* 2007;**24**:1160–3.
54. Bolen S, Feldman L, Vassy J *et al.* Systematic review: comparative effectiveness and safety of oral medications for type 2 diabetes mellitus. *Ann Intern Med* 2007;**147**:386–99.
55. Salpeter S, Greyber E, Pasternak G, *et al.* Risk of fatal and nonfatal lactic acidosis with metformin use in type 2 diabetes mellitus. *Cochrane Database Syst Rev* 2006;**1**:CD002967.
56. Evans J, Ogston S, Emslie-Smith A, Morris A. Risk of mortality and adverse cardiovascular outcomes in type 2 diabetes: a comparison of patients treated with sulphonylureas and metformin. *Diabetologia* 2006;**49**:930–6.
57. Tzoulaki I, Molokhia M, Curcin V, *et al.* Risk of cardiovascular disease and all cause mortality among patients with type 2 diabetes prescribed oral antidiabetes drugs: retrospective cohort study using UK general practice research database. *BMJ*, 2009;**339**:b4731.
58. The ADVANCE Collaborative Group. Intensive blood glucose lowering in type 2 diabetes. *N Engl J Med* 2008;**358**:2560–72.
59. The Action to Control Cardiovascular Risk in Diabetes Study Group. Effects of intensive glucose lowering in type 2 diabetes. *N Engl J Med* 2008;**358**:2545–59.
60. Kahn SE, Haffner SM, Heise MA, *et al.* Glycemic durability of rosiglitazone, metformin, or glyburide monotherapy. *N Engl J Med* 2006;**355**:2427–43.
61. Yki-Jarvinen H. Drug therapy: thiazolidinediones. *N Engl J Med* 2004;**351**:1106–10.
62. Dargie HJ, Hildebrandt PR, Riegger GAJ, *et al.* A randomised, placebo-controlled trial assessing the effects of rosiglitazone on echocardiographic function and cardiac status in type-2 diabetic patients with NYHA functional class I/II heart failure. *J Amer Coll Cardiol* 2007;**49**:1696–704.
63. Juurlink DN, Gomes T, Lipscombe LL, Austin PC, Hux JE, Mamdani MM. Adverse cardiovascular events during treatment with pioglitazone and rosiglitazone: population based cohort study. *BMJ* 2009;**339**:2942–8.
64. Jamieson A, Abousleiman Y. Thiazolidinedione-associated congestive heart failure and pulmonary edema. *Mayo Clin Proc* 2004;**79**:571–577.
65. Dormandy J, Charbonnel B, Eckland D, *et al.* Secondary prevention of macrovascular events in patients with type 2 diabetes in the PROactive Study (PROspective pioglitAzone Clinical Trial In macroVascular Events): a randomised controlled trial. *Lancet* 2005;**366**:1279–89.
66. Nissen SE, Wolski K. Effect of rosiglitazone on the risk of myocardial infarction and death from cardiovascular causes. *N Engl J Med* 2007;**356**:2457–71.
67. *Summary of Revisions for the 2009 Clinical Practice Recommendations. Diabetes Care 2009;32(Suppl 1):S3–5.*
68. Domanski M, Krause-Steinrauf H, Deedwania P, *et al.* The effect of diabetes on outcomes of patients with advanced heart failure in the BEST trial. *J Am Coll Cardiol* 2003;**42**:914–22.
69. Smooke S, Horwich TB, Fonarow GC. Insulin-treated diabetes is associated with a marked increase in mortality in patients with advanced heart failure. *Am Heart J* 2005;**149**:168–74.
70. Karter AJ, Ahmed AT, Liu J, Moffet HH, Parker MM. Pioglitazone initiation and subsequent hospitalisation for congestive heart failure. *Diabet Med*, **22**:986–93.
71. Pocock SJ, Wang D, Pfeffer MA, *et al.* Predictors of mortality and morbidity in patients with chronic heart failure. *Eur Heart J* 2005;**27**:65–75.
72. Erdmann E, Lechat P, Verkenne P, Wiemann H. Results from post-hoc analyses of the CIBIS II trial: effect of bisoprolol in high-risk patient groups with chronic heart failure. *Eur J Heart Fail* 2001;**3**:469–79.
73. Packer M, Fowler MB, Roecker EB, *et al.* Effect of carvedilol on the morbidity of patients with severe chronic heart failure. *Circulation* 2002;**106**:2194–9.
74. Moye LA, Pfeffer MA, Wun CC, *et al.* Uniformity of captopril benefit in the SAVE Study: subgroupanalysis. Survival and Ventricular Enlargement Study. *Eur Heart J* 1994;**15**(Suppl B):2–8; discussion 26–30.
75. Gustafsson I, Torp-Pedersen C, K ber L, Gustafsson F, Per Hildebrandt P, on behalf of the Trace Study Group. Effect of

the angiotensin-converting enzyme inhibitor trandolapril on mortality and morbidity in diabetic patients with left ventricular dysfunction after acute myocardial infarction. *J Am Coll Cardiol* 1999;**34**:83–9.

76. Shindler DM, Kostis JB, Yusuf S, *et al.* Diabetes mellitus, a predictor of morbidity and mortality in the Studies of Left Ventricular Dysfunction (SOLVD) Trials and Registry. *Am J Cardiol* 1996;**77**:1017–20.
77. Arnold JM, Yusuf S, Young J, *et al.* Prevention of heart failure in patients in the Heart Outcomes Prevention Evaluation (HOPE) study. *Circulation* 2003;**107**:1284–90.
78. Fox KM. Efficacy of perindopril in reduction of cardiovascular events among patients with stable coronary artery disease: randomised, double blind, placebo-controlled, multicentre trial (the EUROPA study). *Lancet* 2003;**362**:782–8.
79. Pitt B, Zannad F, Remme WJ, *et al.* The effect of spironolactone on morbidity and mortality in patients with severe heart failure. Randomized Aldactone Evaluation Study Investigators. *N Engl J Med* 1999;**341**:709–17.
80. Pitt B, Remme W, Zannad F, *et al.* Eplerenone, a selective aldosterone blocker, in patients with left ventricular dysfunction after myocardial infarction. *N Engl J Med* 2003;**348**:1309–21.
81. Conn JN, Tognoni G. A randomized trial of the angiotensin-receptor blocker valsartan in chronic heart failure. *N Engl J Med* 2001;**345**:1667–75.
82. Pfeffer MA, Swedberg K, Granger CB, *et al.* Effects of candesartan on mortality and morbidity in patients with chronic heart failure: the CHARM-Overall programme. *Lancet* 2003;**362**:759–66.
83. Yusuf S, Ostergren JB, Gerstein HC, *et al.* Effects of candesartan on the development of a new diagnosis of diabetes mellitus in patients with heart failure. *Circulation* 2005;**112**:48–53.
84. Massie BM, Carson PE, McMurray JJV, *et al.* Irbesartan in patients with heart failure and preserved ejection fraction. *N Engl J Med* 2008;**359**:2456–67.
85. Parving HH, Lehnert H, Brochner-Mortensen J, Gomis R, Andersen S, Arner P. The effect of irbesartan on the development of diabetic nephropathy in patients with type 2 diabetes. *N Engl J Med* 2001;**345**:870–8.
86. Julius S, Kjeldsen SE, Weber M, *et al.* Outcomes in hypertensive patients at high cardiovascular risk treated with regimens based on valsartan or amlodipine: the VALUE randomised trial. *Lancet* 2004;**363**:2022–31.
87. Brenner BM, Cooper ME, de Zeeuw D, *et al.* Effects of losartan on renal and cardiovascular outcomes in patients with type 2 diabetes and nephropathy. *N Engl J Med* 2001;**345**:861–9.
88. Lindholm LH, Ibsen H, Borch-Johnsen K, *et al.* Risk of new-onset diabetes in the Losartan Intervention For Endpoint reduction in hypertension study. *J Hypertens* 2002;**20**:1879–86.
89. Taylor AL, Ziesche S, Yancy C, *et al.* Combination of isosorbide dinitrate and hydralazine in blacks with heart failure. *N Engl J Med* 2004;**351**:2049–57.
90. Shekelle PG, Rich MW, Morton C, *et al.* Efficacy of angiotensin-converting enzyme inhibitors and beta blockers in the management of left ventricular systolic dysfunction according to race, gender, and diabetic status: a meta-analysis. *J Am Coll Cardiol* 2003;**41**:1529–38.
91. Shorr RI, Ray WA, Daugherty JR, Griffin MR. Antihypertensives and the risk of serious hypoglycaemia in older persons using insulin or sulphonylureas. *JAMA* 1997;**278**:40–3.

33

Valvular heart disease

Gregory Ducroq, Bernard Iung, and Alec Vahanian

Valvular heart disease (VHD), although not as common as coronary disease or hypertension, is an important, and challenging, clinical entity. The prevalence of VHD is still high, increasing with age,[1] affecting 13.2% of people over the age of 75. There have been important changes in the distribution of the aetiologies of VHD in Western countries over the last 50 years and the degenerative aetiology is now the most frequent. Increased age is associated with a higher frequency of comorbidity, rendering decision-making for intervention more complex.[1–3]

The presence of VHD is of interest in patients with heart failure (HF) because the treatment of the causative VHD may cure HF, which stresses the importance of its detection and appropriate treatment.[3,4] However, decision-making for surgery may be difficult in patients with VHD and HF because of higher operative mortality and concerns over late results, which may be worsened by progression of the underlying disease.

The present chapter will concentrate on adult patients either with acquired VHD or with a valve prosthesis, focusing specifically on the patient with HF.

General considerations

There is a significant burden of VHD in large cohorts of patients with HF: at least moderate VHD was present in 29% in the Euro Heart Survey on HF[5] and in 17% of patients in a prospective American cohort.[6]

HF in patients with VHD may occur at the endstage of a chronic disease due to continued deterioration of the underlying HF or may be precipitated by cardiac complications such as atrial fibrillation, acute myocardial ischaemia, endocarditis, or noncardiac complications such as respiratory infection. HF may alternatively occur in acute settings in patients without previous significant VHD, mainly due to endocarditis, or more rarely myocardial infarction, or trauma. In such cases, acute valve regurgitation is poorly tolerated because of the absence of prior adaptative mechanisms.

VHD leads predominantly to breathlessness, which has an important prognostic value. Other than in very disabled patients, shortness of breath may be difficult to assess because of its subjective component, in particular in elderly people, who often adapt their activity to their functional capacity or may complain of fatigue rather than breathlessness. Breathlessness may be due to associated disease.

Although there are other clinical signs of HF, the detection of a murmur is the most frequent way of detecting VHD or of relating symptoms to a valvular cause. Auscultation often gives the first clue to the severity of VHD. It should, however, be noted that murmurs in patients with HF can be of low intensity because of low cardiac output despite severe underlying valve disease. Clinical examination also contributes to the search for comorbidities, particularly in elderly patients.

An ECG and chest radiograph are generally done along with the clinical examination. Analysis of pulmonary vascular distribution is useful in the interpretation of dyspnoea.

Echocardiography is the cornerstone of investigations of VHD. It is indicated in patients with a cardiac murmur.[2,3] The aim of echocardiography is to confirm the diagnosis of VHD; to assess its severity, mechanisms, and consequences; and to search for associated lesions. It is important to recognize that that the variability of loading conditions in acute regurgitation decreases the value of the quantitative criteria.

Measurements of left ventricular enlargement and systolic function are important in decision-making for intervention in regurgitant valve diseases. They should be indexed to body surface area (BSA). Echocardiography also enables the measurement of pulmonary pressures and the assessment of combined lesions.

CT and MRI can quantitate accurately the severity of valvular diseases or left ventricular volumes. MRI provides additional information on the size and function of the right ventricle, but in practice, the limited availability of these techniques restricts such application. Cardiac catheterization is indicated only in the rare instances when noninvasive investigations are inconclusive or discordant with clinical findings. On the other hand, coronary angiography should be performed preoperatively according to guidelines.[2,3]

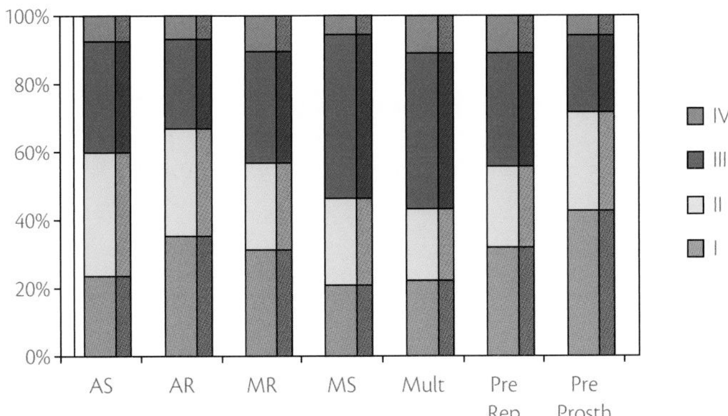

Fig. 33.1 Distribution of New York Heart Association class (I–IV) in the EuroHeart Survey on valvular heart disease.[1]

The final aim of the assessment of VHD is to estimate the patient's prognosis and to compare outcome with operative mortality and the late results of interventions. This comparison remains the rationale for the recommendations of interventions given the lack of randomized trials in patients with VHD. Multivariate risk scores, such as logistic Euroscore or STS score,[7–9] are increasingly used to estimate operative mortality, but the scores have limitations in the highest-risk patients.[8] Final decision-making relies on the clinical judgement of the physician—which should combine components of risk stratification, analysis of patient's quality of life, and the patient's wishes after appropriate information.[9]

Across the spectrum of VHD, patients with HF have a dismal prognosis without intervention and a worse postoperative outcome than those who are at an earlier stage of the disease, which supports the notion of early intervention.

Valvular heart disease and heart failure in the EuroHeart Survey

The EuroHeart Survey on VHD is a good way of illustrating the current presentation and management of VHD patients with HF.[1] The survey was conducted in 2001 in 92 centres from 25 countries, and it included 5001 patients: 3547 with moderate or severe native valve disease and 1454 with heart valve prosthesis. The distribution of New York Heart Association (NYHA) class in the 5001 patients is shown in Fig. 33.1. Clinical or radiological signs of left and/or right HF were present at admission in 1149 patients (23%).

A comparison of patient characteristics according to the presence or absence of signs of HF is detailed in Table 33.1. Patients with HF were older and were more likely to have diabetes and other comorbidities than patients without HF. Patients with HF also had more important left ventricular remodelling, lower ejection fraction (EF), and higher pulmonary artery pressures.

A decision to operate was taken in 435 patients (38%) with HF versus 1515 patients (39%) without. The 30-day mortality was 8.5% in patients with HF versus 2.4% in those without ($p < 0.0001$). The 1-year survival is illustrated in Fig. 33.2 and shows a a higher mortality in medically treated patients. Predictors of 1-year survival in the 1149 patients with HF were age (HR 1.3; 95% CI 1.2–1.5), male sex (HR 1.6; 95% CI 1.2–2.1), ≥1 comorbidity (HR 1.9; 95% CI 1.4–2.6), and decision not to operate (HR 1.4; 95% CI 1.0–1.9).

Thus, almost one-quarter of patients with VHD present with HF. Only 38% of the patients with HF were considered to be candidates for valvular surgery. This highlights the need for guideline implementation to allow for intervention more often and at an earlier stage.

Aortic stenosis

Aortic stenosis (AS) is the most common valve disease in Europe[1] and it is increasing in prevalence because the population is ageing.

Diagnosis

The most common initial symptom is exertional dyspnoea. Later, dyspnoea may progress to overt HF. In practice, AS may be discovered during investigations for unexplained HF. The intensity of the murmur has poor sensitivity for diagnosing AS, since it may be soft if cardiac output is low. The physical examination may be misleading in patients with low output since there is no slow rising pulse; the murmur may become softer or even disappear and findings on auscultation may be limited to a soft murmur of functional mitral regurgitation (MR) and S3 sound at the apex.

Overall cardiac silhouette and pulmonary vascular distribution are abnormal if cardiac decompensation is present. Fluoroscopy will detect calcification of the valve (found in almost all elderly patients with severe AS). Left ventricular hypertrophy (LVH), with or without repolarization abnormalities, is seen on ECG in approximately 80% of patients with severe AS. Other nonspecific signs include left atrial enlargement, left axis deviation, and left bundle branch block. Atrial fibrillation can be seen at a late stage and may suggest coexisting mitral valve disease.

Doppler echocardiography confirms the presence of AS, and is the preferred technique for assessing its severity. For clinical decision-making, valve area should be considered in combination with flow velocity, pressure gradient and ventricular function, as well as functional status. The thresholds generally recommended for the definition of severe AS are aortic jet velocity greater than 4 m/s; mean gradient >40–50 mmHg; aortic valve area less than 1 cm^2. Indexing to BSA, with a cut-off value of 0.6 cm^2/m^2 BSA, is helpful in patients with either unusually small or large BSA.[2,3]

Low flow is common in patients with HF due to AS, usually due to depressed left ventricular function: it may be associated with low pressure gradients even with severe AS. If the mean gradient is less than 40 mmHg, even if the calculated valve area is small, there may not be severe AS since mild to moderately diseased valves may not open fully due to the low cardiac output, resulting in a 'functionally small' valve area (pseudosevere AS). Stress echocardiography, using low-dose dobutamine, is helpful in low-flow, low-gradient AS. Truly severe AS shows only small changes in valve area (increase <0.2 cm^2) which remains less than 1 cm^2 with increasing flow rate but significant increase in gradients (maximum value of mean gradient >40 mmHg). In contrast, patients with 'pseudosevere AS' have a marked increase in valve area with dobutamine with a final value over 1 cm^2 but only minor changes in gradients.[10] In addition, this test may detect the presence of contractile reserve, which has prognostic implications.[10]

Natriuretic peptides, in particular B-type natriuretic peptide (BNP) and NT-proBNP, are increased in relation to the severity of symptoms and the degree of left ventricular dysfunction. These measurements may also be a helpful adjunct in identifying patients with equivocal symptoms.[2]

Table 33.1 Characteristics of patients with or without signs of congestive heart failure at admission in the EuroHeart Survey on valvular heart disease

	CHF (n=1149) mean ± SD (%)	No CHF (n=3842) mean ± SD (%)	p
Age (years)	65 ± 14	63 ± 14	<0.0001
Previous valve surgery	27	30	0.11
Previously known valvular disease	80	84	0.002
Atrial fibrillation	47	24	<0.0001
Comorbidities			
Coronary artery disease	44	38	0.04
Previous myocardial infarction	18	12	<0.0001
Carotid artery disease	3.9	3.5	0.47
Lower limb arteritis	6.4	4.3	0.002
Serum creatinin >200 μmol/L	6.2	2.5	<0.0001
Dialysis	10	6.1	<0.0001
Neurological dysfunction	20	13	<0.0001
Chronic obstructive pulmonary disease	44	31	<0.0001
≥1 comorbidity			<0.0001
Valve disease			
Aortic stenosis	16	27	
Aortic regurgitation	6	8	
Mitral stenosis	9	6	
Mitral regurgitation	19	17	
Multiple valve disease	23	12	
Right-sided valve disease	1	1	
Previous valve surgery	26	29	
Investigations			
LVEF (%)	49 ± 15	58 ± 12	0.0001
LVEF <50%	44	18	
Systolic pulmonary artery pressure (mmHg)	46 ± 21	26 ± 19	<0.0001

CHF, congestive heart failure, LVEF, left ventricular ejection fraction.

Natural history

Outcome in patients with AS is poor when any symptoms are present, with survival rates of only 15–50% at 5 years.[11] The strongest predictors of poor outcome are NYHA class III/IV, associated mitral regurgitation, and left ventricular dysfunction. The combination of these three factors identifies a group at particularly high risk since survival is only 30% at 3 years.[12]

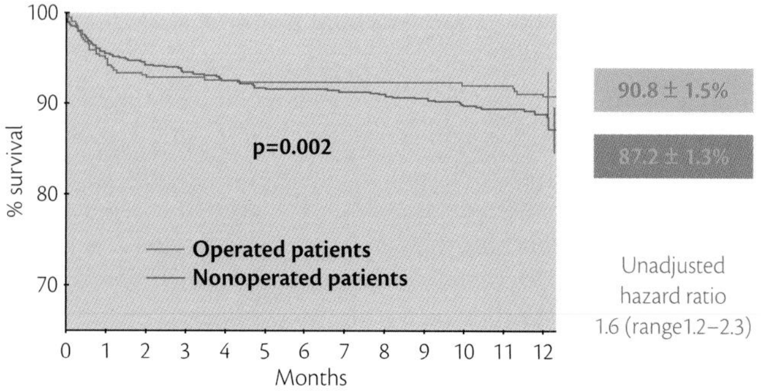

Fig. 33.2 One-year survival according to intervention in 1149 patients with congestive HF at admission in the in the EuroHeart Survey on valvular heart disease.

Treatment strategy

Given that patients with severe AS are often elderly with comorbidities, the selection of candidates for surgery, and especially risk assessment, should involve multidisciplinary consultation between cardiologists, surgeons, and anaesthetists. Early valve replacement should be strongly recommended soon after symptom onset in all symptomatic patients with severe AS who are otherwise candidates for surgery.[2,3,13,14] Unfortunately, repeated observations worldwide show that a large proportion of potentially suitable candidates are not referred for surgery.[15] If the mean transaortic gradient is above 40 mmHg, there is virtually no lower limit of left ventricular ejection fraction for surgery. Surgery may also be considered in low-flow, low-gradient AS even in the absence of contractile reserve on dobutamine echography, but in such cases decision-making should take into account the presence of comorbidity and the feasibility of revascularization.[16]

If the patient has a contraindication for surgery, or if surgery is judged to be at high risk, transcatheter aortic valve implantation (TAVI) can be considered (Fig. 33.3). Current knowledge shows that TAVI is feasible and provides significant clinical and haemodynamic improvement up to 2 years, but the technique is still under evaluation with questions remaining on safety and long-term results. TAVI can be considered only if the patient's life expectancy is more than 1 year, and if there are no contraindications. Contraindications are mostly related to the size of the aortic annulus and/or size and disease of the peripheral arteries when using the transfemoral approach [9,17,18]

Indications for balloon aortic valvuloplasty are very limited: it may be considered as a bridge to surgery, or to TAVI, in haemodynamically unstable patients who are at high risk for intervention, or in patients with symptomatic severe AS who require urgent major noncardiac surgery.[19]

Finally, it seems reasonable to manage medically patients whose life expectancy is less than 1 year, or whose quality of life is comprimised by comorbidities, while acknowledging that management should be tailored to the individual patient's condition. Patients may be treated with digitalis, diuretics, angiotensin converting enzyme (ACE) inhibitors, or angiotensin receptor blockers if they have HF. β-Blockers should be avoided. In selected patients with pulmonary oedema, nitroprusside can be used under haemodynamic monitoring.

Aortic regurgitation

Aortic regurgitation (AR) is seen in 13% of patients with native valve disease. Degenerative valve disease is the most common aetiology in Western countries, followed by bicuspid aortic valve, rheumatic disease, endocarditis, and aortitis.[1] Acute AR may be due to active endocarditis, trauma (either blunt chest or more rarely after percutaneous intervention), dissection of the ascending aorta, or prosthetic valve dysfunction.[20,21]

Diagnosis

Acute AR rapidly leads to disabling dyspnoea or pulmonary oedema as a result of the rapid rise of left ventricular end-diastolic pressures in the nondilated, noncompliant left ventricle. In chronic AR, there is a long latent period and exertional dyspnoea occurs at a late stage of the disease process.

When left ventricular decompensation occurs, the pulse pressure narrows and S3 sound may be heard at the apex. In acute AR, patients are tachycardic and may present with clinical signs of pulmonary oedema. The diastolic murmur and peripheral signs are attenuated because the pulse pressure is narrow. Left ventricular hypertrophy is the main ECG feature in chronic AR, and cardiomegaly is the main abnormality found on chest radiograph. Signs of left HF are frequent in acute AR and are seen in advanced chronic AR.

Transthoracic and/or transoesophageal echocardiography enable the anatomy of the aortic leaflets and the aortic root to be accurately assessed, thereby contributing to the identification of the aetiology and mechanisms of AR (Fig. 33.4). Quantitative measurements are helpful, but are less well validated than for MR. The criteria for defining severe AR are an effective regurgitant orifice area (ERO) greater than 0.30 cm^2, regurgitant volume greater than 60 mL, or a regurgitant fraction of over 50%.[2,3] The most frequent echo features of severe acute AR are vena contracta greater than 6 mm, pressure half-time less than 200 ms, holodiatolic flow reversal in the abdominal aorta, and premature mitral valve closure.[20]

Natural history

In chronic AR, the onset of symptoms carries a poor prognosis and is frequently preceded by left ventricular enlargement.[2,3] Acute AR has a dismal prognosis; HF is the most frequent complication of active endocarditis and moderate to severe HF is the most important predictor of in-hospital and 6-month mortality.[20,21]

Treatment strategy

Chronic AR

The presence of symptoms or left ventricular dysfunction is an indication for surgery even if there appears to be a transient improvement after medical therapy. Operative mortality is relatively low, and surgery improves symptoms and late outcome favourably compared with the natural history.[22] In patients with severe left ventricular dysfunction and severe AR, the current trend is to favour aortic valve replacement over heart transplantation: recent case series have shown reasonable postoperative outcomes

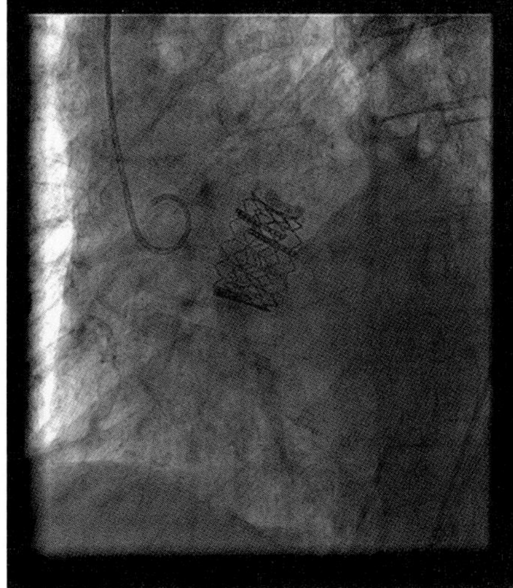

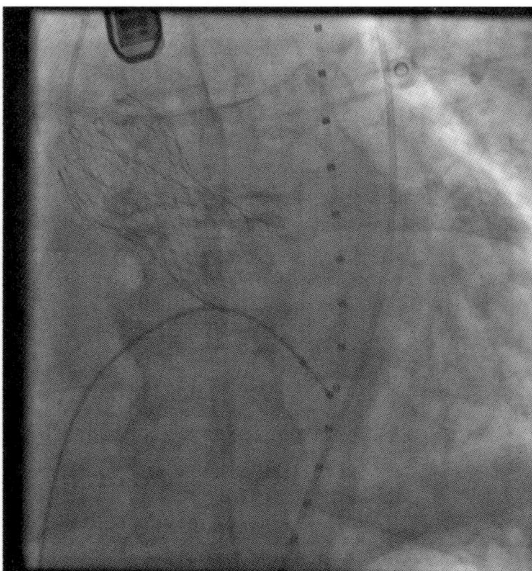

Fig. 33.3 Percutaneous aortic valve implantation. On the left; left anterior oblique view. Balloon expandable prosthesis. On the right; anteroposterior view, self-expandable prosthesis.

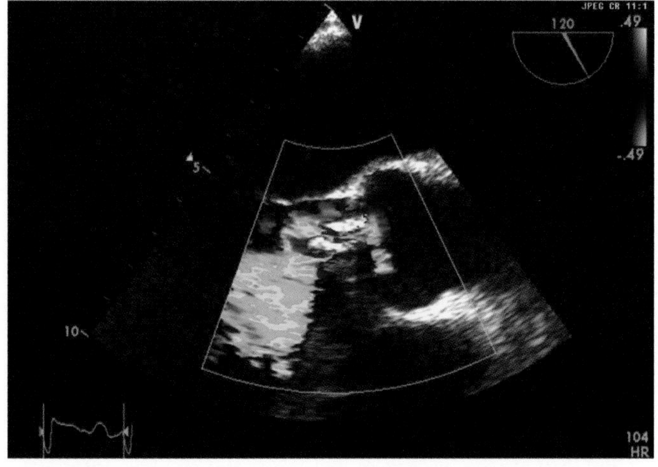

Fig. 33.4 Acute aortic regurgitation due to active endocarditis. Acute aortic regurgitation colour Doppler showing a severe regurgitation and vegetations on the aortic valve.

which are likely to be better than the dismal natural prognosis.[23,24] The final choice between valve replacement, heart transplantation, or medical therapy, is made on an individual basis.

After surgery, patients with persisting left ventricular systolic dysfunction (LVSD) should also receive optimal medical therapy according to HF guidelines, including ACE inhibitors and β-blockers.[4]

Acute AR

Urgent intervention is indicated in acute AR because of poor haemodynamic tolerance.[20] Surgery should not be delayed in favour of efforts at medical management. Nitroprusside and inotropic agents are useful in poorly tolerated acute AR to stablize the clinical condition en route to surgery.

Surgery is indicated during active endocarditis in the presence of HF in the majority of patients and is the principal indication for urgent surgery (Table 33.2).[25] Surgery must be performed on an emergency basis irrespective of the status of infection, in cases with pulmonary oedema or shock despite medical therapy. Surgery is urgent if there are signs of left ventricular failure with echocardiographic signs of unfavourable outcome. Surgery should be considered after healing of infective endocarditis according to the recommendations on the management of VHD (Table 33.2).[26]

Mitral stenosis

Although the prevalence of rheumatic fever has greatly decreased in Western countries, mitral stenosis (MS) still results in significant morbidity and mortality worldwide.[1]

Diagnosis

Usually symptoms appear gradually over years, with patients first reporting dyspnoea on exertion. Patients frequently adapt their level of functional capacity and deny dyspnoea despite objective effort limitation. Pregnancy, emotional stress, sexual intercourse, infection, or the onset of atrial fibrillation may all be precipitating factors of marked dyspnoea or pulmonary oedema. At a more advanced stage, patients may complain of fatigue due to low cardiac output, weakness, or abdominal discomfort due to hepatomegaly when right ventricular failure is present.

Table 33.2 Indications for surgery in acute native valve endocarditis

Recommendations: indications for surgery	Timing	Class	Level
Heart failure			
Aortic or mitral IE with severe acute regurgitation or valve obstruction causing refractory pulmonary oedema or shock	Emergency	I	B
Aortic or mitral IE with fistula into a cardiac chamber or pericardium causing refractory pulmonary oedema or shock	Emergency	I	B
Aortic or mitral IE with severe acute regurgitation or valve obstruction and persisting HF or echocardiographic signs of poor haemodynamic tolerance (early mitral closure or pulmonary hypertension)	Urgent	I	B
Aortic or mitral IE with severe regurgitation and no HF	Elective	IIa	B

Emergency, <24 h; urgent, within a few days; elective, after 7–10 days of antibiotic treatment.

HF, heart failure; IE, infective endocarditis.

Adapted from the ESC guidelines: Task Force on the Prevention, Diagnosis, and Treatment of Infective Endocarditis of the European Society of Cardiology (ESC). Guidelines on the prevention, diagnosis, and treatment of infective endocarditis (new version 2009). *Eur Heart J* 2009;30(19):2369–413.

In patients with HF, the diastolic murmur of MS may be of low intensity or even inaudible in patients with low output. Pulmonary hypertension causes both a louder second heart sound at the base and a murmur of tricuspid regurgitation located at the xyphoid. Pulmonary crackles are present in patients with severe symptoms. At an advanced stage, mitral facies with intermittent malar flushes, jugular distension, and peripheral cyanosis may be seen. Respiratory failure, cachexia, and severe pulmonary hypertension may dominate examination. Atrial fibrillation is frequent at this stage. Signs of right ventricular hypertrophy are usually present in cases of severe pulmonary hypertension.

As the disease progresses, radiological signs of right ventricular enlargement appear. Redistribution of pulmonary vascular flow towards the upper lung fields, a progressively enlarged pulmonary trunk, and signs of interstitial pulmonary and alveolar oedema are all indicative of raised pulmonary pressures.

Echocardiography is the main method to assess the severity and consequences of MS, as well as the extent of the anatomical lesions. Severity of MS should be quantified using two-dimensional planimetry and the pressure half-time method, which are complementary. MS is significant when valve area is less than $1.5cm^2$ or less than $1cm^2/m^2$ BSA. A transthoracic approach provides sufficient information for routine management and decision-making. Transoesophageal examination should also be performed when transthoracic images are suboptimal or to exclude left atrial thrombus (particularly in the appendage) either before percutaneous mitral commissurotomy (PMC) or if there is suspicion after an embolic complication.

Natural history

Symptomatic patients have a poor prognosis, with a 5-year survival rate of only 44%.[27] Progression is highly variable with gradual deterioration in one-half of patients, and sudden deterioration, precipitated by a complication, in the rest.

Treatment strategy

Diuretics or long-acting nitrates transiently ameliorate dyspnoea. β-Blockers or calcium channel blockers are useful to slow the heart rate. Anticoagulant therapy with a target international normalized ratio (INR) in the upper half of the range 2–3 is indicated in patients with atrial fibrillation. In patients with sinus rhythm, anticoagulation is recommended when there has been prior embolism or a thrombus is present in the left atrium, and it should be considered in patients who have an enlarged left atrium (>50–55 mm in diameter) or dense spontaneous echo contrast in the left atrium.[2,3] Cardioversion is not indicated before intervention in patients with severe MS, as it does not durably restore sinus rhythm. If atrial fibrillation is of recent onset and the left atrium only moderately enlarged, cardioversion should be performed soon after successful intervention.

Intervention is indicated in symptomatic patients with severe MS. PMC is the procedure of choice when surgery is contraindicated or in high-risk patients, such as pregnant women, in whom PMC may be appropriate after 20 weeks' gestation in experienced teams (Fig. 33.5). PMC is also indicated for patients with favourable characteristics, particularly young patients with sinus rhythm and favourable anatomy.[28,29]

The decision to intervene in patients with unfavourable anatomy is more complex and should take into account the results in individual institutions. PMC may achieve good long-term results and may be useful to defer surgery in selected patients with mild to moderate calcification or severe impairment of the subvalvular apparatus, who have otherwise favourable characteristics.[2,3,30]

Surgery is the only alternative when PMC is contraindicated, the most important contraindication being left atrial thrombosis. Other contraindications for PMC include more than mild MR, severe calcification, absence of commissural fusion, combined severe aortic or tricuspid valve disease, or coronary disease requiring bypass surgery. In such patients valve replacement is most often performed. PMC can staill be carried out in patients with coexisting moderate aortic valve disease and those with functional tricuspid regurgitation.

Special populations

After previous surgical commissurotomy, PMC can delay the need for reoperation in patients with favourable characteristics in whom the predominant mechanism of restenosis is commissural refusion. Similarly, repeat PMC can be successful in patients with the same characteristics if restenosis occurs several years after an initially successful PMC.[2,3,30]

In elderly patients, it is probably better to avoid intervention in endstage disease in those for whom surgery is contraindicated and all the predictors of poor results of PMC, both clinical and anatomical, are present. On the other hand, PMC can be attempted first in patients with still favourable anatomy, resorting to surgery if results are unsatisfactory.[30] In other patients, surgery is preferable as the first option.

Mitral regurgitation

MR is the second most frequent valve disease after AS in hospitalized patients.[1] It is essential to distinguish between primary organic MR, in which abnormalities of the mitral valve apparatus are the cause of the disease, and secondary MR, which results from left ventricular disease and remodelling. Degenerative MR is the most common aetiology of primary MR in Europe, followed by rheumatic and postendocarditis aetiologies. Severe acute MR is most commonly due to rupture of chordae in degenerative disease, endocarditis, traumatic lesions, prosthetic valve dysfunction, and (rarely in Western countries) acute rheumatic fever. Papillary muscle rupture complicating acute myocardial infarction is less frequent with the use of immediate reperfusion strategies.

Ischaemic MR is increasingly prevalent as a cause of secondary MR, but frequently unrecognized or underestimated. Functional MR, which is frequent in patients with HF, is the consequence of annular dilatation and papillary muscle displacement tethering one or both leaflets, and of LVSD decreasing the mitral valve closing force.

Diagnosis

Acute severe MR usually results in severe dyspnoea, acute pulmonary oedema, or congestive HF. In patients with papillary muscle rupture during acute myocardial infarction, the presence of shock contrasts with a hyperdynamic heart on echocardiography. In patients with severe chronic primary MR, symptoms such as fatigue or dyspnoea occur late when contractile dysfunction develops or with the onset of atrial fibrillation. In secondary MR, symptoms are related to the underlying disease process. MR is a dynamic condition and its severity may vary over time in relation to arrhythmias, ischaemia, hypertension, or exercise. Dynamic chronic ischaemic MR can lead to acute pulmonary oedema in the absence of acute myocardial ischaemia.[32]

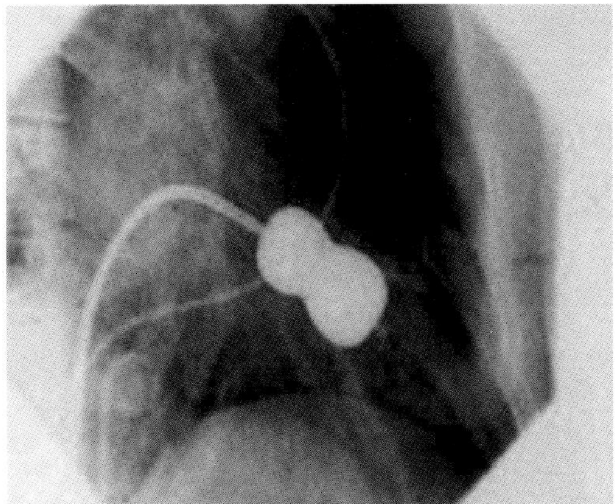
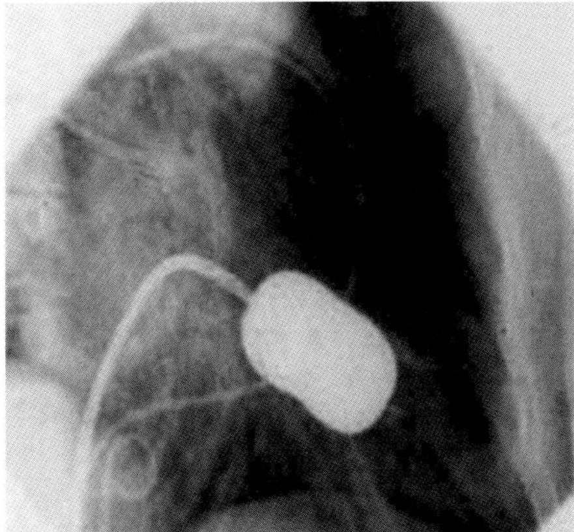

Fig. 33.5 Percutaneous mitral commissurotomy. Right anterior oblique 30°: inflation of the Inoue balloon across the stenotic mitral valve.

In chronic severe primary MR the loudness of the murmur correlates somewhat with the severity of regurgitation. In severe MR, an S3 and a short diastolic rumble reflect the rapid and voluminous left ventricular filling. The loudness of the pulmonary component of S2 increases when pulmonary hypertension is present. In secondary MR, auscultatory signs are highly dynamic; the murmur is usually of low intensity and peak intensity is usually heard in early systole. S3 is frequent. In acute MR, the murmur is shortened by a rapid reduction in the pressure gradient between left ventricular and the left atrium, and it may even be inaudible in papillary muscle rupture with low output.

Evidence of pulmonary congestion or of congestive HF is seen only in patients with decompensated disease.

Chronic MR patients in sinus rhythm may present with left ventricular and left atrial hypertrophy, but atrial fibrillation is common. In ischaemic MR, Q waves may be seen, most frequently in the inferior and/or lateral leads; and there may be left bundle branch block. Chronic severe MR leads to cardiomegaly due to left ventricular and left atrial enlargement, and radiological signs of left HF when cardiac dysfunction is present. In acute MR, the heart volume may be normal, with evidence of interstitial or alveolar pulmonary oedema. In acute MR, pulmonary oedema may be localized to one segment and confused with pneumonia.

Echocardiography helps establish the aetiology and mechanisms of MR, quantifies severity, and assesses the reparability of the valve. In experienced hands, transthoracic echocardiography is highly accurate for precise localization of the involved scallops in cases of degenerative MR. In ischaemic MR, the apical displacement of the leaflets can be quantitated by measuring the tenting area and the distance between the annulus and the coaptation point. Finally, in functional MR, the localization and extent of regional left ventricular dyssynchrony should be analysed.

The assessment of MR severity requires an approach integrating blood flow data from Doppler with morphological information, and careful cross-checking of the validity of such data against the consequences on left ventricular and pulmonary pressures.[2,3,33] Organic MR is considered severe when the regurgitant orifice area is 40 mm^2 or more and the regurgitant volume is at least 60 mL (Fig. 33.6).[13] In secondary MR, the corresponding thresholds of severity are 20 mm^2 and 30 mL respectively.[34] In acute MR, the most frequent signs are vena contracta in excess of 7 mm, reversed pulmonary vein flow, and decreased aortic valve opening.

Preliminary series have suggested that BNP is helpful in evaluating the consequences of MR and as a predictor of long-term outcome, but this also needs to be investigated further.[35]

Natural history

In mitral active endocarditis, HF is observed in 20% of cases and carries a poor prognosis. Acute MR secondary to papillary muscle rupture has a dismal short-term prognosis. In chronic MR, progression is observed in all clinical and anatomic subsets and is associated with more severe left ventricular and atrial remodelling and worse outcome. In symptomatic patients with flail leaflets and severe MR, there is an excess mortality overall.[36]

The natural history of patients with functional MR is less well known. Overall, patients with ischaemic MR have a poor prognosis.[34,37,38] Besides the prognostic importance of coronary artery disease, left ventricular dysfunction, and comorbidity, which are frequent in these patients, the presence and severity of MR, as

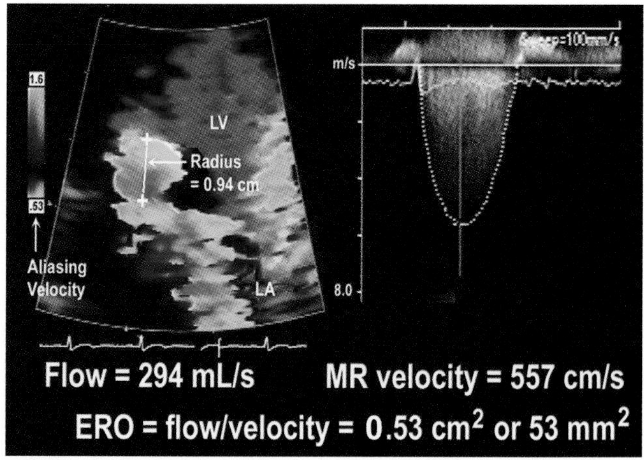

Fig. 33.6 Quantitative evaluation of severe primary mitral regurgitation. ERO, effective regurgitant orifice; MR, mitral regurgitation.

well as its progression, is independently associated with increased mortality. The clinical outcome of functional MR due to cardiomyopathy is less well defined, but data suggest that MR also plays a role in the poor outcome of these patients.[39]

Treatment strategy

Chronic primary MR

Intervention is indicated only in patients with severe MR (Fig. 33.7).[2,3] Surgery is indicated in patients who have symptoms due to chronic MR, no contraindications to surgery, and when left ventricular ejection fraction (LVEF) is above 30%. When LVEF is below 30%, the decision to operate should take into account the response to medical therapy, comorbidity, and the likelihood of valve repair. It is surprising that almost 50% of symptomatic patients with severe MR are not referred for surgery in current practice.[40]

Functional MR

Limited data in the field of ischaemic MR results in less evidence-based management. In patients with left ventricular dysfunction, medical therapy should be the first-line treatment following the guidelines for HF with systolic dysfunction.[4] In functional MR associated with systolic dysfunction and HF, ACE inhibitors and β-blockers, which reduce MR by progressive reverse remodelling, are indicated. Sublingual nitrates are useful for treating acute dyspnoea secondary to any dynamic component.

Patients with persistent or paroxysmal atrial fibrillation should receive drugs for controlling heart rate and anticoagulant therapy with an INR between 2 and 3.[2,3] Anticoagulant therapy is also needed if there is a history of systemic embolism, or left atrial thrombus during the first 3 months after mitral valve repair. In severe MR, maintenance of sinus rhythm after cardioversion is not possible in the absence of surgery.

There is a continuing debate on the indications for surgery in functional MR because there are no data from randomized trials suggesting that treatment of MR reduces mortality and HF.[41–45] In patients with severe MR, surgery is indicated if coronary bypass is performed. Surgery is more likely to be considered if myocardial viability is present and if comorbidity is low. The preferred surgical procedure remains controversial, although there is a trend in favour of repair even if results are less satisfactory than in other aetiologies.[41,42] The limited data available suggest that

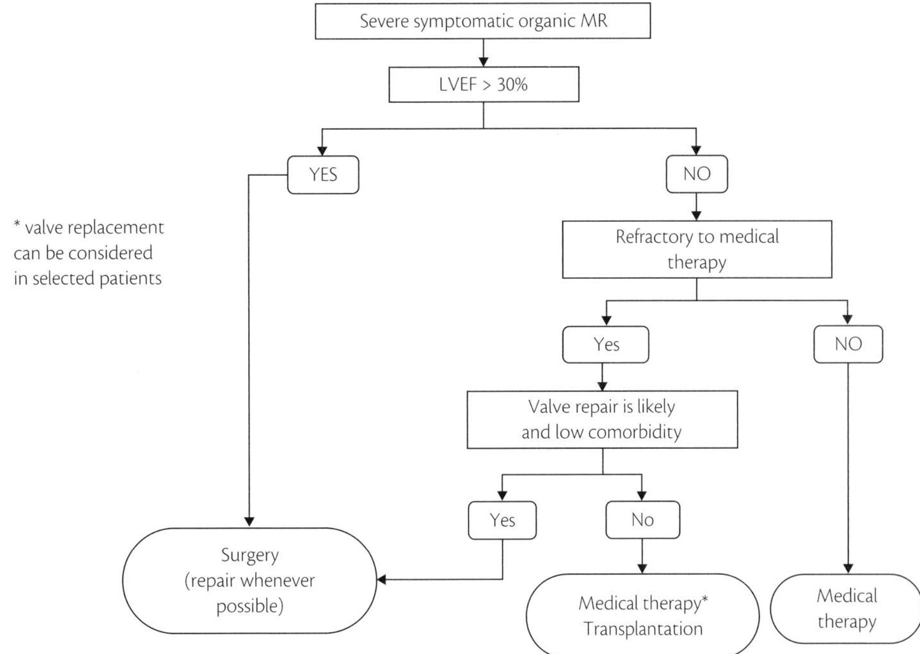

Fig. 33.7 Management of symptomatic severe chronic organic mitral regurgitation.
Adapted from the ESC guidelines: Task Force on the Management of Valvular Heart Disease of the European Society of Cardiology. Guidelines on the management of valvular heart disease. *Eur Heart J* 2007;**28**:230–68.

isolated mitral valve surgery, in combination with left ventricular reconstruction techniques, may be considered in selected patients with severe functional MR and severely depressed left ventricular function.[43,44,46] Such patients include those with coronary disease where bypass surgery is not indicated, who remain symptomatic despite optimal medical therapy, and where comorbidity is low—the aim being to avoid or postpone transplantation. Ongoing trials are expected to define appropriate strategies better. In other patients, medical therapy followed by transplantation when therapy fails is probably the best option. Surgery on the regurgitant mitral valve should not be considered in patients *in extremis* with low output, severe right ventricular failure, and high comorbidity.

In patients with moderate MR, surgery can be considered. Mitral valve repair is preferable, and the decision must be made preoperatively since intraoperative echocardiographic assessment underestimates the severity of ischaemic MR.

Finally, cardiac resynchronization therapy with or without a defibrillator may decrease MR severity, and should be performed according to the classical recommendations.[47] The techniques of percutaneous mitral valve repair are at an early stage and it is not possible to make any recommendations for their use today.[48]

Acute MR

Urgent surgery is indicated in patients with acute MR.[2,3,20] In acute endocarditis resulting in severe MR, the indications for surgery and their timing are the same as in acute AR. The feasibility of mitral valve repair depends on tissue quality and the expertise of the surgeon.[2,3,20,26,49] Rupture of a papillary muscle requires urgent surgical treatment, and inotropic agents. In addition to coronary artery bypass grafting, surgery usually consists of valve replacement. In patients with systemic hypotension, intraaortic balloon pump, vasodilators, and inotropic agents help to stabilize the patient en route to surgery.[50] Finally traumatic mitral valve injury is commonly associated with severe haemodynamic compromise and the majority of cases are operated within hours of the injury. Mitral replacement is often used.[21]

Tricuspid stenosis

Tricuspid stenosis (TS), although still present in developing countries, is rarely seen in Western countries. Detection requires careful attention, as it is almost always associated with left-sided valve lesions that dominate the presentation.

Diagnosis

The main symptoms are those of the other valvular lesions. Liver pain on exercise or after meals may be more directly a consequence of TS. Low cardiac output causes fatigue. Clinical signs are often masked by those of the combined valvular lesions, especially MS. Presystolic jugular distension, systemic venous congestion, oedema, or even anasarca may be seen in the most severe cases. Echocardiography provides the most useful information, but requires careful evaluation. Although there is no consensus, severe TS is generally defined by a mean gradient greater than 5 mmHg.[2,3]

Treatment strategy

Diuretics are useful, but of limited efficacy. Percutaneous balloon dilatation can be performed in the rare cases of isolated and pure TS. In most cases, surgical intervention is carried out at the time of intervention on other valves.[2,3] Conservative surgery is possible with favourable anatomy and appropriate surgical expertise, but prosthetic valve replacement may be needed because of the lack of pliable tissue.[51]

Tricuspid regurgitation

Pathological tricuspid regurgitation (TR) is more often functional than primary. Functional TR is the consequence of right ventricular pressure and/or volume overload in the presence of structurally normal leaflets, and is often caused by pulmonary hypertension resulting from left-sided heart disease. Less commonly, it is casued by cor pulmonale, pulmonary arterial hypertension, and ventricular volume overload (sometimes due to atrial septal defects) or rarely, intrinsic disease of the right ventricle (ischaemic or cardiomyopathy).

Possible causes of primary TR are infective endocarditis, rheumatic heart disease, carcinoid syndrome, myxomatous disease, endomyocardial fibrosis, Ebstein's anomaly, drug-induced valve diseases, and thoracic trauma.

Diagnosis

The dominant symptoms are those of associated diseases. Dyspnoea and fatigue are common. Symptoms more specifically related to TR are right-sided congestion and liver pain. Anorexia and weight loss may occur at a later stage. Three signs are typical: (1) a soft holosystolic murmur best heard along the left sternal border and in the xyphoid region, increasing with inspiration; (2) systolic jugular vein expansion, and (3) a pulsatile and enlarged liver with hepatojugular reflux. The murmur may be mild, or even absent in severe TR when turbulent flow disappears. Peripheral cyanosis, leg oedema, or even ascitis due to the increased right atrial pressure may be seen.

Atrial fibrillation and incomplete right bundle branch block are frequent. Marked cardiomegaly is usually present on chest radiograph due to enlargement of the right cavities. Echocardiography is the ideal technique to quantify TR and distinguish between functional and primary forms. The severity of TR is based on the integration of different indices, taking into account their particularly high sensitivity to loading conditions. The proximal flow convergence method has been validated in only one study: criteria for severe TR were an ERO over 40 mm^2 and a regurgitant volume above 45 mL.[2,3] Measurement of the systolic velocity of the TR jet allows an estimate of the systolic pulmonary arterial pressure but may be inaccurate in the presence of severe TR, which leads to equalization of right ventricular and atrial pressures.

Natural history

Primary TR has a poor prognosis, even when isolated. Functional TR may diminish or disappear as right ventricular failure improves following the treatment of its cause. However, TR may persist or worsen even after successful correction of primary or functional MR, which may have a negative impact on survival.

Treatment strategy

Diuretics improve signs of congestion. Specific therapy of the underlying disease is indicated. The timing of surgical intervention and the appropriate technique remain controversial. Surgery for TR is usually only performed at the time of surgical correction of left-sided valvular lesions.[51,52] In these circumstances, severe TR should be corrected. In patients with moderate TR, whether to operate at the time of surgery for left-sided lesion is controversial. There is a trend to combine the correction of TR and left-heart valve surgery if there is pulmonary hypertension or important dilatation of the tricuspid annulus, particularly if the TR is of primary origin.[51] If technically possible, valve repair is preferable to replacement. Reoperation on the tricuspid valve when TR develops, or persists after mitral valve surgery, carries a high risk related to previous operations and/or irreversible right ventricular dysfunction.

Surgery limited to the tricuspid valve may be required in symptomatic patients with severe primary TR, or for persistent or recurrent TR after mitral valve surgery in the absence of other significant cardiac dysfuction.

Patients after prosthetic valve surgery

The late outcome following valvular surgery depends mainly on the stage of heart disease before surgery, the type of intervention, and the prosthesis. The specific complications associated with cardiac valve prostheses which may lead to HF are structural valve degeneration, nonstructural dysfunction, thromboembolism and thrombosis, and prosthetic valve endocarditis. In such patients HF often has a multifactorial origin.

Clinical evaluation is the cornerstone of follow-up after valve surgery. Functional deterioration or change in auscultation during late follow-up raises the question of valve dysfunction and requires prompt echocardiographic examination.

Treatment of specific prosthetic complications

Prosthetic thrombosis

Occlusive prosthetic thrombosis is characterized by impaired motion of the mobile part of the prosthesis. It is more frequent in patients with mechanical prostheses and should be suspected promptly in any patients with any type of prosthetic valve who present with a recent increase in shortnsess of breath or embolic event. Inadequate anticoagulation is the most important risk factor. The diagnosis should be immediately confirmed by echocardiography and cinefluoroscopy.[53] Clinical examination is often difficult because of frequent pulmonary oedema.

Prosthetic thrombosis is of high risk whatever the option taken. The risk–benefit analysis of the strategy should be adapted to the individual patient's characteristics and local resources.[2,3] Fibrinolysis carries a risk of bleeding, systemic embolism, and recurrent thrombosis. Emergency valve replacement is the treatment of choice in obstructive thrombosis in critically ill patients without serious comorbidities (Fig. 33.8). Fibrinolysis should be considered in critically ill patients unlikely to survive surgery because of comorbidities or severely impaired cardiac function, situations in which surgery is not immediately available, and thrombosis of tricuspid valve because of the high success rate and low incidence of embolism.

Bioprosthesis failure

Reoperation is indicated in symptomatic patients in whom there is an increase in transprosthetic gradient or new significant regurgitation.[2,3] Surgery should be considered early, since its risk rapidly increases in patients in NYHA class III or IV. In the future, percutaneous implantation of a valve in a degenerating prosthetic valve may be a potentially attractive alternative to reoperation.[54]

Nonstructural dysfunction

Reoperation should be considered in patients with paraprosthetic regurgitation leading to severe symptoms or causing severe haemolysis requiring repeated blood transfusions.[55] Reoperation can be associated with a prohibitive risk in cases of multiple previous operations or severe comorbidity. Transcatheter closure of paravalvular regurgitations is feasible[56] but complex, and there are concerns about its efficacy.

Endocarditis

Surgery for prosthetic valve endocarditis follows the same general principles as in native valve endocarditis. Prosthetic valve endocarditis frequently requires surgery, which should not be delayed in patients with HF to avoid intervening in a patient in poor haemodynamic condition.[26]

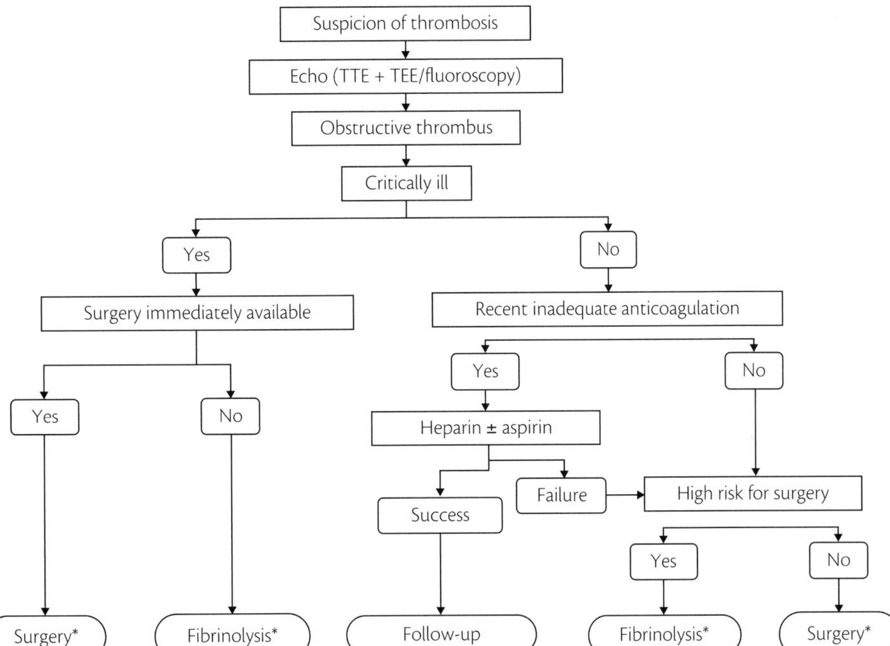

Fig. 33.8 Management of left-sided obstructive prosthetic thrombosis. Risks and benefits of surgery versus fibrinolysis should be individualized. The presence of a first-generation prosthesis is an incentive to surgery. Adapted from the ESC guidelines: Task Force on the Management of Valvular Heart Disease of the European Society of Cardiology. Guidelines on the management of valvular heart disease. *Eur Heart J* 2007;**28**:230–68.

Postoperative heart failure from other causes

If HF occurs postoperatively and is not related to prosthetic dysfunction, one should consider first other causes, such as systemic hypertension, coronary disease, sustained arrhythmias, anaemia, or thyrotoxicosis. If these causes are eliminated, then left ventricular dysfunction should be considered. It is most often due to LVSD resulting from late operation (in particular after correction of a regurgitation) with or without additional perioperative myocardial damage. In such cases, medical treatment, cardiac resynchronization, and cardiac transplantation should follow the guidelines on the management of HF.

Conclusion

The key to successful management of a patient with VHD and HF is establishing a rapid diagnosis, based mainly on echocardiography, followed by early intervention. In the future improvement in patient outcomes will be made possible by better education of patients and physicians in order to decrease the incidence of prosthesis-related complications and earlier indications for intervention when symptoms or objective signs of left ventricular dysfunction are observed in patients with known VHD.

References

1. Iung B, Baron G, Butchart EG, *et al.* A prospective survey of patients with valvular heart disease in Europe: the Euro Heart Survey on valvular heart disease. *Eur Heart J* 2003;**24**:1231–43.
2. The Task Force on the Management of Valvular Heart Disease of the European Society of Cardiology. Guidelines on the management of valvular heart disease. *Eur Heart J* 2007;**28**:230–68.
3. A Report of the American College of Cardiology/American Heart Association Task Force on Practice Guidelines. (Writing committee to revise the 1998 guidelines for the management of patients with valvular heart disease). Focused update incorporated into the ACC/AHA 2006 guidelines for the management of patients with valvular heart disease. *Circulation* 2008;**118**:e523–661.
4. The Task Force for the Diagnosis and Treatment of Acute and Chronic Heart Failure 2008 of the European Society of Cardiology. ESC guidelines for the diagnosis and treatment of acute and chronic heart failure 2008. *Eur Heart J* 2008;**29**:2388–442.
5. Cleland JGF, Swedberg K, Follath F, *et al.* The EuroHeart Failure survey programme—a survey on the quality of care among patients with heart failure in Europe: Part 1: patient characteristics and diagnosis. *Eur Heart J* 2003;**24**:442–63.
6. Bursi F, Weston SA, Redfield MM, Jacobsen SJ, Pakhomov S, Nkomo VT *et al.* Systolic and Diastolic Heart Failure in the Community. *JAMA* 2006;**296**:2209–16.
7. Roques F, Nashef SAM, Michel P, and the Euroscore study group. Risk factors for early mortality after valve surgery in Europe in the 1990s: Lessons from the Euroscore pilot program. *J Heart Valve Dis* 2001;**10**:572–8.
8. Dewey TM, Brown D, Ryan WH, Herbert MA, Prince SL, Mack MJ. Reliability of risk algorithms in predicting early and late operative outcomes in high-risk patients undergoing aortic valve replacement. *J Thorac Cardiovasc Surg* 2008;**135**:180–7.
9. Vahanian A, Alfieri O, Al-Attar N, *et al.* Transcatheter valve implantation for patients with aortic stenosis: a position statement from the European Association of Cardio-Thoracic Surgery (EACTS) and the European Society of Cardiology (ESC), in collaboration with the European Association of Percutaneous Cardiovascular Interventions (EAPCI). *Eur Heart J* 2008;**29**:1463–70.
10. Monin JL, Quere JP, Monchi M, *et al.* Low-gradient aortic stenosis, operative risk stratification and predictors for long-term outcome: a multicenter study using dobutamine stress hemodynamics. *Circulation* 2003;**108**:319–41.
11. Horstkotte D, Loogen F. The natural history of aortic stenosis. *Eur Heart J* 1988;**9**(Suppl E):57–64.
12. Bouma BJ, Van den Brink RBA, Van der Meulen JHP, *et al.* To operate or not on elderly patients with aortic stenosis: the decision and its consequences. *Heart* 1999;**82**:143–8.
13. Melby SJ, Zierer A, Kaiser YP, *et al.* Aortic valve replacement in octogenarians. Risk factors for early and late mortality. *Ann Thorac Surg* 2007;**83**:1651–7.

14. Kolh P, Kerzmann A, Honore C, Comte L, Limet R. Aortic valve surgery in octogenarians: predictive factors for operative and long-term results. *Eur J Cardiothorac Surg* 2007;**31**:600–6.
15. Iung B, Cachier A, Baron G, *et al.* Decision-making in elderly patients with severe aortic stenosis: why are so many patients denied surgery. *Eur Heart J* 2005;**26**:2714–20.
16. Levy F, Laurent M, Monin JL, *et al.* Aortic valve replacement for low-flow/low-gradient aortic stenosis operative risk stratification and long-term outcome : a European multicenter study. *J Am Coll Cardiol* 2008;**51**:1466–72.
17. Webb JG, Altwegg L, Boone RH, Cheung A, Ye J, Lichtenstein S *et al.* Transcatheter aortic valve implantation: impact on clinical and valve-related outcomes. *Circulation* 2009;**119**:3009–16.
18. Walther T, Simon P, Dewey T, *et al.* Transapical minimally invasive aortic valve implantation: multicenter experience. *Circulation* 2007;**116**(11 Suppl):I240–5.
19. Vahanian A, Palacios IF. Percutaneous approaches to valvular disease. *Circulation* 2004;**109**:1572–9.
20. Stout KK, Verrier ED. Acute valvular regurgitation. *Circulation* 2009;**119**:3232–41.
21. Kan CD, Yang YJ. Traumatic aortic and mitral valve injury following blunt chest injury with a variable clinical course. *Heart* 2005;**91**:568–70.
22. Tornos P, Sambola A, Permanyer-Miralda G, Evangelista A, Gomez Z, Soler-Soler J. Long-term outcome of surgically tretaed aortic regurgitation. Influence of guideline adherence toward early surgery. *J Am Coll Cardiol* 2006;**47**:1012–17.
23. Chaliki H, Mohty D, Avierinos J, Scott CG, Schaff HV, Tajil AJ. Outcomes after aortic valve replacement in patients with severe aortic regurgitation and markedly reduced left ventricular function. *Circulation* 2002;**106**:2687–93.
24. Bhudia AK, McCarthy PM, Kumpati GS *et al.* Improved outcomes after aortic valve surgery for chronic aortic regurgitation with severe left ventricular dysfunction. *J Am Coll Cardiol* 2008;**49**:1465–71.
25. Murdoch DR, Corey GR, Hoen B, *et al.* Clinical presentation, etiology, and outcome of infective endocarditis in the 21st century: the International Collaboration on Endocarditis Prospective Cohort Study. *Arch Intern Med* 2009;**169**:463–73.
26. The Task Force on the Prevention, Diagnosis, and Treatment of Infective Endocarditis of the European Society of Cardiology (ESC). Guidelines on the prevention, diagnosis, and treatment of infective endocarditis (new version 2009). *Eur Heart J* 2009;**30**(19):2369–413.
27. Horskötte D, Niehaus R, Strauer BE. Pathomorphological aspects, aetiology and natural history of acquired mitral valve stenosis. *Eur Heart J* 1991;**12**(Suppl B):55–60.
28. Iung B, Cormier B, Ducimetiere P, *et al.* Immediate results of percutaneous mitral commissurotomy. *Circulation* 1996;**94**:2124–30.
29. Palacios IF, Sanchez PL, Harrell LC, Weyman AE, Block PC. Which patients benefit from percutaneous mitral balloon valvuloplasty? Prevalvuloplasty and postvalvuloplasty variables that predict long-term outcome. *Circulation* 2002;**105**:1465–71.
30. Fawzy ME, Hassan W, Shoukri M *et al.* Immediate and long-term results of mitral balloon valvotomy for restenosis following previous surgical or balloon mitral commissurotomy. *Am J Cardiol* 2005;**96**:971–5.
31. Iung B, Garbarz E, Doutrelant L, *et al.* Late results of percutaneous mitral commissurotomy for calcific mitral stenosis. *Am J Cardiol* 2000;**85**:1308–14.
32. Piérard LA, Lancellotti P. The role of ischemic mitral regurgitation in the pathogenesis of acute pulmonary edema. *N Engl J Med* 2004;**35**:1627–34.
33. Enriquez-Sarano M, Avierinos JF, *et al.* Quantitative determinants of the outcome of asymptomatic mitral regurgitation. *N Engl J Med* 2005;**352**:875–83.
34. Grigioni F, Enriquez-Sarano M, Zehr KJ, Bailey KR, Tajik AJ. Ischemic mitral regurgitation: long-term outcome and prognostic implications with quantitative Doppler assessment. *Circulation* 2001;**103**:1759–64.
35. Detaint D, Messika-Zeitoun D, Avierinos JF, *et al.* B-type natriuretic peptide in organic mitral regurgitation : determinants and impact on outcome. *Circulation* 2005;**111**:2391–7.
36. Tribouilloy CM, Enriquez-Sarano M, Schaff HV, *et al.* Impact of preoperative symptoms on survival after surgical correction of organic mitral regurgitation : rationale for optimizing surgical implications. *Circulation* 1999;**99**:400–5.
37. Lancellotti P, Gérard P, Piérard LA. Long-term outcome of patients with heart failure and dynamic functional mitral regurgitation. *Eur Heart J* 2005;**26**:1528–32.
38. Amigoni M, Meris A, Thune JJ, *et al.* Mitral regurgitation in myocardial infarction complicated by heart failure, left ventricular dysfunction, or both : prognostic significance and relation to ventricular size and function. *Eur Heart J* 2007;**28**:326–33.
39. Trichon BH, Felker M, Shaw LK, Cabell CH, O'Connor CM. Relation of frequency and severity of mitral regurgitation to survival among patients with left ventricular systolic dysfunction and heart failure. *Am J Cardiol 2003;***91**:538–43.
40. Mirabel M, Iung B, Baron G, *et al.* What are the characteristics of patients with severe, symptomatic, mitral regurgitation who are denied surgery? *Eur Heart J* 2007;**28**:1358–65.
41. Grossi EA, Goldberg JD, Lapietra, X, *et al.* Ischemic mitral valve reconstruction and replacement : comparison of long-term survival and complications. *J Thorac Cardiovasc Surg* 2001;**122**:1107–24.
42. Braun J, Van der Weire N, Klautz RJN, *et al.* Restrictive mitral annuloplasty cures ischemic mitral regurgitation and heart failure. *Ann Thorac Surg* 2008;**85**:430–7.
43. Acker MA, Bolling S, Shemin R, *et al.* Mitral valve surgery in heart failure: insights from the Acorn Clinical Trial. *J Thorac Cardiovasc Surg* 2006;**132**:568–77.
44. Suma H, Tanabe H, Uejima T, Suzuki S, Horii T, Isomura T. Selected ventriculoplasty for idiopathic dilated cardiomyopathy with advanced congestive heart failure: midterm results and risk analysis. *Eur J Cardiothorac Surg* 2007;**32**:912–16.
45. Mihaljevic T, Lam B-K, Rajeswaran J, *et al.* Impact of mitral valve annuloplasty combined with revascularization in patients with functional ischemic mitral regurgitation. *Am Coll Cardiol* 2007;**49**:2191–201.
46. Gummert JF, Rahmel A, Bucerius, T *et al.* Mitral valve repair in patients with end stage cardiomyopathy: who benefits? *Eur J Cardiothoracic Surg* 2003;**23**:1017–22.
47. Ypenburg C, Lancellotti P, Tops LF, *et al.* Acute effects of initiation and withdrawal of cardiac resynchronisation therapy on papillary muscle dyssynchrony and mitral regurgitation. *J Am Coll Cardiol* 2007;**50**:2071–7.
48. Clark AL, Alamgir MF, Nair RK, Thackray ST. Percutaneous surgery for mitral valve disease. *Heart* 2009;**95**:1850.
49. Iung B, Rousseau-Pauziaud J, Cormier B, *et al.* Contemporary results of mitral valve repair for infective endocarditis. *J Am Coll Cardiol* 2004;**43**:386–92.
50. Russo A, Suri RM, Grigioni F, *et al.* Clinical outcome after surgical correction of mitral regurgitation due to papillary muscle rupture. *Circulation* 2008;**118**:1528–34.
51. Filsoufi F, Anyanwu AC, Salzberg SP, Frankel T, Cohn LH, Adams DH. Long-term outcomes of tricuspid valve replacement in the current era. *Ann Thorac Surg* 2005;**80**:845–50.
52. Dreyfus G, Corbi PJ, John CKM, Bahrami T. Secondary tricuspid regurgitation or dilation: which should be the criteria for surgical repair? *Ann Thorac Surg* 2005;**79**:127–32.

53. Laplace G, Lafitte S, Labeque JN, *et al.* Clinical significance of early thrombosis after prosthetic mitral valve replacement: a postoperative monocentric study of 680 patients. *J Am Coll Cardiol* 2004;**43**:1283–90.
54. Walther T, Kempfert J, Borger MA, *et al.* Human minimally invasive off-pump valve-in-a-valve implantation. *Ann Thorac Surg 2008;* **85**:1072–3.
55. Ionescu A, Fraser AG, Butchart EG. Prevalence and clinical significance of incidental paraprosthetic valvar regurgitation: a prospective study using transesophageal echocardiography. *Heart* 2003;**89**:1316–21.
56. Hein R, Wunderlich N, Robertson G, Wilson N, Sievert H. Catheter closure of paravalvular leak. *Eurointervention* 2006;**2**:318–25.

34

Sleep-disordered breathing

Anita K. Simonds

Introduction

Erratic breathing during sleep in heart failure (HF) patients has been observed for centuries, with Cheyne–Stokes respiration (CSR) being the classic example.[1,2] A rapid increase of knowledge in sleep medicine over the last few decades has identified a range of sleep-disordered breathing conditions, all of which have relevance to the cardiac patient. Sleep-disordered breathing (SDB) is a generic term used to cover the respiratory disturbances during sleep that include obstructive sleep apnoea (OSA), central sleep apnoea (CSA), CSR/periodic breathing, and obstructive and central hypoventilation. In adults, an apnoea is defined by 10 s of cessation in airflow; obstructive apnoeas are accompanied by respiratory effort; and in central events, effort is absent (Fig. 34.1). Hypopnoeas are partial events and are variously defined: most definitions include a reduction of more than 30% in respiratory airflow or thoracoabdominal excursion together with arterial desaturation of 2–4%, or more than 50% reduction in airflow without desaturation.

The syndrome of OSA is defined by the presence of more than 15 obstructive apnoeas and hyponoeas an hour; or more than 5 obstructive apnoeas and hyponoeas an hour associated with symptoms such as daytime sleepiness and fatigue, nocturnal choking, or unrefreshing sleep. The apnoea–hyponoea index (AHI) is the total number of these events per hour of sleep. Severe SDB is considered to be present if there are more than 30 apnoea and hyponoeas per hour. The respiratory disturbance index (RDI) is used to express the total number of respiratory events per hour of study time and therefore may differ from the AHI as any episodes of wakefulness during the monitoring period will be included in the RDI.

Sleep in heart failure

The prevalence of SDB has been examined in a variety of studies over the last decade (Table 34.1).[3–9] Some studies are very small and the prevalence will vary according to whether results are derived from community screening or referrals to a sleep laboratory: subjects in the latter group are likely to have symptoms. More recent findings in optimally medically treated HF patients, however, suggest that SDB is present in around 50% of patients with chronic HF. In the most recent study, by Bitter *et al.*[6] an AHI greater than 15 was found in 47% of patients with HF and normal left ventricular ejection fraction (LVEF). These results compare to a prevalence of obstructive apnoea syndrome in 4% of males and 2% of females in the general population.[10] Previously it was assumed that SDB, particularly CSR, was a marker or epiphenomenon of endstage HF, but it is becoming clearer that SDB is found in patients with mild HF[5] and is likely to contribute to functional cardiac decline through a range of mechanisms including hypoxaemia, increased sympathetic drive and oxidative stress.[11] Treatment to control SDB is therefore an important potential management tool.

Diagnosis of sleep-disordered breathing

Establishing the diagnosis of SDB almost always involves a sleep study to determine whether respiratory disturbances are present and to determine their nature, frequency, and pathophysiological consequences. It is often asserted that detailed polysomnography (assessment of ECG, electro-oculogram, and chin electromyogram to establish sleep stage and arousals, chest and abdominal effort sensors, airflow detection, oximetry, periodic limb and snoring monitoring) is the gold standard technique. However, the diagnosis can usually be secured by monitoring of respiratory variables such as pulse oximetry, airflow, respiratory effort, snoring, and position monitoring. Oximetry alone may establish the diagnosis in severe OSA and can be used to screen heart failure patients for SDB but cannot differentiate between obstructive and central sleep apnoeas. Further trials are in progress to establish the most effective method to screen patients including use of the simple 'ApneaLink' device (ResMed Co., Abingdon, UK) which detects airflow, and heart rate variation analysis from 24-h ECG monitoring.[12] Clearly screening becomes more relevant if therapy is available. This is the case in OSA, but the management of CSA in HF remains controversial (see 'Central sleep apnoea', below).

In many patients, a mixture of obstructive and central apnoeas and hyponoeas is present. OSA is diagnosed if more than 50% of

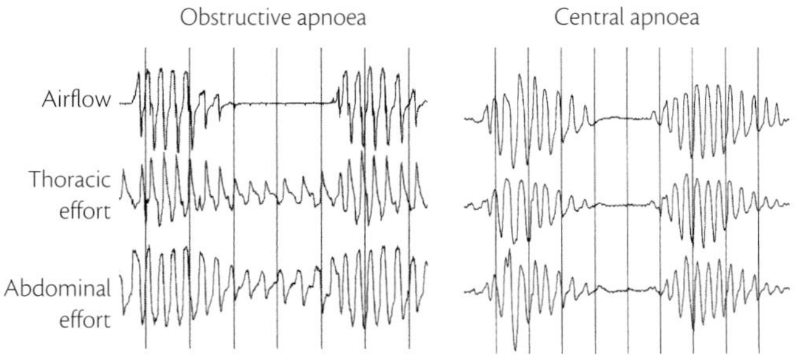

Fig. 34.1 Classification of obstructive and central sleep apnoea.

the events are obstructive and CSA diagnosed when more than 50% of the events are central.

Night-to-night variation in sleep-disordered breathing

In one study examining stable HF patients over four consecutive nights in the home, Vazir *et al.*[13] showed that there was minimal change in the AHI, but around 40% of patients demonstrated a shift in the type of events either from OSA to CSA or vice versa. Remarkably, there is also within-night variation in some patients. Tkacova *et al.*[14] carried out polysomnography in 12 stable patients with mean LVEF of 28.4% (±3.2%) NYHA class II or III, mean age 62.5 years. During the night, circulation time and periodic breathing cycle length increased, while transcutaneous $P\text{CO}_2$ level fell. The changes were accompanied by a reduction in obstructive events as the night progressed and increase in central events. As discussed below, the increase in cycle length is likely to reflect worsening HF overnight, which in turn leads to a shift from OSA to CSA.

Obstructive sleep apnoea

Mechanisms

Obstructive apnoea occurs when the pharynx collapses during sleep, usually at nasopharyngeal, oropharyngeal, and/or hypopharyngeal levels. The obstruction is observed as pharyngeal dilator muscle tone is reduced with the onset of sleep. In addition, the supine posture favours airway collapse, and any obesity causing thickening of the neck adds to anatomical narrowing. In the recumbent position, fluid shift from the legs may increase pharyngeal oedema. Muscle tone is at its nadir in rapid eye movement (REM) sleep.

As a result of airway collapse, arterial oxygen saturation falls and the patient makes increasing respiratory efforts to overcome the obstruction. The pulmonary stretch receptors are stimulated, which causes disinhibition of central sympathetic outflow, thereby increasing heart rate. Arousal to a lighter stage of sleep terminates the apnoea but the associated cortical activity also causes a burst of sympathetic activity and loss of vagal tone. The postapnoeic period is thus characterized by a surge in sympathetic outflow and a brisk increase in blood pressure and heart rate. Once arousal has opened the airway, deeper sleep ensues, the pharynx collapses, and the cycle begins again.

Sleep apnoea can directly affect cardiac function. During the respiratory effort against the occluded airway there is a reduction in intrathoracic pressure. In turn, there is a consequent increase in left ventricular transmural pressure and therefore the afterload against which the left ventricle has to eject blood. Venous return is augmented, producing right ventricular distension which may shift the interventricular septum to the left so reducing left ventricular filling.

OSA may also have proinflammatory, oxidative stress and endothelial effects. Patients with OSA have higher plasma C-reactive protein (CRP) levels than controls[15] and increased reactive oxygen species in neutrophils and moncytes.[7] In OSA patients with ischaemic heart disease, raised levels of soluble circulating adhesion molecules and increased expression of CD15 and CD11c have been reported. Patients with OSA treated with continuous positive airways pressure support (CPAP) appear to have down-regulation of the expression of the adhesion molecules CD15 and CD11c in monocytes.[16] Such changes suggest that OSA might be associated with the development of atherosclerosis, but as yet there is no clear evidence that it does. Hypoxaemia increases production of angiogenic promoters such as vascular endothelial growth factor (VEGF). In patients with OSA, VEGF level is proportional to the number of apnoeas and degree of nocturnal hypoxaemia,[17] but again, no direct link has been demonstrated between OSA and angiogenesis.

Pathophysiological consequences

The pathophysiological consequences of sleep apnoea are outlined in Fig. 34.2. In general, they can be divided into the effects of hypoxaemia, the impact of arousals including sympathetic hyperactivity and sleep fragmentation, and the effects on haemodynamics.[18] In practice, the pathophysiological changes have combined

Table 34.1 Prevalence of sleep-disordered breathing in heart failure

Author, year	Number of patients	NYHA class	Male (%)	LVEF (%)	SDB severity (AHI)	OSA (%)	CSA (%)
Lanfranchi, 2003	47	I	89	27(6)	>15/h	11	55
Ferrier, 2005	53	I–II	77	34(9)	>10/h	15	53
Javaheri, 2006	100	II	100	25(7)	>15/h	37	12
Oldenburg, 2007	700	>II	80	28(7)	>15/h	19	33
Schulz, 2007	203	II, III	75	28	>10/h	43	28
Vazir, 2007	55	II	100	31(10)	>15/h	15	38
MacDonald, 2008	108	>II	85	20	>15/h	30	31
Bitter, 2009	244	II–IV	64	>55	>15/h	24	23

AHI, apnoea–hyponoea index; CSA, central sleep apnoea; LVEF, left ventricular ejection fraction; OSA, obstructive sleep apnoea; SDB, sleep-disordered breathing.

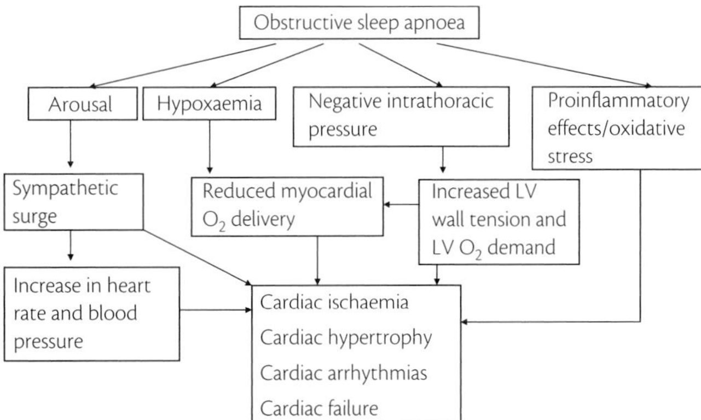

Fig. 34.2 Pathophysiological consequences of obstructive sleep apnoea. LV, left ventricle.

consequences which are likely to converge to exacerbate the progression of cardiac failure and increase mortality.

A prospective epidemiological study has shown that OSA is an independent risk factor for the development of systemic hypertension, and nocturnal blood pressure in patients with hypertension who also have OSA is higher than those without SDB.[19] In patients with HF, elevated daytime blood pressure is increased in proportion to the AHI (in other words, daytime blood pressure is increased in relation to the severity of OSA). In a related effect, OSA diminishes or prevents the usual fall in heart rate and blood pressure that occurs during sleep, and heightened sympathetic tone may predispose individuals to arrhythmia.

Each deep inspiratory effort to open the occluded airway during an apnoea can be associated with very marked swings in intrathoracic pressure. Negative intrathoracic pressures of more than 60 cmH_2O have been recorded. These frequent pressure swings are associated with an increase in afterload and large falls in stroke volume can be seen as a consequence. The repetitive falls in stroke volume occur on a background of arterial hypoxaemia. The repetitive stimuli every night could play a role in myocyte and contractile dysfunction setting up a progressive cycle of cardiac decline.

The presence of OSA has an impact on survival in patients with HF. Kasai et *al.*[20] studied 88 patients with HF (NYHA II or III, LVEF 36%) and moderate to severe OSA to establish outcome in those who either were untreated, received CPAP therapy, or were provided with CPAP but did not comply. During an average follow-up period of 25 months, 44.3% of patients died or were hospitalized. On multivariate analysis, the risk of death and hospitalization was increased in the untreated group (hazard ratio 2.03, 95%CI 1.07–3.68, p = 0.030) and in the poorly compliant CPAP group (hazard ratio 4.02, 95 CI 1.33–12.3, p = 0.014). However, this was a nonrandomized observational study. The results are supported by other work, although Roebuck *et al.*[21] showed no impact of CPAP on survival in HF patients with OSA. Compliance with CPAP was not documented in the latter study, however, so it is possible that patients in the treatment limb did not receive effective CPAP. Further randomized studies looking at the impact of CPAP are likely to be unethical: most patients with OSA are symptomatic, particularly with daytime sleepiness, which CPAP consistently addresses, and it would be unethical to randomize them to no treatment, particularly as they are not allowed to drive without CPAP treatment.

Treatment of obstructive sleep apnoea in heart failure

Management strategies include optimization of therapy for HF, weight loss, positional modification during sleep, positive pressure ventilatory devices, mandibular advancement splints, and oxygen therapy. While optimization of cardiac function and achieving ideal body weight are sensible, the burden of evidence concerns CPAP therapy. There are few data on the use of the mandibular advancement splint in HF patients with OSA.

Impact of treatment of heart failure

Interventions to improve cardiac function are likely to prove beneficial by decreasing both upper airway oedema and pulmonary oedema, thereby stabilizing ventilation. It was previously thought that β-blockers could predispose individuals with HF to OSA, but this has not been borne out in treatment comparison studies.[22] A preliminary report by Garrigue and coworkers[23] suggested that atrial overdrive pacing at a rate of 15 beats/min faster than mean nocturnal heart rate reduced AHI in a group of patients with both OSA and CSA. While an impact on CSA is plausible via an improvement in cardiac output leading to a decrease in heart–lung circulation time and left ventricular filling pressure, the effect on obstructive events is more difficult to explain. Subsequent work has not, however, confirmed the finding and thus the role of atrial overdrive pacing has not been convincingly demonstrated.

Of more relevance is cardiac resynchronization therapy (CRT). While again this might be expected to be more effective in HF patients with CSA, Stanchina *et al.*[24] have examined the impact of CRT in HF patients with OSA. They found that mean ejection fraction increased from 22 (±1.7)% to 33.6 (±2.0)% and AHI fell from 40.9 (±6.4) to 29.5 (±5.9) with CRT. As AHI still remained abnormal, it is not surprisingly that there was no improvement in sleep architecture or sleep-related symptoms.

Given that upper airway anatomy and body habitus contributes to OSA, cardiac transplantation might be expected not to reduce this component of SDB compared to potential beneficial effects on CSA. This seems indeed to be the case, and some transplant patients may in fact develop OSA.

Positive airway pressure therapy

In an early uncontrolled study of the effects of CPAP on patients with dilated cardiomyopathy and OSA, CPAP therapy for a month increased LVEF from 37% to 49% and breathlessness was reduced.[25] The improvements were lost when CPAP was withdrawn. In a randomized study of 24 patients with mean LVEF less than 45% and AHI greater than 20, CPAP lowered daytime heart rate and systolic blood pressure and increased LVEF by 9% over 30 days compared to no change in a matched control group who did not receive CPAP.[26] In a further randomized study in congestive HF (CHF) patients with OSA, CPAP improved LVEF more modestly (5%) and peak exercise capacity did not change. There was a reduction in daytime sleepiness.[27] More recent outcome data suggests that there is a decrease in mortality in HF patients with OSA treated with CPAP compared to those who did not receive CPAP.[20] It is important to stress, however, that the patients were not randomized, so the two treatment groups may represent different populations. As outlined above, it would now be problematic ethically to have a control group of patients with proven OSA randomized to no CPAP therapy.

Central sleep apnoea

Mechanisms

CSA and CSR represent forms of periodic breathing. In contrast to OSA, CSA/CSR arises as a consequence of HF itself. Pulmonary congestion and hypoxaemia stimulate receptors within the lung that cause hyperventilation which in turn lead to low arterial CO_2 levels. Lung congestion may be increased on lying flat at night as venous return from the limbs increases. If $P\text{CO}_2$ falls below the threshold required to stimulate breathing, a central apnoea occurs and continues until $P\text{CO}_2$ rises above the apnoeic threshold. Termination of the apnoea may be accompanied by arousal which stimulates breathing and drives down CO_2 again, leading to a self-perpetuating oscillation between apnoea and hyperpnoea. Prolonged circulation time delays information on arterial blood gas tensions from the lungs reaching the central chemoreceptors in particular, and thereby adds to periodicity such that the length of the ventilatory phase is inversely proportional to cardiac output.[11]

Pathophysiological consequences

Like OSA, CSA is associated with cyclical hypoxaemia, arousal from sleep and sympathetic activation. Passive airway collapse may occur at the end of a central event. Risk factors for the development of CSA/CSR are male sex (perhaps because of higher baseline chemosensitivity in males), age, and the presence of atrial fibrillation. It used to be thought that CSA/CSR was a paraphenomenon and simply represented the presence of severe HF. This is unlikely to be the case as new prevalence studies have shown a high prevalence of CSA in patients with mild HF.[5,6] Importantly, patients with HF and CSA/CSR have a worse prognosis than those without this form of SDB.[28]

Treatment

Impact of treatment for heart failure on central sleep apnoea

Therapies that improve cardiac function should also decrease CSA/CSR. Use of angiotensin-converting enzyme (ACE) inhibitor therapy and diuretic therapy to reduce left ventricular filling pressure can produce a decrease in AHI. Vazir *et al.*[29] showed that an left ventricular assist device (LVAD) reduced CSA/CSR. Therefore steps to optimize cardiac function should always be taken first.

Other therapies

A short term trial of aminophylline produced a reduction in CSA but did not change left or right ventricular function or quality of life.[30] Oxygen therapy at night corrects apnoea-related hypoxaemia and decreases nocturnal noradrenaline level while increasing exercise capacity.[31] However, over a month there was no impact on cardiac function or quality of life.[32] Acetazolamide may reduce apnoeas short term but long-term effects have not been examined.

From a theoretical viewpoint, increasing $P\text{CO}_2$ by either inhaling CO_2 or rebreathing dead space might be expected to stabilize periodic breathing by raising $P\text{CO}_2$ above the apnoeic threshold. Simple inhalation of CO_2 does not seem effective: while it may reduce apnoeas, cortical arousals are increased.[33] Similarly, breathing dead space has been shown to reduce central apnoeas but the benefit was offset by an increased work of breathing.[34] Notwithstanding concerns on the safety of asking patients to breathe CO_2 overnight, Mebrate *et al.*[35] have shown in an experimental model that targeted short-burst CO_2 in a small portion of the ventilatory cycle may stabilize ventilation, but this remains a highly exploratory approach.

Positive pressure therapy

Following the success of CPAP therapy in the management of OSA in HF patients, CPAP use has been extended to patients with CSA. However, the mechanisms of OSA and CSA are clearly different and there is no equivalent respiratory endpoint (opening the airway) to titrate therapy against. Furthermore, CPAP therapy can mildly reduce $P\text{CO}_2$ which might destabilize breathing further. Despite these physiological considerations, initial short-term uncontrolled trials suggested benefit from CPAP in treating CSA in terms of control of SDB and a reduction in ventricular ectopics. In a randomized study of 20 patients with HF and CSA, those who complied with CPAP therapy had a significant reduction in the combined rate of mortality/transplantation over 5 years.[36] However, the improved outcome disappeared when outcome was analysed on an intention-to-treat basis.

As a consequence of this work, the Canadian Positive Airway Pressure Trial for patients with congestive cardiac failure and CSA (CANPAP)[14] recruited 258 patients randomized to receive CPAP or usual therapy. In the patients treated with CPAP, mean nocturnal arterial oxygen saturation increased and there was a small improvement in LVEF. There was an early excess of deaths in the CPAP treated limb, but after 2 years the primary endpoint of combined mortality and transplantation was identical in CPAP and control groups. Recruitment and event rate was slowed by advances in medical and device therapy as the trial progressed, leaving it underpowered, and so the trial was terminated prematurely.[37] A post-hoc analysis suggested that there might be improved survival in patients in whom apnoeas/hyponoeas and CSR was suppressed.[38] This might indicate that therapies better able to suppress SDB may be more effective.

Adaptive servoventilation (ASV) is a form of ventilation that has been designed to smooth out periodic breathing in CSA/CSR by providing ventilatory support during apnoeic periods and reducing the support as spontaneous ventilation begins again. Over a relatively short period, breathing is captured and periodicity removed. As a result, arterial $P\text{CO}_2$ is stabilized, in turn stabilizing breathing further (Fig. 34.3) Positive pressure is provided in expiration to maintain upper airway patency and control any mixed or obstructive respiratory events.

Small studies have shown good control of AHI: in a one-night cross-over study ASV was more effective at controlling AHI, reducing arousals, and normalizing sleep quality than oxygen therapy, CPAP, or bilevel noninvasive ventilation.[39] In addition, ASV appears to be better tolerated by patients than CPAP and so more likely to be effective long term.[40] In a 'real world' study, HF patients with CSA/CSR who accepted ASV had a significant improvement in LVEF compared to those who did not receive ASV for 6 months.[41] Conversely, Pepperell *et al.*[42] showed improvement in sleep-related symptoms and nocturnal sympathetic measures but no change in ejection fraction. The multicentre Serve HF trial is now examining the effects on ASV in HF patients with predominant CSA/CSR on hard clinical endpoints including long-term cardiac and all-cause mortality, and hospital admissions. Other studies are planned looking at positive pressure therapy in HF patients with combined OSA and CSA.

Heart failure in neuromuscular disease

It should not be forgotten that some forms of inherited neuromuscular disease have associated cardiac muscle involvement.

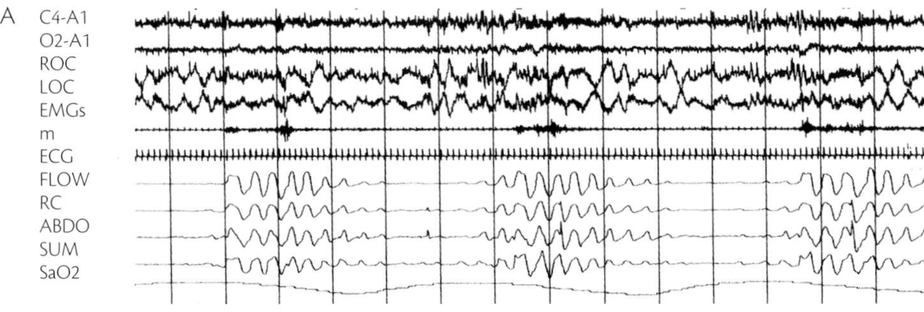

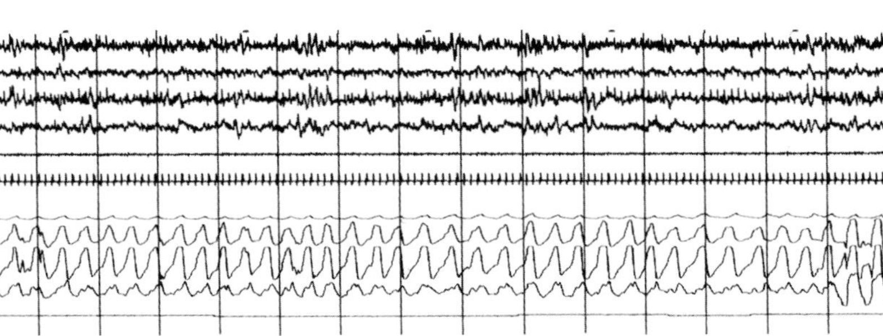

Fig. 34.3 Effect of adaptive servoventilation in Cheyne–Stokes respiration: (A) pretreatment; (B) during adaptive servoventilation (ASV). Abdo, abdominal excursion; C4-A1, O2-A1, electroencephalograms; EMGs electromyogram; Flow, oronasal airflow; Pm, mask pressure; RC, ribcage excursion; ROC, LOC, oculograms; Sum, total respiratory effort; Sa_{O_2}, arterial oxygen saturation.

Cardiomyopathy is almost inevitable in Duchenne muscular dystrophy, and cardiac involvement is seen in Becker and Emery Dreifuss muscular dystrophies, myotonic dystrophy, LGMD 1B, LGMD 1D, LGMD2C-2 sarcoglycanopathy variants of limb girdle muscular dystrophy, and some other myopathies such as acid maltase deficiency. Many of these patients also have respiratory muscle weakness resulting in ventilatory failure.

In some groups the introduction of noninvasive ventilation to control nocturnal hypoventilation has increased survival and reduced respiratory complications so that cardiomyopathy becomes a key prognostic factor. A combination of noninvasive ventilation and optimal cardiac failure therapy means that many patients with Duchenne muscular dystrophy are now living into their 30s. Anticipation of problems with serial monitoring by yearly ECG and echocardiogram is now part of the standard of care in these conditions as the previous nihilistic approach to care is now unjustified.[43]

Duboc[44] has carried out a randomized controlled trial of perindopril in Duchenne patients aged between 9.5 and 13 years (LVEF >55%) for 3 years, after which both perindopril and placebo limbs received open label perindopril 2–4 mg/day as tolerated for a further 2 years. LVEF was similar in both groups after 3 years, but after 5 years a single patient in the phase I perindopril group had an LVEF less than 45%, whereas eight patients had LVEF below 45% in the phase I placebo group ($p = 0.02$). Currently a trial of combined prophylactic ACE inhibitor and β-blocker is in progress in children with Duchenne muscular dystrophy.

Clinical features and implications

It is important to realize that the symptoms of OSA and CSA may differ. While OSA patients are classically sleepy as quantified by Epworth sleepiness score (ESS),[45] patients with CSA (and some HF patients with OSA) do not routinely complain of sleepiness. The ESS is usually within the normal range (<10). Snoring, choking episodes and struggling to breathe are noted by partners of patents with OSA but not those with CSA. The latter may, however, complain of poor quality, fragmented sleep together with tiredness or fatigue. In addition, despite the lack of subjective sleepiness, objective measures of vigilance are reduced, and daytime activity, as measured by actigraphy watches, is reduced in HF patients with all forms of SDB compared to those with no SDB.[46]

Practicalities of assessment in the clinic and therapy

The lack of typical symptoms raises the question of how to identify HF patients with SDB in the clinic. A story of snoring, witnessed apnoea, and daytime sleepiness should be specifically asked for as the symptoms may be present in some, particularly those with higher BMI. SDB occurs in up to three-quarters of CHF patients with chronic atrial fibrillation (AF),[47] so there should be a low threshold for asking about symptoms and carrying out a sleep study in this group. As the presence of SDB cannot be easily predicted in others, a variety of screening mechanisms is being investigated. Screening is, of course, only justified where effective treatment is available for the condition detected. At present, there is good evidence in favour of treating OSA in CHF, but until Serve HF and other trials report, the best management of CSA/CSR is less clear. Screening methods which can be used in the home include oximetry, analysis of heart rate variation, and apnoea detection.

CPAP treatment is best started by experienced teams and a good link between cardiology departments and sleep departments is highly recommended. In patients with labile HF and poor cardiac output, initiating CPAP is more safely done with the patient in hospital with haemodynamic monitoring. In stable CHF patients with OSA, outpatient set-up is usually effective as long as there is careful explanation of the anticipated benefit, the importance of fitting of mask interface, and support in the home.[48] Autoset variable pressure devices can be used to determine the correct pressure setting overnight, but for long-term use, fixed-level standard CPAP machines are usually sufficient. Continued input from the CPAP team to maintain compliance and adherence is helpful. Patients with HF often have other comorbidities. In those with additional severe chronic obstructive pulmonary disease (COPD) or obesity resulting in nocturnal hypoventilation, obstructive hypopnoeas or even obesity–hypoventilation syndrome and daytime hypercapnia, noninvasive ventilation is likely to be preferable to autoset devices.

References

1. Cheyne J. A case of apoplexy in which the fleshy part of the heart was converted into fat. *Dublin Hospital Reports* 1818;**2**:216–23.
2. Stokes W. Fatty degeneration of the heart. In: *The diseases of the heart and aorta*, pp. 320–7. Dublin, 1854.
3. Ferrier K, Campbell A, Yee B, *et al.* Sleep-disordered breathing occurs frequently in stable outpatients with congestive heart failure. *Chest* 2005;**128**:2116–22.
4. Javaheri S, Parker TJ, Liming JD, *et al.* Sleep apnea in 81 ambulatory male patients with stable heart failure: types and their prevalences, consequences and presentations. *Circulation* 1998;**97**:2154–9.
5. Vazir A, Hastings PC, Dayer M, *et al.* A high prevalence of sleep disordered breathing in men with mild symptomatic chronic heart failure due to left ventricular systolic dysfunction. *Eur J Heart Fail* 2007;**9**:243–50.
6. Bitter T, Faber L, Hering D, Langer C, Horstkotte D, Oldenburg O. Sleep disordered breathing in heart failure with normal left ventricular ejection fraction. *Eur J Heart Fail* 2009;**11**:602–8.
7. Schulz R, Mahmoudi S, Hattar K, *et al.* Enhances release of superoxide from polymorphonuclear neutrophils in obstructive sleep apnea: impact of continuous positive airway pressure therapy. *Am J Respir Crit Care Med* 2000;**162**:566–70.
8. MacDonald M, Fang J, Pittman SD, White DP, Malhotra A. The current prevalence of sleep disordered breathing in congestive heart failure patients treated with beta blockers. *J Clin Sleep Med* 2008;**4**:38–42.
9. Lanfranchi PA, Somers VK, Braghiroli A, Corra U, Eleuteri E, Giannuzzi P. Central sleep apnea in left ventricular dysfunction:prevalence and implications for arrhythmic risk. *Circulation* 2003;**107**:727–32.
10. Young T, Palta M, Dempsey J, Skatrud J, Weber S, Badr S. The ocurrence of sleep-disordered breathing among middle-aged adults. *N Engl J Med* 1993;**328**:1230–5.
11. Bradley TD,.Floras JS. Sleep apnea and heart failure. Part I: Obstructive sleep apnea. *Circulation* 2003;**107**:1671–8. Part II Central sleep apnea. *Circulation* 2003;**107**:1822–6.
12. Clark AL, Crabbe S, Aziz A, Reddy P, Greenstone M. Use of a screening tool for the detection of sleep-disordered breathing. *J Laryngol Otol* 2009;**123**:746–9.
13. Vazir A, Hastings PC, Papaioannou I, *et al.* Variation in severity and type of sleep-disordered breathing throughhout 4 nights in patients with heart failure. *Respir Med* 2008;**102**:831–9.
14. Tkacova R, Wang H, Bradley TD. Night to night alterations in sleep apnea type in patients with heart failure. *J Sleep Res* 2006;**15**:321–8.
15. Shamsuzzaman AS, Winnicki M, Lanfranchi P, *et al.* Elevated C-reactive protein in patients with obstructive sleep apnea. *Circulation* 2002;**105**:2462–4.
16. Dyugovskaya L, Lavie P, Lavie L, *et al.* Increased adhesion molecule expression and production of reactive oxygen species in leucocytes of sleep apnea patients. *Am J Respir Crit Care Med* 2002;**165**: 934–9.
17. Schulz R, Hummel C, Heinemann S, *et al.* Serum levels of vascular endothelial growth factor are elevated in patients with obstructive sleep apnea and severe nighttime hypoxia. *Am J Respir Crit Care Med* 2002;**165**:67–70.
18. Somers VK, White DP, Amin R, *et al.* Sleep apnea and cardiovascular disease. AHA/ACCF Scientific Statement. *Circulation* 2008;**118**:1080–111.
19. Peppard PE, Young T, Palta M, Skatrud J. Prospective study of the association between sleep-disordered breathing and hypertension. *N Engl J Med* 2000;**342**:1378–84.
20. Kasai T, Narui K, Dohi T, Yanagisawa N, Ishiwata S, Ohno T. Prognosis of patients with heart failure and obstructive sleep apnea treated with continuous positive airway pressure. *Chest* 2008;**133**:696.
21. Roebuck T, Solin P, Kaye DM, Bergin P, Bailey M, Naughton MT. Increased long-term mortality in heart failure due to sleep apnoea is not yet proven. *Eur Respir J* 2004;**23**:740.
22. Kraiczi H, Hedner J, Peker Y, Grote L. Comparison of atenolol, amlodipine, enalapril, hydrochlorthiazide and losartan for antihypertensive treatment of patients with obstructive sleep apnea. *Am J Respir Crit Care Med* 2000;**161**:1423–8.
23. Garrigue S, Bordier O, Jais P, *et al.* Benefit of atrial pacing in sleep apnea syndrome. *N Engl J Med* 2002;**346**:404–12.
24. Stanchina ML, Ellison K, Malhotra A, *et al.* The impact of cardiac resynchronization therapy on obstructive sleep apnea in heart failure. *Chest* 2009;**132**:433–9.
25 Malone S, Liu PP, Holloway R, Rutherford R, Xie A, Bradley TD. Obstructive sleep apnoea in patients with dilated cardiomyopathy: effects of continuous positive airway pressure. *Lancet* 1991;**338**:1480–4.
26. Kaneko Y, Floras JS, Usui K, *et al.* Cardiovascular effects of continuous positive airway pressure in patinents with heart failure and obstructive sleep apnoea. *New Engl J Med* 2003; **348**:1233–41.
27. Mansfield DR, Gollogly NC, Kaye DM, Richardson M, Bergin P, Naughton MT. Controlled trial of continuous positive airway pressure in obstructive sleep apnoea and heart failure. *Am J Respir Crit Care Med* 2004;**169**:361–6.
28. Lanfranchi PA, Braghiroli A, Bosimini E, Mazzuero G, Colombo R, Donner CF. Prognostic value of nocturnal Cheyne-Stokes respiration in chronic heart failure. *Circulation* 1999;**99**:1435–40.
29. Vazir A, Hastings PC, Morrell MJ, *et al.* Resolution of central sleep apnoea following implantation of a left ventricular assist device. *Int J Cardiol* 2008.
30. Javaheri S, Parker TJ, Wexler L, *et al.* Effect of theophylline on sleep-disordered breathing in heart failure. *N Engl J Med* 1996;**335**:562–7.
31. Andreas S, Clemens C, Sandholzer H, *et al.* Improvement in exercise capacity with treatment of Cheyne-Stokes respiration in patients with congestive cardiac failure. *J Am Coll Cardiol* 1996;**27**:1486–90.
32. Staniforth AD, Kinnear WJ, Starling R, *et al.* Effect of oxygen on sleep quality, cognitive function and sympathetic activity in patients with chronic heart failure and Cheyne Stokes respiration. *Eur Respir J* 1998;**19**:922–8.
33. Szollosi I, Jones M, Morrell M, Helfet K, Coats AJ, Simonds AK. Effect of CO2 inhalation on central sleep apnoea and arousals from sleep. *Respiration* 2004;**71**:493–8.
34. Szollosi I, O'Driscoll DM, Dayer MJ, Coats AJ, Morrell MJ, Simonds AK. Adaptive servo-ventilation and deadspace: effects on central sleep apnoea. *J Sleep Res* 2006;**15**:199–205.
35. Mebrate Y, Willson K, Manisty CH, *et al.* Dynamic CO2 therapy in periodic breathing: a modelling study to determine optimal timing and dosage regimes. *J Appl Physiol* 2009;**107**:696–706.
36. Sin DD, Logan AG, Fitzgerald FS, *et al.* Effects of continuous positive airway pressure on cardiovascular outcomes in heart failure patients with and without Cheyne-Stokes respiration. *Circulation* 2000;**102**:61–6.
37. Bradley TD, Logan AG, Kimoff J, *et al.* Continuous positive airway pressure for central sleep apnea and heart failure. *New Engl J Med* 2005;**353**:2025–33.
38. Artzt M, Floras JS, Logan AG, *et al.* Suppression of central sleep apnea by continuous positive pressure airway pressure and

transplant-free survival in heart failure. A post hoc analysis of the Canadian Continuous Positive Airway Pressure for patients with central sleep apnea and heart failure trial (CANPAP). *Circulation* 2007;**115**:3173–80.

39. Teschler H, Dohring J, Wang YM, Berthon-Jones M. Adaptive pressure support servo-ventilation: a novel treatment for Cheyne-Stokes respiration in heart failure and central sleep apnea. *Am J Resp Crit Care Med* 2001;**164**:614–19.
40. Philippe C, Stoica-Herman M, Druout X, *et al.* Compliance with and effectiveness of adaptive servoventilation versus continuous positive airway pressure in the treatment of Cheyne-Stokes respiration in heart failure over a six month period. *Heart* 2006;**92**:337–42.
41. Hastings PC, Vazir A, Meadows GE, *et al.* Adaptive servo-ventilation in heart failure patients with sleep apnea: a real world study. *Int J Cardiol* 2010;**139**(1):17–24.
42. Pepperell JC, Maskell NA, Jones DR, *et al.* A randomised controlled trial of adaptive ventilation for Cheyne-Stokes breathing in heart failure. *Am J Resp Crit Care Med* 2003;**168**:1109–14.
43. Bushby K, Muntoni F, Bourke JP. 107th International Workshop: the management of cardiac involvement in muscular dystrophy and myotonic dystrophy. *Neuromusc Disord* 2003;**13**:166–72.
44. Duboc D, Meaune C, Lerebours G, Devaux J-Y, Vaksmann G, Becane H-M. Effect of perindopril on the onset and progression of left ventricular dysfunction in Duchenne muscular dystrophy. *J Am Coll Cardiol* 2005;**45**:855–7.
45. Johns MW. A new method for measuring daytime sleepiness: the Epworth sleepiness scale. *Sleep* 1991;**14**(**6**):540–5.
46. Hastings PC, Vazir A, O'Driscoll DM, Morrell MJ, Simonds AK. Symptom burden of sleep-disordered breathing in mild-to-moderate congestive heart failure patients. *Eur Respir J* 2006;**27**:748–55.
47. Stevenson IH, Teichtahl H, Cunnington D, Ciavarella S, Gordon I, Kalman JM. Prevalence of sleep disordered breathing in paroxysmal and persistent atrial fibrillation patients with normal left ventricular function. *Eur J Heart Fail* 2008;**162**:1662–9.
48. Simonds AK. *Non-invasive respiratory support. A practical handbook.* Hodder Arnold, London, 2007.

35

Arthritis

Nicola L. Walker and Anne McEntegart

Introduction

Heart failure (HF) and arthritis are both common in adults, increasing in prevalence with age. The term arthritis covers a wide spectrum of disease (Box 35.1) which may involve the cartilage, bone, tensile structures (ligaments, tendons, and muscles), or synovial tissue, and pathological processes can impact on any of these structures.

Osteoarthritis is the most common arthritis and results from cartilage fragmentation and loss. The major target for inflammatory arthritides, of which rheumatoid arthritis (RA) is the most common, is the synovium. RA affects 1% of the population, and premature death, predominantly from cardiovascular disease, is associated with an 8–15-year reduction in lifespan compared to age-matched controls.[1] The onset of HF is significant in patients with arthritis as there is evidence that deaths are attributed to HF more often for patients with RA than for the general population. However, this difference in mortality results from an increased incidence of HF rather than a worse prognosis overall.[2]

The main focus of this chapter is the interaction of HF with the inflammatory arthritides. As in the general population, the most common cause of HF in inflammatory arthritis is atherosclerotic coronary artery disease. Other causes are now less common. There is less extra-articular disease in inflammatory arthritis as a result of more aggressive management and better control of disease. However, other possible causes of HF include:

- Myocardial disease resulting in ventricular systolic dysfunction (e.g. myocarditis) or ventricular diastolic dysfunction (e.g. amyloidosis).
- Pericardial disease (e.g. pericarditis with effusion).
- Coronary artery disease, due to acute inflammatory arteritis.
- Conduction disease, usually bradyarrhythmias related to myocardial fibrosis.
- Valvular disease, which may occur with the seronegative spondarthropathies such as ankylosing spondylitis, or with endocarditic lesions including the nonbacterial Libman–Sacks endocarditis.

When HF and arthritis coexist, the pharmacotherapy of either condition can impact on the other, to a beneficial or detrimental effect (e.g. gout triggered by diuretic use).

Epidemiology of heart failure and arthritis

Much of the literature on arthritis and HF comes from the extensive study of RA, where the clinical presentation and outcome of HF appears different from that in the general population. The extent of cardiac involvement in arthritis has been a source of ongoing interest for decades. In 1943, Bayles described post-mortem findings in the heart of patients with RA.[3] As early as 1975 it was reported that there was an excess cardiovascular mortality in patients with RA.[4] The prevalence of HF in the RA population increases with age and is greater in men than in women (Fig. 35.1).[5]

There is also a higher incidence of HF in patients with RA compared to those without (37.1% vs 27.7%, $p < 0.001$). In addition, RA patients with HF die sooner than patients with HF and no RA. Mortality rates among patients with and without RA were 39.0 and 29.2 per 1000 person-years, respectively (Fig. 35.2).[2]

As well as being more frequently female, RA patients with HF less frequently suffer from obesity, hypertension, and ischaemic heart disease.[6] Their symptoms and signs at presentation are often more subtle and consequently they are less likely to have an echocardiogram. However, RA patients are more likely to have preserved systolic function (Fig. 35.3) but they have a higher mortality at 1 year (Fig. 35.4). These findings illustrate the difficulties in the assessment and management of this patient group, and highlight the importance and potential benefit in aggressively screening such patients.

Heart failure and arthritis: mechanisms

Ischaemic cardiomyopathy

In the general population, ischaemic cardiomyopathy is the most common cause of HF associated with left ventricular systolic dysfunction (LVSD). The presentation may be obvious, with chest

Box 35.1 Causes of arthritis

Monoarthritis

- Osteoarthritis
- Septic arthritis
- Crystal arthritis (gout and calcium pyrophosphate dihydrate)
- Trauma with haemarthrosis

Polyarthritis

- RA
- Psoriatic arthritis
- Ankylosing spondylitis
- Reactive arthritis (bacterial or viral)
- Osteoarthritis
- Connective tissue disease (e.g. SLE, scleroderma, polymyositis)
- Systemic disease (including malignancy, endocarditis, sarcoidosis, sickle cell disease, familial Mediterranean fever)
- Vasculitis (e.g. Wegener's granulomatosis, Churg–Strauss vasculitis, polyarteritis nodosa)

RA, rheumatoid arthritis; SLE, systemic lupus erythematosus.

pain prompting admission for management of an acute myocardial infarction, or exertional chest pain requiring management of chronic stable angina. However, the presentation may be that of silent ischaemia and insidious development of worsening breathlessness.

It is generally accepted that aggressive management of acute coronary artery occlusion minimizes the impact on systolic function. The optimal reperfusion strategy is currently prompt delivery of primary percutaneous coronary intervention.

As described, there is an excess of cardiovascular disease in many of the arthritides. This often manifests as coronary artery disease. In RA, the risk of coronary artery disease is equally elevated in both men and women and increases with disease severity, disease duration and evidence of extra-articular disease.[7] The increased risk of developing, and dying from, coronary artery disease is significantly higher than in a non-RA individual.[8] A recent meta-analysis of

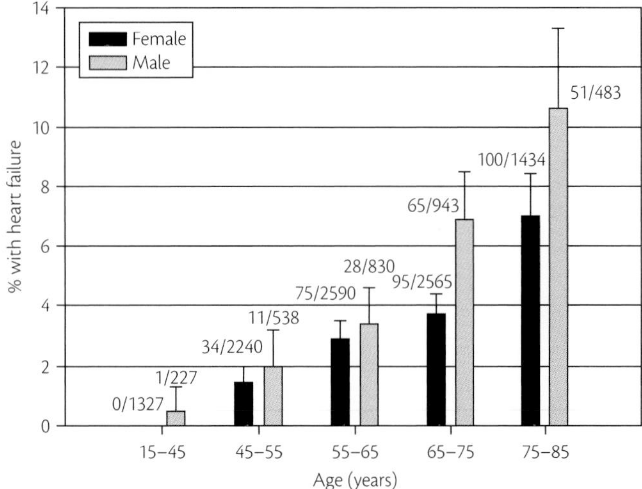

Fig. 35.1 Frequency of heart failure in 13 171 rheumatoid arthritis patients stratified by age and sex. Rates increase with age (p < 0.001) and are always greater in men than in women (p< 0.001).[5]

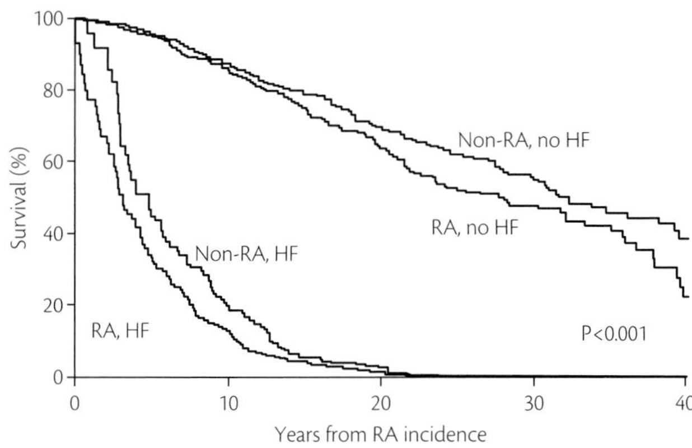

Fig. 35.2 The impact of rheumatoid arthritis on survival, and the cumulative impact of heart failure with rheumatoid arthritis on survival.[2]

24 observational studies, with a total study population of 111 758 patients, described that the risk of mortality related to coronary artery disease was 59% higher in patients with RA than in the general population.[9]

There is a difference in the presentation of coronary artery disease in patients with RA. Patients are twice as likely to experience unrecognized myocardial infarctions and sudden deaths, and less likely to report angina or to undergo coronary artery bypass grafting.[10] The reduction in the presentation of acute myocardial ischaemia impacts on the therapeutic options available to these patients and the unheralded silent ischaemia persists and reduces systolic function. The risk of coronary artery disease in RA patients often precedes the diagnosis of RA, and the risk cannot be explained by an increased incidence of traditional coronary heart disease risk factors in RA patients.

The differential diagnosis of chest pain in patients with systemic inflammatory athritidies includes:

- Costochondral or sternoclavicular joint pain.
- Pericarditis—acute pericarditis causes chest pain with ECG changes, and may be associated with a friction rub. Echocardiography may demonstrate a pericardial effusion; but it should be noted that small effusions are not uncommon in RA or systemic lupus erythematosus (SLE).

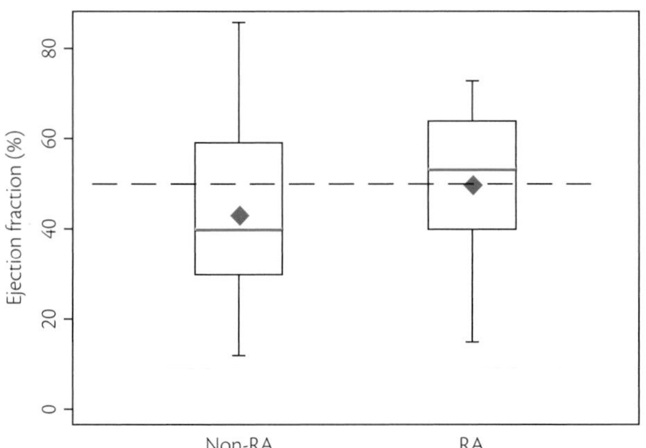

Fig. 35.3 Patients with rheumatoid arthritis are more likely to have preserved systolic function (LVEF >50%) on estimation of ejection fraction by echocardiogram.[6]

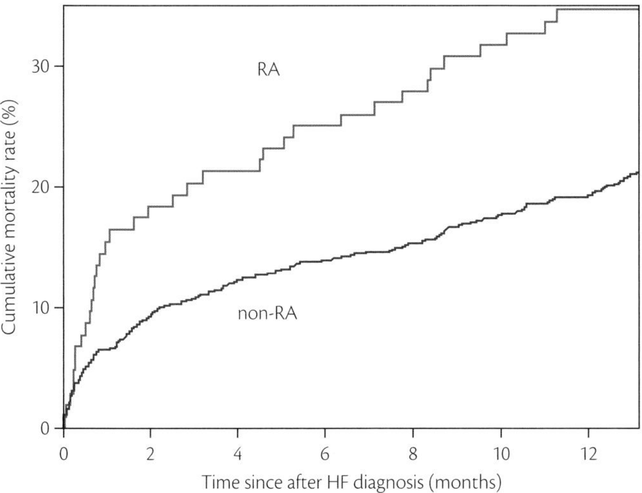

Fig. 35.4 Mortality rates following heart failure are higher in the rheumatoid arthritis group. There is early separation of the curves with 30-day mortality of 15.5% in the rheumatoid arthritis group compared with 6.6% in the non-rheumatoid-arthritis group. The curves continue to separate for at least the first year, and this may persist out to approximately 10 years.[6]

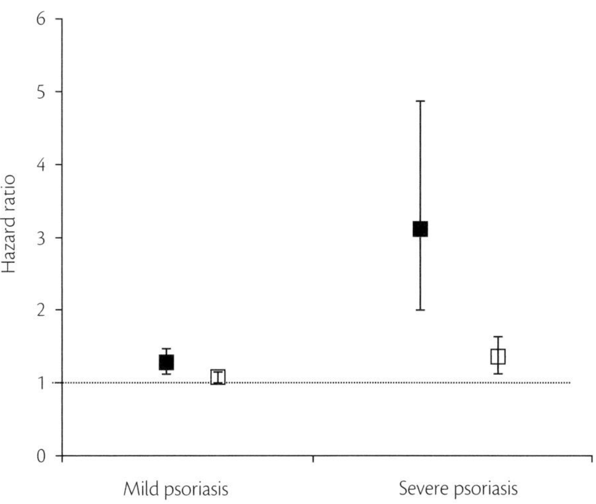

Fig. 35.5 Point estimate for the hazard ratio for myocardial infarction in unadjusted analyses. Filled squares are patients aged 30 and open squares are those aged 60 at the beginning of follow up.
Data from Gelfand JM, Neimann AL, Shin DB, Wang X, Margolis DJ, Troxel AB. Risk of myocardial infarction in patients with psoriasis The data is divided between those with mild or severe psoriasis *JAMA* 2006;**296**:1735–41.

- Coronary arteritis—this is an uncommon manifestation of long-standing, severe RA, often as part of a more general rheumatoid vasculitis. It can present as acute myocardial infarction in children or adolescents with SLE.
- Aortitis with aortic dissection.
- Pulmonary hypertension secondary to arthritis-related interstitial lung disease with exertional chest pain thought to be caused by right ventricular ischaemia.

Arthritis, atherosclerosis and inflammation

It is now well established that RA patients have an increased risk of cardiovascular disease. As a result, classic cardiovascular risk factors (smoking, hypertension, hyperlipidaemia) are increasingly targeted and annual screening for these risk factors is now advocated.[11]

There is a well-described dyslipidaemia in RA, with an inverse association between inflammatory markers (C-reactive protein or ESR) and HDL cholesterol.[12] A reduction in inflammation with RA-modifying drugs correlates with increase in HDL and total cholesterol. Interestingly, the Trial of Atorvastatin in Rheumatoid Arthritis (TARA) study demonstrated that hydroxymethylglutaryl-coenzyme A reductase inhibitor (statin) therapy conferred an improved lipid profile and achieved clinically apparent anti-inflammatory effects with reduction in RA disease activity score.[13] The pleiotropic effects of statins are thought to include anti-inflammatory, antifibrotic, and antioxidant effects;[14] prevention of left ventricular hypertrophy;[15] reduction of endothelial dysfunction;[16,17] inhibition of neurohormonal activation; and prevention of cardiac arrhythmias.[18] These are all potentially beneficial in the management of HF.

Psoriasis is a systemic inflammatory condition that primarily manifests as a skin disorder in 1–3% of the population. Of those affected, 6–11% have psoriatic arthropathy. In the United States, the prevalence of all heart diseases in patients with psoriasis has been estimated at 14.3% compared with 11.3% for the entire US population.[19] There is an increased prevalence of diabetes, hypertension, hyperlipidaemia, smoking, and increased body mass index (BMI) in patients with psoriasis. These key cardiovascular risk factors that comprise the metabolic syndrome are more strongly associated with severe rather than mild psoriasis.[20]

The literature continues to debate whether psoriasis is an independent risk factor for myocardial infarction. Gelfand *et al.*[21] demonstrated that the risk of myocardial infarction associated with psoriasis is greatest in young patients with severe psoriasis, is attenuated with age, and remains increased even after controlling traditional cardiovascular risk factors (Fig. 35.5). In a recent study from the United States, the 10-year risks for coronary heart disease were 28% greater for patients with psoriasis than in the general population.[22] However, a very large Dutch cohort did not find psoriasis to be a clinically relevant risk factor for ischaemic heart disease hospitalizations.[23] It remains to be seen whether aggressive control of the traditional risk factors and of systemic inflammation will impact on the evolution of coronary artery disease in patients with psoriasis and more specifically psoriatic arthropathy.

In RA classic risk factors alone do not explain the excess vascular disease. Del Rincon *et al.*[24] reported a fourfold higher incidence of cardiovascular events relative to a community-dwelling cohort. Adjusting for conventional risk factors, this risk ratio was only minimally attenuated, suggesting that classic risk factors do not fully explain the accelerated atherogenesis in RA.

The role of autoimmune processes is well-described in relation to several arthritic conditions including RA and SLE. A causal association between autoimmune disease and primary heart disease continues to be an area of research. There is increasing evidence that active autoimmune arthritis is associated with heart disease including HF. Sattar *et al.*[25] hypothesized that it is the severity and chronicity of the systemic inflammation that is particularly damaging. Even when the arthritis is clinically quiescent, cytokine production remains high and continues to promote vascular risk.

Inflammatory mediators can be identified in coronary heart disease, but require high-sensitivity assays. Parallels can be drawn between coronary heart disease, with inflammatory molecules and immune cells in the cap region of unstable atheromatous plaques, and the inflammatory process in synovitis. Cytokines, particularly tumour necrosis factor (TNF) α and interleukins IL-1β and IL-6, can be identified in both HF and the inflammatory arthritides. TNFα has been implicated in the pathogenesis of HF and cardiac cachexia.[26] In a follow-up study of the SOLVD (Studies Of Left Ventricular Dysfunction) population levels of TNFα were significantly higher in patients with HF compared with the normal controls.[27] Furthermore, higher cytokine concentrations are associated with a worse prognosis in patients with advanced HF (Fig. 35.7).[28]

TNFα may mediate cardiac myocyte hypertrophy and influence other pathways involved in cardiac remodelling culminating in cardiac dysfunction. TNFα may have time-dependent opposing effects and other cytokines (e.g. IL-1β, IL-10) may also carry independent pathophysiologic importance in HF.[29]

The metabolic effects of cytokines (particularly TNFα, IL-1β, and IL-6) include lipid alterations and peripheral insulin resistance. These effects can be seen as beneficial in the acute-phase response to acute inflammation, but chronic cytokine activity and related metabolic effects are proatherogenic.

The end result of the inflammatory process on cardiac structure and function has recently been described with cardiac magnetic resonance (CMR) imaging.[30] Compared with non-RA patients, RA patients demonstrate a markedly lower left ventricular mass, and a modest decrease in ejection fraction and stroke volume. Disease severity, suggested by higher titres of antibodies to cyclic citrullinated peptide (anti-CCP) and the use of biologic agents, probably correlates with lower left ventricular mass, left ventricular stroke, and end-diastolic volumes.

Inflammatory cardiomyopathy

Myocarditis is an uncommon presentation of inflammatory arthritis. In patients with SLE it is often asymptomatic and can affect between 8–25% of patients,[31,32] particularly in African-American patients. Myocarditis should be considered if there is a persistent tachycardia with nonspecific ST and T wave abnormalities. Echocardiography is indicated and may show systolic or diastolic dysfunction. Establishing the diagnosis of myocarditis can be challenging and may require endomyocardial biopsy. Histology demonstrates mononuclear cell infiltration of the myocardium. In established cases with a more prolonged myocarditic process the inflammation may lead to fibrosis, which may be present clinically as dilated cardiomyopathy, or cause conduction abnormalities. These may present as bradycardia or tachyarrhythmias, both of which may further impact on HF. Myocarditis and HF is also described in other non-ANCA-associated vasculilides, e.g. Takayasu's arteritis.

Churg–Strauss syndrome (CSS) is the ANCA-associated vasculitis most likely to involve the heart, with 14% of patients developing myocardial involvement and HF. Chronic HF is a significant cause of death in CSS.[33]

Pericarditis is described in a number of inflammatory arthritides including RA, ankylosing spondylitis, SLE, scleroderma, and vasculitis. In RA clinical symptoms of pericarditis are infrequent (3%); however, echo studies have reported up to 50% of patients affected and at autopsy up to 30% of patients are found to have had pericardial disease. If effusions are present they are usually small and do not require treatment.[34]

Valvular disease—in particular mitral and aortic insufficiency—is documented in RA. In ankylosing spondylitis aortic regurgitation is more common. Patients with SLE can develop valve thickening or Libman–Sacks endocarditis. Valvular heart disease due to scleroderma is rare. In Takayasu's vasculitis aortic dilatation may involve the aortic valve and in Wegener's granulomatosis both aortic and mitral regurgitation are documented.

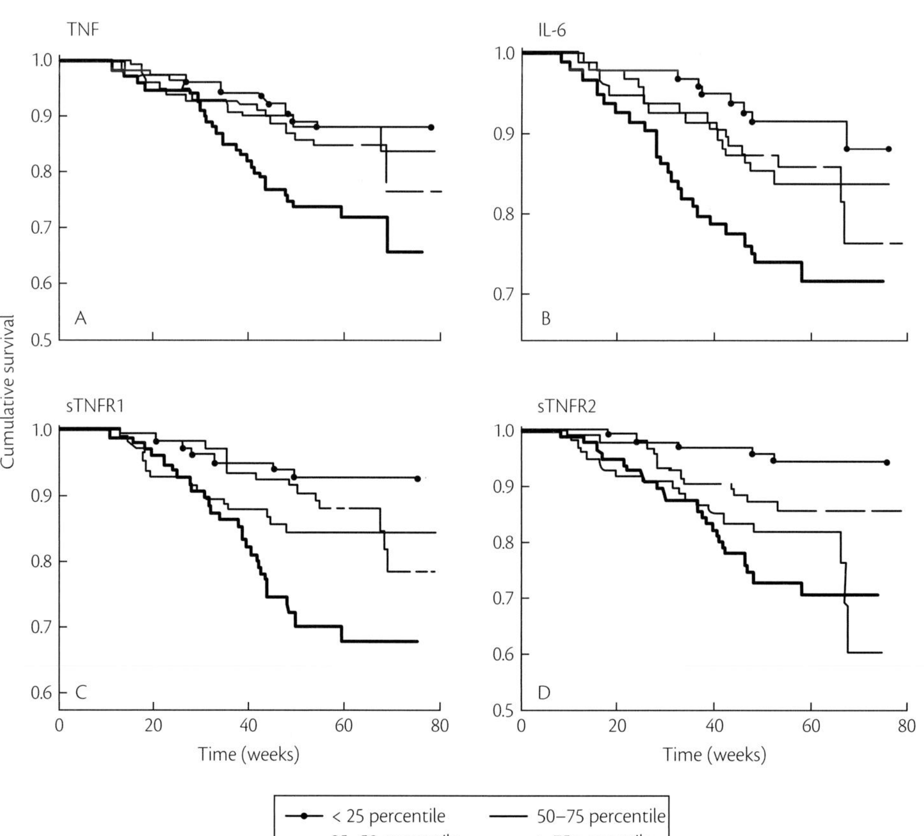

Fig. 35.6 Circulating levels of TNFα, IL-6, soluble TNF receptor 1, and soluble TNF receptor 2 in relation to patient survival during follow-up. Circulating levels of cytokines and cytokine receptors were arbitrarily divided into quartiles.[28]

Diastolic dysfunction

Diastolic dysfunction is more common with increasing age. Impaired ventricular filling and other measures of diastolic dysfunction, including transmitral blood flow velocities and valve annulus velocities, have been assessed in patients with arthritis. These echocardiographic findings are more common in patients with RA than in the general population,[35,36] and a correlation with RA disease duration, perhaps due to subclinical myocardial involvement, has been demonstrated.

Diastolic dysfunction may predate clinically apparent HF. In a study of patients with SLE without clinically evident cardiovascular disease, no significant difference in systolic function was identified, but there was evidence of diastolic dysfunction.[37]

Amyloidosis

Reactive or secondary (AA) amyloidosis refers to predominantly extracellular tissue deposition of fibrils composed of fragments of serum amyloid A protein, an acute-phase reactant. In poorly controlled chronic inflammatory arthritis, mainly seropositive RA and ankylosing spondylitis, cardiac AA amyloidosis can occur. In the context of RA, it has been reported that up to 40% of patients have cardiac involvement,[38] although significant deposition of AA amyloid in the heart is uncommon and is therefore rarely the cause of death.

Cardiac involvement may be suspected by low-voltage complexes in the limb leads or a pseudo-infarct pattern on ECG. Amyloid infiltration of the heart results in increased echogenicity, and therefore echocardiography is the noninvasive test of choice. Early features include left ventricular wall thickening and evidence of diastolic dysfunction. Right ventricular diastolic dysfunction can also occur. If AA amyloidosis is clinically suspected and suggested on noninvasive tests then it can be diagnosed by rectal, subcutaneous abdominal fat, skin, or, if necessary, cardiac biopsies.

However, in the current era of arthritis care, with more aggressive disease control, it is very unusual for patients to develop HF related to AA amyloidosis. A recent study of the natural history and outcome in systemic AA amyloidosis found that cardiac failure attributable to AA amyloidosis was present in only 1 of the 374 patients assessed (60% of whom had chronic inflammatory arthritis as the cause of AA amyloidosis); 224 patients underwent echocardiography and only 2 of them had findings consistent with cardiac infiltration.[39]

Pharmacology-related heart failure

The management of arthritis and HF involves polypharmacy. Many of the agents used to treat arthritis can negatively impact on HF, and in some cases may be the cause of HF.

Nonsteroidal anti-inflammatory drugs

Nonsteroidal anti-inflammatory drugs (NSAIDs) are at the front line of disease control. NSAIDs offer both analgesic and anti-inflammatory properties, but do not slow disease progression. NSAIDs have several potential adverse cardiovascular effects, including interference with the antiplatelet action of aspirin, an increase in cardiovascular events including myocardial infarction, and exacerbation of established HF.

The attenuation of the antiplatelet effect of aspirin is well described with both ibuprofen and naproxen.[40,41] The presumed mechanism is competitive binding at the cyclooxygenase (COX)-1 receptor. The impact of this interaction is the potential for increased thrombotic coronary events, and subsequent HF. This has yet to be proved.

Studies have not demonstrated an increase in first episodes of HF with NSAID use.[42] However, in established HF NSAIDs are associated with relapse of HF symptoms and increased mortality. The proposed mechanism is an increase in afterload resulting from NSAID-induced systemic vasoconstriction, which can lead to a further reduction in cardiac contractility and cardiac output. This effect is exacerbated by hyponatraemia which is a marker of advanced HF. The adjusted risk of rehospitalization for HF is significantly increased in patients on diclofenac or ibuprofen.[43] There was a dose-dependent increase in risk of death, which was highest with diclofenac (adjusted hazard ratio 2.08). Higher doses of ibuprofen (>1200 mg/day) and naproxen (>500 mg/day), but not lower doses, were also associated with an increased risk of death.

COX-2 selective inhibitors

In an attempt to overcome the gastrointestinal adverse effects of nonselective NSAIDS, COX-2 selective inhibitors were developed. Unfortunately, because of significant cardiovascular toxicity many of the agents have been withdrawn. There is an increase in ischaemic coronary events that are presumed to be due to the reduced prostacyclin production by vascular endothelium without inhibition of production of the prothrombotic platelet thromboxane A_2.

In a cohort study to assess the impact of COX-2 selective inhibitors on the incidence of HF, crude rates of hospitalization for HF per 100 patient-years of exposure were 0.9 for the controls, 2.4 for the patients treated with rofecoxib, and 1.3 for the patients treated with celecoxib.[44] Adjusting for potential confounding risk factors, the risk of hospitalization with HF was significantly higher in patients treated with rofecoxib (compared to controls), but not celecoxib. The rate of death was considered in another study that identified that there was a dose-dependent increase in risk of death that was highest with rofecoxib, celecoxib, and diclofenac.[43] A recent meta-analysis looking at both conventional NSAIDs and COX-2 selective inhibitors concluded that the risk of cardiac failure, albeit small, was similar with both types of NSAIDs and that pre-existing cardiac failure increased the risk.[45]

The current evidence therefore suggests that both selective and nonselective NSAIDs should be used with caution in patients with established HF. If new HF develops, the potential cardiovascular adverse effects of these drugs, including myocardial infarction, should be considered as a potential mechanism.

Glucocorticoids

Glucocorticoids are frequently used to achieve inflammatory control in the acute flare of arthritis. However, their use has been associated with increased rates of HF, myocardial infarction, stroke, and all-cause mortality in a dose-dependent manner.[46] The risk of HF increases with the daily dose of glucocorticoids, with a relative risk of 3.72 for prednisolone doses of 7.5 mg/day or more. Ongoing steroid use was associated with a higher risk, than intermittent courses.

Disease-modifying antirheumatic drugs

A number of disease-modifying antirheumatic drugs (DMARDs) are used to treat RA, SLE, and other inflammatory arthritides. Cardiac toxicity secondary to DMARDs is uncommon. Methotrexate is the most commonly prescribed DMARD.

Sulphasalazine is also frequently used particularly in the UK. Potential cardiac side-effects listed for these agents are pericarditis (Methotrexate and Sulphasalazine) and myocarditis (Sulphasalazine). In practice this is very uncommon. Treatment would include withdrawal of the drug and steroids if required.

Chloroquine and hydroxychloroquine have a beneficial effect on the lipid profile in SLE. However, toxicity from either agent can cause a generalized myopathy, conduction abnormalities, and rarely a cardiomyopathy. In the cardiomyopathy, the ECG shows non-specific T-wave changes, and echocardiography or invasive catheterization demonstrates a restrictive physiology.[47] Endomyocaridal biopsy may show myocyte degeneration.[48] Importantly, withdrawal of the agents achieves reversal of the HF syndrome.

Leflunomide and ciclosporin used in the management of RA and psoriatic arthritis can cause hypertension, and regular blood pressure monitoring is done for both these agents along with blood monitoring.

TNFα inhibitors

TNFα is a key agent in systemic inflammation coordinating the stimulation and release of the inflammatory cytokines (including IL-1β, IL-6, IL-8); up-regulation of endothelial adhesion molecules and chemokines; and the migration of leucocytes to targeted organs. The failing heart produces TNFα, but the normal heart does not. Clinical trials of TNFα blockers in advanced HF have been negative.[49,50]

There is ongoing debate as to whether anti-TNFα therapy, which is being used increasingly in the treatment of systemic inflammatory diseases including arthritis, affects the risk of HF in these patients.[51] The current evidence base to assess the risk include clinical trials and registry data. A German register of RA patients reported no increased risk of HF related to TNFα inhibition.[52] On the other hand, Setoguchi *et al.*[53] found an adjusted hazard ratio of 1.70 for HF hospitalization in TNFα-treated patients versus those on methotrexate. All RA patients in this cohort were aged 65 or over and therefore the risk of HF in the elderly RA patient treated with TNFα antagonist may be greater. On the other hand, TNFα antagonist therapies in RA may ameliorate the deleterious cardiac effects of circulating TNFα. A recent study demonstrated that blocking TNFα in RA patients without evident HF decreases NT-proBNP levels by around 18%, suggesting no treatment-induced deterioration in cardiac function, and a potential cardiovascular risk benefit.[54] Despite this the current recommendation is to avoid use of anti-TNFα agents in patients with HF, especially in those with NYHA classes III or IV.[55]

TNFα antagonists offer a significant advance in the management of inflammatory arthritis and so it is important that such a therapy be available to as many patients as appropriate. In patients with NYHA class I or II, TNFα antagonists can be considered but a baseline echo should be performed and careful clinical and echocardiographic follow-up should be employed. High doses of the agents should be avoided. If clinical HF symptoms develop or deteriorate then the TNFα antagonists should be stopped.

Arthritis resulting from heart failure

Gout

Gout is a clinical syndrome that results from the deposition of urate crystals in the joints. Granulocytes phagocytize the crystals and then secrete inflammatory mediators that modulate an intense inflammatory reaction, which can result in an intensely painful acute arthritis and lead to joint destruction. The inflammatory process becomes self-perpetuating with increased lactic acid production reducing the synovial fluid pH, which favours further deposition of urate crystals.[56]

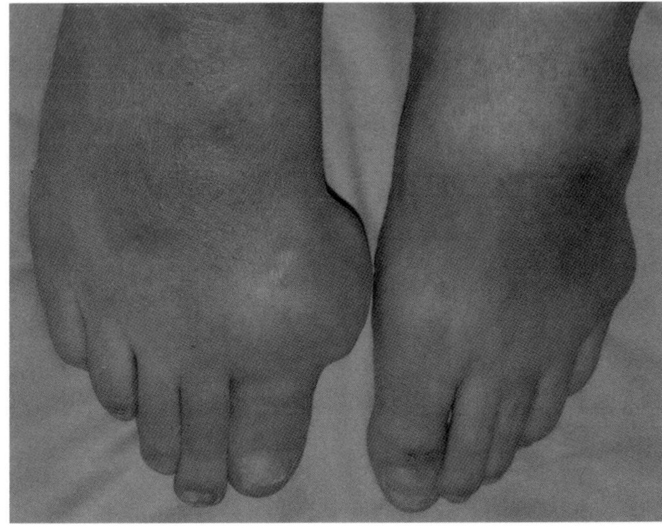

Fig. 35.7 Chronic trophaceous gout in a patient with chronic heart failure treated with loop diuretic.

The diagnosis is made by aspirating urate crystals from the joint. Serum urate levels are less helpful. Patients with acute gout can have a normal serum urate and patients with an elevated serum urate can be asymptomatic. Serum urate levels vary with age and sex, and also blood pressure, renal function, diet, and alcohol intake. However, the incidence of gouty arthritis among men with urate levels exceeding 540 μmol/L (9.0 mg/dL) is less than 5% per year.[57]

Patients with chronic HF frequently present with gout (Fig 35.7). There are multiple factors that contribute to the hyperuricaemia seen in HF. These include hypertension and hyperlipidemia, which may be key in the aetiology of the HF; chronic renal failure, which may reflect a more extensive vascular disease or be consequent to the pharmacotherapy of HF; and diuretics, which are the cornerstone in the management of fluid status of HF patients. All diuretics can cause hyperuricaemia, but loop diuretics are the most likely, then thiazide diuretics;[58] spironolactone is the least likely to cause elevated uric acid levels.[59] Diuretic-induced hyperuricaemia can be minimized by the concurrent prescription of angiotensin converting enzyme (ACE) inhibitors or an angiotensin II receptor blocker (ARB),[60,61] possibly by inhibition of the proximal sodium and urate reabsorption induced by angiotensin II.

Interestingly, serum urate concentrations correlate with maximal oxygen uptake and NYHA functional class,[62] as well as circulating markers of inflammation in patients with chronic HF.[63]

The management of gout in the context of HF can be challenging. Usually, acute gout is managed with NSAIDs. However, as discussed above, NSAIDs are detrimental in HF because of sodium and volume retention, hyperkalaemia, and renal failure. Therefore, a modified approach has been described using a combination of NSAIDs and colchicine, which facilitates the early withdrawal of the NSAID (Fig. 35.8). In the context of acute gout with HF, naproxen is probably the NSAID of choice at as low a dose as is achievable.

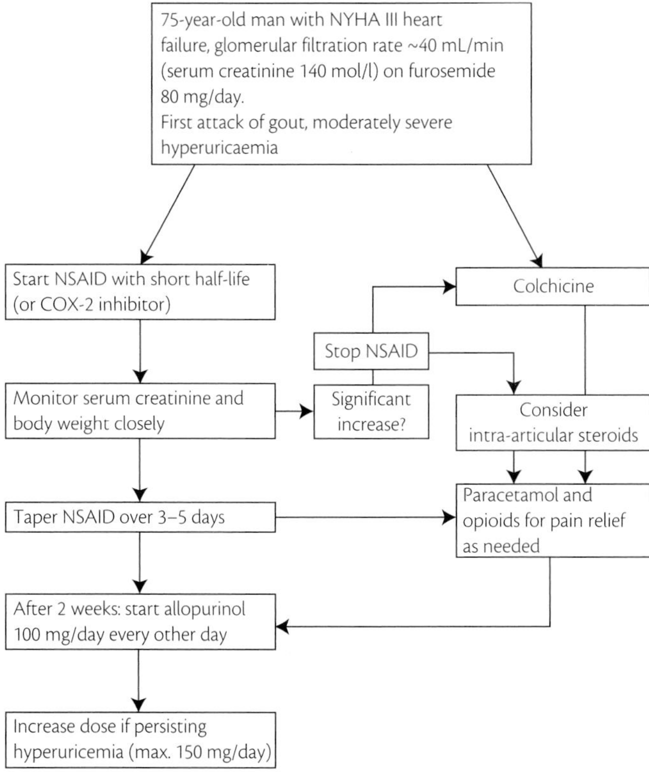

Fig. 35.8 Suggested management of acute gout in a typical heart failure patient.[68]

The use of colchicine was established as a therapy for acute gout almost 250 years ago. If given soon after the onset of symptoms, it almost invariably achieves resolution of symptoms. Colchicine is an antimitotic agent that decreases the functional activity of locally infiltrating granulocytes and inhibits the release of pro-inflammatory mediators.[64] However, the serum urate levels are unchanged. It is best used for short (3–4 day) courses to a maximum dose of 6 mg per course. It can be very effective and has the advantages that unlike NSAIDs it does not induce fluid retention or interact with warfarin. If used for longer, however, it has the almost universal side effects of diarrhoea and vomiting.

Glucocorticoids can be used in acute gout both as anti-inflammatory agents and to reduce the serum urate concentration. Oral glucocorticoids are problematic in HF because of the mineralocorticoid effect of fluid retention. However, local joint aspiration and then injection with glucocorticoid targets the site of inflammation and reduces the systemic dose, as well as relieving the tense hot swollen joint by removing some of the synovial fluid. This is a particularly useful adjuvant in patients who are struggling with painful acute gout despite NSAID and colchicine.

In the longer term the serum urate level should be addressed. Patient education about diet modification, reducing the amount of meat, pulses, and alcohol, is important but usually fails to achieve adequate urate reduction. Therefore, pharmacological modification should be considered. This should be cautiously introduced 2 weeks after the acute episode and then up-titrated over the following weeks to reduce the likelihood of a further acute attack. Two classes of drugs are available in the management of hyperuricaemia: uricosuric agents (e.g. probenicid) and xanthine oxidase inhibitors (allopurinol). Allopurinol is the agent of choice and inhibits the synthesis of uric acid. The dose of allopurinol is titrated up from a starting dose of 100 mg/day by 100 mg increments to achieve a serum urate level below 0.3 mmol/L. The dose of allopurinol needs to be modified if renal failure coexists or develops. An additional potential benefit of allopurinol is its effect in reducing oxidative stress by inhibiting xanthine oxidase in the vascular endothelium, and thus preventing the formation of superoxide free radicals. In patients with HF, allopurinol has been shown to reduce markers of oxidative stress and improve endothelium-dependent vasodilatation.[65] There are also studies demonstrating that allopurinol improves left ventricular efficiency[66] and reverses ventricular remodelling.[67]

Pseudogout

The term 'pseudogout' describes an acute synovitis precipitated by calcium pyrophosphate dihydrate (CPPD) crystal deposition in joints. Clinically such an episode resembles gout caused by urate crystal deposition. The diagnosis of pseudogout is achieved by aspiration of the affected joint, and demonstration of positively birefringent CPPD crystals by polarized light microscopy.

The management of an acute episode of pseudogout is similar to gout, with NSAID and colchicine being the first-line agents and then local glucocorticoid if required. Long-term prophylaxis is different from that of gout. There are several reports of patients suffering recurrent attacks of pseudogout successfully treated using colchicine 0.6 mg twice daily as oral prophylaxis.[69]

The importance of pseudogout in the context of HF is that it may reveal the underlying cause of HF. The majority of cases of CPPD crystal deposition are idiopathic, and it is more common in elderly people (mean age at symptomatic presentation is 72 years). However, CPPD crystal deposition is associated with several metabolic and endocrine conditions that may cause symptoms from the crystal deposition at a younger age, the best-characterized of which is haemachromatosis. The other accepted association of relevance is hypothyroidism. Both of these conditions may offer a reversible cause of HF.[70]

Investigations

In the assessment of patients with HF and arthritis there are several possible presentations:

Established heart failure with new presentation of arthritis

The onset of arthritis in patients with HF may be the evolution of an incidental arthritis, or a complication of the aetiology of, or pharmacotherapy for, HF.

Established arthritis with asymptomatic left ventricular systolic dysfunction

At present, there is no evidence to support screening the asymptomatic patient for evidence of cardiac dysfunction. However, there is a role for risk assessment with the established risk models. The recent European League Against Rheumatism (EULAR) recommendations state:

> Annual cardiovascular risk assessment using national guidelines is recommended for all patients with RA and should be considered for all patients with ankylosing spondylitis and psoriatic arthropathy. Any cardiovascular risk factors identified should be managed according to local guidelines. If no local guidelines are available, cardiovascular risk

management should be carried out according to the SCORE function. In addition to appropriate cardiovascular risk management, aggressive suppression of the inflammatory process is recommended to further lower the cardiovascular risk.[11]

Established arthritis with new-onset heart failure

New-onset HF may be the first manifestation of incidental heart disease, or it may be either a consequence of the arthritic process, or the result of pharmacotherapy. The cause of the HF may be myocardial, pericardial, valvular, rhythm, or coronary artery related. Irrespective of the presentation, the assessment is similar. As usual, detailed history taking and clinical examination may provide many of the clues. Investigations may then include:

- Blood tests targeted to identify the aetiology of the clinical presentation. Anaemia is a common finding in chronic diseases, including HF and arthritis. In acute HF or decompensated HF it may be appropriate to treat this anaemia.
- ECG, which may document rhythm abnormalities or ST-T or T wave abnormalities.
- Chest radiograph, which may demonstrate whether there is cardiomegaly or lung changes.
- Echocardiogram.

In some cases further assessment is appropriate, such as CMR or invasive investigation. For example, the distinction between constrictive pericarditis and restrictive cardiomyopathy often requires cardiac catheterization with simultaneous right and left heart pressures. Cardiac biopsy can provide tissue to identify potentially treatable causes such as antimalarial-induced cardiomyopathy.

Management options

Heart failure

The management of HF in patients with arthritis is similar to that in the general population. There is some evidence that inhibition of angiotensin II with ACE inhibitors or ARBs is associated with benefit in reducing the systemic inflammation.[71] Caution should be used in the prescription of diuretics in patients with HF, as acute gout may be precipitated. Statin therapy is indicated by the risk of coronary heart disease, not by absolute cholesterol levels. Risk is estimated using national risk tables (multiplied by 1.7 to account for the increased vascular risk associated with RA and SLE, and probably ankylosing spondylitis).[8,11]

Arthritis

The management of arthritis in the presence of established HF can be challenging. As discussed previously, TNF inhibition, glucocorticoids, and both selective and nonselective NSAIDs are associated with deterioration of HF status. These agents should therefore be avoided whenever possible. If they are introduced, patients should be advised of symptoms to recognize and report. If symptoms develop, the agent should be withdrawn: in the case of chronic glucocorticoid therapy this will require down-titration and gradual withdrawal. Each patient requires individualized care. If arthritis control is poor despite conventional therapies, TNF inhibition may be considered and cautiously introduced. It may even improve cardiac status.

Summary

The interactions between HF and arthritis are complex. With an ageing population, it is becoming more common to have patients whose lives are limited by both conditions. Teasing apart the cause and effect of the disease processes and the impact of the various therapies can be challenging. However, as the trend towards earlier disease recognition and more aggressive management of both HF and arthritis persists, hopefully the negative impact of each condition on the other will be attenuated. In both HF and arthritis there are also significant physical and psychological benefits achievable by maintaining the patient's physical activity and independence.

References

1. Wolfe F, Freundlich B, Straus WL. Increase in cardiovascular and cerebrovascular disease prevalence in rheumatoid arthritis. *J Rheumatol* 2003;**30**:36–40.
2. Nicola PJ, Crowson CS, Maradit-Kremers H, *et al.* Contribution of congestive heart failure and ischemic heart disease to excess mortality in rheumatoid arthritis. *Arthritis Rheum* 2006;**54**:60–7.
3. Bayles TB. Rheumatoid arthritis and rheumatic heart disease in autopsied cases. *Ann Intern Med* 1943;**19**:113–14.
4. Isomäki HA, Mutru O, Koota K. Death rate and causes of death in patients with rheumatoid arthritis. *Scand J Rheumatol.* 1975;**4**:205–8.
5. Wolfe F and Michaud K. Heart failure in rheumatoid arthritis: rates, predictors, and the effect of anti–tumor necrosis factor therapy. *Am J Med* 2004;**116**:305–11.
6. Davis JM, Roger VL, Crowson CS, Kremers HM, Therneau TM, Gabriel SE. The presentation and outcome of heart failure in persons with rheumatoid arthritis differs from that of the general population. *Arthritis Rheum* 2008;**58**:2603–11.
7. van Doornum S, McColl G, Wicks IP. Accelerated atherosclerosis: an extra-articular feature of rheumatoid arthritis? *Arthritis Rheum* 2002;**46**:862–73.
8. Sattar N, McInnes IB. Vascular comorbidity in rheumatoid arthritis: potential mechanisms and solutions. *Curr Opin Rheum* 2005;**17**:286–92.
9. Avina-Zubieta JA, Choi HK, Sadatsafavi M, Etminan M, Esdaile JM, Lacaille D. Risk of cardiovascular mortality in patients with rheumatoid arthritis: a meta-analysis of observational studies. *Arthritis Rheum* 2008;**59**:1690–7.
10. Maradit-Kremers H, Crowson CS, Nicola PJ, *et al.* Increased unrecognized coronary heart disease and sudden deaths in rheumatoid arthritis:a population-based cohort study. *Arthritis Rheum* 2005;**52**(2):402–11.
11. Peters MJL, Symmons DPM, McCarey D, *et al.* EULAR evidence-based recommendations for cardiovascular risk management in patients with rheumatoid arthritis and other forms of inflammatory arthritis. *Ann Rheum Dis* 2010;**69**:325–31.
12. Munro R, Morrison E, McDonald AG, Hunter JA, Madhok R, Capell HA. Effect of disease modifying agents on the lipid profiles of patients with rheumatoid arthritis. *Ann Rheum Dis* 1997;**56**:374–7.
13. McCarey DW, McInnes IB, Madhok R, *et al.* Trial of Atorvastatin in Rheumatoid Arthritis (TARA): double-blind,randomised placebo-controlled trial. *Lancet* 2004;**363**:2015–21.
14. Mathur N, Ramasubbu K, Mann DL. Spectrum of pleiotropic effects of statins in heart failure. *Heart Fail Clin* 2008;**4**:153–61.
15. Jain MK, Ridker PM. Anti-inflammatory effects of statins: clinical evidence and basic mechanisms. *Nat Rev Drug Discov* 2005;**4**:977–87.
16. Laufs U, La Fata V, Plutzky J, Liao JK. Upregulation of endothelial nitric oxide synthase by HMG CoA reductase inhibitors. *Circulation* 1998;**97**:1129–35.
17. Dilaveris P, Giannopoulos G, Riga M, Synetos A, Stefanadis C. Beneficial effects of statins on endothelial dysfunction and vascular stiffness. *Curr Vasc Pharmacol* 2007;**5**:227–37.

18. Levantesi G, Scarano M, Marfisi R, *et al.* Meta-analysis of effect of statin treatment on risk of sudden death. *Am J Cardiol* 2007;**100**:1644–50.
19. Pearce DJ, Morrison AE, Higgins KB, *et al.* The comorbid state of psoriasis patients in a university dermatology practice. *J Dermatol Treat* 2005;**16**:319–23.
20. Neimann AL, Shin DB, Wang X, Margolis DJ, Troxel AB, Gelfand JM. Prevalence of cardiovascular risk factors in patients with psoriasis. *J Am Acad Dermatol* 2006;**55**:829–35.
21. Gelfand JM, Neimann AL, Shin DB, Wang X, Margolis DJ, Troxel AB. Risk of myocardial infarction in patients with psoriasis. *JAMA* 2006;**296**:1735–41.
22. Kimball AB, Guerin A, Latremouille-Viau D, *et al.* Coronary heart disease and stroke risk in patients with psoriasis: retrospective analysis. *Am J Med* 2010;**123**:350–357.
23. Wakkee M, Herings RM, Nijsten T. Psoriasis may not be an independent risk factor for acute ischemic heart disease hospitalizations: results of a large population-based Dutch cohort. *J Invest Dermatol* 2010;**130**:962–7.
24. del Rincón ID, Williams K, Stern MP, Freeman GL, Escalante A. High incidence of cardiovascular events in a rheumatoid arthritis cohort not explained by traditional cardiac risk factors. *Arthritis Rheum* 2001;**44**:2737–2745.
25. Sattar N, McCarey DW, Capell H and McInnes IB. Explaining how 'high-grade' systemic inflammation accelerates vascular risk in rheumatoid arthritis. *Circulation* 2003;**108**:2957–963.
26. Feldman AM, Combes A, Wagner D, *et al.* The role of tumor necrosis factor in the pathophysiology of heart failure. *J Am Coll Cardiol* 2000;**35**:537–44.
27. Torre-Amione G, Kapadia S, Benedict C, Oral H, Young JB, Mann DL. Proinflammatory cytokine levels in patients with depressed left ventricular ejection fraction: a report from the Studies of Left Ventricular Dysfunction (SOLVD). *J Am Coll Cardiol* 1996;**27**:1201–6.
28. Deswal A, Petersen NJ, Feldman AM, Young JB, White BG, Mann DL. Cytokines and cytokine receptors in advanced heart failure: an analysis of the cytokine database from the Vesnarinone trial (VEST). *Circulation* 2001;**103**:2055–9.
29. Danilaa MI, Patkara NM, Curtisa JR, Saaga KG, Teng GG. Biologics and heart failure in rheumatoid arthritis:are we any wiser? *Curr Opin Rheumatol* 2008;**20**:327–333.
30. Giles JT, Malayeri AA, Fernandes V, *et al.* Left ventricular structure and function in patients with rheumatoid arthritis, as assessed by cardiac magnetic resonance imaging. *Arthritis Rheum* 62;**2010**:940–51.
31. Mandell BF. Cardiovascular involvement in systemic lupus erythematosus. *Semin Arthritis Rheum* 1987;**17**:126–41.
32. Apte M, McGwin G Jr, Vila LM, Kaslow RA, Alarcon GS, Reveille JD. Associated factors and impact of myocarditis in patients with SLE from LUMINA, a multiethnic US cohort (LV). *Rheumatology (Oxford)* 2008;**47**:362–7.
33. Guillevin L, Durand-Gasselin B, Cevallos R, *et al.* Microscopic polyangiitis: clinical and laboratory findings in eight-five patients. *Arthritis Rheum* 1999;**42** (3):421.
34. Maione S, Valentini G, Giunta A, *et al.* Cardiac involvement in rheumatoid arthritis: an echocardiographic study. *Cardiology* 1993;**83**:234–9.
35. Gonzalez-Juanatey C, Testa A, Garcia-Castelo A, *et al.* Echocardiographic and Doppler findings in long-term treated rheumatoid arthritis patients without clinically evident cardiovascular disease. *Semin Arthritis Rheum* 2004;**33**:231.
36. Di Franco M, Paradiso M, Mammarella A, *et al.* Diastolic function abnormalities in rheumatoid arthritis. Evaluation By echo Doppler transmitral flow and pulmonary venous flow: relation with duration of disease. *Ann Rheum Dis* 2000;**59**:227.
37. Wislowska M, Deren D, Kochmanski M, Sypula S, Rozbicka J. Systolic and diastolic heart function in SLE patients. *Rheum Int* 2009;**29**:1469–76.
38. Okuda Y, Takasugi K, Oyama T, Onuma M, Oyama H. ([Amyloidosis in rheumatoid arthritis—clinical study of 124 histologically proven cases]. *Ryumachi* 1994;**34**:939–46.
39. Lachmann HJ, Goodman HJB, Gilbertson JA, *et al.* Natural history and outcome in systemic AA amyloidosis. *N Engl J Med* 2007;**356**:2361–71.
40. Catella-Lawson F, Reilly MP, Kapoor SC, *et al.* Cyclooxygenase inhibitors and the antiplatelet effects of aspirin. *N Engl J Med* 2001;**345**:1809–17.
41. Capone ML, Sciulli MG, Tacconelli S, *et al.* Pharmacodynamic interaction of naproxen with low-dose aspirin in healthy subjects. *J Am Coll Cardiol* 2005;**458**:1295–301.
42. Feenstra J, Heerdink ER, Grobbee DE, Stricker BH. Association of nonsteroidal anti-inflammatory drugs with first occurrence of heart failure and with relapsing heart failure:the Rotterdam Study. *Arch Intern Med* 2002;**162**:265–70.
43. Gislason GH, Rasmussen JN, Abildstrom SZ, *et al.* Increased mortality and cardiovascular morbidity associated with use of nonsteroidal anti-inflammatory drugs in chronic heart failure. *Arch Intern Med* 2009;**169**:141–9.
44. Mamdani M, Juurlink DN, Lee DS, *et al.* Cyclo-oxygenase-2 inhibitors versus non-selective non-steroidal anti-inflammatory drugs and congestive heart failure outcomes in elderly patients:a population-based cohort study. *Lancet* 2004;**363**:1751–6.
45. Scott PA, Kingsley GH, Scott DL. Non-steroidal anti-inflammatory drugs and cardiac failure: meta analyses of observational studies and randomised controlled trials. *Eur J Heart Fail* 2008;**10**:1102–7.
46. Wei L, MacDonald TM, Walker BR. Taking glucocorticoids by prescription is associated with subsequent cardiovascular disease. *Ann Intern Med* 2004;**141**:764–70.
47. Iglesias Cubero G, Rodriguez Reguero JJ, Rojo Ortega JM. Restrictive cardiomyopathy caused by chloroquine. *Br Heart J* 1993;**69**:451–2.
48. Ratliff, NB, Estes, ML, Myles, JL, Shirey EK, McMahon JT. Diagnosis of chloroquine cardiomyopathy by endomyocardial biopsy. *N Engl J Med* 1987;**316**:191–3.
49. Mann DL, McMurray JJ, Packer M, *et al.* Targeted anticytokine therapy in patients with chronic heart failure: results of the Randomized Etanercept Worldwide Evaluation (RENEWAL). *Circulation* 2004;**109**:1594–602.
50. Chung ES, Packer M, Lo KH, Fasanmade AA, Willerson JT. Randomized, double-blind, placebo-controlled, pilot trial of infliximab, a chimeric monoclonal antibody to tumor necrosis factor-alpha, in patients with moderate-to-severe heart failure: results of the anti-TNF Therapy Against Congestive Heart Failure (ATTACH) trial. *Circulation* 2003;**107**:3133–40.
51. Wolfe F, Michaud K. Heart failure in rheumatoid arthritis: rates, predictors, and the effect of anti–tumor necrosis factor therapy. *Am J Med* 2004;**116**:305–11.
52. Listing J, Strangfeld A, Kekow J, *et al.* Does tumour necrosis factor alpha inhibition promote or prevent heart failure in patients with rheumatoid arthritis? *Arthritis Rheum* 2008;**58**:667–77.
53. Setoguchi S, Schneeweiss S, Avorn J, Katz JN, Weinblatt ME, Levin R, Soloman DH. Tumour necrosis factor-alpha antagonist use and heart failure in elderly patients with rheumatoid arthritis. *Am Heart J* 2008;**156**:336–41.
54. Peters MJ, Welsh P, McInnes IB, Wolbink G, Dijkmans BA, Sattar N, Nurmohamed MT. Tumour necrosis factor α blockade reduces circulating N-terminal pro-brain natriuretic peptide levels in patients with active rheumatoid arthritis: results from a prospective cohort study. *Ann Rheum Dis* 2010;**69**(7):1281–5.

55. Danilaa MI, Patkara NM, Curtisa JR, Saaga KG, Teng GG. Biologics and heart failure in rheumatoid arthritis: are we any wiser? *Curr Opin Rheumatol* 2008;**20**:327–333.
56. Spieker LE, Ruschitzka FT, Luscher TF, Noll G. The management of hyperuricemia and gout in patients with heart failure. *Eur J Heart Fail* 2002;**4**:403–10.
57. Lin KC, Lin HY, Chou P. The interaction between uric acid level and other risk factors on the development of gout among asymptomatic hyperuricemic men in a prospective study. *J Rheumatol* 2000;**27**:1501–5.
58. Waller PC, Ramsay LE. Predicting acute gout in diuretic-treated hypertensive patients. *J Hum Hypertens* 1989;**3**:457–61.
59. Schrijver G, Weinberger MH. Hydrochlorothiazide and spironolactone in hypertension. *Clin Pharmacol Ther* 1979;**25**:33–42.
60. Weinberger MH. Influence of an angiotensin converting enzyme inhibitor on diuretic-induced metabolic effects in hypertension. *Hypertension* 1983;**5**:III132.
61. Shahinfar S, Simpson RL, Carides AD, *et al.* Safety of losartan in hypertensive patients with thiazide-induced hyperuricaemia. *Kidney Int* 1999;**56**:1879–85.
62. Leyva F, Anker S, Swan JW, Godsland IF, Wingrove CS, Chua TP, Stevenson JC, Coats AJ. Serum uric acid as an index of impaired oxidative metabolism in chronic heart failure. *Eur Heart J* 1997;**18**:858–65.
63. Leyva F, Anker SD, Godsland IF, *et al.* Uric acid in chronic heart failure: a marker of chronic inflammation. *Eur Heart J* 1998;**19**:1814–22.
64. Spilberg I, Mandell B, Mehta J, Simchowitz L, Rosenberg D. Mechanism of action of colchicine in acute urate crystal induced arthritis. *J Clin Invest* 1979;**64**:775–80.
65. Farquharson CA, Butler R, Hill A, Belch JJ, Struthers AD. Allopurinol improves endothelial dysfunction in chronic heart failure. *Circulation* 2002;**106**:221–6.
66. Cappola TP, Kass DA, Nelson GS, *et al.* Allopurinol improves myocardial efficiency in patients with idiopathic dilated cardiomyopathy. *Circulation* 2001;**104**:2407–11.
67. Minhas KM, Saraiva RM, Schuleri KH, *et al.* Xanthine oxide reductase inhibition causes reverse remodelling in rats with dilated cardiomyopathy. *Circ Res* 2006;**98**:271–9.
68. Spieker LE, Ruschitzka FT, Luscher TF, Noll G. The management of hyperuricemia and gout in patients with heart failure. *Eur J Heart Fail* 2002;**4**:403–10.
69. Alvarellos, A, Spilberg, I. Colchicine prophylaxis in pseudogout. *J Rheumatol* 1986;**13**:804–5.
70. Jones, AC, Chuck, AJ, Arie, EA, Green DJ, Doherty M. Diseases associated with calcium pyrophosphate deposition disease. *Semin Arthritis Rheum* 1992;**22**:188–202.
71. Perry ME, Chee MM, Ferrell WR, Lockhart JC, Sturrock RD. Angiotensin receptor blockers reduce erythrocyte sedimentation rate levels in patients with rheumatoid arthritis. *Ann Rheum Dis* 2008;**67**:1646–7.[25]

36

Arrhythmias

Ashley M. Nisbet and Derek T. Connelly

Introduction

Both atrial and ventricular arrhythmias are common in patients with heart failure (HF), regardless of the underlying aetiology. Arrhythmias contribute significantly to symptoms, and lead to an increase in morbidity and mortality. In particular, ventricular arrhythmias can cause sudden cardiac death (SCD). Therefore, the diagnosis and treatment of arrhythmias is an important element in the clinical management of patients with HF.

Atrial fibrillation in heart failure

Epidemiology

Atrial fibrillation (AF) and HF are common and often coexist. They have been called the 'two new epidemics of cardiovascular disease'[1] and the burden of each is growing as the population ages, with the incidence of both doubling for each successive decade of age. AF is estimated to occur in 15–30% of patients with HF, with the prevalence increasing with advancing New York Heart Association (NYHA) class (Fig. 36.1): 4–15% in NYHA I–III,[2–4] rising to 25–50% in patients with NYHA class III–IV symptoms.[5–7]

The association of AF and HF relates, in part, to the similar disease processes that predispose to each condition.[8] These include hypertension, coronary artery disease, valvular heart disease, and diabetes mellitus. Furthermore, there is a propensity for AF in patients with structural abnormalities commonly found in patients with HF, such as left atrial enlargement, left ventricular hypertrophy, left ventricular dilatation, and left ventricular systolic dysfunction (LVSD).[9]

Haemodynamic consequences

AF is associated with adverse haemodynamic consequences, which may exacerbate HF.[10] The reduction in cardiac output often seen with the onset of AF is multifactorial. In particular, the loss of atrioventricular synchrony impairs diastolic filling of the left ventricle, reducing stroke volume, as well as increasing mean atrial diastolic pressure, further contributing to atrial enlargement and perpetuating the substrate for the arrhythmia. The irregular ventricular rate and rapid ventricular response in AF also contribute to the adverse haemodynamics by decreasing cardiac output, increasing right atrial pressure, and elevating pulmonary artery capillary wedge pressure irrespective of heart rate. This impairs volume homeostasis and thus exacerbates fluid retention, which ultimately further elevates filling pressures. Furthermore, the presence of mitral regurgitation results in left atrial volume and pressure overload, resulting in dilatation providing the substrate for the development of AF, which then perpetuates the problem by further increasing left atrial pressures.

Electrophysiological consequences

There is evidence that cellular electrophysiological remodelling in HF predisposes to AF. Volume and pressure overload in the atria result in stretch-induced reductions in atrial myocyte refractory periods, reduced conduction velocity, and increased triggered activity.[11] This increases automaticity and heterogeneity of depolarization and repolarization within the atria resulting in an environment able to initiate and sustain spontaneous re-entrant atrial arrhythmias. In HF, there is a reduction in atrial myoctye L-type calcium current, and this can both contribute to AF and occur as a result of AF.[12]

Neurohormonal alterations in HF, such as activation of the renin–angiotensin–aldosterone system, result in extracellular matrix fibrosis.[13] Atrial fibrosis results in further areas of slow conduction, again predisposing to AF. Furthermore, alterations in connexin expression and activity have been observed in rapid pacing models of AF.[14] The resultant changes in atrial conducting properties contribute to the maintenance of the arrhythmia.

Effect on mortality and prognosis

The presence of AF is associated with an increased mortality regardless of age or gender, with a 50–90% increased risk of death observed in the Framingham Heart Study.[15–16] The coexistence of AF and HF is associated with an increased risk of mortality and HF progression. In a retrospective review of the SOLVD trials, the

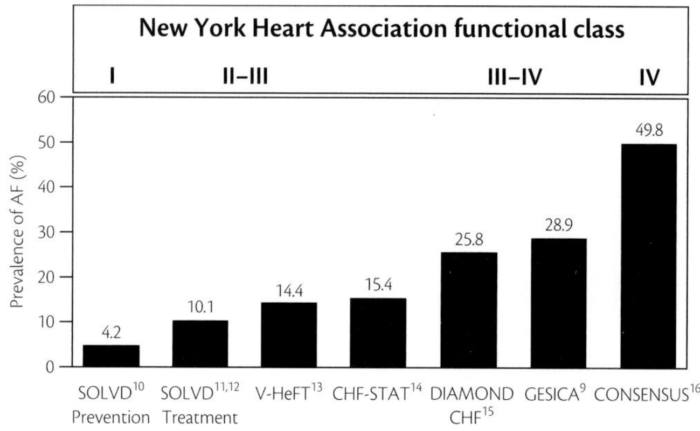

Fig. 36.1 Prevalence of atrial fibrillation with NYHA class.
From Maisel WH, Stevenson LW. Atrial fibrillation in heart failure: epidemiology, pathophysiology, and rationale for therapy. *Am J Cardiol* 2003;**91**(6A):2D–8D.

increase in all-cause mortality occurred in the presence of both symptomatic and asymptomatic LVSD, and resulted from an increased risk of pump-failure death.[2] Furthermore, AF was also associated with an increased risk of the composite endpoint of death from any cause or hospitalization for worsening HF. This confirmed the findings of earlier studies of the negative prognostic effect of AF in HF. However, there has been some debate over the years about this issue, with some studies suggesting the coincidence of AF in HF may be neutral[3] or indeed beneficial.[17] The reasons for the apparent beneficial effect of AF in HF are not clear. It may be a spurious effect as a consequence of underestimation of the left ventricular ejection fraction (LVEF) while in AF with a rapid ventricular response, with a resultant improvement of a greater magnitude compared with the absence of AF. Alternatively, if the LVSD is a consequence of the tachycardia (sometimes known as a tachycardiomyopathy), effective treatment of the arrhythmia would result in an improvement in LVEF and a better outcome.

In the V-HEFT trials, the presence of AF at baseline was not related to either all-cause mortality or sudden death.[3] The disparities in the findings of these studies were addressed using the Framingham Heart Study population,[15] which addressed the temporal relationship of AF and HF and their joint effect on mortality. In individuals who developed AF or HF during the study period, the subsequent onset of the other condition was associated with an increase in mortality.

The mechanism by which AF results in an increase in mortality is not clear. The presence of AF in HF may simply be a marker of the severity of the left ventricular dysfunction. The presence of paroxysmal AF may reflect underlying sinus node disease, and this population may be predisposed to an increased risk of fatal bradyarrhythmias. Furthermore, the increase in mortality in HF with AF may reflect an increase in fatal thromboembolic events.

Aims of treatment of atrial fibrillation in heart failure

The adverse haemodynamic and prognostic effects of AF in HF underpin the rationale for treatment. The reduction in cardiac output and exercise capacity in individuals with HF and AF would suggest that restoration of sinus rhythm should be the target of treatment, but there is currently little evidence in favour of this strategy. The AF-CHF study showed no mortality benefit from a rhythm control versus a rate control strategy in HF patients.[18] Overall the aim of treatment of AF in HF is to improve symptoms and quality of life, to improve prognosis if possible, and reduce the risk of thromboembolic complications. This may be by either the restoration and maintenance of sinus rhythm, or control of ventricular rate, and anticoagulation.

Rhythm control

The maintenance of sinus rhythm may be achieved by means of direct current cardioversion and/or the use of antiarrhythmic drugs. The rationale for this 'rhythm control' approach includes the possibility of fewer symptoms, better exercise tolerance, a lower risk of stroke, eventual discontinuation of long-term anticoagulant therapy, and better quality of life if sinus rhythm can be maintained. However, the recent AF-CHF study has failed to demonstrate any survival benefit from adopting a rhythm control strategy in AF in the context of HF. Furthermore, AF is often poorly responsive to antiarrhythmic drugs, which may also have serious adverse effects. Class I antiarrhythmic drugs are proarrhythmic and therefore contraindicated in the presence of HF. If a rhythm control strategy is adopted, the first-line antiarrhythmic drug is amiodarone, with sotalol or dofetilide suitable alternatives. However, in both AFFIRM[19] and AF-CHF,[18] a rhythm control strategy resulted in more frequent hospitalizations, whether for recurrence of AF, repeat cardioversions, or bradyarrhythmias.

A further strategy for restoration of sinus rhythm is catheter ablation of AF via pulmonary vein isolation (PVI), with or without more extensive left atrial ablation. Several studies have shown that this is an effective method of restoring sinus rhythm with success rates of 50–70%, with possible improvements in LVEF with restoration of sinus rhythm, as well as improvement in symptoms and quality of life scores.[20–22] Furthermore, the PABA-CHF study showed that PVI for AF was superior to atrioventricular (AV) node ablation and biventricular pacing in improving LVEF and symptoms in HF patients.[22] However, this procedure is technically challenging in patients with HF and may be associated with an increased risk of complications such as thromboembolism and cardiac tamponade.

Rate control

A strategy of controlling the ventricular rate in AF via the use of AV nodal blocking drugs may be desirable in HF. Drugs used to control the ventricular rate may be less toxic than antiarrhythmic agents used to restore or maintain sinus rhythm, although in HF some commonly used agents may be contraindicated. Calcium channel blockers should be avoided in the context of HF as a result of their negative inotropic effects, which may result in hospital admissions for worsening HF. First-line therapy for rate control in AF in the context of LVSD should be β-blocker (if no evidence of decompensation), plus or minus digoxin if required. The therapeutic target should be control of the ventricular rate to not more than 80 beats/min at rest and 110 beats/min during exercise.

An alternative to drug therapy for ventricular rate control is ablation of the AV node and permanent pacemaker implantation.[23] This strategy may be appropriate if drug therapy is ineffective or poorly tolerated. The use of biventricular pacemakers has been found to be superior to right ventricular pacing.[24] However, there is a lack of clinical trial evidence for the use of these devices in the presence of AF, and therefore this is not included in the NICE or ESC guidelines for cardiac resynchronization therapy (CRT) device implantation at present.[25]

Anticoagulation

Patients with AF are at increased risk of thromboembolic events. This risk is further increased in the presence of LVSD—the risk of stroke is 2.5 times greater in a patient with moderate-to-severe left ventricular dysfunction.[16] In order to reduce the risk of thromboembolic complications, warfarin is recommended (target INR range 2.0–3.0), whether AF is persistent or paroxysmal. Warfarin does have a number of limitations, however: there is a very narrow therapeutic window, and, at the high end of the therapeutic range, there is a significantly increased risk of intracranial bleeding; it has a slow onset of action; there is significant genetic variation in the response to the drug, and some individuals are resistant to its effects. Furthermore, there are multiple food and drug interactions. Dabigatran is a new oral direct thrombin inhibitor which is as effective as warfarin in reducing the risk of thromboembolic events in AF.[26] It does not require regular INR monitoring and is associated with a reduced risk of bleeding complications in effective doses comparable to warfarin. However, dabigatran is not yet licensed for use.

Atrial flutter

Atrial flutter is a common supraventricular tachyarrhythmia encountered in HF patients. It is a macro re-entrant arrhythmia, in either the right (typical atrial flutter) or left (atypical atrial flutter) atrium. It is typically initiated by a premature impulse within the atrium, and propagated as a result of differences in the conduction properties and refractory periods of the atrial tissue. The atrial rate in atrial flutter is typically between 240 and 350/minute.

In typical atrial flutter, the macro re-entrant circuit is confined to the right atrium. The wavefront can occur in either a clockwise or counter-clockwise direction around the right atrium. The activation wavefront emerges from a zone of slow conduction between the tricuspid valve annulus and the os of the coronary sinus and then, in the case of counter-clockwise flutter, ascends the interatrial septum, spreads to the posterior right atrium, and then downwards and laterally between the tricuspid valve and crista terminalis. The wavefront then crosses via an isthmus between the inferior vena cava and the tricuspid valve annulus. This isthmus is the target for radiofrequency ablation, to create a line of functional conduction block in the circuit, terminating and preventing recurrence of the tachycardia.

Treatment of atrial flutter

The treatment goals in atrial flutter are essentially the same as those of AF: either rate or rhythm control, and anticoagulation. In atrial flutter, the re-entrant nature of the arrhythmia makes it more readily amenable to catheter ablation and this is an effective treatment, even in the HF population. Radiofrequency ablation for atrial flutter has a high long-term success rate (around 90%), and patients with HF and atrial flutter should be prioritized for this treatment, particularly if they have recurrent atrial flutter despite antiarrhythmic drug therapy.

Atypical or left atrial flutter is much less common. It may occur as a complication of radiofrequency ablation in the left atrium for AF. It can be difficult to control with antiarrhythmic drugs. Radiofrequency ablation of the left atrial circuit is feasible, but tends to be technically more challenging than ablation for right atrial flutter, with a lower success rate.

Tachycardiomyopathy

Tachycardiomyopathy is a rare but potentially curable cause of HF (see Chapter 4). However, arrhythmias are frequently a consequence of HF and can therefore be easily overlooked as the potential cause. Incessant AF, ectopic atrial tachycardia, atrial flutter, AV re-entrant tachycardia, AV nodal re-entrant tachycardia, atrial flutter, and ventricular tachycardia have all been shown to cause tachycardiomyopathy. In cases of tachycardiomyopathy, the eventual recognition and treatment of the tachyarrhythmia can lead to complete resolution of the cardiomyopathy.[27–29] This diagnosis should be considered in patients with HF and persistent tachycardia, particularly when the tachycardia persists despite β-blocker therapy. Careful and expert analysis of the ECG is required, since some atrial tachycardias may be very difficult to distinguish from sinus tachycardia (Fig. 36.2).

Ventricular arrhythmias

Prevalence and effect on mortality

Despite recent advances in the treatment of chronic HF, mortality remains high, and sudden arrhythmic death is accepted to be the cause in around 40% of cases. Of these, approximately 80% appear secondary to ventricular tachyarrhythmias.[30] HF patients with a high prevalence of ventricular arrhythmias, including complex ventricular premature beats, nonsustained VT (NSVT), and sustained VT appear to be at a higher risk of death.[31] In the GESICA study,[6] ventricular couplets were found in 59% of the population and in over 90% of the patients with NSVT. Couplets and/or NSVT were detected in 62.7% of the study population, with a 50.8% mortality rate. The remaining 37.3% without couplets had a lower mortality rate of 26.3%. The presence of ventricular premature complexes constituted a significant marker of sudden death, with a sensitivity and specificity of 89% and 42% respectively. Furthermore, the negative predictive value was 95.5%. The incidence of NSVT in HF is 28–80%. The GESICA-GEMA study[32] concluded that the presence of NSVT correlates with total mortality, with a persistent increased risk of 1.63 after adjustment with other variables. However, NSVT was also associated with higher doses of diuretic therapy, lower systolic blood pressure, higher creatinine levels, and faster heart rates, all of which tend to indicate an association between the presence of NSVT and worsening of clinical status. In the UK-HEART study,[33] the presence of NSVT was associated with a twofold increase in the risk of sudden death, particularly in the presence of left ventricular dilatation. Therefore it is unclear whether the presence of ventricular arrhythmias confers an increased mortality risk *per se* or is simply indicative of worse left ventricular systolic function.

Mechanisms and pathogenesis of ventricular arrhythmias in heart failure

Multiple factors are responsible for the initiation and maintenance of ventricular arrhythmias in HF (see Table 36.1). The mechanisms differ with aetiology, although re-entry, which is thought to be responsible for most ventricular arrhythmias, is common to both ischaemic and nonischaemic aetiologies. Furthermore, HF is often characterized by ventricular hypertrophy, which manifests as an increase in left ventricular mass, cellular hypertrophy, alterations in cellular ionic currents, and changes in the histological features of the

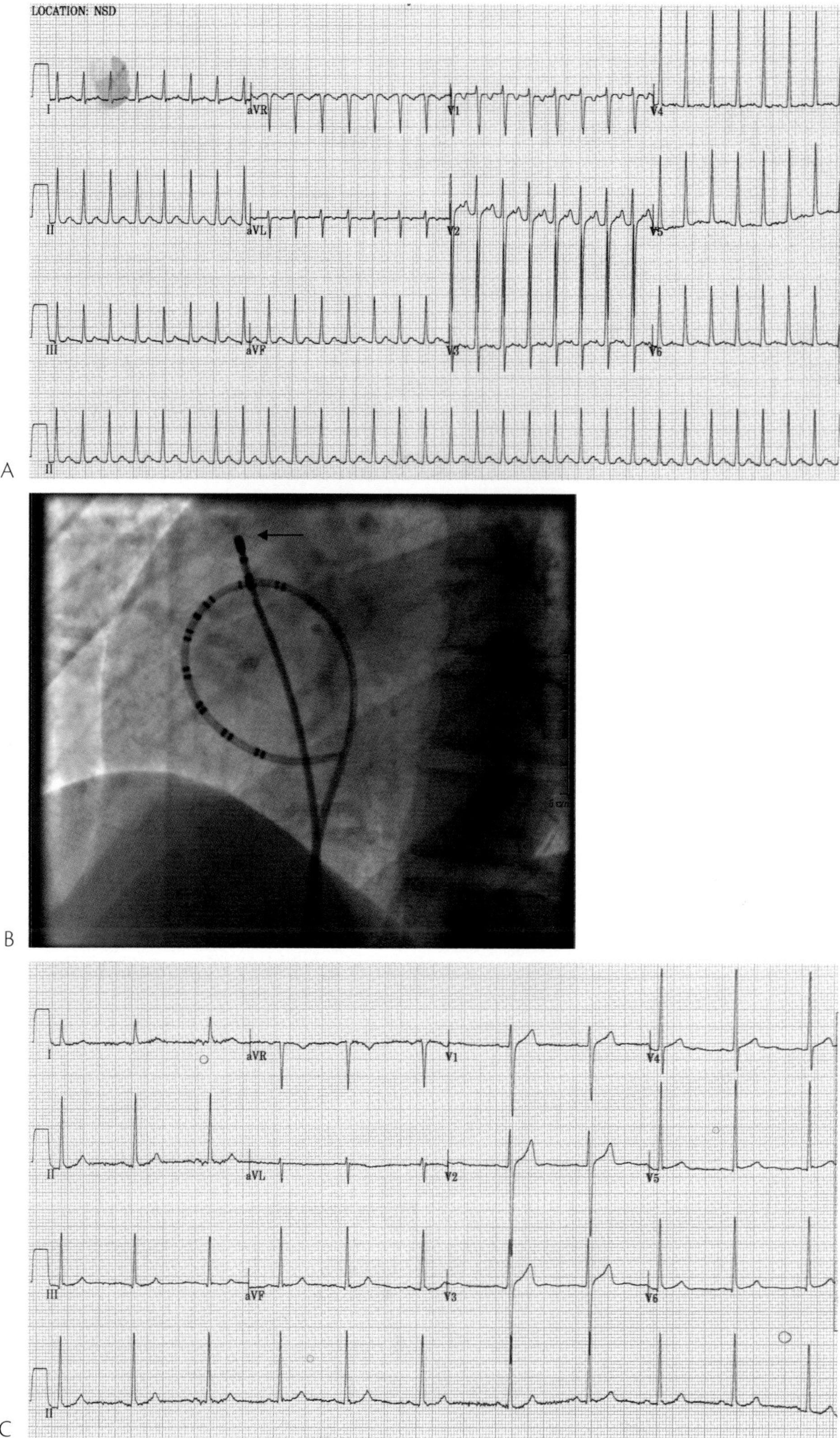

Fig. 36.2 (A) 12-lead ECG of incessant atrial tachycardia in a 16-year-old boy who presented with severe heart failure resistant to medical therapy. (B) Catheter position (arrowed) at which this arrhythmia was successfully ablated (*c.*2 cm from the sinoatrial node). (C) 12-lead ECG in sinus rhythm after successful ablation of atrial tachycardia. Thereafter his rhythm remained normal, his symptoms resolved, and his left ventricular function soon returned to normal.

Table 36.1 Cellular electrophysiological changes linked to arrhythmia mechanisms in heart failure

Arrhythmogenic mechanism	Molecular changes in hypertrophy/HF	
Abnormal automaticity		
Reduced resting membrane potential	Enhanced phase 4 diastolic depolarization	$\uparrow I_{Ca-T}$, $\downarrow I_{K1}$, $\uparrow I_f$
	Reduced maximum diastolic potential	
Triggered activity		
EAD-mediated	AP duration	↓K currents, ↑NCX,
	(↑AP duration and altered profile)	Altered I_{Ca-L} density and kinetics,
Late EAD-mediated and DAD-mediated	Increased $[Ca^{2+}]_i$	Slowed Ca^{2+} transient, ↑NCX
Re-entry		
Reactivation	Prolonged APD	
Slowed conduction and block	Anisotropic conduction	Microfibrosis in the interstitium

APD, action potential duration; DAD, delayed afterdepolarizations; EAD, early afterdepolarizations; HF, heart failure; NCX, Na^+-Ca^{2+} exchanger.

ventricular interstitium. Also, the presence of coronary artery disease increases the risk of myocardial ischaemia, which is proarrhythmic.

Re-entry

In ischaemic cardiomyopathy, patients have typically had a prior myocardial infarction with an area of scarring in the ventricular myocardium, and a remodelled and often dilated left ventricle. In such patients, it is often possible to induce ventricular tachycardia at electrophysiological study due to a macro-re-entrant circuit in the border zone of the infarction. Thus scar-related re-entry is the key mechanism for maintenance of the arrhythmia in ischaemic cardiomyopathy.

In nonischaemic cardiomyopathy, extensive myocardial damage and fibrosis, or the loss of cell-to-cell coupling, provide the substrates for re-entry. New re-entrant wave fronts may be initiated by epicardial breakthrough of the impulse followed by a line of conduction block parallel to the epicardial fibre orientation, suggesting the importance of increased fibrosis with a resultant increase in tissue anisotropy.

Automaticity and triggered activity

Abnormal automaticity may arise in hypertrophied and failing hearts in the setting of a reduction in resting membrane potential or acceleration of phase 4 diastolic depolarization, such that the threshold for activation of the Na^+ current is reached rapidly. Triggered activity, arising from either early afterdepolarizations (EADs) or delayed afterdepolarizations (DADs), also contribute to ventricular arrhythmias in patients with both ischaemic and nonischaemic cardiomyopathy. The cellular electrophysiological mechanisms underlying these principles are discussed in detail below.

Cellular electrophysiology in heart failure

The duration of the action potential is primarily responsible for the time course of repolarization of the heart. Prolongation of the action potential produces delays in cardiac repolarization, manifest as QT interval prolongation on the surface ECG, which can be proarrhythmic. Prolongation of the action potential is characteristic of cells and tissues isolated from ventricles of animals and human subjects with HF independent of the mechanism. A change in the duration of the action potential occurs as a result of alterations in the profiles of the depolarizing and repolarizing currents (Fig. 36.3). Furthermore, heterogeneity of action potential duration across the transmural surface of the ventricular wall may be an important contributor to arrhythmogenesis.[34] Experimental models finding enhanced spatial and temporal dispersion of monophasic action potential duration, refractoriness and ECG QT intervals in humans and animals with HF are consistent with an exaggerated dispersion of action potential duration that may predispose to ventricular arrhythmias.[35–36]

Repolarization in the mammalian heart is achieved primarily by the activity of K^+-selective ionic currents. Functional down-regulation of K^+ currents is a recurring theme in hypertrophied and failing ventricular myocardium with reduction in the current density of the transient outward K^+ current (I_{to}) arguably the most consistent ionic current change. Down-regulation of I_{to}, without a significant change in the voltage dependence or kinetics of the current, has also been observed in cells isolated from terminally failing human hearts. I_{to} is a transient current and as such down-regulation itself may not produce large effects on the action potential duration. However, it does profoundly influence phase 1 and the level of the plateau thereby affecting all of the currents that are active later in the action potential.

HF is characterized by a reduction in the developed force, prolongation of relaxation, and blunting of the frequency-dependent

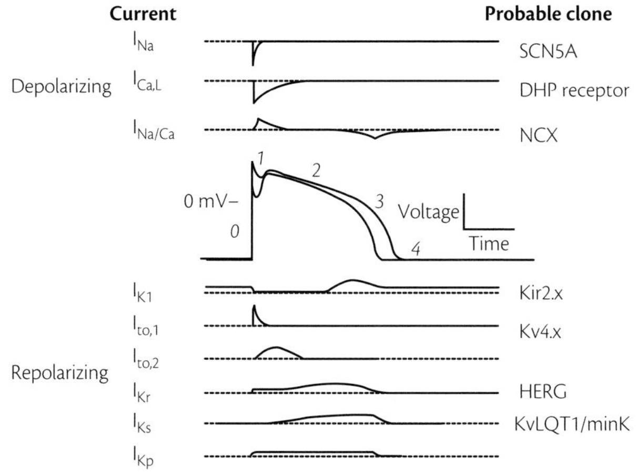

Fig. 36.3 Ionic currents contributing to the ventricular action potential.

facilitation of contraction. The abnormalities in excitation–contraction coupling in HF are a consequence of fundamental changes in Ca^{2+} handling within ventricular myocytes.[37–39] The L-type Ca^{2+} current is the primary source of Ca^{2+} entry, triggering release of Ca^{2+} from the sarcoplasmic reticulum and initiating actin–myosin crossbridge cycling. Studies of L-type Ca^{2+} current in cells isolated from failing human hearts exhibit either no change, or a decrease in current density or dihydropyridine binding sites. Ventricular myocytes isolated from failing hearts exhibit attenuated augmentation of the L-type Ca^{2+} current by β-adrenergic stimulation and depression of rate-dependent potentiation compared to cells isolated from control hearts. Depression of the L-type Ca^{2+} current results in slowing of the decay of the whole-cell current, a change that could alter excitation–contraction coupling and would tend to prolong the action potential duration, the latter of which is proarrhythmic. The amplitude of the intracellular Ca^{2+} transient and its rate of decay are reduced in intact muscles and cells isolated from failing ventricles compared with normal controls. The changes in the Ca^{2+} transient are the result of defective function of the sarcoplasmic reticulum, but the precise molecular mechanism(s) of this defect is controversial. The sarcoplasmic reticulum Ca^{2+}-ATPase (SERCA2a) and the Na^+-Ca^{2+} exchanger (NCX) are primary mediators of Ca^{2+} removal from the cytoplasm. SERCA2a is inhibited by unphosphorylated phospholamban (PLB) by direct protein–protein interaction; when PLB is phosphorylated SERCA2a inhibition is relieved. Ca^{2+} entry into the cell through the L-type Ca^{2+} channel stimulates release of Ca^{2+} from the SR by the ryanodine receptor (RyR) in a process known as Ca^{2+}-induced Ca^{2+} release. The level of ventricular RyR mRNA decreases in some studies of terminal human HF. The NCX importantly contributes to control of $[Ca^{2+}]_i$, extruding cytoplasmic Ca^{2+} by electrogenically exchanging it for extracellular Na^+. Most studies from hypertrophied and failing hearts have demonstrated an increase in both NCX mRNA and protein, suggesting that enhanced NCX function compensates for defective SR removal of Ca^{2+} from the cytoplasm in the failing heart. The characteristic slow decay of the Ca^{2+} transient and increased diastolic $[Ca^{2+}]$ can predispose to oscillatory release of Ca^{2+} from the SR and DAD-mediated triggered arrhythmias. The slow decay of the Ca^{2+} transient will influence ion flux through the NCX and may also predispose to late phase 3 EAD-mediated triggered arrhythmias.

The Na^+,K^+-ATPase (Na, K pump) transports K^+ into the cell and Na^+ out with a stoichiometry of 2:3, thus generating an outward repolarizing current. The expression and function of the Na^+,K^+-ATPase are reduced in failing hearts, which may have arrhythmogenic consequences. This reduction in the outward repolarizing current would tend to prolong action potential duration. Furthermore reduced function of the Na^+,K^+-ATPase would lead to an increase in intracellular $[Na^+]$ and enhanced reversed-mode NCX, increasing depolarizing current.

The hyperpolarization-activated 'funny' or pacemaker current (I_f) in the heart is a nonselective cation current that was originally described in automatic tissues such as the sinoatrial node. More recently I_f has been demonstrated in ventricular cells from animal and human hearts, activating at very negative voltages outside the physiological range. Although I_f is found in higher density in ventricular myocytes from failing human hearts, the difference from controls did not reach statistical significance. It is therefore unclear whether this current has a role to play in abnormal automaticity and the induction of ventricular arrhythmias in HF.

Conduction delay and re-entry

Alterations in anisotropic conduction may contribute to the production of arrhythmias in hypertrophic and failing hearts. Alterations in intracellular $[Ca^{2+}]$ and redistribution of gap junctions affect intercellular conduction. Microfibrosis separates myocytes and myocyte bundles, altering anisotropic conduction and leading to spatial nonuniformities of electrical activation. Diminished intercellular coupling slows conduction, which predisposes to re-entry. Slowed ventricular conduction is manifest on the surface ECG as QRS prolongation, which is an independent risk factor for SCD.[40–41] Furthermore, QRS duration is a major criterion for risk stratification and identification of patients suitable for advanced therapies for HF, namely CRT (biventricular pacemakers) and implantable cardioverter-defibrillators (ICDs).[25,42–43]

Neurohormonal modulation and the pathogenesis of arrhythmias

In the presence of impaired cardiac function, the body attempts to maintain circulatory homeostasis through a complex series of neurohormonal changes. These changes in neurohormonal signalling have prominent effects on the electrophysiology of the failing heart.

The β_1, β_2, and α_1 adrenergic receptors mediate the effects of increased circulating adrenaline and noradrenaline released from cardiac nerve terminals. These receptor subtypes are coupled to different signalling systems. The β_1 and β_2 receptors are coupled by stimulatory G proteins to adenylyl cyclase; activation results in increased cellular levels of cAMP. The α_1 receptor is coupled by a G protein to phospholipase C (PLC) which hydrolyses inositol phospholipids, increasing cellular inositol 1,4,5-trisphosphate (IP3) and diacylglycerol (DAG). Angiotensin II (AT1) receptors are also coupled to PLC. Activation of the AT1 receptor or the α-adrenergic pathway initiates a kinase cascade triggering cell growth and altering the intracellular $[Ca^{2+}]$. This increases the cellular Ca^{2+} load, with possible adverse consequences that include activation of phospholipases, proteases, and endonucleases, culminating in cell necrosis or apoptosis and progression of HF.

The β and α signalling pathways significantly affect the function of a number of ion channels and transporters. The net effect of β-adrenergic stimulation is to shorten the ventricular action potential duration. This is due to an increase in the current density and a hyperpolarizing shift of the activation of I_K, despite β_1 receptor stimulation of depolarizing current through the L-type Ca^{2+} channel. α_1-Adrenergic receptor stimulation inhibits several K^+ currents in the mammalian heart, including I_{to}, I_{K1}, and I_K, with the net effect of prolonging action potential duration.

Mechanical load is an important modulator of excitability in the heart. The effect of altered haemodynamic load may be exaggerated in the failing compared with the normal ventricle. In doxorubicin-induced HF in the rabbit increased load produced exaggerated shortening of the action potential duration and enhanced arrhythmia susceptibility in failing hearts.[44] The effect of load is not likely to be distributed uniformly across the ventricular wall or throughout the myocardium, and thus has the potential to increase dispersion in action potential duration with arrhythmogenic consequences.

The role of myocardial ischaemia in the pathogenesis of arrhythmias in heart failure

Myocardial ischaemia is proarrhythmic and has a role in increasing the risk of sudden death. Ischaemia results in QT interval prolongation and polymorphic ventricular tachycardia, which can degenerate into ventricular fibrillation. The presence of electrolyte abnormalities, sympathetic stimulation, and ventricular hypertrophy all increase the risk of arrhythmias in myocardial ischaemia and are often coexistent in HF. The potential for myocardial ischaemia precipitating ventricular tachyarrhythmia is well recognized in patients with ischaemic cardiomyopathy; however, there is a significant incidence of undiagnosed coronary artery disease in 'nonischaemic' cardiomyopathy with one study reporting a 40% incidence of 'acute' coronary lesions in individuals with a SCD but no previous documented history of ischaemic heart disease.[45] This emphasizes the importance of optimal anti-ischaemic therapies in individuals with ischaemic and perhaps also nonischaemic cardiomyopathies.

Electrolyte abnormalities

Electrolyte abnormalities, in particular hypo- or hyperkalaemia or hypomagnesaemia, are associated with an increased risk of ventricular tachyarrhythmias. Hypokalaemia and hypomagnesaemia may occur as a result of diuretic therapy and predispose to QT interval prolongation. The presence of hypomagnesaemia impairs the repletion of potassium stores and appears to be implicated in ventricular tachyarrhythmias. Conversely, hyperkalaemia may predispose to bradyarrhythmias or sinusoidal ventricular tachycardia, and may occur as a result of impaired renal function or secondary to drug therapy (e.g. ACE inhibitors, ARBs, aldosterone antagonists, or potassium supplements).

Types of ventricular arrhythmias

Ventricular premature beats

Ventricular premature beats (VPBs) are single ventricular impulses caused by re-entry within the ventricle or abnormal automaticity of ventricular cells. VPBs—also called premature ventricular contractions or complexes (PVCs)—may occur erratically or at predictable intervals, e.g. every second (bigeminy), third (trigeminy), or fourth (quadrigeminey) beat. VPBs may increase with stimulants (e.g. anxiety, stress, alcohol, caffeine, sympathomimetic drugs), hypoxia, or electrolyte abnormalities. VPBs may be asymptomatic, or cause palpitations, or may be experienced as missed or skipped beats; the VPB itself is not sensed but rather the following augmented sinus beat. When VPBs are very frequent (e.g. in bigeminy), mild haemodynamic symptoms are possible because the sinus rate has been effectively halved. Diagnosis is by ECG showing a wide QRS complex without a preceding P wave, typically followed by a fully compensatory pause.

Unifocal VPBs occur where the depolarizations are triggered from a single ventricular site, resulting in a single ectopic QRS morphology. Multifocal VPBs arise from more than one ventricular site, resulting in VPBs with more than one QRS morphology. VPBs are of variable prognostic importance, and may be associated with an increased risk of sustained ventricular tachyarrhythmias and SCD. One report evaluated intracardiac electrograms in patients with an ICD. Among those with a reduced LVEF, monomorphic ventricular tachycardia was most often initiated by multiple VPBs, which had morphology different from the ventricular tachycardia.[46] There is, however, little evidence that suppression of VPBs improves mortality in the presence of HF, and in fact the use of class I antiarrhythmic drugs may be proarrhythmic in this patient group, resulting in increased mortality.

Ventricular tachycardia

Three or more ventricular consecutive beats at a rate of more than 100/min (cycle length <600 ms) constitutes ventricular tachycardia (VT). If the rhythm self-terminates within 30 s, it is defined as non-sustained ventricular tachycardia (NSVT). Ventricular tachycardia lasting more than 30 s or requiring cardioversion (either pharmacological, electrical, or by overdrive pacing) for haemodynamic compromise within that time is defined as sustained VT. Occasionally an atrial impulse arrives when the AV node and the His–Purkinje system are not refractory and AV conduction can occur. This results in a capture beat in which normal ventricular conduction occurs with a normal-appearing (narrow) QRS complex. A capture beat occurs at a shorter RR interval than the RR interval of the VT. AV conduction also may occur simultaneously with depolarization of the ventricular focus. In this instance, the ventricle will be depolarized in part over the normal pathway and in part from the ventricular focus. The resulting QRS complex will be intermediate in morphology between a normal QRS and a QRS of ventricular origin. In this instance, the RR interval will not change. This is called a fusion beat. Ventricular tachycardia may be monomorphic or polymorphic (varying QRS morphology during the tachycardia).

Several algorithms have been derived to assist in the ECG diagnosis of VT, in particular the distinction between VT and SVT with bundle branch block.[47] The Brugada algorithm[48] is commonly used and is summarized in Fig. 36.4. Such algorithms are guidelines and should be used with caution in certain circumstances, such as in the context of acute myocardial infarction, complex congenital heart disease, electrolyte abnormalities, and in patients already on antiarrhythmic drugs, especially class 1C agents.

The prognostic significance of NSVT in HF is uncertain. The GESICA-GEMA study showed that in patients with CHF, NSVT is an independent marker for increased overall mortality rate and sudden death. The absence of NSVT and VPBs in a 24-h Holter indicated a low probability of sudden death. However, on the contrary, the CHF-STAT study reported that NSVT is frequently seen in patients with HF and may be associated with worsened survival by univariate analysis. However, after adjusting other variables, especially for LVEF, NSVT was not an independent predictor of all-cause mortality or sudden death. These results have serious implications in that suppression of these arrhythmias may not improve survival.

Torsades de pointes

Torsades de pointes, or polymorphic VT, is a form of VT in which the QRS morphology is constantly changing. As its name suggests, electrical activity appears to be twisted into a helix or turning about a fixed point. This form of VT may occur due to drug toxicity or an idiosyncratic reaction to type IA antiarrhythmic agents such as quinidine, procainamide, or disopyramide, or other agents that prolong the QT interval. Myocardial ischaemia, hypokalaemia, hypomagnesaemia and bradycardia can also initiate torsades de pointes. This arrhythmia is usually precipitated by prolongation of the QT interval.

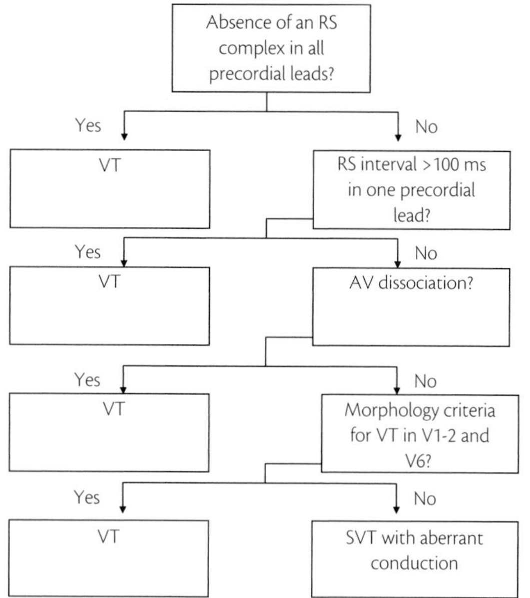

Fig. 36.4 Algorithm for analysis of 12-lead ECG of wide QRS complex tachycardia. Adapted from Brugada P, Brugada J, Mont L, Smeets J, Andries EW. A new approach to the differential diagnosis of a regular tachycardia with a wide QRS complex. *Circulation* 1991;**83**(5):1649–59.

Treatment of ventricular arrhythmias in heart failure

Treatment of modulating factors

As outlined above, the initiation and maintenance of ventricular arrhythmias in HF occur via several mechanisms. Implicit in this are the electrophysiological changes in the failing ventricle in response to changes in myocardial load and stretch. Contemporary HF treatment includes the use of ACE inhibitors which have been shown to confer a survival benefit in HF.[7,49] Furthermore, the V-HEFT-II study showed a significant reduction in sudden death (39% RRR) in patients treated with enalapril compared to a hydralazine and isosorbide dinitrate combination.[50] Of note, this effect was most marked in patient with less severe HF symptoms and may be explained in part by ACE inhibitors preventing the development of myocardial stretch and fibrosis known to be implicated in the genesis of ventricular arrhythmias. This antiarrhythmic effect is evident from the Holter recordings of the patients receiving enalapril, who had fewer complex ventricular arrhythmias compared to the hydralazine and nitrate treated group. Furthermore, ACE inhibitors have some β-blocking properties and also prevent hypokalaemia, further protecting patients with HF from ventricular arrhythmias.

Aldosterone is another neurohumoral agent responsible for some of the deleterious haemodynamic effects of HF. Via its potent mineralocorticoid effects, it results in an imbalance of sodium, potassium, and magnesium, as well as promoting myocardial fibrosis, further adding to the substrate for arrhythmias. Spironolactone is an aldosterone antagonist known to reduce all-cause mortality in HF.[51] Furthermore, spironolactone also reduces SCD, suggesting an effect on the frequency of ventricular arrhythmias. In fact, spironolactone has been shown to reduce the frequency of VPBs and NSVT in Holter monitoring and monitored treadmill testing of HF patients compared to standard medical therapy alone.[52] Further evidence for the antiarrhythmic effect of aldosterone antagonism is provided from the EPHESUS trial of eplerenone for patients with left ventricular dysfunction post myocardial infarction, which reported a significant reduction in sudden cardiac death at 30 days compared to placebo.[53]

Antiarrhythmic drug treatment for ventricular arrhythmias in heart failure

Drug treatment of ventricular arrhythmias in HF presents a difficult challenge. With increasing degrees of left ventricular dysfunction, the efficacy of antiarrhythmic drugs decreases. Furthermore, with increasing degrees of HF, antiarrhythmic drugs demonstrate a greater negative inotropic effect, more frequent proarrhythmic effects, and more frequent bradyarrhythmias. The use of class I antiarrhythmic agents is contraindicated in the presence of LVSD post myocardial infarction.[54] Amiodarone is an iodine-containing benzofuran that is widely used for the prevention of sustained VT and fibrillation. It was originally classified as a class III antiarrhythmic agent with minor class II effects, and later recognized to also have class I and class IV effects. Amiodarone is the drug of choice for HF patients who require antiarrhythmic drug therapy for ventricular arrhythmias, as there is evidence of a reduction in arrhythmic death.[55–57] Interestingly, the SCD-HEFT trial failed to show any reduction in mortality with amiodarone treatment compared to placebo in NYHA class II HF and was in fact associated with decreased survival in NYHA class III.[58] There is no evidence for the prophylactic use of amiodarone in patients with LVSD in the absence of an arrhythmic indication for the drug.[56]

Dronedarone is a novel antiarrhythmic drug which is a noniodinated benzofuran derivative related to amiodarone. Clinical trials of the effectiveness of this drug for the management of AF show promising results. However, its use in HF was investigated in the ANDROMEDA study.[59] This trial was terminated early because of an observed excess of deaths in the dronedarone treatment group, largely due to worsening HF, with an increased risk of death in the presence of severely reduced LVEF. It is therefore contraindicated in severe HF.

Device therapy

There have been several studies of ICD therapy for the primary or secondary prevention of SCD. SCD occurs in approximately 50 000–70 000 people annually in the United Kingdom and represents the largest proportion of the deaths attributable to coronary heart disease. Approximately 85–90% of SCD is due to the first recognized arrhythmic event; the remaining 10–15% is due to recurrent events. The survival rates for out-of-hospital sudden cardiac episodes are less than 5% in most industrialized countries, including the United Kingdom. People who survive a first episode of a life-threatening ventricular arrhythmia are at high risk of further episodes. Prevention of SCD is either primary, defined as prevention of a first life-threatening arrhythmic event, or secondary, which refers to the prevention of an additional life-threatening event in survivors of sustained VT or ventricular fibrillation (VF) or patients with recurrent unstable rhythms. Apart from a history of previous VT or VF, risk factors for SCD include a prior myocardial infarction, coronary artery disease, HF, LVEF of less than 35%, prolonged QRS duration, and certain familial cardiac conditions (including long QT syndrome, Brugada syndrome, hypertrophic cardiomyopathy and arrhythmogenic right ventricular cardiomyopathy). The incidence of SCD increases with age.

The use of the ICD in secondary prevention has been extensively investigated. Three trials involving a total of 1850 survivors of cardiac arrest (AVID,[60] CASH,[61] and CIDS[62]) have since been the subject of three different meta-analyses. These meta-analyses reported that, compared with amiodarone or another antiarrhythmic drug, treatment with ICDs resulted in a 50% reduction in the risk of cardiac death and a 25–28% risk reduction in all-cause mortality.

There is also evidence that primary prevention ICDs have a mortality benefit in HF patients with a reduced LVEF. MADIT II reported a significant reduction in mortality (31% relative risk reduction at 20 months) in patients with LVEF less than 30% post myocardial infarction with ICD therapy compared to conventional medical therapy alone.[63] SCD-HEFT was a primary prevention trial of amiodarone versus ICD therapy and found that ICD therapy led to a 23% relative reduction in mortality after 5 years in patients with HF (NYHA class II–III and LVEF <35%).[58] Furthermore, in patients with advanced HF and a prolonged QRS interval, CRT, with or without an defibrillator significantly reduces mortality.[42–43] The role of the ICD in the primary and secondary prevention of sudden arrhythmic death is discussed in Chapter 47.

Role of electrophysiological studies and radiofrequency ablation for ventricular arrhythmias

In the HF patient, VT is often related to re-entry around a scar most often a consequence of myocardial infarction. Monomorphic VT can be studied in the electrophysiology laboratory by conventional methods, and may be amenable to radiofrequency ablation. The purpose of mapping in ventricular tachycardia is to identify an area of slow conduction (usually the exit point of the re-entrant circuit)—this isthmus is the target for ablation. Electrophysiological testing is of much less value in patients with NSVT, polymorphic VT, or primary VF.

Conventional mapping of VT requires the arrhythmia to be both electrically and haemodynamically stable. This can be a limitation of VT mapping and ablation in HF patients, who often decompensate as a consequence of the ventricular arrhythmia. In order to limit the time spent in tachycardia, a number of strategies may be used to approximate the location of the re-entrant circuit. The 12-lead ECG during tachycardia can provide the initial clues to the location via the QRS morphology and axis. Thereafter, mapping in sinus rhythm can be used to identify areas of low amplitude, fractionated potentials in the peri-infarct zone. Pace-mapping identifies the region of the exit site of the circuit. Thereafter, following induction of VT, activation mapping confirms the exit site and zone of slow conduction, i.e. the target region for ablation.

The role of ablation for VT occurring in the context of structural heart disease or HF has not been established, and ICD therapy is currently recommended as first-line therapy to most such patients.[64–66] The decision as to whether and when to offer catheter ablation to patients with VT and structural heart disease varies between hospitals and even between individual clinicians. Most would agree, however, that VT ablation should be considered in patients with ICDs *in situ* who experience multiple shocks despite appropriate antiarrhythmic drug therapy, particularly if there is a single morphology of haemodynamically well-tolerated VT (or more than one morphology, but likely to be utilizing a single diastolic circuit[66]) and no major contraindications to the procedure. Furthermore, VT ablation may need to be considered on an urgent or emergency basis in cases of incessant VT resistant to medical therapy (Fig. 36.5).

Recent studies have investigated whether VT ablation should be more widely used in patients with ICDs *in situ*, in order to reduce the frequency of subsequent ICD shocks. The SMASH-VT Trial[64] has demonstrated that VT ablation can decrease appropriate ICD therapy rates from 33% to 15% ($p = 0.022$) over only 2-year follow-up and prevent VT storms. However, the study was not powered to look for differences in mortality and so could not establish the superiority of VT ablation over ICD therapy in the patients with VT in the context of structural heart disease. Further research is therefore required to clarify the role of VT ablation in patients with HF. Furthermore, there has been recent evidence to indicate that catheter ablation of stable VT before ICD implantation may prolong the time to VT recurrence.[67]

The main contraindications to VT ablation are problems with either vascular access or access to the left ventricle (e.g. bilateral femoral arterial stenoses, severe aortic stenosis, contraindication to trans-septal puncture) and other potential hazards such as left ventricular thrombus. Previously, the presence of haemodynamically unstable VT or multiple morphologies of VT were considered to be contraindications to ablation, but now with the use of electroanatomical or nonfluoroscopic mapping systems and the use of 'substrate-based' ablation (which aims to target abnormal electrical activity in sinus rhythm) some of these more complex arrhythmias may be amenable to ablation.

Bradycardia in heart failure

Disorders of sinus node function and AV nodal conduction are common, especially in the elderly population, and many patients with HF will be prone to these conditions. Furthermore, sinus node dysfunction and AV nodal conduction disorders can both be exacerbated by β-blockers, which are a cornerstone of HF therapy. In addition, HF itself is often associated with PR interval prolongation and bundle branch block.[68,40–41] In many cases where there is symptomatic bradycardia (even bradycardia induced or exacerbated by drugs, when it is necessary to continue that drug therapy)[69] or life-threatening conduction disturbances, the standard treatment is implantation of a permanent pacemaker. HF is an important comorbidity in many patients undergoing pacemaker implantation, although in the United Kingdom is it the primary reason for pacemaker implantation in only a small minority of cases.[70]

Careful individual decision-making is required in selecting the optimum pacing mode[25] in patients with HF. Those with sinus node dysfunction but intact AV conduction (normal PR interval, normal QRS duration, and no AV block with atrial pacing at rates up to 100–120 beats/min), atrial pacing alone (AAI mode) might be considered. However, despite these selection criteria, there is a finite incidence of AV block of between 0.5% and 3% per year.[71–72] Modern dual-chamber pacemakers with algorithms to limit unnecessary ventricular pacing are likely to be more appropriate than AAI pacemakers in this population.[73]

Patients with HF and AV block (actual or threatened) will require ventricular pacing. There is no strong evidence from clinical trials that dual-chamber pacing (DDD or DDDR) is superior to single-chamber ventricular pacing (VVI or VVIR), even in the HF population.[74] Clinical trials of pacing modes in patients without HF have been inconclusive; the MOST study in patients with sinus

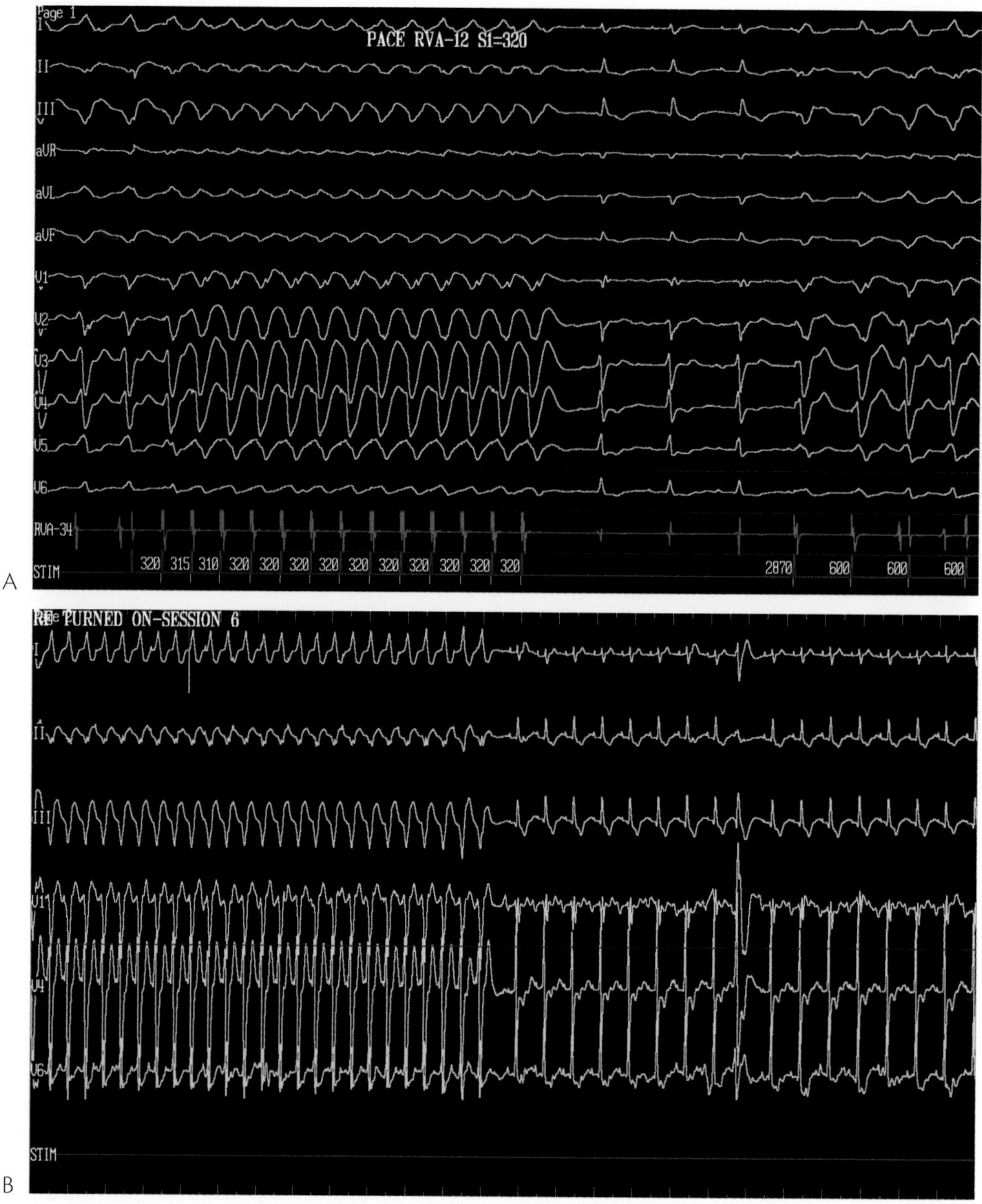

Fig. 36.5 (A) Incessant ventricular tachycardia (VT) in a 73-year-old man with prior myocardial infarction and heart failure. The VT persisted despite treatment with high-dose amiodarone and β-blockade. A burst of antitachycardia pacing (arrows) terminated the tachycardia, but spontaneous reinitiation occurred within 3 s. (B) Treatment with radiofrequency catheter ablation resulted in termination of the VT and improvement in the patient's symptoms.

node disease showed better 'HF scores' in patients randomized to dual-chamber pacing than to single-chamber ventricular pacing,[75] but the UK-PACE study in elderly patients with AV block showed a trend towards less HF during follow-up in patients randomized to fixed-rate ventricular pacing (VVI mode) than in those randomized to rate-adaptive ventricular pacing (VVIR mode) or dual-chamber pacing (DDD mode).[76] A meta-analysis of mode selection studies showed no significant reduction in HF mortality with atrial-based pacing than with ventricular pacing.[74]

However, there is ample evidence that right ventricular pacing *per se* is deleterious in patients with left ventricular dysfunction[77] (and may be deleterious even in the normal heart[78–79]). Atrio-biventricular pacing (CRT—see Chapter 48) is therefore often considered in patients with HF and severe left ventricular dysfunction who are likely to require long-term ventricular pacing. It is worth emphasizing that all the major clinical trials of CRT deliberately excluded patients with either significant sinus node disease or AV conduction disease,[43,80–81] so a strategy of implantation of biventricular pacemakers in patients with LVSD and AV block is not strictly 'evidence-based'.

Conclusions

The treatment of cardiac arrhythmias in patients with HF is complex and difficult, and close collaboration is often needed among different cardiology subspecialties. Treatment can do more harm than good: several antiarrhythmic drugs, both old and new, are known to be potentially hazardous in the patient with severe HF, because of proarrhythmia, negative inotropism, or other factors. Even drugs which are known to be beneficial, such as certain β-blockers, must be used initially in low dosages and titrated gradually in order to avoid clinical deterioration in patients with HF.

When treating arrhythmias in these patients, physicians are reminded to consider carefully the significance of the arrhythmia and the aims of treatment. Specifically, one should ask whether the intended treatment is aimed at improving symptoms or improving prognosis. If it is the former, one should be certain that the arrhythmia is the cause of the symptoms and not merely an epiphenomenon. If it is the latter, one should have good evidence that the treatment has been proven to improve the patient's prognosis. If neither of these criteria is fulfilled, then treatment may not be required. Finally, if the arrhythmia itself does require treatment, one should always consider the different modalities of treatment (drugs, ablation, devices) in order to ensure the optimum outcome for the patient.

References

1. Braunwald E. Shattuck lecture—cardiovascular medicine at the turn of the millennium: triumphs, concerns, and opportunities. *N Engl J Med* 1997;**337**(19):1360–9.
2. Dries DL, Exner DV, Gersh BJ, Domanski MJ, Waclawiw MA, Stevenson LW. Atrial fibrillation is associated with an increased risk for mortality and heart failure progression in patients with asymptomatic and symptomatic left ventricular systolic dysfunction: a retrospective analysis of the SOLVD trials. Studies of Left Ventricular Dysfunction. *J Am Coll Cardiol* 1998;**32**(3):695–703.
3. Carson PE, Johnson GR, Dunkman WB, Fletcher RD, Farrell L, Cohn JN. The influence of atrial fibrillation on prognosis in mild to moderate heart failure. The V-HeFT Studies. The V-HeFT VA Cooperative Studies Group. *Circulation* 1993;**87**(6 Suppl):VI102–10.
4. Deedwania PC, Singh BN, Ellenbogen K, Fisher S, Fletcher R, Singh SN. Spontaneous conversion and maintenance of sinus rhythm by amiodarone in patients with heart failure and atrial fibrillation: observations from the veterans affairs congestive heart failure survival trial of antiarrhythmic therapy (CHF-STAT). The Department of Veterans Affairs CHF-STAT Investigators. *Circulation* 1998;**98**(23):2574–9.
5. Torp-Pedersen C, Moller M, Bloch-Thomsen PE, *et al.* Dofetilide in patients with congestive heart failure and left ventricular dysfunction. Danish Investigations of Arrhythmia and Mortality on Dofetilide Study Group. *N Engl J Med* 1999;**341**(12):857–65.
6. Doval HC, Nul DR, Grancelli HO, Perrone SV, Bortman GR, Curiel R. Randomised trial of low-dose amiodarone in severe congestive heart failure. Grupo de Estudio de la Sobrevida en la Insuficiencia Cardiaca en Argentina (GESICA). *Lancet* 1994;**344**(8921):493–8.
7. Effects of enalapril on mortality in severe congestive heart failure. Results of the Cooperative North Scandinavian Enalapril Survival Study (CONSENSUS). The CONSENSUS Trial Study Group. *N Engl J Med* 1987;**316**(23):1429–35.
8. Benjamin EJ, Wolf PA, D'Agostino RB, Silbershatz H, Kannel WB, Levy D. Impact of atrial fibrillation on the risk of death: the Framingham Heart Study. *Circulation* 1998;**98**(10):946–52.
9. Vaziri SM, Larson MG, Benjamin EJ, Levy D. Echocardiographic predictors of nonrheumatic atrial fibrillation. The Framingham Heart Study. *Circulation* 1994;**89**(2):724–30.
10. Maisel WH, Stevenson LW. Atrial fibrillation in heart failure: epidemiology, pathophysiology, and rationale for therapy. *Am J Cardiol* 2003;**91**(6A):2D–8D.
11. Solti F, Vecsey T, Kekesi V, Juhasz-Nagy A. The effect of atrial dilatation on the genesis of atrial arrhythmias. *Cardiovasc Res* 1989;**23**(10):882–6.
12. Nattel S. Ionic determinants of atrial fibrillation and Ca^{2+} channel abnormalities : cause, consequence, or innocent bystander? *Circ Res* 1999;**85**(5):473–6.
13. Li D, Shinagawa K, Pang L, *et al.* Effects of angiotensin-converting enzyme inhibition on the development of the atrial fibrillation substrate in dogs with ventricular tachypacing-induced congestive heart failure. *Circulation* 2001;**104**(21):2608–14.
14. Li D, Fareh S, Leung TK, Nattel S. Promotion of atrial fibrillation by heart failure in dogs: atrial remodeling of a different sort. *Circulation* 1999;**100**(1):87–95.
15. Wang TJ, Larson MG, Levy D, *et al.* Temporal relations of atrial fibrillation and congestive heart failure and their joint influence on mortality: the Framingham Heart Study. *Circulation* 2003;**107**(23):2920–5.
16. Wang TJ, Massaro JM, Levy D, *et al.* A risk score for predicting stroke or death in individuals with new-onset atrial fibrillation in the community: the Framingham Heart Study. *JAMA* 2003;**290**(8):1049–56.
17. Takarada A, Kurogane H, Hayashi T, *et al.* Prognostic significance of atrial fibrillation in dilated cardiomyopathy. *Jpn Heart J* 1993;**34**(6):749–58.
18. Roy D, Talajic M, Nattel S, *et al.* Rhythm control versus rate control for atrial fibrillation and heart failure. *N Engl J Med* 2008;**358**(25):2667–77.
19. Wyse DG, Waldo AL, DiMarco JP, *et al.* A comparison of rate control and rhythm control in patients with atrial fibrillation. *N Engl J Med* 2002;**347**(23):1825–33.
20. Hsu LF, Jais P, Sanders P, *et al.* Catheter ablation for atrial fibrillation in congestive heart failure. *N Engl J Med* 2004;**351**(23):2373–83.
21. Chen MS, Marrouche NF, Khaykin Y, Gillinov AM, Wazni O, Martin DO *et al.* Pulmonary vein isolation for the treatment of atrial fibrillation in patients with impaired systolic function. *J Am Coll Cardiol* 2004;**43**(6):1004–1009.
22. Khan MN, Jais P, Cummings J, *et al.* Pulmonary-vein isolation for atrial fibrillation in patients with heart failure. *N Engl J Med* 2008;**359**(17):1778–85.
23. Brignole M, Menozzi C, Gianfranchi L, *et al.* Assessment of atrioventricular junction ablation and VVIR pacemaker versus pharmacological treatment in patients with heart failure and chronic atrial fibrillation: a randomized, controlled study. *Circulation* 1998;**98**(10):953–60.
24. Hay I, Melenovsky V, Fetics BJ, *et al.* Short-term effects of right-left heart sequential cardiac resynchronization in patients with heart failure, chronic atrial fibrillation, and atrioventricular nodal block. *Circulation* 2004;**110**(22):3404–10.
25. Bernstein AD, Daubert JC, Fletcher RD, *et al.* The revised NASPE/BPEG generic code for antibradycardia, adaptive-rate, and multisite pacing. North American Society of Pacing and Electrophysiology/British Pacing and Electrophysiology Group. *Pacing Clin Electrophysiol* 2002;**25**(2):260–4.
26. Connolly SJ, Ezekowitz MD, Yusuf S, *et al.* Dabigatran versus warfarin in patients with atrial fibrillation. *N Engl J Med* 2009;**361**(12):1139–51.
27. Noe P, Van D, V, Wittkampf F, Sreeram N. Rapid recovery of cardiac function after catheter ablation of persistent junctional reciprocating tachycardia in children. *Pacing Clin Electrophysiol* 2002;**25**(2):191–4.
28. Aguinaga L, Primo J, Anguera I, *et al.* Long-term follow-up in patients with the permanent form of junctional reciprocating tachycardia treated with radiofrequency ablation. *Pacing Clin Electrophysiol* 1998;**21**(11 Pt 1):2073–8.
29. Walker NL, Cobbe SM, Birnie DH. Tachycardiomyopathy: a diagnosis not to be missed. *Heart* 2004;**90**(2):e7.
30. Nikolic G, Bishop RL, Singh JB. Sudden death recorded during Holter monitoring. *Circulation* 1982;**66**(1):218–25.

31. de Sousa MR, Morillo CA, Rabelo FT, Nogueira Filho AM, Ribeiro AL. Non-sustained ventricular tachycardia as a predictor of sudden cardiac death in patients with left ventricular dysfunction: a meta-analysis. *Eur J Heart Fail* 2008;**10**(10):1007–14.
32. Doval HC, Nul DR, Grancelli HO, *et al.* Nonsustained ventricular tachycardia in severe heart failure. Independent marker of increased mortality due to sudden death. GESICA-GEMA Investigators. *Circulation* 1996;**94**(12):3198–203.
33. Kearney MT, Fox KA, Lee AJ, *et al.* Predicting sudden death in patients with mild to moderate chronic heart failure. *Heart* 2004;**90**(10):1137–43.
34. Akar FG, Rosenbaum DS. Transmural electrophysiological heterogeneities underlying arrhythmogenesis in heart failure. *Circ Res* 2003;**93**(7):638–45.
35. Sicouri S, Antzelevitch C. A subpopulation of cells with unique electrophysiological properties in the deep subepicardium of the canine ventricle. The M cell. *Circ Res* 1991;**68**(6):1729–41.
36. Akar FG, Yan GX, Antzelevitch C, Rosenbaum DS. Unique topographical distribution of M cells underlies reentrant mechanism of torsade de pointes in the long-QT syndrome. *Circulation* 2002;**105**(10):1247–53.
37. Tomaselli GF, Marban E. Electrophysiological remodeling in hypertrophy and heart failure. *Cardiovasc Res* 1999;**42**(2):270–83.
38. McIntosh MA, Cobbe SM, Smith GL. Heterogeneous changes in action potential and intracellular Ca^{2+} in left ventricular myocyte sub-types from rabbits with heart failure. *Cardiovasc Res* 2000;**45**(2):397–409.
39. Pogwizd SM, Schlotthauer K, Li L, Yuan W, Bers DM. Arrhythmogenesis and contractile dysfunction in heart failure: Roles of sodium-calcium exchange, inward rectifier potassium current, and residual beta-adrenergic responsiveness. *Circ Res* 2001;**88**(11):1159–67.
40. Shamim W. Intraventricular conduction delay: a prognostic marker in chronic heart failure. *Int J Cardiol* 1999;**70**:171–8.
41. Shamim W, Yousufuddin M, Cicoria M, Gibson DG, Coats AJS, Henein MY. Incremental changes in QRS duration in serial ECGs over time identify high risk elderly patients with heart failure. *Heart* 2002;**88**(1):47–51.
42. Cleland JGF, Daubert JC, Erdmann E, *et al.* The CARE-HF study (CArdiac REsynchronisation in Heart Failure study): rationale, design and end-points. *Eur J Heart Fail* 2001;**3**(4):481–9.
43. Bristow MR, Saxon LA, Boehmer J, *et al.* Cardiac-resynchronization therapy with or without an implantable defibrillator in advanced chronic heart failure. *N Engl J Med* 2004;**350**(21):2140–50.
44. Pye MP, Cobbe SM. Arrhythmogenesis in experimental models of heart failure: the role of increased load. *Cardiovasc Res* 1996;**32**(2):248–57.
45. Uretsky BF, Thygesen K, Armstrong PW, *et al.* Acute coronary findings at autopsy in heart failure patients with sudden death: results from the Assessment of Treatment With Lisinopril and Survival (ATLAS) trial. *Circulation* 2000;**102**(6):611–16.
46. Saeed M, Link MS, Mahapatra S, *et al.* Analysis of intracardiac electrograms showing monomorphic ventricular tachycardia in patients with implantable cardioverter-defibrillators. *Am J Cardiol* 2000;**85**(5):580–7.
47. Wellens HJ. Ventricular tachycardia: diagnosis of broad QRS complex tachycardia. *Heart* 2001;**86**(5):579–85.
48. Brugada P, Brugada J, Mont L, Smeets J, Andries EW. A new approach to the differential diagnosis of a regular tachycardia with a wide QRS complex. *Circulation* 1991;**83**(5):1649–59.
49. Campbell RW. ACE inhibitors and arrhythmias. *Heart* 1996;**76**(3 Suppl 3):79–82.
50. Cohn JN, Johnson G, Ziesche S, *et al.* A comparison of enalapril with hydralazine-isosorbide dinitrate in the treatment of chronic congestive heart failure. *N Engl J Med* 1991;**325**(5):303–10.
51. Pitt B, Zannad F, Remme WJ, *et al.* The effect of spironolactone on morbidity and mortality in patients with severe heart failure. Randomized Aldactone Evaluation Study Investigators. *N Engl J Med* 1999;**341**(10):709–17.
52. Ramires FJ, Mansur A, Coelho O, *et al.* Effect of spironolactone on ventricular arrhythmias in congestive heart failure secondary to idiopathic dilated or to ischemic cardiomyopathy. *Am J Cardiol* 2000;**85**(10):1207–11.
53. Pitt B, Remme W, Zannad F, *et al.* Eplerenone, a selective aldosterone blocker, in patients with left ventricular dysfunction after myocardial infarction. *N Engl J Med* 2003;**348**(14):1309–21.
54. Greene HL, Roden DM, Katz RJ, Woosley RL, Salerno DM, Henthorn RW. The Cardiac Arrhythmia Suppression Trial: first CAST… then CAST-II. *J Am Coll Cardiol* 1992;**19**(5):894–8.
55. Cairns JA, Connolly SJ, Roberts R, Gent M. Randomised trial of outcome after myocardial infarction in patients with frequent or repetitive ventricular premature depolarisations: CAMIAT. Canadian Amiodarone Myocardial Infarction Arrhythmia Trial Investigators. *Lancet* 1997;**349**(9053):675–82.
56. Julian DG, Camm AJ, Frangin G, *et al.* Randomised trial of effect of amiodarone on mortality in patients with left-ventricular dysfunction after recent myocardial infarction: EMIAT. European Myocardial Infarct Amiodarone Trial Investigators. *Lancet* 1997;**349**(9053):667–74.
57. Effect of prophylactic amiodarone on mortality after acute myocardial infarction and in congestive heart failure: meta-analysis of individual data from 6500 patients in randomised trials. Amiodarone Trials Meta-Analysis Investigators. *Lancet* 1997;**350**(9089):1417–24.
58. Bardy GH, Lee KL, Mark DB, *et al.* Amiodarone or an implantable cardioverter-defibrillator for congestive heart failure. *N Engl J Med* 2005;**352**(3):225–37.
59. Kober L, Torp-Pedersen C, McMurray JJV, *et al.* Increased mortality after dronedarone therapy for severe heart failure. *N Engl J Med* 2008;**358**(25):2678–87.
60. The Antiarrhythmics versus Implantable Defibrillators (AVID) Investigators. A comparison of antiarrhythmic-drug therapy with implantable defibrillators in patients resuscitated from near-fatal ventricular arrhythmias. *N Engl J Med* 1997;**337**(22):1576–84.
61. Kuck KH, Cappato R, Siebels J, Ruppel R. Randomized comparison of antiarrhythmic drug therapy with implantable defibrillators in patients resuscitated from cardiac arrest : the Cardiac Arrest Study Hamburg (CASH). *Circulation* 2000;**102**(7):748–54.
62. Connolly SJ, Gent M, Roberts RS, *et al.* Canadian implantable defibrillator study (CIDS) : a randomized trial of the implantable cardioverter defibrillator against amiodarone. *Circulation* 2000;**101**(11):1297–302.
63. Moss AJ, Zareba W, Hall WJ, *et al.* Prophylactic implantation of a defibrillator in patients with myocardial infarction and reduced ejection fraction. *N Engl J Med* 2002;**346**(12):877–83.
64. Reddy VY, Reynolds MR, Neuzil P, *et al.* Prophylactic catheter ablation for the prevention of defibrillator therapy. *N Engl J Med* 2007;**357**(26):2657–65.
65. Estes NA, III. Ablation after ICD implantation—bridging the gap between promise and practice. *N Engl J Med* 2007;**357**(26):2717–19.
66. Wilber DJ, Kopp DE, Glascock DN, Kinder CA, Kall JG. Catheter ablation of the mitral isthmus for ventricular tachycardia associated with inferior infarction. *Circulation* 1995;**92**(12):3481–9.
67. Kuck KH, Schaumann A, Eckardt L, *et al.* Catheter ablation of stable ventricular tachycardia before defibrillator implantation in patients with coronary heart disease (VTACH): a multicentre randomised controlled trial. *Lancet* 2010;**375**(9708):31–40.
68. Schoeller R, Andresen D, Buttner P, Oezcelik K, Vey G, Schroder R. First or second degree atrioventricular block as a risk factor in idiopathic dilated cardiomyopathy. *Am J Cardiol* 1993;**71**(8):720–6.
69. Epstein AE, DiMarco JP, Ellenbogen KA, *et al.* ACC/AHA/ HRS 2008 Guidelines for Device-Based Therapy of Cardiac Rhythm

Abnormalities: a report of the American College of Cardiology/American Heart Association Task Force on Practice Guidelines (Writing Committee to Revise the ACC/AHA/NASPE 2002 Guideline Update for Implantation of Cardiac Pacemakers and Antiarrhythmia Devices): developed in collaboration with the American Association for Thoracic Surgery and Society of Thoracic Surgeons. *Circulation* 2008;**117**(21):e350–408.

70. Cunningham AD. *National pacemaker and ICD annual report 2007*. Available at: http://www.ic.nhs.uk/webfiles/Services/NCASP/audits%20and%20reports/Annual%20Report%202007.pdf.
71. Sutton R, Kenny RA. The natural history of sick sinus syndrome. *Pacing Clin Electrophysiol* 1986;**9**(6 Pt 2):1110–14.
72. Clarke KW, Connelly DT, Charles RG. Single chamber atrial pacing: an underused and cost-effective pacing modality in sinus node disease. *Heart* 1998;**80**(4):387–9.
73. Sweeney MO, Shea JB, Fox V, *et al.* Randomized pilot study of a new atrial-based minimal ventricular pacing mode in dual-chamber implantable cardioverter-defibrillators. *Heart Rhythm* 2004;**1**:160–7.
74. Healey JS, Toff WD, Lamas GA, *et al.* Cardiovascular outcomes with atrial-based pacing compared with ventricular pacing: meta-analysis of randomized trials, using individual patient data. *Circulation* 2006;**114**:11–17.
75. Lamas GA, Lee KL, Sweeney MO, *et al.* Ventricular pacing or dual-chamber pacing for sinus-node dysfunction *N Engl J Med* 2002;**346**:1854–62.
76. Toff WD, Camm AJ & Skehan JD. Single-chamber versus dual-chamber pacing for high-grade atrioventricular block. *N Engl J Med* 2005;**353**:145–55.
77. Wilkoff BL, Cook JR, Epstein AE. Dual-chamber pacing or ventricular backup pacing in patients with an implantable defibrillator: the Dual Chamber and VVI Implantable Defibrillator (DAVID) Trial. *JAMA* 2002;**288**:3115–23.
78. Lindsay BD. Deleterious effects of right ventricular pacing. *N Engl J Med* 2009;**361**:2183–85.
79. Yu CM, Chan JYS, Zhang Q, *et al.* Biventricular pacing in patients with bradycardia and normal ejection fraction. *N Engl J Med* 2009;**361**:2123–34.
80. Bradley DJ, Bradley EA, Baughman KL, *et al.* Cardiac resynchronization and death from progressive heart failure: a meta-analysis of randomized controlled trials. *JAMA* 2003;**289**:730–9.
81. Cleland JG, Daubert JC, Erdmann E, *et al.* The effect of cardiac resynchronization on morbidity and mortality in heart failure. *N Engl J Med* 2005;**352**:1539–40.

PART XI

Medical therapy for chronic heart failure

37

Angiotensin converting enzyme inhibitors and vasodilators

Iain Squire and Andrew L. Clark

Introduction

Heart failure (HF) is a complex syndrome, characterized by neurohumoral activation. That increased activation of the renin–angiotensin–aldosterone system (RAAS) plays a central role in the pathophysiology of chronic HF, has been recognized for many years.[1] However, until the latter part of the 20th century, the pharmacological management of chronic HF was limited to correction of fluid and electrolyte disturbances (diuretics) and augmentation of myocardial contractility (cardiac glycosides).

The situation is very different now; physicians caring for patients with HF have at their disposal an armamentarium of powerful pharmacological therapies, encompassing angiotensin converting enzyme (ACE) inhibitors, angiotensin receptor antagonists, aldosterone receptor antagonists, and β-receptor blockers, in addition to our old friends diuretics and digoxin. To a greater or lesser extent, the newer agents act to inhibit activity of the RAAS, emphasizing the crucial role of this system in the HF syndrome. Among the agents with proven efficacy in the management of HF, ACE inhibitors have the most extensive evidence base, and, in head-to head comparisons with alternative RAAS inhibitors, remain unsurpassed in terms of clinical benefit.[2–4]

This chapter considers briefly the development and pharmacology of ACE inhibitors, their physiological actions, and the evidence base for their prescription to patients with HF. It also discusses the side effect profile of ACE inhibitors.

Development of ACE inhibitors

It is little remembered that ACE inhibitors for oral administration were designed for the purpose of inhibiting angiotensin converting enzyme, based on the ACE-inhibiting action of peptides from South American pit viper venom, and on similarities between ACE and the pancreatic digestive enzyme carboxypeptidase A. The known zinc dependence of ACE led Ondetti and Cushman[5] to incorporate a sulphydryl moiety in their original dipeptide ACE inhibitor, captopril. Subsequent ACE inhibitor molecules were developed to bind to sites on the ACE molecule other than the zinc atom, with varying aims of increasing duration of action or potency, or to increase absorption. Of currently available ACE inhibitors, only captopril binds via a sulphydryl ligand, fosinopril via a phosphinyl group, and the remainder via a carboxyl ligand.[6] These differences are associated with pharmacokinetic and pharmacodynamic differences, the clinical significance of which is unclear in the management of patients with HF.

Physiology

The RAAS is a ubiquitous endocrine system, and ACE is found in the circulation as well as in many tissues. The enzyme has a number of potential substrates, the most relevant to the use of ACE inhibitors in HF being angiotensin I and bradykinin.

A number of claims has been made for one or other ACE inhibitor having properties of high affinity for, and inhibition of, tissue ACE. In reality, ACE inhibitors block tissue ACE and plasma ACE with the same rank-order of potency. Again, the clinical relevance of differences among ACE inhibitors in this context is unclear. In HF, ACE inhibition leads to reduced plasma angiotensin II and aldosterone levels, with subsequently lower systemic blood pressure via reduction in peripheral vascular resistance. In contrast to other vasodilator drugs, the fall in systemic vascular resistance is not accompanied by reflex tachycardia, possibly due to interaction between angiotensin II and the sympathetic nervous system. Plasma potassium concentrations increase. Left-sided cardiac pressures fall rapidly after ACE inhibition, as does pulmonary artery pressure, and cardiac index increases. Importantly, these changes, beneficial in the setting of HF, are maintained with chronic dosing and in exercise. Cardiac work and myocardial oxygen demand is reduced, and left ventricular ejection fraction (LVEF) tends to increase, at least with chronic treatment.

The magnitude of the blood pressure response to ACE inhibition is often a concern to physicians caring for patients with HF. Indeed, in the early years of ACE inhibitor use, it was common practice for patients to be admitted to hospital for initiation of therapy.

This seldom, if ever, happens now. Prediction of the magnitude of blood pressure response in an individual patient is very difficult, and we will return to this clinical issue later in the chapter.

In clinical practice, ACE inhibitor therapy is well tolerated in the vast majority of patients. Measured changes in systemic blood pressure are seldom associated with clinically meaningful symptoms, although they do occur in a minority of patients. While accumulation of bradykinin appears to contribute to the fall in blood pressure after ACE inhibition in normal individuals,[7] it is not known whether the accumulation occurs in people with HF. Moreover, the relevance to the survival benefits of ACE inhibition is doubtful, given the consistent equivalence or superiority of ACE inhibitors over angiotensin receptor blockers (ARBs) in clinical studies to date. Importantly, the acute haemodynamic response to ACE inhibition is poor predictor of clinical benefit.[8]

ACE inhibitors in clinical practice

Captopril, the first orally administered ACE inhibitor, was demonstrated in 1979 to lower left ventricular filling pressure and systemic vascular resistance in HF.[9] Sustained beneficial haemodynamic effects were demonstrated soon afterwards.[10]

The earliest evidence of survival benefit from vasodilators in HF came from two studies in the mid 1980s,[11,12] with the first evidence for benefit of ACE inhibitors coming from a trend to survival in the captopril multicenter research trial.[13] Since then, ACE inhibitors have become perhaps the most extensively investigated class of drug in any branch of medicine, and certainly in HF, with tens of thousands of patients enrolled in clinical trials, and many millions treated in clinical practice.

Clinical trials of ACE inhibitors in chronic heart failure

The first randomized, controlled trial to show a clear benefit from ACE inhibition in CHF was the CONSENSUS study.[14] In what would now be considered a very small trial, 127 patients were randomized to receive enalapril at a dose of 2.5–40 mg once daily, and 126 received matching placebo. The patient group chosen for this trial was at high risk, being a population of patients with advanced HF and New York Heart Association (NYHA) class IV symptoms. Over an average follow-up of 6 months, crude mortality of 44% in the placebo group was reduced to 26% in those treated with enalapril, a relative risk reduction of 40%, which was ascribed entirely to reduction in death from progressive HF.

Perhaps the magnitude of benefit in this trial was fortuitous, but case-fatality in the placebo group was indeed representative of that seen in such patients at the time. An important point is that a consistent finding in trials of ACE inhibition in HF is that those patients with the most severe disease have the greatest relative benefit from intervention.

CONSENSUS was one of two landmark trials which demonstrated the benefit of enalapril in patients with chronic, symptomatic HF. The other was the Studies of Left Ventricular Dysfunction (SOLVD) treatment trial,[15] which recruited patients with less symptomatic HF, mostly NYHA II–III. In SOLVD, 2569 patients were randomized to receive enalapril 2.5–10 mg twice daily (n = 1285) daily or placebo (n = 1284). The summary statistics for the results of these two trials are shown in Table 37.1.

The absolute and relative risk reductions seen in these trials, and the numbers of patients needed to treat to achieve one event saved, are clear and consistent, and it is on the basis of these result that we base our use of ACE inhibitors in chronic HF. The observations are also supported by a meta-analysis of smaller randomized trials, which also reported improved survival, reduced hospitalization, and improvement in quality of life and exercise capacity.[16]

ACE inhibitors in asymptomatic heart failure

Between them, CONSENSUS (NYHA IV) and SOLVD treatment (NYHA II–III) addressed the efficacy of patients with symptomatic HF and reduced LVEF. As ACE inhibition produces benefit primarily by interfering with pathophysiological processes, rather than with symptoms, the SOLVD prevention trial examined the effect of enalapril, in the same doses as used in the treatment trial, in patients with asymptomatic left ventricular systolic dysfunction (LVSD).[17] As shown in Table 37.1, the effects on mortality were of lesser magnitude than in the other trials, but there was a statistically

Table 37.1 Summary statistics from CONSENSUS and SOLVD (Treatment) trials

	Deaths				NNT	Additional findings
	Number		RRR	ARR		
CONSENSUS NYHA IV LVEF ≤40%	Enalapril n = 127	33 (26%)	40%[a] (p = 0.002)	18%	7 (over average of 6 months)	Reduced NYHA class; reduced heart size
	Placebo n = 126	55 (44%)				
SOLVD-T NYHA II–III LVEF ≤35%	Enalapril n = 1285	452 (35.2%)	16% (p = 0.0036)	4.5%	22 (over average of 41 months)	26% reduction HF hospitalization
	Placebo n = 1284	510 (39.7%)				
SOLVD-P NYHA I LVEF ≤35%	Enalapril n = 2111	313 (14.8%)	8% (p = 0.30)	1%	N/A	20% RRR in risk of death or HF hospitalization
	Placebo n = 2117	334 (15.8%)				

[a] 6-month mortality RRR. 1-year RRR was 31%

ARR, absolute risk reduction; HF, heart failure; LVEF, left ventricular ejection fraction; NNT, number needed to treat to delay one death; NYHA, New York Heart Association; RRR, relative risk reduction.

significant benefit in the composite of death or HF hospitalization. Thus, there is evidence or the use of ACE inhibitors in chronic LVSD irrespective of symptom severity.

Why might the benefit in asymptomatic patients be so much less than in those with symptoms, in the context of similar LVEF? There are of course a myriad of potential explanations, but the observation perhaps demonstrates the limitations of assessing the severity of HF using LVEF as a dichotomized variable. In the current era, we have much more sensitive tools by which we may make this assessment, in particular plasma biomarkers such as natriuretic peptides. However, great reliance continues to be put upon (usually echocardiographic) assessment of LVEF. The potential usefulness of contemporary measures should be borne in mind when assessing an individual patient with HF.

Clinical trials of ACE inhibitors after acute myocardial infarction

For patients with chronic HF, starting treatment with an ACE inhibitor is secondary prevention therapy introduced at very variable time points in the natural history of an individual's disease progression. As the single largest contributing cause of chronic HF is coronary artery disease, starting ACE inhibitors in patients with acute myocardial infarction (AMI) in the coronary care unit represents an opportunity to start treatment early in the course of the disease. Following the results of CONSENSUS and SOLVD, it was logical that the impact of ACE inhibition should be investigated in patients early following AMI.

The randomized, placebo-controlled clinical trials of ACE inhibition following AMI have varied in terms of eligibility criteria, timing of initiation of therapy in relation to the index event, and duration of follow-up. Overall, the trials can be divided helpfully into (1) those which initiated ACE inhibition in the acute phase of AMI, recruited patients irrespective of evidence of HF or LVSD, and continued therapy for a relatively short period of time and (2) those which initiated therapy more remote from the index MI, recruited patients with evidence of impaired left ventricular function, and continued therapy over a longer period.

Early ACE inhibition

Four major trials have investigated the effects of ACE inhibition initiated 0–36 h after the onset of symptoms of myocardial infarction (MI), together including nearly 100 000 patients.[18–21] These trials—CONSENSUS II,[18] GISSI-3,[19] ISIS-4,[20] and CCS-1[21]—enrolled patients within 24 h [18–20] or 36 h[21] of onset of symptoms, and investigated captopril,[20,21] lisinopril,[19] or enalapril[18] administered over 28 days [20,21], 42 days,[19] or 6 months.[18]

Reassuringly, in a meta-analysis, there was no evidence of heterogeneity among the results of the four trials.[22] Over the first 30 days of follow-up, mortality was 7.1% in patients allocated to ACE inhibitor, and 7.6% in patients allocated to comparator treatment, a 7% relative risk reduction (p = 0.004), and corresponding to approximately 5 fewer deaths per 1000 patients treated for 30 days. Remarkably, 80% of these deaths were avoided in the first 7 days of treatment, corresponding to 4 fewer deaths per 1000 treated patients. The incidence of nonfatal HF was also reduced over the first 30 days.[22]

The CONSENSUS II study[18] is unique among outcome studies of ACE inhibition in HF in that treatment was initiated with intravenous enalaprilat, followed by oral enalapril. It is also the only randomized, controlled trial of ACE inhibition in which the point estimate of the magnitude of effect was indicative of harm. The implications of this are discussed below.

Across the four trials, the absolute and proportional benefits of ACE inhibition were similar in men and women, and across age groups. It is important to note that absolute benefits were greater in patients at higher risk of adverse outcome; thus, patients with high heart rate, high Killip class at entry, with anterior MI or with prior MI or diabetes had greater absolute benefit.

Later ACE inhibition

Several randomized controlled trials have studied the efficacy of initiation of ACE inhibition after AMI but commenced beyond the very early phase. The trials have also been characterized by restriction of eligibility to patients with clinical or echocardiographic evidence of left ventricular dysfunction, and have observed the effects of therapy over at least a year.

The three largest such trials were SAVE,[23] AIRE,[24] and TRACE,[25] which respectively studied captopril, ramipril, and trandolapril, each started at least 3 days after the acute event. As with the trials of early ACE inhibition, meta-analysis indicates the absence of heterogeneity among the results, with significant overall benefit.[26] Across the three trials, median duration of treatment was 31 months, during which case-fatality in patients receiving ACE inhibitor was 23.4% compared to 29.1% for placebo, an absolute reduction of 5.7% and an odds ratio for mortality of 0.74 (95% CI 0.66–0.83). This equates to 60 fewer deaths per 1000 patients treated for 30 months. Survival benefit was evident within a few weeks of initiation of treatment (Fig. 37.1).

In the longer-term trials in patients with impaired left ventricular function, ACE inhibition was also associated with reduced risk of hospitalization with HF, and of reinfarction.

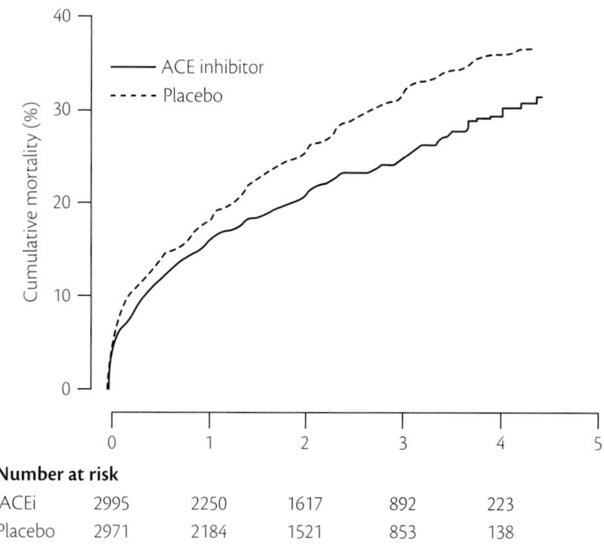

Fig. 37.1 Combined Kaplan–Meier mortality curve for the SAVE, AIRE, and TRACE trials of ACE inhibition (ACEi) in patients with heart failure or echocardiographic left ventricular systolic dysfunction following AMI.
From Flather MD,Yusuf S, Køber L, *et al.* Long-term ACE-inhibitor therapy in patients with heart failure or left-ventricular dysfunction: a systematic overview of data from individual patients *Lancet* 2000;**355**:1575–81.

Adverse events in post myocardial infarction ACE inhibitor trials

The potential benefits of ACE inhibition after MI are clear; treatment is associated with statistically, and clinically, significant benefits. The benefits were not achieved without unwanted effects. In the short-term early-treatment trials[18–21] persistent hypotension occurred in 17.6% and 9.3% of ACE inhibitor and control patients respectively, an excess of 84 per 1000 patients treated. Although there were more cases of cardiogenic shock and renal dysfunction in ACE inhibitor-treated patients compared with placebo (4.6 and 6.2 per 1000 respectively), absolute event rates were very small.

In the trials in which an ACE inhibitor was started rather later and continued for longer,[23–25] hypotension (14.7% in ACE inhibitor-treated patients compared with 8.7% in placebo-treated patients; OR 1.86, $p < 0.0001$) and renal dysfunction (5.2% ACE inhibitor compared with 3.6% placebo; OR 1.49, $p < 0.0001$) were more common with active therapy, but again the absolute rates were low.

ACE inhibition after acute myocardial infarction—which patients?

The studies of early (<36 h) initiation show a relatively small overall benefit using an all-inclusive, unselective approach to treatment; the benefit is seen within the first 7 days, and is of greater absolute magnitude in patients with higher baseline risk. The benefits are countered (to some degree) by a greater likelihood of important adverse events within the same time frame, including cardiogenic shock.[22] The adverse events were particularly evident in the CONSENSUS II trial, which addressed the hypothesis that very early ACE inhibition with intravenous enalaprilat would be of clinical benefit. That CONSENSUS II refuted the hypothesis serves as a caution against the introduction of powerful pharmacological therapy in the very early period after AMI.

The studies of later introduction of ACE inhibition, recruiting patients with evidence of left ventricular impairment followed for longer periods, showed greater absolute benefit as the studies included only higher risk patients. Benefit was again evident from an early time after initiation of treatment.

Overall, the data support the prescription of ACE inhibitor from around day 3 after MI, in patients with evidence of left ventricular dysfunction. In patients without evidence of significant LVSD, additional criteria suggesting that there is likely to be benefit from treatment should be considered; prior or concomitant conditions (e.g. diabetes or prior MI, hypertension), the site (anterior) or extent of MI (high cardiac enzymes or troponin) should encourage the use of ACE inhibitor.

In Europe, current guidelines[27] recommend prescription of ACE inhibitor for patients with LVEF below 40%.[27] Other (UK national) guideline documents recommend that ACE inhibition should be considered for all patients with HF due to LVSD.[28] In reality, in many countries ACE inhibition is prescribed to the majority of patients after MI, or with a diagnosis of HF, irrespective of left ventricular function. This is pragmatic, and safe for the vast majority of patients, but caution should be exercised; after AMI, very early treatment should be avoided, and care should be taken in patients with impaired renal function and in haemodynamically compromised individuals. In the future, more sophisticated methods may be used to identify patients likely to benefit from therapy, such as the circulating concentration of one or more biomarker.

The patients at highest risk have the most to gain from treatment. However, such patients are often the most challenging to treat with ACE inhibition, and indeed with other pharmacological therapies; they may present with extensive infarction or severe HF, low blood pressure, and renal impairment. It is in the management of these individuals that physicians best demonstrate their clinical expertise. In practice a clinically pragmatic approach may be adopted; if the patient has sufficient blood pressure to maintain cerebral (i.e. no, or minimal, symptoms of hypotension), and renal (maintenance of appropriate renal function) perfusion, then that patient has adequate blood pressure. This avoids the often knee-jerk response to low brachial blood pressure which leads to withdrawal of disease-modifying therapy.

An alternative to ACE inhibitor in chronic heart failure? Comparative studies

A number of studies have compared the clinical efficacy of ACE inhibitors to alternative pharmacological therapy. Indeed, one of the earliest trials to investigate the clinical effects of ACE inhibitors in HF was a comparison of enalapril against the combination of hydralazine and isosorbide dinitrate, the second Veterans Administration Heart Failure Trial, VHeFT II.[29]

More recent studies have investigated the comparative benefits of ACE inhibitors and angiotensin receptor antagonists, the class of agent which has become the alternative RAAS inhibitor. The first such trial, ELITE, Evaluation of Losartan in The Elderly, suggested that losartan in a target dose of 50 mg once daily was associated with over 40% improved survival compared to captopril.[30] Unsurprisingly, this result stimulated enormous interest in the angiotensin receptor antagonists, and led to a number of large, properly powered studies. ELITE was a safety and tolerability study in only approximately 700 patients, and the subsequent definitive outcome trial, ELITE II, showed no superiority of losartan over captopril.[31]

ACE inhibitors have also stood up to the test of comparison with ARBs . Losartan has once again been compared with captopril, in the OPTIMAAL (Optimal Trial In Myocardial Infarction with the angiotensin II antagonist Losartan) trial.[32] The results of this trial, summarized in Table 37.2, confirmed the (statistically nonsignificant) superiority of the ACE inhibitor captopril, at a mean dose of 45 mg three times daily, compared to losartan at a mean dose of 44 mg once daily. A later post MI trial, VALIANT, studied the comparative survival benefits of captopril, valsartan, or the combination of the two agents. VALIANT demonstrated very similar survival benefit for captopril compared to valsartan, with no evidence of added benefit, and greater side effects, from the combination of the two.[33]

Overall, the evidence is compelling for the use of ACE inhibitors in patients with LVSD in patients with HF or following AMI. No alternative single agent has been shown to be superior to ACE inhibitors in improving both mortality and morbidity.

Side effect profile

The ACE inhibitors are generally very well tolerated and have a side effect profile predictable from their pharmacology; they lower blood pressure and glomerular perfusion in the kidney, and inhibition of neutral endopeptidase leads to accumulation of bradykinin. The resulting potential effects are: symptomatic hypotension, renal impairment, and cough. It is important to remember that each of

Table 37.2 Summary of clinical endpoints for treatment with losartan or with captopril in the OPTIMAAL trial[32]

	Losartan	Captopril	RR losartan vs captopril	p value
All-cause mortality	499 (18.2%)	447 (16.4%)	1.13 (0.99–1.28)	0.069
Myocardial reinfarction	384 (14.0%)	379 (13.9%)	1.03 (0.89–1.18)	0.722
Cardiovascular mortality	420 (15.3%)	363 (13.3%)	1.17 (1.01–1.34)	0.032
First all-cause hospitalization	1806 (65.8%)	1774 (64.9%)	1.03 (0.97–1.10)	0.362
First HF hospitalization	306 (11.2%)	For 265 (9.7%)	1.16 (0.98–1.37)	0.072

HF, heart failure; RR, relative risk.

these side effects is commonly found in patients with HF irrespective of ACE inhibitor therapy.

Renal impairment is a common accompaniment to HF, and there is a small absolute risk of significant worsening following initiation of ACE inhibitor therapy. In the SAVE, TRACE, and SOLVD studies, renal impairment was recorded in 5.2% of patients treated with ACE inhibitor compared to 3.6% of patients receiving placebo.[26] In clinical practice patients at risk of developing renal dysfunction are not easy to identify, but renovascular disease is more prevalent among patients with peripheral vascular disease. Thus, the finding of reduced or absent peripheral (foot) pulses indicates a patient at risk of renovascular disease. It is important to remember that a degree of deterioration in renal function is to be expected after introduction or up-titration of ACE inhibitor therapy. A small increase in urea and creatinine should not lead to withdrawal of ACE therapy. Changes in renal function should always be considered in the context of the patient's quality of life and prognosis, and in the context of the potential consequences of denial of disease-modifying ACE inhibitor treatment.

Cough is common in patients with HF, and is often incorrectly assumed to be secondary to the patient's ACE inhibitor. The clinical response to withdrawal of treatment should always be monitored.

A lowering of blood pressure is an expected consequence of ACE inhibitor therapy, and this alone should not raise concerns of health care professionals caring for those with HF. In contrast, hypotension leading to symptoms is of more concern and may limit therapy. While often described as 'first-dose hypotension', and considered by many to occur only at the initiation of treatment, the blood pressure response to an individual dose of a given ACE inhibitor is the same after many months of treatment as it is to the very first dose.[33,34]

The variation in the blood pressure response to the very first dose of ACE inhibitor can be gauged from Fig. 37.2, which shows the individual mean arterial pressure responses to the first dose of oral enalapril 2.5 mg in 24 patients with HF.[35] While the maximum average fall in mean arterial pressure was 15 mmHg, it ranged from zero to over 40 mmHg; importantly the time to the maximum fall varied enormously, from 2 to 8 h.

Although a number of physiological variables have been reported to be associated with the magnitude of the blood pressure response to ACE inhibition, it is in reality very difficult to predict in an individual patient with HF. Murray *et al.*[35] attempted to identify clinical variables predicting the magnitude of the blood pressure fall in response to initiation of ACE inhibition in 144 patients with HF. Age, sex, NYHA class, diuretic dose, sodium, potassium, creatinine concentration, serum ACE activity, and plasma renin concentration were not predictive of the fall in blood pressure. At best, the combination of plasma renin activity, creatinine, age, the ACE inhibitor, and baseline blood pressure explained less than 25% of the blood pressure response. It is of note that in these patients with HF, higher baseline blood pressure was associated with a greater fall in response to ACE inhibition.

Finally, a small fall in haemoglobin may be observed during ACE inhibitor treatment, possibly as a consequence of the role of angiotensin II in the formation of erythroid precursors. The magnitude of fall in haematocrit is seldom more than 5%; the overall risk of a clinically significant change is very small and is associated with higher creatinine and with concurrent weight loss,[36] both of which are more common in advanced HF.

Initiation and titration

It is clear from the above that adverse events in response to initiation of ACE inhibition, while rare, are potentially important and are unpredictable. On this background, all national[28] and international[27] guidelines for the management of HF recommend initiation of therapy at a low dose of the individual agent, and careful monitoring of the response of both blood pressure and renal function. This is simple, sound advice.

Hydralazine and nitrates

Hydralazine is a direct-acting vasodilator acting predominantly on the arterial side of the circulation. Nitrates are vasodilators with marked effects on the venous circulation. Used together, the combination therapy potentially offers balanced vasodilation, reducing both preload and afterload for the failing heart.

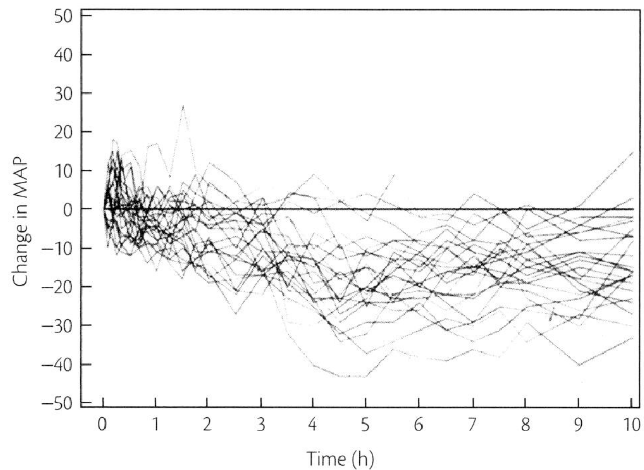

Fig. 37.2 Individual change in mean arterial blood pressure in 24 patients with heart failure following the first oral dose of enalapril 2.5 mg.

In the earliest large-scale mortality study for patients with chronic HF, 652 patients were randomized to receive combination therapy with the combination of hydralazine and isosorbide dinitrate, prazosin (an α-blocker), or placebo.[37] The study, known as VHeFT 1, showed a small benefit from the hydralazine and isosorbide dinitrate combination over the other limbs of the study.

The next step was VHeFT 2, in which 804 men with chronic HF were randomized to either the hydralazine and isosorbide dinitrate combination or enalapril.[38] Two-year mortality was significantly lower in patients randomized to enalapril than hydralazine/isosorbide dinitrate, although a striking finding was that combination therapy led to a greater improvement in exercise capacity than did enalapril.

Interest in the hydralazine/nitrate combination largely waned with the results of VHeFT 2. Hydralazine is a difficult drug to use, particularly as some subjects metabolize it slowly (slow acetylators) and are at risk of developing a lupus-like syndrome with its use. Both hydralazine and nitrates are metabolized rapidly and have to be given frequently to have an effect.

However, reviews of the VHeFT programme suggested that black patients may have more to gain from hydralazine/nitrate therapy than white patients.[39] The AHeFT (African-American Heart Failure Trial) was thus constructed.[40] Over 1000 black patients were randomized to receive isosorbide dinitrate plus hydralazine or placebo in addition to standard therapy for HF. All the patients had dilated left ventricles, and nearly 80% were taking either an ACE inhibitor or angiotensin receptor antagonist at baseline. There was a significant improvement in outcome in patients treated with isosorbide dinitrate plus hydralazine.

The practical consequences are not clear-cut. The results lend support to the common practice of using hydralazine/isosorbide dinitrate in patients with chronic HF who for some reason cannot tolerate an ACE inhibitor or ARB. However, there is no clear-cut evidence that such an approach is appropriate in white patients. Equally, it is not clear whether all people with HF who identify themselves as being black should be offered hydralazine/isosorbide dinitrate.

Other vasodilators

An important finding from VHeFT 2[38] was that hydralazine/isosorbide dinitrate had a greater effect on exercise capacity than enalapril although a lesser effect on mortality. The finding emphasizes the importance of the neurohormonal hypothesis for HF—ACE inhibitors are not mediating their benefit primarily through vasodilatation. Drugs with more pure vasodilating activity, such as flosequinan, do improve exercise capacity quite strikingly,[41] but are associated with a worse outcome.[42]

Amlodipine, a dihydropyridine calcium antagonist, has been extensively tested in HF. The PRAISE trial[43] suggested that amlodipine might be beneficial for patients with HF due to causes other than ischaemic heart disease. PRAISE-2 studied 1652 patients with severe HF and a normal coronary angiogram randomized to amlodipine or placebo.[44] There was no difference in outcome between the two groups. It is possible that the difference between PRAISE and PRAISE-2 is explained by a beneficial effect of amlodipine in patients with HF due to occult coronary heart disease: such patients in PRAISE would have been analysed together with patients with dilated cardiomyopathy as there was no requirement for coronary angiography on PRAISE, only PRAISE-2.

The general conclusion from the PRAISE study programme is that there is no role for specific vasodilators in patients with chronic HF, but that if a patient has angina or blood pressure difficult to control with standard HF medication, then amlodipine is a safe additional therapy.

Summary

The ACE inhibitors are among the most investigated groups of drugs in cardiovascular medicine. Twenty-five years after the first inkling that ACE inhibitors may have a place in the management of HF, they remain a central component of the physician's armamentarium. As a class, ACE inhibitors have transformed not only the management of patients with HF, but also our understanding of this complex syndrome. All efforts should be made to initiate, and maintain at appropriate doses, treatment with ACE inhibitors in all patients with LVSD. We, and our patients, are fortunate to have them.

References

1. Nicholls GG, Riegger AJG. Renin in cardiac failure. In: Robertson JIS, Nicholls MG (eds.) *The renin angiotensin system,* pp 76.1–76.21. Gower Medical Publishing, London, 1993.
2. Pitt B, Poole-Wilson PA, Segal R, *et al.* Effects of losartan compared with captopril on mortality in patients with symptomatic heart failure: the Losartan Heart Failure Survival Study ELITE II. *Lancet* 2000;**355**:1582–7.
3. Dickstein K, Kjekshus J, and the OPTIMAAL Steering Committee Effects of losartan and captopril on mortality and morbidity in high-risk patients after acute myocardial infarction: the OPTIMAAL randomised trial. *Lancet* 2002;**360**:752–60.
4. Pfeffer MA, McMurray JJ, Velazquez EJ, *et al.* Valsartan, captopril or both in myocardial infarction complicated by heart failure, left ventricular dysfunction, or both. *N Engl J Med* 2003;**349**(20):1893–906.
5. Cushman DW, Ondetti MA. Personal and historical perspectives: history of the design of captopril and related inhibitors of angiotensin converting enzyme. *Hypertension* 1991;**17**:589–592.
6. Johnston CI. Angiotensin converting enzyme inhibitors. In Robertson JIS, Nicholls MG (eds.) *The renin angiotensin system,* pp 87.1–87.15. Gower Medical Publishing, London, 1993.
7. Squire IB, O'Kane KPJ, Anderson N, Reid JL. Bradykinin B2 receptor antagonism attenuates the blood pressure response to acute ACE inhibition in normal man. *Hypertension* 2000;**36**:132–6.
8. Packer M, Medina N, Yushak M, Meller J. Haemodynamic patterns of response during long-term captopril therapy for severe chronic heart failure. *Circulation* 1983;**68**:803–12.
9. Turini GA, Gribic M, Brunner HR, Waeber B, Gavras H. Improvement of chronic congestive heart failure by oral captopril. *Lancet* 1979;**i**:1213–15.
10. Dzau VJ, Colucci WS, Williams GH, Curfman G, Meggs L, Hollenberg NK. Sustained effectiveness of converting enzyme inhibition in patients with severe congestive heart failure. *N Engl J Med* 1980;**302**:1373–9.
11. Furberg CD, Yusuf S. Effect of vasodilators on survival in chronic congestive heart failure. *Am J Cardiol* 1985;**55**:1110–13.
12. Cohn J, Archibald DG, Ziesche S, *et al.* Effect of vasodilator therapy on mortality in chronic congestive heart failure. *N Engl J Med* 1986;**314**:1547–55.
13. Captopril Multicenter Research Group. A placebo controlled trial of captopril in refractory chronic congestive heart failure. *J Am Coll Cardiol* 1983;**2**:755–63.

14. The CONSENSUS Trial Study Group. Effects of enalapril on mortality in severe congestive heart failure. Results of the cooperative North Scandinavian Enalapril Survival Study (CONSENSUS). *N Engl J Med* 1987;**316**:1429–35.
15. The SOLVD Investigators. Effects of enalapril on survival in patients with reduced left ventricular ejection fractions and congestive heart failure. *N Engl J Med* 1991;**325**:293–302.
16. McAlister FA, Stewart S, Ferrua S, McMurray JJ. Multidisciplinary strategies for the management of heart failure patients at high risk of admission: a systematic review of randomised trials. *J Am coll Cardiol* 2004;**44**:810–19.
17. The SOLVD Investigators. Effect of enalapril on mortality and the development of heart failure in asymptomatic patients with reduced left ventricular ejection fractions. *N Engl J Med* 1992;**327**:685–91.
18. Swedberg K, Held P, Kjekshus J, *et al.*, on behalf of the CONSENSUS II Study Group. Effects of the early administration of enalapril on mortality in patients with acute myocardial infarction: results of the Cooperative New Scandinavian Enalapril Survival Study II (CONSENSUS II). *N Engl J Med.* 1992;**327**:678–84.
19. Gruppo Italiano per lo Studio della Sopravvivenza nell'Infarto Miocardico. GISSI-3: effects of lisinopril and transdermal glyceryl trinitrate singly and together on 6-week mortality and ventricular function after acute myocardial infarction. *Lancet* 1994;**343**:1115–22.
20. ISIS-4 Collaborative Group. ISIS-4: a randomised factorial trial assessing early oral captopril, oral mononitrate, and intravenous magnesium sulphate in 58050 patients with suspected acute myocardial infarction. *Lancet* 1995;**345**:669–85.
21. Chinese Cardiac Study Collaborative Group. Oral captopril versus placebo among 13,634 patients with suspected acute myocardial infarction: interim report from the Chinese Cardiac Study (CCS-1). *Lancet* 1995;**345**:686–7.
22. ACE Inhibitor Myocardial Infarction Collaborative Group. Indications for ACE Inhibitors in the Early Treatment of Acute Myocardial Infarction; systematic overview of individual data from 100 000 patients in randomized trials. *Circulation* 1998;**97**:2202–12.
23. Pfeffer MA, Braunwald E, Moyé L, *et al.* Effect of captopril on mortality and morbidity in patients with left ventricular dysfunction after myocardial infarction: results of the survival and ventricular enlargement trial. *N Engl J Med* 1992;**327**:669–77.
24. Acute Infarction Ramipril Efficacy (AIRE) Study Investigators. Effect of ramipril on mortality and morbidity of survivors of acute myocardial infarction with clinical evidence of heart failure. *Lancet* 1993;**342**:821–28.
25. Kober L, Torp-Pedersen C, Carlsen JE, *et al.* A clinical trial of the angiotensin-converting-enzyme inhibitor trandolapril in patients with left ventricular dysfunction after myocardial infarction. *N Engl J Med* 1995;**333**:1670–76.
26. Flather MD,Yusuf S, Køber L, *et al.* Long-term ACE-inhibitor therapy in patients with heart failure or left-ventricular dysfunction: a systematic overview of data from individual patients. *Lancet* 2000;**355**:1575–81.
27. The Task Force for the diagnosis and treatment of acute and chronic heart failure 2008 of the European Society of Cardiology ESC Guidelines for the diagnosis and treatment of acute and chronic heart failure 2008. *Eur Heart J* 2008;**29**:2388–442.
28. National Institute for Health and Clinical Excellence. *Chronic heart failure.* NICE Guideline Document 5, 2003.
29. Cohn JN, Johnson G, Ziesche S, *et al.* A comparison of enalapril with hydralazine-isosorbide dinitrate in the treatment of chronic congestive heart failure. *N Engl J Med* 1991;**325**:303–10.
30. Pitt B, Segal R, Martinez FA, *et al.* Randomised trial of losartan versus captopril in patients over 65 with heart failure. *Lancet* 1997;**349**:747–52.
31. Pitt B, Poole-Wilson PA, Segal R, *et al.* Effect of losartan compared with captopril on mortality in patients with symptomatic heart failure: randomised trial—the Losartan Heart Failure Survival Study ELITE II. *Lancet* 2000;**355**:1582–7.
32. Dickstein K, Kjekshus J,. and the OPTIMAAL Steering Committee Effects of losartan and captopril on mortality and morbidity in high-risk patients after acute myocardial infarction: the OPTIMAAL randomised trial. *Lancet* 2002;**360**:752–60.
33. McLay JS, McMurray J, Bridges A, Struthers AD. Practical issues when initiating captopril therapy in chronic heart failure. *Eur Heart J* 1992;**13**:1521–1527.
34. Packer M, Lee WH, Yushak M, Medina N. Comparison of captopril and enalapril in patients with severe chronic heart failure. *N Engl J Med* 1986;**315**:847–53.
35. Murray L, Squire IB, Reid JL, Lees KR. Determinants of the blood pressure response to the first dose of ACE inhibitor in mild to moderate congestive heart failure. *Br J Clin Pharmacol* 1998;**45**:559–66.
36. Ishani A, Weinhandl E, Zhao Z, *et al.* Angiotensin converting enzyme inhibitor as a risk factor for the development of anaemia, and the impact of incident anaemia on mortality in patients with left ventricular dysfunction. *J Am Coll Cardiol* 2005;**45**:391–9.
37. Cohn JN, Archibald DG, Ziesche S, *et al.* Effect of vasodilator therapy on mortality in chronic congestive heart failure. Results of a Veterans Administration Cooperative Study. *N Engl J Med* 1986;**314**:1547–52.
38. Cohn JN, Johnson G, Ziesche S, *et al.* A comparison of enalapril with hydralazine-isosorbide dinitrate in the treatment of chronic congestive heart failure. *N Engl J Med* 1991;**325**:303–10.
39. Carson P, Ziesche S, Johnson G, Cohn JN. Racial differences in response to therapy for heart failure: analysis of the vasodilator heart failure trials. *J Card Fail* 1999;**5**:178–87.
40. Taylor AL, Ziesche S, Yancy C, *et al.*; African-American Heart Failure Trial Investigators. Combination of isosorbide dinitrate and hydralazine in blacks with heart failure. *N Engl J Med* 2004;**351**:2049–57.
41. Cowley AJ, Wynne RD, Stainer K, Fullwood L, Rowley JM, Hampton JR. Flosequinan in heart failure: acute haemodynamic and longer term symptomatic effects. *BMJ* 1988;**297**:169–73.
42. Packer M, Rouleau J, Swedberg K, *et al.* Effect of flosequinan on survival in chronic heart failure: preliminary results of the PROFILE study. *Circulation* 1993;**88**(suppl 1):301.
43. Packer M, O'Connor CM, Ghali JK, *et al.* Effect of amlodipine on morbidity and mortality in severe chronic heart failure. Prospective Randomized Amlodipine Survival Evaluation Study Group. *N Engl J Med* 1996;**335**:1107–14.
44. Thackray S, Witte K, Clark AL, Cleland JG. Clinical trials update: OPTIME-CHF, PRAISE-2, ALL-HAT. *Eur J Heart Fail* 2000;**2**:209–12.

38

β-Adrenoreceptor antagonists and heart failure

Henry J. Dargie and Desmond Fitzgerald

Background

Sir James Black's quest for a substance that would block the potentially harmful effects of adrenaline on the ischaemic heart led to his invention of the β-adrenoceptor (AR) antagonists pronethalol and propranalol between 1959 and 1962.[1] The ubiquitous nature of adrenaline ensured that these β-AR antagonists, commonly referred to in clinical practice as β-blockers, found a role in multiple aspects of cardiovascular therapeutics.[2] Sir James could not have predicted the colossal impact his discovery of β-blockers subsequently would have in improving the lives and preventing the deaths of countless patients over the subsequent 50 years. Regarded by basic scientists as the father of analytical pharmacology, he was also a committed exponent of what we now regard as translational medical research. James Black's achievement in discovering β-blockers followed by histamine type 2 antagonists (H_2 blockers), the first effective treatment for peptic ulcer, was recognized by the award of the Nobel Prize in 1986.

Black's original hypothesis was that patients with stable angina pectoris might benefit by reducing the work of the heart, rather than increasing the blood flow. So the first clinical study with the initial β-blocker pronethalol was carried out in angina pectoris by Pritchard.[3] In a careful dose–response study he showed that there was clinical improvement in 16 of 17 patients. Pritchard also noted that during the dose–response period there was also a fall in blood pressure. This serendipitous observation was confirmed in a subsequent study with propranolol showing a significant fall in blood pressure in 17 of 18 patients. Subsequent clinical studies showed that propranolol had antiarrhythmic properties, and much later reduced mortality in patients with myocardial infarction (MI).[4] Most recently β-blockers have conclusively been shown to be of great benefit in heart failure (HF), clearly demonstrating the extensive role of sympathetic nervous activity in cardiovascular disease.[5,6] The pharmacological properties of β-blockers that have been used in heart failure studies are summarized in Table 38.1.

Using β-blockers in HF seems counter-intuitive given that the increased sympathetic activity that occurs in patients with HF is required to support the failing heart. Early experimental studies of propranolol in experimental HF in calves[7,8] fuelled a natural concern at inhibiting the very system on which the heart appeared to depend for support. Based on such clinical considerations, there was a universally agreed view that the use of the nonselective β-blockers available at that time was contraindicated in HF.[9]

Despite these experimental findings and clinical anecdotage, the early published studies of β-blockade in patients with HF in the United Kingdom and Sweden did point tantalizingly to potential benefit in selected patients, but it was not until the 1970s that the somewhat counter-intuitive notion of using β-blockers to treat patients with HF began to be taken seriously. The initial clinical studies of the effects of β-blockade in HF were performed both by Gibson *et al.* at the National Heart Institute, London[9] and by Waagstein and colleagues in Gothenburg.[10,11] Both groups studied the β_1 cardioselective blocker practolol (ICI50172), and the Swedish workers also used alprenolol, which has partial agonist activity, in patients with idiopathic dilated cardiomyopathy. The initial studies from both groups involved the parenteral administration of practolol to patients in severe HF with supraventricular tachycardia. The marked reduction in heart rate was accompanied by significant clinical improvement without side effects. A subsequent long-term study with the β_1-selective blocker metoprolol in patients with dilated cardiomyopathy showed that after 3 years of treatment, the survival in the β-blocker-treated group was 52%, compared to only 10% for matched controls.[12]

The idea that β-blockers might be of value in HF was consistent with the developing 'neuroendocrine hypothesis' of HF. This was prompted when the CONSENSUS study showed a huge 60% reduction in mortality by the angiotensin converting enzyyme (ACE) inhibitor enalapril.[13] Subsequently it was suggested that several neurohormonal systems, principally the renin–angiotensin–aldosterone system (RAAS) and the sympathetic nervous system, could be responsible for the apparently inexorable deterioration of cardiac function and high mortality in HF.

Thereafter, inhibition of this neuroendocrine response by ACE inhibitors,[13,14] selective inhibition of angiotensin II receptors by angiotensin receptor blockers (ARBs),[15] and of aldosterone

Table 38.1 Pharmacological properties of β-blockers evaluated in CHF trials

Component	In vitro K_D[33]		β_1/β_2 Ratio	MSP	Partial agonism	$t_{1/2}$ (h)	Dose (mg)	Vasodilation
β_1-Selective								
Atenolol	β_1–6.66	β_2–5.99	4.7	No	No		50–100	No
Bisoprolol	–7.83	–6.70	13.5	No	No	10–12	10–20	No
Nebivolol	0.88	48	55	–	No	10.3–31.9	5–10	Yes
Xamoterol	–	–	40	No	Yes (43% of isoprenaline)	13	200 bd	No
Nonselective								
Bucindolol	–	–	?	No	Yes	3.6–9.0	50–200	Yes weak AR_1
Carvedilol	–8.75	–9.40	4.5 (β_2)	Yes	No	2–4	15–50	Yes (AR_1)[a]
β_2-Selective								
ICI 118551	–6.52	–9.26	549.5	Yes	No	3	25–50	No

[a] α-AR blockade.
AR, adrenoceptor; bd, twice daily.

receptors[16] together with β-blockers has become the standard evidence-based approach to the medical treatment of HF. This combination of treatments markedly improves survival by reducing both sudden cardiac death and death due to worsening HF. It also leads to improved ventricular function due to amelioration of ventricular remodelling consequent upon myocardial cell loss from MI or other heart muscle disorders.

The evidence

There can be few medicines whose efficacy in HF has been so clearly demonstrated as β-blockers insofar as the two major outcomes of survival and need for hospital admission are concerned. Following the early pioneering and hypothesis-generating studies of the potential value of β-blockers in MI and HF performed in the United Kingdom and Sweden with practolol, alprenolol, and metoprolol, there are now data from over 15 000 patients from randomized placebo controlled trials that, collectively, demonstrate impressive statistically and clinically important reductions in death and unscheduled admissions to hospital for worsening HF. A summary of the major trials can be found in Table 38.2.

Survival

Additional interest in the use of β-blockers in chronic HF dramatically increased more than 15 years ago when the results of the US Carvedilol Heart Failure Trial Programme on survival in just over 1000 patients with NYHA class II–IV HF were disclosed.[17] This was a series of double-blind randomized controlled trials in HF which individually investigated dose, haemodynamics, exercise capacity, and symptoms while collectively assessing the impact of β-blockade on mortality. The reduction in mortality reported in this programme greatly strengthened the hypothesis that β-blockers could indeed improve survival to a similar extent as had been demonstrated in the definitive ACE inhibitor studies in HF of the previous decade. It also lent even greater credence to the neuroendocrine hypothesis of HF promulgated in the wake of the early ACE inhibitor studies—that activation of a number of neural and endocrine systems, notably the RAAS and sympathetic nervous system, was not simply a reflection of the presence and severity of HF, but also directly contributed to poor outcomes in patients with HF through deleterious effects on the myocardium, blood vessels, and kidney.

Published in 1996, the carvedilol HF programme was an ambitious enterprise of great significance to the development of a comprehensive evidence base for the use of β-blockers together with ACE inhibitors in patients with HF due to left ventricular systolic dysfunction (LVSD). Nevertheless the survival benefit was based on a relatively small number of deaths, 31 (7.8%) on placebo versus 22 (3.2%) on carvedilol, representing absolute and relative reductions in mortality of 4.6% and 65% respectively. The overall mortality in the carvedilol programme was relatively low and it was clear that the results of further ongoing and new studies in larger and more diverse patient groups were required to establish as securely as with ACE inhibitors a strong evidence base for the safety and efficacy of β-blockers to improve clinical status and outcome in HF.

In 1998 the results of the CIBIS II trial of bisoprolol (β_1 selective) in over 2000 patients, essentially the first large single randomized controlled trial of β-blockade in HF, showed a survival advantage for patients in the bisoprolol arm with an increase in survival of 5.5% in a trial where the mortality rate in the placebo group was 17.3%, the highest studied thus far in a large clinical trial.[18] The trial patients included patients in NYHA classes II–IV. CIBIS II also drew attention to the remarkable relative reduction of 54% in the sudden death rate and the important reductions not only on hospital admission for worsening HF but also on all-cause hospital admissions.

Later that year the MERIT trial of metoprolol in an even larger study of almost 4000 patients essentially completed the evidence base for the impressive improvement in outcome in terms of survival and admission to hospital afforded by chronic treatment with β-blockers.[19] It also confirmed the marked reduction in sudden cardiac death demonstrated by the preceding trials. Thus in the short space of 3 years the cumulative evidence for the efficacy of β-blockers raised the profile of β-blockers as having at least as salutary an additional beneficial effect on morbidity and mortality as ACE inhibitors when given in conjunction with them.

Remodelling

Unfavourable changes to the geometry, structure, and function of the left (or right) ventricles accompany several disease processes affecting the myocardium, among which MI is the most typical and frequent cause. Myocyte loss or dysfunction can set in train a series of cellular processes including myocyte hypertrophy and renewal,

Table 38.2 Major β-blocker trials

(a)

	CIBIS II	BEST	MERIT-HF	MDC	SENIORS	GAXST	XAMOTEROL in Severe Heart Failure Study Group
Patients (n)	2647	2708	3991	383	2128	433	352
β-Blocker	Bisoprolol	Bucindolol	Metoprolol CR/XL	Metoprolol	Nebivolol	Xamoterol	Xamoterol
NYHA class	III–IV	III–IV	II–IV	I–IV	II–IV	II–III	III–IV
LVEF	≤35%	≤35%	≤40%	<40%	33%	N/A	N/A
Mean follow-up (months)	14	24	12	12	21	3	13 weeks
Mean dose achieved (mg/day)	7.5	152	159	100–150	1.25–10	200mg BD	200mg TID
Primary endpoint	All-cause mortality	All-cause mortality	All-cause mortality	Exercise LV function	All-cause mortality Hospitalization	Effort tolerance improved 37%	9.2% died vs 3.7% placebo
Results	All-cause mortality reduced 34%	All-cause mortality reduced 10%	All-cause mortality reduced 34%	EF increased Exercise increased	All-cause mortality reduced	Reduced oedema/ pulmonary congestion	Trial suspended
p value	<0.001	0.13	0.0062	0.0001 0.046	0.039	N/A	N/A

BEST, β-Blocker Evaluation of Survival Trial; CIBIS II, Cardiac Insufficiency Bisoprolol Study II; CR/XL, controlled release/extended release; GASXT, German and Austrian Xamoterol Trial; MDC, Metoprolol in Dilated Cardiomyopathy; MERIT-HF, Metoprolol CR/XL Randomized Intervention Trial in Congestive Heart Failure.

(b)

	USCTP	COPERNICUS	CAPRICORN	CARMEN[a]	COMET[b]	MOCHA	PRECISE	COLUCCI *et al.*
Patients (n)	1094	2289	1959	479	3029		278	366
NYHA class	II–IV	NA	NA	I–III	II–IV	II–III	II–III	II
LVEF	≤35%	<25%	Post-MI ≤40%	≤39%	26%	23%	22%	23%
Mean follow-up (months)	6.5	10.4	15	18	58	6	6	12
Mean dose achieved (mg/day)	45	37	20	CAR: 47.9[c] CAR: 48.7[d]	CAR: 41.8 MET: 85.0	6.25 12.5 bd 25.0	6.25 bd upwards	6.25 bd
Primary endpoint	Safety	All-cause mortality	All-cause mortality or all-cause mortality or CV hospitalization combined	LV remodelling	All-cause mortality	Exercise tolerance Quality of life	Improved EF	CHF progression^
Results	All-cause mortality reduced 65%[e]	All-cause mortality reduced 35%	All-cause mortality reduced 23%	LVESVI reduced in combination with enalapril	17% relative risk reduction in favour of carvedilol	All-cause mortality reduced 73%	Morbidity and mortality reduced	Mortality Hospitalization EF^^ all reduced
p value	0.0001	0.00013	0.031	<0.002	0.0017	0.001 Hospitalization rate 0.01	0.001/0.029	^0.008 ^^0.03

[a] Compared with enalapril alone or in combination with enalapril.

[b] Carvedilol vs metoprolol.

[c] Dose of carvedilol achieved as monotherapy.

[d] Dose of carvedilol achieved as part of combination therapy with enalapril.

[e] Endpoint.

CAPRICORN, Carvedilol Postinfarct Survival Controlled Evaluation; CAR, carvedilol; CARMEN, Carvedilol Ace Inhibitor Remodelling Mild Heart Failure Evaluation; COMET, Carvedilol or Metoprolol European Trial; COPERNICUS, Carvedilol Prospective Randomized Cumulative Survival; LVEF, left ventricular ejection fraction; LVESVI, left ventricular end-systolic volume index; MET, metoprolol; MI, myocardial infarction; NYHA, New York Heart Association class; RRR, relative risk reduction; USCTP, US Carvedilol Heart Failure Study Programme.

as well as interstitial fibrosis and dilatation of the left ventricle, causing the chamber to become more spherical than elliptical. This results in increased wall tension, reduced contractility, impaired filling, and ultimately the clinical syndrome of HF.[20]

In 1997 the Australia and New Zealand (ANZ) trial in 415 patients convincingly demonstrated that carvedilol improved left ventricular systolic function although exercise capacity did not change.[21] The ANZ trial also contributed to the evidence that clinical outcomes improved on β-blockers. Subsequently the CAPRICORN trial of carvedilol showed that similar benefits can occur with β-blockers in conjunction with ACE inhibitors in patients with post-MI left ventricular dysfunction or HF.[22,23] The totality of data from these and other mechanistic trials indicate that β-blockers have a clinically important beneficial effect on remodelling in HF.

Arrhythmia

It is said that it was the sudden unexpected death of the young James Black's father following a very stressful day at work that caused him to consider the possibility that high levels of adrenaline from excess sympathetic nervous activity could have been responsible and that blocking these effects of adrenaline on the heart might prevent such tragedies. Perspicacious in the extreme, perhaps, but there is no doubt that a major feature of β-blocker therapy is the reduction in sudden death observed both after MI and in HF. Given the proarrhythmic effects of catecholamines, the major antiarrhythmic effects of β-blockers is scarcely surprising. This is a singular benefit of β-blockers, for no other medicine currently available in the entire pharmacopoeia has conclusively been shown to reduce sudden death. The precise mechanism by which β-blockers achieve this effect is unclear, but substantial reductions in serious ventricular arrhythmias including ventricular tachycardia and ventricular fibrillation were noted during ambulatory ECG monitoring in CAPRICORN, a trial in which a marked reduction in sudden death was a feature in the carvedilol-treated group.[22,23]

Of considerable importance also is the suppression of supraventricular arrhythmias, especially atrial fibrillation and atrial flutter, which in patients with HF often precipitate acute HF and decompensation in patients with known chronic HF.

The down side of the antiarrhythmic properties of β-blockers is bradycardia, which may limit the maximum tolerated dose in individual patients and lead to various degrees of heart block, most commonly first degree but occasionally second degree and complete heart block. In the latter it is usually in the context of preexisting conduction disturbance and in such cases permanent pacing may be required.

Specific patient subgroups

Severe heart failure

Despite the impressive results of the US Carvedilol programme and the CIBIS and MERIT trials, many questions still remained to be answered about β-blocking therapy, including its safety and efficacy in very severe HF. For, although patients with NYHA classes III and IV were included in the preceding trials, they were relatively few in number and had to have been clinically stable for some time before entry to these trials. This question has best been addressed in the COPERNICUS trial of carvedilol in over 2000 patients with NYHA class III or IV HF in which there was a total of over 500 deaths, the largest yet recorded in a HF trial. Carvedilol reduced all-cause mortality,[24] but, overall, significant survival benefit was also derived by patients in a prespecified subgroup at even higher risk due to, among other criteria, recent decompensation or a severely depressed ejection fraction of 14% or less. In this subgroup the annualized mortality rate was 24%. COPERNICUS indicated that, far from being hazardous, it is in the highest-risk groups of patients that β-blockers can exert their greatest effects. It must be stressed, however, that these benefits of β-blockers were obtained in the context of a standard of patient care as near optimal as possible.

Heart failure after myocardial infarction

The powerful effects of β-blockers on survival in patients with cardiovascular disease was first demonstrated in the β-blocker trials in MI in the previous decade. The first of these trials, and still the most impressive in terms of outcome benefits, the Norwegian multicentre trial of timolol published 15 years previously in 1980, was followed by several other trials with metoprolol, propranolol, practolol, oxprenolol, sotalol, and alprenolol in which the results on survival and recurrent MI, though more variable, were directionally similar to those of the timolol trial. Subsequent meta-analyses confirmed the powerful beneficial effects of β-blockers in the post-MI patient on survival and recurrent MI.[4] Patients with HF were included in some of these studies but generally they were excluded because of safety concerns. Consequently it soon became apparent that, in clinical practice, the prescription rate of β-blockers in patients whose MI was complicated by HF remained low. This was the reason for carrying out a specific trial in post-MI patients with significant left ventricular dysfunction and/or HF, the CAPRICORN trial with carvedilol in approximately 2000 patients.[24] The impact on survival reflected in a relative risk reduction of 23% (absolute reduction 3%) was identical to that calculated in meta-analyses of the previous MI trials, and the effects on sudden death and recurrent MI were also statistically and clinically highly significant. The CAPRICORN trial therefore completed the spectrum of post-MI trials by indicating that patients with HF or severe left ventricular dysfunction post MI should definitely and specifically be considered for β-blocker therapy. An important practical contribution was the experience gained in initiating β-blocker treatment safely in patients with acute HF guided by specific clinical indicators which could be applied for the safe use of β-blockers in patients with HF however caused.

Heart failure with preserved systolic function (HeFNEF)

Over many years the main experimental and clinical focus of interest in HF encompassing particularly the neuroendocrine hypothesis for the development and progression of HF has been on LVSD. It is now recognized that while patients in this category who are characterized by a reduced ejection fraction (REF), a significant proportion of patients who present with all the typical clinical features of HF have a 'preserved' or normal ejection fraction (PEF or NEF). These patients more often are older, with a history of hypertension and evidence of left ventricular hypertrophy.[25] Although they are not rare there is debate on whether they are as numerous as those with a reduced ejection fraction. This has led to the introduction of numerous acronyms by which patients with HF may be described, HeFREF and HeFNEF being, currently, among the most frequently employed. Most of the 'landmark' clinical trials of β-blockers in HF have been in patients with HeFREF while such data in patients with HeFNEF are few. Theoretically the risk/benefit ratio could be more favourable with less myocardial depression and improved ventricular filling from a slower heart rate.

Although no large trial specifically in HeFNEF has been reported, the SENIORS trial studied nebivolol, a β_1-selective β-blocker with a nitric oxide based vasodilator activity, in a large trial of patients aged 70 or older. A secure clinical diagnosis of HF but no specific value of ejection fraction was required.[26] The composite 1-year endpoint of all-cause mortality or cardiovascular hospitalizations was significantly reduced by nebivolol regardless of ejection fraction. Nebivolol is licensed for the treatment of HF in some countries but it has not been approved in the United States. Thus there is insufficient evidence to say confidently that nebivolol is more effective in HF or that other β-blockers would have a similar effect in the SENIORS patient group. Nevertheless it is common practice to prescribe β-blockers in clinically stable patients with HeFNEF according to the same safety specifications applied to patients with HeFREF.

Chronic obstructive pulmonary disease

It is always a significant clinical disappointment when contraindications prevent the use of life-enhancing and life-saving medicines. With respect to β-blockers, one of the most common is reversible airways obstruction. In patients who have a firm diagnosis of asthma based on appropriate investigations β-blockers, including those that are said to be β_1 selective, are firmly contraindicated. In those with confirmed chronic obstructive pulmonary disease (COPD) without significant reversibility, clinical trials and meta-analyses suggest that the risk–benefit ratio remains favourable.[27] In the presence of diagnostic doubt it is advisable to seek a formal opinion from a respiratory specialist as to the correct underlying diagnosis. Ultimately the decision lies with the physician who, aware of the balance of risks of exacerbating bronchoconstriction and of withholding a most effective treatment for HF and preventing sudden cardiac death, can give an informed opinion.

Gender

Men and women do not always respond equally to medicines. but as far as β-blockers are concerned a meta-analysis involving the major trials (USCTP, CIBIS II, MERIT-HF, and COPERNICUS) confirms equal benefit in terms of major outcomes.[28]

Pharmacological differences among β-blockers

Selective and nonselective β-blockers

The human heart contains both β_1 and β_2 ARs in a ratio of approximately 4:1. It is commonly believed that the harmful effects of increased sympathetic activity are mediated by the β_1 receptor through G-protein-coupled stimulation of cyclic AMP (cAMP) leading to activation of a number of downstream signalling pathways associated with ventricular and vascular remodelling.

Nevertheless, there has been prolonged debate as to the relative merits clinically of β_1 'selective' and 'nonselective' β_1 and β_2 AR antagonists in cardiovascular disease generally. Insofar as HF is concerned this issue seemed to be resolved when the β_1-selective β-blockers bisoprolol and metoprolol and the nonselective β-blocker carvedilol were all shown to reduce all-cause death substantially and to the similar extent of about one-third in, respectively, the CIBIS II, MERIT-HF, and COPERNICUS trials. But interest in potential differences, initiated by the remarkable two-thirds reduction in mortality in the US carvedilol trials, was dramatically heightened by the results of the COMET trial, in which the nonselective β-blocker carvedilol was associated with a statistically and clinically significant lower mortality than the β_1-selective β-blocker metoprolol.[29] Although carvedilol has other potentially valuable ancillary properties, including α_1 AR blockade, there is no supportive outcome data from large clinical trials in HF for benefit of α_1 blockade[30] or antioxidant activity.

For these reasons, the question of dose was questioned in COMET in which the aim was to effect comparable reductions in heart rate between the two groups since the molecular effects in the myocardium are similar when equipotent doses of carvedilol and metoprolol, in terms of inhibition of exercise-induced tachycardia, are compared.[31]

The resting heart-rate reduction of 13 beats/min in COMET with carvedilol 50 mg/day was very similar to that achieved with the same dose in the US carvedilol studies on which the dose was based. The heart-rate reduction with the dose of 100 mg/day metoprolol tartrate, however, was only 11.7 beats/min compared with 15 beats/min achieved with 150 mg/day in the Metoprolol in Dilated Cardiomyopathy trial (MDC) on which the dose of metoprolol in COMET was based. Moreover, the major study of metoprolol in HF that addressed outcome was the MERIT-HF study in which the preparation of metoprolol used was metoprolol succinate, a controlled/extended release formulation (metoprolol CR/XL) in a target dose of 200 mg/day. The mean dose actually taken and the mean reduction in heart rate achieved were 106 mg and 14 beats/min, both very similar to that found in the MDC trial. Thus the greater benefit in outcomes with carvedilol over metoprolol in the COMET trial might suggest that equivalent blockade of cardiac β_1 receptors may not have been achieved in the metoprolol arm.

Recent experimental data on β-blocker pharmacology (Fig. 38.1) challenge the conventional wisdom regarding the primacy of the β_1 receptor in health and disease and HF in particular. First, receptor-binding studies using cultured human cells have questioned the validity of previous clinical classifications of β-blockers as 'selective' or 'nonselective'.[32] For example, carvedilol in human tissue is a more potent blocker of β_2 than of β_1 receptors, while the β_2 effects of drugs formerly classified as 'selective' β_1 antagonists such as bisoprolol and metoprolol could be clinically more significant than previously appreciated.[32] Secondly, in health, the β_1 ARs are located on the cell crests, ensuring their wide distribution over the entire cell surface (Fig. 38.2).[33] This facilitates, following their stimulation, wide diffusion of the Gs-protein-coupled production of the second messenger cAMP throughout the cytoplasm where it increases the strength and frequency of myocyte contraction. The effects of cAMP following stimulation of the β_2 ARs, residing in the base of the T tubules of the cell membrane, are more localized. Recent studies show, however, that this compartmentalization of β-AR function is disrupted, leading to relocation of β_2 ARs to the cell surface where their subsequent stimulation causes a pattern of cAMP release similar to that of β_1 receptor stimulation. Thirdly, β_1 but not β_2 receptors are down-regulated in HF,[34,35] thereby changing the effective ratio of functioning β_1 and β_2 activity from 4:1 to 3:2.

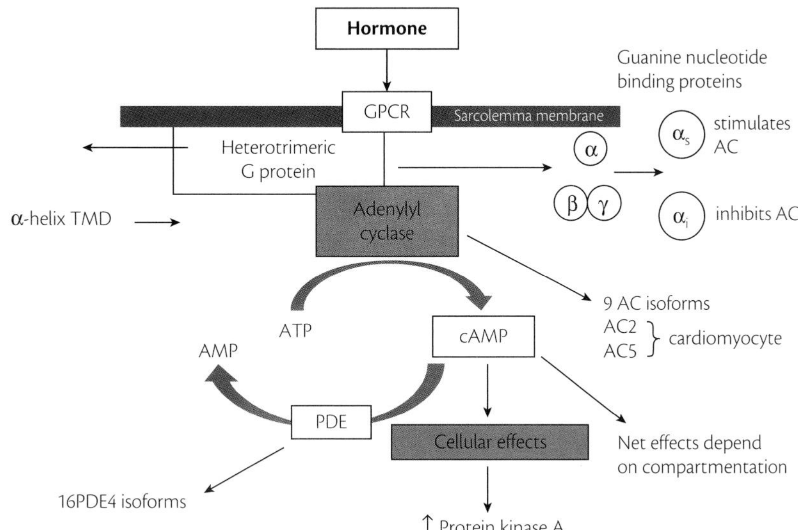

Fig. 38.1 Different β_1/β_2 coupling mechanisms to downstream effectors. Note that β_2 adrenoceptors, when phosphorylated, can activate the Gi proteins which in turn activate various kinases to initiate apoptotic, fibrotic, and inflammatory processes. The original model pathway in shown in green; subsequent discoveries of cAMP modulation are in red. ·

It has also been hypothesized that carvedilol may have a protective effect by stimulating the β-arrestin signalling pathway in the presence of chronic catecholamine stimulation leading to inhibition of mycocyte apoptosis, as is the case in HF. In contrast, G-protein-dependent signalling may be cardiotoxic under these same conditions.[36] Thus there remains a place for further investigation of the relative roles of β_1 and β_2 receptor function in HF.

Intrinsic sympathomimesis (partial agonism)

Several β-adrenoceptor antagonists have partial agonist activity, which it was hoped might protect against β-blocker-induced myocardial depression while also ameliorating or preventing some common side effects including excessive bradycardia due to either β_1 or β_2 antagonism, cold hands, and bronchoconstriction due to β_2 antagonism. Partial agonism has never been shown conclusively to have beneficial effects, however, and in terms of outcome no improvement has been seen in post-MI trials.

The role of partial agonism in HF was investigated through the clinical development programme of the β_1 selective partial agonist xamoterol (CORWIN).[37,38] It was hypothesized that xamoterol would be useful in protecting the heart from the adverse effects of increased sympathetic stimulation during daytime activities while providing support for the heart through expression of partial agonism during periods of low sympathetic traffic during rest. Ambulatory ECG monitoring showed a clear reduction of the heart rate during the day and a substantial increase nocturnally, in keeping with its significant degree of β_1 agonism. The clinical trials that led to the licensing of xamoterol for mild to moderate HF demonstrated clear evidence of benefit by improving quality of life and increasing exercise capacity.[37] Unfortunately the large trial set up to investigate its efficacy and safety in severe HF was stopped by the data monitoring committee because of excess mortality in the xamoterol arm.[38] There was no pattern to the mode of death and no plausible explanation for the adverse outcome could be discerned from all the data collected. Despite the ambulatory

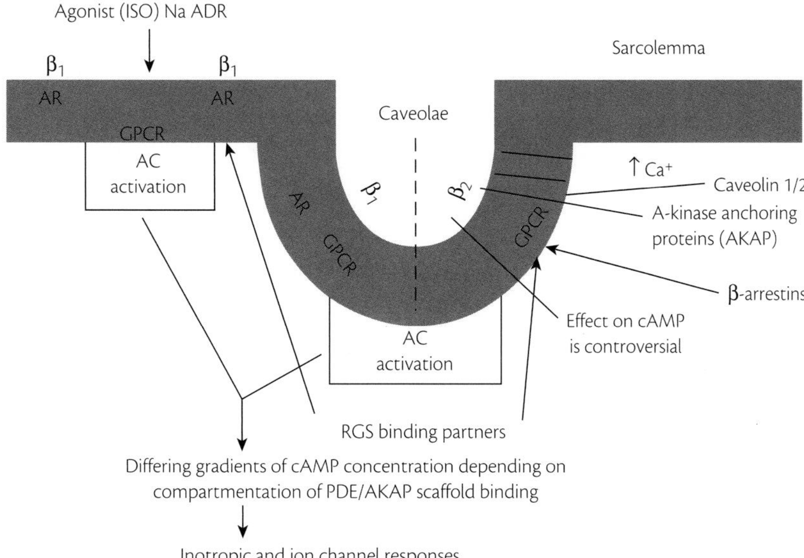

Fig. 38.2 The differing downstream effects of activation of protein kinase A by cAMP. Note the complex effects of phosphorylation of different cardiomyocyte cytosolic mediators and its role in β_2 adrenoceptor down-regulation.

monitoring studies no definite association between the heart rate findings and mortality could be determined. It remains tantalizing to speculate that had xamoterol been introduced at a very small dose and titrated slowly to the target dose, in keeping with modern β-blocking therapy in HF, the outcome of that trial might have been very different.

The only other β-blocker with partial agonism to be studied in a large randomized controlled trial in HF is bucindolol. Unlike all the other recent landmark trials of β-blockers, the BEST trial of bucindolol failed to show a convincing increase in survival[39,40] by being detrimental in black Americans but beneficial in white subjects. It cannot be concluded that partial β-receptor partial agonism was culpable, but it has been suggested that genetic polymorphisms among the subjects could have influenced the result. Bucindolol is known to be strongly sympatholytic and in BEST, as in the MOXCON study of moxonidine in heart failure, sympatholysis was associated with poor survival. Polymorphism of two genes concerned with β_1 AR function, the glycine moiety of the β-arginine/glycine 389 and the preadrenergic junctional α_2c-Del 3222–3225 AR, were linked to sympatholysis and poorer survival.[41,42]

Practical aspects of β-blocker use

Who should receive β-blockers?

β-Blockers are a class 1 (A) recommendation in the major guidelines on HF treatment because of the overwhelming evidence of benefit, especially in patients with LVSD (HeFREF).[43,44] The evidence for benefit in patients with a preserved ejection fraction (HeFNEF) is much less complete at present, due not to adverse results but to a relative dearth of trials similar to those on which the secure evidence base for β-blockers in HeFREF has been built. The data in SENIORS,[26] the only large trial to address this issue, is consistent with the trials in HeFREF and their meta-analyses. In SENIORS, the most recent of the large trials on β-blockers, a pragmatic, more modern, approach was taken by including patients with 'heart failure' or 'HeF' in the acronymic parlance of the present times, as determined by a clinical diagnosis made in a specialist setting. The results revealed no heterogeneity of effect between those with impaired or significantly unimpaired left ventricular systolic function. Since the overarching view of the progression of HF and its pharmacological treatment is based on antagonizing the putative deleterious effects of neuroendocrine systems, especially the RAAS and the sympathetic nervous system,[45] it is not unreasonable to believe that inhibitors of these systems should be beneficial in HF *per se*, both HeFREF and HeFNEF, to an extent depending on the degree of activation of these systems. There are also other reasons for prescribing β-blockers due to the protean nature of their indications, including hypertension and angina pectoris, conditions which are present in many patients either as a comorbidity or a cause of their HF. The antiarrhythmic effects of β-blockers are particularly relevant in HF for preventing or gaining rate control of atrial fibrillation and for preventing sudden cardiac death from serious ventricular arrhythmia. In the specific case of HeFPEF there may also be pathophysiological justification for β-blockade including the promotion of better filling by reducing the heart rate.[46] For all these reasons β-blockers should be considered in all patients with HF in the absence of a specific disease related or other standard contraindication.

Research and especially clinical trials of medications has been almost completely dominated by studies in LVSD, although more recently complemented by studies of angiotensin receptor antagonists in patients with preserved systolic function. Very little is known about the effects of the major 'heart failure' medications including β-blockers in patients with other forms of specific heart disease such as valvular heart diseases and specific heart muscle disorders, apart from their indication for rate control in atrial fibrillation. In those circumstances clinical judgement is required to identify those patients with characteristics that might suggest benefit from β-blockers. in whom all of these issues consistently arise in individual patients.

Which β-blocker should be prescribed and at what dose?

In both Europe and the United States bisoprolol, carvedilol, and metoprolol are approved by the relevant regulatory bodies for the treatment of heart failure due to LVSD because of the strong evidence for benefit for all three medicines. In the United Kingdom but not in the United States nebivolol is also licensed for the treatment of HF in patients over the age of 70 years. Currently it has not been approved for HF by either the European Medicines Agency or the US Food and Drug Administration. No other β-blocker has been licensed in the HF indication because of the absence of large trials confirming safety and efficacy. In these circumstances it is recommended that, where possible, licensed medicines should be prescribed at a dose and in a manner that was tested in the relevant clinical trials.

Recent pharmacoepidemiological data[47,48] provide a perspective on outcomes of different classes of β-blockers from managed care databases—DECIDE and the North Carolina Medicaid/Medicare patients. The objective was to determine the outcomes of patients using either β-blockers approved by the FDA, namely carvedilol, metoprolol succinate, and bisoprolol fumarate, which are considered to have evidence-based treatment for HF, or atenolol. In DECIDE, there was no difference between atenolol and carvedilol in either mortality or rehospitalization rates, whereas there appeared to be an increased risk using short-acting metoprolol tartrate.[47] The Medicare/Medicaid study showed that there was no difference between outcomes in either approved or nonapproved β-blockers, and both showed a substantial benefit compared with no β-blocker treatment.[48]

Pharmacoepidemiology data is available for atenolol—one of the most widely prescribed β-blockers in the world—for many other indications, which suggests that long-term outcomes were similar in patients on licensed β-blockers and atenolol. This is by no means equivalent to data on safety and efficacy but does give some comfort to patients and clinicians practising in economically challenged countries throughout the world.

At what stage of heart failure should β-blockers be prescribed?

The data from the large trials were obtained in patients in with NYHA class II–IV HF who were clinically stable at the time of initiation of treatment. The earlier trials recruited largely ambulant outpatients of milder severity and greater stability, while studies such as CAPRICORN[22] and COPERNICUS[24] included inpatients recovering from an acute MI or recent decompensation of chronic

HF respectively. These trials demonstrated the safety of inpatient prescribing in an environment where the availability of specialist expertise in HF and adherence to a clear protocol for initiation and up-titration allowed the safe introduction and continuation of β-blockade. Subsequently the additional benefit obtained from initiating treatment during an acute admission has been confirmed in clinical practice.[49]

How should β-blockers be used?

A detailed exposition of initiation, titration, and chronic dosing is beyond the scope of this chapter but it is crucially important that patients are clinically stable at the time of initiation even though this may be only a few days after an episode of decompensation or of an acute MI. Beta blockers are normally commenced following ACE inhibition. There is difference in outcomes between the two approaches of ACE inhibitor first versus beta-blocker first.[50] Recognition of 'stability' is a matter of clinical judgement but cardinal signs include absence of fluid retention and of other signs of circulatory failure such as hypotension (systolic blood pressure ≥90 mmHg), peripheral hypoperfusion, and oliguria. These criteria are a matter for local implementation guidelines ideally in the context of a multidisciplinary heart failure programme within which the safe and effective use of β-blockers is best achieved (Chapter 54).

The clinical trials all have had detailed initial dose titration schedules and a final target dose and these are a practical guide to management.

What is the optimum prescription rate for β-blockers in heart failure?

Adherence to medication and doses achieved in clinical trials are generally much higher than in 'real life' clinical practice for several very good reasons related to the selection criteria of the former circumstance and the clinical status and frailty of unselected patients in the latter. In clinical audits of HF prescription rates vary from around 80% in the US 'ADHERE' Registry[51] to 49% in the EuroHeart Study[52] and 40–50% in various audits in the United Kingdom.[53] These data may represent an apparently wide variation in practice but, more likely, they are simply reflecting a direct relationship between the degree of selectivity of patients enrolled in the individual studies and the rate of prescription and doses achieved. Nevertheless, in clinical practice it is possible to achieve target doses in a high percentage of patients depending on the skill, patience and time available to the health professionals concerned. Medical therapy in heart failure is complex for many reasons and should be conducted in a multidisciplinary setting such as in the clinical trials within which the data on safety and efficacy were obtained.

When should β-blockers be withdrawn or reduced?

'Withdrawal' effects due to excess sympathetic stimulation have been noted after abrupt cessation of β-blockers in circumstances other than heart failure. In hypertension this has led to loss of control of blood pressure and in angina pectoris to acute exacerbations.[54] There has therefore been concern over the possible consequences of sudden withdrawal of β-blockers in patients with HF, especially in the situation of acute decompensation. In order to avoid this potential hazard many have simply reduced the dose to that of initiation with up-titration when stabilization has occurred. Recently no detriment has been reported by continuing with the maintenance dose.[55] Nevertheless, no hard and fast rule need apply and there will be clinical situations in which acute, partial, or no withdrawal will be appropriate according to the individual circumstances.

Reduction or withdrawal of β-blockers can be necessary in very advanced HF associated with hypotension and deteriorating renal function as part of a general review of the overall medicines prescription since all 'evidence-based medicines' for HF can lower the blood pressure to an extent that renal function is compromised. This is often temporary, but in the state of terminal care it is reasonable to continue only those medicines that will contribute positively to the palliative care of the patient.

Conclusions

The use of β-blockers in HF has been both a revelation and a revolution. Sir James Black, the inventor of by far the most successful class of medicines for cardiovascular disease, died earlier this year at the age of 82. Modest to the end about his immense contribution to cardiovascular science and medicine, his quests for new mechanisms and medicines had never ceased. Without prejudice to his many colleagues with whom he was still working, it may be said that the β-blocker odyssey of discovery has not ended.

References

1. Fitzgerald D. The importance of chance and the prepared mind in the discovery of beta blockers. *Dialog Cardiovasc Med* 2000;**5**:172–5.
2. Cruickshank JM, Pritchard BNC. *β-Blockers in clinical practice.* Churchill Livingstone, London, 1994.
3. Pritchard BNC, Dickinson CJ, Alleyne GAO, *et al.* Effect of pronethalol in angina pectoris. *Br Med J* 1963;**ii**:1226–7.
4. Yusuf S, Peto R, Lewis J, Collins R, Sleight I. Beta blockade during and after myocardial infarction: an overview of the randomized trials. *Prog Cardiovasc Dis* 1985;**27**:335–71.
5. McMurray J. Major β blocker mortality trials in chronic heart failure: a critical review. *Heart* 1999;**82**(suppl IV):IV14–22.
6. Chidsey CA, Vogel JHK. Adrenergic mechanisms in heart failure. In Kattus AA, Ross G, Hall VE (eds) *Cardiovascular β-adrenergic responses: UCLA Forum in Medical Sciences 13*, pp. 81–92. University of California Press, Berkeley, 1970.
7. Chidsey CA, Braunwald E. Sympathetic activity and neurotransmitter depletion in congestive heart failure. *Pharmacol Rev* 1966;**18**:685–700.
8. Epstein SE, Braunwald E. Circulatory effects and clinical a pplications of β-adrenergic receptor inhibition. In Kattus AA, Ross G, Hall VE (eds) *Cardiovascular β-adrenergic responses: UCLA Forum in Medical Sciences 13*, pp. 139–49. University of California Press, Berkeley, 1970.
9. Gibson DG, Balcon R, Souten E. Clinical use of ICI 50172 as an anti-dysrhythmic agent in heart failure. *Br Med J* 1968;**3**:161–3.
10. Waagstein F, Hjalmaison A, Vernauskas E, Wallentin I. Effects of chronic β-adrenergic receptor blockade in congestive cardiomyopathy. *Br Heart J* 1975;**37**:1022–36.
11. Swedberg K, Hjalmarson A, Waagstein F, Wallentin I. Beneficial effects of long-term β-blockade in congestive cardiomopathy. *Br Heart J* 1980;**44**:117–33.
12. Waagstein F, Bristow MR, Swedberg K, *et al.* Beneficial effects of metoprolol in idiopathic dilated cardiomyopathy. Metoprolol in Dilated Cardiomyopathy (MDC) Trial Study Group. *Lancet* 1993;**342**(8885):1441–6.
13. CONSENSUS Trial Study Group. Effects of enalapril on mortality in severe congestive heart failure. Results of the Cooperative North Scandinavian Enalapril Survival Study (CONSENSUS). *New Engl J Med* 1987;**316**:1429–35.

14. Effect of enalapril on survival in patients with reduced left ventricular ejection fractions and congestive heart failure. The SOLVD Investigators. *N Engl J Med* 1991;**325**:293–302.
15. Granger CB, McMurray JJ, Yusuf S, *et al.* Effects of candesartan in patients with chronic heart failure and reduced left-ventricular systolic function intolerant to angiotensin-converting-enzyme inhibitors: the CHARM-Alternative trial. *Lancet* 2003;**362**:772–6.
16. Pitt B, Zannad F, Remme WJ, *et al.* The effect of spironolactone on morbidity and mortality in patients with severe heart failure. Randomized Aldactone Evaluation Study Investigators. *N Engl J Med* 1999;**341**:709–717.
17. Packer M, Bristow MR, Cohn JN, *et al.* The effects of carvedilol on morbidity and mortality in chronic heart failure. *N Engl J Med* 1996;**334**:1249–55.
18. CIBIS II investigators and committees. The Cardiac Insufficiency Bisoprolol Study: a randomized trial. *Lancet* 1999;**353**:9–13.
19. MERIT HF Study Group. Effect of metoprolol CR/XL in chronic heart failure: CR/XL Randomised Intervention Trial in Congestive Heart Failure (MERIT HF). *Lancet* 1999;**353**:2001–7.
20. Mann DL. Basic mechanisms of left ventricular remodeling: the contribution of wall stress. *J Card Fail* 2004;**10**(6 Suppl): S202–6.
21. Australia/New Zealand Heart Failure Research Collaborative Group. Randomised, placebo-controlled trial of carvedilol in patients with congestive heart failure due to ischaemic heart disease. *Lancet* 1997;**349**:375–80.
22. Dargie HJ. Effect of carvedilol on outcome after myocardial infarction in patients with left-ventricular dysfunction: the CAPRICORN randomised trial. *Lancet* 2001;**357**(9266):1385–90.
23. Doughty RN, Whalley GA, Walsh HA, Gamble GD, Lopez-Sendon J, Sharpe N. Effects of carvedilol on left ventricular remodeling after acute myocardial infarction: the CAPRICORN Echo Substudy. *Circulation* 2004;**109**(2):201–6.
24. Packer M, Coats AJ, Fowler MB, *et al.* Effect of carvedilol on survival in severe chronic heart failure. *N Engl J Med* 2001;**344**:1651–8.
25. Zile M. Heart failure with preserved ejection fraction: is this diastolic heart failure? *J Am Coll Cardiol* 2003;**41**:1519–1522.
26. Flather MD, Shibata MC, Coats AJ, *et al.* Randomized trial to determine the effect of nebivolol on mortality and cardiovascular hospital admission in elderly patients with heart failure. (SENIORS). *Eur Heart J* 2005;**26**:215–25.
27. Andrus MR, Holloway KP, Clark DB. Use of beta-blockers in patients with COPD. *Ann Pharmacother* 2004;**38**(1):142–5.
28. Fonarow GC. A review of evidence-based beta-blockers in special populations with heart failure. *Rev Cardiovasc Med* 2008;**9**(2):84–95.
29. Poole-Wilson P, Swedberg K, Cleland JG, *et al.* Comparison of carvedilol and metoprolol on clinical outcomes in patients with chronic heart failure in the Carvedilol Or Metoprolol European Trial (COMET): randomised controlled trial. *Lancet* 2003;**362**:7–13.
30. Cohn JN, Archibald DG, Ziesche S, *et al.* Effect of vasodilator therapy on mortality in chronic congestive heart failure. *N Engl J Med* 1986;**314**:1547–52.
31. Dargie HJ Beta blockers in heart failure. *Lancet* 2003;**362**(9377):2–3.
32. Baker JG. The selectivity of β-adrenoceptor antagonists at the human β_1, β_2, and β_3 adrenoceptors. *Br J Pharmacol* 2005;**144**:317–22.
33. Nikolaev VO, Moshkov A, Lyon AR, *et al.* Beta2-Adrenergic receptor redistribution in heart failure changes cAMP compartmentation. *Science* 2010;**327**:1653–7.
34. Bristow MR, Ginsburg R, Umans V, *et al.* Beta 1- and beta 2-adrenergic-receptor subpopulations in nonfailing and failing human ventricular myocardium: coupling of both receptor subtypes to muscle contraction and selective beta 1-receptor down-regulation in heart failure. *Circ Res* 1986;**59**:297–309.
35. Brodde O-E. β_1-and β_2-Adrenoceptors in the human heart: properties, function and alterations in chronic heart failure. *Pharmacol Rev* 1991;**43**:203–41.
36. Wisler JW, DeWire SM, Whalen EJ, *et al.* A unique mechanism of β-blocker action: Carvedilol stimulates β-arrestin signaling. *Proc Natl Acad Sci U S A* 2007;**104**:16659–62.
37. Marlow HF. Review of clinical experience with xamoterol. Effects on exercise capacity and symptoms in heart failure. *Circulation* 1990;**81**(2 Suppl):III93–8.
38. The Xamoterol in Severe Heart Failure Study Group. Xamoterol in severe heart failure. *Lancet* 1990;**336**(8706):1–6.
39. The BEST Investigators. A trial of the β-adrenergic blocker bucindolol in patients with advanced chronic heart failure. *N Engl J Med* 2001;**344**:1659–67.
40. Domanski MJ, Krause-Steinrauf H, Massie BM, *et al.* A comparative analysis of the results from 4 trials of beta-blocker therapy for heart failure: BEST, CIBIS-II, MERIT-HF, and COPERNICUS. *J Card Fail* 2003;**9**(5):354–63.
41. Cohn JN, Pfeffer MA, Rouleau J, *et al.* Adverse mortality effect of central sympathetic inhibition with sustained-release moxonidine in patients with heart failure (MOXCON). *Eur J Heart Fail* 2003;**5**(5):659–67.
42. Bristow MR, Murphy GA, Krause-Steinrauf H, *et al.* An alpha2C-adrenergic receptor polymorphism alters the norepinephrine-lowering effects and therapeutic response of the beta-blocker bucindolol in chronic heart failure. *Circ Heart Fail* 2010;**3**(1):21–8.
43. Dickstein K, Cohen-Solal A, Filippatos G, *et al.* ESC guidelines for the diagnosis and treatment of acute and chronic heart failure 2008: the Task Force for the diagnosis and treatment of acute and chronic heart failure 2008 of the European Society of Cardiology. Developed in collaboration with the Heart Failure Association of the ESC (HFA) and endorsed by the European Society of Intensive Care Medicine (ESICM). *Eur J Heart Fail* 2008;**10**(10):933–89.
44. Hunt SA, Abraham WT, Chin MH, *et al.* 2009 focused update incorporated into the ACC/AHA 2005 Guidelines for the Diagnosis and Management of Heart Failure in Adults: a report of the American College of Cardiology Foundation/American Heart Association Task Force on Practice Guidelines: developed in collaboration with the International Society for Heart and Lung Transplantation. *Circulation* 2009;**119**(14):e391–479.
45. Mann DL. Basic mechanisms of disease progression in the failing heart: the role of excessive adrenergic drive. *Prog Cardiovasc Dis* 1998;**41**(1 Suppl 1):1–8.
46. Zile MR. Diastolic heart failure. Diagnosis, prognosis, treatment. *Minerva Cardioangiol* 2003;**51**(2):131–42.
47. Go AS, Yang J, Gurwitz JH, Hsu J, Lane K, Platt R. Comparative effectiveness of different beta-adrenergic antagonists on mortality among adults with heart failure in clinical practice. *Arch Intern Med* 2008;**168**(22):2415–21.
48. Kramer JM, Curtis LH, Dupree CS, Pelter D, Hernandez A, Massing M, *et al.* Comparative effectiveness of beta-blockers in elderly patients with heart failure. *Arch Intern Med* 2008;**168**(22):2422–8; discussion 8–32.
49. Martinez-Selles M, Datino T, Alhama M. Rapid carvedilol up-titration in hospitalized patients with left ventricular systolic dysfunction—data from the Carvedilol in Hospital: Up-titration Limits after Acute Patients Admission registry. *J Cardiovasc Med (Hagerstown)* 2010;**11**(5):352–8.
50. Dobre D, van Veldhuisen DJ, Goulder MA, Krumr H, Willenheimer R. Clinical effects of initial 6 months monotherapy with bisoprolol versus enalapril in the treatment of patients with mild to moderate chronic heart failure. Data from the CIBIS III Trial. *Cardiovasc Drugs Ther* 2008 oct;**22**(5):399–405.

51. Yancy CW, Lopatin M, Stevenson LW, De Marco T, Fonarow GC. Clinical presentation, management, and in-hospital outcomes of patients admitted with acute decompensated heart failure with preserved systolic function: a report from the Acute Decompensated Heart Failure National Registry (ADHERE) Database. *J Am Coll Cardiol* 2006;**47**(1):76–84.
52. Nieminen MS, Brutsaert D, Dickstein K, *et al.* EuroHeart Failure Survey II (EHFS II): a survey on hospitalized acute heart failure patients: description of population. *Eur Heart J* 2006;**27**(22):2725–36.
53. Nicol ED, Fittall B, Roughton M, Cleland JG, Dargie H, Cowie MR. NHS heart failure survey: a survey of acute heart failure admissions in England, Wales and Northern Ireland. *Heart* 2008;**94**(2):172–7.
54. Teichert M, de Smet PA, Hofman A, Witteman JC, Stricker BH. Discontinuation of beta-blockers and the risk of myocardial infarction in the elderly. *Drug Saf* 2007;**30**(6):541–9.
55. Fonarow GC, Abraham WT, *et al.* Influence of beta-blocker continuation or withdrawal on outcomes in patients hospitalized with heart failure: findings from the OPTIMIZE-HF program. *J Am Coll Cardiol* 2008;**52**(3):190–9.

39

Aldosterone antagonists

Sushma Rekhraj, Benjamin R. Szwejkowski, and Allan Struthers

Background

Heart failure (HF) is a condition which is associated with a high morbidity and mortality rate despite advancements in treatment options such as angiotensin converting enzyme (ACE) inhibitors and β-blockers. Half of all HF patients are dead within 4 years. Numerous neurohormonal mechanisms are involved in the pathophysiology of HF including the renin–angiotensin–aldosterone system (RAAS), the sympathetic nervous system, and arginine vasopressin (AVP). With regards to the RAAS, plasma aldosterone levels are 20-fold higher in HF than in normal individuals. In normal individuals with normal sodium intake, plasma aldosterone levels are 5–15 ng/dL (139–416 pmol/L) compared to plasma levels up to 300 ng/dL (8322 pmol/L) in HF patients.[1] Aldosterone has been confirmed to play a pivotal role in the HF syndrome as highlighted by two landmark studies, RALES and EPHESUS. In the past, the importance of aldosterone was underappreciated as it was falsely assumed that ACE inhibitors will block aldosterone synthesis. However, further studies have found this not to be true.

Aldosterone

Aldosterone is a mineralocorticoid secreted mainly by the zona glomerulosa of the adrenal cortex. It is also produced in the heart, brain, and blood vessels. The main stimulus for aldosterone secretion is angiotensin II. However, other stimuli include increased serum potassium levels, corticotropin, catecholamines, AVP, and endothelin. Only 60% of aldosterone is bound to plasma proteins, thereby resulting in a short half-life of 20 min.

Aldosterone acts on the mineralocorticoid receptor which is located within the cytoplasm, leading to genomic effects. Aldosterone, independently and by potentiating the cardiovascular damaging effects of angiotensin II, contributes towards the HF syndrome and increases a patient's risk of sudden death. Aldosterone can act within the kidneys to retain sodium and water which increases blood volume and blood pressure and causes peripheral oedema. Aldosterone also renders a patient susceptible to arrhythmias by stimulating renal excretion of potassium and magnesium, stimulating sympathetic activity, inhibiting parasympathetic activity, and reducing the baroreceptor reflex. Aldosterone causes endothelial dysfunction and can increase the tendency to thrombosis which increases the risk of cardiovascular events. It also stimulates collagen deposition resulting in perivascular and myocardial fibrosis, cardiac hypertrophy and remodelling (Fig. 39.1).[2]

Aldosterone has been known for a long time to be a predictor of poor prognosis in HF patients. Hormonal data from the CONSENSUS study found that HF patients with higher aldosterone levels had a worse prognosis.[3] In the neurohormonal substudy of the SAVE study, which looked at post myocardial infarction (MI) patients with asymptomatic impaired left ventricular function, aldosterone levels at 3 months were associated with patients developing severe HF or the combined endpoint of cardiovascular death, MI, or severe HF.[4] In view of its various deleterious effects, it is important to block aldosterone in HF.

'Aldosterone escape'

Chronic ACE inhibitor and angiotensin II receptor blocker (ARB) therapy does not completely suppress aldosterone production. In fact these drugs only reduce aldosterone levels for a brief period and it gradually returns back to baseline in the medium to long term. Staessen *et al.*[5] found that suppressing angiotensin II using captopril resulted in a reduction in aldosterone levels for 1 month (74–21 pg/mL, $p < 0.05$) but this then gradually increased and peaked at 165 pg/mL after a year. This well-known phenomenon is called 'aldosterone escape'. It occurs in up to 40% of HF patients[6] and 50% of hypertensive patients[7] on chronic ACE inhibitor therapy. This phenomenon even occurs in patients despite taking the highest recommended doses of ACE inhibitors or on combination therapy (ACE inhibitor and ARB) which agrees with the fact that aldosterone is not only under control by angiotensin II.

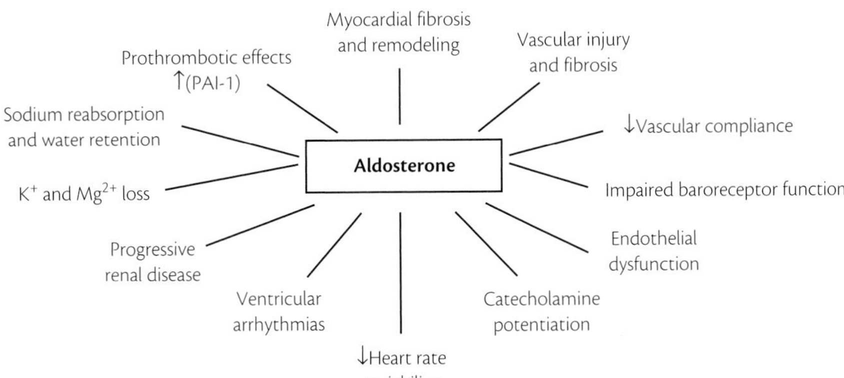

Fig. 39.1 Multiple mechanisms by which aldosterone dysregulation may contribute to cardiovascular disease. PAI-1, plasminogen activator inhibitor-1.
Adapted with permission from Struthers AD, MacDonald TM. Review of aldosterone and angiotensin II-induced target organ damage and prevention. *Cardiovasc Res* 2004;**61**(4):663–70.

Possible reasons for the aldosterone escape phenomenon include

- production of angiotensin II by non-ACE pathways
- aldosterone produced by non-angiotensin-II related secretagogues such as high potassium levels, catecholamines, corticotrophin, and AVP.

Aldosterone escape has been associated with a significantly reduced exercise capacity in HF patients.[8]

The two currently available aldosterone antagonists are spironolactone and eplerenone. Aldosterone antagonists are licensed in the United Kingdom and Europe only to treat HF, whereas in the United States they are licensed in the treatment of both HF and hypertension.

Spironolactone

Spironolactone is a nonselective mineralocorticoid receptor antagonist that was synthesized by researchers in Chicago in 1959. As it also acts as an antagonist against androgen, glucocorticoid, and progesterone receptors, spironolactone is associated with numerous sexual side effects.

In the plasma, more than 90% of spironolactone is bound to albumin. It is then metabolized by the liver into three main active metabolites including 7-α thiomethylspironolactone (TMS), canrenone, and 6-β-hydroxy-7-α-thiomethylspironolactone (HTMS). The half-life of spironolactone is only 1.4 h although the half-life of the active metabolites is much longer at 14–22 h.

Systolic dysfunction

The Randomized Aldactone Evaluation Study (RALES) study was a landmark study assessing the use of spironolactone in severe HF patients.[9] It involved 1663 severe HF patients with a mean left ventricular ejection fraction (LVEF) of 25% on medical treatment including ACE inhibitor, loop diuretic, and in most cases digoxin. Patients were excluded if baseline bloods indicated a serum creatinine in excess of 220 μmol/L or potassium in excess of 5 mmol/L. Patients were commenced on 25 mg spironolactone which was up-titrated to 50 mg after 2 months if there was no evidence of hyperkalaemia.

This study was stopped prematurely at a mean follow-up period of 24 months in view of the significant benefits of using spironolactone in this patient group. Patients on spironolactone were noted to have a 30% reduced mortality rate compared to the placebo group. A reduction was seen in both deaths due to HF and to sudden cardiac deaths. These patients also had a 35% reduced risk of HF admissions and 41% had an improvement in NYHA class (compared to 33% in placebo group). Although these are very impressive results, it must be noted that in this study only a small number of patients were on β-blocker therapy (11% in the spironolactone group compared to 10% in the placebo group) compared to our current HF population. Nevertheless this small subgroup on β-blockers appeared to benefit equally from spironolactone. Since the publication of RALES, there have been numerous HF studies highlighting the benefit of prescribing β-blockers in this patient group.

Most HF studies using spironolactone have been carried out on patients with severe HF symptoms. However, it is important to assess if spironolactone plays a role in treating patients with milder HF symptoms. Spironolactone prescribed to HF patients with LVEF 40% or less and mild HF symptoms (NYHA class I/II) has been found to reduce B-type natriuretic peptide (BNP) and procollagen type III N-terminal peptide (PIIINP) levels [10] and to lead to a statistically nonsignificant 32% reduction in major cardiac events and HF rehospitalizations.[11] Further work is ongoing to see if aldosterone blockade is really effective in mild systolic dysfunction.

Diastolic dysfunction

Diastolic HF is a subset of HF that is not well treated at the present moment because of the lack of therapeutic options. Spironolactone (25 mg) has been found to improve diastolic dysfunction parameters in hypertensive heart disease[12] while also increasing exercise capacity (peak exercise Vo_2 increased by 8.3%, p = 0.001), and improving NYHA class (p = 0.004) in a group of elderly women with diastolic HF.[13] These are small-scale studies only and therefore it is important to assess the efficacy of spironolactone in treating diastolic dysfunction in larger numbers. The Treatment Of Preserved Cardiac function HF with an Aldosterone anTagonist (TOPCAT) is an ongoing randomized multicentre study funded by the US National Heart, Lung and Blood Institute (NHLBI) assessing the use of spironolactone in HF patients with LVEF of 45% or greater. It is hoping to recruit 4500 patients and to complete the study in 2011.

Are we prescribing spironolactone as evidence suggests?

Three years after publication of RALES, a review of medical documentation of HF patients in four urban hospitals found that only 14% of NYHA class III and IV HF patients were prescribed spironolactone as recommended by the guidelines.[14] Nevertheless, Juurlink and colleagues found that following the RALES study, prescription of spironolactone increased fivefold in the HF population of 65 years or older in Ontario.[15] They also highlighted a high incidence of adverse effects such as hyperkalaemia, but these were often due to the wrong high dose of spironolactone being given to the wrong patients.

Eplerenone

Eplerenone is a selective aldosterone receptor antagonist that was derived from spironolactone in 1984 to avoid the sexual side effects associated with spironolactone. The 9,11-epoxy group of the drug is responsible for its selective property (Fig. 39.2).

Eplerenone has a 67% oral bioavailability and lower protein binding than spironolactone (approximately 50% of the drug is protein bound). It is an active drug that is metabolized in the liver by cytochrome P450 3A4 into inactive metabolites. It is therefore important to reduce the dosage of eplerenone in patients also taking cytochrome P450 inhibitors such as ketoconazole and erythromycin, as eplerenone levels will be increased. The half-life of eplerenone is 4–6 h which is much shorter than the half-life of spironolactone active metabolites. The shorter half-life could in theory be beneficial when adverse effects like hyperkalaemia occur since the adverse event should reverse quicker. The main benefit of eplerenone is that it is less associated with sexual side effects than spironolactone, because of its reduced affinity to bind to androgen receptors (1000 times less) and progesterone receptors (100 times less).

Systolic dysfunction

The Eplerenone Post-acute MI Heart failure Efficacy and Survival Study (EPHESUS) was a randomized multicentre double-blinded placebo-controlled study that assessed the use of a selective aldosterone antagonist in 6632 patients who were 3–14 days post MI with left ventricular systolic dysfunction (LVSD) in the presence of either coincidental diabetes or symptoms of HF. The patients were recruited over a period of 2 years (1999–2001) and were already on maximal therapy which included drugs such as β-blockers, ACE inhibitors, ARBs, and diuretics, and coronary revascularization. In comparison to RALES, EPHESUS recruited more patients (6632 vs 1663) with a higher LVEF (33% vs 25.6%) and a higher usage of β-blockers (75% vs 11%). Although the results were not quite as impressive as RALES, there was noted to be a significant reduction in all-cause mortality (15%) and cardiovascular mortality (17%) and a 15% relative risk reduction in HF hospitalization.[17] A retrospective subanalysis of diabetic patients in the EPHESUS study noted that eplerenone therapy in diabetics was associated with a greater absolute risk reduction of all-cause and cardiovascular mortality or cardiovascular hospitalization compared to nondiabetics.[18]

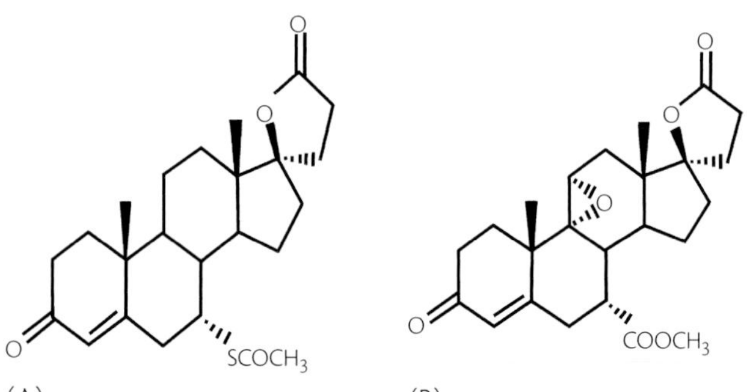

Fig. 39.2 Molecular structure of spironolactone (A) and eplerenone (B). Adapted with permission from Garthwaite S, McMahon E. The evolution of aldosterone antagonists. Mol Cell Endocrinol 2004;**217**:27–31. Copyright © 2004 Elsevier. All rights reserved.

Diastolic dysfunction

Animal studies have noted a benefit in administering eplerenone in diastolic dysfunction.[19] This maybe due to its effects on left ventricular mass regression and reduced collagen deposition and myocardial fibrosis.

Effects of aldosterone antagonists

Antihypertensive effects

Both spironolactone (25–100 mg) and eplerenone (50–200 mg) have been found to be effective in lowering blood pressure. The ASCOT-Blood Pressure Lowering Arm found that adding spironolactone at a median dose of 25 mg to 1411 study participants who were already prescribed three other antihypertensives led to a mean reduction in blood pressure of 21.9/9.5 mmHg (95% CI 20.8 to 23/ 9 to 10.1 mmHg; $p < 0.001$).[20] Eplerenone has been found to be not inferior to amlodipine as an antihypertensive [21] and has led to a significantly greater reduction in mean blood pressure in a predominantly black population compared to losartan or placebo.[22] The antihypertensive effect of eplerenone is dose-related. Weinberger and colleagues found that in a population of mild–moderate hypertensives, 100 mg spironolactone had 25% greater mean reduction in blood pressure compared to eplerenone 100 mg.[23]

Reduced remodelling

Aldosterone production is stimulated post MI and in congestive HF. This has implications for left ventricular remodelling as aldosterone increases left ventricular mass, stimulates cardiac collagen synthesis, and increases both the effect of angiotensin II itself and the expression of the angiotensin 1 receptor. PIIINP is a biomarker of collagen synthesis which is associated with a poor prognosis in cardiac patients. Experimental animal and human studies have shown that spironolactone and eplerenone are associated with a significant improvement in LVEF and diastolic function as well as improvements in left ventricular dilatation (left ventricular end-diastolic volume index and left ventricular end-systolic volume index), left ventricular mass index (LVMI), and PIINP plasma levels.[24,25]

Left ventricular mass regression

Left ventricular hypertrophy (LVH) is known to be an independent risk factor for cardiac events and mortality. Aldosterone causes cardiac hypertrophy by its direct action on cardiac mineralocorticoid receptors and indirectly through its effects on blood pressure.

A study on hypertensive patients with LVH found that patients given spironolactone with an ACE inhibitor had a statistically significant greater regression of LVMI compared to the group just treated with an ACE inhibitor, and this was independent of blood pressure reduction.[26] The 4E study has also shown eplerenone to be as effective as enalapril in LVH regression, although combination therapy led to the greatest LVH regression.[27]

Electrolytes

Aldosterone antagonists, through their action on the distal and collecting tubules of the kidneys, can result in excretion of sodium and retention of potassium. It remains uncertain whether such effects really occur at the kind of low doses that these drugs are used at in HF.

Antiarrhythmic effects

HF patients are at an increased risk of ventricular arrhythmias and sudden cardiac death. Aldosterone antagonists reduce ventricular arrhythmias and sudden cardiac death by a number of mechanisms which include maintaining serum potassium and magnesium levels, regressing LVH, reducing left ventricular remodelling, and improving LVEF. They also reduce cardiac sympathetic activity by increasing myocardial noradrenaline uptake and increasing parasympathetic activation as well as heart rate variability.[28,29] QT dispersion, which is a marker of sudden cardiac death in HF patients, has also been noted to reduce in patients prescribed aldosterone antagonists.[29] In HF patients, spironolactone has been shown to significantly reduce the frequency of ventricular ectopics and nonsustained ventricular tachyarrhythmias (VT) on 24-h Holter monitor.[30] Eplerenone has also been noted to reduce atrial tachyarrhythmias in HF-induced dogs.[31]

Exercise capacity

HF failure patients treated with 50 mg spironolactone achieve a significant improvement in peak oxygen consumption.[32]

Improved endothelial function

HF is associated with endothelial dysfunction due to increased levels of oxidative stress. The increased levels of superoxide anion (O_2^-) reduces the bioavailability of nitric oxide (NO) in the vessel wall. Experimental and human studies have found aldosterone antagonists to reduce the production of superoxide anions in HF patients which results in increased endothelial NO bioavailability and endothelial NO synthase expression and suppresses the conversion of angiotensin I into angiotensin II.[33,34] This results in an improvement in endothelial dysfunction in chronic HF patients. Such an effect may contribute to the ability of aldosterone antagonists to reduce sudden deaths since improved endothelial function may reduce atherothrombotic events in the coronary arteries.

Side effects

Side effects associated with spironolactone include hyperkalaemia, renal deterioration, gastrointestinal disturbances, gynaecomastia in men, and sexual disturbances (impotence in men and menstrual irregularities in women). The nonselective action of spironolactone is responsible for causing gynaecomastia and sexual disturbances. The side effects seem to be related to medication dosage and to the treatment duration. In the RALES study, 8% of spironolactone patients discontinued taking the medication as a result of adverse events compared to 5% in the placebo group.[9] This discontinuation rate is found to be much higher in real life. Eplerenone is associated with the same side effects as spironolactone except it produces no gynaecomastia because of its more selective pharmacological profile.

Hyperkalaemia

Aldosterone acts at the renal distal tubules by reabsorbing sodium and excreting potassium. Hence, aldosterone antagonists are associated with hyperkalaemia. In the RALES pilot study, the risk of developing hyperkalaemia with spironolactone was dose dependent. The incidence of hyperkalaemia (potassium ≥5.5 mmol/L) was 5% (12.5 mg spironolactone), 13% (25 mg spironolactone), 20% (50 mg spironolactone), and 24% (75 mg spironolactone) compared to 5% for placebo group.[35] For risk factors for developing hyperkalaemia, see Box 39.1

Baseline renal function is key to determining the risk of hyperkalaemia. A study by Shah and colleagues found that in HF patients treated with spironolactone, 35% of patients with creatinine 132 μmol/L or more developed hyperkalaemia compared to 63% with creatinine 220 μmol/L or more.[36]

Cavallari and colleagues have suggested that there maybe a racial discrepancy in the ability of spironolactone to cause hyperkalaemia They found that 25 mg spironolactone increased potassium levels by a median of 0.5 mEq/L in white patients but only 0.1 mEq/L in African Americans ($p < 0.01$).[37]

In the RALES study, the incidence of serious hyperkalaemia (serum potassium ≥6 mmol/L) was 2% in spironolactone patients and 1% in placebo patients ($p = 0.42$).[9] This was not statistically significant. This low incidence may be related to its exclusion in the trial of patients with baseline serum creatinine in excess of 220μmol/L and serum potassium in excess of 5 mmol/L and undertaking close, regular blood test monitoring.

Svensson and colleagues noted that in HF patients taking spironolactone, a serum potassium level in excess of 5 mmol/L

Box 39.1 Risk factors for developing hyperkalaemia on aldosterone antagonists

- Elderly population
- Higher dosage of aldosterone antagonists
- Diabetes—associated hyporeninaemic hypoaldosteronism
- Baseline renal dysfunction
- Higher baseline serum potassium levels
- Concomitant medication:
  - ACE inhibitors, ARBs
  - β-Blockers
  - Potassium supplements
  - Potassium-sparing diuretics
  - NSAIDs

occurred in 36% whereas 10% attained serum potassium in excess of 6 mmol/L.[38] This much higher incidence of hyperkalaemia in daily practice compared to the RALES study may be due to inappropriate prescribing of spironolactone (especially in elderly patients, those with impaired renal function, or those using concomitant medication), prescribing of larger doses compared to that used in RALES study, and inadequate patient monitoring. Shah and colleagues found that 34% of the patients did not have a follow-up potassium and creatinine blood test at 3 months.[36]

In the EPHESUS, serious hyperkalaemia (serum K ≥6 mmol/L) occurred in 5.5% eplerenone patients compared to 3.9% placebo patients, which was statistically significant.[17]

Renal deterioration

In the RALES study, there was a small, clinically nonsignificant increase in serum creatinine levels.[9] In the EPHESUS study, there was a statistically significant increase in serum creatinine levels in patients treated with eplerenone (5.3 μmol/L) compared to placebo (1.8 μmol/L).[17]

Patients who are at increased risk of developing renal deterioration whilst taking aldosterone antagonists include elderly people, especially those with LVEF less than 20%, lower baseline body weight, increased baseline creatinine level, and concomitant diuretic therapy.

Gynaecomastia

Male patients taking spironolactone develop gynaecomastia as a result of the drug's actions at the androgen receptor, increased testosterone metabolism, and increased peripheral conversion of testosterone to oestradiol. In the RALES study, 9% of men on spironolactone had gynaecomastia compared to 1% in the placebo group ($p < 0.001$). Breast pain in men was also noted in 0.1% in the placebo group compared to 1% in the spironolactone group.[9] This is not a problem with eplerenone. In the EPHESUS study, eplerenone therapy did not have a statistically significant increased risk of developing gynaecomastia (0.5% vs 0.6%; $p = 0.70$) or breast pain (0.1% vs 0.3%; $p = 0.63$).[17]

Dosage/prescribing

Appropriately selected HF patients should be commenced on either low-dose spironolactone (25 mg) or eplerenone (25 mg) which can be gradually up-titrated to 50 mg. Aldosterone antagonists should be contraindicated in patients with GFR less than 30 mL/min or hyperkalaemia (K^+ ≥5.0 mmol/L). Patients should have a monitoring blood test done at least monthly for the first 3 months and then 3-monthly for 1 year and then 6-monthly from then onwards. Patients with renal dysfunction should have blood tests done more frequently. If serum potassium level increases to more than 5 mmol/L or creatinine more than 220 μmol/L, then either reduce concomitant medication such as diuretics or NSAIDS or reduce dosage of aldosterone antagonist by half and repeat blood test after 3–4 days. If potassium is in excess of 6 mmol/L or creatinine in excess of 310 μmol/L then stop aldosterone antagonist, commence potassium-lowering therapy, and then repeat blood test next day.

Cost

Eplerenone is much more expensive than spironolactone. In the United Kingdom, the cost of a packet of 28 spironolactone tablets is £1.76 for 25-mg tablets and £2.53 for 50-mg tablets, whereas eplerenone (25 mg or 50 mg) costs £42.72.

Conclusion

HF is a condition still associated with a high morbidity and mortality rate despite advances in therapy. Experimental animal and human studies, especially the RALES and EPHESUS studies, have shown the benefit of aldosterone antagonist therapy in HF patients and HF patients post MI when added to maximal medical HF therapy (Table 39.1). Spironolactone is effective and cheap but is associated with unwanted sexual side effects and hyperkalaemia, which affect patient's tolerability of the drug. Eplerenone, on the other hand, is indicated in post MI HF patients and is also useful in patients who develop sexual side effects on spironolactone. However, eplerenone is much more costly than spironolactone. The evidence base for each drug is different in that spironolactone was studied in moderate to severe chronic HF whereas eplerenone was studied in post MI

Table 39.1 Comparison of RALES and EPHESUS studies

Study	RALES[9]	EPHESUS[17]
Year published	1999	2003
Drug	Spironolactone	Eplerenone
Dosage (mg)	25–50	25–50
Patient no.	1663	6632
Mean age (years)	65	64
Patient group	Severe chronic HF	Post MI
	NYHA class III–IV	NYHA I–IV
	LVEF≤35%	LVEF≤40%
Mean LVEF (%)	25.6	33
Mean follow-up (months)	24	16
ACE inhibitors/ARB (%)	95	86
Beta blocker (%)	11	75
RR all-cause death	0.70*	0.85*
RR cardiac death	0.69*	0.83*
RR sudden cardiac death	0.71*	0.79*
RR hospitalization for worsening HF	0.65*	0.85*
Drug discontinuation due to adverse events (vs placebo)	8% vs 5%	4.4% vs 4.5%
Gynaecomastia (vs placebo)	9% vs 1%	0.5% vs 0.6%
Breast pain (vs placebo)	2% vs 0.1%	0.1% vs 0.3%
Serious hyperkalaemia (vs placebo)	2% vs 1%	5.5% vs 3.9%

ACE, angiotensin converting enzyme; ARB, angiotensin II receptor blocker; EPHESUS, Eplerenone Post acute Myocardial Infarction Heart Failure Efficacy and Survival Study; HF, heart failure; MI, myocardial infarction; LVEF, left ventricular ejection fraction; NYHA, New York Heart Association; RALES, Randomized Aldactone Evaluation Study; RR, relative risk.

p value <0.05 indicated by *.

left ventricular dysfunction. It is very important to select patients carefully and monitor them regularly while on the medication. The TOPCAT trial is currently ongoing to assess the use of an aldosterone antagonist in diastolic dysfunction.

References

1. Weber KT. Aldosterone in congestive heart failure. *N Engl J Med* 2001;**345**(23):1689–97.
2. Struthers AD, MacDonald TM. Review of aldosterone- and angiotensin II-induced target organ damage and prevention. *Cardiovasc Res* 2004;**61**(4):663–70.
3. Swedberg K, Eneroth P, Kjekshus J, Wilhelmsen L. Hormones regulating cardiovascular function in patients with severe congestive heart failure and their relation to mortality. CONSENSUS Trial Study Group. *Circulation* 1990;**82**(5):1730–6.
4. Vantrimpont P, Rouleau JL, Ciampi A, *et al.* Two-year time course and significance of neurohumoral activation in the Survival and Ventricular Enlargement (SAVE) Study. *Eur Heart J* 1998;**19**(10):1552–63.
5. Staessen J, Lijnen P, Fagard R, Verschueren LJ, Amery A. Rise in plasma concentration of aldosterone during long-term angiotensin II suppression. *J Endocrinol* 1981;**91**(3):457–65.
6. MacFadyen RJ, Lee AF, Morton JJ, Pringle SD, Struthers AD. How often are angiotensin II and aldosterone concentrations raised during chronic ACE inhibitor treatment in cardiac failure? *Heart* 1999;**82**(1):57–61.
7. Sato A, Saruta T. Aldosterone escape during angiotensin-converting enzyme inhibitor therapy in essential hypertensive patients with left ventricular hypertrophy. *J Int Med Res* 2001;**29**(1):13–21.
8. Cicoira M, Zanolla L, Franceschini L, *et al.* Relation of aldosterone 'escape' despite angiotensin-converting enzyme inhibitor administration to impaired exercise capacity in chronic congestive heart failure secondary to ischemic or idiopathic dilated cardiomyopathy. *Am J Cardiol* 2002;**89**(4):403–7.
9. Pitt B, Zannad F, Remme WJ, *et al.* The effect of spironolactone on morbidity and mortality in patients with severe heart failure. Randomized Aldactone Evaluation Study Investigators. *N Engl J Med* 1999;**341**(10):709–17.
10. Berry C, Murphy NF, De Vito G, *et al.* Effects of aldosterone receptor blockade in patients with mild-moderate heart failure taking a beta-blocker. *Eur J Heart Fail* 2007;**9**(4):429–34.
11. Baliga RR, Ranganna P, Pitt B, Koelling TM. Spironolactone treatment and clinical outcomes in patients with systolic dysfunction and mild heart failure symptoms: a retrospective analysis. *J Card Fail* 2006;**12**(4):250–6.
12. Mottram PM, Haluska B, Leano R, Cowley D, Stowasser M, Marwick TH. Effect of aldosterone antagonism on myocardial dysfunction in hypertensive patients with diastolic heart failure. *Circulation* 2004;**110**(5):558–65.
13. Daniel KR, Wells G, Stewart K, Moore B, Kitzman DW. Effect of aldosterone antagonism on exercise tolerance, Doppler diastolic function, and quality of life in older women with diastolic heart failure. *Congest Heart Fail* 2009;**15**(2):68–74.
14. Trujillo JM, Gonyeau MJ, DiVall MV, Alexander SL. Spironolactone use in patients with heart failure. *J Clin Pharm Ther* 2004;**29**(2):165–70.
15. Juurlink DN, Mamdani MM, *et al.* Rates of hyperkalemia after publication of the Randomized Aldactone Evaluation Study. *N Engl J Med* 2004;**351**(6):543–51.
16. Garthwaite SM, McMahon EG. The evolution of aldosterone antagonists. *Mol Cell Endocrinol* 2004;**217**(1–2):27–31.
17. Pitt B, Remme W, Zannad F, *et al.* Eplerenone, a selective aldosterone blocker, in patients with left ventricular dysfunction after myocardial infarction. *N Engl J Med* 2003;**348**(14):1309–21.
18. O'Keefe JH, Abuissa H, Pitt B. Eplerenone improves prognosis in postmyocardial infarction diabetic patients with heart failure: results from EPHESUS. *Diabetes Obes Metab* 2008;**10**(6):492–7.
19. Masson S, Staszewsky L, Annoni G, *et al.* Eplerenone, a selective aldosterone blocker, improves diastolic function in aged rats with small-to-moderate myocardial infarction. *J Card Fail* 2004;**10**(5):433–41.
20. Chapman N, Dobson J, Wilson S, *et al.* Effect of spironolactone on blood pressure in subjects with resistant hypertension. *Hypertension* 2007;**49**(4):839–45.
21. White WB, Duprez D, St Hillaire R, *et al.* Effects of the selective aldosterone blocker eplerenone versus the calcium antagonist amlodipine in systolic hypertension. *Hypertension* 2003;**41**(5):1021–6.
22. Flack JM, Oparil S, Pratt JH, Roniker B, Garthwaite S, Kleiman JH, *et al.* Efficacy and tolerability of eplerenone and losartan in hypertensive black and white patients. *J Am Coll Cardiol* 2003;**41**(7):1148–55.
23. Weinberger MH, Roniker B, Krause SL, Weiss RJ. Eplerenone, a selective aldosterone blocker, in mild-to-moderate hypertension. *Am J Hypertens* 2002;**15**(8):709–16.
24. Tsutamoto T, Wada A, Maeda K, *et al.* Effect of spironolactone on plasma brain natriuretic peptide and left ventricular remodeling in patients with congestive heart failure. *J Am Coll Cardiol* 2001;**37**(5):1228–33.
25. Fraccarollo D, Galuppo P, Schmidt I, Ertl G, Bauersachs J. Additive amelioration of left ventricular remodeling and molecular alterations by combined aldosterone and angiotensin receptor blockade after myocardial infarction. *Cardiovasc Res* 2005;**67**(1): 97–105.
26. Sato A, Suzuki Y, Saruta T. Effects of spironolactone and angiotensin-converting enzyme inhibitor on left ventricular hypertrophy in patients with essential hypertension. *Hypertens Res* 1999;**22**(1):17–22.
27. Pitt B, Reichek N, Willenbrock R, *et al.* Effects of eplerenone, enalapril, and eplerenone/enalapril in patients with essential hypertension and left ventricular hypertrophy: the 4E-left ventricular hypertrophy study. *Circulation* 2003;**108**(15):1831–8.
28. MacFadyen RJ, Barr CS, Struthers AD. Aldosterone blockade reduces vascular collagen turnover, improves heart rate variability and reduces early morning rise in heart rate in heart failure patients. *Cardiovasc Res* 1997;**35**(1):30–4.
29. Yee KM, Pringle SD, Struthers AD. Circadian variation in the effects of aldosterone blockade on heart rate variability and QT dispersion in congestive heart failure. *J Am Coll Cardiol* 2001;**37**(7):1800–7.
30. Ramires FJ, Mansur A, Coelho O, *et al.* Effect of spironolactone on ventricular arrhythmias in congestive heart failure secondary to idiopathic dilated or to ischemic cardiomyopathy. *Am J Cardiol* 2000;**85**(10):1207–11.
31. Shroff SC, Ryu K, Martovitz NL, Hoit BD, Stambler BS. Selective aldosterone blockade suppresses atrial tachyarrhythmias in heart failure. *J Cardiovasc Electrophysiol* 2006;**17**(5):534–41.
32. Cicoira M, Zanolla L, Rossi A, *et al.* Long-term, dose-dependent effects of spironolactone on left ventricular function and exercise tolerance in patients with chronic heart failure. *J Am Coll Cardiol* 2002;**40**(2):304–10.
33. Farquharson CA, Struthers AD. Spironolactone increases nitric oxide bioactivity, improves endothelial vasodilator dysfunction, and suppresses vascular angiotensin I/angiotensin II conversion in patients with chronic heart failure. *Circulation* 2000;**101**(6):594–7.
34. Schafer A, Fraccarollo D, Hildemann SK, Tas P, Ertl G, Bauersachs J. Addition of the selective aldosterone receptor antagonist eplerenone to ACE inhibition in heart failure: effect on endothelial dysfunction. *Cardiovasc Res* 2003;**58**(3):655–62.

35. Effectiveness of spironolactone added to an angiotensin-converting enzyme inhibitor and a loop diuretic for severe chronic congestive heart failure (the Randomized Aldactone Evaluation Study [RALES]). *Am J Cardiol* 1996;**78**(8):902–7.
36. Shah KB, Rao K, Sawyer R, Gottlieb SS. The adequacy of laboratory monitoring in patients treated with spironolactone for congestive heart failure. *J Am Coll Cardiol* 2005;**46**(5):845–9.
37. Cavallari LH, Groo VL, Momary KM, Fontana D, Viana MA, Vaitkus P. Racial differences in potassium response to spironolactone in heart failure. *Congest Heart Fail* 2006;**12**(4):200–5.
38. Svensson M, Gustafsson F, Galatius S, Hildebrandt PR, Atar D. Hyperkalaemia and impaired renal function in patients taking spironolactone for congestive heart failure: retrospective study. *BMJ* 2003;**327**(7424):1141–2.

40

Angiotensin receptor blockers

John J.V. McMurray

Angiotensin receptor blockers (ARBs) were developed to provide an alternative approach to interrupting the renin–angiotensin system (RAS), which was pharmacologically distinct from that of angiotensin converting enzyme (ACE) inhibitors.[1] By selectively blocking the angiotensin II type 1 (AT_1) receptor, ARBs were thought to offer the potential for more complete blockade of the RAS. Evidence had accumulated that angiotensin II could be generated through enzymes other than ACE (e.g. chymase) and ARBs block the action of angiotensin II, regardless of its source, at the receptor level (Fig. 40.1). Another fundamental difference between the two approaches is the lack of effect of ARBs on bradykinin which is metabolized by ACE (also known as kininase II). Accumulation of bradykinin with ACE inhibitors is responsible for cough and angioedema. Consequently, it was hoped that ARBs would be better tolerated than ACE inhibitors. Bradykinin, however, may also have beneficial effects, including vasodilatation, antithrombotic activity, and inhibition of pathological tissue remodelling. This latter perspective, that bradykinin might have beneficial actions, underpinned the hypothesis that the combination of an ACE inhibitor and ARB might be better than an ACE inhibitor alone in heart failure (HF). In other words, the ARB would maximize RAS inhibition and the ACE inhibitor would augment bradykinin.

Less tangible differences between ARBs and ACE inhibitors were also postulated. Because an ARB displaces angiotensin II from the AT_1 receptor, ligand is available to bind to other AT receptor subtypes, the number and activity of which remain uncertain in humans (Fig. 40.1). One theory is that stimulation of an AT_2 receptor leads to biological actions that oppose those resulting from AT_1 receptor activation, i.e. actions that might be beneficial in HF.

These considerations led to the hypothesis that ARBs might be more effective, better tolerated or both, compared with ACE inhibitors. The challenge, however, was to prove this in randomized controlled trials, a challenge made much more difficult by the fact that the clinical development of ARBs did not begin until about 15 years after that of ACE inhibitors. By that time, ACE inhibitors were established as the cornerstone of treatment of patients with HF and a low ejection fraction. Consequently, only four options were available: (1) demonstrate superiority or 'comparability' (noninferiority) of the new treatment to an ACE inhibitor in a head-to-head comparison, (2) demonstrate additional benefit when an ARB is added to an ACE inhibitor, (3) demonstrate benefit from ARBs in patients intolerant of an ACE inhibitor, and (4) demonstrate benefit from ARBs in new patient groups in which ACE inhibitors had not been shown to be of value.

Head-to head comparison of an ARB and ACE inhibitor

This approach was pursued in the second Evaluation of Losartan in the Elderly (ELITE-2) trial which compared losartan 50 mg once daily with captopril 50 mg three times daily (Table 40.1).[2] The design and dosing used in ELITE-2 was based on the smaller ELITE pilot study designed to compare the renal tolerability of the same two drugs used in the same doses.[3] Although the proportion of patients experiencing a rise in creatinine of 26.5 μmol/L (0.3 mg/dL) was similar in the two treatment arms, another, unexpected, finding in ELITE caused enormous excitement. Although there were few deaths overall in this relatively small and short-term study, their distribution between treatment groups was unequal, with 17/353 (4.8%) deaths in patients assigned to losartan and 32/370 (8.7%) deaths in those assigned to captopril, giving a relative risk reduction in death for losartan compared with captopril of 46% (95% CI 5–69%, $p = 0.035$).

With 3152 patients and over 530 deaths (greater than 10 times ELITE 1), occurring over a median follow-up of 18 months, ELITE-2 was statistically powered to provide a much more reliable comparison of losartan with captopril. In ELITE-2 the mortality difference between the two treatments was not significant, although there was a trend in favour of the ACE inhibitor with 250/1574 (15.9%) deaths in the captopril group and 280/1578 (17.7%) deaths in the losartan group, hazard ratio 1.13 (97.5% CI 0.95–1.35, $p = 0.16$) (Fig. 40.2).[2] With the trend toward better survival in the captopril group it was not even possible to conclude

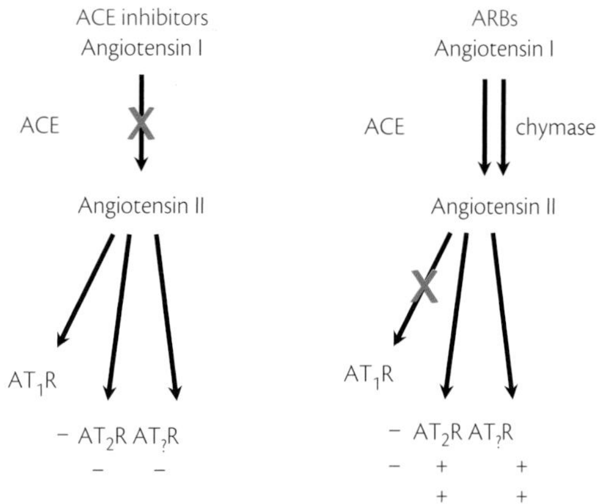

Fig. 40.1 ARBs versus ACE inhibitors. ACE inhibitors only block ACE, reducing the availability of angiotensin II to interact with any of its receptors. However, angiotensin II is still produced via the action of chymase. ARBs block the angiotensin II, type 1 receptor, but allow angiotensin II still to interact with its other receptors.

that losartan was 'as good as' (not inferior to) an ACE inhibitor in this patient population. With hindsight, it is possible to speculate that the design of ELITE-2 and a sister study, Optimal Therapy in Myocardial Infarction with the Angiotensin II Antagonist Losartan (OPTIMAAL), in acute myocardial infarction (MI) using the same drugs and dosing strategy, was fatally flawed because the dose of losartan used was too low (although this would not have been obvious at the time, given the apparent benefit of 50 mg daily in ELITE). That 50 mg daily may have been an inadequate dose was suggested by the two subsequent trials in patients with hypertension and diabetic nephropathy where losartan used in a target dose of 100 mg daily led to a statistically significant clinical benefit.[4,5]

To test this hypothesis, a further trial in HF was set up. In that trial, Heart failure Endpoint evaluation of Angiotensin II Antagonist Losartan (HEAAL), patients with HF and a low ejection fraction who were intolerant of ACE inhibitors, were randomly assigned to treatment with losartan 50 mg once daily or losartan 150 mg once daily (Table 40.1).[6] After a median follow-up of 4.7 years, patients assigned to the higher dose of losartan were significantly less likely to have died or been admitted to hospital for worsening HF (828/1927, 43%) than those randomized to the lower dose (889/1919. 46%), hazard ratio 0.90 (95% CI 0.82–0.99), p = 0.027 (Fig. 40.3). The numbers experiencing a cardiovascular death or HF hospitalization were 698 and 771, respectively, giving a hazard ratio of 0.88 (95% CI 0.79–0.97), p = 0.011. Of interest was the finding that the incremental benefits of higher-dose losartan were obtained with few additional serious adverse effects.

The story of losartan in HF illustrates many of the pitfalls in drug development including the importance of dose selection and the potential for misleading findings (or the misinterpretation of findings) from small studies. Although we shall never know, it is interesting to speculate what the result of ELITE-2 (and the history of ARBs) might have been if 150 mg of losartan had been used instead of 50 mg.

Adding an ARB to an ACE inhibitor

This was the second approach to the use of ARBs tested in a large outcome trial and was clearly an approach testing a completely different hypothesis than ELITE-2. The first of the two trials to adopt the strategy was the Valsartan Heart Failure Trial (Val-HeFT) (Table 40.1).[7]

Val-HeFT was designed with the coprimary outcomes of death from any cause and the combination of death or any of hospitalization for heart failure, administration of intravenous inotropic or vasodilator drugs for 4 h or more without hospitalization or cardiac arrest with resuscitation. The 'alpha' was split between the two endpoints. With a total of 979 deaths occurring during a mean follow-up of 23 months, survival was not improved with the addition of the ARB to conventional therapy: 495/2511 (19.7%) deaths in the valsartan group and 484/2499 (19.4%) deaths in the placebo group, relative risk 1.02; (98% CI 0.88–1.18, p = 0.80) (Fig. 40.4). On the other hand, the rate of composite coprimary outcome was reduced by valsartan (RR 0.87; 97.5% CI 0.77–0.97, p = 0.009) (Fig. 40.5). The major contributor to the reduction was fewer hospitalizations for HF in the valsartan group (13.8% valsartan vs 18.2% placebo). The benefit was obtained at the cost of a small increase in renal dysfunction and hyperkalaemia.

A small subgroup of patients (7%, n = 366) were not treated with an ACE inhibitor at baseline. In this subgroup, the reduction in the mortality/morbidity composite outcome with valsartan was 44%.[8]

A second trial also tested the strategy of adding an ARB to an ACE inhibitor, this time candesartan (in a target daily dose of 32 mg once daily). This Candesartan in Heart failure: Assessment of Reduction in Mortality and morbidity (CHARM)-Added, differed from Val-HeFT in several important respects (Table 40.1).[9] First, by design, patients were at higher risk because those in NYHA class II had to have been hospitalized for a cardiac reason in the previous 6 months. Secondly, and also by design, all patients had to be taking an ACE inhibitor, and investigators were encouraged to optimize patients' dose of ACE inhibitor based on evidence-based guidelines and tolerability. Because CHARM-Added began enrolling after Val-HeFT, use of β-blockers had become more prevalent and treatment with these drugs (and spironolactone) was considerably more frequent in CHARM-Added than Val-HeFT.

In CHARM-Added, after a median follow-up of 41 months, 483/1276 (38%) patients in the candesartan group experienced a cardiovascular death or HF hospitalization compared with 538/1272 (42%) patients in the placebo group, hazard ratio 0.85 (95% CI 0.75–0.96), p = 0.011 (Fig. 40.6). As in Val-HeFT, there was also a more striking reduction in both the total number of patients hospitalized (17%) and in the number of admissions, for worsening HF (27%).

The results of Val-HeFT and CHARM-Added led to much debate about adequacy of background ACE inhibitor dosing, and the US Food and Drug Administration requested subgroup analyses of CHARM-Added to examine the effect of candesartan according to baseline ACE inhibitor dose.[10] These analyses showed that the effect of candesartan was consistent, irrespective of baseline ACE inhibitor dose, and even patients taking very large doses of ACE inhibitor seemed to obtain the same benefit from candesartan as that observed in the overall CHARM-Added trial population (Fig. 40.7). However, as this conclusion is based on retrospective subgroup analyses, it is open to criticism and, with hindsight, a better design for both of these trials would have been to mandate treatment with an evidence-based dose of a proven ACE inhibitor for all patients.

Table 40.1 Randomized controlled mortality/morbidity trials with angiotensin receptor blockers in heart failure

	ELITE-2	Val-HeFT	CHARM-Alternative	CHARM Added	HEAAL	CHARM-Preserved	I-Preserve
	(n = 3152)	(n = 5010)	(n = 2028)	(n = 2548)	(n = 3846)	(n = 3023)	(n = 4128)
Key entry criteria							
Age (yr)	≥60	≥18	≥18	≥18	≥18	≥18	≥60
EF (%)	≤40	<40	≤40	≤40	≥40	>40	≥45
NYHA class	II—IV	II—IV	II—IV	II—IV and II if cardiac hosp. in prior 6 mo.	II—IV	II—IV and prior cardiac hosp.	III–IV[a] and II if HF hosp. in prior 6 mo.
Creatinine (μmol/L)	≤220	≤221	<265	<265	≤220	<265	≤221
Key baseline characteristics							
Age (yr)	72	63	67	64	66	67	72
NYHA class							
II	52	62	48	24	70	61	22
III	43	36	48	73	30	37	76
IV	5	2	4	3	1	2	3
EF (%)	31	27	30	28	33	54	60
Systolic BP (mmHg)	134	124	130	125	125	136	137
Creatinine (μmol/L)	104[b]	108	113[b]	103[b]	97	99	88
Baseline treatment							
ACE inhibitor (%)	NA	93	NA	100	NA	19	26
β blocker (%)	22	35	55	55	72	56	59
Spironolactone/ Aldo. antagonist (%)	22[c]	5	24	17	38	12	15
Treatment comparison							
	Losartan 50 mg qd	Valsartan 160 mg bid	Candesartan 32 mg qd	Candesartan 32 mg qd	Losartan 50 mg qd	Candesartan 32 mg qd	Irbesartan 300 mg qd
	Captopril 50 mg tid	Placebo	Placebo	Placebo	Losartan 150 mg qd	Placebo	Placebo
Primary/coprimary endpoint							
	All-cause mortality	(i) All-cause mortality (ii) All-cause mortality, cardiac arrest with resuscitation, hosp. for HF or >4 h IV inotropic/ vasodilator therapy for HF	CV mortality or HF hosp.	CV mortality or HF hosp.	CV mortality or HF hosp.	All-cause mortality or HF hosp.	All-cause mortality or CV hosp. (HF, MI, stroke, UA or arrhythmia)
Mean/median follow-up (months)							
	19	23	34	41	56	37	50
Results							
	Losartan not superior to captopril; losartan not inferior to captopril	No reduction in mortality 13% RRR mortality/ morbidity composite (p = 0.009)	23% RRR in primary endpoint (p = 0.0004)	15% RRR in primary endpoint (p = 0.011)	10% RRR in primary endpoint (150 mg vs. 50 mg losartan) (p = 0.027)	No reduction in primary endpoint	No reduction in primary endpoint

[a] If no HF hospitalization in prior 6 months, must have supporting findings: abnormal chest radiograph (pulmonary congestion), ECG (left ventricular hypertrophy or bundle branch block) or echocardiogram (left ventricular hypertrophy or enlarged left atrium)

[b] From substudies.

[c] Potassium-sparing diuretic.

ACE, angiotensin converting enzyme; aldo., aldosterone; CV, cardiovascular; EF, ejection fraction; HF, heart failure; hosp., hospitalization; NYHA, New York Heart Association functional class; RRR, relative risk reduction; UA, unstable angina.

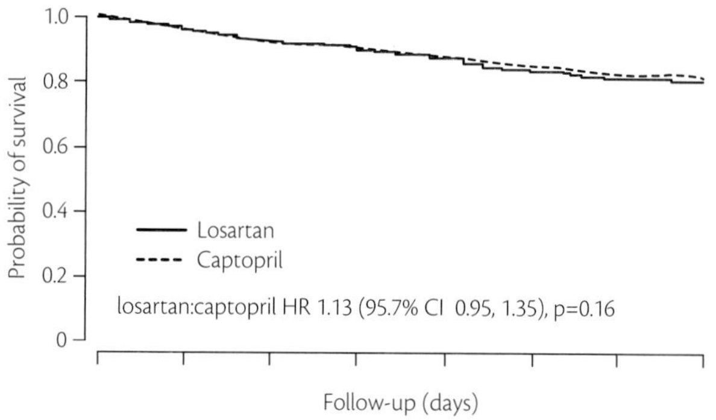

Fig. 40.2 Mortality in ELITE-2.[2] There was no difference between the ARB, losartan, and the ACE inhibitor, captopril.

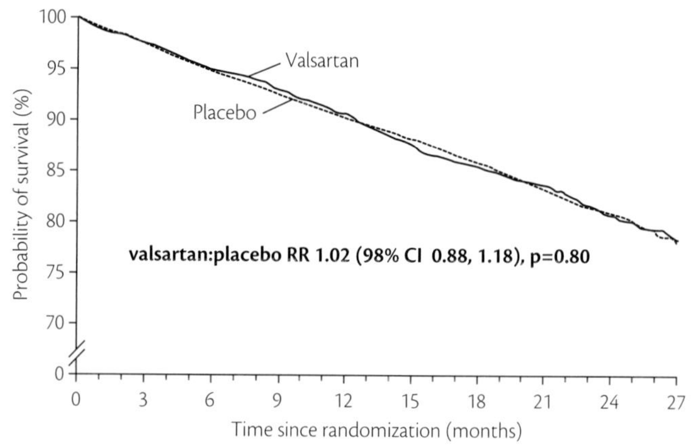

Fig. 40.4 Mortality in the Val-HeFT study.[7] Survival was not improved with the addition of the ARB to conventional therapy.

Such as design was used in subsequent trials in patients with acute infarction (Valsartan in Acute Myocardial Infarction Trial Investigators. VALsartan In Acute myocardial iNfarcTion trial, VALIANT) and in patients with atherosclerotic arterial disease (Ongoing Telmisartan Alone and in Combination with Ramipril Global Endpoint Trial, ONTARGET).[11,12] In both of the latter trials, addition of an ARB to a 'full dose' of ACE inhibitor resulted in no additional clinical benefit (but did cause more adverse effects). These findings have led many to doubt the value of adding an ARB in patients with HF taking a full dose of ACE inhibitor. While it is possible that Val-HeFT and CHARM-Added might not have shown any benefit from adding an ARB if designed like VALIANT and ONTARGET, it is also possible that HF is different and that greater RAS activation occurs in this condition and that more intense RAS blockade leads to greater clinical benefit. One piece of evidence supports this latter hypothesis. The Randomized Evaluation of Strategies for Left Ventricular Dysfunction (RESOLVD) pilot study was a precursor of CHARM in which patients were randomized to various doses of candesartan, enalapril 20 mg per day, or the combination of enalapril and candesartan (and also subsequently rerandomized to placebo or metoprolol).[13] In RESOLVD, addition of candesartan to full-dose enalapril led to greater reverse left ventricular remodelling and neurohumoral suppression, compared with placebo, providing mechanistic support for the findings of CHARM-Added.

Another question that is frequently asked is much more difficult to answer, namely what should be added next after an ACE inhibitor (and β-blocker)—an ARB or an aldosterone antagonist? Until recently, for patients with milder heart failure, the only direct evidence was for an ARB as aldosterone antagonists had not been studied in mild chronic heart failure. At the time of writing, however, a trial filling this gap, the Eplerenone in Mild Patients Hospitalization And SurvIval Study in Heart Failure (EMPHASIS-HF) has just been reported, showing an impressive effect of eplerenone on death from any cause and all-cause hospitalization. These new findings make aldosterone antagonism the preferred next treatment-step after use of an ACE inhibitor and beta-blocker; i.e, an ACB should only be the third neurohumoral antagonist if a patient cannot tolerate an aldosterone blocker.[14] Given the very different mechanism of action of the two types of treatment, perhaps the most pertinent question now is whether both drugs should be added, although there is no evidence to support this suggestion and such an approach must carry a significant risk of renal dysfunction and hyperkalaemia.

As an aside, it is worth mentioning that early termination of trials for benefit is likely to exaggerate the effect of treatment. Indeed, if CHARM-Alternative or Added (or the pooled low ejection fraction cohort) had been stopped early, highly statistically significant

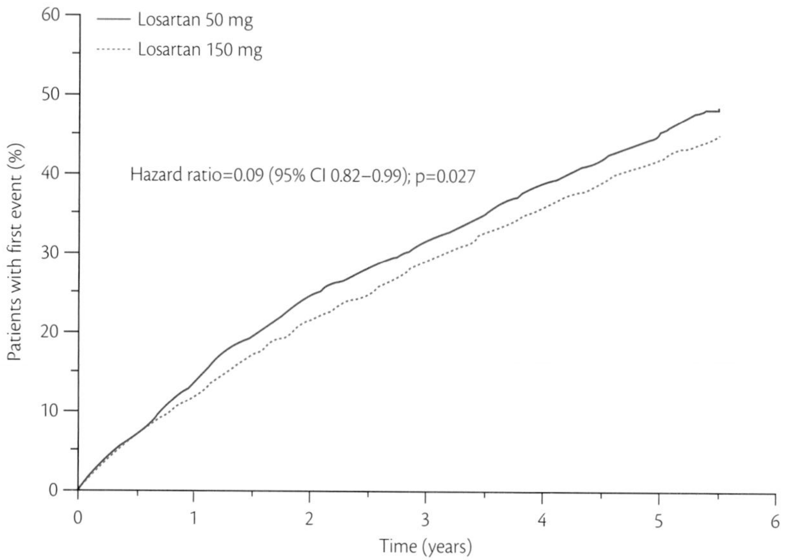

Fig. 40.3 Death or hospitalization for heart failure in the HEAAL study.[6] Higher-dose losartan was more effective than lower.

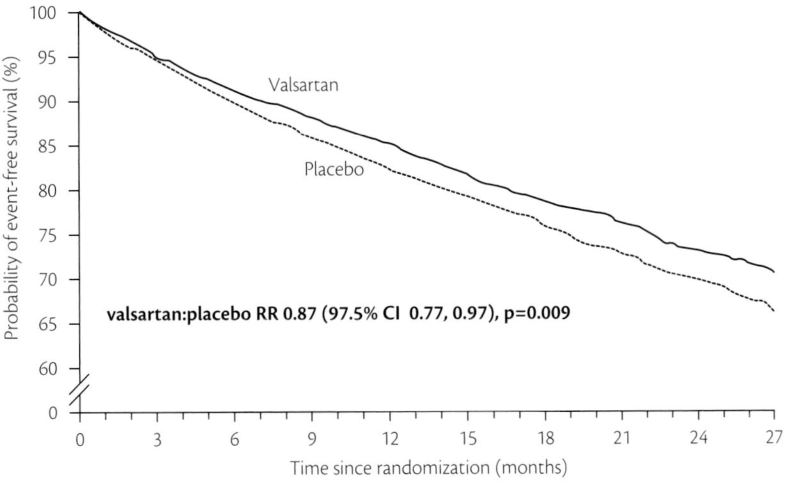

Fig. 40.5 Data from Val-HeFT.[7] For the combined endpoint event-free survival (an event being death or heart failure morbidity) there was a modest effect of valsartan, driven by a reduction in hospitalizations for heart failure.

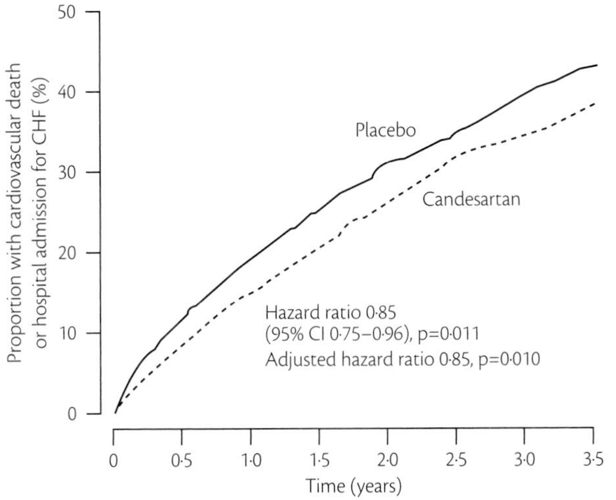

Fig. 40.6 Data from CHARM-Added.[9] Cardiovascular death or hospitalization for heart failure was reduced by candesartan in addition to ACE inhibitor therapy.

and substantial reductions in the primary endpoint and death from any cause would have been reported.[15] Both the CHARM-Programme and the SOLVD-Treatment trial[16] before it, show that with long-term follow-up, the early benefit of treatment becomes less prominent over time.

Use of ARBs in patients intolerant of an ACE inhibitor

A minority of patients cannot tolerate an ACE inhibitor because of cough, and in such patients an ARB may be a useful alternative. Proof of this is provided by the findings of the CHARM-Alternative trial in which 334/1013 (33%) of patients with low-ejection-fraction HF assigned to candesartan experienced a cardiovascular death or HF hospitalization over a median follow-up of 33.7 months compared with 406/1015 (40%) of patients assigned to placebo, hazard ratio 0.77 (95% CI 0.67–0.89), p = 0.0004 (Table 40.1 and Fig. 40.8).[17] Similarly large benefits were seen with valsartan in the

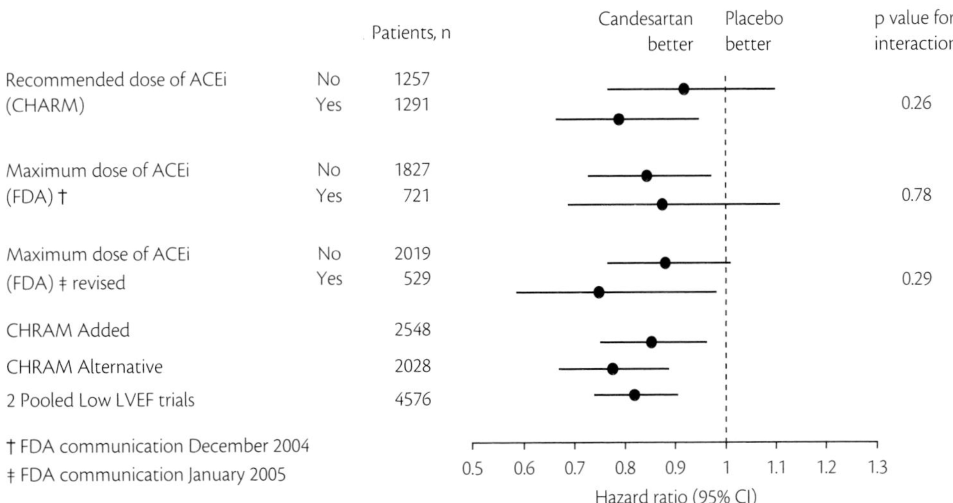

Fig. 40.7 CHARM-Added: risk of cardiovascular death or hospitalization for heart failure according to background ACE inhibitor dose. Even patients taking very large doses of ACE inhibitor seemed to obtain the same benefit from candesartan.[10] The primary outcome was cardiovascular death of heart failure hospitalization for patients in Charm-Added at recommended or higher dose of ACEi or maximum dose of ACEi as defined by the US Food and Drug Administration in the communication of December 2004 and revised in January 2005. Also presented are the results for Charm-Alternative (no ACEi) and the pooled results for these two trials in patients with low left ventricular ejection fraction.

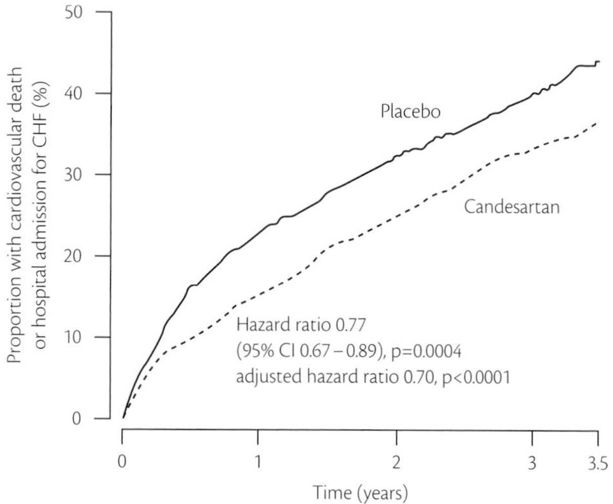

Fig. 40.8 Data from CHARM-Alternative.[17] Candesartan reduced the combined edn-point of cardiovascular death or hospitalization for heart failure in patients unable to tolerate ACE inhibitor.

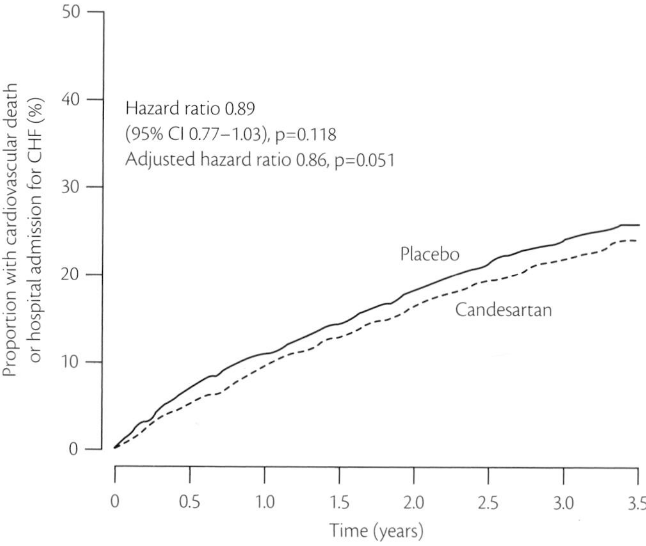

Fig. 40.9 CHARM-Preserved:[18] candesartan had no effect on the endpoint of cardiovascular death or hospitalization for heart failure in patients with heart failure and normal left ventricular ejection fraction.

small subset (7%, n = 366) of patients not treated with an ACE inhibitor at baseline in Val-HeFT.[8]

It is important to point out that a 'full', evidence-based, dose of ARB is just as likely to cause hypotension and renal dysfunction as an ACE inhibitor—the best evidence for this comes from VALIANT.[11] Consequently, if patients have genuinely been unable to tolerate an ACE inhibitor because of these adverse effects, they are unlikely to tolerate an ARB either. It is only cough and angio-oedema that are less likely with an ARB than an ACE inhibitor.

Additional patient groups in which ACE inhibition is not of proven benefit

The last strategy adopted during the development of ARBs was to examine the potential role of the drugs in patient populations where ACE inhibition had not been tested. For heart failure, this meant patients with preserved ejection fraction (HeFPEF) or so called 'diastolic' heart failure. Two trials addressed this question.[18,19] The first was one component trial of the CHARM-Programme (Table 40.1). During screening of patients with heart failure, CHARM investigators could enrol patients with LVEF over 40% into CHARM-Preserved.[18] In this trial, 333/1514 (22%) patients assigned to candesartan experienced a cardiovascular death or HF hospitalization over a median follow-up of 36.6 months compared with 366/1509 (24%) patients assigned to placebo, hazard ratio 0.89 (95% 0.77–1.03), p = 0.118 (Fig. 40.9). Although the primary outcome did not differ significantly between treatments, there were reductions in the proportion of patients admitted to hospital with worsening HF (15%) and in the number of hospitalizations for this problem (29%) with candesartan. So, while not a 'positive' trial, CHARM-Preserved did suggest that RAS blockade might be of benefit in patients with HeFPEF.

A second study sought to confirm or refute this possibility. I-PRESERVE, randomized patients to placebo or 300 mg of irbesartan, a dose previously used successfully in a trial in patients with diabetic nephropathy.[20] Patients were required to have an ejection fraction of 45% or above (Table 40.1).[19] The primary outcome in I-PRESERVE was the composite of death or hospitalization for a cardiovascular cause (heart failure, myocardial infarction, unstable angina, arrhythmia, or stroke). During a mean follow-up of 49.5 months, 742/2067 (35.9%) patients in the irbesartan group and 763/2061 (37.0%) patients in the placebo group experienced the primary outcome, hazard ratio 0.95 (95% CI 0.86–1.05), p = 0.35 (Fig. 40.10). No other outcome was favourably affected either.

These disappointing findings led to much discussion about the similarities and differences of CHARM-Preserved and I-PRESERVE and why the two trials appeared to give a different result (of course, strictly speaking, CHARM-Preserved showed no between treatment-difference in its primary outcome and, therefore, interpreted rigorously, did not differ from I-PRESERVE). If there is a difference, there are at least two possible explanations. First, the dose of irbesartan used was probably only half as effective as blocking the action of angiotensin II as 32 mg of candesartan

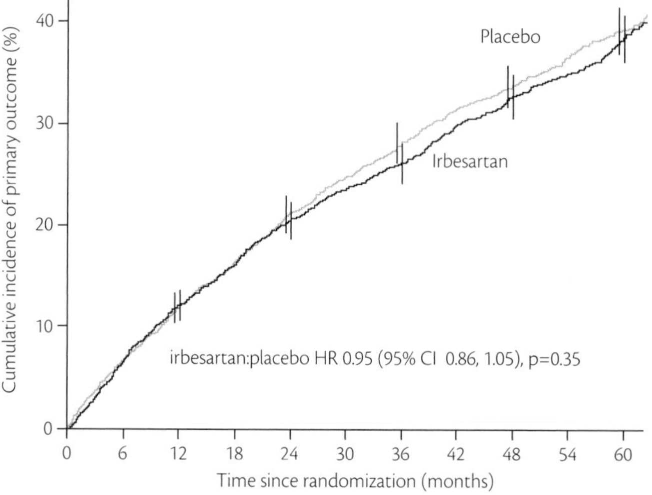

Fig. 40.10 I-Preserve:[20] Irbesartan had no effect on the endpoint of death or cardiovascular hospitalization in patients with heart failure and normal left ventricular ejection fraction.

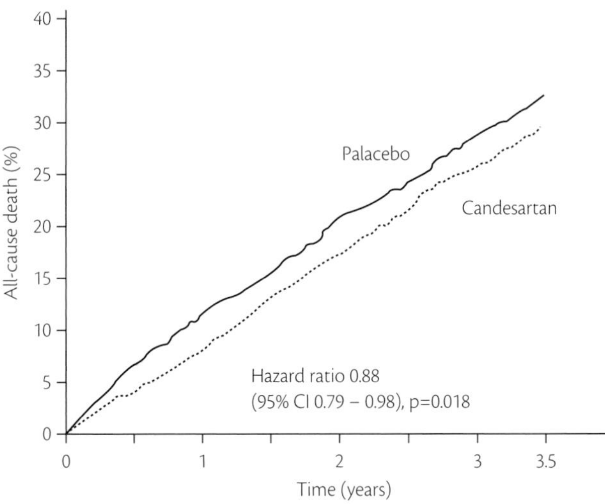

Fig. 40.11 CHARM-Low LVEF trials:[22] patients with heart failure and low left ventricular ejection fraction from CHARM-Alternative and CHARM-Added were pooled. Death from any cause was reduced by candesartan.

(and the blood pressure reduction in I-PRESERVE was about half that in CHARM-Preserved).[21] On the other hand, CHARM-Preserved enrolled a segment of patients with what might be called 'mild systolic dysfunction', i.e. those with a LVEF of 41–45% who might have had more to gain from RAS blockade. Whatever the correct perspective is, it is certain that ARBs are of unproven value in HeFPEF, unlike low-LVEF heart failure.

Other observations on ARBs in heart failure

A prespecified analysis of the CHARM-Programme that received less attention than it might have done was the planned pooling of the two low-LVEF trials (CHARM-Alternative and -Added).[22] This was done because, although neither had the statistical power to look at all-cause mortality individually, when combined there was sufficient power to look at this outcome. Among patients randomly assigned to candesartan, followed for a median of 40 months, 642/2289 (28.0%) died compared with 708/2287 (31.0%) in the placebo group, hazard ratio 0.88 (95% CI 0.79–0.98), p = 0.018 (Fig. 40.11).

It is interesting to compare this finding to the SOLVD-Treatment trial in which enalapril 20 mg daily given for a mean of 41.4 months reduced mortality (452/1285, 35.2%) compared with placebo (510/1284, 39.7%), relative risk reduction 16% (95% CI 5–26%), p = 0.0036. The approximate relative risk reduction with candesartan 12% (95% CI 2–21%) compares favourably with (and completely overlaps) that of enalapril, although, of course, 56% of patients in the CHARM low EF population were taking an ACE inhibitor (compared with 0% in the placebo group of SOLVD-T) and 55% were taking a β-blocker (compared with 8% in SOLVD-T).[16]

Table 40.2 Classification of guideline recommendations and level of evidence

Class	
I	Conditions for which there is evidence and/or general agreement that a given procedure/therapy is beneficial, useful, and/or effective
II	Conditions for which there is conflicting evidence and/or a divergence of opinion about the usefulness/efficacy of a procedure/therapy
II	Weight of evidence/opinion is in favour of usefulness/efficacy
IIb	Usefulness/efficacy is less well established by evidence/opinion
Level of evidence	
A	Data are derived from multiple randomized clinical trials or meta-analyses
B	Data are derived from a single randomized trial, or non-randomized studies
C	Only consensus opinion of experts, case studies, or standard of care

What do the guidelines advise?

The most current guidelines show some inconsistency in their recommendations about the role of ARBs in the treatment of low-LVEF HF (Table 40.2 and Table 40.3).[23–27] Although most guidelines give a level A recommendation for the use of ARBs in patients intolerant of an ACE inhibitor, this level of evidence requires data from 'multiple randomized trials or meta-analyses' (Table 40.2): multiple trials do not exist—unless the subset of Val-HeFT patients not treated with an ACE inhibitor at baseline is equated to a second trial, in addition to CHARM-Added.

There is more heterogeneity in the recommendations regarding use of ARBs in addition to an ACE inhibitor and the recommendation also varies between the summary and full guideline in certain cases (and has changed between the 2006 and 2009 American College of Cardiology/American Heart Association guideline). It is also not clear what outcome the recommendation refers to. The European Society of Cardiology (ESC) guideline is more precise in this respect, indicating that with both Val-HeFT and CHARM-Added showing a reduction in admissions for worsening heart

Table 40.3 Guideline recommendations for ARBs in low ejection fraction heart failure

	ESC (2008)		ACC/AHA (2009)		CCS (2006)		A/NZ (2006)		HFSA (2010)	
	Level	Class	Level	Class	Level	Class	Level	Class	Level	Class
ACE inhibitor intolerant	B	I	A	I	A	I	A	I	A	AI
ACE inhibitor treated	–	–	B	IIb	A	I	A	IIa	A	IIa
– to reduce mortality	B	IIa								
– to reduce HF hospitalization	A	I								

A/NZ, Cardiac Society of Australia & New Zealand; ACC/AHA, American College of Cardiology/American Heart Association; CCS, Canadian Cardiovascular Society; ESC, European Sociey of Cardiology; HFSA, Heart Failure Society of America.

Terms 'is recommended', 'should be considered' and 'may be considered' have been equated to classes I, IIa, and IIb respectively.

Box 40.1 Practical guidance on the use of ARBs in patients with heart failure due to LVSD

Why?

Added to standard therapy, including an angiotensin converting enzyme (ACE) inhibitor, in patients with all grades of symptomatic heart failure, the angiotensin receptor blockers (ARBs) valsartan and candesartan have been shown, in two major randomized trials (Val-HeFT and CHARM), to reduce HF hospital admissions, to improve NYHA class, and to maintain quality of life. The two CHARM low-left ventricular ejection fraction trials (CHARM-Alternative and CHARM-Added) also showed that candesartan reduced all-cause mortality. In patients previously intolerant of an ACE inhibitor, candesartan has been shown to reduce the risk of the composite outcome of cardiovascular death or HF hospitalization, to reduce the risk of HF hospital admission and to improve NYHA class. These findings in HF are supported by another randomized trial in patients with left ventricular systolic dysfunction, HF or both complicating acute myocardial infarction (VALIANT) in which valsartan was as effective as the ACE inhibitor captopril in reducing mortality and cardiovascular morbidity.

In whom and when?

Indications

- Potentially all patients with heart failure.
- First-line treatment (along with β-blockers) in patients with NYHA class II–IV HF intolerant of an ACE inhibitor.
- Second-line treatment (after optimization of ACE inhibitor and β-blocker[a]) in patients with NYHA class II–IV heart failure.

Contraindications

- Known bilateral renal artery stenosis.

Cautions/seek specialist advice

- Significant hyperkalaemia (K^+ >5.0 mmol/L).
- Significant renal dysfunction (creatinine 221 μmol/L or >2.5 mg/dL).
- Symptomatic or severe asymptomatic hypotension (systolic blood pressure <90 mmHg).

Drug interactions to look out for:

- K^+ supplements/K^+ sparing diuretics e.g. amiloride and triamterene (beware combination preparations with furosemide).
- Aldosterone antagonists (spironolactone, eplerenone), ACE inhibitors, NSAIDs[b].
- 'Low salt' substitutes with a high K^+ content.

Where?

- In the community for most patients.
- Exceptions—see Cautions/seek specialist advice.

Which ARB and what dose?

- Candesartan: starting dose 4 or 8 mg once daily, target dose 32 mg once daily.
- Valsartan: starting dose 40 mg twice daily, target dose 160 mg twice daily.

How to use?

- Start with a low dose (see above).
- Double dose at *not less than* 2 weekly intervals.
- Aim for target dose (see above) or, failing that, the highest tolerated dose.
- Remember *some* ARB is better than no ARB.
- Monitor blood pressure and blood chemistry (urea/blood urea nitrogen, creatinine, K^+).
- Check blood chemistry 1–2 weeks after initiation and 1–2 weeks after final dose titration.
- When to stop up-titration/reduce dose/stop treatment—see 'Problem solving'.
- A specialist HF nurse may assist with education of the patient, follow-up (in person or by telephone), biochemical monitoring and dose up-titration.

Advice to patient?

- Explain expected benefits (see 'Why?').
- Treatment is given to improve symptoms, prevent worsening of HF leading to hospital admission and to increase survival.
- Symptoms improve within a few weeks to a few months of starting treatment.
- Advise patients to principal adverse effect (i.e. report dizziness/ symptomatic hypotension)—see 'Problem Solving'.
- Advise patients to avoid NSAIDs[b] not prescribed by a physician (self purchased 'over the counter') and salt substitutes high in K^+—see 'Problem solving'.

Problem solving

Asymptomatic low blood pressure

- Does not usually require any change in therapy.

Symptomatic hypotension

- If dizziness, light-headedness or confusion and a low blood pressure reconsider need for nitrates, calcium channel blockers[c] and other vasodilators.
- if no signs/symptoms of congestion consider reducing diuretic dose.
- if these measures do not solve problem seek specialist advice.

Worsening renal function

- Some rise in urea (blood urea nitrogen), creatinine and potassium is to be expected after initiation of an ARB; if the increase is small and asymptomatic, no action is necessary.
- An increase in creatinine of up to 50% above baseline, or 266 µmol/L (3 mg/dL), whichever is the smaller, is acceptable.
- An increase in potassium to < 5.5 mmol/L is acceptable.
- If urea, creatinine or potassium does rise excessively consider stopping concomitant nephrotoxic drugs (eg NSAIDs[b]) and potassium supplements or retaining agents (triamterene, amiloride, spironolactone-eplerenone[a]) and, if no signs of congestion, reducing the dose of diuretic.
- If greater rises in creatinine or potassium than those outlined above persist despite adjustment of concomitant medications, the dose of the ARB should be halved and blood chemistry rechecked within 1–2 weeks; if there is still an unsatisfactory response specialist advice should be sought.
- If potassium rises to >5.5 mmol/L or creatinine increases by >100% or to above 310 µmol/L (3.5 mg/dL) the ARB should be stopped and specialist advice sought.
- Blood chemistry should be monitored frequently and serially until potassium and creatinine have plateaued.
- NB: it is very rarely necessary to stop an ARB and clinical deterioration is likely if treatment is withdrawn—ideally, specialist advice should be sought before treatment discontinuation.

[a] The safety and efficacy of an ARB used with an ACE inhibitor *and* spironolactone (as well as β-blocker) is uncertain and the use of all three inhibitors of the RAAS together is not recommended.
[b] Avoid nonsteroidal anti-inflammatory drugs (NSAIDs) unless essential.
[c] Calcium channel blockers should be discontinued unless absolutely essential (e.g. for angina or hypertension).
Adapted from 28. McMurray J, Cohen-Solal A, Dietz R, *et al.* Practical recommendations for the use of ACE inhibitors, beta-blockers, aldosterone antagonists and angiotensin receptor blockers in heart failure: putting guidelines into practice. *Eur J Heart Fail* 2005;**7**:710–21.

failure, the level of evidence of clinical benefit is greater than for reducing cardiovascular mortality: Val-HeFT did not show a mortality benefit but it was observed in CHARM-Added.

Practical guidance

The use of an ARB should follow the same principles as that of an ACE inhibitor and the starting doses, target doses, and approach to dose up-titration should be guided by the relevant clinical trials, as summarized in Box 40.1.[28]

Summary and conclusions

ARBs provide an alternative to ACE inhibitors in patients intolerant of the latter because of cough or angio-oedema. When added to an ACE inhibitor in patients with low ejection fraction HF, ARBs reduce hospital admission for worsening HF and candesartan has also been shown to reduce death from cardiovascular causes when used in this way. Use of both an ACE inhibitor and ARB together, however, necessitates careful biochemical surveillance for renal dysfunction and hyperkalaemia and is no longer the preferred next treatment-step after an ACE inhibitor and beta-blocker (an aldosterone antagonist is now preferred).

References

1. McMurray JJ, Pfeffer MA, Swedberg K, Dzau VJ. Which inhibitor of the renin-angiotensin system should be used in chronic heart failure and acute myocardial infarction? *Circulation* 2004;**110**:3281–8.
2. Pitt B, Poole-Wilson PA, Segal R, *et al.* Effect of losartan compared with captopril on mortality in patients with symptomatic heart failure: randomised trial—the Losartan Heart Failure Survival Study ELITE II. *Lancet* 2000;**355**:1582–7.
3. Pitt B, Segal R, Martinez FA, *et al.* Randomised trial of losartan versus captopril in patients over 65 with heart failure (Evaluation of Losartan in the Elderly Study, ELITE). *Lancet* 1997;**349**:747–52.
4. Dahlöf B, Devereux RB, Kjeldsen SE, *et al.*; LIFE Study Group. Cardiovascular morbidity and mortality in the Losartan Intervention For Endpoint reduction in hypertension study (LIFE):a randomised trial against atenolol. *Lancet* 2002;**359**:995–1003.
5. Brenner BM, Cooper ME, de Zeeuw D, *et al.*; RENAAL Study Investigators. Effects of losartan on renal and cardiovascular outcomes in patients with type 2 diabetes and nephropathy. *N Engl J Med* 2001;**345**:861–9.
6. Konstam MA, Neaton JD, Dickstein K, *et al.*; HEAAL Investigators. Effects of high-dose versus low-dose losartan on clinical outcomes in patients with heart failure (HEAAL study): a randomised, double-blind trial. *Lancet* 2009;**374**:1840–8.
7. Cohn JN, Tognoni G, Valsartan Heart Failure Trial Investigators. A randomised trial of the angiotensin-receptor blocker valsartan in chronic heart failure. *N Engl J Med* 2001;**345**:1667–75.
8. Maggioni AP, Anand I, Gottlieb SO, Latini R, Tognoni G, Cohn JN; Val-HeFT Investigators (Valsartan Heart Failure Trial). Effects of valsartan on morbidity and mortality in patients with heart failure not receiving angiotensin-converting enzyme inhibitors. *J Am Coll Cardiol* 2002;**40**:1414–21.
9. McMurray JJ, Ostergren J, Swedberg K, *et al.*; CHARM Investigators and Committees. Effects of candesartan in patients with chronic heart failure and reduced left-ventricular systolic function taking angiotensin-converting-enzyme inhibitors:the CHARM-Added trial. *Lancet* 2003;**362**:767–71.
10. McMurray JJ, Young JB, Dunlap ME, *et al.* CHARM Investigators. Relationship of dose of background angiotensin-converting enzyme inhibitor to the benefits of candesartan in the Candesartan in Heart failure:Assessment of Reduction in Mortality and morbidity (CHARM)-Added trial. *Am Heart J* 2006;**151**:985–91.
11. Pfeffer MA, McMurray JJ, Velazquez EJ, *et al.*; Valsartan in Acute Myocardial Infarction Trial Investigators. Valsartan, captopril, or

both in myocardial infarction complicated by heart failure, left ventricular dysfunction, or both. *N Engl J Med* 2003;**349**:1893–906.

12. ONTARGET Investigators, Yusuf S, Teo KK, Pogue J, *et al.* Telmisartan, ramipril, or both in patients at high risk for vascular events. *N Engl J Med* 2008;**358**:1547–59.
13. McKelvie RS, Yusuf S, Pericak D, *et al.* Comparison of candesartan, enalapril, and their combination in congestive heart failure: randomized evaluation of strategies for left ventricular dysfunction (RESOLVD) pilot study. The RESOLVD Pilot Study Investigators. *Circulation* 1999;**100**:1056–64.
14. Zannad F, McMurray JJ, Krum H, van Veldhuisen DJ, Swedberg K, Shi H, Vincent J, Pocock SJ, Pitt B; the Emphasis-HF Study Group. Eplerenone in Patients with Systolic Heart Failure and Mild Symptoms. *N Engl J Med. 2010* Nov 14. [Epub ahead of print] PubMed PMID: 21073363.
15. Pocock S, Wang D, Wilhelmsen L, Hennekens CH. The data monitoring experience in the Candesartan in Heart Failure Assessment of Reduction in Mortality and morbidity (CHARM) program. *Am Heart J* 2005;**149**:939–43.
16. Effect of enalapril on survival in patients with reduced left ventricular ejection fractions and congestive heart failure. The SOLVD Investigators. *N Engl J Med* 1991;**325**:293–302.
17. Granger CB, McMurray JJ, Yusuf S, *et al.*; CHARM Investigators and Committees. Effects of candesartan in patients with chronic heart failure and reduced left-ventricular systolic function intolerant to angiotensin-converting-enzyme inhibitors:the CHARM-Alternative trial. *Lancet* 2003;**362**:772–6.
18. Yusuf S, Pfeffer MA, Swedberg K, *et al.*; CHARM Investigators and Committees. Effects of candesartan in patients with chronic heart failure and preserved left-ventricular ejection fraction: the CHARM-Preserved Trial. *Lancet* 2003;**362**:777–81.
19. Lewis EJ, Hunsicker LG, Clarke WR, *et al.*; Collaborative Study Group. Renoprotective effect of the angiotensin-receptor antagonist irbesartan in patients with nephropathy due to type 2 diabetes. *N Engl J Med* 2001;**345**:851–60.
20. Massie BM, Carson PE, McMurray JJ, *et al.*; I-PRESERVE Investigators. Irbesartan in patients with heart failure and preserved ejection fraction. *N Engl J Med* 2008;**359**:2456–67.
21. Belz GG, Butzer R, Kober S, Mutschler E. Pharmacodynamic studies on the angiotensin II type 1 antagonists irbesartan and candesartan based on angiotensin II dose response in humans. *J Cardiovasc Pharmacol* 2002;**39**:561–8.
22. Young JB, Dunlap ME, Pfeffer MA, *et al.*; Candesartan in Heart failure Assessment of Reduction in Mortality and morbidity (CHARM) Investigators and Committees. Mortality and morbidity reduction with Candesartan in patients with chronic heart failure and left ventricular systolic dysfunction: results of the CHARM low-left ventricular ejection fraction trials. *Circulation* 2004;**110**:2618–26.
23. Arnold JM, Liu P, Demers C, *et al.*; Canadian Cardiovascular Society. Canadian Cardiovascular Society consensus conference recommendations on heart failure 2006:diagnosis and management. *Can J Cardiol* 2006;**22**:23–45.
24. Krum H, Jelinek MV, Stewart S, Sindone A, Atherton JJ, Hawkes AL; CHF Guidelines Core Writers. Guidelines for the prevention, detection and management of people with chronic heart failure in Australia, 2006. *Med J Aust* 2006;**185**:549–57.
25. Heart Failure Society Of America. Lindenfeld J, Albert NM, Boehmer JP, *et al.* HFSA 2010 Comprehensive Heart Failure Practice Guideline. *J Card Fail.* 2010;**16**:e1–194.
26. European Society of Cardiology; Heart Failure Association of the ESC (HFA); European Society of Intensive Care Medicine (ESICM), Dickstein K, Cohen-Solal A, Filippatos G, *et al.* ESC guidelines for the diagnosis and treatment of acute and chronic heart failure 2008: the Task Force for the diagnosis and treatment of acute and chronic heart failure 2008 of the European Society of Cardiology. Developed in collaboration with the Heart Failure Association of the ESC (HFA) and endorsed by the European Society of Intensive Care Medicine (ESICM). *Eur J Heart Fail* 2008;**10**:933–89.
27. Hunt SA, Abraham WT, Chin MH, *et al.*; American College of Cardiology Foundation; American Heart Association. 2009 Focused update incorporated into the ACC/AHA 2005 Guidelines for the Diagnosis and Management of Heart Failure in Adults A Report of the American College of Cardiology Foundation/American Heart Association Task Force on Practice Guidelines Developed in Collaboration With the International Society for Heart and Lung Transplantation. *J Am Coll Cardiol* 2009;**53**:e1–90.
28. McMurray J, Cohen-Solal A, Dietz R, *et al.* Practical recommendations for the use of ACE inhibitors, beta-blockers, aldosterone antagonists and angiotensin receptor blockers in heart failure: putting guidelines into practice. *Eur J Heart Fail* 2005;**7**:710–21.

41

Therapeutic control of fluid balance in chronic heart failure

Andrew L. Clark, Alison P. Coletta, and John G.F. Cleland

One of the cardinal clinical features of chronic HF (CHF) is fluid retention. Ankle swelling is one of the commonest presentations leading to the diagnosis of heart failure (HF), and oedema is the state that leads to the diagnosis of 'congestive' HF. Until the arrival of thiazide and loop diuretics, the management of fluid retention in HF was very limited. Tourniquets could be used to reduce preload, and Southey's tubes,[1] introduced by direct skin incision, were used to drain fluid. Venesection was a further option, and HF is perhaps one of the few instances where venesection proved helpful,[2] at least in the short term.

Digoxin provided some diuretic effect, particularly in those patients with atrial fibrillation and a rapid ventricular response, but the first specific diuretics available for use were the mercurials when mercury treatment for syphilis was noted to have a diuretic effect.[3,4] Thiazide diuretics became available in the late 1950s[5] and the loop diuretic furosemide in the 1960s,[6,7] revolutionizing the management of HF.

Diuretics

Data from the SOLVD registry showed that diuretics were the most commonly prescribed treatment[8] for HF, and the EuroHeart Failure Survey reported that 86.9% of patients with HF were prescribed diuretic therapy.[9] However, unlike the situation with angiotensin converting enzyme (ACE) inhibitors and β-blockers, whose clinical efficacy in HF has been clearly demonstrated in large randomized studies, there is relatively little clinical trial evidence to guide the use of diuretics in HF. Clinical experience and small-scale studies have shown that diuretics are effective in providing symptomatic relief of HF, but there are no data from large-scale clinical trials. A favourable effect on mortality has never been demonstrated in an individual clinical trial. For ethical reasons, it is now unlikely that there will be any large-scale, randomized, placebo-controlled studies to evaluate the effect of diuretic therapy on the prognosis of HF.

Guidelines suggest that diuretics are essential for the symptomatic treatment of HF in patients with fluid overload. However, it has been suggested that in the absence of fluid overload, the use of diuretics should be decreased where possible and in some cases treatment may be discontinued.[10]

Mechanism of action

Cardiac oedema is due to sodium and water retention, and is a major cause of hospitalization in patients with HF[11] due to progressive cardiac or renal dysfunction, excessive dietary intake, noncompliance with diuretics, or variable diuretic absorption.

The success of diuretic therapy depends on the ability of the diuretic drug to reduce sodium reabsorption in the kidney. In the normal kidney, more than 99% of filtered sodium is usually reabsorbed; 60–70% in the proximal tubule, 20–25% in the loop of Henle, 5–10% in the distal tubule, and 3% in the collecting duct.[12] In HF, low cardiac output, activation of the renin–angiotensin–aldosterone system (RAAS) and sympathetic stimulation can affect the pattern of renal absorption of sodium, causing sodium (and hence water) retention and thus oedema. To complicate matters, renal dysfunction is a common comorbidity in patients with HF[13] and as renal function deteriorates, so the response to diuretics falls.[14]

There are four classes of diuretic commonly used in the treatment of HF: (1) loop diuretics (furosemide, bumetanide, torasemide, and ethacrynic acid); (2) thiazides (including hydrochlorthiazide, bendrofluazide, and the thiazide-like metolazone); (3) directly acting potassium-sparing diuretics (amiloride and triamterene); and (4) aldosterone antagonists (spironolactone, canrenoate, and eplerenone). Each of these has a different site of action in the renal tubule as illustrated in Fig. 41.1. In addition, newer agents are becoming available that are not diuretics but help induce fluid loss, namely vasopressin antagonists and adenosine antagonists.

Loop diuretics

Loop diuretics are also called fast-acting, high ceiling, or high-potency diuretics and are the most widely used diuretics for HF. The principal site of action of loop diuretics is the thick ascending limb of the loop of Henle, where they inhibit the sodium, potassium, and

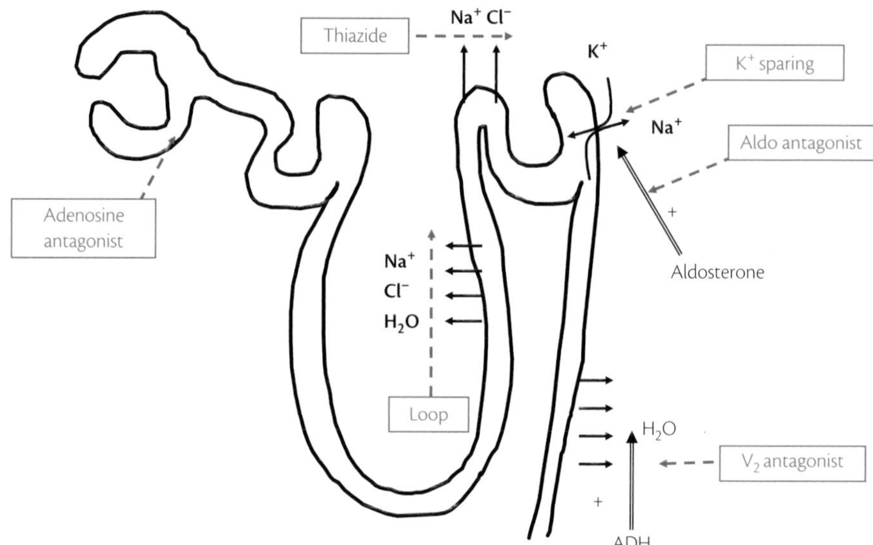

Fig. 41.1 Sites of action of different diuretics in the renal tubule.

chloride cotransporter. Since approximately 20–30% of filtered sodium is reabsorbed at the ascending loop of Henle, these are potent diuretics. The drugs work from the luminal surface and are reliant on renal function being sufficient to reach the lumen.

Loop diuretics have a rapid onset of action, and diuresis occurs within minutes following intravenous administration and within 30 min after oral administration.[15] However, loop diuretics have a short half-life so their duration of action is brief but intense. Loop diuretics may therefore need to be administered more than once a day in order to maintain the diuretic effect and to minimize rebound sodium reabsorption.

The newer loop diuretic torasemide has a longer half-life (3–4 h) than other loop diuretics and can therefore be administered less frequently. Unlike furosemide, which undergoes renal elimination, torasemide and bumetanide undergo substantial hepatic elimination and therefore should not accumulate in patients with renal insufficiency.[16]

The oral bioavailability of furosemide is extremely variable, with values between 12% and 112% reported.[17] In an open crossover study to compare the bioavailability of furosemide from five different commercially available preparations, the variability in absorption between patients was greater than any inter-product differences in bioavailability.[17] Absorption can be delayed by food,[18] and non-steroidal anti-inflammatory drugs (NSAIDs) blunt the response to loop diuretics.[19] Compared to furosemide, torasemide and bumetanide have a much higher and more predictable oral bioavailability.

Thiazide and thiazide-like diuretics

Thiazide diuretics act on the cortical diluting segment of the distal tubule, where they inhibit sodium and chloride reabsorption. The distal tubule reabsorbs only about 10–15% of filtered sodium and thus thiazides can only have a smaller diuretic effect than loop diuretics. The diuretic effect occurs within 1–2 h of oral administration, but thiazides have a longer duration of action (12–24 h) than loop diuretics so rebound sodium retention is less likely to occur. Although thiazide diuresis is less intense at peak effect, the long duration of action means that 24-h sodium excretion may be similar to that observed with standard doses of loop diuretics, so that hydrochlorothiazide 100 mg/day and furosemide 40 mg/day have a similar 24-h natriuretic effect. The prolonged diuresis makes thiazides more likely to cause hypokalaemia and nocturia than loop diuretics.[20,21]

Thiazide diuretics have reduced efficacy in renal impairment; in patients with a creatinine clearance less than 50 mL/min, the response to thiazides is poor and a loop diuretic is the treatment of choice.[16] Thiazides should not be used in patients with a GFR (glomerular filtration rate) of less than 30 mL/min, except in combination with a loop diuretic (see below).

Metolazone acts principally like a thiazide; however it also has a mild effect on the proximal tubule. Since 60–70% of filtered sodium is reabsorbed in the proximal tubule, metolazone may cause a considerable diuresis and is intermediate in potency between thiazide and loop diuretics. Unlike other thiazides, metolazone is effective in patients with moderate renal impairment.[22]

Potassium-sparing diuretics

Potassium-sparing diuretics produce only a mild diuresis. They inhibit the sodium:potassium exchange in the distal convoluted tubule, which is typically highly active in patients with HF because of the use of loop and thiazide diuretics. The potassium-sparing diuretics thus produce increased excretion of sodium with decreased loss of potassium. Potassium-sparing diuretics are rarely used as sole therapy, but are administered in combination with loop or thiazide diuretics to reduce potassium loss.[30,31] Potassium-sparing diuretics are more effective than potassium supplements in maintaining serum potassium and magnesium and total body potassium.[32]

Aldosterone antagonists

The aldosterone antagonists spironolactone and eplerenone have beneficial effects in the treatment of CHF beyond that of simple diuresis and are considered elsewhere (Chapter 40). They should be prescribed in preference to the other potassium-sparing diuretics.

Side effects

Side effects of both loop and thiazide diuretics are common. Both groups necessarily increase the delivery of sodium distally in the nephron, which causes increased potassium excretion as the activity of the sodium:potassium exchanger in the distal tubule is increased.

Hypokalaemia is more likely with thiazides.[23] Acute increases in lipid levels have also been reported with furosemide, and both groups can cause impaired glucose tolerance. Hyponatraemia is more common with thiazides than with loop diuretics.[24]

High-dose intravenous furosemide can cause deafness, particularly if it is administered rapidly. Gout is a common side effect, which can be difficult to treat in patients who should not receive NSAIDs.

Hyperkalaemia can be a problem with potassium-sparing diuretics, particularly in elderly people, which is potentially hazardous in patients taking concomitant ACE inhibitors.

Potentially the most important long-term side-effect of diuretics is activation of the RAAS and sympathetic nervous system (Fig. 41.2).[25–27] Neurohormonal activation is, of course, related to progression of left ventricular dysfunction and increased morbidity and mortality. If they are used in the absence of fluid overload, diuretics may reduce stroke volume and blood pressure, again resulting in neurohormonal activation.[28] To what extent neurohormonal activation is actually iatrogenic is difficult to be certain: although noradrenaline, renin, and aldosterone are, on average, substantially increased prior to diuretic therapy, they are not all activated in all patients.[29]

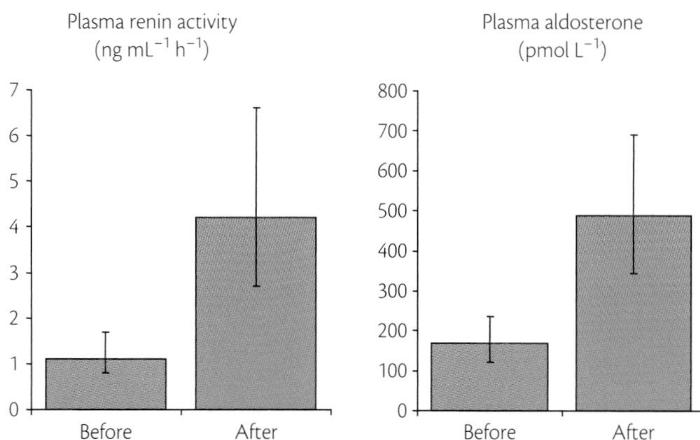

Fig. 41.2 The effect of diuretic therapy on neurohormonal activation in resting patients with CHF. Even more striking effects were seen after exertion.
Data taken from Bayliss J, Norell M, Canepa-Anson R, Sutton G, Poole-Wilson P. Untreated heart failure clinical and neuroendocrine effects of introducing diuretics. *Br Heart J* 1987:**57**:17–22.

Clinical trials of diuretic use

Placebo-controlled studies

The available randomized placebo-controlled studies evaluating diuretic therapy in HF are summarized in Table 41.1. Only small numbers of patients have been included, but the results show that diuretics are effective in reducing symptoms in HF patients.[33–38] A meta-analysis has suggested that conventional diuretics can reduce the risk of death and worsening HF compared with placebo.[39]

Diuretic withdrawal

Given the potential side effects of diuretics, one possible approach to long-term treatment is to consider withdrawing diuretic once any fluid retention has been treated. Studies of diuretic withdrawal are shown in Table 41.2.[40–48] A large (if variable) proportion of patients might be able to come off diuretics (or perhaps use them only on an 'as needed' basis), but at a cost of some increase risk of deterioration.[40] The largest single study (202 elderly patients in primary care) suggested that perhaps half of patients could successfully stop taking diuretic.[46] Elderly HF patients with normal left ventricular ejection fraction (LVEF) are particularly likely to tolerate diuretic withdrawal.[49]

Thiazide versus loop diuretic

Trials comparing thiazide with loop diuretics are all small (none has over 100 participants: see Table 41.3).[38,50–63] Both classes of drug are approximately equally effective in managing patients with HF, with a trend in favour of loop diuretics.[38,59,61] The risk of hypokalaemia is greater with thiazides,[38,54,55,57] but there is no

Table 41.1 Randomized placebo-controlled diuretic studies in heart failure

Author (year)	No of patients/ HF severity	Treatment	Duration	Outcome compared with placebo
Kourouklis (1976)	10	Bumetanide Furosemide Placebo	14 days XO	Both diuretics increased diuresis, and had similar effects on electrolytes
Sherman (1986)	38 NYHA II-III	Piretanide Placebo	28 days DB/PG	Improved NYHA class (p<0.05 compared to baseline), no increase in 24-h K excretion
Haerer (1990)	60 NYHA II-III	Piretanide Placebo	21 days SB	44 patients reported subjective improvement, decreased systolic and diastolic diameters on echo, decreased heart volume on CXR. Serum K unchanged
Kleber (1990)	247 mild HF	Hydrochlorothiazide Ibopamine HCZ plus IB Placebo	8 weeks DB/PG	Weight loss with all active treatments Hypokalaemia greater with HCZ
Patterson (1994)	66 NYHA II-III	Torasemide 5 mg Torasemide 10 mg Torasemide 20 mg Placebo	7 days DB/R/PG	Weight loss with 10-mg and 20-mg doses
Stewart (1965)	3	Furosemide Bendrofluazide Ethacrynic acid	2 days treatment XO for 32 days	Diuresis

CXR, chest radiograph; DB, double blind; HCZ, hydrochlorthiazide; HF, heart failure; IB, ibopamine; K, potassium; NYHA, New York Heart Association classification; PG, parallel group; SB, single blind; XO, crossover.

Table 41.2 Studies of withdrawal of diuretic therapy in heart failure

Author (year)	N	Treatment	Duration	Outcome
Taggart (1983)	42	Diuretic W/D in patients on moderate doses, with no HT, active HF, renal or hepatic oedema	12 weeks	71% completed the study. 29% deteriorated clinically or radiologically. 1 patient died
Richardson (1987)	14	All patients on diuretic at baseline, then W/D DB, rand, to captopril or furosemide plus amiloride, then XO	16 weeks	10 patients remained stable on captopril alone, 4 patients developed pulmonary oedema or breathlessness and required diuretic therapy
Magnani (1988)	94	Diuretic W/D if used and patients randomized to captopril or placebo	1 year	After 1 year, 25% of patients required diuretic in captopril group vs 36% in placebo group
Walma (1993)	15	Diuretic W/D	Pilot study 6 months	Reinstatement of diuretic therapy required in 9 patients
Grinstead (1994)	41	Diuretic W/D and substituted with either lisinopril or placebo	12 weeks	71% of patients required reinitiation of diuretic therapy. There was no difference between lisinopril and placebo
Walma (1997)	202	Patients on long-term diuretics rand DB to diuretic W/D or continuation	6 months	50 patients in the W/D group required diuretic compared with 13 patients in the continuation group
van Kraaj (2000)	32	Patients rand DB to continuation of furosemide therapy or placebo (diuretic W/D)	Pilot study 3 months	W/D successful in 90% of patients
Braunschweig (2002)	4	Haemodynamic study of diuretic W/D	Pilot study 2 weeks	Deterioration in ventricular pressure parameters with signs and symptoms of worsening HF following diuretic W/D
Galve (2005)	26	Diuretic W/D in stable HF patients	3 months	17 patients were able to tolerate W/D with improvements in renal function and glucose metabolism, but ANP increased

ANP, atrial natriuretic peptide; DB, double blind; rand, randomized; W/D, withdrawal.

conclusive evidence of a differential effect on glucose tolerance and diabetes between loop and thiazide diuretics.[58,64]

Thiazide diuretics are often preferred by patients as they cause less rapid diuresis and less frequent micturition than loop diuretics; this may also have an impact on patient compliance with therapy.[60]

Comparisons between loop diuretics

Comparisons between different loop diuretics are shown in Table 41.4a. Only studies with N over 100 are shown. Nonrandomized studies suggest that torasemide might reduce hospital days compared with furosemide,[65] and TORIC, an observational study in 2303 patients with chronic congestive HF, suggested that there might be a mortality benefit for torasemide compared with furosemide.[66]

Randomized studies comparing one loop diuretic with another in HF are listed in Table 41.4b.[67–71] Several smaller studies have failed to find large consistent differences between loop diuretics, but inasmuch as there is any trend, torasemide appears to be associated with better outcomes.

Loop diuretic versus ACE inhibitor

ACE inhibitors may have made diuretics redundant, at least when there is no overt fluid retention. Some studies of patients with HF uncontrolled with moderate diuretic therapy alone treated with either higher doses of diuretics or the introduction of ACE inhibitor therapy show that both treatments produce similar results,[72,73] but others have found that increasing diuretic dose gives a better symptomatic response.[74]

Diuretic resistance

As CHF progresses, patients often require higher doses of diuretic to achieve a given therapeutic effect, and commonly reach a state of diuretic resistance when the diuretic response is either diminished or lost before the therapeutic goal is reached. A number of mechanisms potentially contribute.

- Worsening renal perfusion: as HF progresses, venous pressure tends to rise and arterial pressure to fall, thus reducing the potential perfusion pressure across the glomerulus.
- Worsening renal function:[13] intrinsic renal dysfunction prevents diuretics from exerting their beneficial effect. Furosemide has to be secreted by the organic acid transporter in the proximal tubule to reach its site of action.
- Renal adaptation: chronic diuretic use results in increased delivery of sodium to the distal convoluted tubule (DCT), which hypertrophies in consequence.[75,76] The hypertrophied DCT is able to retain more sodium (and hence water) than in a diuretic-naive patient.
- Braking: with bolus diuretic dosing, there are times when there is no diuretic at the site of action. There can be rebound excessive sodium resorption from the DCT during such times.
- Decreased drug bioavailability: with increasing generalized oedema, there is increased bowel wall oedema, and potentially failure of drug absorption from the bowel lumen, particularly with furosemide.[77,78]
- Drug interactions: NSAIDs, including aspirin, can interfere with the renal response to diuretic.[79]

Approaches to managing diuretic resistance include changing the route of delivery of diuretic and the use of combination therapy—so-called 'sequential nephron blockade'.

Route of administration

Parenteral administration of diuretic overcomes the problems of variation in bioavailability. Several small studies have suggested that

Table 41.3 Randomized studies of loop versus thiazide diuretics in heart failure

Author (date)	Number of patients/HF severity	Diuretics used	Design and duration	Outcome
Stewart (1965)	11	Furosemide Ethacrynic acid Bendrofluazide Mersalyl		Furosemide had greater natriuretic effect than bendrofluazide. More K loss on bendrofluazide
Peltola (1970)	8	Furosemide HCZ	XO Single dose	Both treatments produced similar diuresis. Na and aldosterone excretion greater with HCZ
Levy (1977)	32 NYHA II–III	HCZ + spironolactone Furosemide	DB 16 weeks	Both treatments produced similar control of HF symptoms. Increased plasma renin activity and aldosterone excretion with HCZ
Coodley (1979)	30	Diapamide Furosemide	O/XO 4 days	Urine output greater with furosemide (p value not stated)
Levy (1979)	32 NYHA II–III	HCZ + spironolactone HCZ + triamterene Furosemide	Open 16 weeks	No clinical benefit of combinations over furosemide. Changes in BUN, plasma renin and aldosterone excretion were greater with HCZ
Gillies (1980)	?	Piretanide Chlorothiazide	3 days	Similar diuresis and weight loss. Greater K loss with thiazide
Gabriel (1981)	18	Bendrofluazide Bumetanide Furosemide	XO 9 months	Patients remained stable with no significant changes in body weight. Bendrofluazide had greater effect on plasma K
Pothuizen (1982)	23 NYHA II–III	Furosemide SR HCZ	R/DB 6 weeks	Both treatments produced similar improvement in functional class, less nocturia with furosemide, small reduction in K in both groups
Vermeulen (1982)	38 NYHA I-III	Furosemide HCZ	DB/R 6 weeks	Similar improvement in functional class. More hypokalaemia with HCZ
Pehrsson (1985)	86 NYHA II–III	Furosemide SR Bendroflumethiazide	R/DB 12 weeks	Similar clinical response with both treatments
Gonska (1985)	30 NYHA II–III	Piretanide HCZ + triamterene	O/R 14 days	More patients fully recompensated, and LVEDD and LVESD less on piretanide. Piretanide caused small fall in serum K
Funke-Kupper (1986)	37 NYHA II–III	HCZ + triamterene Furosemide + triamterene	R/XO 16 weeks	Equivalence on maintenance of body weight and symptoms, but patient preference for HCZ due to less acute diuresis
Crawford (1988)	47 General practice	Furosemide + amiloride Cyclopenthiazide + KCl	Open 3 months	Furosemide superior on patient symptom assessment
Heseltine (1988)	70 NYHA II	Furosemide Thiazide	Obs	Postural hypotension and hypokalaemia with thiazide
Allman (1990)	71 mild HF	Furosemide + amiloride Cyclopenthiazide + K^+	O/R 12 weeks	Similar improvement in oedema, crepitations, orthopnoea, and self-assessed dyspnoea of effort

DB, double blind; HCZ, hydrochlorothiazide; HF, heart failure; O, open; Obs, observational study; R, randomized; SR, slow release; XO, crossover.

continuous furosemide or bumetanide infusion may avoid braking,[80–85] and continuous dosing may reduce the potential ototoxic effects of large boluses of furosemide.[80] Continuous bumetanide infusion may be associated with a high rate of side effects.[86] There is very little evidence to favour continuous infusion of torasemide,[87] and given its high oral bioavailability, it is unlikely that there is much difference between oral and intravenous torasemide.

Combination therapy

That combination diuretic therapy might be helpful in diuretic resistance has been known since the early days of effective diuretic therapy (Fig. 41.3).[38] The enhanced sodium resorbtion arising from hypertrophy of the cells in the DCT after prolonged use of loop diuretics can be blocked with the addition of a thiazide—sequential nephron blockade. The combination can cause a profound diuresis. Many small observational studies[88,89] and two randomized trials[90,91] have reported the synergistic effects of combining loop diuretics with thiazides or thiazide-like diuretics in HF (Table 41.5 and Fig. 41.4). Most studies of combination therapy have used metolazone, which by virtue of its additional action on the proximal tubule is possibly more potent than other thiazides. However, Channer *et al.*[91] showed that metolazone and bendrofluazide were equally effective in inducing diuresis in patients with resistant oedema when added to intravenous furosemide. Combination of loop and potassium-sparing diuretics seems to be of limited benefit, probably because potassium-sparing diuretics act on the collecting duct where the potential for limiting sodium reabsorption is small.

There are few data comparing the relative efficacy of different thiazides in combination therapy, but there is no reason to believe that one is better than another. Sequential nephron blockade is effective in patients with diuretic resistance, even when the patient has significant renal impairment.[89]

Table 41.4 Studies comparing one loop diuretic with another in HF

Author (date)	N	Diuretics used	Design and duration	Outcomes
Nonrandomized studies				
Cosin (TORIC) (2002)	1377	Torasemide Furosemide or other diuretics	Open, nonrandomized, post marketing. 1 year	Morbidity & mortality benefit for torasemide
Spannheimer (1998)	400	Torasemide Furosemide	Observational pharmaco-economic study 1 year	80% reduction in hospital days on torasemide
Randomized studies				
Stauch (1990)	104	Torasemide 5 or 10 mg Furosemide 40 mg	4 weeks db/mc/rand	All treatments were effective in reducing body weight and improving NYHA class and cardiac symptoms
Noe (PEACH) (1999)	240	Torasemide Furosemide	6 months rand/open/mc	Similar efficacy and treatment costs
Stroupe (2000)	193	Torasemide Furosemide	1 year rand/open	Fewer hospital admissions with torasemide
Murray (2001)	234	Torasemide Furosemide	1 year rand/open	Fewer cardiovascular readmissions and less fatigue with torasemide
Muller (2003)	237	Torasemide Furosemide	9 months open/rand	Trend to greater clinical improvement and QoL benefit with torasemide

db, double blind; KCl(sr), slow release potassium chloride; mc, multicentre; pg, parallel group; QoL, quality of life; rand, randomized; xo, crossover.

However, combination therapy should be monitored closely as unpredictably large diuretic effects may occur, leading to unwanted effects such as electrolyte disturbances, hypotension, dehydration, and renal dysfunction. It may take several days before the effect of combination therapy reaches a maximum.

Other therapies

There is some emerging evidence that steroid therapy might be helpful in patients with diuretic resistance,[92,93] perhaps by up-regulating responses to natriuretic hormones.[94]

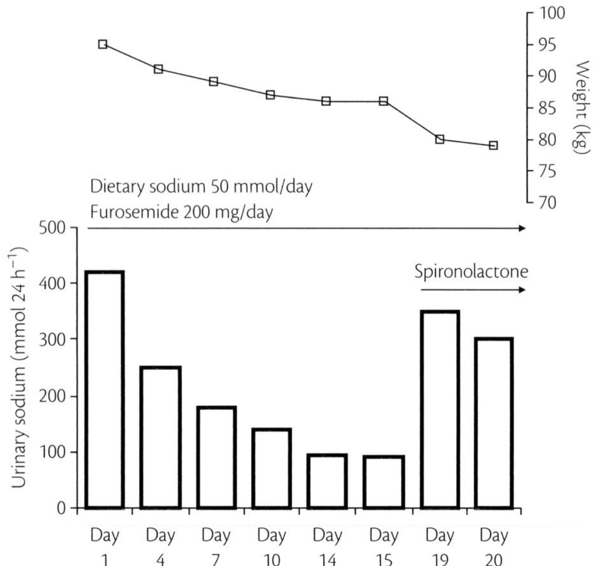

Fig. 41.3 Effect of adding spironolactone to furosemide on daily urinary sodium levels.

Adapted from Stewart JH, Edwards KDG. Clinical comparison of frusemide with bendrofluazide, mersalyl and ethacrynic acid. *Br Med J* 1965;**2**:1277–81.

Aquaretics

Antidiuretic hormone (ADH), also known as arginine vasopressin (AVP), is raised in many patients with CHF,[95,96] although not all studies have found raised values to be universal.[29] The primary physiological role of AVP is to modulate body water content to maintain plasma osmolality constant. AVP is released from the posterior pituitary in response to a fall in osmolality or a fall in blood pressure. Its effects are mediated through two main receptor subtypes, V_1 and V_2. V_1 receptors are predominantly vascular and mediate vasoconstriction. V_2 receptors are found in the collecting ducts of nephrons. Stimulation of the V_2 receptors results in the translocation of preformed and stored aquaporin molecules from the interior of collecting duct cells to the apical membrane of the cells where they allow water molecules to leave the urine along an osmotic gradient back to the circulation. There are many human aquaporins: aquaporin-2 is the one involved in renal osmoregulation.

AVP antagonists have two potential beneficial effects. V_1 antagonists cause vasodilation, and V_2 antagonists cause an 'aquaresis': that is, unlike diuretics which cause simultaneous loss of sodium and water, aquaretics cause loss of water only by increasing free water clearance. There are currently three AVP antagonists being evaluated for use in HF; of these conivaptan is a dual V_1 and V_2 antagonist, whereas tolvaptan and lixivaptan are selective for the V_2 receptor.

In normal subjects, conivaptan causes an increase in urine flow with fall in urine osmolality.[97] In HF patients,[98] intravenous conivaptan caused a fall in right atrial and pulmonary capillary wedge pressures together with substantial increases in urine output without causing hyponatraemia or worsening the serum creatinine. Tolvaptan also increases free water clearance, increases urine flow, and causes acute weight loss in patients with CHF.[99,100] Lixivaptan is also in development and causes similar effect.[101] Excessive thirst is a very common side effect of all the AVP antagonists.

Table 41.5 Randomized controlled trials of addition of thiazide to loop diuretic in heart failure patients with diuretic resistance

Author (date)	Number of patients	Diuretics used	Design and duration	Outcome
Sigurd (1975)	18	Bumetanide Add: bendroflumethiazide	Single dose, R/XO	Increased diuresis on addition of thiazide Hypokalaemia
Channer (1994)	33 NYHA III/IV	Furosemide (IV) Add bendrofluazide or metolazone	R/C 3 days or indefinite	Diuresis on addition of thiazide, which continued after withdrawal

C, controlled; NYHA, New York Heart Association class; R, randomized; XO, crossover.

The role of the routine use of AVP antagonists is not yet clear. In the major trial of AVP antagonists to date, EVEREST,[102,103] 4133 patients admitted with HF were randomized to receive tolvaptan or placebo in addition to standard therapy. Tolvaptan had no effect on total mortality or HF hospitalization, but did lead to an improvement in breathlessness and weight loss in the first day and weight loss at 1 week. The ADVANCE study, testing the effects of conivaptan on exercise capacity,[104] is yet to report.

A particular role for AVP antagonists will be in the management of patients with hyponatraemia. Low serum sodium is common in end-stage HF and is associated with a very bleak outlook. In EVEREST, patients with hyponatraemia had a significant increase in serum sodium.[102] In a more general population of patients, tolvaptan, at least, causes a marked increase in serum sodium in patients with hyponatraemia during 30 days of administration (Fig. 41.5).[105] There were associated small improvements in mental function.

Whether the beneficial effects of AVP antagonists on serum sodium persist in the longer term is not known. Further trials will be needed to establish their role in managing fluid balance.

Adenosine antagonists

Within individual nephrons, the distal tubule lies very close to the vascular pole of the glomerulus. At this point, metabolically active cells in the distal tubule, the macula densa, act as detectors of the nephron's GFR. When the sodium load in the distal tubule is increased, as in patients with HF treated with diuretics, the macula densa cells 'interpret' the rise as being due to an increased GFR. The response is to reduce GFR by inducing constriction of the afferent arteriole of the glomerulus. This homeostatic mechanism is known as tubuloglomerular feedback.

The precise mediators of tubuloglomerular feedback are not known, but involve adenosine, perhaps being formed from the cleavage of ATP. Adenosine released by the macula densa causes afferent arteriolar constriction through binding to A_1 receptors in the mesangium.

A fall in GFR is particularly associated with a poor outlook in CHF,[106] and adenosine antagonists may potentially improve renal function by increasing GFR, and perhaps enhance the diuresis induced by standard diuretics. Gottlieb and colleagues showed that a single dose of the adenosine antagonist BG9719 increased both urine output and GFR.[107] By contrast, furosemide produced an increase in urine output but decreased GFR. When BG9719 and furosemide were administered together, there was a further increase in urine volume with no reduction in GFR, suggesting that the adenosine antagonist may protect against the adverse effects of loop diuretics.

In a combined analysis of two studies of patients hospitalized with fluid overload, KW-3902 showed diuretic properties and appeared to enhance response to loop diuretics compared to placebo.[108] A pilot study of KW-3902,[109] now named rolofylline, confirmed the findings of an apparent protective effect against decline in renal function, However, in the PROTECT study, in 2033 patients with heart failure and renal impairment, rolofylline showed no beneficial effect. Its use is associated with a risk of seizures.[110]

Ultrafiltration

Although the physical removal of oedema fluid can be achieved by venesection or Southey's tubes, another approach is to use ultrafiltration. In dialysis, blood is run against another fluid, dialysate, separated by a semipermeable membrane. Solutes pass along a concentration gradient, and the fluid compartment of blood is removed by ultrafiltration, that is, by the hydrostatic pressure of the blood relative to the dialysate.

For treating patients with HF and fluid retention, only the ultrafiltration is needed: fluid is removed from blood by pressure gradient alone. As fluid passes across the membrane, some solutes (including sodium, potassium, and some larger molecules) are 'dragged' along simultaneously. In practice, blood is removed, usually via a large bore tube, pumped through a filter where filtrate is removed, and 'concentrated' blood is returned to the patient (Fig. 41.6). The flow rate can be adjusted to remove fluid at the required rate: depending upon the equipment, large volumes (at least 1 L h^{-1}) can be removed rapidly.

That filtration or dialysis might work for patients with CHF predates the availability of loop diuretics,[111] and even peritoneal dialysis can work.[112,113] The recent advances in understanding of ultrafiltration have been driven by the availability of veno-venous ultrafiltration systems which avoid the more invasive alternatives. Ultrafiltration removing around 5 L in 24 h can restore central

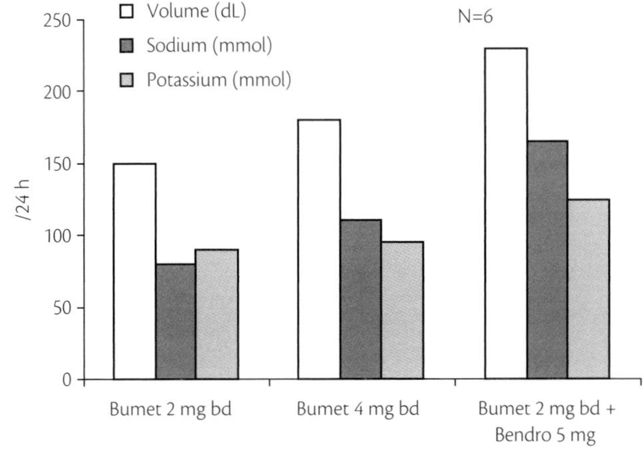

Fig. 41.4 Effect of adding a thiazide (bendrofluazide) to a low-dose loop diuretic (bumetanide) compared with increasing the dose of loop diuretic, on urine volume and sodium and potassium excretion, measured in six patients over 24 h.[90]

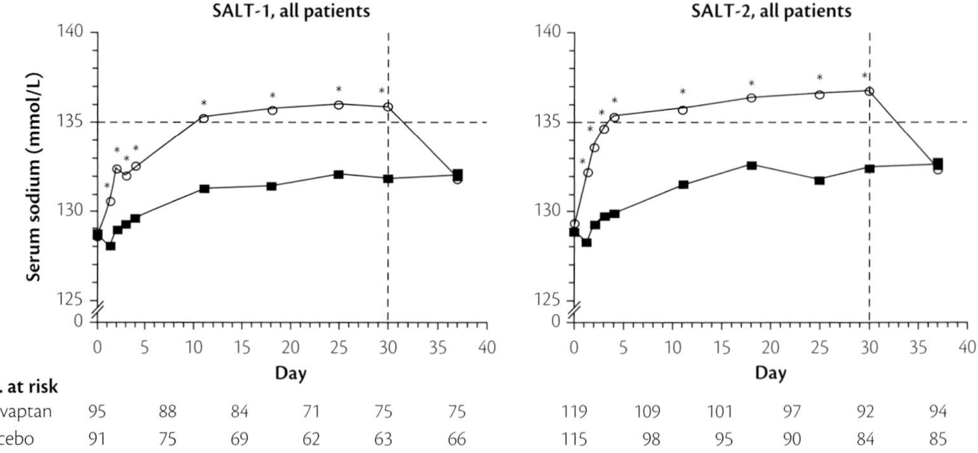

Fig. 41.5 Effect of tolvaptan given for 30 days in two studies of patients presenting with fluid retention and hyponatraemia due to a variety of causes. Approximately one-third had HF. Open circles, patients treated with tolvaptan; closed circles, patients treated with placebo.
From Schrier RW, Gross P, Gheorghiade M, *et al.*, for the SALT Investigators. Tolvaptan, a selective oral vasopressin V2-receptor antagonist, for hyponatremia. *N Eng J Med* 2006;**355**:2099–112, with permission.

haemodynamics towards normal rapidly with reduction in filling pressures and an increase in cardiac output,[114] and even more rapid removal of over 3 L in 8 h is safe and effective.[115]

Ultrafiltration used even before intravenous diuretics have been tried can be successful.[116] Such an approach may allow early discharge from hospital of patients admitted with severe fluid retention, and intermittent outpatient use[117] may maintain selected patients in a euvolaemic state and prevent recurrent admissions even in those with refractory fluid retention. Another important possible benefit is that ultrafiltration can lead to an increase in serum sodium in those with hyponatraemia.[116] Ultrafiltration is effective in patients refractory to diuretics and can initiate a diuresis (Fig. 41.7).[118]

There is some evidence that ultrafiltration can have potentially beneficial neurohormonal effects, such as the reduction of BNP[118] as well as interleukins and tumour necrosis factor.[119]

In the largest trial of ultrafiltration in CHF to date, 200 patients admitted to hospital with fluid overload due to HF were randomized to receive ultrafiltration or standard intravenous diuretic therapy.[120] Weight and fluid loss was slightly greater in the ultrafiltration group. Although it was not a primary endpoint in the study, HF-related hospitalization at 90 days was reduced.

The role of ultrafiltration in the standard management of HF is not yet clear. There is no definitive evidence that it is better than standard diuretic management, although it appears to have some beneficial effects in patients refractory to treatment. It is at least possible that well-designed studies may show advantages for ultrafiltration, if only in the rate of removal of fluid made possible with the consequent reduction in length of hospital stay.

Practical approach to managing fluid balance

Day-to-day management

Most patients with clinical HF will need diuretic therapy during the course of their illness. At presentation, the majority have symptoms at least partly attributable to fluid retention and will need diuretic treatment. The standard approach is to use a loop diuretic, usually furosemide (although an argument could be made that bumetanide is the better choice) at a dose of 40–80 mg/day. At the

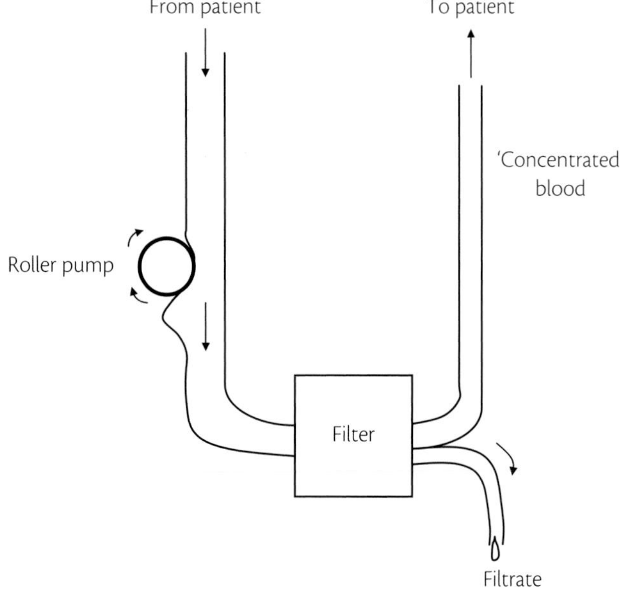

Fig. 41.6 Basic ultrafiltration circuit.

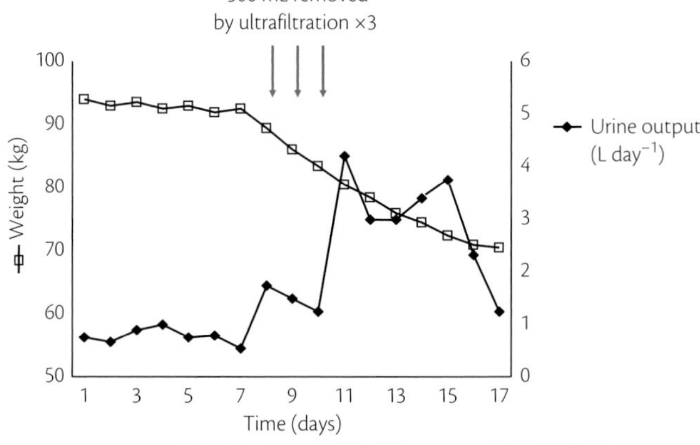

Fig. 41.7 Effect of ultrafiltration in restoring urine flow. The patient was a 57-year-old woman with underlying ischaemic heart disease (ejection fraction 18%) and intractable fluid retention. Three episodes of ultrafiltration to remove 500 mL of fluid on each occasion were sufficient to restore urine flow. Before filtration, the patient had been receiving 20 mg/h furosemide, bendrofluazide, spironolactone, and digoxin for 1 week and dopamine and dobutamine for 72 h.

same time, depending on the clinical scenario, ACE inhibitor therapy will also be started.

Once the patient has reached clinical euvolaemia—in other words, when the jugular venous pressure has returned to normal and any ankle oedema has resolved—the diuretic is often simply continued without further consideration.

A better way is to involve patients in actively managing their own fluid retention. Patients should be taught to weight themselves regularly (preferably with the same scales at the same time of day), preferably in kilograms, and taught (or reminded) that 1 kg is the mass of 1 L of water. Patients should learn that diuretics have a different purpose from the rest of their medication: whereas β-blockers, ACE inhibitors, and aldosterone antagonists are disease-modifying agents, diuretics are for the relief of symptoms due to fluid retention.

Patients are then in a position to modify their diuretic management. In general, the lowest dose of diuretic needed to control symptoms should be used, and for many patients, this may mean complete withdrawal from diuretic therapy. For others, it may mean that diuretic need only be taken every few days if weight increases 2–3 kg. Even in more severely affected cases with greater reliance on diuretic, it is important that the patient understands that missing a dose of diuretic is perfectly reasonable when the diuresis might be inappropriate (e.g. before a long car or coach trip). Similarly, education should include what to do if visiting a hot country (reduce diuretic dose as there will be increased fluid loss due to sweating) or how to manage an episode of diarrhoea.

Many elderly patients find that a very brisk diuresis is very difficult to manage, and may benefit from a trial of thiazide rather than loop therapy as the diuresis, although longer lived, is more gentle. Similarly, torasemide may have a less dramatic effect.

Any patient on long-term diuretic therapy should have their renal function assessed on a regular basis. The finding that renal function is impaired is almost 'normal' for patients with CHF and should not be seen as an indication for reducing therapy unless the deterioration is large or rapid.

If the patient is still not well controlled with 80 mg furosemide or 2 mg bumetanide, then rather than increasing the dose of loop diuretic still further, starting combination therapy with a thiazide, such as bendroflumethiazide (bendrofluazide) 2.5 mg once daily may be more effective. Some patients may need even more diuretic, with bumetanide 2 mg twice a day or its equivalent being common. With this level of diuretic use, monthly checks of renal function should be made. Patients should be told not to take their second dose later than mid-afternoon to avoid interrupting sleep.

Anasarca

During the course of their illness, many patients with CHF need admission to hospital with fluid retention. As fluid retention worsens to cause abdominal wall oedema, ascites, and pleural effusions, the condition is known as anasarca (see Chapters 2 and 27). It is often managed very conservatively, with resulting prolonged patient stays in hospital.

The patient should be confined to bed with the legs raised. Appropriate antithrombotic prophylaxis is important as patients with anasarca are at particularly high risk of thromboembolic complications. Intravenous diuretics should be used, especially if furosemide is the agent used, with an intravenous infusion circumventing the problem of braking. Strict monitoring of fluid balance is vital: unless fluid balance is known, it is very difficult to track progress. Fluid intake and urine output must be measured accurately and charted, together with daily weights. The daily weight should be measured at the same time of day with the same scales with the patient wearing similar clothing.

Urea and electrolytes should be measured daily with careful replacement of potassium as necessary. Fluid restriction to 1.5 L in 24 h is probably helpful without being draconian. Salt restriction is usually not necessary and is very unpalatable.

Which (if any) medication should be stopped if a patient is admitted with anasarca remains controversial. Unnecessary medication should certainly be stopped, as should agents likely to worsen renal function, particularly NSAIDs (including aspirin). Standard advice is to stop β-blocker therapy when patients are admitted, but there is some provisional evidence that those patients who continue with β-blockers once they are admitted have a better outcome.[121]

The aim should be to get the patient to lose around 2 kg each day (equivalent to around 2 L of fluid loss) until achieving dry weight. Assessment by an experienced clinician is probably adequate to determine fluid status.[122] Careful daily assessment is vital. If the patient is not making the expected progress, then treatment needs to be modified. If the patient is not losing weight, then increasing loop diuretic therapy (to 20 mg/h of furosemide) and adding a thiazide and spironolactone are next steps. If this is insufficient, then consideration should be given to ultrafiltration.

As the patient is reaching dry weight, ACE inhibitor and β-blocker should be started. As a rule of thumb, the patient will need to be discharged on more diuretic than they were taking before admission: education for the patient on the effects of diuretics and how to manipulate them is of great importance to avoid rapid readmission.

References

1. Southey R. Chronic parenchymatous nephritis of right kidney. Left kidney small, atrophied. Old scrofulous pyelitis. *Trans Clin Soc London* 1877;**10**:152–6.
2. Krishnakumar N, Harikrishnan S, Tharakan JM. Self-blood letting in congestive cardiac failure. *Int J Cardiol* 2007;**114**:135–6.
3. Vogl A. The discovery of the organic mercurial diuretics. *Am Heart J* 1950;**39**:881–3.
4. Ventura HO, Mehra MR,Young JB. Treatment of heart failure according to William Stokes: the enchanted mercury. *J Card Fail* 2001;**7**:277–82.
5. Novello FC, Sprague JM. Benzothiadiazine dioxides as novel diuretics. *J Am Chem Soc* 1957;**79**:2028.
6. Robson AO, Kerr DN, Ashcroft R, Teasdale G. The diuretic response to frusemide. *Lancet* 1964;**2**:1085–8.
7. Verel D, Stentiford NH, Rahman F, Saynor R. A clinical trial of frusemide. *Lancet* 1964;**ii**:1088–9.
8. Young JB, Weiner DH, Yusuf S, *et al.* Patterns of medication use in patients with heart failure: a report from the Registry of studies of left ventricular dysfunction (SOLVD) *South Med J* 1995;**88**:514–23.
9. Komajda M, Follath F, Swedberg K *et al.* Study Group on Diagnosis of the Working Group on Heart Failure of the European Society of Cardiology. The EuroHeart Failure Survey programme—a survey on the quality of care among patients with heart failure in Europe. Part 2: treatment. *Eur Heart J* 2003;**24**:464–74.
10. van Veldhuisen DJ, van Gilst WH. The pharmacological management of heart failure: too many treatments? *Eur J Heart Fail* 2003;**5**:5–8.
11. Bennett SJ, Huster GA, Baker SL, *et al.* Characterisation of the precipitants of hospitalisation for heart failure decompensation. *Am J Crit Care* 1998;**7**:168–74.

12. Dormans TPJ, Gerlag PGG, Russel FGM, Smits P. Combination diuretic therapy in severe congestive heart failure. *Drugs* 1998;**2**:165–172.
13. de Silva R, Nikitin NP, Witte KKA, *et al.* Incidence of renal dysfunction over 6 months in patients with chronic heart failure due to left ventricular systolic dysfunction: contributing factors and relationship to prognosis. *Eur Heart J* 2006:**27**:569–581.
14. Maxwell AP, Ong HY, Nicholls DP. Influence of progressive renal dysfunction in chronic heart failure. *Eur J Heart Fail* 2002;**4**:125–130.
15. Brater DC. Pharmacology of diuretics. *Am J Med Sci* 2000;**319**:38–50.
16. Brater DC. Drug therapy: diuretic therapy. *N Eng J Med* 1998;**339**:387–97.
17. Murray MD, Haag KM, Black PK, Hall SD, Brater DC. Variable furosemide absorption and poor predictability of response in elderly patients. *Pharmacother* 1997;**17**:98–106.
18. McCrindle JL, Li Kam Wa TC, Barron W, Prescott LF. Effect of food on the absorption of frusemide and bumetanide in man. *Br J Clin Pharmacol* 1996;**42**:743–746.
19. Kramer BK, Schweda F, Reigger GAJ. Diuretic treatment and diuretic resistance in heart failure. *Am J Med* 1999;**106**:90–96.
20. Pothuizen LM, Chada DR. Treatment of congestive cardiac failure in elderly patients: randomised study of hydrochlorothiazide and slow release furosemide. *Curr Ther Res* 1982;**32**:513–19.
21. Vermeulen A, Chada DR. Slow-release furosemide and hydrochlorothiazide in congestive cardiac failure: A controlled trial. *J Clin Pharmacol* 1982;**22**:513–19.
22. Dargie HJ, Allison MEM, Kennedy AC, Gray MHJ. High dose metolazone in chronic renal failure. *Br Med J* 1972;**4**:196.
23. Robertson JIS. Diuretics, potassium depletion and the risk of arrhythmias. *Eur Heart J* 1984;**5**(Suppl A):25–8.
24. Spital A. Diuretic induced hyponatremia. *Am J Nephrol* 1999;**19**:447–52.
25. Francis GS, Siegel RM, Goldsmith SR, Olivari MT, Levine TB, Cohn JN. Acute vasoconstrictor response to intravenous furosemide in patients with chronic congestive heart failure. *Ann Int Med* 1985;**103**:1–6.
26. Ikram H, Chan W, Espiner EA, Nicholls MG. Haemodynamic and hormone responses to acute and chronic frusemide therapy in congestive heart failure. *Clin Sci* 1980;**59**:443–449.
27. Bayliss J, Norell M, Canepa-Anson R, Sutton G, Poole-Wilson P. Untreated heart failure clinical and neuroendocrine effects of introducing diuretics. *Br Heart J* 1987:**57**:17–22.
28. Anand IS, Florea VG. Diuretics in chronic heart failure- benefits and hazards. *Eur Heart J* 2001;**3**(suppl):G8–18.
29. Anand IS, Ferrari R, Kalra GS, Wahi PL, Poole-Wilson PA, Harris PC. Edema of cardiac origin. Studies of body water and sodium, renal function, hemodynamic indexes, and plasma hormones in untreated congestive cardiac failure. *Circulation* 1989;**80**:299–305.
30. Ghosh AK, Mankikar G, Strouthidis T, Windsor A, Long C, Glover DR. A single-blind, comparative study of hydrochlorothiazide/amiloride (Moduret 25) and hydrochlorothiazide/triamterene (Dyazide) in elderly patients with congestive heart failure. *Curr Med Res Opin* 1987;**10**:573–9.
31. Townsend HA, Waddy AL, Eason CT, Richards HH. Frusemide/amiloride combination in heart failure: an open mulit-centre study in general practice. *Curr Med Res Opin* 1984;**9**:132–40.
32. Kohvakka A. Maintenance of potassium balance during long-term diuretic therapy in chronic heart failure patients with thiazide induced hypokalemia. *Int J Clin Pharmacol Ther Toxicol* 1988;**26**:273–7.
33. Kourouklis CC, Christensen O, Augoustakis D. Bumetanide in congestive heart failure. *Curr Med Res Opinion* 1976;**4**:422–431.
34. Sherman LG, Liang CS, Baumgardner S, Charuzi Y, Chardo F, Kim CS. Piretanide a potent diuretic with potassium sparing properties, for the treatment of congestive heart failure. *Clin Pharmacol Ther* 1986;**40**:587–94.
35. Haerer W, Bauer U, Sultan N, *et al.* Acute and chronic effects of a diuretic monotherapy with piretanide in congestive heart failure A placebo controlled trial. *Cardiovasc Drug Ther* 1990;**4**:515–22.
36. Kleber FX, Thyroff-Freisinger U. Treatment of mild chronic congestive heart failure with ibopamine, hydrochlorthiazide, ibopamine plus hydrochlorthiazide or placebo. *Cardiology* 1990;**77**:67–74.
37. Patterson JH, Kirkwood FA, Applefield MM, Corder CN, Masse BR for the Torasemide Investigators group. Oral torasemide in patients with chronic congestive heart failure: effects on body weight, edema and electrolyte excretion. *Pharmacotherapy* 1994;**14**:514–21.
38. Stewart JH, Edwards KDG. Clinical comparison of frusemide with bendrofluazide, mersalyl and ethacrynic acid. *Br Med J* 1965;**2**:1277–81.
39. Faris R, Flather M, Purcell H, Henein M, Poole Wilson P, Coats A. Current evidence supporting the role of diuretics in heart failure; a meta analysis of randomised controlled trials. *Int J Cardiol* 2002;**82**:149–58.
40. Taggart AJ, McDevitt DG. Diuretic withdrawal a need for caution. *Curr Med Res Opin* 1983;**8**:501–8.
41. Richardson A, Bayliss J, Scriven AJ, Parameshwar J, Poole-Wilson PA, Sutton GC. Double-blind comparison of captopril alone against frusemide plus amiloride in mild heart failure. *Lancet* 1987;**ii**:709–11.
42. Magnani B. Converting enzyme inhibition and heart failure. *Am J Med* 1988;**84**:87–91.
43. Grinstead WC, Francis MJ, Marks GF, Tawa CB, Zoghbi WA, Young JB. Discontinuation of chronic diuretic therapy in stable congestive heart failure secondary to coronary artery disease or to idiopathic dilated cardiomyopathy. *Am J Cardiol* 1994;**73**:881–6.
44. Braunschweig F, Linde C, Eriksson MJ, Hofman-Bang C, Ryden L Continuous haemodynamic monitoring during withdrawal of diuretics in patients with congestive heart failure. *Eur Heart J* 2002;**23**:59–69.
45. Walma EP, Hoes AW, Prins A, Boukes FS, van der Does E. Withdrawing long-term diuretic therapy in the elderly: a study in general practice in The Netherlands. *Fam Med* 1993;**25**:661–4.
46. Walma EP Hoes AW, van Dooren C, Prins A, van der Does E. Withdrawal of long term diuretic medication in elderly patients: a double-blind randomised trial. *BMJ* 1997;**315**:464–8.
47. Galve E, Mallol A, Catalan R, Palet J, *et al.* Clinical and neurohormonal consequences of diuretic withdrawal in patients with chronic stabilised heart failure and systolic dysfunction. *Eur J Heart Fail* 2005;**7**:892–8.
48. Van Kraaij DJW, Jansen RWMM, Gribnau FWJ, Hoefnagels WHL. Diuretic therapy in elderly heart failure patients with and without left ventricular systolic dysfunction. *Drugs Aging* 2000;**16**:289–300.
49. Van Kraaij DJW, Jansen RWMM, Bouwels LHR, Gribnau FWJ, Hoefnagels WHL. Furosemide withdrawal in elderly patients with preserved left ventricular systolic function. *Am J Cardiol* 2000;**85**:1461–6.
50. Peltola P, Lahovaara S, Paasonen MK Effect of furosemide and hydrochlorothiazide on plasma renin activity in man. *Ann Med Exp Fenn* 1970;**48**:122–124.
51. Levy B. The efficacy and safety of furosemide and a combination of spironalactone and hydrochlorothiazide in congestive heart failure. *J Clin Pharmacol* 197;**17**:420–30.
52. Coodley EL, Nandi PS, Chiotellis P. Evaluation of a new diuretic diapamide in congestive heart failure. *J Clin Pharmacol* 1979;**19**:127–36.
53. Levy B. Fixed-dose combination diuretics in congestive heart failure: an evaluation. *J Clin Pharmacol* 1979;**19**:743–6.
54. Gillies A, Morgan T, Myers J. Comparison of piretanide and chlorothiazide in the treatment of cardiac failure. *Med J Aust* 1980;**1**:170–2.

55. Gabriel R, Baylor P. Comparison of the chronic effects of bendrofluazide, bumetanide and frusemide on plasma biochemical variables. *Postgrad Med J* 1981;**57**:71–4.
56. Pothuizen LM, Chada DR. Treatment of congestive cardiac failure in elderly patients: randomised study of hydrochlorothiazide and slow release furosemide. *Curr Ther Res* 1982;**32**:513–19.
57. Vermeulen A, Chada DR. Slow-release furosemide and hydrochlorothiazide in congestive cardiac failure: A controlled trial. *J Clin Pharmacol* 1982;**22**:513–19.
58. Pehrsson SK. Multicentre comparison between slow release furosemide and bendroflumethiazide in congestive heart failure. *Eur J Clin Pharmacol* 1985;**28**:235–9.
59. Gonska BD, Kreuzer H. Diuretic monotherapy in heart failure. Comparison of piretanide and hydrochlorothiazide-triamterene. *Dtsch Med Ewochenschr* 1985;**110**:1812–16.
60. Funke Kupper AJ, Fitelman H, Huige MC, Koolen JJ, Liem KL, Lustermans FA. Cross-over comparison of the fixed combination of hydrochlorothiazide and triamterene and the free combination of furosemide and triamterene in the maintenance treatment of congestive heart failure. *Eur J Clin Pharmacol* 1986;**30**:341–3.
61. Crawford RJ, Allman S, Gibson W, Kitchen S, Richards HH. A comparative study of frusemide-amiloride and cyclopenthiazide-potassium chloride in the treatment of congestive cardiac failure in general practice. *Int J Med Res* 1988;**16**:143–149.
62. Heseltine D, Bramble MG. Loop diuretics cause less postural hypotension than thiazide diuretics in the frail elderly. *Curr Med Res Opin* 1988;**11**:232–5.
63. Allman S, Norris RJ. An open parallel group study comparing frusemide/amiloride diuretic and a diuretic containing cyclopenthiazide with sustained release potassium in the treatment of congestive cardiac failure-a multicentre general practice study. *Int J Med Res* 1990;**18**:17–23B.
64. Suter PM, Vetter W. Metabolic effects of antihypertensive drugs. *J Hypertens Suppl* 1995;**13**:S11–17.
65. Spannheimer A, Goertz A, Dreckmann-Behrendt B. Comparison of therapies with torasemide or furosemide in patients with congestive heart failure from a pharmacoeconomic viewpoint. *Int J Clin Pract* 1998;**52**:467–71.
66. Cosin J, Diez J, on behalf of the TORIC investigators. Torasemide in chronic heart failure: results of the TORIC study. *Eur J Heart Fail* 2002;**4**:507–13.
67. Stauch M, Stiehl L. Controlled double blind clinical trial on the efficacy and tolerance of torasemide in comparison with furosemide in patients with congestive heart failure a multicentre study. *Prog Pharmacol Clin Pharmacol* 1990;**8**:121–6.
68. Noe LL, Vreeland MG, Pezzella SM, Trotter JP. A pharmacoeconomic assessment of torsemide and furosemide in the treatment of patients with congestive heart failure. *Clin Ther* 1999;**21**:854–66.
69. Stroupe KT, Forthofer MM, Brater DC, Murray MD. Healthcare costs of patients with heart failure treated with torasemide or furosemide. *Pharmacoeconomics* 2000;**17**:429–40.
70. Murray MD, Deer MM, Ferguson JA, *et al.* Open label randomised trial of torasemide compared with furosemide therapy for patients with heart failure. *Am J Med* 2001;**111**:513–19.
71. Muller K, Gamba G, Jaquet F, Hess B. Torasemide vs furosemide in primary care patients with chronic heart failure NYHA II to IV—efficacy and quality of life. *Eur J Heart Fail* 2003;**5**:793–801.
72. Boccanelli A, Zachara E, Liberatore SM, Carboni GP, Prati PL. Addition of captopril versus increasing diuretics in moderate but deteriorating heart failure: a double-blind comparative trial. *Postgrad Med J* 1986;**62**:184–7.
73. Lewis SJ, Roberts CJC. Double-blind comparison of high-dose bumetanide and half-dose bumetanide together with captopril in heart failure. *Curr Ther Res* 1991;**50**(Suppl A):3–13.
74. Cowley AJ, Stainer K, Wynne RD, Rowley JM, Hampton JR. Symptomatic assessment of patients with heart failure; double-blind comparison of increasing doses of diuretics and captopril in moderate heart failure. *Lancet* 1986;**2**:770–2.
75. Kaissling B, Stanton BA. Adaptation of distal tubule and collecting duct to increased sodium delivery: I Ultrastructure. *Am J Physiol* 1988;**255**:F1256–75.
76. Stanton BA, Kaissling B. Adaptation of distal tubule and collecting duct to increased Na delivery II. Na and K transport. *Am J Physiol* 1988;**255**:1269–75.
77. Brater DC, Day B, Burdette A, Anderson S. Bumetanide and furosemide in heart failure. *Kidney Int* 1984;**26**:183–189.
78. Vasko MR, Cartwright DB, Knochel JP. Furosemide absorption altered in decompensated congestive heart failure. *Ann Intern Med* 1985;**102**:314–18.
79. Bartoli E, Arras S, Faedda R, Soggia G, Satta A, Olmeo NA. Blunting of furosemide diuresis by aspirin in man. *J Clin Pharmacol* 1980;**20**:452–8.
80. Van Meyel JJ, Smits P, Dormans T, Gerlag PG, Russel FG, Gribnau FW. Continuous infusion of furosemide in the treatment of patients with congestive heart failure and diuretic resistance. *J Intern Med* 1994;**235**:329–34.
81. Dormans TPJ, Meyel JJM, Gerlag PGG, Tan Y, Russel FGM, Smits P. Diuretic efficacy of high dose furosemide in severe heart failure: bolus versus continuous infusion. *J Am Coll Cardiol* 1996;**28**:376–82.
82. Lahav M, Regev A, Ra'anani P, Theodor E. Intermittent administration of furosemide vs continuous infusion preceded by a loading dose for congestive heart failure. *Chest* 1992;**102**:725–31.
83. Pivac N, Rumboldt Z, Sardelic S, Bagatin J, Polic S, Ljutic D, *et al.* Diuretic effects of furosemide infusion versus bolus injection in congestive heart failure. *Int J Clin Pharmacol Research* 1998;**18**:121–8.
84. Paterna S, Di Pasquale P, Parrinello G, *et al.* Effects of high dose furosemide and small volume hypertonic saline solution infusion in comparison with a high dose of furosemide as a bolus, in refractory congestive heart failure. *Eur J Heart Fail* 2000;**2**:305–13.
85. Rudy DW, Voelker JR, Greene PK, Esparza FA, Brater DC. Loop diuretics for renal insufficiency: a continuous infusion is more efficacious than bolus therapy. *Ann Intern Med* 1991;**115**:360–6.
86. Howard PA, Dunn MI. Severe musculoskeletal symptoms during continuous infusion of bumetanide. *Chest* 1997;**111**:359–64.
87. Kramer WG, Smith WB, Ferguson J, *et al.* Pharmacodynamics of torsemide administered as an intravenous injection and as a continuous infusion to patients with congestive heart failure. *J Clin Pharmacol* 1996;**36**:265–70.
88. Kiyingi A, Field MJ, Pawsey CC, Yiannikas J, Lawrence JR, Arter WJ. Metolazone in treatment of severe refractory congestive cardiac failure. *Lancet* 1990;**335**:29–31.
89. Dormans TPJ, Gerlag PGG. Combination of high-dose furosemide and hydrochlorothiazide in the treatment of refractory congestive heart failure. *Eur Heart J* 1996;**17**:1867–74.
90. Sigured B, Olesen KH, Wennevold A. The supra-additive natriuretic effect of addition of bendroflumethiazide and bumetanide in congestive heart failure. *Am Heart J* 1975;**89**:163–70.
91. Channer KS, McLean KA, Lawson-Matthew P, Richardson M. Combination diuretic treatment in severe heart failure: a randomised controlled trial. *Br Heart J* 1994;**71**:146–50.
92. Liu C, Liu G, Zhou C, Ji Z, Zhen Y, Liu K. Potent diuretic effects of prednisone in heart failure patients with refractory diuretic resistance. *Can J Cardiol* 2007;**23**:865–8.
93. Zhang H, Liu C, Ji Z, *et al.* Prednisone adding to usual care treatment for refractory decompensated congestive heart failure. *Int Heart J* 2008;**49**:587–95.
94. Lanier-Smith KL, Currie MG. Effect of glucocorticoids on the binding of atrial natriuretic peptide to endothelial cells. *Eur J Pharmacol* 1990;**178**:105–9.

95. Szatalowicz VL, Arnold PE, Chaimovitz C, Bichet D, Berl T, Schrier RW. Radioimmunoassay of plasma arginine vasopressin in hyponatremic patients with congestive heart failure. *New Engl J Med* 1981;**305**:263–6.
96. Francis GS, Benedict C, Johnstone DE, *et al.* Comparison of neuroendocrine activation in patients with left ventricular dysfunction with and without congestive heart failure: a substudy of the Studies of Left Ventricular Dysfunction (SOLVD). *Circulation* 1990;**82**:1724–9.
97. Burnier M, Fricker AF, Hayoz D, *et al.* Pharmacokinetic and pharmacodynamic effects of YM087, a combined V1/V2 vasopressin receptor antagonist in normal subjects. *Eur J Clin Pharmacol* 1999;**55**:633–7.
98. Udelson JE, Smith WB, Hendrix GH, *et al.* Acute hemodynamic effects of conivaptan, a dual V1a and V2 vasopressin receptor antagonist, in patients with advanced heart failure. *Circulation* 2001;**104**:2417–23.
99. Gheoghiade M, Niazi I, Ouyang J *et al.* Vasopressin V2-receptor blockade with tolvaptan in patients with chronic heart failure. *Circulation* 2003;**107**:2690–6.
100. Gheorghiade M, Gattis WA, O'Conner C, *et al.* Effects of tolvaptan vasopressin antagonist, in patients hospitalized with worsening heart failure. *JAMA* 2004;**291**:1963–71.
101. Abraham WT, Shamshirsaz AA, McFann K, Oren RM, Schrier RW. Aquaretic effect of lixivaptan an oral non-peptide selective V2 receptor vasopressin antagonist in New York Heart Association functional class iI and III chronic heart failure. *J Am Coll Cardiol* 2006;**47**:1615–21.
102. Konstam MA, Gheorghiade M, Burnett JC Jr, *et al.*; Efficacy of Vasopressin Antagonism in Heart Failure Outcome Study With Tolvaptan (EVEREST) Investigators. Effects of oral tolvaptan in patients hospitalized for worsening heart failure: the EVEREST Outcome Trial. *JAMA* 2007;**297**:1319–31.
103. Gheorghiade M, Konstam MA, Burnett JC Jr, *et al.*; Efficacy of Vasopressin Antagonism in Heart Failure Outcome Study With Tolvaptan (EVEREST) Investigators. Short-term clinical effects of tolvaptan, an oral vasopressin antagonist, in patients hospitalized for heart failure: the EVEREST Clinical Status Trials. *JAMA* 2007;**297**:1332–43.
104. Russell SD, Selaru P, Pyne DA, *et al.* Rationale for use of an exercise end point and design for the ADVANCE (A Dose evaluation of a Vasopressin ANtagonist in CHF patients undergoing Exercise) trial. *Am Heart J* 2003;**145**:179–86.
105. Schrier RW, Gross P, Gheorghiade M, *et al.*, for the SALT Investigators. Tolvaptan, a selective oral vasopressin V2-receptor antagonist, for hyponatremia. *N Eng J Med* 2006;**355**:2099–112.
106. Hillege HL, Girbes ARJ, de Kam PJ, *et al.* Renal function neurohormonal activation and survival in patients with chronic heart failure. *Circulation* 2000;**102**:203–210.
107. Gottleib SS, Brater C, Thomas I, Havranek E, Bourge R, Goldman S, *et al.* BG9719 (CVT-124) an adenosine receptor antagonist protects against the decline in renal function observed with diuretic therapy. *Circulation* 2002;**105**:1348–53.
108. Givertz MM, Massie BM, Fields TK, Pearson LL, Dittrich HC; CKI-201 and CKI-202 Investigators. The effects of KW-3902, an adenosine A1-receptor antagonist,on diuresis and renal function in patients with acute decompensated heart failure and renal impairment or diuretic resistance. *J Am Coll Cardiol* 2007;**50**:1551–60.
109. Cotter G, Dittrich HC, Weatherley BD, *et al.*; Protect Steering Committee, Investigators, and Coordinators. The PROTECT pilot study: a randomized, placebo-controlled, dose-finding study of the adenosine A1 receptor antagonist rolofylline in patients with acute heart failure and renal impairment. *J Card Fail* 2008;**14**:631–40.
110. Massie BM, O'Connor CM, Metra M, *et al.* PROTECT Investigators and Committees. Rolofylline, an adenosine A1-receptor antagonist, in acute heart failure. *N Engl J Med* 2010;**363**:1419–28.
111. Kolff WJ, Leonards JR. Reduction of otherwise intractable edema by dialysis or filtration. *Cleveland Clin Q* 1954;**21**:61–71.
112. Mailloux LU, *et al.* Peritoneal dialysis for refractory congestive heart failure. *J Am Med Assoc* 1967;**199**:873–8.
113. Cairns KB, Porter GA, Kloster FE, Bristow JD, Griswold HE. Clinical and hemodynamic results of peritoneal dialysis for severe cardiac failure. *Am Heart J* 1968;**76**:227–34.
114. Marenzi G, Lauri G, Grazi M, Assanelli E, Campodonico J, Agostoni P. Circulatory response to fluid overload removal by extracorporeal ultrafiltration in refractory congestive heart failure. *J Am Coll Cardiol* 2001;**38**:963–8.
115. Bart BA, Boyle A, Bank AJ, *et al.* Ultrafiltration versus usual care for hospitalized patients with heart failure: the Relief for Acutely Fluid-Overloaded Patients With Decompensated Congestive Heart Failure (RAPID-CHF) trial. *J Am Coll Cardiol* 2005;**46**:2043–6.
116. Costanzo MR, Saltzberg M, O'Sullivan J, Sobotka P. Early ultrafiltration in patients with decompensated heart failure and diuretic resistance. *J Am Coll Cardiol* 2005;**46**:2047–51.
117. Sheppard R, Panyon J, Pohwani AL, *et al.* Intermittent outpatient ultrafiltration for the treatment of severe refractory congestive heart failure. *J Card Fail* 2004;**10**:380–3.
118. Libetta C, Sepe V, Zucchi M, *et al.* Intermittent haemodiafiltration in refractory congestive heart failure: BNP and balance of inflammatory cytokines. *Nephrol Dial Transplant* 2007;**22**:2013–19.
119. Bellomo R, Tipping P, Boyce N. Continuous veno-venous hemofiltration with dialysis removes cytokines from the circulation of septic patients. *Crit Care Med* 1993;**21**:522–6.
120. Costanzo MR, Guglin ME, Saltzberg MT, *et al.*; UNLOAD Trial Investigators. Ultrafiltration versus intravenous diuretics for patients hospitalized for acute decompensated heart failure. *J Am Coll Cardiol* 2007;**49**:675–83 (Erratum in: *J Am Coll Cardiol* 2007;**49**:1136).
121. Cleland JG, Coletta AP, Torabi A, Clark AL. Clinical trials update from the European Society of Cardiology heart failure meeting 2009: CHANCE, B-Convinced, CHAT, CIBIS-ELD, and Signal-HF. *Eur J Heart Fail* 2009;**11**:802–5.
122. Anand IS, Veall N, Kalra GS, *et al.* Treatment of heart failure with diuretics: body compartments, renal function and plasma hormones. *Eur Heart J* 1989;**10**:445–50.

42

Digoxin

Andrew J.S. Coats

Introduction

Digoxin is the oldest drug in use in cardiovascular medicine. William Withering (Fig. 42.1), a physician working in Birmingham in the second half of the 18th century, first described in the scientific literature the use of extracts of the foxglove plant (*Digitalis purpurea*), [1] which he said had been used as a cure for dropsy, now recognized as including a description of a disease of peripheral oedema probably caused by heart failure (HF) in many cases. Foxglove extract includes digitalis alkaloids and thus digoxin, a pure alkaloid, which has a consecutive use going back nearly a quarter of a millennium. That it is still in regular use and that it remains one of the most debated and argued about of all cardiovascular drugs says a lot about the changes in our processes for evaluating and accepting therapeutic advances in cardiovascular medicine over the last half century.

As we enter a discussion of the risks and benefits of using digoxin and consider the correct dosing and indications, it is salutary to read what Withering himself said:

> After being frequently urged to write upon this subject, and as often declining to do it, from apprehension of my own inability, I am at length compelled to take up the pen, however unqualified I may still feel myself for the task. The use of the Foxglove is getting abroad, and it is better the world should derive some instruction, however imperfect, from my experience, than that the lives of men should be hazarded by its unguarded exhibition, or that a medicine of so much efficacy should be condemned and rejected as dangerous and unmanageable. It is now about 10 years since I first began to use this medicine. Experience and cautious attention gradually taught me how to use it. For the last two years I have not had occasion to alter the modes of management; but I am still far from thinking them perfect. It would have been an easy task to have given select cases, whose successful treatment would have spoken strongly in favour of the medicine, and perhaps been flattering to my own reputation. But Truth and Science would have condemned the procedure. I have therefore mentioned every case in which I have prescribed the Foxglove, proper or improper, successful or otherwise. . . .
>
> I seldom prescribed it, but when the failure of every other method compelled me to do it; so that upon the whole, the instances I am going to adduce, may truly be considered as cases lost to the common run of practice, and only snatched from destruction, by the efficacy of the Digitalis; and in this so remarkable a manner, that, if the properties of that plant had not been discovered, by far the greatest part of these patients must have died.

It was thus a comprehensive case series with an imputed historical control as there was no effective therapy at the time. Withering reported all 156 cases he had seen in his private practice where he had used Digitalis, and seven whom he had treated at the Birmingham Hospital.[2] It was thus one of the largest case series of his, or previous, times ever reported.

With the development of powerful diuretics after the 1950s, the unique role of digoxin in the treatment of HF ended; it remained an adjunct to diuretic therapy, and although some questioned whether it was still necessary, the consensus remained in favour of its use. The long-established use of digoxin goes some way to explain why there are so few controlled clinical trials evaluating its use. In modern practice we expect several randomized controlled trials (RCTs) attesting to the value of a new drug, prior to its adoption. The previous detailed case series with historical or contemporaneous but nonrandomized controlled groups are no longer seen as adequate. As we have seen, however, digoxin went through this phase 200 years ago and it was already in established practice, so that new RCTs were not conducted.

Prior to the important trials of the 1990s (especially the DIG trial) the only modern trial design for digoxin was a withdrawal trial in which patients who were already receiving digoxin were randomly taken off the drug and then either continued or not in a double-blind manner. Although this may seem to fulfil the requirement of a modern RCT, there are some inherent biases. Several groups of patients are not included in such trials, and by their exclusion one can never say the true value of starting digoxin to a group of digoxin-naive patients. The excluded groups include those who cannot tolerate digoxin (and hence were never continued on it in the first place) and those who died because they were commenced on it. Another potential bias is that there may be particular risks in ceasing digoxin once it has been started even if no benefit was seen with

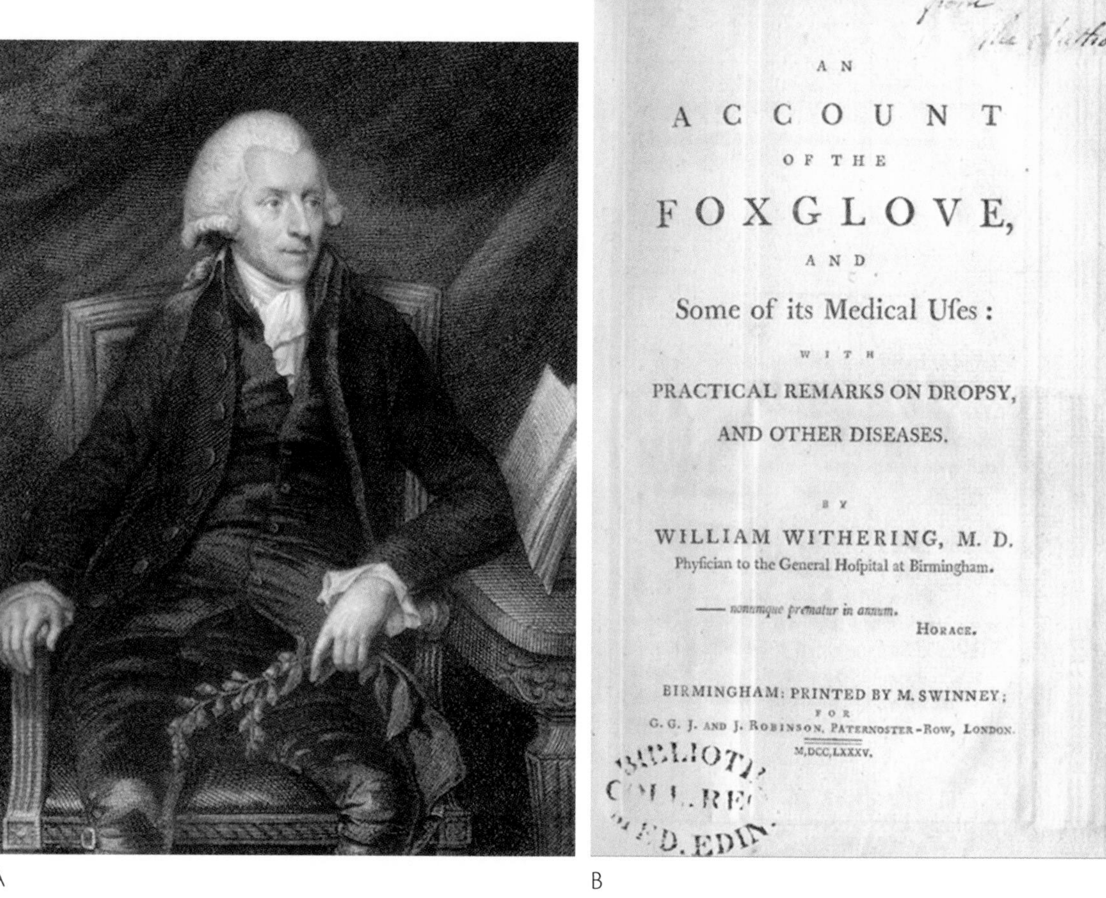

AN

ACCOUNT

OF THE

FOXGLOVE,

AND

Some of its Medical Ufes:

WITH

PRACTICAL REMARKS ON DROPSY,
AND OTHER DISEASES.

BY

WILLIAM WITHERING, M. D.
Phyfician to the General Hofpital at Birmingham.

—— *nonumque prematur in annum.*
HORACE.

BIRMINGHAM: PRINTED BY M. SWINNEY;
FOR
G. G. J. AND J. ROBINSON, PATERNOSTER-ROW, LONDON.
M,DCC,LXXXV.

Fig. 42.1 (A) Dr William Withering (1741–1799) (B) Title page of the first scientific description of the use of digitalis alkaloids in the treatment of heart disease.
Source: http://www.jameslindlibrary.org/trial_records/17th_18th_Century/withering/withering_portrait.html

commencement; such might be the case with rapid withdrawal of a β-blocker even for a patient who never needed it in the first place.

An important but more subtle concern is that it is possible that digoxin permanently damages the patient but acutely covers the damage with short-term benefit; when digoxin is stopped, the damage is thereby uncovered. There is no evidence for this last effect, but it cannot be excluded. Thus, although it might be that there is a greater deterioration in a group randomized to go from digoxin therapy to placebo than in a group continued on digoxin, such a finding is certainly not proof that digoxin is beneficial. With this warning in mind there is, however, a degree of consensus from a number of relatively small withdrawal trials that stopping digoxin in HF patients already stabilized on this therapy is probably ill advised, as it appears, in the short term at least, to be harmful so to do.

Therapeutic uses of digoxin

Withering listed a range of conditions for which digitalis had been suggested as offering an effective cure, including those as diverse as epilepsy, episodic asthma, hydrocephalus, and insanity, but only two uses survive today: the treatment of atrial fibrillation (AF) or flutter and the treatment of HF, regardless of rhythm. Although other drugs and electrophysiological methods exist to convert AF and even to stabilize an excessively fast ventricular response in AF, digoxin retains a role in the treatment of established AF with a fast ventricular response. As this rhythm is common in patients with chronic HF (CHF) (afflicting one-third or more of all patients) many CHF patients will be prescribed digoxin because of their coincident AF. Its role in CHF with sinus rhythm is the more controversial and it is this that will form the bulk of the following discussion.

Mechanism of action

Digoxin has two major cardiovascular effects useful in clinical practice. It has a positive inotropic effect, shown as a shift in the Frank–Starling curve upwards and to the left. Thus, for a given preload, the work of the contracting myocyte is increased in the presence of digoxin. The effect is mediated via blockade of the Na^+, K^+ -ATPase at cell membranes (see Fig. 42.2). The consequence is a rise in intracellular sodium. A second membrane protein, the Na^+–Ca^{2+} exchanger, is stimulated to extrude the increased intracellular sodium in exchange for calcium, thereby increasing the intracellular calcium, which ultimately mediates the positive inotropic effect.

The second major effect of digoxin is less well understood. It has 'vagotonic' and antiadrenergic effects, as well as direct effects on the electrical properties of atrial, and particularly AV nodal, tissues. The consequence is a slowing of AV nodal conduction, particularly valuable in controlling ventricular rate in patients with AF.

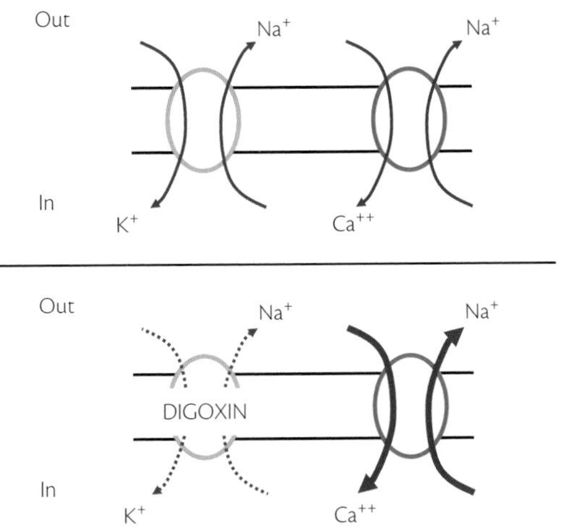

Fig. 42.2 Mechanism of the positive inotropic effect of digoxin. Digoxin blocks the Na^+, K^+-ATPase (left), thereby increasing the intracellular sodium concentration. The Na^+-Ca^{2+} exchanger exchanges the sodium for calcium, increasing intracellular calcium, leading to positive inotropy.

In over-dosage, however, digoxin can cause an increase in spontaneous depolarizations, so that as well as causing excessive bradycardia, digoxin can precipitate dangerous tachyarrhythmia.

The early clinical trials

There were several early trials, the majority of digoxin withdrawal versus continuation, using a placebo-controlled design. The results were variable and usually of minor clinical importance and would not be considered compelling by today's standards. In 1977 Dobbs *et al.*[3] assessed the need for continuation of digoxin in a double-blind, variable-dose, crossover comparison with placebo in 46 CHF outpatients (33 in sinus rhythm and13 in AF) who had been prescribed the drug for HF. Sixteen of the 46 patients deteriorated on placebo, with 8 completely recovering when digoxin was reintroduced; in the remainder additional diuretics were required temporarily. The study reported apparent benefits in spirometry and in left ventricular ejection time, neither of which would be considered targets reliably predictive of clinical benefit in CHF nowadays.

In 1982 Fleg *et al.*[4] performed a double-blind crossover study with digoxin and placebo in 30 patients on stable digoxin for chronic clinically compensated congestive HF and normal sinus rhythm. No patient's clinical condition deteriorated during 3 months of placebo administration. Discontinuation of digoxin resulted in a small increase in echocardiographically determined resting left ventricular end-diastolic dimension (1.8 ± 0.6 mm, $p < 0.001$). Maximal exercise capacity was unchanged. The authors concluded that long-term digoxin therapy had only a minor effect on cardiac performance that was without apparent clinical importance.

That same year Lee[5] performed a randomized, double-blind, crossover protocol of placebo versus digoxin in 25 CHF patients in sinus rhythm. According to a clinico-radiographic scoring system, the severity of HF was reduced by digoxin in 14 patients. In 9 of these 14, improvement was confirmed by repeated trials (5 patients) or right-heart catheterization (4 patients). The other 11 patients had no detectable improvement from digoxin. Patients who responded to digoxin had more chronic and more severe HF, greater left ventricular dilatation, and more severe HF.

Taggart[6] performed a double-blind placebo-controlled crossover trial of digoxin withdrawal in 22 patients with sinus rhythm who had a previous history of frank HF and were taking therapeutic doses of the drug. During the course of the study, 14 patients showed no clinical change whether taking digoxin or placebo, 5 patients deteriorated on placebo (4 with HF and 1 with supraventricular tachycardia), and 3 deteriorated on digoxin (2 with HF and 1 with digoxin toxicity). These differences were not statistically significant. Compared to placebo, while taking digoxin patients had lower resting heart rates and significant shortening of systolic time intervals. The authors concluded digoxin appeared to exert a sustained positive inotropic effect during maintenance therapy, but this was not of clinically meaningful benefit in the majority of patients.

In 1988 Guyatt[7] performed a placebo-controlled crossover trial of digoxin in CHF patients in sinus rhythm: 20 patients received 7 weeks of digoxin titrated to a level of 1.54 to 2.56 nmol/L and 7 weeks of matching placebo. In patients with deteriorating condition, the treatment period was terminated and outcome measures were obtained. If deterioration occurred during the first period, the patient was crossed over without the code being broken. Seven patients required premature termination of study periods because of increasing symptoms of CHF. All 7 were taking placebo at the time ($p = 0.016$). Small differences in dyspnoea ($p = 0.044$), walking test score ($p = 0.055$), clinical assessment of CHF ($p = 0.036$), and ejection fraction ($p = 0.004$) favoured the digoxin treatment group. Patients with more severe CHF were more likely to benefit from digoxin administration. It was concluded that oral digoxin, in doses titrated to produce a serum level of 1.54–2.56 nmol/L, improved quality of life and functional exercise capacity in some patients with CHF in sinus rhythm.

A year later, Pugh *et al.*[8] performed a randomized, double-blind, placebo-controlled, crossover study of digoxin withdrawal and reintroduction over two periods of 8 weeks each after long-term digoxin treatment: 44 patients with stable HF in sinus rhythm and plasma digoxin concentrations over 0.8 ng/ml were studied. Their progress was assessed by clinical criteria and by haemodynamic measurements (systolic time intervals and echocardiography). After withdrawal of digoxin clinical deterioration occurred in 25% of the patients (in 9% of cases digoxin reintroduction was thought to be necessary) compared to 11% of the patients during digoxin treatment.

In 1993 the most definitive evidence to date was published with the two largest of these withdrawal trials (PROVED and Radiance). In PROVED, Uretsky *et al.*[9] compared withdrawal of digoxin (placebo group, n = 46) with its continuation (digoxin group, n = 42) in a prospective, randomized, double-blind, placebo-controlled multicentre trial of patients with chronic, stable mild to moderate HF secondary to left ventricular systolic dysfunction who had normal sinus rhythm and were receiving long-term treatment with diuretic drugs and digoxin. Patients withdrawn from digoxin therapy showed worsened maximal exercise capacity (median change in exercise time –96 s) compared with that of patients who continued to receive digoxin (change in exercise time +4.5 s, $p = 0.003$). Patients withdrawn from digoxin therapy showed an increased incidence of treatment failures ($p = 0.039$, 39%, digoxin withdrawal group vs 19%, digoxin maintenance group) and a decreased time to treatment failure ($p = 0.037$). In addition, patients who continued to receive digoxin had a lower body weight ($p = 0.044$) and heart rate ($p = 0.003$) and a higher left ventricular ejection fraction (LVEF) ($p = 0.016$). In probably the only borderline convincing trial of its kind, the authors concluded there was worthwhile clinical efficacy of digoxin in patients with normal sinus rhythm and mild to moderate chronic HF secondary to systolic dysfunction who were already being treated with diuretics.

In the Radiance trial[10] the investigators studied 178 patients with CHF (NYHA class II or III, LVEF ≤35% in normal sinus rhythm) who were clinically stable while receiving digoxin, diuretics, and an ACE inhibitor. The patients were randomly assigned in a double-blind fashion either to withdrawing digoxin (93 patients) or continuing (85 patients) for 12 weeks. Worsening HF necessitating withdrawal from the study developed in 23 patients switched to placebo, but in only 4 patients who continued to receive digoxin ($p < 0.001$, relative risk of worsening HF = 5.9, 95% CI 2.1–17.2). In addition, all measures of functional capacity deteriorated in the patients receiving placebo as compared with those continuing to receive digoxin ($p = 0.033$ for maximal exercise tolerance, $p = 0.01$ for submaximal exercise endurance, and $p = 0.019$ for NYHA class). In addition, the patients switched from digoxin to placebo had lower quality-of-life scores ($p = 0.04$), decreased LVEF ($p = 0.001$), and increased heart rate ($p = 0.001$) and body weight ($p < 0.001$). The authors concluded that withdrawal of digoxin carries considerable risks for patients with chronic HF and impaired systolic function who have remained clinically stable while receiving digoxin and ACE inhibitors.

The larger (confounded) pre-DIG trials

Several larger trials which were not pure digoxin versus placebo-controlled studies were performed in the 1990s. In 1989, DeBianco[11] randomly assigned 230 patients in sinus rhythm with moderately severe HF to treatment with digoxin, milrinone, both, or placebo for 12 weeks. Treatment with milrinone or digoxin significantly increased treadmill exercise time as compared with placebo (by 82 s and 64 s respectively; 95% confidence limits, 44 and 123, and 30 and 100 respectively). Both treatments reduced the frequency of decompensation from HF, from 47% with placebo to 34% with milrinone ($p < 0.05$; 95% CI 22–46) and 15% with digoxin ($p < 0.01$; 95% CI 7–26). However, the clinical condition of 20% of the patients taking milrinone deteriorated within 2 weeks after treatment was begun, as compared with only 3% of those taking digoxin ($p < 0.05$). LVEF was increased by digoxin (+1.7%; $p < 0.01$; 95% CI 0.03–3.4) but not milrinone, and decreased on placebo (–2.0%; 95%CI –3.8–0.1). Mortality was not affected by digoxin but an adverse trend for milrinone nearly reached significance ($p = 0.064$). Perhaps unfairly, this study is better remembered for showing milrinone might aggravate ventricular arrhythmias and adversely affect survival than for any clinically important benefit of digoxin.

The Captopril Digoxin study[12] compared captopril and digoxin with placebo. Captopril significantly improved exercise time (mean increase, 82 s vs 35 s on placebo) and NYHA class (41% vs 22%), whereas digoxin did not. Digoxin treatment, however, led to a greater increase in LVEF (+4.4%) than captopril therapy (1.8% increase) or placebo (0.9% increase). Treatment failures, increased requirements for diuretic therapy, and hospitalizations were significantly more frequent in patients receiving placebo compared to either active drug. The fact that digoxin led to improvement in a measurement (LVEF) rather than any clinically useful change for the patient, and doubt about the relevance of the composite treatment failure definitions, limit the importance of the finding, at least as far as digoxin is concerned. In an other comparison, the German and Austrian Xamoterol study[13] randomized 433 mild to moderate CHF patients to the partial β-agonist xamoterol (subsequently withdrawn due to increased mortality in severe CHF), digoxin 0.125 mg twice daily, or placebo. After 3 months, xamoterol significantly increased exercise capacity whereas digoxin did not. Digoxin did not improve the severity of the majority of symptoms.

The results of these studies taken together with the early studies suggest that there is an inconsistent and modest beneficial effect of digoxin on symptoms and little to suggest a clinical benefit on major outcomes such as mortality.

The DIG trial

The most important study performed in two and a half centuries of digoxin use was published in 1997: the DIG trial.[14] In one of the largest ever HF trials, 6800 patients with systolic HF (LVEF ≤45%, nearly 85% class II or III, all in sinus rhythm, <50% previously taking digoxin) were randomized to digoxin (median dose 0.25 mg/day) or matching placebo on top of diuretics and ACE inhibitors for an average of 37 months. The primary endpoint was total mortality and it was not affected by digoxin (34.8% died on digoxin vs 35.1% on placebo, risk ratio 0.99; 95%CIs 0.91–1.07; Fig. 42.3), so that the trial was negative: further analyses for other types of outcomes or effects in subgroups should be treated with caution. Nevertheless, it has been widely reported (and mostly accepted) that the secondary endpoint, total hospitalizations, was significantly reduced by digoxin and the combination of the size of the trial and the statistical significance of the effect made this a reliable and true finding. There were 2184 (64.3%) patients hospitalized for any reason on digoxin compared to 2282 (67.1%) on placebo, risk ratio 0.92, 95% CIs 0.87–0.98, $p < 0.006$. The effect was mainly due to a reduction in the number of hospitalizations for congestive HF. DIG was, as mentioned above, a negative study and on the background of the inconsistent, albeit numerous, earlier trials, there is little to suggest a need for digoxin therapy in patients with HF in sinus rhythm. Nevertheless, the hospitalization reduction still leads some experts and some guidelines to offer digoxin as a possible treatment for HF in selected cases.

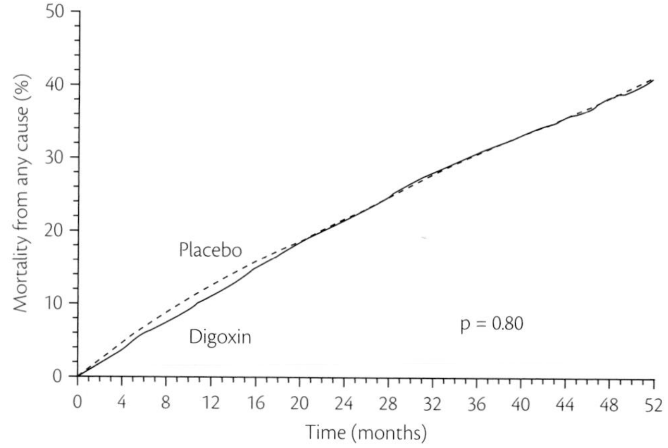

Fig. 42.3 Digoxin had no effect on mortality in the DIG trial.
From Digitalis Investigation Group. The effect of digoxin on mortality and morbidity in patients with HF. *N Engl J Med* 1997;**336**:525–533.

The DIG trial design incorporated a prespecified plan to examine the influence of digoxin on both the relative and the absolute reduction in the risk of a secondary outcome in prespecified subgroups. With regard to the combined outcome of mortality from worsening HF or a hospitalization related to that diagnosis, the benefit of digoxin appeared to be greater among higher–risk patients—lower LVEF, larger hearts, and those in NYHA class III or IV. In addition, there was an ancillary trial to DIG with the same design which recruited 988 patients with CHF and LVEF >45%, now often termed HF with normal ejection fraction (HeFNEF). In the ancillary trial, there were 115 deaths in the digoxin group (23.4%) and 116 deaths in the placebo group (23.4%) giving a risk ratio of 0.99, 95% CIs 0.76 to 1.28. The authors reported that the primary combined outcome of death or hospitalization due to worsening HF was associated with a risk ratio of 0.82 (95% CIs 0.63–1.07) and said this was consistent with the findings of the main trial: however, the result is not robust enough to depend on and no effect can be assumed in the HeFNEF patients.

Despite the fact the main and ancillary trials were both negative and the trial design prespecified only certain subgroups to determine differential digoxin effects, some authors have subsequently attempted to report different results in other subgroups. These should be considered speculative and not a true or reliable finding. They include suggestions that digoxin was associated with a higher risk of death compared to placebo in women (but not men)[15] and that the serum level of digoxin affected both the overall effect of digoxin and the supposed harmful effect in women, with harm only being seen when the serum digoxin concentrations were more than 1.2 ng/mL when measured 6–30 h after the last dose of study drug 4 weeks into the trial in men[16] or in women.[17] In one of the most outrageously misleading figures in a major trial report, the authors present the results of death due to worsening HF or hospitalization due to worsening HF showing a big reduction due to digoxin, but ignoring the fact that other cardiovascular deaths showed an increase with digoxin and other cardiovascular hospitalizations were also increased. The figure in the DIG paper was also misleadingly entitled 'Death or Hospitalization due to Worsening Heart Failure', suggesting it included all deaths, and giving this endpoint disproportionate weighting. The misleading effect was compounded by the selective use of this secondary post-hoc analysis in a negative trial as the only reproduced figure in a supposedly balanced review of the topic.[18] If only one figure from the trial is to be reproduced, it should be the negative primary outcome shown in Figure 2, not a misleadingly titled and excessively positive-looking tertiary analysis.

More patients had suspected digoxin toxicity in the digoxin group than in the placebo group (11.9% vs 7.9%). Among these patients, 16.5% of those in the digoxin group were hospitalized, as compared with 11.4% of those in the placebo group. The most common manifestations of digoxin toxicity were ventricular fibrillation or tachycardia, supraventricular arrhythmia, and second- or third-degree atrioventricular block. The increase in the risk of digoxin toxicity in the digoxin group was similar for all subgroups.

The weakest form of evidence: retrospective series

The controversy over digoxin shows no sign of abating. A report of a transplant waiting list analysis[19] showed in 455 advanced HF patients referred for transplant evaluation that after a median of 27 months, 83 of 277 (36.6%) of the patients treated with digoxin versus 36 of 228 (15.8%) of the patients without digoxin met primary outcome of death (n = 101), urgent transplantation (n = 14), or ventricular assist device implantation (n = 4) (HR 2.28; 95% CI, 1.51–3.43; $p < 0.001$). This was, of course, biased, as sicker or higher-risk patients may be more likely to be prescribed digoxin, and the fact that a significant but lesser hazard (HR 1.73; 95% CI, 1.09–2.75; $p = 0.021$) was seen compared to a propensity score-matched cohort does not overcome the criticism that such analyses are biased by unknown factors. It does not, however, give much support to the notion that digoxin is being particularly beneficial, although the main benefit seen if DIG that of prevention of hospitalization was not in the composite primary outcome of this report.

What the guidelines say

The European Society of Cardiology guidelines[20] recommend that in patients with symptomatic HF and AF, digoxin may be used to slow a rapid ventricular rate. In patients with AF and an LVEF of 40% or less, it should be used to control heart rate in addition to, or prior to, a β-blocker. In addition, the guidelines recommend that in patients in sinus rhythm with symptomatic HF and an LVEF of 40% or less, treatment with digoxin (in addition to an ACE inhibitor) improves ventricular function and patient well-being and reduces hospital admission for worsening HF, but with no effect on survival. The American College of Cardiology and the American Heart Association guidelines[21] for the management of patients with HF recommend the use of digoxin for symptoms and to prevent HF-related hospitalizations. A similar role for digoxin is also endorsed by the Heart Failure Society of America.[22]

Clinical use of digoxin

If initial treatment with digoxin is considered necessary, its use and effects should be carefully monitored to check it that continues to be necessary. Loading doses of digoxin are generally not required for patients in sinus rhythm. A single daily maintenance dose of 0.25 mg is recommended in adults with normal renal function. In the elderly and in those with renal impairment, a reduced dose of 0.125 mg or 0.0625 mg daily should be used instead. Digoxin blood levels should be checked early during chronic therapy and repeated after a few weeks in those with renal impairment. Regular digoxin concentration measurements have not been shown to be clinically necessary. The therapeutic serum concentration should be between 0.6 and 1.2 ng/mL. Care should be taken when digoxin is coprescribed with drugs which increase plasma digoxin levels. These include amiodarone, quinidine, diltiazem, verapamil, and some antibiotics.

Side effects and cautions

Side effects with digoxin are common and diverse and are more likely with elevated serum drug levels such as may be seen in elderly people and in those with poor renal function. They include atrial and ventricular arrhythmias (especially in the presence of hypokalaemia), sinoatrial and AV block, gynaecomastia, disturbances in colour vision, confusion, nausea, anorexia, and vomiting. Serious toxicity can be treated with digoxin-specific Fab antibody fragments.

Contraindications to digoxin use include second- or third-degree heart block (in the absence of a permanent pacemaker), pre-excitation syndromes (where there is a risk of precipitating rapid ventricular responses), and previous evidence of digoxin intolerance.

Summary

Digoxin is the oldest drug in use in cardiovascular medicine and probably still the most controversial. Its use for over 200 years is extremely well established, yet the modern clinical trial evidence of benefit is quite disappointing. It has worrying side effects, has been proven not to reduce mortality, and its stated benefits—reduction in the risk of HF-related hospitalization and improvement in symptoms—are softer and more difficult to quantify. When we have so many other effective treatments, some argue we should finally abandon its use. Yet it has several unique features. It is the only safe and probably efficacious positive inotropic agent, it is the only agent in common use that does not reduce blood pressure or risk worsening renal function, and has a particular role in stabilizing ventricular response rates in patients with AF, so a permanent moratorium on its use is not likely for the foreseeable future. Its use is declining, however, as we have so many better-studied and more efficacious agents. It is an old friend that should be allowed to slide into graceful retirement, being called on only in certain restricted circumstances for limited tasks; the first part-time semi-retired treatment for HF.

References

1. Withering W. *An account of the foxglove and some of its medical uses: with practical remarks on dropsy and other diseases.* J & J Robinson, London, 1785. Accessible at: http://www.gutenberg.org/files/24886/24886-h/24886-h.htm.
2. Lee MR. *William Withering (1741–1799): a biographical sketch of a Birmingham Lunatic,* 2005. In: The James Lind Library (www.jameslindlibrary.org). Accessed 22 February 2010.
3. Dobbs SM, Kenyon WI, Dobbs RJ. Maintenance digoxin after an episode of heart failure: placebo-controlled trial in outpatients. *BMJ* 1977;**i**:749–52.
4. Fleg JL, Gottlieb SH, Lakatta EG. Is digoxin really important in treatment of compensated heart failure? A placebo-controlled crossover study in patients with sinus rhythm. *Am J Med* 1982;**73**:244–50.
5. Lee DC, Johnson RA, Bingham JB, *et al.* Heart failure in outpatients. A randomized trial of digoxin versus placebo. *N Engl J Med* 1982;**306**:699–705.
6. Taggart AJ, Johnston GD, McDevitt DG. Digoxin withdrawal after cardiac failure in patients with sinus rhythm. *J Cardiovasc Pharmacol* 1983;**5**:229–34.
7. Guyatt GH, Sullivan MJJ, Fallen EL, Tihal H, Rideout E, Halcrow S, *et al.* A controlled trial of digoxin in congestive heart failure. *Am J Cardiol* 1988;**61**:371–5.
8. Pugh SE, White NJ, Aronson JK, Grahame-Smith DG, Bloomfield JG. Clinical, haemodynamic, and pharmacological effects of withdrawal and reintroduction of digoxin in patients with heart failure in sinus rhythm after long term treatment. *Br Heart J* 1989;**61**:529–39.
9. Uretsky BF, Young JB, Shahidi FE, Yellen LG, Harrison MC, Jolly MK. Randomized study assessing the effect of digoxin withdrawal in patients with mild to moderate chronic congestive heart failure: results of the PROVED Trial. *J Am Coll Cardiol* 1993;**22**:955–62.
10. Packer M. Gheorghiade M. Young JB. Costantini PJ. Adams KF. Cody RJ. Smith LK. Van Voorhees L. Gourley LA. Jolly MK. Withdrawal of digoxin from patients with chronic heart failure treated with angiotensin-converting-enzyme inhibitors. RADIANCE Study. *N Engl J Med* 1993;**329**(1):1–7.
11. DiBianco R, Shabetai R, Kostuk W, Moran J, Schlant RC, Wright R, for the Milrinone Multicenter Trial Group. A comparison of oral milrinone, digoxin, and their combination in the treatment of patients with chronic heart failure. *N Engl J Med* 1989;**320**:677–83.
12. The Captopril-Digoxin Multicenter Research Group. Comparative effects of therapy with captopril and digoxin in patients with mild to moderate heart failure. *JAMA* 1988;**259**:539–44.
13. German and Austrian Xamoterol Study Group. Double-blind placebo-controlled comparison of digoxin and xamoterol in chronic heart failure. *Lancet* 1988;**1**:489–93.
14. Digitalis Investigation Group. The effect of digoxin on mortality and morbidity in patients with heart failure. *N Engl J Med.* 1997;**336**:525–33.
15. Rathore SS, Wang Y, Krumholz HM. Sex-based differences in the effect of digoxin for the treatment of heart failure. *N Engl J Med.* 2002;**347**:1403–11.
16. Rathore SS, Curtis JP, Wang Y, Bristow MR, Krumholz HM. Association of serum digoxin concentration and outcomes in patients with heart failure. *JAMA.* 2003;**289**:871–8.
17. Adams KF, Patterson JH, Gattis WA, *et al.* Relationship of serum digoxin concentration to mortality and morbidity in women in the Digitalis Investigation Group trial: a retrospective analysis. *J Am Coll Cardiol.* 2005;**46**:497–504.
18. Gheorghiade M, van Veldhuisen DJ, Colucci WS. Contemporary use of digoxin in the management of cardiovascular disorders. *Circulation* 2006;**113**:2556–64.
19. Georgiopoulou VV, Kalogeropoulos AP, Giamouzis G, *et al.* Digoxin therapy does not improve outcomes in patients with advanced heart failure on contemporary medical therapy. *Circ Heart Fail* 2009;**2**:90–7.
20. Authors/Task Force Members. ESC Guidelines for the diagnosis and treatment of acute and chronic heart failure 2008: The Task Force for the Diagnosis and Treatment of Acute and Chronic Heart Failure 2008 of the European Society of Cardiology. Developed in collaboration with the Heart Failure Association of the ESC (HFA) and endorsed by the European Society of Intensive Care Medicine (ESICM). *Eur Heart J* 2008;**29**:2388–442.
21. Jessup M, Abraham WT, Casey DE, *et al.* 2009 focused update: ACCF/AHA Guidelines for the Diagnosis and Management of Heart Failure in Adults: a report of the American College of Cardiology Foundation/American Heart Association Task Force on Practice Guidelines: developed in collaboration with the International Society for Heart and Lung Transplantation. *Circulation* 2009;**119**(14):1977–2016.
22. Heart Failure Society of America (HFSA) practice guidelines. HFSA guidelines for management of patients with heart failure caused by left ventricular systolic dysfunction–pharmacological approaches. *J Card Fail* 1999;**5**:357–82.

43

Antithrombotic agents

John G.F. Cleland, Azam Torabi, Jufen Zhang, and Raj K. Chelliah

Introduction

Heart failure (HF) and the causes of HF provide, theoretically, a powerful pathophysiological substrate for thrombosis but there is remarkably little evidence that the rate of thrombotic events can be reduced by antithrombotic therapy.[1–4] HF is often associated with coronary artery disease and with atrial fibrillation,[5,6] two conditions for which long-term antithrombotic agents are traditionally given. Accordingly, many consider it unnecessary to investigate whether antithrombotic agents are effective in HF, since they consider the result a foregone conclusion. Some would even consider it unethical to withhold antithrombotic agents in patients with HF. Such an opinion reflects a general lack of rigour in the analysis and interpretation of long-term trials of antithrombotic agents for cardiovascular disease, undermining the scientific basis of medicine.

It is widely perceived that patients with HF have high rates of vascular occlusive events, including myocardial infarction (MI) and stroke,[7] but this may not be true. Reported rates of MI and stroke are certainly low compared to mortality in patients with HF.[1] Moreover, treatment directed at reducing the risk of vascular events, including aspirin,[8,9] statins,[10] and coronary revascularization,[11] has not yet been shown to reduce mortality in patients with HF, even though statins reduce the rate of nonfatal vascular events.

In summary, the contribution of vascular occlusive events to the morbidity and mortality of HF is uncertain. Too many opinions have been based on too few facts, resulting in recommendations about management that are only weakly supported by evidence. A lot of this stems from misinterpretation of the effects of aspirin in long-term trials of patients with atherosclerotic vascular disease.[12]

Pathophysiology of vascular occlusion: Virchow's triad revisited

While the precise history and components of Virchow's triad are disputed, in principle it describes the three categories of factors that contribute to thrombosis: blood stasis; reduced integrity of the walls of chambers and vessels containing blood; and hypercoagulability of the blood itself (Fig. 43.1).[13] Changes in one factor will affect the others.

Blood stasis or turbulence

Cardiac output is usually normal at rest until HF is advanced. Low cardiac output is unlikely to play a role in vascular occlusive events in most patients. Myocardial disease may cause ventricular dilatation, regional wall motion abnormalities and, more rarely, aneurysm formation, which may cause local stasis and increase thrombotic risk. However, the atria are likely to be a more common source of thrombi. The atria dilate and hypertrophy in response to atrial hypertension secondary to valve disease or ventricular dysfunction, either systolic or diastolic. This is a powerful stimulus to the development of atrial fibrillation, which further contributes to sluggish flow around the atrial walls and left atrial appendage, greatly increasing the risk of stroke.[14] Devices to occlude the left atrial appendage have been advocated as means to avoid blood stasis as an alternative to anticoagulation. Further research is required before this approach can be recommended as a mainstream therapy, although it might be considered for patients who cannot receive anticoagulants.

In the arterial system, atheroma and aneurysms may cause turbulence and pockets of stasis, provoking changes in the vessel wall that promote atherogenesis and predisposing to thrombotic risk. High venous pressure combined with reduced mobility will increase the propensity to venous stasis and thrombosis.

Integrity of vessel and chamber walls

Atheroma will affect most patients with HF, even if coronary artery disease is not the primary cause of cardiac dysfunction, and will alter vascular compliance, create turbulent flow, and contribute to focal arterial endothelial dysfunction. However, there are other causes of systemic arterial and venous endothelial dysfunction in patients with HF, including oxidative stress, and activation of neuroendocrine, inflammatory, and haemostatic systems. Endothelial dysfunction is complex and reflects activation of systems likely

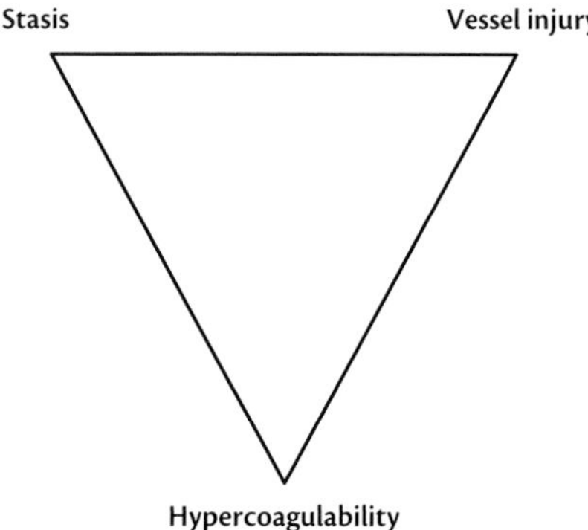

Fig. 43.1 Virchow's triad.

both to promote and retard thrombosis. Keeping the activation of these countervailing systems in balance is important.[15–17] Dysfunctional endothelium secretes more endothelin, von Willebrand factor, and adhesion molecules that may cause vasoconstriction and thrombosis.[15] Nitric oxide metabolism is compromised, leading to impaired flow-mediated dilatation and increased platelet adhesion.[18] On the other hand, there is marked activation of vasodilator prostaglandins in HF that mitigates the thombotic tendency, provided clumsy physicians do not intervene. Inhibition of vasodilator prostaglandin synthesis by nonsteroidal anti-inflammatory drugs (NSAIDs), including aspirin in doses as low as 75 mg/day, may cause arteriolar and venous constriction (Fig. 43.2),[16,17] enhance endothelin-induced vasoconstriction,[19] exacerbate renal dysfunction,[20] accelerate atherosclerosis,[21,22] and might also increase the risk of vascular occlusion.[23]

There is a widespread view that the primary event causing arterial vascular occlusion is thrombotic. This may not be true. Histology suggests that haemorrhage into plaque may often be the primary occlusive event, with thrombosis a secondary feature.[24,25] Clearly, antithrombotic drugs could increase the risk of plaque haemorrhage, accelerating plaque growth[25] or causing acute events. This may be why there is so little evidence that long-term antiplatelet or antithrombotic therapy reduces mortality in patients with (or at risk of) cardiovascular disease. In the acute setting the haemorrhage has already occurred and the main risk is thrombosis, whereas in the chronic setting the increased risk of haemorrhage into plaque may negate any benefit acquired from inhibition of thrombosis.

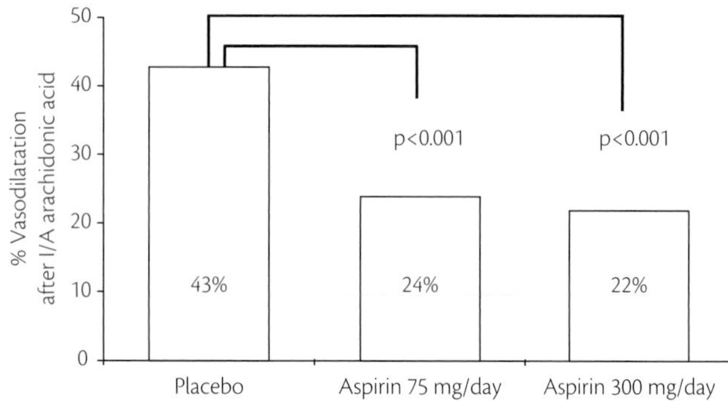

Fig. 43.2 Effects of low-dose aspirin on prostanoid-mediated arterial vasodilatation.[17]

Hypercoagulable state

As with the endothelium, there is evidence of activation of both pro- and antithrombotic factors.[26–28] The most consistently elevated haemostatic factors are D-dimer and von Willebrand factor, the former reflecting increased breakdown of crosslinked fibrin and the latter a manifestation of endothelial dysfunction. Both are independently related to an adverse prognosis in patients with HF and are similarly affected in patients with or without ischaemic heart disease. The severity of HF, particularly right HF leading to hepatic congestion, is an important determinant of haemostatic dysfunction. Disturbance of other haemostatic factors has been investigated less often, but is generally consistent with a prothrombotic state held in check by increases in thrombolytic activity.

While knowledge of the factors that predispose to thrombosis may be of value in deciding theoretically which interventions might be of value for patients with HF, the clinical setting is sufficiently complex that theory should be put to the clinical test before making firm recommendations.

Epidemiology of vascular events in HF

As with all received wisdom, the perception that patients with HF are at increased risk of many different types of arterial and venous occlusive events should be questioned. Indeed, careful scrutiny of clinical trial data indicates that patients with HF have somewhat lower rates of nonfatal vascular events than those who do not. This may be deceptive. Sudden death could be the most common manifestation of vascular events in patients with HF.[29–31] Alternatively, vascular events may be less likely to be diagnosed in patients with HF.

The low rate of MI in patients with HF could be explained by a change in its presentation and the shortened life expectancy of HF. A patient who dies of an arrhythmia or of HF is no longer at risk of having a vascular event. Alternatively, patients with HF may be at increased risk of both painless MI and of sudden death as manifestations of vascular events.[32] Increases in troponin are common during exacerbation of HF and augur a poor outcome.[33] Although raised troponin may reflect myocardial stress due to HF, it also probably reflects coronary vascular occlusion. Prior MI, comorbid diabetes, and HF itself may all conspire to denervate the heart and reduce the pain associated with myocardial ischaemia and infarction. In studies of hypertension and diabetes that included few patients with HF, about one-third of all MIs diagnosed were silent.[3,34,35] Presumably, many more silent infarcts remained undiagnosed and the rate of undiagnosed MI in patients with HF may be substantially higher than in other patients. Vascular occlusion may also be more likely to trigger ventricular arrhythmias as a result of either worsening ventricular function or increased electrical instability, resulting in sudden death.[29] An effective treatment for reducing vascular occlusion might reduce the rate of worsening HF and sudden death but might have little impact on the rate of classical MI.

The rate of clinically overt strokes is similar in patients with vascular disease with and without HF. Thus the ratio of stroke to MI in patients with HF is higher than in those without. This is probably because strokes are difficult to conceal, whether or not HF is present. The origin of strokes in HF is uncertain. Some will be cardioembolic and some due to cerebrovascular disease, but atherosclerosis in the aortic arch may also be an important source. Age, atrial fibrillation, diabetes, and atheroma are common risk factors for stroke and HF. Well-treated patients with HF are now unlikely to have a high arterial pressure and this, as well as improved management of atrial fibrillation, may account for the decline in the rate of stroke in patients with HF over the last 30 years.[1] Patients with more severe HF or left ventricular dysfunction are at greater risk of stroke.[7,36] The risk of haemorrhagic stroke will be increased by either aspirin or warfarin. MRI suggests a high prevalence of subclinical cerebral infarction in patients with HF,[37] but similar rates might exist in age-matched patients with vascular disease but not HF.

Deep venous thrombosis and pulmonary embolism are rare diagnoses in ambulant patients with HF, but common in patients confined to bed because of worsening HF or concomitant illness.[38] The proportion of sudden deaths due to pulmonary embolism is hard to quantify but is generally considered low.

Ultimately, the two most common manifestations of vascular events in HF may be worsening cardiac function and sudden death. Autopsy data show a high rate of fresh coronary occlusion amongst patients who have died in either of these ways.[31,39]

Evidence for antithrombotic agents

After myocardial infarction

MI is an important cause of ventricular dysfunction leading to HF. Surprisingly, no substantial, long-term trial of aspirin after MI at doses less than 300 mg/day exists, and no long-term trial of aspirin at any dose has ever shown a reduction in mortality(Fig. 43.3).[3] Among patients with HF after MI, the two largest long-term trials showed trends to a higher mortality in patients assigned to aspirin compared to placebo.[3,40,41] The validity of the meta-analysis of trials of aspirin is undermined by strong evidence of publication bias.[12] Many patients stop their aspirin therapy within a few months of a MI, perhaps because the patients have a better grasp of the evidence than their doctors! Indeed, a large trial of older patients likely to have stable coronary disease showed that aspirin increased the risk of fatal or nonfatal MI.[23]

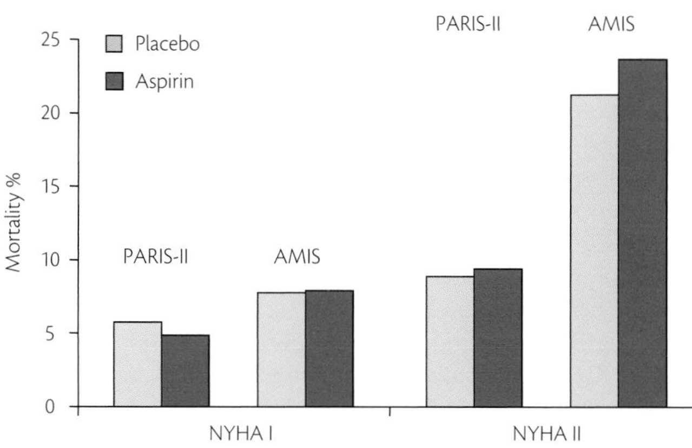

Fig. 43.3 Mortality on aspirin and placebo in the two largest long-term randomized trials after MI. Adapted from[40,41]

The data on warfarin after MI are only slightly more encouraging. Trials of warfarin conducted in the 1960s were widely considered to be neutral because they failed to reduce mortality by more than 75%—they reduced mortality only by 60%, with mortality dropping from 9.9% to 4.0% amongst the 4814 patients enrolled.[42] How times and expectations have changed in clinical trials! The landmark WARIS trial was conducted in only two hospitals and using one central laboratory.[43] Although the study was positive, it is not clear that the results can be replicated. Indeed, the WARIS-II trial failed to show that aspirin, warfarin, or their combination had substantially different effects on outcome.[44]

In atrial fibrillation

Atrial fibrillation (AF) is another common condition that commonly complicates, and is complicated by, HF.[45–47] There have been numerous trials of antithrombotic agents in patients with AF. There are two reasons why the findings are relevant to HF. Firstly, most of these patients probably had HF,[45–47] although many protocols paid insufficient attention to the diagnosis. Moreover, the event rates for patients without HF were low and probably not that much above the background population risk for stroke or other cardiovascular events (Fig. 43.4).[46] The risk of events and of death resided almost entirely in the patients who had some manifestation of HF. Although there is a lot of evidence that HF confers increased risk on patients with AF, the converse is far from certain.[48] Indeed, it might be considered that the trials were really trials of HF among patients who just happened to have AF. In other words, people have jumped to the conclusion that anticoagulants should be used for AF, but it might be that AF is just a surrogate marker for HF and the trials could be interpreted as evidence for an effect of anticoagulants in HF.

Aspirin generally failed to reduce thromboembolic events in patients with AF and was inferior to warfarin in patients with concomitant major ventricular dysfunction or HF.[49] Aspirin did not reduce mortality in these trials. Although recent trials have shown that the combination of aspirin and clopidogrel is inferior to warfarin, the combination is superior to aspirin alone for patients with AF who are ineligible for treatment with warfarin.[50,51] On the other hand, clopidogrel alone might be a better choice than

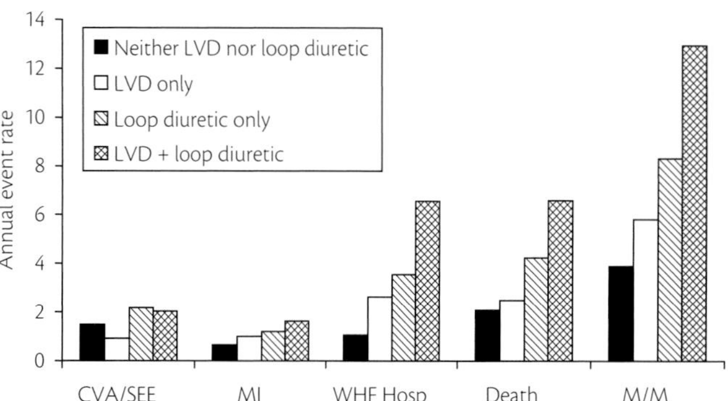

Fig. 43.4 Event rates in two trials of antithrombotic treatment in patients with atrial fibrillation, SPORTIF III and SPORTIF V. Patients are divided by treatment with or without loop diuretic, and by diagnosis of left ventricular dysfunction (LVD). CVA, cerebrovascular accident; M/M, morbidity (i.e. all of the nonfatal events illustrated) and mortality; SEE, systemic embolic event; WHF, worsening HF.[46]

in combination with aspirin for patients with vascular disease.[52] More recently, direct thrombin antagonists proved as, or more, effective than warfarin in reducing stroke and death in studies of AF that included many patients with HF.[53]

Observational data and mechanistic trials of antiplatelet agents in heart failure

There are biologically plausible reasons why aspirin may have adverse effects in patients with HF.[3] Neuroendocrine systems that cause vasoconstriction and other adverse effects are activated in patients with HF, but so too are systems that could be considered defence mechanisms, including natriuretic peptides and vasodilator prostaglandins.[54] Although aspirin might reduce platelet activation associated with HF, it may also reduce vascular prostaglandin production leading to an increase in vascular resistance, sodium retention, worsening renal function, and reduced vascular defences against platelet adhesion.[16,20,55,56] Also, ACE inhibitors may exert some of their benefit through increased prostaglandin synthesis which aspirin may counteract. Even small doses of aspirin may be sufficient to block both the arteriolar and venous response to a variety of prostaglandin-mediated vasodilator agents and such effects may last for 24 h or more,[16,55,56] suggesting that assertions, largely based on *in vitro* evidence, that 75 mg/day affects only platelets and not vessel wall prostaglandins, are wrong.

Aspirin remains the most widely used antithrombotic agent in patients with HF and in sinus rhythm.[10] Small randomized controlled trials have generally, but not always, shown that aspirin impairs the haemodynamic response to ACE inhibitors.[3,57,58] Small randomized studies also suggest that plasma concentrations of natriuretic peptides (cardiac stress hormones) are lower when patients take clopidogrel rather than aspirin,[59,60] that arterial function is better on clopidogrel than aspirin,[61] and that oxygen uptake during exercise is impaired by aspirin[62,63] and is better on clopidogrel.[64]

Observational trials can be used to argue any preferred point of view about the effect of aspirin on outcomes in HF, but such an approach to the prediction of drug effects is now generally discredited. Retrospective analysis of the SOLVD study suggested that aspirin use was associated with a lower morbidity and mortality,[65] with more prominent effects observed in the prevention arm rather than the treatment arm of the study, despite the poorer prognosis of the latter group. However, these observations many not be evidence of a therapeutic benefit from aspirin but simply reflect the fact that aspirin was given to patients at lower risk. Patients treated with aspirin had higher baseline ejection fraction, were less likely to have New York Heart Association (NYHA) class III/IV HF and more likely to be on a β-blocker. Other observational datasets have reported conflicting results.[3]

Cardiovascular prophylactic aspirin is a powerful risk factor for gastrointestinal bleeding, increasing with age and accounting for 30% or more of all major gastrointestinal haemorrhage in patients aged over 60 years.[66] There is little evidence that the risk is altered by reducing the dose of aspirin[66] or switching to enteric-coated preparations.[67] Compared to patients who do not have HF, those with HF are at markedly increased risk (odds ratio 5.9; 95% CI 2.3–13.1) of a major gastrointestinal haemorrhage when taking aspirin.[68]

Evidence for an aspirin–ACE inhibitor interaction

In large randomized trials of ACE inhibitors in patients with HF or ventricular dysfunction, the effect of ACE inhibitors on mortality was reduced in the presence of aspirin (from 26% to 14%, test for interaction p = 0.04)[69]. In the most relevant trial, SOLVD (n = 6512),[65] patients taking aspirin derived no mortality benefit from enalapril (hazard ratio for death with enalapril compared to placebo if taking aspirin 1.10 [0.93–1.30] compared to 0.77 [0.67–0.87] if not taking aspirin; a striking p = 0.0006 for the interaction. There was a similar trend for the composite of death or hospitalization for HF (HR 0.81 vs 0.71; p = 0.09). More recently, a meta-analysis of the HOPE and EUROPA studies (n = 25 515) suggested that the reduction of fatal and nonfatal vascular events by ACE inhibitors was halved (from about 40% to 17%) in the presence of aspirin (test for interaction p = 0.003) (Fig. 43.5).[70]

The reason for the interaction between aspirin and ACE inhibitors is unclear. It could reflect a reduction in the benefit of ACE inhibitors by aspirin. ACE inhibitors block the production of angiotensin II and impede the breakdown of bradykinin. The latter action may enhance the production of vasodilator prostaglandins and this action may be lost in patients taking aspirin. Alternatively, aspirin and ACE inhibitors may exert benefits by a similar pathway and therefore the benefits of the treatments could be less than additive.[3] Aspirin has also been reported to reduce the improvement in ventricular function with carvedilol,[71] although this may just reflect the association between aspirin and aetiology of ventricular function.[72]

The most important aspect of managing an adverse interaction between therapies is to be sure that both components are required. We do not know that long-term aspirin has ever been effective for the management of vascular disease. With the concurrent use of ACE inhibitors, aspirin may have been rendered worse than useless or, less likely, may finally be in an environment in which it works. This needs clarification. In the meantime, there is no evidence to support its long-term use in patients who require ACE inhibitors.

Alternative antiplatelet agents

Antiplatelet agents that do not block cyclooxygenase, such as dipyridamole and clopidogrel, may be preferred in patients with HF (Fig. 43.6).

One small randomized trial of 28 patients followed for 1 year suggested that dipyridamole was associated with better cardiovascular function.[73] Another study suggested that aspirin plus dipyridamole was associated with a slightly lower incidence of HF compared to clopidogrel.[74] This could reflect a benefit from the vasodilator effects of dipyridamole. However, the incidence of HF was so low that it suggests many cases were missed.

Clopidogrel exerts its actions by inhibiting the binding of ADP to platelet receptors, thereby reducing activation of the glycoprotein GPIIb/IIIa which is the binding site for fibrinogen. As noted above, compared to aspirin, treatment with clopidogrel is associated with better exercise capacity, lower serum creatinine and lower plasma natriuretic peptide concentrations. A post-hoc analysis of the CAPRIE study conducted on patients with ischaemic heart disease who had had cardiac surgery and who had a much higher prevalence of ventricular dysfunction and HF, suggested a strikingly greater effect of clopidogrel, compared to aspirin, on vascular morbidity and mortality.[75]

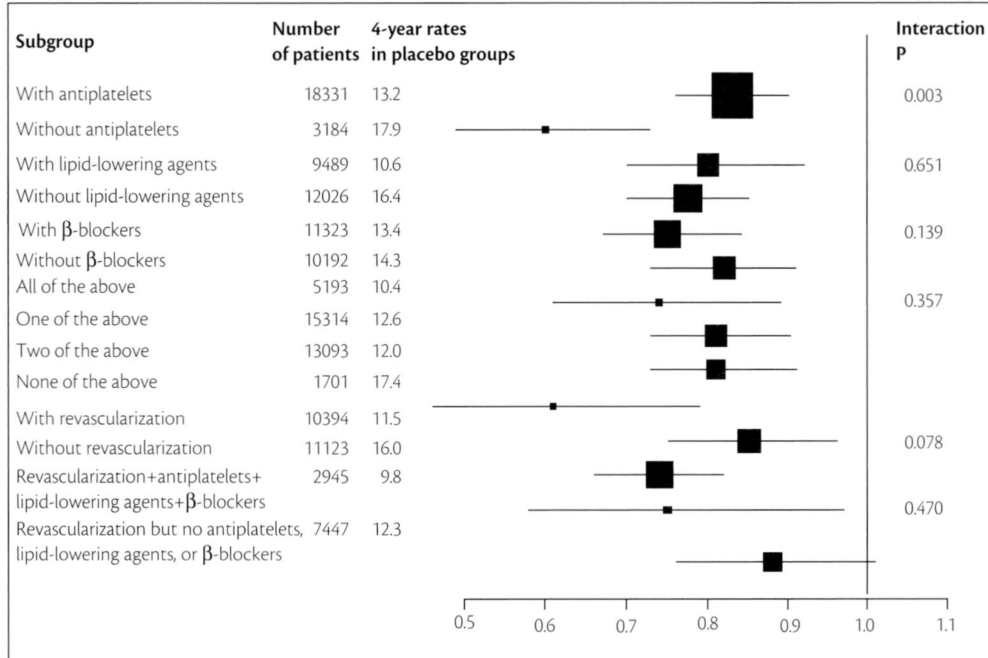

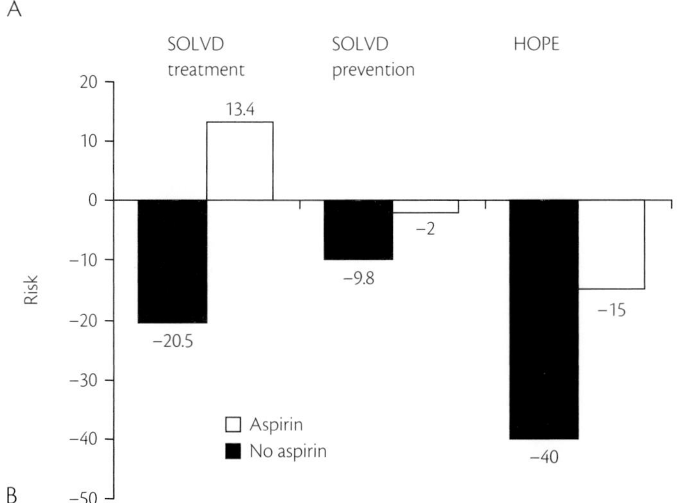

Fig. 43.5 (A) Effects of ramipril or perindopril on cardiovascular mortality, nonfatal MI, or stroke in patients taking antiplatelet, agents, lipid-lowering agents, or β-blockers individually or together. Data from [70]. (B) The effect of ACE inhibitors on mortality (SOLVD) and on mortality plus morbidity (HOPE) in the presence of absence of aspirin. Adapted from [3].

Observational data and mechanistic trials of oral anticoagulants in heart failure

Coumadin anticoagulants act specifically on vitamin-K dependent clotting factors. They are not known to have direct effects on the vasculature, renal function, or electrolytes and do not appear to interact with neuroendocrine systems (Fig. 43.7). By reducing thrombin formation and fibrin deposition, anticoagulants may additionally reduce platelet activation. Anticoagulants may reduce the risk of dying from cancer, either by acting as an early warning system for bowel and bladder tumours, which are picked up earlier because of the increased risk of bleeding, or because of the more intense haematological surveillance associated with anticoagulant monitoring.[76]

For decades there have been strong advocates, supported by guidelines, for the routine use of anticoagulants in patients with HF, and surveys and trials in patients with HF suggest that more than 20% of patients in sinus rhythm receive such therapy.[5,6] In SOLVD, warfarin was associated with a reduction in both morbidity and mortality without evidence of any interactions with ACE inhibitor therapy.[77] Anticoagulants are inconvenient because they require regular monitoring: they gained a reputation as dangerous drugs before modern monitoring techniques were introduced, and there were few conclusive trials to support their use other than in AF. Aspirin was 'sold' as a more convenient, safer alternative that was just about as effective. In the context of HF, warfarin was thought to be an agent only to reduce the risk of stroke, a relatively uncommon event, and for the management of ventricular thrombus, although there is no evidence to support such practice.[1]

HF complicates the management of vitamin-K-dependent anticoagulants. Hepatic congestion reduces the synthesis of clotting factors and may result in over-anticoagulation. Amiodarone and other drugs interfere with warfarin metabolism. Intercurrent illness requiring antibiotics, and procedures that require treatment to be stopped, also make accurate control more difficult, adding to the hazard of therapy. Direct thrombin antagonists may give rise to fewer problems.

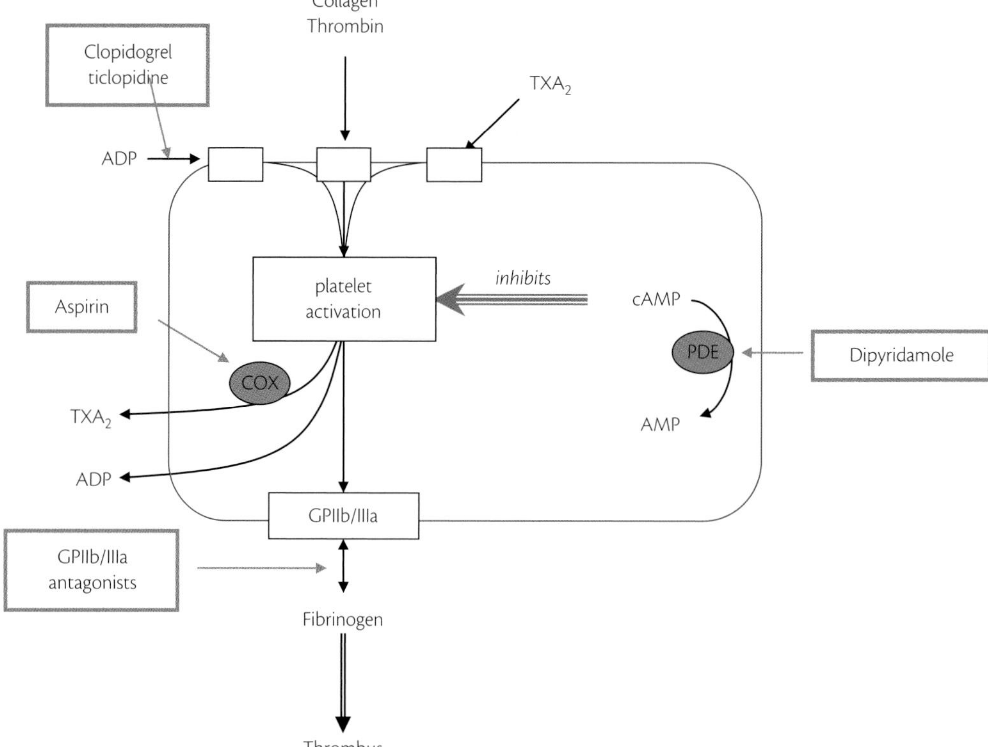

Fig. 43.6 The mechanism of action of orally active antiplatelet agents. Once a platelet is activated, it releases ADP and TXA2, thereby recruiting more platelets. The final common pathway of platelet activation is formation of the GPIIb/IIIa complex. cAMP is a powerful inhibitor of platelet activation, the breakdown of which is catalysed by PDE. cAMP, cyclic AMP; COX, cyclooxygenase; PDE, phosphodiesterase; TXA2, thromboxane A_2.

Randomized trials of antithrombotic agents in heart failure

Warfarin-Aspirin Study in Heart Failure

The Warfarin-Aspirin Study in Heart Failure (WASH)[8,78] was the first substantial randomized controlled trial of antithrombotic therapy for HF. It compared no antithrombotic therapy, aspirin (300 mg/day), or warfarin (target INR 2.5) in patients with HF who also had left ventricular systolic dysfunction (LVSD) and required diuretic therapy. The study was not blinded and was designed as a pilot study to address the feasibility of doing a trial that included a placebo or no-antithrombotic therapy group. The trial was slow to recruit, afflicted by concerns (on the part of patients as well as investigators) not only about withholding antithrombotic therapy but also about randomization to warfarin without a compelling reason, given the perceived risk and inconvenience. The concerns influenced the design of the WATCH and WARCEF studies (see below) which both avoided the problem of a no-antithrombotic treatment group but still struggled to recruit patients, who were reluctant to accept warfarin without a strong mandate.

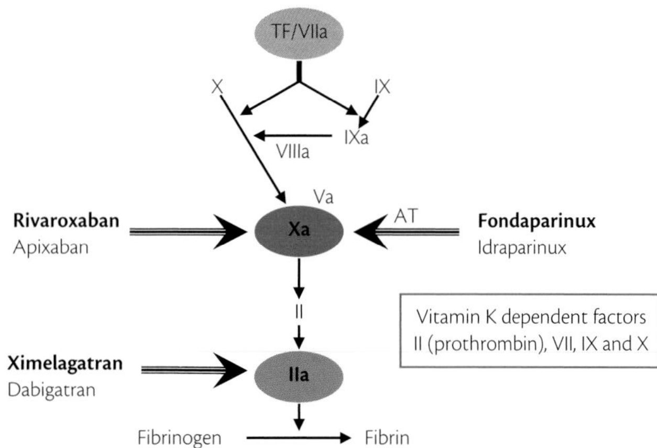

Fig. 43.7 Mechanisms of action of anticoagulants.
Adapted from Weitz JL, Bates SM, New anticoagulants. *J Thromb Haemost* 2005;**3**:1843–53.

About 60% of patients in WASH had definite ischaemic heart disease and only 15% of patients were proven to be free of coronary disease. Over a mean follow-up of 27 months, 70 (25%) of the 279 patients enrolled died but only 18 had a MI and only 4 had a stroke (Fig. 43.8). There were no significant differences in these outcomes amongst assigned groups but a trend to a worse outcome in those assigned to aspirin. Similar proportions of patients were hospitalized in those assigned to no antithrombotic treatment (48%) and warfarin (47%) but a higher proportion of those assigned to aspirin (64%; $p = 0.044$). The difference was driven by an increase in hospitalizations for HF (19%, 20%, and 34% of patients were hospitalized for HF respectively; $p = 0.032$). When the endpoint of both hospitalization for cardiovascular reasons and haemorrhage was considered, then the group randomized to no antithrombotic therapy fared better than either active intervention (22%, 25%, and 40% of patients were hospitalized, respectively; $p = 0.019$).

Clearly, WASH is not large enough to be definitive but does question the received wisdom that patients with HF should generally be on an antithrombotic agent, especially if they have coronary artery disease. The rate of overt atherothrombotic events was much lower than the rate of death, suggesting that the primary target of antithrombotic therapy in HF is to reduce mortality. It is possible that the dose of aspirin in WASH was too high, but there are no long-term trials of aspirin at lower doses in patients with ventricular dysfunction.

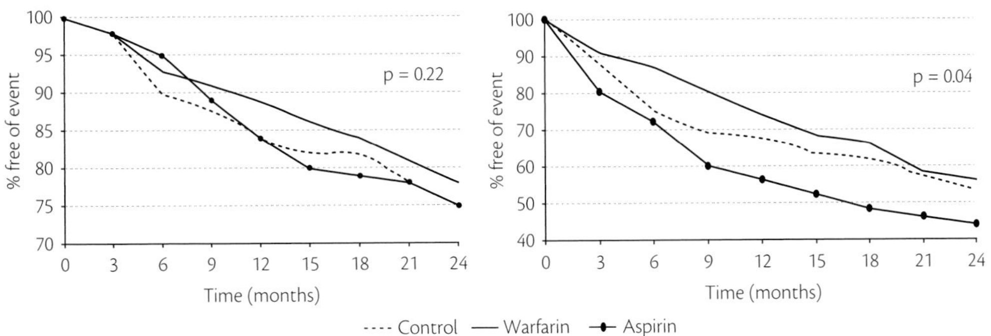

Fig. 43.8 Results of the WASH trial. The left-hand panel shows the primary endpoint cluster of death, nonfatal MI, or nonfatal stroke. The right-hand panel shows the time to first hospitalization for any reason. Data from [8].

HELAS

HELAS had a complex design to try and circumvent the issue of withholding antithrombotic agents in patients with coronary artery disease.[79] It enrolled a cohort of 115 patients with HF and LVSD due to ischaemic heart disease, who were then assigned to aspirin (325 mg/day) or warfarin, and a cohort of 82 patients who were not considered to have coronary artery disease, who were then assigned to placebo or warfarin. Over 22 months, 28 patients (14%) died, but only 2 had a MI (one a patient who was thought not to have coronary artery disease who had been assigned to warfarin) and only 5 had a stroke (4 of these on antithrombotic therapy). There was no difference in outcome depending on assigned group, with patients who had ischaemic heart disease assigned to aspirin doing marginally worse than other groups. Overall, the limited tconclusions that can be drawn from HELAS support those from WASH.

WATCH

The WATCH trial compared aspirin, at a lower dose than the above trials (162.5 mg/day), to clopidogrel 75 mg/day double-blind and, open-label, to warfarin titrated to an INR of between 2.5 and 3.0.[9] The study was stopped prematurely because of slow recruitment and showed no difference between aspirin, clopidogrel, and warfarin for the primary endpoint (20.7% on aspirin, 21.6% on clopidogrel, and 19.6% on warfarin) which was a composite of death, MI, or stroke. The reasons for slow recruitment mainly reflected the reluctance of patients with HF to consent to warfarin. However, patients assigned to warfarin had a lower rate of stroke (2.3%, 2.3%, and 0.6% respectively; p = 0.01) and of hospitalization for HF (22.2%, 18.5%, and 16.5% respectively; p = 0.0186), very similar to the WASH trial (Fig. 43.9). Clopidogrel was not quite as good as warfarin and not quite as bad aspirin. Whether lower doses of aspirin would have produced a different result is unclear.

The WATCH study result is unsatisfactory because, although it suggests that warfarin is the best option, warfarin is not sufficiently superior to aspirin to warrant its being the clear preferred option. Indeed, given the neutral primary outcome of WATCH, the preferred option could be considered to be aspirin, since it is not inferior, most convenient and, arguably,[80] the least expensive option.

SPORTIF

SPORTIF was a study in patients with AF, half of whom had HF, comparing warfarin and ximelagatran, a direct thrombin antagonist.[46] The risks of hospitalization for HF or of death were both strongly related to the presence of markers of HF at baseline. Ximelagatran was associated with a lower risk of the composite outcome of a vascular event, hospitalization for HF, or death (HR = 0.84, CI 0.72–0.98). This was driven by a 27% reduction in hospitalization for worsening HF (p = 0.02) (Fig. 43.10). Patients with HF were also less likely to develop abnormal liver function tests on ximelagatran than patients who did not have HF.

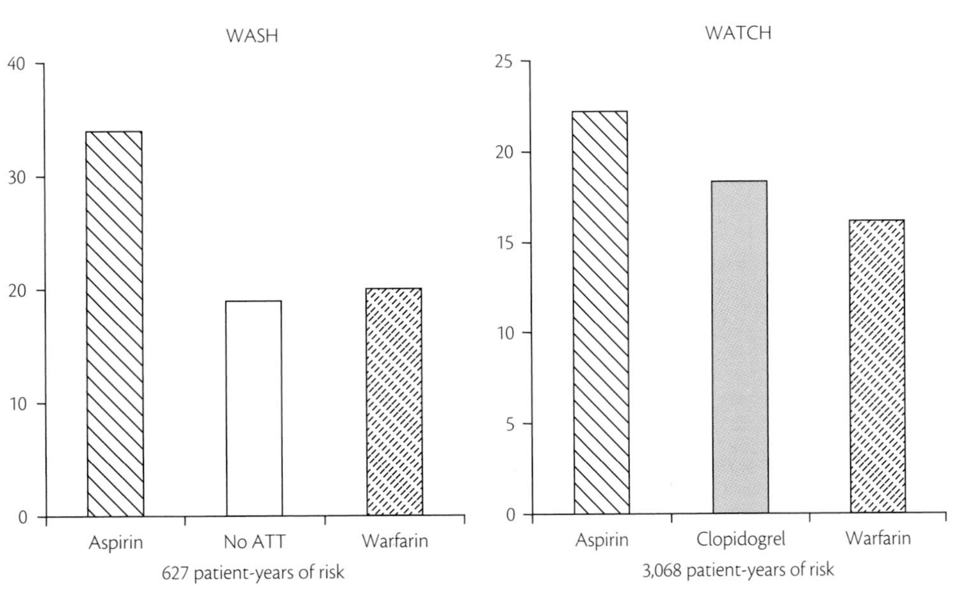

Fig. 43.9 Hospitalization for HF in the WASH and WATCH trials. In WASH, there were 41% fewer patients (p = 0.032) and 31% fewer events in the warfarin group compared with aspirin, and in WATCH, 27% fewer patients (p = 0.01) and 31% fewer events.[8,9]

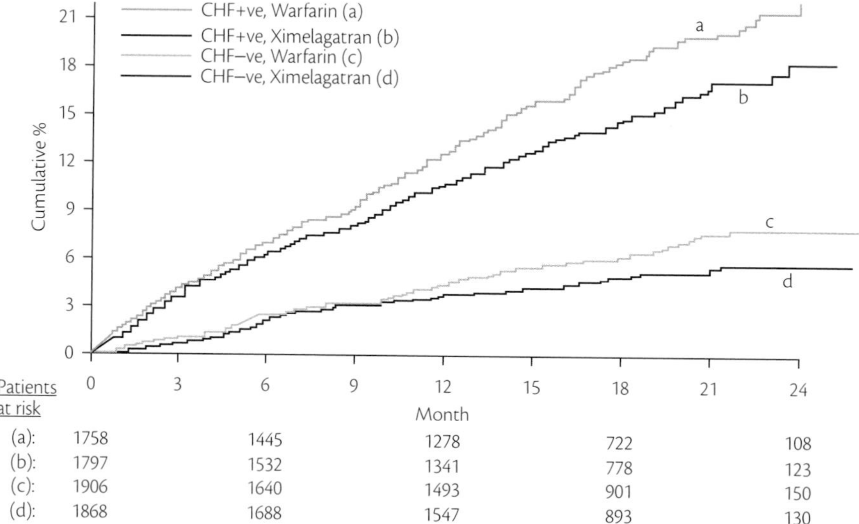

Fig. 43.10 Death or worsening heart failure in the SPORTIF trials.[46]

WARCEF

WARCEF is an ongoing study comparing aspirin 325 mg/day with warfarin at a target INR of 2.5–3 in patients with HF regardless of symptom severity, in sinus rhythm and with a left ventricular ejection fraction below 35%.[81] The study is double-blind which, for warfarin, is complex to manage. The study aims to recruit 2860 patients, of whom 70% or more have already been recruited.

CACHE

The CACHE study intends to compare open-label aspirin 75 mg/day with clopidogrel 75 mg/day in 3000 patients with HF and an NT-proBNP level greater than 400 pg/mL. Most of the patients should be treated with diuretics, ACE inhibitors, and β-blockers. The hypothesis is that aspirin and clopidogrel will both inhibit platelet aggregation but that clopidogrel will not inhibit cyclooxygenase. If cyclooxygenase inhibition leads to adverse effects on renal function, sodium retention, and lung, neuroendocrine, arteriolar, and venous function, then this should translate into a clinical difference between aspirin and clopidogrel. The primary outcome is all-cause mortality with hospitalization for HF, vascular events, and quality of life as key secondary outcomes.

Conclusion

For patients with HF and in sinus rhythm, the weight of evidence suggests that doctors should generally avoid using any antithrombotic agent. If they feel compelled to treat, then there is less evidence of harm with clopidogrel or warfarin than with aspirin, and yet aspirin is most widely used. It is likely to be several years before this therapeutic mess is sorted out. For those who have the opportunity, engaging with a randomized controlled trial is clinically, ethically, and scientifically appropriate.

References

1. Cleland JGF. anticoagulant and antiplatelet therapy in heart failure. *Curr Opinion Cardiol* 1997;**12**:276–87.
2. Cleland JGF. Management of thrombosis in heart failure. In: Mann DL (ed.) *Heart Failure: a companion to Braunwald's Heart Disease*, pp. 653–82. WB Saunders, Philadelphia, 2003.
3. Cleland JGF. Is aspirin 'the weakest link' in cardiovascular prophylaxis? The surprising lack of evidence supporting the use of aspirin for cardiovascular disease. *Prog Cardiovasc Dis* 2002;**44**:275–92.
4. Cleland JGF. Chronic aspirin therapy for the prevention of cardiovascular events: a waste of time or worse? *Nat Clin Pract Cardiovasc Med* 2006;**3**:234–5.
5. Cleland J.G.F., Swedberg K, Follath F, *et al.* The EuroHeart Failure Survey Programme: survey on the quality of care among patients with heart failure in Europe. Part 1: patient characteristics and diagnosis. *Eur Heart J* 2003;**24**:422–63.
6. Cleland JGF, Cohen-Solal A, Cosin-Aguilar J, *et al.* An international survey of the management of heart failure in primary care. The Improvement of Heart Failure Programme. *Lancet* 2002;**360**:1631–9.
7. Loh E, Sutton MS, Wun C-CC, *et al.* Ventricular dysfunction and the risk of stroke after myocardial infarction. *N Engl J Med* 1997;**336**:251–7.
8. Cleland JGF, Findlay I, Jafri S *et al.* The Warfarin/Aspirin Study in Heart Failure (WASH): A randomized trial comparing antithrombotic strategies for patients with heart failure. *Am Heart J* 2004;**148**:157–64.
9. Massie B, Collins JF, Ammon SE *et al.* Randomized trial of warfarin, aspirin and clopidogrel in patients with chronic heart failure. The Warfarin and Antiplatelet Therapy in Chronic Heart Failure (WATCH) Trial. *Circulation* 2009;**119**:1616–24.
10. Kjekshus J, Apetrei E, Barrios V, *et al.* Rosuvastatin in older patients with systolic heart failure. *New Engl J Med* 2007;**357**:2248–61.
11. Coletta AP, Cleland JGF, Cullington D, Clark AL. Clinical trials update from Heart Rhythm 2008 and Heart Failure 2008: ATHENA, URGENT, INH study, HEART and CK-1827452. *Eur J Heart Fail* 2008;**10**:917–20.
12. Cleland JGF. For debate: Preventing atherosclerotic events with aspirin. *BMJ* 2002;**324**:103–5.
13. Lip GYH, Gibbs CR. Does heart failure confer a hypercoagulable state? Virchow's triad revisited. *J Am Coll Cardiol* 1999;**33**:1424–6.
14. Wolf PA, Abbott RD, Kannel WB. Atrial fibrillation as an independent risk factor for stroke. The Framingham Study. *Stroke* 1991;**22**:983–9.
15. Good JM, Nihoyannopoulos P, Ghatei MA, *et al.* Elevated plasma endothelin concentrations in heart failure; an effect of angiotensin II? *Eur Heart J* 1994;**15**:1634–40.
16. Jhund PS, Davie AP, McMurray JJ. Aspirin inhibits the acute venodilator response to furosemide in patients with chronic heart failure. *J Am Coll Cardiol* 2001;**37**:1234–8.
17. Davie AP, Love MP, McMurray JJV. Even low-dose aspirin inhibits arachidonic acid-induced vasodilation in heart failure. *Clin Pharmacol Ther* 2000;**67**:530–7.

18. Habib F, Dutka D, Crossman D, Oakley CM, Cleland JGF. Enhanced basal nitric oxide production in heart failure: another failed counter regulatory vasodilator mechanism? *Lancet* 1994;**344**:371–3.
19. Haynes G, Webb DJ. Endothelium-dependent modulation of responses to endothelin-1 in human veins. *Clin Sci* 1993;**84**:427–33.
20. de Silva R, Nikitin NP, Witte KK *et al.* Effects of applying a standardised management algorithm for moderate to severe renal dysfunction in patients with chronic stable heart failure. *Eur J Heart Failure* 2007;**9**:415–23.
21. Ranke C, Hecker H, Creutzig A, Alexander K. Dose-dependent effect of aspirin on carotid atherosclerosis. *Circulation* 1993;**87**:1873–9.
22. Knottenbelt C, Brennan PJ, Meade TW, for the MRC general practice research framework. Antithrombotic treatment and the incidence of angina pectoris. *Ann Intern Med* 2002;**162**:881–6.
23. Pulmonary Embolism Prevention (PEP) Trial Collaborative Group. Prevention of pulmonary embolism and deep vein thrombosis with low dose aspirin: Pulmonary Embolism Prevention (PEP) trial. *Lancet* 2000;**355**:1295–302.
24. van Dantzig JM, Becker AE. Sudden cardiac death and acute pathology of coronary arteries. *Eur Heart J* 1986;**7**:987–91.
25. Burke AP, Kolodgie FD, Farb A, *et al.* Healed plaque ruptures and sudden coronary death: evidence that subclinical rupture has a role in plaque progression. *Circulation* 2001;**103**:934–40.
26. Sbarouni E, Bradshaw A, Andreotti F, Tuddenham E, Oakley CM, Cleland JGF. Relationship between hemostatic abnormalities and neuroendocrine activity in heart failure. *Am Heart J* 1994;**127**:607–12.
27. Loh PH, Goode K, Tin L, *et al.* Prognostic values of laboratory markers for haemostasis, rheology, inflammation and endothelial function in patients with left ventricular systolic dysfunction. *Eur Heart J* 2006;**27**(suppl):P513.
28. Gibbs CR, Blann AD, Watson RD, Lip GY. Abnormalities of hemorheological, endothelial, and platelet function in patients with chronic heart failure in sinus rhythm: effects of angiotensin-converting enzyme inhibitor and beta-blocker therapy. *Circulation* 2001;**103**:1746–51.
29. Cleland JGF, Massie BM, Packer M. Sudden death in heart failure: vascular or electrical? *Eur J Heart Fail* 1999;**1**:41–5.
30. Cleland JGF, Thygesen K, Uretsky BF, *et al.* Cardiovascular critical event pathways for the progression of heart failure. A report from the ATLAS study. *Eur Heart J* 2001;**22**:1601–12.
31. Uretsky B, Thygesen K, Armstrong PW, *et al.* Acute coronary findings at autopsy in heart failure patients with sudden death: Results from the assessment of treatment with lisinopril and survival study (ATLAS) trial. *Circulation* 2000;**102**:611–16.
32. Kannel WB, Abbott RD. Incidence and prognosis of unrecognised myocardial infarction: An update on the Framingham Study. *N Engl J Med* 1984;**311**:1144–7.
33. Perna ER, Macin SM, Parras JI, *et al.* Cardiac troponin T levels are associated with poor short-and long-term prognosis in patients with acute cardiogenic pulmonary oedema. *Am Heart J* 2002;**143**:814–20.
34. Dormandy JA, Charbonnel B, Eckland DJA, *et al.* Secondary prevention of macrovascular events in patients with type 2 diabetes in the PROactive Study (PROspective pioglitAzone Clinical Trial In macroVascular Events): a randomised controlled trial. *Lancet* 2005;**366**:1279–89.
35. Hansson L, Zanchetti A, Carruthers SG, *et al.* Effect of intensive blood pressure lowering and low-dose aspirin in patients with hypertension: principal results of the hypertension optimal treatment (HOT) randomised trial. *Lancet* 1998;**351**:1755–62.
36. Cleland JGF, Thackray S. Antiplatelet therapy for ACS: a house in need of a spring clean. *Prescriber* 2009;**20**:7–10.
37. Schmidt R, Fazekas F, Offenbacher H, Dusleag J, Lechner H. Brain magnetic resonance imaging and neuropsychological evaluation of patients with idiopathic dilated cardiomyopathy. *Stroke* 1991;**22**:195–9.
38. Levine M, Gent M, Hirsh J, *et al.* A comparison of low-molecular -weight heparin administered primarily at home with unfranctionated heparin administered in the hospital for proximal deep-vein thrombosis. *N Engl J Med* 1996;**334**:677–81.
39. Orn S, Cleland JG, Romo M, Kjekshus J, Dickstein K. Recurrent infarction causes the most deaths following myocardial infarction with left ventricular dysfunction. *Am J Med* 2005;**118**:752–8.
40. The aspirin myocardial infarction study research group. The aspirin myocardial infarction study: final results. *Circulation* 1980;**62**(suppl V): V79–84.
41. Klimt CR, Knatterud GL, Stamler J, Meier P. Persantine-Aspirin Reinfarction Study. Part II. Secondary coronary prevention with persantine and aspirin. *J Am Coll Cardiol* 1986;**7**:251–69.
42. Anand SS, Yusuf S. Oral anticoagulant therapy in patients with coronary artery disease: a meta-analysis. *JAMA* 1999;**282**:2058–67.
43. Smith P, Arnesen H, Holme I. The effect of warfarin on mortality and reinfarction after myocardial infarction. *New Engl J Med* 1990;**323**:147–51.
44. Hurlen M, Abdelnoor M, Smith P, Erikssen J, Arnesen H. Warfarin, aspirin, or both after myocardial infarction. *New Engl J Med* 2003;**347**:969–74.
45. Shelton RJ, Clark AL, Kaye GC, Cleland JGF. The atrial fibrillation paradox of heart failure. *Congest Heart Fail* 2010;**16**:3–9.
46. Cleland JGF, Shelton R, Nikitin NP, Ford S, Frison L, Grind M. Prevalence of markers of heart failure in patients with atrial fibrillation and the effects of ximelagatran compared to warfarin on the incidence of morbid and fatal events: A report from the SPORTIF III and V trials. *Eur J Heart Fail* 2007;**9**:730–9.
47. Khand A, Rankin AC, Kaye GC, Cleland JGF. Systematic review of the management of atrial fibrillation in patients with heart failure. *Eur Heart J* 2000;**21**:614–32.
48. Carson PE, Johnson GR, Dunkman WB, Fletcher RD, Farrell L, Cohn JN. The influence of atrial fibrillation on prognosis in mild to moderate heart failure: The V-HeFT studies. *Circulation* 1993;**87**:VI102–10.
49. Cleland JGF, Cowburn PJ, Falk RH. Should all patients with atrial fibrillation receive warfarin? Evidence from randomised clinical trials. *Eur Heart J* 1996;**17**:674–81.
50. Connolly S, pogue J, Hart R, *et al.* Clopidogrel plus aspirin versus oral anticoagulation for atrial fibrillation in the Atrial fibrillation Clopidogrel Trial with Irbesartan for prevention of Vascular Events (ACTIVE W): a randomised controlled trial. *Lancet* 2006;**367**:1903–12.
51. Connolly SJ, pogue J, Hart RG *et al.* Effect of clopidogrel added to aspirin in patients with atrial fibrillation. *N Engl J Med* 2009;**360**:2066–78.
52. Diener H-C, Bogousslavsky J, Brass LM, *et al.* Aspirin and clopidogrel compared with clopidogrel alone after recent ischaemic stroke or transient ischaemic attack in high-risk patients (MATCH): randomised, double-blind, placebo-controlled trial. *Lancet* 2004;**364**:331–7.
53. Connolly SJ, Ezekowitz MD, Yusuf S, *et al.* Dabigatran versus warfarin in patients with atrial fibrillation. *N Engl J Med* 2009;**361**:1139–51.
54. Cleland JGF, Oakley CM. Vascular tone in heart failure: The neuroendocrine-therapeutic interface. *Br Heart J* 1991;**66**:264–7.
55. MacIntyre IM, Jhund PS, McMurray JJ. Aspirin inhibits the acute arterial and venous vasodilator response to captopril in patients with chronic heart failure. *Cardiovasc Drugs Ther* 2005;**19**:261–5.
56. Davie AP, Love MP, McMurray JJV. Even low-dose aspirin inhibits arachidonic acid-induced vasodilatation in heart failure. *Clin Pharmacol Ther* 2000;**67**:530–7.
57. Meune C, Mahe I, Mourad JJ, *et al.* Aspirin alters arterial function in patients with chronic heart failure treated with ACE inhibitors: a dose-mediated deleterious effect. *Eur J Heart Fail* 2003;**5**:271–9.

58. Hall D, Zeitler H, Rudolph W. Counteraction of the vasodilator effects of enalapril by aspirin in severe heart failure. *J Am Coll Cardiol* 1992;**20**:1549–55.
59. Meune C, Wahbi K, Fulla Y, *et al.* Effects of aspirin and clopidogrel on plasma brain natriuretic peptide in patients with heart failure receiving ACE inhibitors. *Eur J Heart Fail* 2007;**9**:197–201.
60. Jug B, Sebestjen M, Sabovic M, Keber I. Clopidogrel is associated with a lesser increase in NT-proBNP when compared to aspirin in patients with ischemic heart failure. *J Card Fail* 2006;**12**:446–51.
61. Meune C, Mahe I, Cohen-Solal A. Comparative effect of aspirin and clopidogrel on artrial function in CHF. *Int J Cardiol* 2006;**106**:61–6.
62. Guazzi M, Pontone G, Agostoni P. Aspirin worsens exercise performance and pulmonary gas exchange in patients with heart failure who are taking angiotensin-converting enzyme inhibitors. *Am Heart J* 1999;**138**:254–60.
63. Guazzi M, Marenzi G, Alimento M, Contini M, Agostoni P. Improvement of alveolar-capillary membrane diffusing capacity with enalapril in chronic heart failure and counteracting effect of aspirin. *Circulation* 1997;**95**:1930–6.
64. Kindsvater S, Leclerc K, Ward J. Effects of coadministration of aspirin or clopidogrel on exercise testing in patients with heart failure receiving angiotensin-converting enzyme inhibitors. *Am J Cardiol* 2003;**91**:1350–2.
65. Al-Khadra AS, Salem DN, Rand WM, Udelson JE, Smith JJ, Konstam MA. Antiplatelet agents and survival: a cohort analysis from the studies of left ventricular dysfunction (SOLVD) trial. *J Am Coll Cardiol* 1998;**31**:419–25.
66. Weil J, Colin-Jones D, Langman M *et al.* Prophylactic use of aspirin and risk of peptic ulcer bleeding. *Br Med J* 1995;**310**:827–30.
67. Kelly MJ, Kaugman DW, Jurgelon JM, Sheehan J, Koff RS, Shapiro S. Risk of aspirin-associated major upper-gastrointestinal bleeding with enteric-coated or buffered product. *Lancet* 1996;**348**:1413–6.
68. Weil J, Langman MJS, Wainwright P, *et al.* Peptic ulcer bleeding: accessory risk factors and interactions with non-steroidal anti-inflammatory drugs. *Gut* 2000;**46**:27–31.
69. Teo K, Yusuf S, Pfeffer M, *et al.* Effects of long-term treatment with angiotensin-converting-enzyme inhibitors in the presence or absence of aspirin: a systematic review. *Lancet* 2002;**360**:1037–43.
70. Dagenais GR, Pogue J, Fox K, Simoons ML, Yusuf S. Angiotensin-converting-enzyme inhibitors in stable vascular disease without left ventricular systolic dysfunction or heart failure: a combined analysis of three trials. *Lancet* 2006;**368**:581–8.
71. Lindenfeld J, Robertson AD, Lowes BD, Bristow MR, for the MOCHA Investigators. Aspirin impairs reverse myocardial remodeling in patients with heart failure treated with beta-blockers. *J Am Coll Cardiol* 2001;**38**:1950–6.
72. Cleland JGF, Pennell DJ, Ray SG, *et al.* Myocardial viability as a determinant of the ejection fraction response to carvedilol in patients with heart failure (CHRISTMAS trial): randomised controlled trial. *Lancet* 2003;**362**:14–21.
73. Sanada S, Asanuma H, Koretsune Y, *et al.* Long-term oral administration of dipyridamole improves both cardiac and physical status in patients with mild to moderate chronic heart failure: a prospective open-randomized study. *Hypertens Res* 2007;**30**:913–9.
74. Sacco RL, Diener HC, Yusuf S, *et al.* Aspirin and extended-release dipyridamole versus clopidogrel for recurrent stroke. *N Engl J Med* 2008;**359**:1238–51.
75. Bhatt DL, Chew DP, Hirsch AT, Ringleb PB, Hacke W, Topol EJ. Superiority of clopidogrel versus aspirin in patients with prior cardiac surgery. *Circulation* 2001;**103**:363–8.
76. Tagalakis V, Tamim H, Blostein M, Collet JP, Hanley JA, Kahn SR. Use of warfarin and risk of urogenital cancer: a population-based, nested case-control study. *Lancet Oncol* 2007;**8**:395–402.
77. Al-Khadra AS, Salem DN, Rand WM, Udelson JE, Smith JJ, Konstam MA. Warfarin anticoagulation and survival: A cohort analysis from the studies of left ventricular dysfunction. *J Am Coll Cardiol* 1998;**31**:749–53.
78. The WASH study steering committee and investigators. The WASH study (Warfarin /Aspirin Study in Heart failure): rationale, design and endpoints. *Eur J Heart Fail* 1999;**1**:95–9.
79. Cokkinos DV, Haralabopoulos GC, Kostis JB, Toutouzas PK. Efficacy of antithrombotic therapy in chronic heart failure: the HELAS study. *Eur J Heart Fail* 2006;**8**:428–32.
80. Morant SV, McMahon AD, Cleland JGF, Davey PG, MacDonald TM. Cardiovascular prophylaxis with aspirin: costs of supply and management of upper gastrointestinal and renal toxicity. *Br J Clin Pharmacol* 2004;**57**:188–98.
81. Pullicino P, Thompson JL, Barton B, Levin B, Graham S, Freudenberger RS. Warfarin versus aspirin in patients with reduced cardiac ejection (WARCEF): rationale, objectives, and design. *J Card Fail* 2006;**12**:39–46.

PART XII

Medical therapy for acute heart failure

44

Inotropes, pressors, and vasodilators

Susanna Price and Shahana Uddin

Introduction

There has been a perceptible change in the approach to the management of chronic heart failure (CHF) from focusing on inotropy, to a predominantly neurohormonal approach to therapeutic intervention. By contrast, in acute heart failure (AHF) the critical inability of the myocardium to maintain a cardiac output sufficient to meet the demands of the peripheral circulation demands urgent intervention to restore adequate perfusion.[1] Thus, haemodynamic considerations are pivotal, and the use of inotropes, pressors, and vasodilators remains widespread.[2,3] This is despite concerns about the potential of inotropic agents to increase mortality in some patient populations.[4,5] Current recommendations are therefore that inotropes should be used only in selected patients, and withdrawn as soon as adequate organ perfusion is restored. The present chapter reviews the pharmacology of positive inotropic drugs, the principles underlying the choice of vasoactive drugs in AHF, and potential future developments in the field.

General mechanisms of action

Mechanisms of inotropic effects

Classically, direct inotropic effects are mediated via release of calcium ions from the myocyte sarcoplasmic reticulum and other subsarcolemmal sites, and subsequent interaction between calcium and contractile proteins. The release of calcium is effected via cyclic AMP (cAMP)-dependent or -independent mechanisms (Fig. 44.1). cAMP increases phosphokinase A (PKA) activity which promotes opening of the cell membrane L-type calcium channels, in turn promoting intracellular calcium entry, and then increasing calcium release via the ryanodine receptor in the sarcoplasmic reticulum. PKA also phosphorylates phospholamban and calmodulin, promoting uptake of calcium into the sarcoplasmic reticulum, and may potentially additionally promote sarcoplasmic reticulum calcium release independently via a voltage sensitive release mechanism. There are numerous cell membrane receptors on the human myocardium, many of which are linked to G proteins (Gs, Gi, Gq). The different G proteins have a number of specific effects, including the modulation of cAMP formation (Gs, Gi), and production of diacylglycerol and inositol triphosphate (Gq), with resultant changes in intracellular calcium ion concentration. More novel inotropic agents act by increasing the sensitivity of the contractile process.[6]

cAMP-dependent mechanisms

The β_1- and β_2-adrenergic receptors found on the surface of cardiomyocytes (Fig. 44.1, Table 44.1) mediate cardiac responses to endogenous and exogenous catecholamines via coupling to the G_s proteins resulting in production of cAMP.[7] Stimulation of β_1-receptors (but not β_2-receptors) results in PKA-mediated phosphorylation of phospholamban and cardiac contractile proteins[8] and promotes cardiomyocyte apoptosis.[9,10] In heart failure, there is a redistribution in the proportions of β_1- and β_2-receptors on the cardiomyocyte surface modulating the responses of the myocyte to adrenergic stimulation.[11] The redistribution, together with the relative desensitization of β-receptor pathways found in heart failure, and down-regulation of receptor numbers with prolonged administration of β-agonists, may additionally alter the clinical effects of inotropic agents, although the precise implications are not yet fully understood. β-Receptor agonists include the catecholamines (adrenaline, noradrenaline, dopamine, dobutamine, isoprenaline, and dopexamine) which contain a benzene ring with different ethylamine side chains. They all activate different adrenoreceptors to varying degrees depending on the dosage used (Table 44.1).

Phosphodiesterase (PDE) is a ubiquitous enzyme that catalyses the hydrolysis of both cAMP and cGMP. A number of drugs inhibit the different subtypes of the enzyme with varying degrees of specificity (Table 44.2): however, those most relevant to positive inotropic effects relate to PDE III or IV (the biguanides amrinone and milrinone, and the imidazolone derivative enoximone).

cAMP-independent mechanisms

A number of drugs increase intracellular calcium levels via cAMP-independent mechanisms, or exert their positive inotropic effect

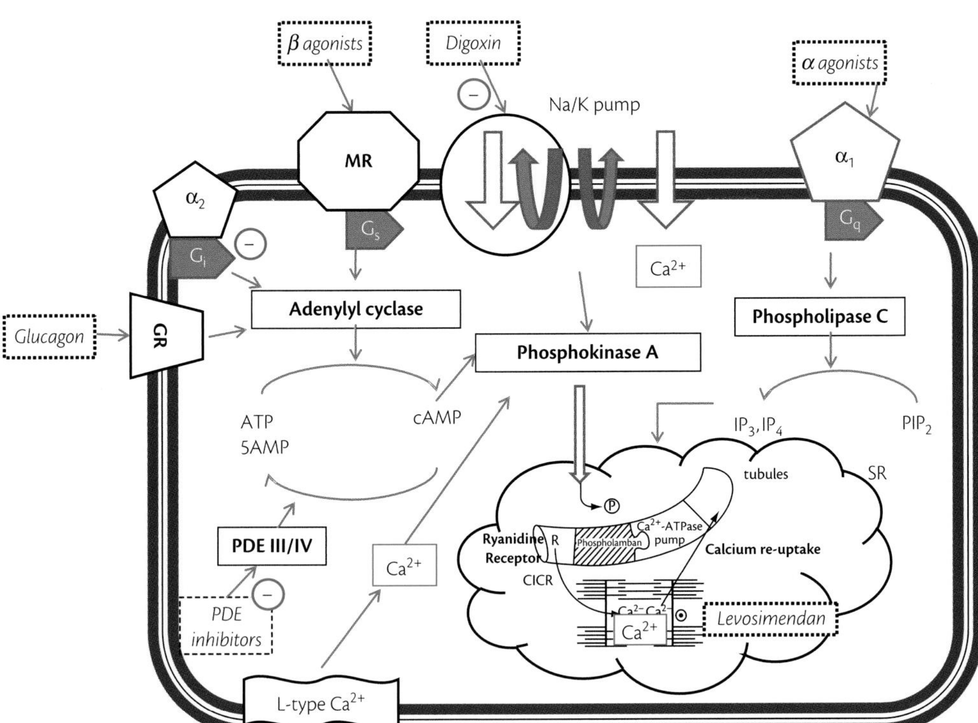

Fig. 44.1 Schematic representation of mechanism of action of inotropes on cardiac myocytes. Stimulation/inhibition of cell receptors alters enzyme (in black boxes) activity which in turn alters the availability of substrates to facilitate calcium entry into the sarcoplasmic reticulum and subsequent force of myocardial contraction. Agents affecting receptor or pump activity are shown in dotted boxes. α_1, alpha 1 adrenoreceptor; α_2, alpha 2 adrenoreceptor; Gx, various G proteins (s, i, q); MR, various myocyte receptors (including beta adrenoreceptors 5HT receptors, VIP, somatostatin, M2 muscurinic); GR, glucagon receptor; Na/K pump, sodium potassium exchange pump; θ, inhibits; Ca^{2+}, calcium; PDE, phosphodiesterase; SR, sarcoplasmic reticulum.

by increasing sensitivity to calcium. Inhibition of the ATPase-dependent Na^+/K^+ pump leads to a gradual increase in intracellular sodium. This in turn leads to a reduction in the exchange of intracellular calcium with extracellular sodium, thus increasing calcium stores in the sarcoplasmic reticulum (Fig. 44.1). The only currently used inotrope with such an action is the cardiac glycoside digoxin.[12] α_1-Receptor agonists (phenylephrine, methoxamine) act on myocardial α_1 receptors resulting in an increase in contractility via Gq protein-mediated increases in inositol phosphatase 3 and calcium release from the sarcoplasmic reticulum, additionally acting to sensitize the contractile proteins (Fig. 44.1). Finally, the myofilament calcium sensitizers (pimobendan, levosimendan) augment calcium binding to the calcium-specific regulatory site of cardiac troponin C, stabilizing calcium-induced conformational changes and thus inducing positive inotropy with no related change in intracellular calcium (Fig. 44.1).

Mechanisms of vascular dilatation and constriction

The vascular endothelium is highly complex, with synthetic and metabolic capabilities. It reacts to a variety of substances to produce vasodilatation or constriction (Fig. 44.2). The drugs used in the management of heart failure may have simultaneous dilator and constrictor effects depending upon the pathological process and the vascular bed studied, and differential effects on the arterial/venous and pulmonary/systemic circulations depending upon the distribution of receptors and the downstream signalling pathways. A number of mechanisms have been implicated in the mechanism of action of drugs used to modify vascular reactivity in heart failure including cAMP-dependent, cGMP-dependent and hyperpolarization-mediated dilatation/constriction. These mechanisms depend upon changes in intracellular calcium concentrations and/or myosin light chain phosphorylation, with an increase in intracellular calcium resulting in myosin light chain phosphorylation and thus sustained constriction.[6]

β_2-Adrenergic receptors mediate their dilatory effects on vascular tone by coupling to the Gs proteins resulting in an increase in adenylyl cyclase activity, and an increase in cAMP. The resultant PKA-mediated phosphorylation of myosin light chain kinase reduces the phosphorylation of myosin light chains themselves. α_1-Receptor agonists and vasopressin (via vascular V_1 receptors) mediate their effects by coupling with the G proteins. An increase in smooth muscle contractility results from Gq and Gi protein-mediated increase in inositol phosphatase 3, and calcium release from the sarcoplasmic reticulum. Nitric oxide donors (inducible NO, nitrates, and nitroprusside) reduce vascular tone via an increase in intracellular cGMP and protein kinase G activity, resulting in the dephosphorylation of myosin light chains. Neseritide acts by binding to the particulate guanylyl cyclase receptor of vascular smooth muscle and endothelial cells leading to increased intracellular cGMP and thus smooth muscle cell relaxation. Of note, the differential effects on the venous and arterial circulation reflect the relative concentration of guanylyl cyclase in the different vascular beds.

Inotropic agents

Inotropic agents are those which act predominantly by increasing cardiac contractility, although many have combined vasodilator or constrictor effects, depending upon the dosage used (Table 44.1). Numerous studies have failed to show reduced mortality with their use in AHF with some showing actual harm.[4,5] Routine administration of the drugs in AHF is thus not recommended, in particular where there is ongoing myocardial ischaemia. However, on occasion their transient use may be life-saving for individual, selected patients. Current guidelines recommend that their use be considered in patients with a low cardiac output state, in the presence of signs of

Table 44.1 Pharmacology of differing inotropes, vasodilators, and vasopressors

Agent	Site of action Receptor/ enzymes	Dosage		Onset	Duration	Metabolism	Elimination $t_{1/2}$	Clearance	Side effects/cautions
		Bolus	Infusion						
Vasodilators									
Nitroglycerines	NO donor (indirect via thiol) Catalyses cGMP Venous > arterial	Nil	10–20 μg/min Titrate up to 200 μg/min	Minutes	Short	Hepatic nitrate reductase & thiols	3 min	Liver	Hypotension, headache
Nitroprusside	NO donor (direct) Catalyses cGMP Arterial = venous	Nil	1 mg/hr Titrate upto 10 mg/hr	Minutes	Short	See text	Thiocyanate 2–7 days	Urine	Toxicity Metabolic acidosis ↑ScVO2
Nesiritide	Particulate GC	2 μg/kg	0.015–0.03 μg/kg/min	10 min	Short	See text	18 min	Urine Endopeptidase	Hypotension
Inotropes									
Dobutamine	$\beta_1\beta_2$	Nil	2–20 μg/kg/min	5 min	Short	COMT	2 min	Urine	Include: tachycardia arrhythmia hypotension hypertension myocardial ischaemia
Dopamine	DA1 DA2 $\beta_1\beta_2$ α	Nil	1–10 μg/kg/min	5 mins	10 min	MAO/ COMT Liver, kidney, blood	3 min	Urine	As Dobutamine plus: Vasoconstriction Bradycardia
Milrinone	PDE III/IV	25–75 μg/kg over 10–20 min	0.375–0.75 μg/kg/min	30 min	Medium	12% hepatic	1–2.5 h	Urine	As Dobutamine
Enoximone	PDE III/IV	0.25–0.75 mg/kg	1.25–7.5 μg/kg/min	30 min	Medium	Hepatic	4.5 h	Urine	As Dobutamine
Isoprenaline	$\beta_1\beta_2$		0.5–10 μg/min	Minutes	Short	COMT	2 h	Urine	
Levosimendan	Myofilaments Contractile proteins in SR	12 μg/kg over 10 min	0.1 μg/kg/min 0.05–0.2 μg/kg/min	12 min (bolus) 4 h (infusion)	Long	Hepatic Small bowel	80 h	Urine Faeces	Tachycardia Arrhythmia Hypotension
Vasopressors									
Noradrenaline	$\beta_1\alpha_1$	Nil	0.02–1 μg/kg/min	Minutes	Short	Uptake 1-MAO Circulation MAO/ COMT	2 mins	Urine	Hypertension Bradycardia Arrhythmia Vasoconstriction Decreased CO
Metaraminol	$\alpha_1 > \beta$	1–5 mg	5 μg/kg/min	Seconds	Short	Hepatic Unknown	Unknown	Urine Tissue uptake	As Noradrenaline
Phenyephrine	α_1 Partial	50–100 μg	40–180 μg/min	Seconds	10 min	Hepatic MAO GIT	2–3 h	Urine	As Noradrenaline
Methoxamine	α_1	1 mg	0.1–0.3 mg/min	Seconds	Minutes	Hepatic	Unknown	Unknown?urine	As Noradrenaline
Adrenaline	Cardiac β_1 Peripheral $\alpha_2\beta_2$	Nil Except in cardiac arrest	0.05–0.5 μg/kg/min	Minutes	Short	MAO/COMT Liver, kidney, blood	2 min	Urine	As Dobutamine and Noradrenaline plus: Lactic acidosis

α, alpha adrenoceptor; β, beta adrenoceptor; COMT, catechol-*O*-methyl transferase; DA, dopamine receptor; GC, guanylate cyclase; MAO, monoamine oxidase, NO, nitric oxide; PDE, phosphodiesterase; $ScVo_2$, mixed central venous oxygen saturations.

Table 44.2 Differing phosphodiesterase isoforms, target enzyme system, tissues expressing receptors, and inhibitor drugs (those shown in **bold** are directly relevant to the heart, and detailed further in the text)

Isoenzyme	Target	Tissues	Inhibitors
I	Calmodulin cGMP > cAMP	**Heart**, brain, kidney, liver, skeletal muscle, smooth muscle	Vinpocetine Phenothiazines
II	cGMP, cAMP	Adrenal cortex, brain, corpus cavernosum, **heart**, liver, kidney, airway smooth muscle, platelets	ENHA
III	cAMP>cGMP	**Heart**, corpus cavernosum, platelets, smooth muscle, liver, kidney, inflammatory cells (T&B lymphocytes, basophils, mast cells, monocytes, macrophages)	**Amrinone** Cilostamide Cilostazol Imadazodan **Milrinone** Motapizone Olprinone Pimobendam Piroximone
IV	cAMP	Kidney, lung, **heart**, skeletal muscle, smooth muscle (vascular, visceral, airway), platelets, inflammatory cells (T&B lymphocytes, basophils, mast cells, monocytes, macrophages, endothelial cells, eosinophils, neutrophils)	**Enoximone** Rolipram
III & IV	cAMP, CGMP	As above	Benafentrine Piclmilast Tibenelast Tolafentrine Zardavarine
VII	cAMP	Skeletal muscle, **heart**, kidney, airways, T&B lymphocytes, monocytes, eosinophils	Dipyridamole
Nonspecific	cAMP, adenosine		Caffeine Papaverine Theophylline

hypoperfusion or congestion despite the use of diuretics and/or dilators.[1,13,14] Additional recommendations are that inotropic drugs should be administered as early as possible and reduced or stopped as soon as adequate organ perfusion is restored. Such guidance demands a rapid diagnosis of inadequate cardiac output and of the presence of potentially reversible cause for deterioration.[1,3] Treatment algorithms based on the systolic blood pressure and estimated left-sided filling pressures are shown in Fig. 44.3.

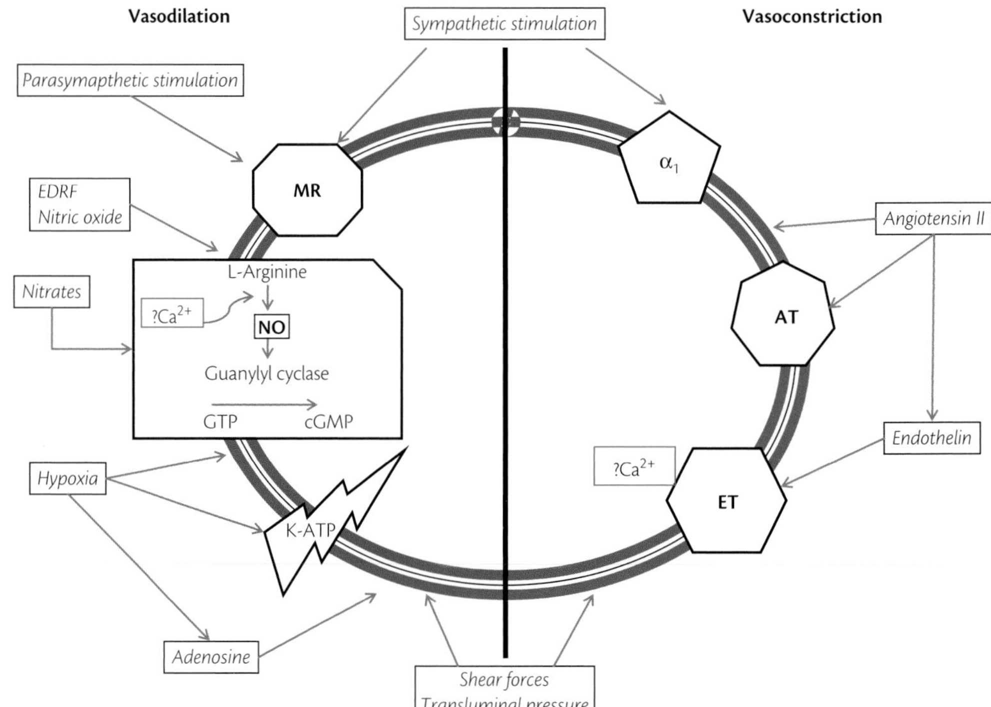

Fig. 44.2 Schematic representation of action of agents on vascular smooth muscle.
Vasomotor tone results from a balance between vasodilating and vasoconstricting factors which are secreted from and / or act upon vascular endothelial cells.
α_1, alpha 1 adrenoreceptor; MR, various myocyte receptors (including beta adrenoreceptors, 5HT receptors, VIP, somatostatin, M2 muscurinic); K-ATP, potassium ATPase channels; θ, inhibits; Ca^{2+}, calcium; AT, angiotensin receptors; ET, endothelin receptors

Dobutamine

A structural analogue of isoprenaline, dobutamine acts as an agonist at β_1- and β_2-receptors. It thus acts as an inotrope increasing cardiac output while also decreasing vascular resistance. Dobutamine can exacerbate tachycardia and tachyarrhythmias, and in the presence of hypovolaemia can result in profound hypotension. Dosage should be titrated up to 15 µg/kg/min according to clinical effect. When used in patients receiving concomitant β-blocker therapy, the dose may need to be increased to 20 µg/kg/min. Therapy should be weaned gradually while simultaneously optimizing oral therapy.[1]

Dopamine

A naturally occurring precursor of noradrenaline, at low doses (0.5–3 µg/kg/min) dopamine has its predominant activity on the doperminergic DA_1 and DA_2 receptors. At higher doses (3–10 µg/kg/min), its β_1 effects predominate, with some β_2-mediated peripheral vasodilatation, thus maintaining mean arterial pressure, venous capacitance and preload. Higher doses of dopamine should be used with caution as they are associated with an increasing risk of tachycardia, tachyarrhythmias, and α stimulation resulting in increased systemic vascular resistance.[1]

Milrinone and enoximone

Milrinone and enoximone are predominantly phosphodiesterase III inhibitors (PDEIs), acting as inodilators: that is, their use results in an increase in cardiac output and stroke volume with a concomitant reduction in pulmonary artery pressure, pulmonary capillary wedge pressure (PCWP), and systemic/pulmonary vascular resistance. As their site of action is downstream from the β receptors, they may be used in patients treated with concomitant use of β-blocker therapy. Milrinone and other PDEIs should be used with caution in patients with coronary artery disease (CAD) as there may be an increase in medium-term mortality.[4,15] Although milrinone has similar haemodynamic effects to dobutamine, there are some important differences. Milrinone has more significant vasodilatory effects, and appears to cause less tachycardia and increase in myocardial oxygen demand. Further, milrinone is renally cleared and has a longer half-life. It should, therefore, be used with caution in renal impairment. In certain circumstances, a loading dose can be used, although this is rarely done in practice because of the potential for provoking profound haemodynamic instability.[1]

Levosimendan

Levosimendan is a calcium sensitizer that exerts its inotropic effect by binding to troponin C in cardiomyocytes. It additionally causes significant vasodilatation through its action on ATP-sensitive potassium channels and has mild PDE inhibitory action at higher doses. Its haemodynamic effects are to increase cardiac output and stroke volume, and reduce PCWP and systemic/pulmonary vascular resistance. Because of metabolism to active metabolites, its haemodynamic effects persist for several days after discontinuation of treatment. Levosimendan should be used with caution in those with a relatively low systemic vascular resistance. As with milrinone, the drug may be loaded (although in the presence of haemodynamic instability the bolus should be omitted), and is effective even in the presence of β-blockade.

Adrenaline

An endogenous catecholamine formed by the methylation of noradrenaline, adrenaline acts on cardiac β_1- and peripheral α_1-receptors resulting in inotropic and vasoconstrictor effects. Adrenaline additionally acts as a constrictor of venous beds causing an increase in preload; however, peripheral β_2-receptor activation results in vasodilator activity. The net effect of adrenaline on systemic vascular resistance is thus less predictable than with noradrenaline. Adrenaline is also dromotropic (speeds conduction in the AV node), and bathmotropic (makes myocytes more electrically excitable). The potential adverse effects of adrenaline are thus (1) to increase myocardial work and oxygen consumption significantly, (2) to have proarrhythmogenic effects, and (3) to induce/exacerbate myocardial ischaemia. Further, stimulation of the Embden–Meyerhof pathway resulting in pyruvate production increases lactic acid, especially in the presence of an impaired citric acid cycle. Although adrenaline is not recommended for the routine treatment of AHF in current guidelines, it is frequently used at low doses in patients with severe refractory haemodynamic instability as a potentially life-saving measure, and as part of current advanced life support (ALS) guidelines in the management of cardiac arrest.[16]

Isoprenaline

Isoprenaline is a synthetic derivative of dopamine, with potent β_1 and β_2 effects. Its chronotropic effects predominate and it is therefore infrequently used as an inotrope, being more frequently used to provide a temporary increase in heart rate pending institution of definitive pacing, or whilst awaiting resolution of the bradycardia. One exception is in the presence of significant pulmonary hypertension where isoprenaline acts both as an inotrope and a pulmonary vasodilator.

Vasodilator agents

Vasodilators are recommended early in the treatment of AHF in the absence of hypotension (systolic blood pressure <90 mmHg) or severe obstructive valvular disease. However, there is a high incidence of side effects (Table 44.1). The effects of vasodilators are to reduce both right- and left-sided filling pressures and systemic vascular resistance, resulting in improved haemodynamics and symptoms. Coronary artery flow is usually not compromised unless either a steal phenomenon occurs, or the left ventricular end-diastolic pressure remains high despite a fall in diastolic blood pressure. Dosage and administration of the principal vasodilators used in AHF are shown in Table 44.1.

Organic nitrates

These are prodrugs that undergo complex biotransformation, predominantly in smooth muscle,[17] to form nitric oxide (NO) or S-nitrosothiol, which, via cGMP, result in venous and arterial vasodilatation. Clearance is by extraction, blood hydrolysis, or glutathione–nitrate reductase in the liver. Nitrates are administered as detailed in Table 44.1 and should be titrated up to maximum tolerated dosage. Potential haemodynamic effects include: reduction in right- and left-sided filling pressures; a fall in systemic and pulmonary vascular resistance; and a fall in systolic blood pressure. Therapy is usually associated with little or no change in heart rate, but results in an increase in cardiac output due to reduction in afterload, reversal in ischaemia and reduction in severity of any mitral regurgitation. Other effects are shown in Table 44.3. The limitations of nitrates include the development of resistance, with a marked attenuation of initial effects within hours of starting therapy in up to 50% of patients.[18–20]

Nitroprusside

Sodium nitroprusside is a potent vasodilator and is generally considered the standard against which other vasodilators are assessed. Comprising the sodium (or potassium) salt of a complex molecule containing a ferrous iron atom bound to five cyanide molecules and nitric acid, nitroprusside mediates its effects by decomposition to produce nitrosothiol on contact with red blood cells. This in turn generates cGMP in the vascular smooth muscle, resulting in NO-mediated vasodilatation. Clearance is via hepatic metabolism to thiocyanate, which is then renally excreted with a half-life of 3–4 days. The administration and dosage of nitroprusside is shown in Table 44.1. The haemodynamic effects of nitroprusside are to reduce systemic and pulmonary vascular venous tone, increase vascular compliance, and reduce afterload and any atrioventricular valvular regurgitation, with the net effect of increasing cardiac output. The main limitation of the drug relates to the toxicity of its metabolites (cyanide and thiocyanate), the presence of which are related to the dose and duration of therapy. Where toxicity is suspected (lactic acidosis, confusion, fits) thiocyanate toxicity should be suspected, and treated using haemofiltration.

Nesiritide

This recombinant DNA preparation of human ventricular brain natriuretic peptide (BNP) has an elimination half-life of 18 min.[21] Clearance is via binding to cell surface receptors, uptake and intracellular proteolysis, proteolytic cleavage via neutral endopeptidases within renal tubular and vascular cells, and renal filtration. The administration and dosage of nesiritide is shown in Table 44.1. The haemodynamic effects are to reduce venous tone, increase vascular compliance, and reduce systemic and pulmonary vascular resistance, with an increase in cardiac output. Other effects of nesiritide are shown in Table 44.3. The main limitations of its usage are hypotension and availability.

Although nesiritide has been widely used in the United States, it has not been licensed for use by the European regulatory authorities, at least partly because some preliminary studies suggest that it may worsen outcome.[22,23]

Vasopressin antagonists

The vasoconstrictor effects of arginine vasopressin have led to development of antagonists proposed for the use in AHF. A dual $V_{1a/2}$ vasopressin receptor antagonist (conivaptan) reduces PCWP and right atrial pressure, with no significant change in blood pressure, heart rate, cardiac output and pulmonary/systemic vascular resistance.[24] The use of vasopressin antagonists is not currently recommended routinely in the treatment of AHF.

Vasopressor agents

Vasopressor agents are not generally recommended in the management of AHF, but the use of vasodilator/inodilators drugs and/or the concomitant presence of sepsis in the critically ill patient with AHF may demand their use. Care must always be exercised to avoid an excessive increase in systemic vascular resistance resulting in a critical deterioration in cardiac output. Further, regional vasoconstriction in key vascular beds may result in life-threatening hypoperfusion which must be rapidly recognized.

Noradrenaline

Noradrenaline is a potent β_1- and α_1-agonist, causing peripheral vasoconstriction especially in the pulmonary and splanchnic beds. The α-mediated increase in systemic vascular resistance opposes its β-mediated inotropic effects, manifesting clinically with an increase in mean arterial pressure and a minor increase in heart rate, but little change in cardiac output. The effects of noradrenaline are dose related; in low doses the β effects are apparent, whereas in higher doses vasoconstrictive α effects predominate. The dose of noradrenaline should therefore be titrated to achieve a mean arterial pressure consistent with adequate end-organ perfusion, as excessive doses result in tissue ischaemia, progressive metabolic acidosis, and excessive systemic vascular resistance, resulting in a fall in cardiac output.

Table 44.3 Effects of agents on physiological variables

	CI	SV	HR	PCWP	MPAP	PVR	SBP	SVR	CSBF	MOC
Dopamine	↑	↑	↑↑	↔	↔	↔	↑↓	↓	↑	↑
Isoprenaline	↑	↑/↔	↑↑	↓	↓	↓	↓	↓↓	↓	↑
Noradrenaline	↑	↑	↓	↑	↑	↑↑	↑↑	↑↑	↑	↑
Adrenaline	↑	↑	↑	↑↓	↑	↑↓	↑	↑↓	↑	↑↑
Milrinone	↑	↑	↑	↓↓	↓↓	↓↓	↓	↓↓	↔	↑
Enoximone	↑	↑	↑	↓↓	↓↓	↓↓	↓	↓↓	↔	↑
Dobutamine	↑	↑	↑↑	↓	↓	↓	↓/↑	↓	↑	↑↑
Levosimendan	↑	↑	↑	↓	↓↓	↓↓	↓↓	↓	↑	↔
Nitroprusside	↑	↑	↑	↓	↓	↓	↓	↓	↑↓	↓
Neseritide	↑	↑	↔	↓	↓	↓	↓↓	↓	↑	↓
Phenylephrine	↑↓	↑	↓	↑	↑	↑	↑	↑	↓	↓
Metaraminol	↑↓	↑↓	↓	↓	↑	↑	↑	↑	↑	↑

CI, cardiac index; CSBF, coronary sinus blood flow; HR, heart rate; MOC, myocardial oxygen consumption; MPAP, mean pulmonary artery pressure; PCWP, pulmonary capillary wedge pressure; PVR, pulmonary vascular resistance; SBP, systolic blood pressure; SV, stroke volume; SVR, systemic vascular resistance; ↑, increase; ↔, equivocal; ↓, decrease.

Metaraminol/phenylephrine

These α-agonists cause a rise in systolic and diastolic pressures, a marked increase in systemic and pulmonary vascular resistance, and a concomitant decrease in cardiac output. Because of the profound constrictor effects and the fall in cardiac output associated with their administration, the only use of these drugs in AHF is in the emergency and short-term support of blood pressure in the periarrest situation or in cardiogenic shock, while definitive life-saving treatment is initiated.

Vasopressin

Arginine vasopressin is released from the posterior pituitary in response to increased serum osmolality or reduced plasma volume. Vasopressin becomes a constrictor in shock states, where its actions are to produce constriction in some vascular beds, and dilatation in others (renal, pulmonary, mesenteric, and vascular). The precise mechanisms are not well understood, but may include blockade of activated ATP-sensitive K^+ channels in vascular smooth muscle, a decrease in the NO second messenger cGMP, and stimulation of endothelin-1 synthesis. As with other constrictors, the use of vasopressin in AHF is generally limited to the short-term support of the circulation of the critically ill patient in whom there is profound and life-threatening vasodilatation, resistant to other agents.

Choice of vasoactive agent

Intravenous vasoactive agents may be indicated in patients with a low cardiac output state determined either clinically and/or by cardiac output monitoring. Their use should also be considered in the presence of significant pulmonary or peripheral congestion despite the appropriate use of diuretics and/or vasodilators. Algorithms to guide the institution of therapy and the potential choice of inotropic drug have been published,[1] but the choice and dose of inotropic drug must be tailored to the individual patient's circumstances (Fig. 44.3, Table 44.3). When considering the choice of vasoactive agent, several important principles apply. First, the heart should be considered as two pumps in series, with the effects of reducing and increasing the filling pressures of each considered independently. This is particularly relevant when a wide discrepancy exists between the stroke work equations of the right and left hearts. Second, the underlying pathophysiology of AHF must be considered and the precipitant or cause reversed where possible. Where ischaemia is present, positive inotropic agents which increase myocardial oxygen consumption should be avoided if the haemodynamics allow, and mechanical support maybe more beneficial. Finally, repeated re-evaluation of global and regional perfusion is required in order to optimize organ perfusion.

Future directions

There are marked limitations in the management of AHF using currently available vasoactive agents due to their many adverse effects. Novel agents with potential for short-term alternative pharmacological support are at varying stages of investigation. Istaroxime is a prototype of a new class of drug with two actions: it increases sarcoplasmic reticular calcium ATPase isoform 2a (SERCA 2a) activity and inhibits the Na^+,K^+-ATP pump. It thereby has inotropic and lusitropic activity with no increase in myocardial oxygen demand, and no adverse haemodynamic consequences.[25] Cardiovascular effects are to increase systolic blood pressure and reduce heart rate and PCWP, while increasing cardiac output.

Cinaciguat is a haem-independent activator of soluble guanylate cyclase, with a potentially more predictable vasodilator response

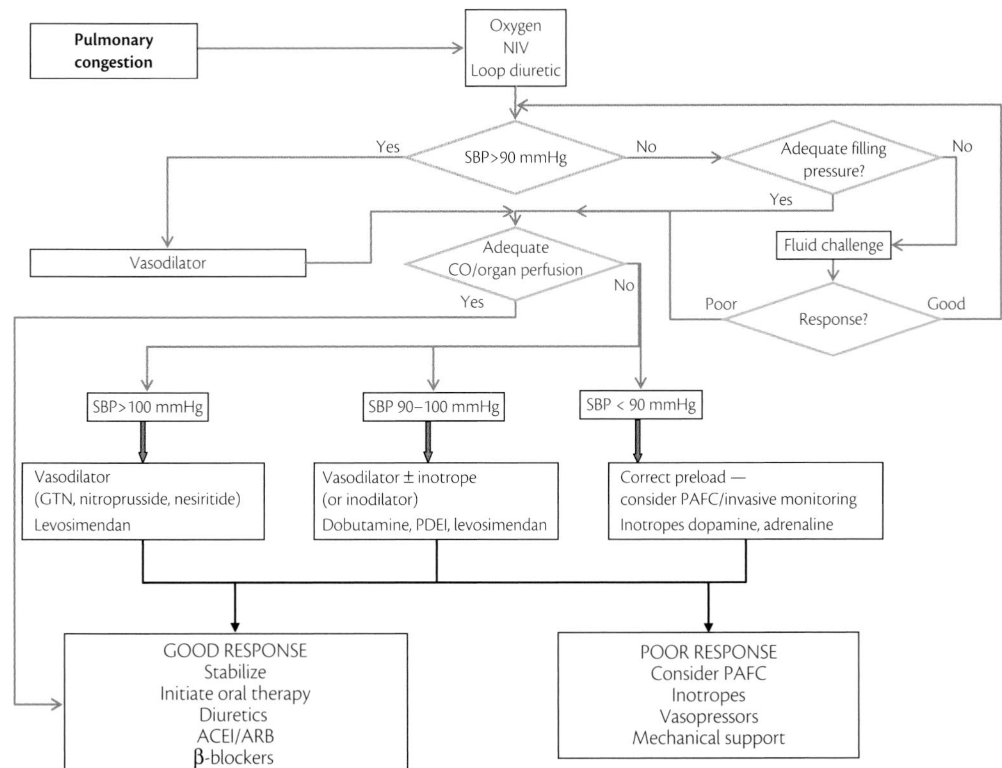

Fig. 44.3 Flowchart to aid selection of inotropic or vasodilator therapy depending on clinical status (systolic blood pressure, left atrial filling pressure, end organ perfusion) in pulmonary oedema due to acute heart failure or acute exacerbation of chronic heart failure.
NIV, Non Invasive Ventilation; SBP, systolic blood pressure; CO, cardiac output; PAFC, pulmonary artery flotation catheter; GTN, glyceral tri nitrate; PDEI, phosphodiesterase inhibitor; ACEI, Angiotensin converting enzyme inhibitor; ARB, angiotensin receptor blocker.

than established nitrate-based vasodilator therapies.[26] Chimeric natriuretic peptides are being developed, proposed to combine the beneficial effects of the different natriuretic peptides while avoiding their potentially detrimental effects, and reducing the risk of hypotension. Cardiac myosin activators are cardiac-specific myosin ATPase activators that may increase myocardial contractility by accelerating the phosphate-release step of the crossbridge cycle, thereby improving efficiency of the contractile apparatus.[27] Finally, peptide hormones, the urocortins, have been shown to exert inotropic and lusitropic effects by their binding to the CRH-R2 receptor on the myocardium and vascular endothelium.[28–31]

Although these drugs may offer alternative methods of positive inotropic support, they are all limited to short-term use in order to support the failing circulation while more definitive therapy is instigated. Further, their adverse side-effect profile, and requirement for close patient monitoring, demand that therapy be reduced as soon as the haemodynamic status of the patient allows, whilst instituting more standard oral therapy. Although some of the newer agents in development seem promising, modern demands for a high level of evidence showing outcome benefit will undoubtedly prove a significant hurdle in their widespread usage.

References

1. Dickstein K, Cohen-Solal A, *et al.* ESC Guidelines for the diagnosis, treatment of acute and chronic heart failure 2008: the Task Force for the Diagnosis and Treatment of Acute and Chronic Heart Failure 2008 of the European Society of Cardiology. Developed in collaboration with the Heart Failure Association of the ESC (HFA) and endorsed by the European Society of Intensive Care Medicine (ESICM). *Eur Heart J* 2008;**29**(19):2388–442.
2. Adams KF Jr, Fonarow GC, *et al.* Characteristics and outcomes of patients hospitalized for heart failure in the United States: rationale, design, and preliminary observations from the first 100,000 cases in the Acute Decompensated Heart Failure National Registry (ADHERE). *Am Heart J* 2005;**149**(2):209–16.
3. Abraham WT, Adams KF, *et al.* In-hospital mortality in patients with acute decompensated heart failure requiring intravenous vasoactive medications: an analysis from the Acute Decompensated Heart Failure National Registry (ADHERE). *J Am Coll Cardiol* 2005;**46**(1):57–64.
4. Felker GM, Benza RL, *et al.* Heart failure etiology and response to milrinone in decompensated heart failure: results from the OPTIME-CHF study. *J Am Coll Cardiol* 2003;**41**(6):997–1003.
5. Gheorghiade M, Gattis WA, *et al.* OPTIME in CHF trial: rethinking the use of inotropes in the management of worsening chronic heart failure resulting in hospitalization. *Eur J Heart Fail* 2003;**5**(1):9–12.
6. Evers AS, Maze M. *Anesthetic pharmacology: physiologic principles and clinical practice: a companion to Miller's Anesthesia.* Churchill Livingstone, Philadelphia, 2004.
7. Xiang Y, Kobilka BK. Myocyte adrenoceptor signaling pathways. *Science* 2003;**300**(5625):1530–2.
8. Xiao RP. Beta-adrenergic signaling in the heart: dual coupling of the beta2-adrenergic receptor to G(s) and G(i) proteins. *Sci STKE* 2001(104):re15.
9. Communal C, Singh K, *et al.* Opposing effects of beta(1)- and beta(2)-adrenergic receptors on cardiac myocyte apoptosis : role of a pertussis toxin-sensitive G protein. *Circulation* 1999;**100**(22):2210–12.
10. Zhu WZ, Zheng M, *et al.* Dual modulation of cell survival and cell death by beta(2)-adrenergic signaling in adult mouse cardiac myocytes. *Proc Natl Acad Sci U S A* 2001;**98**(4):1607–12.
11. Nikolaev VO, Moshkov A, *et al.* Beta2-adrenergic receptor redistribution in heart failure changes cAMP compartmentation. *Science* 2010;**327**(5973):1653–7.
12. Gheorghiade M, Pang PS. Acute heart failure syndromes. *J Am Coll Cardiol* 2009;**53**(7):557–73.
13. Jessup M, Abraham WT, *et al.* 2009 focused update: ACCF/AHA Guidelines for the Diagnosis and Management of Heart Failure in Adults: a report of the American College of Cardiology Foundation/ American Heart Association Task Force on Practice Guidelines: developed in collaboration with the International Society for Heart and Lung Transplantation. *Circulation* 2009;**119**(14):1977–2016.
14. Teerlink JR, Metra M, *et al.* Agents with inotropic properties for the management of acute heart failure syndromes. Traditional agents and beyond. *Heart Fail Rev* 2009;**14**(4):243–53.
15. Metra M, Nodari S, *et al.* Beta-blocker therapy influences the hemodynamic response to inotropic agents in patients with heart failure: a randomized comparison of dobutamine and enoximone before and after chronic treatment with metoprolol or carvedilol. *J Am Coll Cardiol* 2002;**40**(7):1248–58.
16. Nolan JP, Deakin CD, *et al.* European Resuscitation Council guidelines for resuscitation 2005. Section 4. Adult advanced life support. *Resuscitation* 2005;**67**(Suppl 1):S39–86.
17. Khot UN, Novaro GM, *et al.* Nitroprusside in critically ill patients with left ventricular dysfunction and aortic stenosis. *N Engl J Med* 2003;**348**(18):1756–63.
18. Elkayam U, Roth A, *et al.* Hemodynamic and volumetric effects of venodilation with nitroglycerin in chronic mitral regurgitation. *Am J Cardiol* 1987;**60**(13):1106–11.
19. Dupuis J, Lalonde G, *et al.* Tolerance to intravenous nitroglycerin in patients with congestive heart failure: role of increased intravascular volume, neurohumoral activation and lack of prevention with N-acetylcysteine. *J Am Coll Cardiol* 1990;**16**(4):923–31.
20. Elkayam U. Nitrates in the treatment of congestive heart failure. *Am J Cardiol* 1996;**77**(13):41–51C.
21. Elkayam, U., M. Janmohamed, *et al.* Vasodilators in the management of acute heart failure. *Crit Care Med* 2008;**36**(1 Suppl): S95–105.
22. Sackner-Bernstein JD, Kowalski M, Fox M, Aaronson K. Short-term risk of death after treatment with nesiritide for decompensated heart failure: a pooled analysis of randomized controlled trials. *JAMA* 2005;**293**:1900–5.
23. Sackner-Bernstein JD, Skopicki HA, Aaronson KD. Risk of worsening renal function with nesiritide in patients with acutely decompensated heart failure. *Circulation* 2005;**111**:1487–91.
24. Udelson JE, Smith WB, *et al.* Acute hemodynamic effects of conivaptan, a dual V(1A) and V(2) vasopressin receptor antagonist, in patients with advanced heart failure. *Circulation* 2001;**104**(20):2417–23.
25. Gheorghiade M, Blair JE, *et al.* Hemodynamic, echocardiographic, and neurohormonal effects of istaroxime, a novel intravenous inotropic and lusitropic agent: a randomized controlled trial in patients hospitalized with heart failure. *J Am Coll Cardiol* 2008;**51**(23):2276–85.
26. Lapp H, Mitrovic V, *et al.* Cinaciguat (BAY 58–2667) improves cardiopulmonary hemodynamics in patients with acute decompensated heart failure. *Circulation* 2009;**119**(21):2781–8.
27. Coletta AP Cleland JG, *et al.* Clinical trials update from Heart Rhythm 2008 and Heart Failure 2008: ATHENA, URGENT, INH study, HEART and CK-1827452. *Eur J Heart Fail* 2008;**10**(9):917–20.
28. Rademaker MT, Cameron VA, *et al.* Integrated hemodynamic, hormonal, and renal actions of urocortin 2 in normal and paced sheep: beneficial effects in heart failure. *Circulation* 2005;**112**(23):3624–32.
29. Davis ME, Pemberton CJ, *et al.* Urocortin 2 infusion in healthy humans: hemodynamic, neurohormonal, and renal responses. *J Am Coll Cardiol* 2007;**49**(4):461–71.
30. Davis ME, Pemberton CJ, *et al.* Urocortin 2 infusion in human heart failure. *Eur Heart J* 2007;**28**(21):2589–97.
31. Davidson SM, Rybka AE, *et al.* The powerful cardioprotective effects of urocortin and the corticotropin releasing hormone (CRH) family. *Biochem Pharmacol* 2009;**77**(2):141–50.

PART XIII

Nonpharmacological management

45

Cardiac rehabilitation and chronic heart failure

Massimo F. Piepoli and Andrew L. Clark

Introduction

All patients with established chronic heart failure (CHF), with or without an implantable cardioverter defibrillator (ICD) and with or without cardiac resynchronization therapy (CRT), require a multifactorial cardiac rehabilitation (CR) approach. The role of the multidisciplinary approach is considered elsewhere (see Chapter 54).

The traditional model of care delivery is thought to contribute to frequent hospitalizations. During these brief episodic encounters, little attention is paid to the numerous barriers to effective CHF treatment and the possible treatment of the common modifiable factors that are the cause of disease progression and thus hospital readmissions. To face these limitations, a CHF disease multidimensional management programme is necessary to curb the rising cost of management and to improve morbidity and mortality for individual patients.[1]

CR is the ideal comprehensive structured disease intervention since it best addresses the complex interplay of medical, psychological, and behavioural factors facing CHF patients. It is a co-ordinated multidimensional intervention designed to stabilize or slow disease progression, alleviate symptoms, improve exercise tolerance, and enhance quality of life, thereby reducing morbidity and mortality.[2] In CHF populations, such a programme has been proven to improve functional capacity, recovery and emotional well-being and to reduce hospital admissions in CHF patients.

Exercise training as a key component in a CR programme may improve survival and reduce hospitalization in stable heart failure (HF) patients. It is recommended for all stable CHF patients. There is no evidence that it should be limited to any particular HF patient subgroup based on aetiology, NYHA class, left ventricular function, or medication (class of recommendation I, level of evidence A).[3]

Despite the virtues of CR, only a small percentage of eligible HF patients ever get referred, due to barriers such as lack of physician and patient-family awareness of its benefits, and logistical or financial constraints. Patients with CHF are a patient population that challenges CR with the need to employ active strategies to disseminate and implement appropriate standards of care.

Core components of cardiac rehabilitation in chronic heart failure

Box 45.1 lists the core components of cardiac rehabilitation.

Clinical assessment and risk stratification

Careful history, physical examination, cardiac imaging, and biochemical assays are essential to describe fluid status and functional capacity accurately. Defining the severity of HF is vital before an appropriate rehabilitation programme can be started.[4,5] In particular, the following must be considered:

- Clinical history, including screening for cardiovascular risk factors, comorbidities, and disabilities. Likely concurrent problems such as claudication or cerebrovascular disease should be identified.
- Symptoms: what limits the patient on exertion—as well as using the NYHA class for dyspnoea severity, it is vital to know whether other symptoms are limiting the patient.
- Adherence to the medical regime and self-monitoring (weight, blood pressure, symptoms).
- Physical examination: general health status with particular care for haemodynamic and fluid status. Signs of congestion, or peripheral and central oedema suggest that further manipulation of diuretic therapy is necessary before an exercise regime can be prescribed safely. Blood pressure, heart rate and rhythm are also essential. Signs of cachexia should be sought: reduced muscle mass, muscle strength, and endurance will limit exercise capacity at least initially.
- ECG: heart rate, rhythm, QRS width, repolarization abnormalities, arrhythmias (particularly atrial fibrillation, AF).
- Blood testing for routine biochemical assay: serum electrolytes, urea, and creatinine should be monitored as part of usual care.
- Usual physical activity level is an important consideration. For some patients with a sedentary lifestyle, the idea of an exercise

Box 45.1 Core components of cardiac rehabilitation in chronic heart failure

- Clinical assessment and risk stratification
- Identification and treatment of causative factors and/or correction of precipitating factors (non-compliance to drug, non-steroidal anti-inflammatory and cyclooxygenase-2 inhibitors drug abuse, nasal decongestants, infection, pulmonary emboli, dietary indiscretion, inactivity, hyperthyroidism)
- Pharmacological therapy optimization
- Physical activity and exercise training programme
- Counselling and education: lifestyle, diet/nutritional, weight control, smoking cessation, self-monitoring
- Psychosocial support
- Planning of a continuum of care through an organized link between hospital and community

programme may be a startling departure. Domestic, occupational, and recreational needs should be explored; readiness to change behaviour and self-confidence should be assessed, together with describing any barriers to increased physical activity. Encouraging social support in making positive changes can be key for some patients.

- Exercise capacity: an assessment of exercise capacity before any exercise training regime is important. Maximal symptom-limited incremental cardiopulmonary exercise tests with metabolic gas exchange measurements are gold standard tools commonly used in research or in assessing patients for possible advanced therapies such as transplantation. Protocols with small increments (such as 5–10 W/min on a cycle ergometer or modified Bruce or Naughton protocols on a treadmill) are indicated. Other tests such as the six- or twelve-minute walk tests are perfectly reasonable in daily practice to assess exercise tolerance and have the merit of perhaps more resembling normal life for the patient.
- Education: clear, comprehensible information on the basic purpose of the CR programme and the role of each component should be provided to each patient.

The assessment should lead to the formulation of a tailored, patient-specific, treatment plan and document short-term goals within the core components of care that guide intervention strategies.

Identification and treatment of causative factors and/or correction of precipitating factors

Coexisting conditions are responsible for 40% of preventable hospital readmission. Causative factors (which include hypertension, coronary artery disease, arrhythmias), and precipitating factors (such as noncompliance with drug treatment; abuse of non-steroidal anti-inflammatory drugs (NSAIDs), cyclooxygenase-2 inhibitors; and nasal decongestants; infection; pulmonary emboli; dietary indiscretion; inactivity; hyperthyroidism) must be clearly identified. As the disease progresses and the patient ages, medication and remedies directed at the underlying pathology may be less relevant and the need for treatment of coexisting symptoms may outweigh the possible adverse consequences of some therapies for HF care.

Pharmacological therapy optimization

According to clinical assessment, medical therapy should be oriented to achieve normal jugular venous pressure, resolution of orthopnea and oedema, systolic blood pressure of at least 80 mmHg, stable renal function, and the ability to walk the hospital ward without dizziness or dyspnoea.

Attendance at supervised exercise training sessions makes it possible to ensure that the patient is taking appropriate medical therapy. Treatment must be tailored according to the individual characteristics with the goal of prescribing according to international guidelines with adequate doses. A careful upward dosage titration is required in the introduction of both angiotensin converting enzyme (ACE) inhibitors and β-blockers up to the highest tolerated dosages. The up-titration schedule usually extends into the convalescent period after the patient has been discharged from the hospital.

The simultaneous presence of competing comorbidities further complicates pharmacological management. The ever-increasing complexity of polypharmacotherapy is intimidating, meaning that some therapies may not to be used, especially by practitioners who lack the time and expertise to pursue the kind of 'micromanagement' required with complex regimens. Although little evidence is available to guide polypharmacotherapy, collaborative disease management programmes (such as those provided in the CR setting) that include a careful review of medications can be very helpful for patients with chronic HF and multiple comorbidities.[6]

Educating patients about their condition and motivating their adherence to a course of therapy are steps towards success. A clear and comprehensible explanation of the basic purpose and action of each drug is required. Patients' understanding and adherence of drug regiment should be periodically refreshed.

Physical activity and exercise training programme

As the CHF syndrome starts and develops, the natural tendency for patients is to do whatever seems reasonable to avoid symptoms. Hence the recognition that effort induces undue breathlessness leads to progressive inactivity, contributing to skeletal muscle detraining and general unfitness that contribute to further progression of the HF syndrome. A sedentary lifestyle, with little or no physical activity during leisure time or at work, is a risk factor for the development and progress of cardiovascular disease.[7,8]

Rest as therapy in chronic heart failure

For many years, standard medical advice was that exercise should be avoided for patients with CHF, with standard textbooks containing such advice as, 'Reduced physical activity is critical in the care of patients with HF throughout their entire course'.[9] There are some small studies suggesting that rest as a specific intervention may have some modest beneficial effects in terms of reducing heart size,[10–12] but these studies were carried out at a time when modern medical therapy was in its infancy and CHF had an exceptionally high mortality rate. A common problem with long-term rest has been thromboembolic complications and sudden death. Rest as an intervention has not been trialled in the modern therapeutic era.

Safety of exercise training in chronic heart failure

Part of the concern about exercise comes from the possibility that it might be dangerous, particularly in patients with underlying ischaemic heart disease. The increased wall stress imposed by exercise might be expected to result in further cardiac enlargement. An influential paper reported on the effects of training in patients who had had a moderate-sized anterior myocardial infarct.[13] There appeared to be some echocardiographic evidence of worsening cardiac function despite an improvement in exercise capacity. Further work in animal models[14] suggested that training may worsen left ventricular function.

These observations were alarming: no treatment that worsens left ventricular function is likely to confer long-term benefit. However, the Judgutt study was relatively small, uncontrolled, and used a strenuous training programme. A key study was the EAMI trial in which 95 patients were randomized following an anterior myocardial infarction to a training regime or usual therapy. Although patients with a lower left ventricular ejection fraction (LVEF) at study entry showed ventricular enlargement after 6 months, there was no difference between the control and training groups.[15] Similar findings have been reported elsewhere,[16] and data from the longer term ELVD-CHF study suggested that training actually reduced left ventricular volumes and increased LVEF.[17]

Training might, of course, have some other dangerous effects, such as potentially increasing the risk of ventricular arrhythmias. Most of the early studies in the field used carefully supervised training regimes in carefully selected patients. Incremental exercise testing in patients with CHF is safe,[18,19] and now that large studies of relatively unselected and unsupervised patients have been conducted, the safety of training is established.[20]

Training in other patient groups

The benefits of exercise training for patients with ischaemic heart disease,[21] and following myocardial infarction,[22,23] have been known for many years. Training can actually improve left ventricular systolic function in 'normal' older men,[24] and rehabilitation is helpful after cardiac events in older people,[25,26] the population most likely to suffer from CHF. Training apparently improves endurance exercise more than peak exercise capacity,[27] the very improvement likely to have the greatest symptomatic benefit for older patients who rarely if ever need to undertake maximal exercise. Given the effects of ageing on muscle strength and bulk, it is not surprising that training might be more generally helpful in older subjects.[28]

The nature of these studies means that they must have included many patients with significant left ventricular impairment, and the lack of cardiac complication in the studies is further evidence that training is safe.

Rationale for training in patients with chronic heart failure

Although the pathophysiology of CHF is commonly discussed principally in terms of changes to central haemodynamic function, much research over the last 20 years or so has emphasized the fact that CHF is a multisystem disorder with abnormalities affecting many body systems from the central nervous system to bowel wall function to immunological function. The greatest contributor to exercise limitation appears to be changes to skeletal (rather than cardiac) muscle function (see discussions in Chapter 2 and Chapter 33).

A striking feature of the peripheral changes seen is how closely they resemble the effects of detraining in normal subjects. Activation of the renin–angiotensin[29] and sympathetic[30] systems, loss of skeletal muscle bulk, and depletion of oxidative enzymes[31,32] are all seen in both conditions (see Table 45.1). Given the apparent safety of training regimes, the similarity of CHF to detraining, and the beneficial effects of training in very similar patient groups, training as a specific intervention for CHF patients was an inevitable progression.

Early studies

Early uncontrolled work including patients with severe left ventricular dysfunction showed promising results.[33,34] Sullivan and colleagues[35,36] were amongst the first to assess training systematically, and found that a training regimen improved exercise capacity by around 20% (as assessed by peak oxygen consumption). An important observation was that central haemodynamics at matched workloads was unchanged after training, and the changes responsible were presumably peripheral as reflected in a fall in arterial and venous lactate during exertion.

In a crossover trial, Coats and coworkers[37,38] demonstrated that exercise training improved exercise capacity by a similar proportion and helped improve symptoms.

Since these pioneering studies, the beneficial effects of training on peak exercise capacity have been repeatedly confirmed, and, indeed, the effects are greater than (and additive to) the effects of ACE inhibitors.[39]

Benefits of training

Gas exchange and ventilation

Training programmes produce a variety of improvements in HF patients, not simply an improvement in peak exercise capacity. There is improvement in endurance exercise capacity and an increase in both anaerobic and ventilatory thresholds.[36,40] In addition, the increased ventilatory response to exercise (as reflected in the increase in the relation between ventilation and carbon dioxide production) is improved by training,[41] an effect not seen in normal subjects.[42] Ventilation at matched submaximal workloads is reduced by training.[36,43] Peak exercise ventilation is increased, reflecting the increased overall exercise capacity following training.[44]

Table 45.1 Similarities between the chronic heart failure syndrome and detraining in normal subjects

	Detraining	Heart failure
Heart rate	↑	↑
Exercise capacity	↓	↓
Muscle size	↓	↓
Muscle enzymes	↓	↓
Sympathetic	↑	↑
Renin:angiotensin	↑	↑
Heart rate variability	↓	↓

Exercise capacity

As well as increasing maximal exercise capacity, training regimes also improve submaximal exercise capacity. This is perhaps a more important observation, as patients rarely encounter peak exertion in daily life. Training induces an increase both in the duration of exercise at a fixed workload,[36] and an increase in the distance covered in a six-minute walk test.[40,45]

Quality of life

Quality of life measures are consistently improved by training, which is not something necessarily seen with all treatments that improve prognosis. The effect on quality of life may be more important than effects on abstract measures that do not really reflect day-to-day life. Patients self assessment scores during exercise tests are improved,[37,40] and there are improvements in anxiety and depression following training.[46]

The best evidence for the effects of training on quality of life comes from the HF-ACTION study. Using the Kansas City Cardiomyopathy Questionnaire, the investigators found a marked benefit on quality of life persisting through the 3 years of the study (see Fig. 45.1).[47] The effect was the same regardless of the aetiology of the HF.

Sympathovagal balance

The abnormal sympathovagal balance of CHF is improved by training as shown by an increase in heart rate variability and reduction in noradrenaline spillover.[37] There is an improvement in circadian variability of heart rate in some studies,[48] although others have reported that only daytime heart rate variability is increased.[43]

Neurohormonal effects

Training has a beneficial effect on the neurohormonal activation of CHF causing reductions in angiotensin, aldosterone, and arginine vasopressin.[49] It can also reduce sympathetic activation and natriuretic peptide levels.[50]

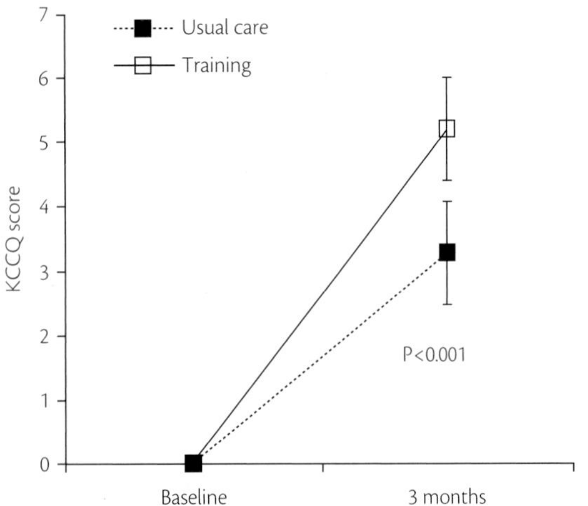

Fig. 45.1 Legend. Improvement in quality of life using the Kansas City Cardiomyopathy Questionnaire (KCCQ) in the HF-ACTION study at three months. The higher the score, the better the quality of life. Error bars indicate standard errors at each time point.

Data from Flynn KE, Piña IL, Whellan DJ, *et al.* Effects of exercise training on health status in patients with chronic heart failure: HF-ACTION randomized controlled trial. *JAMA* 2009;**301**:1439–50.

Haemodynamic effects

As a consequence of increasing exercise performance, training has been found in many studies to increase maximal cardiac output and heart rate. The effects on submaximal cardiac output is not completely clear: most investigators suggest that at matched workload, cardiac output is unchanged by training,[35,43] but some have reported modest increases.[37] It is unlikely that changes to cardiac output mediate any benefit, however, as most patients have normal cardiac output responses to submaximal exercise before training.[51,52]

There is some evidence to suggest that training might improve diastolic cardiac function with improved early diastolic filling and increases in peak filling rates at matched heart rates during exercise.[53,54] Other changes include a reduction in both cardiac volume and systemic vascular resistance together with increased endothelium-dependent vasodilation.[55,56] That arm vasodilation is improved after leg training[57] suggests that there are some structural effects of training on the vasculature.[58]

Effects on skeletal muscle

Studies examining skeletal muscle histology have shown that mitochondrial density is increased by training, along with a shift back towards type I muscle fibres and an increase in the ratio of capillaries to myocytes.[59–61] Many of these changes correlate with the improvement in exercise capacity seen, suggesting that the mechanism for improvement lies with changes to skeletal muscle rather than in any haemodynamic changes. Additional effects include a decrease in myocyte phosphocreatine depletion during exercise, and a shortening in the recovery time of phosphocreatine following exercise.[62] Selective training of ventilatory muscle can also be beneficial.[63]

Other effects in skeletal muscle include an increase in insulin-like growth factor,[64] suggesting that the insulin resistance of HF may be partially reversible by training. In addition, training also has a general antioxidant effect in skeletal muscle with an increase in skeletal muscle antioxidant enzymes.[65] A potential link to the improvement in exercise capacity and reduction in ventilatory response induced by training is via the abnormal activation of the ergoreflexes[66] closely associated with the abnormal exercise physiology of patients with CHF: the ergoreflex is reduced by training.[67]

Type and intensity of exercise

Formal studies of training have generally used quite strenuous training stimuli. Different studies have used different techniques ranging from home cycle training to supervised rowing (Table 45.2).

The effects of isometric exercise seem to be broadly unfavourable in CHF, with adverse haemodynamic consequences.[68,69] However, a resistive component of a training regime does seem to produce benefits above what is gained from endurance training alone.[70] It may even be possible to achieve some benefits with very localized training,[71] including of respiratory muscle alone.[63]

The strenuous endurance approach is reasonably easy to follow for supervised patients in short-term clinical trials, but is not be broadly applicable for most patients with CHF. There is some evidence that rather more gentle regimes can have a beneficial effect.

Table 45.2 Early studies of exercise training in chronic heart failure to show the type and intensity of exercise typically used

Lead author	Type of training	Intensity of training	Frequency	Duration	S/U	↑Peak Vo_2
Sullivan[35]	Cycle, walking	75%	60 min, 3–5/week	16–24 w	S	23%
Coats[37]	Cycle	60–80%	20 min, 5/week	8 w	U	18%
Meyer[40]	Cycle, walking (interval[a])	50%	45 min, 11/week	3 w	S	20%
Kiilavuori[43]	Walking, cycling	55%	30 min, 3/week	6 mo	S, 3 mo U, 3 mo	12%
Keteyian[44]	Treadmill, cycle, rowing	60–80%	45 min, 3/week	24 w	S	16%
Kavanagh[76]	Walking	55%	10–21 km/week	52 w	Initially S[b]	17%
Hambrecht[59]	Cycle	near max	40 min daily	6 mo	S, 3w U, 6 mo[c]	33%
Belardinelli[72]	Cycle	40%	30 min, 3/week	8 w	S	17%
Demopoulos[45]	Cycle	<50%	60 min, 4/week	12 w	S	22%

[a] Interval training is characterized by repeated short bursts of exercise with recovery periods between.
[b] Initially supervised, but then mainly home based with regular review visits.
[c] Additional twice weekly supervised group sessions.
S, supervised; U, unsupervised.

Belardinelli *et al.*[72] found beneficial effects in patients with mild CHF with low-intensity training at only 40% of peak oxygen consumption, a finding confirmed in patients with more severe HF who trained at low workloads (<50% of maximal) using supine cycle exercise in a deliberate attempt to minimize ventricular wall stress.[45]

A further consideration is that most patients with CHF are elderly, and many have comorbidities that will greatly limit their capacity to take part in formal training programmes. One possible alternative approach is that of electrical muscle stimulation. It is possible to induce painless muscle contraction using large electrode plates, and devices can be programmed to deliver stimulation to several large muscle groups in the legs (quadriceps, gluteals, and hamstrings).[73] In normal subjects, such a device can have a training effect,[74] and we have shown that electrical muscle stimulation can have a beneficial training effect in patients with CHF (Fig. 45.2).[75] Whether programmed electrical muscle stimulation leads to prolonged benefits is not yet known.

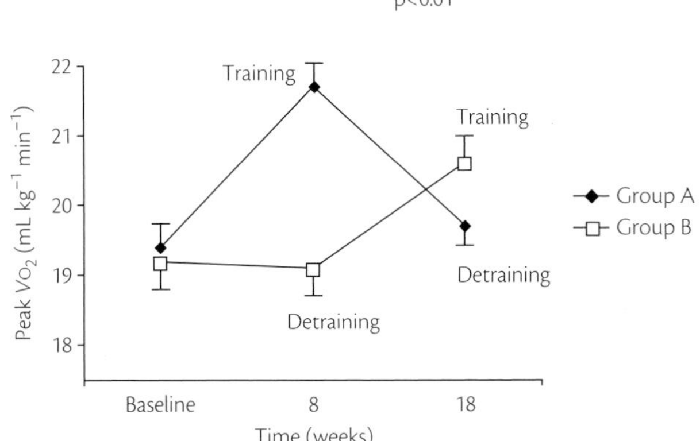

Fig. 45.2 The improvement in peak oxygen capacity (Vo_2) seen after training using programmed muscle stimulation.
Data from Banerjee P, Caulfield B, Crowe L, Clark AL. Prolonged electrical muscle stimulation exercise improves strength, peak Vo_2, and exercise capacity in patients with stable chronic heart failure. *J Card Fail* 2009;**15**:319–26, with permission.

Duration of benefit

An important observation is that the improvement in exercise capacity is proportional to compliance with the training regime.[38] That the benefits are not just short-term gains was confirmed by Kavanagh[76] who demonstrated that the effects lasted for at least a year, reaching a plateau at around 16 weeks–6 months. The HF-ACTION study demonstrates that the benefits of training persist for longer—up to 3 years.[47]

Effect on mortality

A key question has been whether the apparently beneficial changes seen in the multitude of relatively small-scale studies translate into improvements in outcome. The ExTraMATCH collaborative[77] included 801 patients who had been randomized into trials of exercise training. Follow-up was limited to just over 700 days, but there was a strong suggestion that patients randomized to training were not only less likely to be admitted to hospital, but had a better prognosis (Fig. 45.3).

Mounting a sufficiently large study to answer the question definitively has been very difficult, in part because of the problem of sponsorship, and in part because of the difficulty of running the trial. Blinding the intervention is, of course, impossible, and many patients randomized to usual care are likely to take up exercise once included in any study. There are also likely to be problems with drop-outs: compliance with the training regime is difficult to monitor, and it is easier for individual patients to resile from training than, say, from a drug trial—where the randomization and blinding makes it far less likely that crossovers will be a problem.

The HF-ACTION study[20] randomized 2331 patients to receive a training programme or usual care. The training programme consisted of 36 supervised 30-min sessions three times per week followed by home exercise five times per week at moderate intensity for 40 min. The control group was simply encouraged

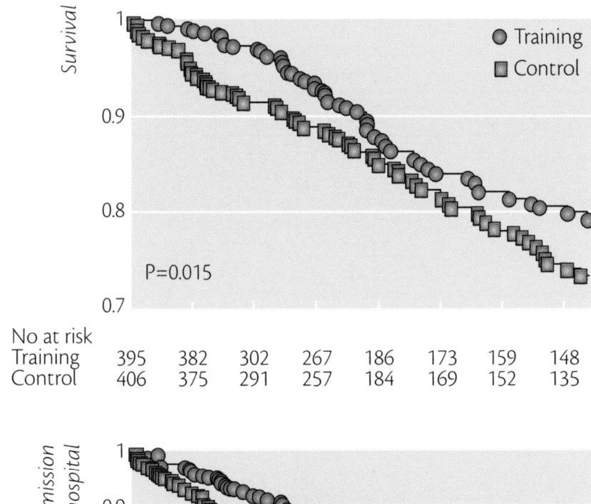

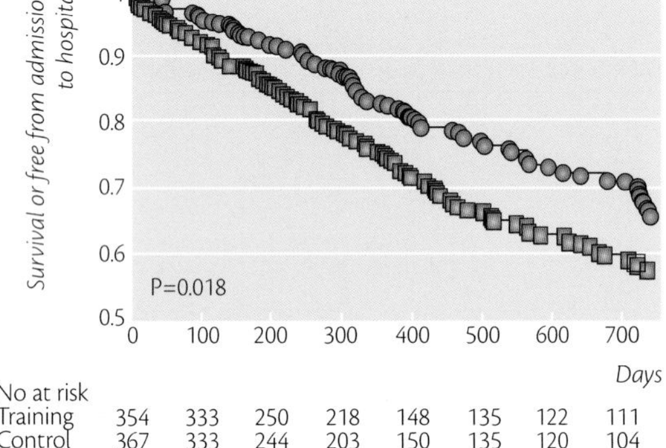

Fig. 45.3 Data from the ExtraMatch collaborative suggesting that exercise training was associated with a better outcome in patients with chronic heart failure.
Reprinted from *BMJ* 2004;**328**:189

to take exercise. The primary endpoint was all-cause death and hospitalization.

Although the training group had a marked improvement in exercise capacity over the course of the trial, there was no effect on the primary endpoint. However, when adjustment was made for other prognostic indicators, there was a modest benefit in favour of training. The effect appears to be modest, but should be set in the context that at 3 years, only 30% of patients in the intervention limb were adhering to the recommended 120 min/week, and the median exercise duration per week was only around 50 min. The additional benefit of striking improvement in long-term quality of life[47] means that a structured exercise programme should now be part of the routine management of patients with CHF.

Approach to the patient

Improving adherence to a physical activity and exercise training programme is vital: without compliance, the programme is worthless. A step-by-step approach is helpful.

Assessment

Assess current physical activity level and determine domestic, occupational, and recreational needs. Evaluate activities relevant to age, sex, and daily life. Assess readiness to change behaviour, self-confidence, barriers to increased physical activity, and social support in making positive changes.

Educational processes and support

- A minimum of 30–60 min/session of moderately intense aerobic activity, preferable daily, or at least 3–4/week. Supervised group activity is helpful initially for many patient to restore confidence (many will have been told by well-meaning friends or family to 'take it easy'), and to allow the mutually supportive atmosphere that comes with having many patients facing the same challenges together.
- Emphasize sedentary lifestyle as risk factor, and benefits of physical activity: any increase in activity has a positive health benefit.
- Recommend gradual increases in daily lifestyle activities over time, and how to incorporate it into daily routine.
- Advise individualize physical activity according to patient's age, past habits, comorbidities, preferences, and goals.
- Reassure regarding the safety of the recommended protocol.
- Encourage involvement in leisure activities which are enjoyable and in a group exercise training programme, as patients tend to revert to previous sedentary habits over time.
- Forewarn patients of the risk of relapses: thus education should underline how benefits may be achieved and the need for its lifelong continuation. If physical activity interruption has occurred, physical, social and psychological barriers to attendance should be explored, and alternative approaches suggested.[78]

Exercise programme

- Initial stage: intensity should be kept at a low level (40–50% of peak exercise capacity), increasing duration from 15 to 30 min, 2–3 times/week according to perceived symptoms and clinical status for the first 1–2 weeks.
- Improvement stage: a gradual increase of intensity (50%, 60%, 70%, to 80% of peak exercise capacity, as tolerated) is the primary aim. Prolongation of exercise session is a secondary goal.

The expected outcomes from exercise training programmes are highlighted in Box 45.2.

Specific issues

Exercise training and β-blockers

There is some obvious difficulty in determining heart rate targets in patients taking β-blockers. Patients on β-blockers benefit to the same extent as those not taking them,[79,80] and in HF-ACTION, nearly 95% of patients were taking a β-blocker at baseline. The

Box 45.2 Expected outcomes from exercise training programmes for patients with chronic heart failure

- Increased participation in domestic, occupational, and recreational activities
- Improved psychosocial well-being, prevention of disability, and enhancement of opportunities for independent self-care, improved aerobic fitness
- Increased cardiorespiratory fitness and enhanced flexibility, muscular endurance, and strength
- Reduction of symptoms and attenuated physiological responses to physical challenges

heart rate at maximum exertion at baseline allows an appropriate target heart rate for training to be determined.

Exercise training and atrial fibrillation

The key here is to make sure that there is adequate control of ventricular rate during exercise. Almost always, a β-blocker will be needed to control heart rate rather than simply digoxin alone. In HF-ACTION, just over one-fifth of the patients had AF at baseline, and there is no reason to exclude patients with AF from a training regime.

Exercise training and patients with an implantable cardioverter-defibrillator

There are only limited data available, but there appear to be no adverse consequences for patients with ICDs undergoing a training programme.[81,82] There is a risk of device discharge from a rapidly accelerating heart rate,[82] and certainly to start with, supervision by qualified staff is important, particularly to monitor the heart rate response to exercise. Training intensity should be determined by the heart rate response and established at a level to increase the heart rate to between 20 and 30 beats below the ICD detection rate.

Counselling and education

The role of the multidisciplinary team in delivering counselling and education is considered elsewhere. In relation to the exercise component, however, some factors are particularly important.

Obesity

Obesity has numerous adverse effects on haemodynamics and cardiac structure and function. On the other hand, obese chronic HF patients have a better prognosis than underweight patients.[83,84] Obesity should not be seen as a contraindication to exercise training, and training may help weight control.

Cigarette smoking

Smoking should be strongly discouraged in CHF patients. In addition to the well-established adverse effects on coronary artery disease, which is the underlying cause in a substantial proportion of patients, smoking has adverse haemodynamic effects in patients with CHF, including increase heart rate and systemic blood pressure, mild increase in pulmonary artery pressure, ventricular filling pressure, and total systemic and pulmonary vascular resistance. Increased peripheral vasoconstriction may contribute to a mild reduction of stroke volume. Finally, in CHF patients, enhanced broncopathic susceptibility and breathing problems precipitate or aggravate HF.

Psychosocial management

Depression is extremely common in the HF population,[40] with a wide range of quoted prevalence rates across studies due to the use of different diagnostic instruments and the inclusion of different patient populations. Treatment of depression is an important clinical strategy as it is associated with more frequent hospital admissions, decline in activities of daily living, worse NYHA functional classification, and increased medical costs. However, depression commonly goes undiagnosed.

The depressed patient is far less likely to comply with a training regimen, and its recognition at an early stage is important. Patients may be unwilling to disclose emotional distress to their physicians for fear of being stigmatized with the label of mental illness. On the other hand, physicians may not address depression because they have not been adequately trained to recognize both typical and atypical depressive symptoms, because of time constraints in high-volume settings, or because they do not know how best to treat the condition. Recognition and management of depression may be enhanced through the use of multidisciplinary team or disease management programmes.[85,86]

Continuum of care

A good cardiac rehabilitation programme is characterized by a continuum of services that spans inpatient and outpatient rehabilitation.

Inpatients

Inpatient rehabilitation should begin as soon as possible after hospital admission and should be part of routine daily care for every HF inpatient. The main elements are appropriate strategies for optimal therapy; education with full participation of patient/caregiver; reassurance and support; mobilization when possible; and group education, according to clinical assessment and risk stratification. Progression of mobilization should be developed according to the patient's clinical condition, functional capacity, age, and comorbidity under careful medical review and supervision.

Outpatients

As the length of stay for acute HF and procedures continues to decrease, patient and family attendance in outpatient cardiac rehabilitation assumes even greater importance. Structured outpatient cardiac rehabilitation is a crucial point for the development of a lifelong approach to prevention. Attendance should start soon after discharge from the hospital. Outpatient cardiac rehabilitation may be provided in a range of settings, such as HF clinics, non-clinic settings (community health centres and general medical practices), or a combination of these. It may also be provided on an individual basis at home, including a combination of home visits, telephone support, telemedicine, and specially developed self-education materials.

The main elements of outpatient cardiac rehabilitation include assessment, review and follow-up, therapy optimization, low or moderate intensity physical activity and exercise training, education, discussion and counselling.

Continued care

Evaluation of ongoing cardiac rehabilitation programme objectives on a regular basis is a key to success.

References

1. Corrà U, Giannuzzi P, Adamopoulos S, *et al.* Executive summary of the position paper of the Working Group on Cardiac Rehabilitation and Exercise Physiology of the European Society of Cardiology (ESC): core components of cardiac rehabilitation in chronic heart failure. *Eur J Cardiovasc Prev Rehabil* 2005;**12**(5):321–5.
2. Piepoli MF, Corrà U, Benzer W, *et al.* Secondary prevention through cardiac rehabilitation: from knowledge to implementation. A Position Paper from the Cardiac Rehabilitation Section of the European Association of Cardiovascular Prevention and Rehabilitation. *Eur J Cardiovasc Prev Rehabil* 2010;**17**(1):1–17.

3. Task Force for Diagnosis and Treatment of Acute and Chronic Heart Failure 2008 of European Society of Cardiology, Dickstein K, Cohen-Solal A, Filippatos G, *et al.* ESC Guidelines for the diagnosis and treatment of acute and chronic heart failure 2008: the Task Force for the Diagnosis and Treatment of Acute and Chronic Heart Failure 2008 of the European Society of Cardiology. Developed in collaboration with the Heart Failure Association of the ESC (HFA) and endorsed by the European Society of Intensive Care Medicine (ESICM). *Eur Heart J* 2008;**29**(19):2388–442.
4. Hunt SA, Baker DW, Chin MH, *et al.* ACC/AHA guidelines for the evaluations and management of chronic heart failure in the adult: a report of the American College of Cardiology/American Heart Association Task Force on Practice Guidelines. *J Am Coll Cardiol* 2001;**38**:2101–13.
5. The 2001 Canadian cardiovascular society consensus guidelines update for the management and prevention of heart failure. *Can J Cardiol* 2001;**17**(suppl E):5–25E.
6. Masoudi FA, Krumholz HM. Polipharmacy and comorbidity in heart failure. *BMJ* 2003;**327**:514–15.
7. Exercise and physical activity in the prevention and treatment of atherosclerotic cardiovascular disease. A statement from the Council on Clinical Cardiology (subcommittee on Exercise, Rehabilitation, and Prevention) and the Council on Nutrition, Physical Activity, and Metabolism (subcommittee on Physical Activity). *Circulation* 2003;**107**:3109–16.
8. Giannuzzi P, Mezzani A, Saner H, *et al.* Physical activity for primary and secondary prevention. Position paper of the Working Group on Cardiac Rehabilitation and Exercise Physiology of the European Society of Cardiology. *Eur J Cardiovasc Prev Rehabil* 2003;**10**(5);319–27.
9. Braunwald E. *Heart disease*, 3rd edition. WB Saunders, Philadelphia, 1988.
10. Burch GE, Walsh JJ, Black WC. Value of prolonged bed rest in management of cardiomegaly. *JAMA* 1963;**183**:81–7.
11. Burch GE, McDonald CD. Prolonged bed rest in the treatment of ischemic cardiomyopathy. *Chest* 1971;**60**:424–30.
12. McDonald CD, Burch GE, Walsh JJ. Prolonged bed rest in the treatment of idiopathic cardiomyopathy. *Am J Med* 1972;**52**:41–50.
13. Jugdutt BI, Michorowski BL, Kappagoda CT. Exercise training after anterior Q wave myocardial infarction: Importance of left ventricular function and topography. *J Am Coll Cardiol* 1988;**12**:362–72.
14. Gaudron P, Hu K, Schamberger R, Budin M, Walter B, Ertl G. Effect of endurance training early or late after coronary artery occlusion on left ventricular remodelling, hemodynamics, and survival in rats with chronic transmural myocardial infarction. *Circulation* 1994;**89**:402–12.
15. Gianuzzi P, Tavazzi L, Temporelli PL, *et al.*, for the EAMI study group. Long-term physical training and left ventricular remodelling after anterior myocardial infarction (EAMI) trial. *J Am Coll Cardiol* 1993;**22**:1821–9.
16. Ehansi AA, Miller TR, Miller TA, Ballard EA, Schechtman KB. Comparison of adaptations to a 12-month exercise program and late outcome inpatients with healed myocardial infarction and ejection fraction <45% and >50%. *Am J Cardiol* 1997;**79**:1258–60.
17. Giannuzzi P, Temporelli PL, Corrà U, Tavazzi L; ELVD-CHF Study Group. Antiremodeling effect of long-term exercise training in patients with stable chronic heart failure: results of the Exercise in Left Ventricular Dysfunction and Chronic Heart Failure (ELVD-CHF) Trial. *Circulation* 2003;**108**:554–9.
18. Tristani FE, Hughes CV, Archibald DG, Sheldahl LM, Cohn JN, Fletcher R. Safety of graded symptom-limited exercise testing in patients with congestive heart failure. *Circulation* 1987;**76**(supplVI):54–8.
19. Keteyian SJ, Isaac D, Thadani U, *et al.*; HF-ACTION Investigators. Safety of symptom-limited cardiopulmonary exercise testing in patients with chronic heart failure due to severe left ventricular systolic dysfunction. *Am Heart J* 2009;**158**(4 Suppl):S72–7.
20. O'Connor CM, Whellan DJ, Lee KL, *et al.*; HF-ACTION Investigators. Efficacy and safety of exercise training in patients with chronic heart failure: HF-ACTION randomized controlled trial. *JAMA* 2009;**301**:1439–50.
21. Clausen JP. Circulatory adjustments to dynamic exercise and effect of physical training in normal subjects and in patients with coronary artery disease. *Prog Cardiovasc Dis* 1976;**18**:459–95.
22. Oldridge NB, Guyatt GH, Fisher ME, Rimm AA. Cardiac rehabilitation after myocardial infarction: Combined experience of randomized clinical trials. *JAMA* 1988;**260**:945–50.
23. O'Connor GT, Buring JE, Yusuf S, *et al.* An overview of randomized trials of rehabilitation with exercise after myocardial infarction. *Circulation* 1989;**80**:234–44.
24. Ehansi AA, Ogawa T, Miller TR, Spina RJ, Jilka SM. Exercise training improves left ventricular systolic function in older men. *Circulation* 1991;**83**:96–103.
25. Lavie CJ, Milani RV. Effects of cardiac rehabilitation and exercise training programs in patients ≥75 years of age. *Am J Cardiol* 1996;**78**:675–7.
26. Levine CJ, Milani RV. Benefits of cardiac rehabilitation and exercise training in elderly women. *Am J Cardiol* 1997;**79**:664–6.
27. Ades PA, Waldmann ML, Poehlman ET, *et al.* Exercise conditioning in older coronary patients: submaximal lactate response and endurance capacity. *Circulation* 1993;**88**:572–5.
28. Fielding RA. Effects of exercise training in the elderly: impact of progressive resistance training on skeletal muscle and whole-body protein metabolism. *Proc Nutr Soc* 1996;**54**:665–75.
29. Hespel P, Lijnen P, Faggard R, *et al.* Effects of physical endurance training on the plasma renin-angiotensin-aldosterone system in normal man. *J Endocrinol* 1988;**116**:443–9.
30. Cooksey JD, Reilly P, Brown S, Bomze H, Cryer PE. Exercise training and plasma catecholamines in patients with ischemic heart disease. *Am J Cardiol* 1978;**42**:372–6.
31. Holloszy JO. Adaptations of muscular tissue to training. *Prog Cardiovasc Dis* 1976;**18**:445–58.
32. Refenberick DH, Gamble JG, Max SR. Response of mitochondrial enzymes to decreased muscular activity. *Am J Physiol* 1973;**225**:1295–9.
33. Lee AP, Ice R, Blessey R, Sanmarco ME. Long term effects of physical training on coronary patients with impaired LV function. *Circulation* 1978;**60**:1519–26.
34. Conn EH, Williams RS, Wallace AG. Exercise responses before and after physical conditioning in patients with severely depressed left ventricular function. *Am J Cardiol* 1982;**49**:296–300.
35. Sullivan MJ, Higginbotham MB, Cobb FR. Exercise training in patients with severe left ventricular dysfunction: hemodynamic and metabolic effects. *Circulation* 1988;**78**:506–16.
36. Sullivan MJ, Higginbotham MB, Cobb FR. Exercise training in patients with chronic heart failure delays ventilatory anaerobic threshold and improves submaximal exercise performance. *Circulation* 1989;**79**:324–9.
37. Coats AJS, Adamopoulos S, Meyer T, Conway J, Sleight P. Physical training in chronic heart failure. *Lancet* 1990;**335**:63–6.
38. Coats AJS, Adamopoulos S, Radaelli A, *et al.* Controlled trial of physical training in chronic heart failure: exercise performance, hemodynamics, ventilation, and autonomic function. *Circulation* 1992;**85**:2119–31.
39. Meyer TE, Casadei B, Coats AJS, *et al.* Angiotensin-converting enzyme inhibition and physical training in heart failure. *J Intern Med* 1991;**230**:407–13.
40. Meyer K, Schwaibold M, Westbrook S, *et al.* Effect of short-term exercise training and activity restriction on functional capacity in patients with severe chronic congestive heart failure. *Am J Cardiol* 1996;**78**:1017–22.
41. Davey P, Meyer T, Coats A, *et al.* Ventilation in chronic heart failure: effects of physical training. *Br Heart J* 1992;**68**:473–7.

42. Clark AL, Skypala I, Coats AJS. Ventilatory efficiency is unchanged after physical training in health persons despite an increase in exercise tolerance. *J Cardiovasc Risk* 1994;**1**:347–351.
43. Kiilavuori K, Toivonen L, Naveri H, Leinonen H. Reversal of autonomic derangements by physical training in chronic heart failure assessed by heart rate variability. *Eur Heart J* 1995;**16**:490–5.
44. Keteyian SJ, Levine AB, Brawner CA, *et al.* Exercise training in patients with heart failure. *Ann Intern Med* 1996;**124**:1051–7.
45. Demopoulos L, Bijou R, Fergus I, Jones M, Strom J, LeJemtel T. Exercise training in patients with severe congestive heart failure: enhancing peak aerobic capacity whilst minimizing the increase in ventricular wall stress. *J Am Coll Cardiol* 1997;**29**: 597–603.
46. Kostis JB, Rosen RC, Cosgrove NM, Shindler DM, Wilson AC. Nonpharmacologic therapy improves functional and emotional status in congestive heart failure. *Chest* 1994;**106**:996–1001.
47. Flynn KE, Piña IL, Whellan DJ, *et al.* Effects of exercise training on health status in patients with chronic heart failure: HF-ACTION randomized controlled trial. *JAMA* 2009;**301**:1439–50.
48. Adamopoulos S, Ponikowki P, Cerqetani E, *et al.* Circadian pattern of heart rate variability in chronic heart failure patients—effects of physical training. *Eur Heart J* 1995;**16**:1380–6.
49. Braith RW, Welsch MA, Feigenbaum MS, Kluess HA, Pepine CJ. Neuroendocrine activation in heart failure is modified by endurance exercise training. *J Am Coll Cardiol* 1999;**34**:1170–5.
50. Passino C, Severino S, Poletti R, *et al.* Aerobic training decreases B-type natriuretic peptide expression and adrenergic activation in patients with heart failure. *J Am Coll Cardiol* 2006;**47**:1835–9.
51. Wilson JR, Mancini DM, Dunkman WB. Exertional fatigue due to skeletal muscle dysfunction in patients with heart failure. *Circulation* 1993;**87**:470–5.
52. Wilson JR, Rayos G, Yeoh TK, Gothard P. Dissociation between peak exercise oxygen consumption and hemodynamic dysfunction in potential heart transplantation candidates. *J Am Coll Cardiol* 1995;**26**:429–35.
53. Belardinelli R, Georgiou D, Cianci G, Berman N, Ginzton L, Purcaro A. Exercise training improves left ventricular diastolic filling in patients with dilated cardiomyopathy. Clinical and prognostic implications. *Circulation* 1995;**91**:2775–84.
54. Belardinelli R, Georgiou D, Cianci G, Purcaro A. Effects of exercise training on left ventricular filling at rest and during exercise in patients with ischemic cardiomyopathy and severe left ventricular dysfunction. *Am Heart J* 1996;**132**:61–70.
55. Katz SD, Yuen J, Bijou R, LeJemtel TH. Training improves endothelium-dependent vasodilation in resistance vessels of patients with heart failure. *J Appl Physiol* 1997;**82**:1488–92.
56. Hambrecht R, Hilbrich L, Erbs S, *et al.* Correction of endothelial dysfunction in chronic heart failure: additional effects of exercise training and oral L-arginine supplementation. *J Am Coll Cardiol* 2000;**35**:706–13.
57. Linke A, Schoene N, Gielen S, Hofer J, Erbs S, Schuler G, Hambrecht R. Endothelial dysfunction in patients with chronic heart failure: systemic effects of lower-limb exercise training. *J Am Coll Cardiol* 2001;**37**:392–7.
58. Hambrecht R, Gielen S, Linke A, *et al.* Effects of exercise training on left ventricular function and peripheral resistance in patients with chronic heart failure: A randomized trial. *JAMA* 2000;**283**:3095–101.
59. Hambrecht R, Niebauer J, Fiehn E, *et al.* Physical training in patients with stable chronic heart failure: Effects on cardiorespiratory fitness and ultrastructural abnormalities of leg muscles. *J Am Coll Cardiol* 1995;**25**:1239–49.
60. Hambrecht R, Fiehn E, Yu J, *et al.* Effects of endurance training on mitochondrial ultrastructure and fiber type distribution in skeletal muscle of patients with stable chronic heart failure. *J Am Coll Cardiol* 1997;**29**:1067–73.
61. Magnusson G, Gordon A, Kaijser L, *et al.* High intensity knee extensor training in patients with chronic heart failure. *Eur Heart J* 1996;**17**:1048–55.
62. Adamopoulos S, Coats AJS, Brunotte F, *et al.* Physical training improves skeletal muscle metabolic abnormalities in patients with chronic heart failure. *J Am Coll Cardiol* 1993;**23**:1101–6.
63. Mancini DM, Henson D, LaManca J, Donchez L, Levine S. Benefit of selective respiratory muscle training on exercise capacity in patients with chronic congestive heart failure. *Circulation* 1995; **91**:320–9.
64. Hambrecht R, Schulze PC, Gielen S, *et al.* Effects of exercise training on insulin-like growth factor-I expression in the skeletal muscle of non-cachectic patients with chronic heart failure. *Eur J Cardiovasc Prev Rehabil* 2005;**12**:401–6.
65. Linke A, Adams V, Schulze PC, *et al.* Antioxidative effects of exercise training in patients with chronic heart failure: increase in radical scavenger enzyme activity in skeletal muscle. *Circulation* 2005;**111**:1763–70.
66. Piepoli M, Clark AL, Coats AJ. Muscle metaboreceptors in hemodynamic, autonomic, and ventilatory responses to exercise in men. *Am J Physiol* 1995;**269**(4 Pt 2):H1428–36.
67. Piepoli M, Clark AL, Volterrani M, Adamopoulos S, Sleight P, Coats AJ. Contribution of muscle afferents to the hemodynamic, autonomic, and ventilatory responses to exercise in patients with chronic heart failure: effects of physical training. *Circulation* 1996;**93**:940–52.
68. Elkayam U, Roth A, Weber L, *et al.* Isometric exercise in patients with chronic advanced heart failure: hemodynamic and neurohormonal evaluation. *Circulation* 1985;**72**:975–81.
69. Reddy HK, Weber KT, Janicki JS, McElroy PA. Hemodynamic, ventilatory and metabolic effects of light isometric exercise in patients with chronic heart failure. *J Am Coll Cardiol* 1988;**12**:353–8.
70. McKelvie RS, McCartney N, Tomlinson C, Bauer R, MacDougall JD. Comparison of hemodynamic responses to cycling and resistance exercise in congestive heart failure secondary to ischemic cardiomyopathy. *Am J Cardiol* 1995;**76**:977–9.
71. Ohtsubo M, Yonezawa K, Nishijima H, Okita K, Hanada A, Kohya T, Murakami T, Kitabatake A. Metabolic abnormality of calf skeletal muscle is improved by localised muscle training without changes in blood flow in chronic heart failure. *Heart* 1997;**78**:437–43.
72. Belardinelli R, Georgiou D, Scocco V, Barstow TJ, Purcaro A. Low intensity exercise training in patients with chronic heart failure. *J Am Coll Cardiol* 1995;**26**:975–82.
73. Banerjee P, Clark A, Witte K, Crowe L, Caulfield B. Electrical stimulation of unloaded muscles causes cardiovascular exercise by increasing oxygen demand. *Eur J Cardiovasc Prev Rehabil* 2005;**12**:503–8.
74. Banerjee P, Caulfield B, Crowe L, Clark A. Prolonged electrical muscle stimulation exercise improves strength and aerobic capacity in healthy sedentary adults. *J Appl Physiol* 2005;**99**: 2307–11.
75. Banerjee P, Caulfield B, Crowe L, Clark AL. Prolonged electrical muscle stimulation exercise improves strength, peak VO2, and exercise capacity in patients with stable chronic heart failure. *J Card Fail* 2009;**15**:319–26.
76. Kavanagh T, Myers MG, Baigrie RS, Mertens DJ, Sawyer P, Shephard RJ. Quality of life and cardiorespiratory function in chronic heart failure: effects of 12 months' aerobic training. *Heart* 1996;**76**:42–49.
77. Piepoli MF, Davos C, Francis DP, Coats AJ; ExTraMATCH Collaborative. Exercise training meta-analysis of trials in patients with chronic heart failure (ExTraMATCH). *BMJ* 2004;**328**:189.
78. Graham I, Atar D, Borch-Johnsen K, *et al.;* Fourth Joint Task Force of the European Society of Cardiology and other societies on cardiovascular disease prevention in clinical practice. *Eur J Cardiovasc Prev Rehabil* 2007;**14**(Suppl 2):S1–113.

79. Forissier JF, Vernochet P, Bertrand P, Charbonnier B, Monpère C. Influence of carvedilol on the benefits of physical training in patients with moderate chronic heart failure. *Eur J Heart Fail* 2001;**3**:335–42.
80. Curnier D, Galinier M, Pathak A, *et al.* Rehabilitation of patients with congestive heart failure with or without beta-blockade therapy. *J Card Fail* 2001;**7**:241–8.
81. Fan S, Lyon CE, Savage PD, Ozonoff A, Ades PA, Balady GJ. Outcomes and adverse events among patients with implantable cardiac defibrillators in cardiac rehabilitation: a case-controlled study. *J Cardiopulm Rehabil Prev* 2009;**29**:40–3.
82. Vanhees L, Kornaat M, Defoor J, *et al.* Effect of exercise training in patients with an implantable cardioverter defibrillator. *Eur Heart J* 2004;**25**:1120–6.
83. Davos CH, Doehner W, Rauchhaus M, *et al.* Body mass and survival in patients with chronic heart failure without cachexia: the importance of obesity. *J Card Fail* 2003;**9**:29–35.
84. Horwich TB, Fonarow GC, Hamilton MA, MacLellan WR, Woo MA, Tillish JH. The relationship between obesity and mortality in patients with advanced heart failure. *J Am Coll Cardiol* 2001; **38**:789–95.
85. Sullivan M, Simon G, Spertus J, Russo J. Depression-related costs in heart failure care. *Arch Intern Med* 2002;**162**:1860–66.
86. Rumsfeld JS, Havranek E, Masoudi FA, *et al.* Depressive symptoms are the strongest predictors of short-term declines in health status in patients with heart failure. *J Am Coll Cardiol* 2003; **42**: 1811–17.
87. Hambrecht R, Niebauer J, Fiehn E, *et al.* Physical training in patients with stable chronic heart failure: Effects on cardiorespiratory fitness and ultrastructural abnormalities of leg muscles. *J Am Coll Cardiol* 1995;**25**:1239–49.

46

Nonpharmacological management

Lynda Blue and Yvonne Millerick

Introduction

Managing heart failure (HF) is not an easy task: the numbers of patients are large and increasing, and many patients have complex needs. This presents a challenge not only to patients and their caregivers but also to health care systems and health care professionals. Patients are asked to take multiple pharmacological agents that often require adjustment; are expected to make lifestyle changes; and a growing number of patients are now being considered for device therapy. At hospital discharge, few patients receive lifestyle and self-management advice in written form[1] and it is therefore not surprising that many patients with HF have poor knowledge about their condition and its management.

Over the last decade, various guidelines have been published on the management of chronic HF. The guidelines have primarily concentrated on pharmacological treatment (and more recently, device therapy) and only briefly address lifestyle advice and self-care management strategies.

Several trials of specialist HF management programmes which adopt a multidisciplinary approach have shown that self-management strategies lead to an improved quality of life.[2] A multidisciplinary approach has also been shown to reduce hospitalizations[2,3] and mortality.[4]

Optimal management of HF requires not only best practice in pharmacological management but also appropriate education strategies, practical advice, and caring support to enable patients and their caregivers to achieve the best possible quality of life, without offering unrealistic expectations of cure. It is important not only that patients and their caregivers are given the opportunity to take greater control of managing their condition, but also that health care professionals should not underestimate the critical role they have in empowering their patients. Much of the present chapter is based on expert advice, rather than robust evidence.

Education

Education is an important component of HF management programmes and can influence the patient's physical and psychosocial well-being and activities of daily living. The goals of HF education should be increasing the patient's and their caregiver's knowledge and their adherence to self-care management, although increased knowledge alone does not necessarily lead to improved adherence.[5]

Knowledge is generally defined as a quality which gives an individual the ability to understand, to reflect, and to reach conclusions that can be used to bring about a change. In contrast, adherence is the extent to which a persons' behaviour concurs with professional health advice. Empowering patients to be knowledgeable about the implementation of appropriate treatment strategies at an early stage is an important educational outcome.

Barriers to effective learning can be wide ranging and difficult to overcome and are commonly associated with functional and cognitive limitations, such as increasing age, dementia, and comorbidities, particularly visual and hearing difficulties. Other common barriers include poor physical capacity, fatigue, anxiety and depression, often resulting in low self-esteem.

By its very nature HF is difficult and obtrusive; combined with its complex treatment regime, this makes it perplexing for some patients and their caregivers, particularly if they have very little or no social support.[5,6] It is therefore essential that any health care professional involved in the development and delivery of patient education is aware of what the barriers to learning are. Furthermore, education programmes need to be individualized to the patient and caregiver and should always be aligned with key health outcomes to bring about long-term success.

Many patients feel anxious and unwell in the inpatient hospital setting and this may not be the most appropriate time to pass on vital information, as the significance of it may not be understood. It is usually only when patients return home that they are able to formulate questions about their condition and seek to clarify treatment options. It is important, however, that at hospital discharge patients and/or caregivers are provided with written instructions and educational materials, in a format which is easily understood, advising on medications, diet, activity levels, follow-up appointments, weight monitoring, and what to do if symptoms worsen.

Patients (especially elderly people) can have difficulty in remembering the details of their condition and their treatment, especially when their medication is adjusted on a frequent basis in response to their HF status. Health care professionals also have difficulty in tracking the progress of the patient and appreciate a concise but accurate summary of both the patient and their treatment. A good way of facilitating the patient's understanding of their condition and treatment (and the health care professional's management of the HF) is to provide the patient with an information book that is both educational and represents a record of their progress and treatment. Ideally, the book should be given before hospital discharge, backing up verbal information the patient has received initially, and giving clear information to patients and carers on when and from whom to seek advice. To address the needs of patients with impaired hearing and vision, it is important that educational materials are also available in audio format or large font, and in other languages.

Computer-based education for HF patients has also been found to be an efficient way of increasing knowledge.[7] The web page heartfailurematters.org represents an Internet tool provided by the Heart Failure Association of the European Society of Cardiology (ESC) that permits patients, their families, and caregivers to obtain useful, practical information in a user-friendly format.

The ESC (2008) identified important educational topics for discussion with patients and their caregivers living with HF (Table 46.1).

Table 46.1 Essential topics in patient education with associated skills and appropriate self-care behaviours

Educational topics	Skills and self-care behaviours
Definition and aetiology of HF	Understand the cause of HF and why symptoms occur
Symptoms and signs of HF	Monitor and recognize signs and symptoms
	Record daily weight and recognize rapid weight gain
	Know how and when to notify health care provider
	Use flexible diuretic therapy if appropriate and recommended
Pharmacological treatment	Understand indications, dosing, and effects of drugs
	Recognize the common side effects of each drug prescribed
Risk factor modification	Understand the importance of smoking cessation
	Monitor blood pressure if hypertensive
	Maintain good glucose control if diabetic
	Avoid obesity
Diet recommendation	Sodium restriction if prescribed
	Avoid excessive fluid intake
	Modest intake of alcohol
	Monitor and prevent malnutrition
Exercise recommendations	Be reassured and comfortable about physical activity
	Understand the benefits of exercise
	Perform exercise training regularly
Sexual activity	Be reassured about engaging in sex and discuss problems with health care professionals
	Understand specific sexual problems and various coping strategies
Immunization	Receive immunization against infections such as influenza and pneumococcal disease
Sleep and breathing disorders	Recognize preventive behaviour such as reducing weight if obese, smoking cessation, and abstinence from alcohol
	Learn about treatment options if appropriate
Adherence	Understand the importance of following treatment recommendations and maintaining motivation to follow treatment plan
Psychosocial aspects	Understand that depressive symptoms and cognitive dysfunction are common in patients with HF and the importance of social support
	Learn about treatment options if appropriate
Prognosis	Understand important prognostic factors and make realistic decisions
	Seek psychosocial support if appropriate

HF, heart failure.

Self-care

Self-care is defined as actions aimed at maintaining physical stability; avoidance of behaviour that can worsen the condition; and detection of the early symptoms of deterioration.[8]

Effective self-care is an essential part of HF management because patients and their caregivers have to live with the consequences of HF and are responsible for the management of their condition in their own homes. For effective self-care, patients not only need to be adherent to prescribed treatment regimes including medication, diet, and exercise, but also to monitor and recognize symptom deterioration and be able to take appropriate action. The action needed may be to increase the prescribed diuretic dose and/or to contact the health care team.

Self-care is complex and can be challenging as it is influenced by individual patient factors, such as the patient's knowledge of HF and its symptoms, previous experiences, ability, coping strategies, and cognitive status.[9] Diminished cognitive function affects 25–50% of patients with HF[10] and is associated with poor self-care.[11]

Comorbidities can complicate symptom management: for example, many patients with HF also have lung disease and may find it difficult to distinguish between dyspnoea caused by HF and that caused by their lung condition. The incidence and prevalence of depression in HF patients is higher than in the general population[12] and negatively influences self-care abilities.[13] Anxiety may be present in up to 50–70% of HF patients and may affect a patient's willingness and ability to engage in self-care, as it impairs cognition, energy, and motivation.[14]

Cultural, social, and geographical factors must also be considered, as they may impact on the patient's willingness to participate in self-care management. Equally important is the relationship between health professionals and the patient and caregiver. Failure to recognize the significance of the above factors may lead to the patient and caregiver losing confidence in health care professionals and the health care system.

A recent study explored the influence individual and contextual factors have on HF self-care, and found that links between knowledge of HF and self-care were weak: long delays in seeking professional care were frequent. The authors concluded that knowledge of HF and its management is a necessary, but not sufficient, determinant of HF self-care. Individual and contextual factors all influence willingness and capacity to undertake HF self-care. Interestingly, the participants in the study did not have access to a specialist HF management programme.[15]

To evaluate the effectiveness of interventions aimed at improving self-care behaviours of HF patients, a valid, reliable and user-friendly scale which can be used in different countries has been developed (Box 46.1).[16] The scale is easy to administer and is practical for use in everyday clinical practice. It reflects the actions that a HF patient undertakes to maintain life, healthy functioning, and well-being. The nine-item scale includes behaviours such as adherence to medication, diet, exercise, as well as self-management of symptoms, daily weighing and response to fluid retention, and when to seek advice. For this reason, it may prove a useful tool for measuring the effectiveness of the education and support that is regularly provided by most HF management programmes.

Adherence to treatment

Good adherence decreases morbidity and mortality and improves well-being,[17] but research suggests that only 20–60% of HF patients adhere to their prescribed pharmacological and nonpharmacological treatment.[18] Adherence to prescribed medications is lower in HF patients who have multiple comorbidities[19,20] and in patients with depression.[21]

A study of 202 HF patients recently discharged from hospital found a high rate of medication nonadherence. The reasons given were a lack of understanding about discharge instructions (57%), confusion regarding conflicting instructions by different physicians (22%), not being convinced of the effectiveness of the medication (9%), and worry about potential side effects (7%). Patients took medications that had not been prescribed because they had previously been taking them (68%), they lacked confidence in the new prescription (19%), they did not realize that two medications were the same (generic vs commercial name, 8%) or they confused their own medication with that of other individuals living in the same house (7%).[19]

A large study monitoring the pharmacy records of nearly 1000 patients with HF for 1 year after hospital discharge found that only 80% of patients who had been prescribed an angiotensin converting enzyme (ACE) inhibitor at discharge continued with the medication during the 30 days after discharge, and the percentage reduced to 60% and remained constant over the remainder of the year after discharge.[22]

After comprehensive education and instruction, it may be possible for many patients to alter their own diuretic regime in response to weight gain and worsening symptoms. A large proportion of patients will need support from a health professional before making a change to their medication regime. Weekly medication boxes are useful, but it is always helpful for the patient to have a separate prescription of diuretics in the house for times when symptoms are exacerbated. The role of the community pharmacist should not be underestimated and is particularly valuable in empowering patients and facilitating medication prescriptions and aids to support medication adherence.

Box 46.1 European Heart Failure Self-Care Behaviour Scale

This scale contains statements about self-care for heart failure. Please respond to each statement by circling the number which you think best applies to you.

		I completely agree				I don't agree at all
1	I weigh myself every day	1	2	3	4	5
2	If my shortness of breath increases, I contact my doctor or nurse	1	2	3	4	5
3	If my feet/legs become more swollen than usual, I contact my doctor or nurse	1	2	3	4	5
4	If I gain 2 kgs in 1 week, I contact my doctor or nurse	1	2	3	4	5
5	I limit the amount of fluids I drink (not more than 1½–2 litres per day)	1	2	3	4	5
6	If I experience increased fatigue, I contact my doctor or nurse	1	2	3	4	5
7	I eat a low salt diet	1	2	3	4	5
8	I take my medication as prescribed	1	2	3	4	5
9	I exercise regularly	1	2	3	4	5

Symptom monitoring/recognition

Patients are not always knowledgeable about the condition of HF, or its associated symptom burden. Several studies have demonstrated that patients delay seeking care when their symptoms worsen.[9,15] The delay may be due to patients not routinely monitoring their symptoms, or not recognizing and appreciating the significance should their symptoms deteriorate.

Although men and women with HF experience similar symptoms, their perception of the symptoms differs: for example, men perceive the impact of physical and social limitations as being more difficult to cope with, while women regard the inability to support family and friends as more problematic.[23,24] Studies have also demonstrated a difference between the assessment of symptoms by patients and their caregivers compared to health care professionals.[25,26] It is, however, worth remembering that many patients are unable to assume an active role in their treatment and overall HF management and therefore the role of the caregiver is crucial.

In the EuroHeart survey, 91% of patients recently hospitalized with HF could recall that they had a heart-related condition, but only 78% realized that the description 'heart failure' applied to them.[27] If patients and their caregivers are to take more control of their condition and its management they need to have a better understanding about the disease and its treatment through tailored education programmes.[29]

Weight monitoring

Previous studies suggests that fewer than one-half of HF patients report weighing themselves daily,[30] including patients recently discharged from hospital for an exacerbation of HF.[19] Even amongst those who do weigh themselves (even intermittently), few consider weight gain to be a significant problem.[11] The EuroHeart Failure survey found that 12 weeks after discharge only 49% of patients with a clinical diagnosis of HF recalled receiving advice to weigh themselves regularly and only 68% of them followed the advice completely.[27]

Educating patients to understand that sudden weight gain or loss can be indicative of early clinical deterioration may encourage incorporating weight monitoring into their daily management routine. Furthermore, by directly linking changes in body weight to clinical deterioration, patients can be empowered to respond accordingly by increasing or decreasing their diuretic dose appropriately with good effect.[25] Patients should also be made aware that routine deterioration in symptoms may also occur in the absence of weight changes.[31]

A key component of weight management is to determine (where possible) the patient's ideal 'dry' weight (when a patient who has had signs of fluid retention after diuretic treatment reaches a steady weight at which there are no further signs of fluid overload). Patients should be encouraged to weigh themselves daily at the same time, usually in the morning in minimal clothes, and record their weight in the chart/diary provided. Patients (or caregivers, where appropriate), should be advised that a steady weight gain over a number of days may indicate that they are retaining too much fluid. If the gain in weight is more than 2 kg (4 lb) in 3 days, patients may increase their diuretic dose and alert the health care team. It is also important that patients are advised that if they lose a similar amount of weight over the same period, they need to contact the health care team in case they are volume depleted due to excessive diuretic usage.

Fluid management

Careful fluid management is a key component of symptom monitoring and control. Careful adherence has the potential to reduce episodes of clinical deterioration associated with either fluid retention or fluid loss. Patients should understand that an intake of more than 2.0 L/day should be avoided and that during episodes of fluid retention and weight gain, the patient should be encouraged to reduce fluid intake to 1.5–2 L/day. To maximize adherence, it is important that the patient and/or caregiver understands what contributes to fluid intake, including, for example, tea, coffee, soups, and alcoholic drinks. Patients should know how much fluid their usual cup, mug, glass, or bowl holds. Keeping a record of the daily fluid intake should be encouraged as this not only enables the patient to pace their daily fluid allowance but also provides them with the opportunity to have some control over their illness and its management.[32] Fluid restrictions may be modified in response to warmer weather. Asymptomatic patients who have noticed a weight decrease may be required to increase their daily fluid intake to maintain their dry weight and avoid potential dehydration.

There is little research available on fluid management. A randomized controlled trial study of fluid intake in stable HF patients demonstrated that it is safe and beneficial to recommend a moderate fluid intake based on body weight.[33] A further small randomized study in acutely decompensated patients who had a hospital admission reported no difference in time of discontinuing parenteral diuretic therapy between the fluid-restricted and non-fluid-restricted groups.[32]

Fluid intake should be restricted to 1.5 L/day in patients with severe symptoms, particularly if hyponatremia coexists.[29] There is no rationale for routine fluid restriction in patients with stable, mild to moderate CHF.

Alcohol

There are few data available to guide restriction of alcohol in HF. Alcohol may have a negative inotropic effect, and may be associated with an increase in blood pressure and greater risk of arrhythmias. Excessive use may be deleterious. Alcohol intake should be limited to 1–2 standard drinks or glasses of wine per day (10–20 g/day).[29]

Prolonged and large intake of alcohol can cause cardiomyopathy. Although the actual course of alcoholic cardiomyopathy is difficult to define, abstinence stops deterioration and may lead to improved cardiac function. Patients with alcohol-induced cardiomyopathy are advised that they should abstain from alcohol completely.[29,34]

Sodium restriction

Guidelines on the recommended intake of sodium are conflicting and there is a lack of evidence from trials in HF patients. In patients with advanced HF, excessive sodium intake can cause diuretic resistance and deteriorations which trigger hospital admission.[35] A randomized trial comparing low versus normal sodium diet in patients receiving high doses of furosemide found that sodium restriction was associated with worse clinical outcomes.[36] Although there is no evidence as to the optimal threshold for restricting sodium intake, published HF guidelines suggest a sodium intake of around 2–3 g/day.[37,38]

In the Euro Heart Failure survey only 58% of patients reported receiving advice to decrease their sodium intake, and only 36% reported following this advice.[27]

Patients and caregivers should be advised to avoid salt-rich foods and advised not to add supplemental salt to food when cooking. It is also important that patients and caregivers are aware that salt substitutes (such as Lo-Salt) that are high in potassium must be avoided because of the risk of hyperkalaemia.[28] Patients should be encouraged to use alternatives such as lemon juice and spices. Where appropriate, patients should be referred for specialist review and advice from a dietitian, to facilitate dietary knowledge and adherence.

Weight reduction

Weight reduction in obese patients (body mass index (BMI) >30 kg/m^2) with HF should be considered in order to prevent the progression of HF, decrease symptoms, and improve well-being.[29]

Nonprescription medication

Many people take nonprescription medications such as herbal remedies, alternative medicines, and over-the-counter preparations. Over-the-counter preparations may exacerbate HF symptoms and must be highlighted to the patient and caregiver. The main drug group of concern is non-steroidal anti-inflammatory drugs (NSAIDs) which can easily be bought over the counter. NSAIDs can lead to fluid retention and worsening renal function, increasing the risk of hospitalization in patients with HF.[39]

A study of the use of nonprescription therapy in patients with HF found that (84.3%) had used at least one drug that had not been recommended by their physician: 75.8% used over-the-counter drugs, 21.3% had used herbal remedies, and 20.9% had used vitamins and minerals. Importantly, the patients were unaware of the possible interaction with HF therapies and rarely informed their physician that they were using these therapies.[40]

Smoking

Smoking is a major risk factor in cardiovascular disease and patients with chronic HF should therefore be encouraged to stop. Smoking cessation strategies are recommended in patients with HF and should be discussed and employed to avoid the harmful effects of continued smoking on the cardiovascular physiology and association with poorer health outcomes. Observational studies support the association between smoking cessation and decreased morbidity and mortality.[41,42]

Pregnancy and contraception

Chronic HF greatly increases the risk of maternal and neonatal morbidity and mortality. Pregnancy may lead to deterioration in HF due to the increase in blood volume, cardiac output, and extravascular fluid. Many of the medications to treat HF are contraindicated during pregnancy. Contraceptive and pregnancy advice should be discussed and tailored on an individual basis with a physician. Potential risks can be assessed and discussed to enable patient and physician to reach an informed decision.[43]

Sexual activity

There is a limited evidence base regarding the influence of sexual activity on patients with mild to moderate symptoms associated with chronic HF. Common problems have, however, been reported by HF patients in connection with their cardiac disease, symptoms of fatigue and depression, and treatment side effects. Symptoms such as dyspnoea, palpitations, or angina during sex rarely occur in patients who do not experience similar symptoms during exercise levels representing moderate exertion.[44]

Fatigue management

Fatigue is a prominent and difficult symptom in HF to manage and can have a profound effect on the patient's quality of life and their ability to perform daily activities. It is important that patients receive optimal medical management and treatment of any underlying conditions that could contribute to worsening fatigue. Nonpharmacological management of fatigue should include attention to nutritional status, tolerance to exercise, and the promotion of energy conservation. Adherence to these factors combined with robust assessment of fatigue will help to ensure that the patient's well-being is optimized.

Management of breathlessness

Nonpharmacological management strategies for breathlessness should include advice on correct positioning of the upper body while sitting on a chair during the day, and advice on sleeping upright supported with pillows to reduce the risk of orthopnoea at night. The role of other team members, such as the physiotherapist and occupational therapist, should not be underestimated as they can provide invaluable information about energy conservation to minimize the risk of breathlessness associated with activities of daily living. They can also demonstrate the potential benefits of relaxation therapy, breathing exercises, and the importance of correct posture. Simple techniques to increase air flow across the face can be helpful: for example, an open window or electric fan can be helpful to breathless patients. The air flow exerts its effects via sensory receptors on the face and/or in the upper respiratory tract.[45] Small scale studies suggest that the use of relaxation, complementary therapy, and distraction therapy may reduce the anxiety that often precipitates an acute breathlessness event. Such therapies are seldom used in HF because of the extremely limited evidence base.

Immunization

Influenza infection is a major public health concern across the world as it is associated with high rates of morbidity and mortality each year.[46] Respiratory infections are a major cause of avoidable HF-related deaths and hospitalizations, particularly during winter months.[47]

Although there is general agreement in recommending that HF patients with no contraindications should be offered an annual influenza vaccine and one pneumococcal vaccination,[29,48,49] the degree of clinical effectiveness is controversial and there are few available studies on the subject.

A large epidemiological study of elderly people found that immunization against influenza was associated with reductions in the risk of hospitalization for heart disease, cerebrovascular disease, and pneumonia or influenza as well as in the risk of death from all causes during influenza season, and recommends that pneumococcal vaccination and annual influenza vaccination should be considered in patients with symptomatic HF without known contraindications.[50]

A more recent observational study researched 1340 individuals aged 65 or older living in the community, who had chronic heart disease (HF or coronary artery disease), and followed them from January 2002 to April 2005. The study found that influenza vaccination was associated with a significant reduction in mortality (37%) during the study period. The authors estimated that one death was prevented for every 122 annual vaccinations.[51]

Previous reports have shown that the uptake of influenza vaccination is low,[20] with approximately one-third of elderly patients with chronic diseases in developed countries remaining nonvaccinated each year.[51,52] The Euro Heart Failure survey analysis 2007 on patients recently hospitalized for HF found that only 38% recalled vaccination advice.[27]

Pneumococcal vaccinations are usually only given once and may be effective for 6–10 years.[50] Pneumococcal vaccination reduces the risk of bacteraemia but has not consistently been shown to reduce the risk of hospitalization for pneumonia.[53]

Travel

Patients with stable compensated HF may be reassured about their safety to travel. However, they should be advised to make sure that they have adequate medical cover included in their travel insurance and that the insurance company is fully aware of their diagnosis and any hospitalizations that have occurred in the previous 12 months. General travel information should always include advice about medication and the importance of carrying extra medication doses in hand luggage in addition to the regular supply. A full list of medications using the generic name will make certain that the exact drug equivalent can be issued overseas if a problem occurs. A brief letter from the primary or secondary care physician describing the traveller's medical problem and treatment may be helpful if illness occurs while travelling.

The safest and most suitable mode of travel should always be considered and where possible discussed with either the general practitioner or physician. Most people with stable HF can travel as safely as everyone else, but the specific method of travel needs to be considered carefully well in advance. Air travel has become a routine feature of modern life and although it can have physiological repercussions, the incidence of traveller-associated events among the healthy flying population is relatively low.

Air travel for short-haul destinations may be preferable to long journeys by other means of transport.[29] Long-haul and high-altitude flights, however, are associated with greater risk for a patient with HF. The aircraft cabin during long-haul flights is pressurized to an equivalent of an altitude of around 2400 m (8000 ft) resulting in a fall in ambient partial pressure of oxygen to around 75% of that at sea level. Such a fall is tolerated without discomfort by most people, and patients with well-controlled HF can usually cope. As a general rule of thumb, if a patient can manage to climb a flight of stairs without discomfort, then long-haul flight is safe. If a patient's HF symptoms are poorly controlled, high-altitude and long-haul flights to very humid or hot destinations should be avoided or discouraged. For those patients who are going to travel by air, anticipatory planning around modification of fluid intake, diuretic adjustment, and the need for oxygen supplementation during the flight should be considered and discussed with the physician in preparation for travelling.

Patients with cardiac pacemakers and implantable defibrillators are safe to fly and will not be affected by airline metal detectors. Travellers with a device should, however, carry a card or a letter with all the relevant details.[54]

Travelling by car has many advantages, particularly for the diuretic user, as it can permit route planning around services while encouraging regular stops and mobilization every 2–3 h which may reduce the development of dependent oedema and deep venous thrombosis. Individuals with a diagnosis of HF may continue to drive provided there are no symptoms that may distract the driver's attention. If drug treatment for any cardiovascular condition including HF is required, any adverse effect from the treatment likely to affect driver performance will result in disqualification.[55]

In the United Kingdom, current regulations (last updated February 2010) advise that drivers who have had an implantable cardioverter defibrillator (ICD) for primary prevention may drive after 1 month. If the ICD is implanted for nonincapacitating sustained ventricular arrhythmia the patient may drive 1 month after implantation if (1) left ventricular ejection fraction (LVEF) is more than 35%; and (2) no fast VT induced on electrophysiological study (minimum RR interval must be less than 250 ms); and (3) any induced VT could be pace-terminated by the ICD twice, without acceleration, during the post implantation study. Drivers who have had an ICD inserted for ventricular arrhythmia associated with incapacity should not drive for a period of 6 months following implantation. If they have shock therapy or symptomatic antitachycardia pacing, they should not drive for a further 6 months. If any therapy following device implantation has been accompanied by incapacity (whether caused by the device or arrhythmia) the patient may not drive for a period of 2 years.[55] For full up-to-date details, consult the DVLA website at http://www.dft.gov.uk/dvla/medical/ataglance.aspx.

Travellers should be aware of the increased risk of dehydration in hot climates. The salt content of food and drink in other countries may be difficult to determine, particularly for restaurant foods. Self-management of daily diuretics can be particularly helpful in these circumstances.

Discussion

Providing effective nonpharmacological advice is an important component of HF care. The consequences of failing to address the issue adequately can be wide-ranging for patients and their caregivers, and incur significant economic costs to the health care system generally.

HF patients need continuous, long-term support in the community and should ideally be seen as soon as possible following hospital discharge. A health care professional can provide advice and support, complementing the information given on hospital discharge. A comprehensive assessment of both patient's and caregiver's needs and knowledge base is essential to inform future education and care requirements.

Deviating from recommended medication and dietary restriction can often lead to exacerbation of symptoms and reduced quality of life, which very often results in hospital admission and associated increased costs. Providing effective education and support for self-care management is therefore essential: however, self-care is a complex process and requires not only implementation of recommendations featured in guidelines, but also the patient's (and caregiver's) ability to interpret symptoms, willingness to participate, and willingness to seek help at an early stage.

A major goal of many HF programmes is to provide education and support for HF patients and to improve self-care behaviour, but the effectiveness of these programmes are generally evaluated on outcomes such as hospital readmissions, health care costs, and quality of life.[38] If a more tailored approach in HF management is to be adopted, it is essential to evaluate programmes on outcomes such as symptom relief and self-care behaviour.[16]

Key areas for further research in HF management include strategies to detect early fluid retention and to encourage improved adherence; investigation of the benefits (if any) of salt and fluid restriction; studies of the impact (and the effect of treatment) of depression, anxiety, and impaired cognition on self-care behaviour and other important outcomes.

Telemonitoring is an emerging area in HF management which may prove to be important in providing support to patients and caregivers. It has the potential to allow individualized care to be given to a larger population, by allowing daily monitoring of symptoms and signs measured by patients, family, or caregivers at home while keeping patients under close supervision.[56]

References

1. Goldberg RJ, Farmer C, Spencer FA, Pezella S, Meyer TE. Use of nonpharmacologic treatment approches in patients with heart failure. *Int J Cardiol* 2006;**110**:348–53.
2. Gonseth J, Guallar-Castillon P, Banegas JR, Rodriguez-Artalejo F. The effectiveness of disease management programmes in reducing hospital re-admissions in older patients with heart failure: a systematic review and meta-analysis of published reports. *Eur Heart J* 2004;**25**:1570–95.
3. Phillips CO, Wright SM, Kern DE, Singa RM, Shepperd S, Rubin HR. Comprehensive discharge planning with postdischarge support for older patients with congestive heart failure—a meta-analysis. *JAMA* 2004;**291**:1358–67.
4. McAlister FA, Stewart S, Ferrua S, McMurray JJV. Multidisciplinary strategies for the management of heart failure patients at high risk for admission: a systematic review of randomized trials. *J Am Coll Cardiol* 2004;**44**:810–19.
5. Stromberg A. The crucial role of patient education in heart failure. *Eur J Heart Fail* 2005;**7**:363–9.
6. Luttik ML, Jaarsma T, Moser D, Sanderman R, van Veldhuisen DJ. The importance and impact of social support on outcomes in patients with heart failure: an overview of the literature. *J Cardiovasc Nurs* 2005;**20**(3):162–69.
7. Stromberg A, Dahlstrom U, Fridlund B. Computer-based education for patients with chronic heart failure. A randomised controlled, multicentre trial of the effects on knowledge, compliance and quality of life. *Patient Educ Couns* 2006;**64**(1–3):128–35.
8. Jaarsma T, Stromberg A, Martensson J, Dracup K. Development and testing of the European Heart Failure Self-care Behaviour scale. *Eur J Heart Fail* 2003;**5**:363–70.
9. Patel H, Shafazand M, Scahaufelberger M, Ekman I. Reasons for seeking acute care in chronic heart failure. *Eur J Heart Fail* 2007;**9**:702–8.
10. Vogels RL, Scheltens P, Schroeder-Tanka JM, Weistein HC. Cognitive impairment in heart failure: a systematic review of the literature. *Eur J Heart Fail* 2007;**9**:440–9.
11. Carlson B, Riegel B, Moser DK. Self-care abilities of patients with heart failure. *Heart Lung* 2001;**30**:351–9.
12. Rutledge T, Reis VA, Linke SE, Greenberg BH, Mills PJ. Depression in heart failure: a meta-analytic review of prevalence, intervention effects, and associations with clinical outcomes. *J Am Coll Cardiol*ogy 2006;**48**:1527–37.
13. Riegel B, Dickson VA. A situation-specific theory of heart failure self care. *J Cardiovasc Nurs* 2002;**23**:287–95.
14. Di Mateo MR, Lepper HS, Croghan TW. Depression is a risk factor for noncompliance with medical treatment: metanalysis of the effects of anxiety and depression on patient adherence. *Arch Intern Med* 2000;**160**:2101–7.
15. Clark AM, Freydberg CN, McAlister, Tsuyuki RT, Armstrong PW, Strain LA. Patient and informal caregivers' knowledge of heart failure: necessary but insufficient for effective self-care. *Eur J Heart Fail* 2009:**11**:617–21.
16. Jaarsma T, Arestedt KF, Martensson J, Dracup K, Stromberg A. The European Heart Failure Heart Failure Self-care Behaviour scale revised into a nine-item scale (EHFScB-9): a reliable and valid international instrument. *Eur J Heart Fail* 2009;**11**:99–105.
17. Granger BB, Swedberg K, Ekman I, *et al.* Adherance to candesartan and placebo on outcomes in chronic heart failure in the CHARM programme: double blind, randomised, controlled clinical trial. *Lancet* 2005;**366**:2005–11.
18. van der Wal MH, Jaarsma T, van Veldhuisen DJ. Non-compliance in patients with heart failure; how can we manage it? *Eur J Heart Fail* 2005;**7**:5–17.
19. Moser DK, Doering LV, Chung ML. Vulnerabilities of patients recovering from an exacerbation of chronic heart failure. *Am Heart J* 2005;**150**:984.
20. Martinez-Selles M, Garcia Robles JA, Munoz R, *et al.* Pharmacological treatments in patients with heart failure: patient's knowledge and occurrence of polypharmacy, alternative medicine and immunisations. *Eur J Heart Fail* 2004;**6**:219–26.
21. Morgan AL, Masoudi FA, Havranek EP, *et al.* For the Cardiovascular Outcomes Research Consortium (CORC). Difficulties taking medications, depression, and health status in heart failure patients. *J Card Fail* 2006;**12**:54–60.
22. Butler J, Arbogast PG, Daugherty J, Jain MK, Ray WA, Griffin MR. Outpatient utilization of angiotensin-converting enzyme inhibitors among heart failure patients after hospital discharge. *J Am Coll Cardiol* 2004;**43**:2036–43.
23. Friedman MM. Gender differences in the health related quality of life in older adults with heart failure. *Heart Lung* 2003;**32**:320–27.
24. Ekman I, Ehrenberg A. Fatigue in chronic heart failure, does gender make a difference? *Eur J Cardiovasc Nurs* 2003;**1**:77–82.
25. Ekman I, Cleland JG, Swedberg K, Charlesworth A, Metra M, Poole-Wilson PA. Symptoms in patients with heart failure are prognostic predictors: insight from COMET. *J Card Fail* 2005;**11**:288–92.
26. Ekman I, Ehrenberg A. Fatigued elderly patients with chronic heart failure: do patient reports and nursing documentation correspond? *Nurse Diagn* 2002;**13**:127–36.
27. Lainscak M, Cleland JGF, Lenzen MJ, *et al.* Recall of lifestyle advice in patients recently hospitalised with heart failure: A EuroHeart Failure Survey analysis. *Eur J Heart Fail* 2007;**9**:1095–103.
28. Hoye A, Clark A. Iatrogenic hyperkalaemia. *Lancet* 2003;**361**:2124.
29. Dickstein K, Cohen-Solal A, Filippatos G, *et al.* ESC guidelines for the diagnosis and treatment of acute and chronic heart failure. *Eur J Heart Fail* 2008;**10**:933–89.
30. Wright SP, Walsh H, Ingley KM, Muncaster SA, *et al.* Uptake of self management strategies in a heart failure management programme. *Eur J Heart Fail* 2003;**5**:371–80.
31. Lewin J, Ledwidge M, O'Loughlin C, McNally C, McDonald K. Clinical deterioration in established heart failure: what is the value of BNP and weight gain in aiding diagnosis? *Eur J Heart Fail* 2005;**7**:953–7.
32. Travers B, O'Loughlin C, Murphy J, *et al.* Fluid restriction in the management of decompensated heart failure: no impact on time to clinical stability. *J Card Fail* 2007;**13**:128–32.
33. Holst M, Stromberg A, Lindholm M, Willenheimer R. Liberal versus restricted fluid prescription in stabilised patients with chronic heart failure: results of a randomised crossover study of the effects on health related quality of life, physical capacity, thirst and morbidity. *Scand Cardiovasc J* 2008;**42**:316–22.
34. Nicolas JM, Fernandez-Sola J, Estruch R, *et al.* The effect of controlled drinking in alcoholic cardiomyopathy. *Ann Intern Med* 2002:**136**:192–200.
35. Kramer BK, Schweda F, Riegger GA, *et al.* Diuretic treatment and diuretic resistance in heart failure. *Am J Med* 1999;**106**:90–6.
36. Paterna S, Gaspare P, Fasullo S, Sarullo FM, Di Pasquale P. Normal-sodium diet compared with low-sodium diet in compensated congestive heart failure: is sodium an old enemy or new friend? *Clin Sci (Lond)* 2008;**114**:221–30.
37. Heart Failure Society of America. HFSA Comprehensive heart failure practice guideline. *J Card Fail* 2006;**12**, e1–2.
38. Swedberg K, Cleland J, Dargie H, *et al.* The Task Force for the Diagnosis and Treatment of Chronic Heart Failure of the European Society of Cardiology. Guidelines for the diagnosis and treatment of chronic heart failure: executive summary (update 2005). *Eur Heart J* 2005;**26**:1115–40.
39. Garcia RLA, Hernandez-Diaz S. Nonsteroidal inflammatory drugs as a trigger of clinical heart failure. *Epidemiology* 2003;**14**:240–6.
40. Dal Corso E, Bondiani AL, Zanolla L, Vassanelli C.. Nurse educational activity on non-prescriptive therapies in patients with chronic heart failure. *Eur J Cardiovasc Nurs* 2007;**6**:314–20.

41. Evangelista LS, Doering LV, Dracup K. Usefulness of a history of tobacco and alcohol use in predicting multiple heart failure readmissions among veterans. *Am J Cardiol* 2000;**86**:1339–42.
42. Suskin N, Sheth T, Negassa A, Yusuf S. Relationship of current and past smoking to mortality and morbidity in patients with left ventricular dysfunction. *J Am Coll Cardiol* 2001;**37**:1677–82.
43. The Task Force of the Working Group on Heart Failure of the European society of Cardiology. The Treatment of Heart Failure. *Eur Heart J* 1997;**18**:736–53.
44. Kostis JB, Jackson G, Rosen R, *et al.* Sexual dysfunction and cardiac risk (the Second Princeton Consensus Conference. *Am J Cardiol* 2005;**26**:85M–M.
45. Manning HL, Scwartztein RM. Pathophysiology of dyspnoea. *N Engl J Med* 2005;**333**:1547–53.
46. Wang CS, Wang ST, Lai CT, Lin LJ, Chou P. Impact of influenza vaccination on major cause specific mortality. *Vaccine* 2007;**25**:1196–203.
47. Stewart S, MacIntyre K, Capewell S, McMurray JJV. Heart failure in a cold climate: seasonal variation in heart failure-related morbidity and mortality. *J Am Coll Cardiol* 2002;**39**:760.
48. Scottish Intercollegiate Guidelines Network. *Guideline 95: Management of chronic heart failure: A National clinical guideline.* SIGN, Edinburgh, 2007.
49. Salisbury DM, Begg NT (eds) *Immunisation against infectious disease.* Department of Health, London, 2006.
50. Nichol KL, Nordin J, Mulhooly J, Lask R, Fillibrandt K, Iwane M. Influenza vaccination and reduction in hospitalizations for cardiac disease and stroke among the elderly. *N Engl J Med* 2003;**348**:1322–32.
51. Diego C, Vila-Corcoles, Ochoa O, *et al.* and Epivac Study Group. Effects of annual influenza vaccination on winter mortality in elderly people with chronic heart disease. *Eur Heart J* 2009;**30**:209–16.
52. Centres for Disease Control and Prevention. Prevention and control of influenza: Recommendations of the Advisory Committee on Immunisation Practices (ACIP). *MMWR Recomm Rep* 2004;**53**:1–40.
53. Prevention of pneumococcal disease: recommendations of the Advisory Committee on Immunization Practices (ACIP). *MMWR Morb Mortal Wkly Rep* 1997;**46**(RR-8):1–24.
54. British Thoracic Society Recommendations. British Thoracic Society Standards of Care Committee. Managing patients with respiratory disease Planning Air Travel http://www.brit-thoracic.org.uk/c2/uploads/FlightRevision04.pdf. Accessed June 2007.
55. *Guide to the Current Medical Standards of Fitness to Drive.* Drivers Medical Group, DVLA, Swansea, 2010.
56. Clark RA, Inglis SC, McAlister FA, Cleland JGF, Stewart S. Telemonitoring or structured telephone support programmes for patients with chronic heart failure: systematic review and meta-analysis. *BMJ* 2007;**334**(7600):942–5.

PART XIV

Device therapy for heart failure

47

Implantable cardioverter-defibrillators in heart failure

Rachel C. Myles and Derek T. Connelly

Introduction

The implantable cardioverter-defibrillator (ICD) is established as an effective therapy for ventricular arrhythmias and is now routinely used for both primary and secondary prevention of sudden cardiac death in at-risk populations. Patients with heart failure (HF) have an increased propensity to arrhythmic sudden death and large randomized trials have demonstrated a clear mortality benefit following ICD implantation in selected HF patients. Despite this, the optimal use of ICDs in patients with HF remains a particularly challenging area of clinical practice. This is primarily because patients with HF are exposed to competing risks, which are both dynamic and difficult to quantify. As the cost and morbidity associated with ICD implantation are not insignificant, careful consideration of the risks and benefits associated with ICD implantation in each individual patient is required.

Sudden cardiac death in heart failure

HF is not only a common condition which is associated with an extremely high mortality, it is a diverse, complex clinical syndrome in which patients are exposed to competing risks, of sudden arrhythmic death or death from progressive pump failure.[1,2] Prevention of arrhythmic sudden cardiac death (SCD) constitutes a particular challenge because accurate risk prediction in such a large and heterogeneous population is extremely difficult.[3] Indeed, achieving effective prevention of SCD in HF is one of the principal challenges facing contemporary cardiovascular medicine.

Incidence and prevalence

Sudden deaths are, by definition, unexpected and are often unwitnessed, making the classification of the exact cause of death difficult in many cases. Estimates of the prevalence of SCD in HF come mainly from observational studies or from clinical trials, in which the definition of SCD is necessarily both arbitrary and pragmatic.[4] The accepted definition is death from a cardiac cause which is sudden and unexpected, in the absence of progressive cardiac deterioration, either within 1 h of cardiac symptoms, in bed during sleep, or within 24 h of last being seen alive.[5] Where these tight definitions in endpoint classification are used, as much as 50% of total mortality in HF is due to SCD.[6,7]

Aetiology

Sudden death may be caused by a number of different underlying pathologies, not all of which are cardiac. However, cardiac causes include ventricular arrhythmia, acute cardiogenic shock, and cardiac tamponade. The relative importance of arrhythmic or vascular events as causes of SCD in HF is debated.[7] Data regarding the specific aetiology of SCD are difficult to gather, but where they are available, recordings from monitored episodes of SCD show that the cause is ventricular arrhythmia in around 85% of cases.[8–11] To what extent these ventricular arrhythmias are primary or secondary to myocardial ischaemia is more difficult to ascertain. Autopsy data from the Assessment of Treatment with Lisinopril and Survival (ATLAS) trial suggested that myocardial infarction (MI) may be implicated in as many as 40% of sudden deaths in patients with HF.[12] However, a review of 157 episodes of ambulatory SCD which occurred during Holter monitoring concluded that the incidence of ST changes prior to ventricular arrhythmias was low.[11] Data from the second Multicenter Automatic Defibrillator Trial (MADIT-II) showed that 51% of deaths in the conventional therapy arm met accepted criteria for SCD, compared with 27% of deaths in the ICD arm,[5] suggesting that around one-quarter of all deaths and around one-half of sudden deaths were due to arrhythmia and amenable to ICD treatment.

Risk stratification for SCD in heart failure

At present, left ventricular ejection fraction (LVEF) is used to risk stratify patients with HF for ICD therapy. Although this method has identified populations in whom significant mortality reductions have been demonstrated, the 7% absolute risk reduction observed with an ICD in the Sudden Cardiac Death in Heart Failure Trial (SCDHeFT) was achieved with only 21% of patients receiving appropriate therapy over 5 years,[13] suggesting that the use of LVEF alone is suboptimal. A number of noninvasive risk stratification

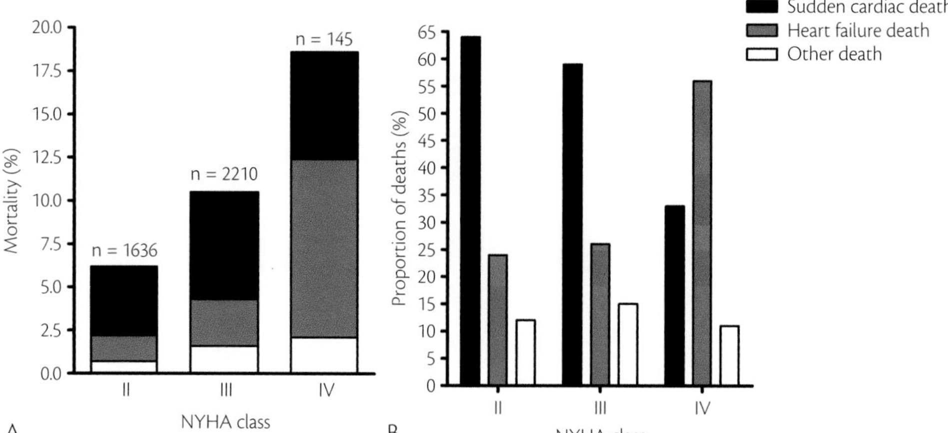

Fig. 47.1 Interaction between cause of death and NYHA class in MERIT-HF.[6]

tools have been proposed as having predictive value for arrhythmic events, but none has the required sensitivity or specificity to predict SCD accurately.[14,15] The search for improved risk stratification tools continues and the challenge of delivering effective population-wide prevention of SCD through ICD therapy is dependent on their development.

Pharmacological therapy to prevent arrhythmic SCD in heart failure

Until recently, attempts to prevent SCD have relied on pharmacological therapy to reverse left ventricular remodelling. Disease-modifying therapy with β-blockers,[16] angiotensin converting enzyme (ACE) inhibitors,[17] angiotensin receptor blockers,[2] and aldosterone antagonists[18] modestly reduces the risk of SCD in patients with HF and after MI. However, even patients on optimal medical therapy remain at high risk of SCD[2,6] and specific antiarrhythmic drug therapy has failed to improve survival.[13,19,20]

Competing risks in heart failure

Patients with HF are exposed to competing risks. HF carries a risk of sudden death along with a risk of death from progressive pump failure. In addition, many patients with HF are elderly and have comorbidities, which will also influence survival. An interaction is recognized between severity of HF symptoms and mode of death, which was exemplified in an analysis of cause-specific mortality by New York Heart Association (NYHA) class at enrolment in the Metoprolol CR/XL Randomized Intervention Trial In Congestive Heart Failure (MERIT-HF) study, which included 3991 patients with NYHA II–IV HF and LVEF 40% or less.[6] As shown in Fig. 47.1, the proportion of sudden deaths reduced with increasing NYHA class (64%, 59%, and 33% respectively), while the proportion of deaths due to worsening HF increased (24%, 26%, and 56% respectively).

As a result of the existence of these competing risks in a population with HF, any treatment which significantly reduces the risk of SCD will be expected to increase the risk of death from worsening HF simply by virtue of the fact that more patients will be alive to be exposed to this risk. For this reason, ICD trials have been designed to assess their impact on overall mortality, assuming that a reduction in arrhythmic sudden death will occur, but accepting that conversion to death from worsening HF within a short timescale is not a desirable outcome. The correct targeting of ICD therapy is crucial to ensure that patients not only gain sufficient survival benefit to justify the risks of implantation but also can enjoy improved survival free of debilitating HF for a reasonable length of time. This reinforces the need for accurate prognostication in patients with HF, such that ICD therapy can be appropriately directed. It also underlines the importance of optimization of medical therapy for HF when ICD therapy is being considered, and following implantation.

The implantable cardioverter-defibrillator

The concept of transvenous defibrillation for ventricular arrhythmias was developed by Mirowski and colleagues in the 1970s[21] and the first ICDs were implanted in patients with recurrent refractory ventricular arrhythmias in 1980.[22,23] These early devices incorporated large pulse generators implanted in the abdomen and connected to epicardial sensing and shocking electrodes, tunnelled from the chest. The implant procedure required thoracotomy and was associated with a considerable complication rate. Since then, significant improvements in technology have resulted in systems with smaller pulse generators which can be implanted prepectorally under local anaesthesia, and which employ transvenous lead systems integrated for pacing, tachycardia detection and administration of therapies. The components of an ICD system are shown in Fig. 47.2.

Pulse generator

An ICD pulse generator consists of a power source, capacitors for storing electrical charge, and the circuits and microprocessors necessary to manage its output. It must combine a pacing capability with the potential to deliver high-energy shocks within seconds of tachycardia detection. This means that specialized anode/cathode configurations are required to allow maintenance of high current and voltage during charging of the high-voltage capacitors for a defibrillation shock. As a consequence, ICD pulse generators are larger than those used in conventional pacemaker systems, and usually have a shorter battery life. The ICD pulse generator also incorporates the circuitry for the monitoring and programming functions necessary for these devices. In most ICD configurations, as described below, the pulse generator or 'can' may also form an active part of the lead system.

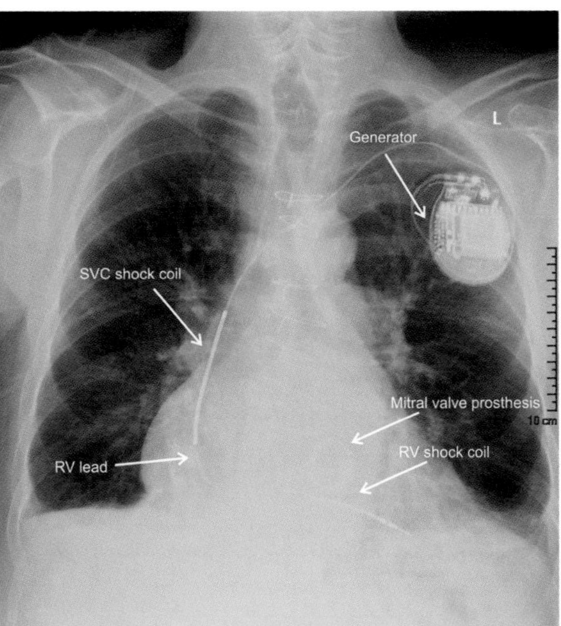

Fig. 47.2 A chest radiograph showing a transvenous ICD in a patient with a prior mitral valve replacements.

Lead systems

ICD lead systems must combine sensing, pacing, and defibrillation functions. In order to achieve this, the right ventricular endocardial lead contains a series of separately insulated conductors running in parallel. Standard coil conductors are required for pacing and sensing: one attached to the distal tip electrode and a second attached to the proximal ring electrode will provide bipolar sensing and stimulation. Delivery of a defibrillation shock is achieved using a high-voltage cable conductor connected to a shock coil on the external surface of the lead. In single-coil systems the coil is positioned on the distal portion of the lead and therefore sits in the right ventricular apex and the shock energy is passed between the coil and the pulse generator (an 'active can' configuration). In a two-coil system, there is a second coil positioned more proximally which sits in the superior vena cava (SVC), with defibrillation energy being passed between the right ventricular coil and both the SVC coil and the can. The Jewel Active Can Study randomized ICD recipients to receive ICDs with either active or passive can configuration and found that the active can system was associated with lower defibrillation thresholds and shorter implant times without any adverse events at 3 months.[24]

Dual-chamber ICD systems incorporate a standard atrial lead in addition to the integrated right ventricular defibrillation lead. The atrial lead can be used for sensing or stimulating in the right atrium and is used when dual-chamber pacing is desirable, or when atrial electrograms will improve tachycardia differentiation. Cardiac resynchronization therapy defibrillator (CRT-D) devices have an additional left ventricular epicardial lead, which is used to provide atrio-biventricular pacing.

Detection algorithms

Rate sensing

The effectiveness of an ICD depends upon its ability to detect the occurrence of those ventricular arrhythmias which require treatment. In a single-chamber system, the determination of ventricular tachyarrhythmia is principally achieved by measuring the rate of the sensed ventricular electrogram. The sensing function of an integrated ICD lead is therefore critical to its function, particularly during ventricular fibrillation (VF). In order to avoid undersensing of small amplitude potentials during VF, ICDs employ automatic algorithms which adjust their sensitivity over the cardiac cycle. Heart rate intervals, usually referred to as detection zones, are set for ventricular tachycardia (VT) and VF. The detection algorithm will stipulate a certain number of consecutive R-R intervals which are within the detection interval before designating a tachycardia to be VT or VF. Following administration of therapy, a series of usually less stringent redetection rate criteria are applied to ascertain whether it has been successful.

SVT discrimination

The major disadvantage with identification of VT or VF by rate sensing algorithms is that atrial fibrillation (AF) or a supraventricular tachycardia (SVT), occurring within the detection zone may trigger clinically inappropriate therapies (Fig. 47.3). A number of different algorithms are available to aid the identification of SVT occurring within the VT detection zone, so that therapy can be appropriately withheld. These include analyses of the R-R interval stability, the timescale of tachycardia onset, and the electrogram morphology. All of these algorithms have potential pitfalls and may result in delayed therapy for VT. As such they are optional and the ICD is generally programmed to deliver therapy if a tachycardia designated as SVT persists within the VT detection zone. In dual-chamber systems, atrial electrograms can be used to improve arrhythmia classification, by identifying atrioventricular dissociation.[25] However, in MADIT-II rates of inappropriate therapies were not different between dual-chamber and single-chamber devices.[26] This comparison may be confounded by the fact that stored electrograms from a dual-chamber device give more information regarding the tachycardia and inappropriate therapies may therefore be identified more often than a single-chamber system. In the Detect Supraventricular Tachycardia Study, the dual-chamber detection group experienced a modest reduction in the proportion of SVTs which were inappropriately detected as VT (30.9% vs 39.5%), but this did not translate into a reduction in inappropriate shocks.[27] Nevertheless, the availability of atrial electrograms can often be invaluable in 'troubleshooting' and in planning subsequent treatment for the patient, including changes in programming, drug therapy and ablation (Fig. 47.4).

Programmable therapies

Modern ICD systems incorporate complex programmable pacing and antitachyarrhythmia therapies. Optimal ICD programming should always be based on the individual's needs and subject to regular review.

Pacing

All ICDs have programmable pacing functions, and depending on the device and lead systems used, pacing capabilities can range from backup VVI pacing with single-chamber systems, though 'physiologic' (DDDR) pacing with dual-chamber ICDs to atrio-biventricular pacing with cardiac resynchronization therapy defibrillators (CRT-D). The rationale for provision of backup VVI capabilities with all ICDs is to protect from postshock bradycardia, which can be sufficient to cause haemodynamic compromise in the absence of bradycardia pacing. In dual-chamber systems, the atrial

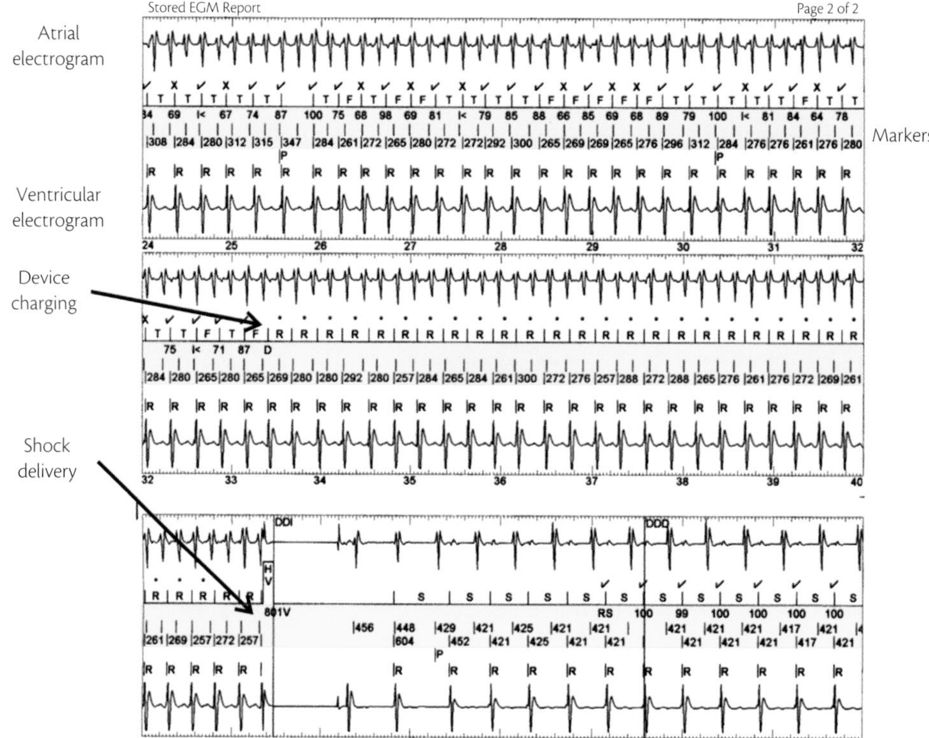

Fig. 47.3 Inappropriate ICD therapy for atrial fibrillation.

lead can sense atrial electrograms and therefore makes improved SVT discrimination possible and will also allow provision of atrially based pacing as a treatment for atrial arrhythmias or in the event that the patient were to develop conducting system disease. Cardiac resynchronization therapy pacing (CRT-P), which employs atrio-biventricular pacing to correct interventricular dyssynchrony, has been shown to improve outcome in patients with severe symptomatic HF despite optimal medical therapy who also have left ventricular dysfunction and QRS prolongation.[28] It can be combined with a defibrillator function (CRT-D) in these patients when an ICD indication also exists.

Antitachycardia pacing

Overdrive or antitachycardia pacing (ATP) is an effective therapy for VT[29] and ICDs can be programmed to administer various types of ATP for tachycardias falling within the VT detection zone. ATP is administered using trains of stimuli, either in a burst (constant cycle length) or a ramp (decremental cycle length) configuration, with the ATP cycle length determined to be a proportion of the tachycardia cycle length (Fig. 47.5). Unlike defibrillation shocks, ATP is seldom uncomfortable for the patient. Successful ATP should therefore improve device tolerability and also has the potential advantage of minimizing the impact of therapies on battery life. However, there is a risk of tachycardia acceleration during ATP and prolonged VT during multiple unsuccessful attempts at ATP may lead to haemodynamic compromise. In addition, rapid VTs (>200 beats/min) are less likely to respond to ATP and more likely to cause haemodynamic compromise, particularly in patients with pre-existing left ventricular dysfunction.[29] In order to optimize ATP delivery, most devices therefore allow programming of two VT detection zones with differential ATP protocols. A slow VT zone can be programmed with less aggressive (and therefore lower risk of acceleration) ATP algorithms and may include more attempts before a shock is eventually delivered. Alternatively, a fast VT zone can be programmed with a lower number of more aggressive ATP protocols before defaulting to defibrillation.

Defibrillation

The mainstay of effective tachycardia treatment by an ICD is the defibrillator capability. In the event of a tachycardia falling within the VF detection zone or the failure of ATP to terminate a tachycardia, the ICD will deliver a defibrillation shock. Defibrillation shocks are effective in terminating spontaneously occurring VT and VF in most cases.[30] An example of successful VF termination

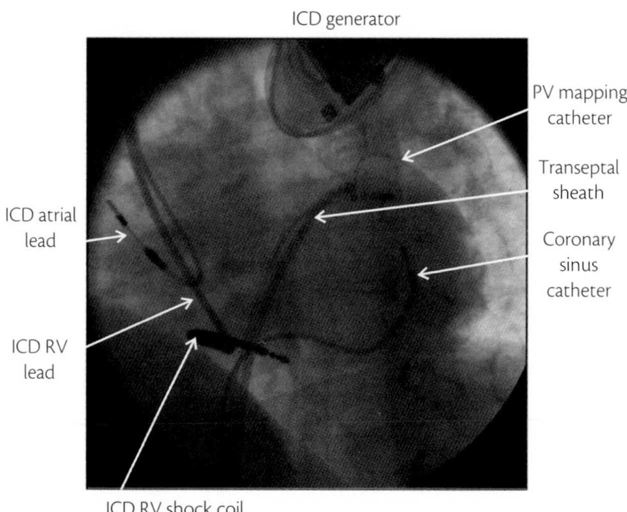

Fig. 47.4 Fluoroscopy image during radio frequency ablation for atrial fibrillation in an ICD patient.

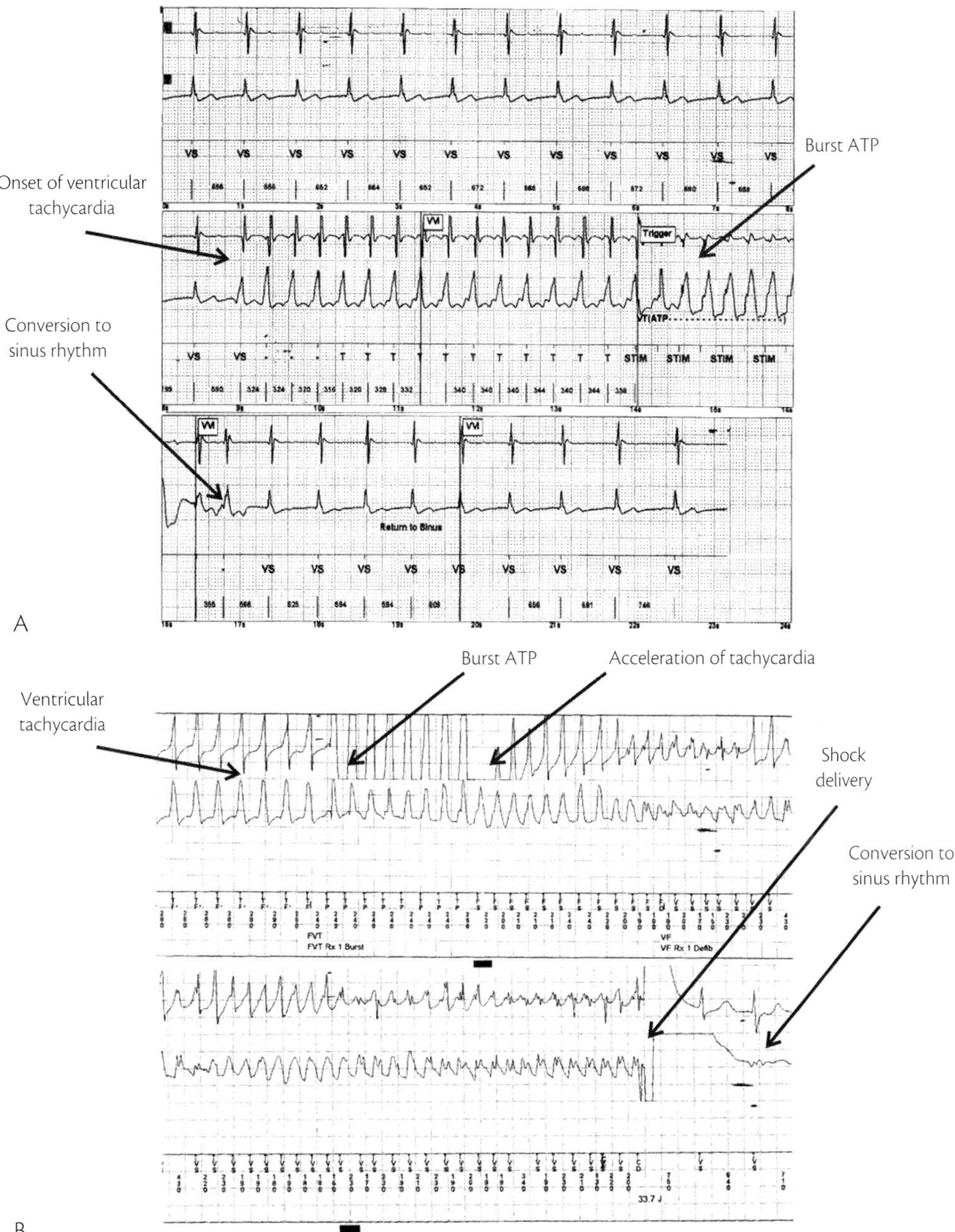

Fig. 47.5 Antitachycardia pacing for ventricular tachycardia.

by an ICD is shown in Fig. 47.6. Effective defibrillation depends on a sufficient voltage (the defibrillation threshold) being delivered to depolarize the bulk of the myocardium. In order to ensure effective defibrillation, the pulse generator must be able to charge the high-voltage capacitor such that the threshold voltage is consistently surpassed. Historically, assessment of the defibrillation threshold has been a critical component of the ICD implant and programming procedure, but prospective data have failed to show clinical benefit associated with this practice.[31]

ICD therapies as endpoints in clinical trials

Appropriate ICD therapies are often used as endpoints in studies of ICD recipients. In interpreting such studies it is important to note that appropriate ICD therapies are not a surrogate for SCD. An analysis from the DEFINITE (Defibrillators in Non-Ischemic Cardiomyopathy Treatment Evaluation) trial suggested that patients in the ICD arm experienced an appropriate ICD shock for VF/VT at a rate twice that of the SCD rate in the medical therapy arm, suggesting that around one-half of the ventricular arrhythmic events treated by an ICD may have been well tolerated or self-terminating and would not have resulted in the patient's death.[32]

Implantation

The implant procedure is usually performed under conscious sedation with local anaesthesia, although in some complex cases general anaesthesia may be preferable. An operating theatre environment is used and strict surgical aseptic techniques are adhered to. A single incision, approximately 5 cm in length, is made inferior to the left clavicle, and a pocket is made for the generator, either subcutaneously or deep to the pectoralis major muscle. A lead is introduced to the subclavian or cephalic vein using a Seldinger

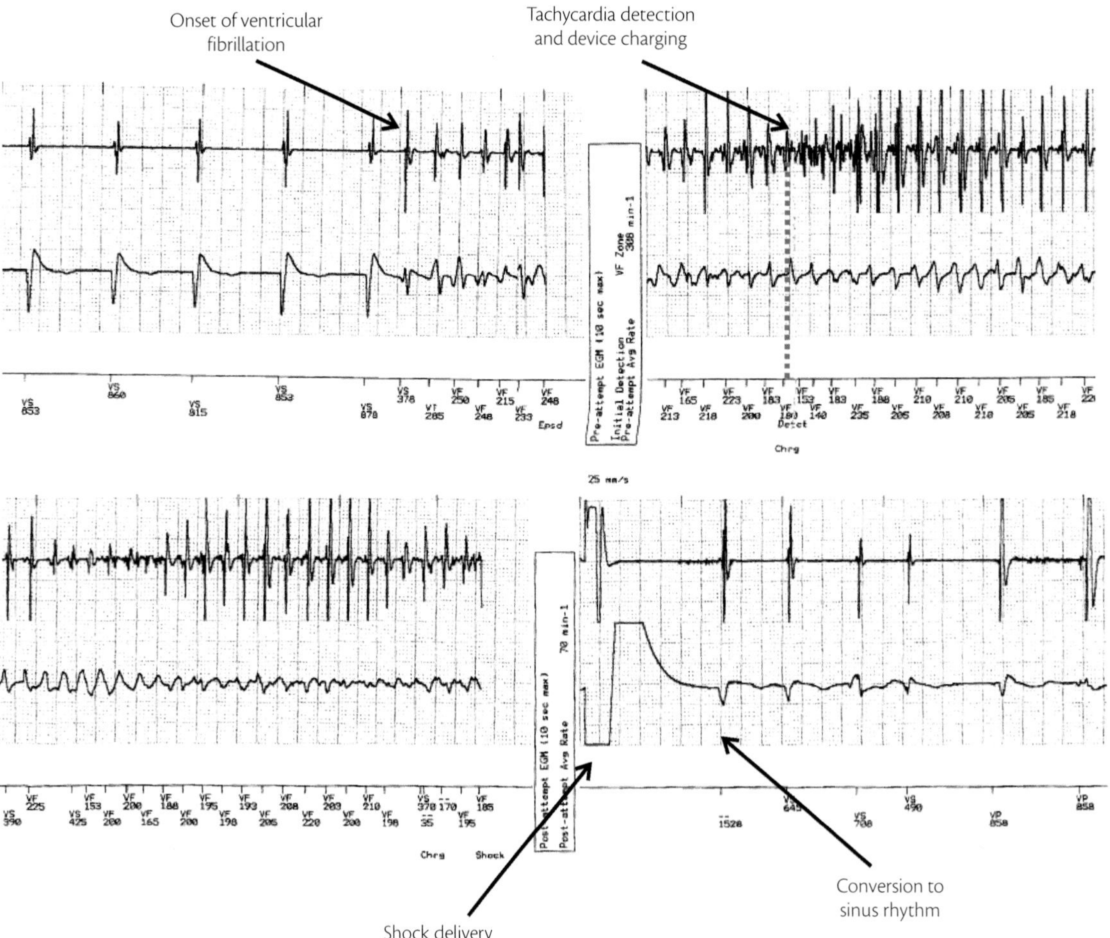

Fig. 47.6 Termination of ventricular fibrillation by an ICD shock.

technique and advanced under fluoroscopy to the apex of the right ventricle. If necessary a right atrial pacing lead may also be implanted. Additionally, if a patient with HF requires CRT, a left ventricular epicardial lead is placed via the coronary veins. As for permanent pacing, accurate lead placement, with close attention to achieving optimal sensing, threshold, impedance, and stability is crucial. Once the leads are secured in place they are connected to the generator which is buried in the subcutaneous or submuscular pocket, which is then closed in layers using absorbable sutures. Where appropriate, defibrillation efficacy is then determined. This is performed by inducing VF (either by delivering a small shock on the T-wave or a short burst of AC or DC current) and programming the device to terminate the arrhythmia. Conventionally, effective shock energy at least 10 J less than the maximum deliverable by the device is acceptable. An external defibrillator is available should the implanted device fail to terminate the arrhythmia. Patients are usually discharged home the following day provided that pacing parameters are satisfactory and a chest radiograph shows satisfactory lead positions and no evidence of pneumothorax (see Fig. 47.4).

Complications

ICD implantation has numerous potential complications and it is estimated that as many as one-quarter of those who receive an ICD will experience a complication over a 5-year period.[33]

Procedure-related complications

The complications of ICD implantation are similar to those associated with pacemaker implantation, and include haematoma, infection, pneumothorax, and lead displacement. A recent study has estimated that an index complication occurs in around 10% of patients, with mechanical complications being the most common.[34] Implant-related mortality is very rare; published rates of 30-day mortality are around 1% and usually related to the severity of the patient's cardiac disease.[35]

Failure of ICD therapy

It is important to recognize that an ICD is not a cure. Patients are still at risk of a ventricular arrhythmia, which may cause syncope or cardiac arrest. In a retrospective analysis of 320 deaths in 4889 patients enrolled in preclinical trials, 28% of 317 classifiable deaths were sudden and for 68 of these 90 sudden deaths a cause was identifiable.[36] 16% of all deaths in patients with a functioning ICD in place were found to be due to VT/VF, in 17 of 50 the ICD failed to terminate the arrhythmia, in 9 there was incessantly recurrent ventricular arrhythmia, and in 20 immediate postshock pulseless electrical activity (PEA—previously known as electromechanical dissociation, EMD) was the terminal rhythm. The mechanism of postshock PEA is unclear, and in some cases factors such as global myocardial ischaemia are likely to be implicated.

Myocardial damage by ICD shocks

Studies in animal models suggest that high-energy defibrillation shocks can cause myocardial damage, although the energies required for damage are significantly higher than those required for effective defibrillation.[37] In MADIT-II, the risk of HF was increased following appropriate shocks but not following inappropriate shocks, suggesting that the effects of the defibrillation shock on the myocardium was not implicated in producing subsequent myocardial dysfunction but rather that the occurrence of a ventricular arrhythmia identified patients at particular risk of developing HF.[38] Conversely, all-cause mortality was increased following an inappropriate shock, but not following ATP,[26] suggesting that under some circumstances the shock may indeed have adverse consequences. Myocardial damage as indicated by troponin elevation is not infrequently detectable following defibrillation threshold testing at ICD implant,[39] during which the duration of VF is minimized. Patients with severe left ventricular dysfunction are most at risk of developing haemodynamic instability during routine defibrillation testing at ICD implantation[40] and in a limited multivariate analysis the only variable which independently predicted postshock PEA was the presence of NYHA class III/IV HF.[36] It is therefore possible that in some patients with severe left ventricular dysfunction and HF, therapeutic defibrillation energy may be sufficient to cause myocardial damage or left ventricular dysfunction, particularly where multiple shocks are administered in close succession.

Inappropriate shocks

In the long term, the commonest adverse event associated with ICD therapy is an inappropriate shock from the device. These are most frequently due to AF or an SVT occurring within the VT/VF detection zones (see Fig. 47.5), but can occur due to abnormal sensing as a result of hardware problems such as conductor fracture or insulation break of the ventricular lead. The reason for inappropriate shocks can usually be diagnosed by interrogation of the device. Inappropriate shocks are not only unpleasant for the patient,[41] they limit battery longevity, may cause myocardial damage,[42] and are associated with an increased risk of mortality.[26,43] Patients with HF have a high incidence of AF, which occurs in up to 30% of patients with NYHA class II/III HF,[44] putting them at particular risk of receiving inappropriate therapies. In MADIT-II, 31% of all shocks administered were judged to be inappropriate and 11.5% of patients in the ICD arm received inappropriate shocks over the 2-year period.[26] Of these, 44% were due to AF, 36% due to SVT and 20% due to abnormal sensing. In the Sudden Cardiac Death in Heart Failure (SCDHeFT) Trial, which implanted single-chamber shock-only devices in patients with symptomatic HF, 32% of shocks were inappropriate and 17% of patients in the ICD arm received inappropriate shocks over 5 years.[43] The PainFree Study showed similar rates of inappropriate shocks, which accounted for 40% of all shocks and occurred in 15% of patients.[40] The occurrence of antitachycardia pacing is not associated with adverse outcomes, suggesting that the increased risk of mortality following defibrillation shocks may relate to the shock rather than the arrhythmia which triggered it. However, it may equally reflect the fact that ATP is generally reserved for slower, less dangerous arrhythmias.

On an individual basis, inappropriate shocks for SVT can be minimized by judicious programming and appropriate use of β-blockers and other antiarrhythmic drugs.[45] There is little evidence that dual-chamber detection algorithms have a significant impact on the rate of inappropriate ICD shocks. In MADIT-II, use of the stability algorithm, designed to prevent inappropriate shocks due to AF, was associated with a lower rate of inappropriate shocks.[26] Clearly, programming of a higher detection rate would likely result in a reduction in inappropriate shocks, the majority of which occur at a rate less than 200 beats/min.[26] However, this would lead to underdetection of slow VTs and may therefore compromise the efficacy of the ICD.

Psychological problems

Although a minority of patients may develop an adverse psychological reaction to ICD implantation, it is important to be aware that these patients often improve over time as they become accustomed to having the device and adapt to their physical limitations. Although clear associations between the underlying condition, the presence of the ICD, delivery of therapies and psychological stress are difficult to establish, it is clear that ICD patients experience a degree of psychological morbidity compared to other patients with cardiovascular disease.[46] Many individual patients tolerate defibrillation shocks very poorly, particularly if they experience multiple shocks (whether appropriate or inappropriate). For this reason, antiarrhythmic drugs and ablation may have a role in reducing the incidence of both ventricular and supraventricular arrhythmias in patients with ICDs.[45]

Lifestyle implications

Inevitably, many patients with ICDs face lifestyle restrictions. The implant procedure is similar to that of a pacemaker, but follow-up of patients with ICDs tends to be more complex. However this may change with the development of systems for remote ICD monitoring.

Quality of life

Patients with HF do not simply live longer with an ICD, but live longer with their HF symptoms and so are at risk of experiencing a deterioration in those symptoms. ICD therapy in HF patients therefore carries a risk of increasing survival but reducing quality of life (QOL). An analysis of health-related QOL from SCDHeFT found that QOL was greater in the ICD arm at 3 and 12 months, but equalled that in the medical therapy arm at 30 months,[47] at least providing reassurance that ICD therapy does not significantly impair QOL in patients with symptomatic HF. It is noteworthy that ICD shocks occurring in the month before interview were associated with a reduction in QOL.

Driving

The regulations regarding fitness to drive in patients with ICDs vary between countries, and are subject to periodic review. In the United Kingdom, the Driver and Vehicle Licensing Agency publishes recommendations on its website.[48] UK patients who have received an ICD for secondary prevention may be allowed to drive provided that the device has been implanted for at least 6 months and has not delivered shock therapy or symptomatic ATP in that period, and if previous discharges have not been accompanied by incapacity. Patients must stop driving for 1 month if the device (lead or generator) is revised, or if any change is made to their antiarrhythmic treatment. Patients who have a primary prevention ICD implanted need only refrain from driving for 1 month, unless they subsequently receive shocks from the device. Patients with ICDs are permanently disqualified from driving commercial vehicles. The guidelines in the United States are largely similar, except that primary prevention ICD patients are only restricted from driving until recovery from the procedure (at least 1 week).[49] The European Heart Rhythm Association guidelines differ in that they recommend that patients need only refrain from driving for 3 months following a secondary prevention implant or an appropriate therapy.[50]

Sources of electromagnetic interference

Modern pacemakers and ICDs are well protected against external sources of electromagnetic interference. Although devices are being developed that will be compatible for use in MRI scanners, at present ICD recipients are advised that they cannot undergo MRI scanning. Cellular telephones (mobile phones) can occasionally interfere with ICDs and pacemakers, but only if the telephone is within 15 cm (6 in) of the generator. There have been occasional reports of interference to pacemakers and ICDs caused by electronic article surveillance gates, but only if the patient is in the vicinity of the gates for several seconds.[51] Very occasionally there are patients with these devices who work in environments where high-intensity electrical or magnetic fields might interfere with the device, and such scenarios require specialist assessment which often involves collaboration between the patient's cardiologist, the engineers employed by the device manufacturer, and the occupational health physician at the place of work.

Evidence for ICD implantation in left ventricular dysfunction and heart failure

Secondary prevention

Rationale

ICD implantation in survivors of life-threatening ventricular tachyarrhythmia is referred to as secondary prevention. For the purposes of clinical trial enrolment, life-threatening ventricular arrhythmias are defined as VF or sustained VT, meaning VT which lasts for at least 30 s or requires emergency intervention to terminate the arrhythmia because of cardiac arrest, syncope, haemodynamic compromise or HF. In the absence of an identifiable and reversible precipitant, these patients are at high risk of recurrent ventricular arrhythmia.[52]

Secondary prevention ICD trials

Three large randomized trials have examined the efficacy of ICD implantation for secondary prevention,[53–55] and the recruited populations are summarized in Table 47.1. Of the three, only the Antiarrhythmics Versus Implantable Defibrillator (AVID) trial demonstrated a statistically significant reduction in mortality associated with ICD use.[53] The Canadian Implantable Defibrillator Study (CIDS) was terminated early after results from AVID were reported[54] and the Cardiac Arrest Study of Hamburg (CASH) trial showed a nonsignificant benefit.[55] However, all three studies reported a similar absolute risk reduction (*c.*6% over 2 years) and a meta-analysis showed a 28% relative reduction in mortality in the ICD group compared to amiodarone therapy.[56] In a nonprespecified subgroup analysis of the AVID trial, patients with LVEF 35% or less had more to gain from ICD implantation than those with preserved LVEF in whom there was no significant difference in mortality compared to amiodarone[57]—a finding which was borne out in the meta-analysis.[56] However, the idea that those patients with preserved LVEF following life-threatening arrhythmias may not benefit from ICD implantation has not been prospectively evaluated and as such is not reflected in the consensus guidelines governing secondary prevention ICD implantation. ICD implantation is recommended for all survivors of life-threatening ventricular arrhythmias, regardless of LVEF,[58] unless a reversible cause is identified (class I, level of evidence A), and remains the only evidence-based therapy for this group of patients. Those ventricular arrhythmias associated with a reversible cause, such as myocardial ischaemia, infarction, electrolyte disturbance, or a proarrhythmic drug effect were excluded from the secondary prevention trials, although data from the AVID registry suggests a poor outcome in these patients.[59] It is common practice not to implant ICDs for VT/VF which occurred during the acute phase of ST segment elevation MI, but whether the same applies to non-ST segment elevation MI is unclear. Perhaps in acknowledgement of this uncertainty, along with the fact that low-grade myocardial ischaemia may be difficult to completely reverse, ischaemia is not listed as a reversible cause in the consensus guidelines.

Table 47.1 Summary of populations enrolled in the main secondary prevention ICD trials

	n	Age (years)	LVEF (%)	NYHA Class I or II/III or IV	ACEi (%)	β-Blocker (%)
AVID[53]	1016	65	~32	50/10	68	~25
CIDS[54]	659	~63	~33	40/10	NA	~25
CASH[55]	288	~58	~45	83/17	~40	~33[a]

[a] Randomized therapy.

ACEi, angiotensin converting enzyme inhibitor; LVEF, left ventricular ejection fraction; NYHA, New York Heart Association.

Primary prevention

Rationale

The majority of victims of SCD do not experience a prior arrhythmic event to identify them as high risk,[15] and because of this, a primary prevention ICD strategy is also required. Such a strategy relies on effective means of identifying patients at high risk. The current method of identifying such patients is the presence of a severely impaired LVEF, usually either as a result of prior MI or idiopathic dilated cardiomyopathy.

Primary prevention ICD trials

A significant mortality benefit has been demonstrated in large randomized trials of prophylactic ICD therapy in patients with left ventricular systolic dysfunction (LVSD) and a history of either chronic HF or MI; the recruited populations are summarized in Table 47.2.

Coronary disease, LVSD and nonsustained/inducible ventricular arrhythmias

The first Multicenter Automatic Defibrillator Implantation Trial (MADIT) recruited patients with prior MI, LVEF 35% or less, spontaneous nonsustained VT and inducible sustained VT at electrophysiological study (EPS) which could not be suppressed acutely using antiarrhythmic therapy, and randomized them to chronic antiarrhythmic therapy (mostly amiodarone) or ICD implantation.[60] The Multicenter UnSustained Tachycardia Trial

Table 47.2 Summary of populations enrolled in the main primary prevention ICD trials

	n	Age (years)	LVEF (%)	NYHA class I/II/III/IV (%)	ACEi (%)	β-Blocker (%)
Coronary disease, LVSD and nonsustained/inducible ventricular arrhythmias						
MADIT[60]	196	~63	~26	~65% II or III	~57	~21
MUSTT[61]	704	~67	~30	35/40/25/0	~75	~40
Coronary disease and LVSD						
MADIT-II[62]	1232	~65	~23	35/35/25/5	70	70
LVSD early after acute MI						
DINAMIT[63]	674	~62	~28	7/30/15/0	95	87
Nonischaemic cardiomyopathy						
DEFINITE[66]	458	~58	~21	22/57/21/0	85	85
Symptomatic HF and LVSD						
SCDHeFT[13]	2521	~60	~25	0/70/30/0	85	69

ACEi, angiotensin converting enzyme inhibitor; HF, heart failure; LVEF, left ventricular ejection fraction; LVSD, left ventricular systolic dysfunction; MI, myocardial infarction; NYHA, New York Heart Association.

(MUSTT) recruited a similar population and was designed to assess the efficacy of EPS-guided pharmacological therapy, but included a provision for patients to receive an ICD in a nonrandomized fashion if antiarrhythmic drugs failed to suppress inducible ventricular arrhythmias.[61] Both of these studies implanted relatively small numbers of ICDs in highly selected patients and demonstrated a sizeable survival advantage with an ICD, the relative reductions in all-cause mortality being 54% and 60% respectively.

Coronary disease and LVSD

More recently, results from larger studies with less stringent, and noninvasive, entry criteria have led to the expansion of primary prevention ICD therapy. MADIT-II randomized 1232 patients with ischaemic cardiomyopathy and LVEF of 30% or less to receive an ICD or be treated with conventional therapy alone.[62] No documentation of spontaneous or inducible ventricular arrhythmia was required for enrollment. The patients were well treated, with 70% receiving ACE inhibitors and β-blockers, and the majority had previously undergone coronary revascularization. The trial was designed to be stopped after a prespecified boundary treatment effect had been observed, which occurred after a mean follow-up of 20 months, with an observed mortality of 14.2% in the ICD group compared to 19.8% in the conventionally treated group. This equates to a relative risk reduction of 31%, less than that achieved in MADIT and MUSTT, but of a similar magnitude to that seen in the secondary prevention trials. The prespecified subgroup analyses did not identify any statistically significant differences in the magnitude of benefit across age (<60 vs 60–69 vs ≥70 years), sex, NYHA class (I vs ≥II), ejection fraction (dichotomized at 25%) and QRS duration (<120 vs 120–150 vs >150 ms), either in terms of reduction in all-cause mortality,[62] or the reduction in SCD.[5] However, there was an observed trend for greater benefit associated with an ICD in patients with a QRS complex width of 120 ms or more.

LVSD early after acute MI

Patients with a history of MI within the preceding 3 months were ineligible for recruitment into MADIT-II. Data from studies of ICD implantation early after MI suggest that the benefit seen in MADIT-II cannot be extrapolated to within 4–6 weeks of acute MI. Indeed, the Defibrillator in Acute Myocardial Infarction Trial (DINAMIT) demonstrated a trend towards harm with an ICD in patients with LVEF 35% or less and abnormal autonomic function in the early phase (6–40 days) following MI.[63] There was a reduction in the rate of arrhythmic death which was offset by an increase in nonarrhythmic death in the ICD arm. The reason for the increase in nonarrhythmic death remains unclear, but was recapitulated in the Immediate Risk Stratification Improves Survival (IRIS) trial. The IRIS protocol identified post-MI patients as high risk on the basis of either resting tachycardia in combination with LVEF ≤40% or the presence of nonsustained VT regardless of LVEF,[64] and so included a proportion (*c.*33%) of patients with ischaemic cardiomyopathy and preserved left ventricular function, a group in whom there was no pre-existing evidence for ICD implantation. However, survival benefit was not demonstrated for either high-risk group despite a significant reduction in arrhythmic mortality.[65] It has been suggested that in this population the occurrence of ventricular arrhythmia identifies a group at such high risk of overall cardiac mortality that the presence of an ICD will simply convert the mode of death within a relatively short timescale, an effect which is not evident in the trials of chronic ischaemic cardiomyopathy. Whether this is the case, or whether some aspect of ICD implantation actively increases cardiac mortality in the early phase following MI remains to be established. Nevertheless, published guidelines have taken account of this in recommending that primary prevention ICDs should not be implanted within 4–6 weeks of MI.[58]

Nonischaemic cardiomyopathy

The DEFINITE trial randomized 458 patients with nonischaemic cardiomyopathy, LVEF 35% or less, and either premature ventricular complexes or nonsustained VT on ambulatory monitoring to receive optimal medical therapy or optimal medical therapy plus an ICD.[66] The entry criteria only specified a history of HF, but the enrolled population had a high prevalence of current symptomatic HF (78% NYHA II/III). The trial did not reach statistical significance but demonstrated a trend towards improved survival in the ICD arm over 2 years.

Heart failure and LVSD

The Sudden Cardiac Death in Heart Failure trial (SCDHeFT) is the largest ICD trial so far published,[13] and the only to mandate current symptomatic HF at entry. In this study, 2521 patients with NYHA class II or III HF were randomized to receive optimal medical therapy with placebo, medical therapy plus amiodarone, or medical therapy with implantation of a single-chamber, shock-only ICD. Approximately one-half of the patients had nonischaemic dilated cardiomyopathy and the majority (70%) were in NYHA class II. After a follow-up period of 5 years the mortality in the medical therapy arm was 36.1% (7.2% per year). Amiodarone had no effect on mortality, but there was a 23% reduction in mortality with ICD therapy, which equated to a 7% absolute risk reduction over 5 years. In subgroup analyses, the benefit from ICD therapy was most pronounced in those with an LVEF of less than 30% and in the patients with relatively mild symptoms (NYHA class II vs. III). Importantly, a similar magnitude of benefit was seen in patients with ischaemic and nonischaemic cardiomyopathy. The mortality benefit was attributable to a 60% reduction in sudden death with no observed effect of ICD therapy on HF deaths.[67]

Indeed, the HF status of surviving patients, as assessed by LVEF and NYHA class, improved over the course of the study, possibly reflecting benefit from optimized medical therapy and regular medical contact.[68]

Guidelines for the use of ICD therapy in heart failure

Guidelines from the United Kingdom, Europe, and the United States all recommend the use of ICDs for secondary prevention in survivors of life-threatening ventricular arrhythmias in the absence of an identifiable reversible cause and where survival with a good QOL of at least 1 year can reasonably be expected. For primary prevention indications, however, consensus guidelines vary (Table 47.3), although each assumes that the patient is established on optimal medical therapy. In the United Kingdom, the National Institute for Health and Clinical Excellence (NICE) published an ICD guidance which was reviewed in 2006, but this specifically did not include patients with nonischaemic DCM.[72] The Scottish Intercollegiate Guidelines Network (SIGN) published a more expansive guidance on the use of primary prevention ICDs in patients with coronary artery disease in 2007.[73]

Patients who do not have a reasonable expectation of survival with a reasonable functional status for a period of 1 year are again specifically excluded from ICD implantation, regardless of the indication. This includes patients with refractory NYHA class IV HF who are not candidates for cardiac transplantation. Other exclusions (class III recommendations) include incessant VT/VF, significant psychiatric illness, or the identification of completely reversible causes for the occurrence of VT/VF.

Table 47.3 Guidelines for primary prevention ICD implantation

	ACC/AHA/HRS 2008[58]	ESC 2006[69–71,99]	NICE 2006[72]	SIGN 2007[73]
Coronary disease, LVSD and inducible arrhythmias				
LVEF ≤40%	Class I[a]	Class I[a]	NR	NR
LVEF ≤35%	Class I[a]	Class I[a]	Recommended[b]	Prioritize[b]
Coronary disease, LVSD and nonsustained arrhythmias				
LVEF ≤40%	NR	Class I[a]	NR	NR
LVEF ≤35%	Class IIa[a]	Class I[a]	Recommended[b]	Prioritize[b]
Coronary disease and LVSD				
LVEF ≤30%	Class I[a]	Class IIa[a]	NR	Consider[b]
LVEF ≤30% and QRSd ≥120 ms	Class I[a]	Class IIa[a]	Recommended[b]	Prioritize[b]
LVEF ≤35% and NYHA II/III	Class I[a]	Class I[a,c]	NR	Consider[b]
Nonischaemic cardiomyopathy				
NYHA I	Class IIb	Class IIb	NR	NR
NYHA II/III	Class I	Class I[c]	NR	NR
Syncope	Class IIa	Class IIb	NR	NR
Symptomatic HF and LVSD				
NYHA II/III	Class I	Class I[a,c]	NR	NR

[a] At least 40 days post acute MI.

[b] At least 4 weeks post acute MI.

[c] Chronic Heart Failure Guideline 2008.

HF, heart failure; LVEF, left ventricular ejection fraction; LVSD, left ventricular systolic dysfunction; MI, myocardial infarction; NR, not recommended; NYHA, New York Heart Association.

Cost-effectiveness of primary prevention ICD therapy in heart failure

The available evidence suggests that improved outcomes can be achieved with primary prevention ICDs in patients with HF and these indications are now included in international consensus guidelines. However, there is a significant cost associated with ICD therapy and because the potential primary prevention population is large, ICD therapy may therefore have major implications for finite health budgets.[74] The cost-effectiveness of ICD therapy depends heavily on the health care system in which it is assessed and the time window over which it is considered, particularly as the majority of the cost is associated with the hardware and implant, and the fact that survival benefit takes some time to manifest.[75] Cost-effectiveness analyses were prespecified in SCDHeFT; cost data were collected prospectively and survival benefit was extrapolated beyond the 5-year follow-up. The incremental cost per quality-adjusted life year (QALY) saved was around $41 000,[76] which is congruent with estimates from other primary prevention studies.[77] The Buxton and Sharples model, used as the basis for the NICE guidance, estimated the incremental cost effectiveness ratio of primary prevention ICD implantation in the United Kingdom as £35 000–45 000 per QALY.[78] However, these figures are dependent on the survival benefit associated with the ICD persisting for around 7–8 years, which in elderly patients with NYHA III HF, may be unrealistic. Using a limit of $50 000 per life year saved as a threshold for an acceptable cost-effectiveness profile,[79] this suggests that the cost of primary prevention ICD therapy in HF is acceptable in economic terms, provided that the real benefits are similar to those observed in SCDHeFT, and persist beyond 5 years.

The importance of heart failure in ICD trials

Although SCDHeFT was the only one of the primary prevention ICD trials to mandate symptomatic HF at enrolment, patients with low ejection fraction HF were also enrolled into the other trials—in DEFINITE and MADIT-II, the prevalence of NYHA II/III HF was around 78%[66] and 60%[62] respectively (see Table 47.2). Moreover, patients with asymptomatic LVSD remain at risk of developing symptomatic HF. Although ICDs reduced mortality overall in HF patients in SCDHeFT, those patients in the ICD arm who received an appropriate shock had a fivefold greater mortality than those who received no shock.[43] Patients receiving inappropriate shocks displayed a doubling of mortality. The most common cause of death in patients who received an ICD shock was progressive HF, which accounted for 40% of all deaths in this group. These findings underline the central confounding factor as regards ICD therapy in patients with HF—the existence of competing risks dictates that a reduction in sudden death will result in an increase in HF death.

The relationship between NYHA class and ICD benefit

The results from randomized trials of ICD therapy have produced conflicting results in terms of the relationship of severity of HF symptoms (as determined by NYHA class) and the magnitude of benefit derived from an ICD. In MADIT-II a similar magnitude of benefit was identified for patients with NYHA I symptoms, who constituted around 35% of the population, compared with those with an NYHA class II or greater.[62] In DEFINITE, patients with NYHA class III HF may have greater benefit from ICD therapy than those in class II.[66] In a prespecified subgroup analysis of SCDHeFT, the benefit seen with an ICD appeared confined to the 70% of the population who had NYHA class II symptoms.[13] The reasons for these contradictory findings are not immediately apparent, and it is important to note both the limitations of NYHA class in grading HF severity and the fact that these studies were not powered to detect differences between subgroups. The numbers of NYHA class IV patients enrolled in ICD trials is sufficiently small that outcomes cannot be extrapolated to this group, and it is likely that in this group the risk of HF death is such that any benefit from an ICD would be offset. Therefore patients with NYHA class IV HF who are not candidates for CRT or cardiac transplantation should not have ICDs implanted.

The relationship between LVEF and benefit in ICD trials

Data from AVID,[53] CIDS,[54] MADIT,[62] and SCDHeFT[13] all suggest that those patients with the most severely depressed ejection fraction have the most to gain from ICD therapy, despite having a higher overall mortality and a higher absolute risk of death from progressive HF. Conversely, data from MADIT-II showed similar benefit across different LVEFs under 35%.[80] There is however evidence to suggest that there may be a lower limit for ICD benefit, with one analysis suggesting that all deaths in patients with prior MI and LVEF below 10% were nonarrhythmic.[81]

The emergence of heart failure following ICD implantation

Although the bulk of the evidence for ICD effectiveness comes from trials which implanted single-chamber devices[13,53–55,60], registry data suggest that a significant proportion of ICDs are dual-chamber devices.[85] However, the Dual Chamber and VVI Defibrillator (DAVID) study raises concerns over the use of dual-chamber pacing in patients with ICDs without standard indications for pacing.[82] The study randomized dual-chamber ICD recipients to receive either DDD rate-responsive pacing at 70/min or VVI pacing at 40/min, and was based on the hypothesis that provision of DDDR pacing in patients with left ventricular dysfunction would suppress atrial arrhythmias, allow optimization of medical therapy and would therefore improve HF outcomes. Enrolment was stopped early after the observation that those randomized to DDDR pacing were significantly more likely to experience the composite primary endpoint of all-cause mortality or hospitalization for HF at 1 year than those receiving VVI pacing. DDDR programming was associated with a significantly higher level of right ventricular apical pacing, with a mean of 58.9% versus 3.5% in the VVI arm.

The subsequent Intrinsic-RV study demonstrated noninferiority of DDDR pacing versus VVI for the same composite primary endpoint when an AV search hysteresis algorithm was used to minimize RV apical pacing during DDDR (10% vs 3% in the VVI arm). Cumulative RV apical pacing greater than 2% was shown to be associated with an increased risk for both subsequent appropriate ICD shocks and for HF events.[83] Similar results were seen in the second Multicenter Automatic Defibrillator Implantation Trial (MADIT-II).[84] This may at least in part explain the greater number of HF events seen in the ICD arm of MADIT-II in which around 40% of the ICDs implanted were dual-chamber devices.[62] The increased risk of first or recurrent HF associated with an ICD in MADIT-II was greatest in those with dual-chamber ICDs where there was a higher proportion of right ventricular pacing.[38] It therefore appears that right ventricular apical pacing in ICD recipients may induce ventricular dysynchrony, worsen left ventricular function, and thereby induce or exacerbate clinical HF. While there are theoretical potential benefits to dual-chamber devices in terms of SVT discrimination and provision of physiologic pacing should conducting system disease develop, there are insufficient data to support routine dual-chamber ICD implantation in patients without standard indications for bradycardia pacing, and concerns regarding dual-chamber pacing are particularly pertinent in patients with pre-existing HF. The evidence certainly supports the use of algorithms to minimize ventricular pacing in ICD recipients, whether single- or dual-chamber devices are used. It is also true that although ICDs reduce mortality, patients who experience an ICD shock experience a worse outcome than those who do not, and in some patients, the occurrence of a ventricular arrhythmia marks the onset of deterioration in their HF, which may result in death from progressive HF. It is therefore particularly important that patients with HF are on optimal medical therapy, in order to prevent or slow such a decline.

Cardiac resynchronization therapy in combination with an ICD

Rationale

QRS prolongation in HF indicates underlying interventricular dysynchrony and is associated with poor prognosis, in terms of HF, sudden death, and overall mortality. CRT pacing employs atrio-biventricular pacing to reduce interventricular dysynchrony and produce improvements in left ventricular function and mortality. CRT is discussed in more detail in Chapter 48, but is discussed briefly here as it can be combined with a defibrillator (CRT-D), when an ICD indication also exists. A CRT-D system is shown in Fig. 47.7.

Evidence for CRT-D in heart failure

The Comparison of Medical Therapy, Pacing and Defibrillators in Chronic Heart Failure (COMPANION) trial enrolled 1520 patients in sinus rhythm with NYHA III/IV HF, LVEF 35% or less, and QRS duration 120 ms or more, and randomized them to optimal medical therapy alone, medical therapy plus CRT-P, or medical therapy plus CRT-D.[87] The primary endpoint, a composite of death or first hospitalization for HF, was reduced by both CRT-P and CRT-D, although all-cause mortality, the secondary endpoint, was only significantly reduced in the CRT-D arm. The subsequent Cardiac Resynchronization in Heart Failure (CARE-HF) study demonstrated that addition of an ICD was not required for survival benefit with CRT.[28,88]

Following the observation of increased HF events with an ICD in MADIT-II, the MADIT-CRT Trial was designed to test the hypothesis that the addition of CRT to an ICD would provide additional benefit for high-risk but minimally symptomatic patients.[89]

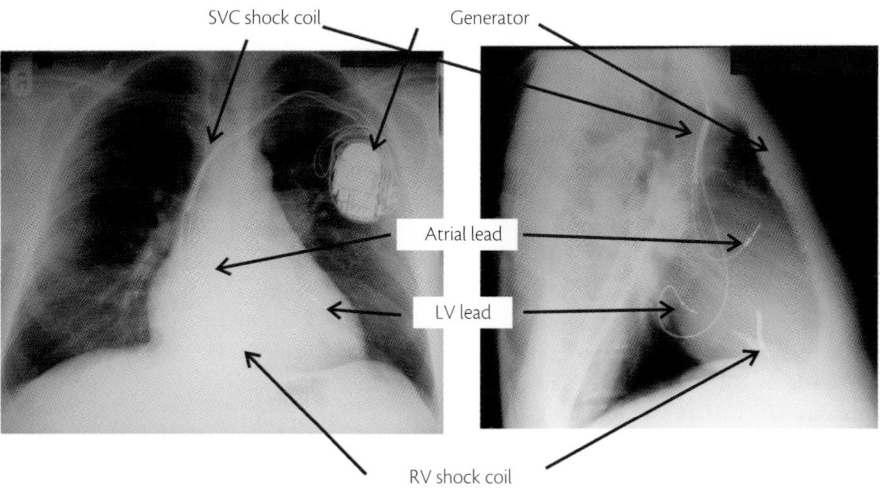

Fig. 47.7 Chest radiographs showing a cardiac resynchronization therapy-defibrillator system.

1820 patients with LVSD (LVEF ≤30%) and QRS prolongation (≥130 ms) who were minimally symptomatic (NYHA I/II HF) were randomized to receive CRT-D or an ICD (programmed to VVI or DDI at 40 beats/min). There was a relative risk reduction of 34% in the primary endpoint of all-cause mortality or a nonfatal HF event with CRT-D over a 4.5-year period. This benefit was driven primarily by a reduction in nonfatal HF events with CRT-D, without any demonstrable survival advantage, particularly in those patients with a QRS duration of 150 ms or more (*c*.65% of the recruited population). CRT-D was also accompanied by an 11% absolute improvement in LVEF at 1 year, as opposed to 3% seen in the ICD arm. These findings are congruent with those seen in trials of CRT-P in minimally symptomatic patients, in which favourable left ventricular reverse remodelling and a reduction in HF events have been observed.[90] A pragmatic interpretation might therefore be that CRT-D is likely to reduce HF morbidity in ICD candidates with NHYA II HF and a very broad QRS complex, particularly those who have a history of more severe HF symptomatology.

Overall, the results from these CRT-D trials once again emphasize the importance of the interplay between HF and sudden death in patients with left ventricular dysfunction, and the limitations of NHYA class as a tool to assess the severity of HF symptoms. The presence of HF indicates a substrate for sudden death which may be modified by medical therapy and CRT and the occurrence of HF is constantly present as a competing risk which cannot be modified by an ICD.

Cost-effectiveness of CRT-D in heart failure

Using estimates of cost and benefit based on data from the COMPANION and CARE-HF trials, the incremental cost from a UK health care perspective, of adding an ICD to CRT-P (i.e. CRT-D) in patients with HF has been estimated.[91] The incremental cost of CRT-D over CRT-P was around €48 000 per QALY saved. This may be around the threshold level for an acceptable cost-effectiveness profile, but it significantly exceeds the estimates for CRT-P over optimal medical therapy, of around €7500 per QALY saved.

Palliative care and device deactivation

HF is a chronic condition associated with a high mortality and, even with optimal medical therapy; some recipients will inevitably experience a progression in the severity of their HF to refractory endstage disease. This may be particularly true of patients with ICDs who have survived ventricular arrhythmias as a result of the device. Patients with endstage HF are recognized as carrying a heavy symptom burden, and effective palliation is therefore extremely important. A key principle of palliative care is withholding treatments which do not improve symptomatology and may produce unpleasant side effects. Both appropriate and inappropriate ICD therapies meet this description, and so, while ventricular arrhythmias may not be a particularly common mode of death in endstage HF, in most circumstances it will be appropriate to disable ICD therapies in the dying patient and this is now included in the Liverpool Care Pathway.[92] Device deactivation requires a sensitive discussion with patients, who have previously accepted the ICD on the basis that it would be a life-saving intervention. Such discussions are best introduced early once a deterioration in HF status is recognized, and for some patients it may be appropriate to raise the possibility of future device deactivation at the time of implantation.[93] Patients may have a preference for device deactivation, and physicians should certainly recognize the need to consider ICD deactivation when death is imminent, when other therapies are withdrawn, or when a decision not to attempt resuscitation has been taken.

Counselling patients with heart failure for an ICD

Patients with HF may overestimate the potential benefit associated with ICD therapy compared with that observed in clinical trials, underlining the importance of appropriate counselling, a task which is made more difficult by the lack of accurate risk stratification algorithms for different modes of death in patients with HF.[94] A useful outline for such discussions has been suggested by Stevenson and Desai and is based on the available clinical trial evidence for ICD benefit in patients with HF and left ventricular dysfunction.[95] It focuses on a 5-year time period and quantifies the risks and benefits associated with an ICD in terms of expected events affecting 100 patients: 7–8 patients will have their life saved as a result of the ICD; 30 will die anyway, some having requested that the device be switched off; 10–20 patients will have a shock they did not need; 5–15 will experience some other complication; and the rest will not experience their device at all.[95] This approach quantifies the risks and benefits in a way which is accessible to patients, and makes clear to the physician the importance of individual choice in this decision-making process.

Future developments in ICD therapy for patients with heart failure

Predicting heart failure death

Effective targeting of ICD therapy to patients with HF who are most likely to benefit depends on identifying two key subpopulations—- those who will die of progressive HF or other causes before receiving a life-saving therapy from their device, and those who are at such low risk from an arrhythmia that they are very unlikely to derive meaningful benefit from an ICD. Ideally then, each potential ICD recipient should undergo two types of assessment which must be combined to give a balanced reflection of whether they would be likely to benefit from ICD implantation. Interest in this approach is increasing with the development of multivariable models which can predict outcome in HF (see Chapter 25). The Seattle Heart Failure Model is one such multivariable model, which uses routine clinical variables to predict mortality risk in patients with HF.[96] When applied to the SCDHeFT population to produce quintiles of risk, this model was able to separate groups with greater benefit from ICD therapy (quintile 2 relative risk 0.48[0.26–0.89, p = 0.019] versus quintile 5 relative risk 0.98[0.71–1.82, p = 0.89]).[96] The development of such models to include powerful risk predictors, such as B-type natriuretic peptides, and to predict cause-specific mortality, may well lead to improvements in our ability to risk stratify patients with HF and in our ability to select ICD candidates in the future.

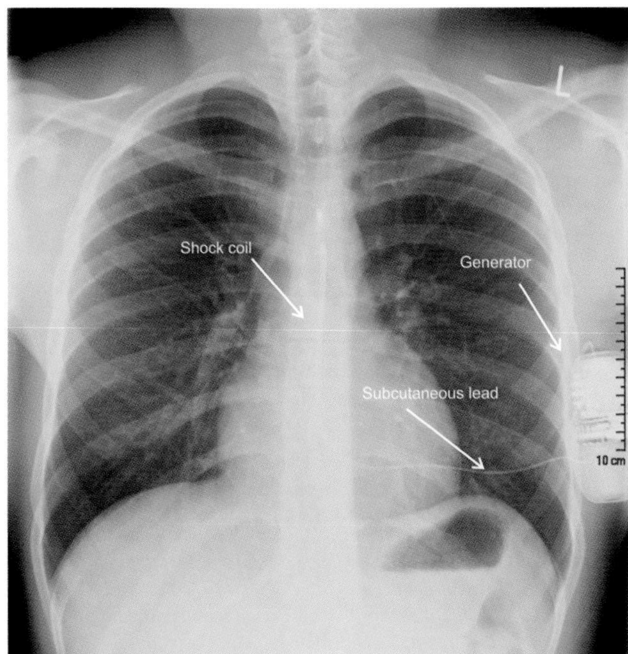

Fig. 47.8 A subcutaneous ICD system.

The impact of noncardiac comorbidities

The effect of noncardiac comorbidities must also be taken into account when trying to quantify risk of death which would not be modifiable by an ICD. In an analysis of the impact of noncardiac comorbidities on outcome in 2500 ICD recipients over 2 years in an Ontario registry, comorbidities such as peripheral vascular disease, pulmonary disease, and renal impairment were significant determinants of mortality following ICD implantation, and risk increased incrementally with increasing numbers of comorbidities.[97]

Subcutaneous implantable cardioverter defibrillators

Although effective at reducing SCD, transvenous ICD systems are costly and associated with potential hazard, and in reality the eligible population is often elderly with significant comorbidity, making physicians reluctant to treat. The subcutaneous ICD is a novel device which offers a number of potential advantages to the traditional transvenous ICD system. It consists of a subcutaneous defibrillation lead, which runs parallel to the left sternal edge and along the inferior border of the heart to a generator implanted in the axilla (see Fig. 47.5). Initial studies of acute sensing and defibrillation capabilities in humans have been performed,[98] although results from chronic implant studies are awaited. It is expected that implant and lead-related complications will be significantly reduced, device infections are likely to be less serious and device explants less hazardous. Whether the associated cost will be significantly lower than for transvenous systems remains to be seen. These devices are shock-only and do not have the capability to perform ATP or bradycardia pacing outside the postshock period. However, this is largely the same profile of therapies to that which produced a mortality benefit in HF patients enrolled in the SCDHeFT trial. If proved safe and effective subcutaneous ICD systems may be an option for providing protection from life-threatening arrhythmias in patients with HF.

Summary

The prevention of arrhythmic sudden death in patients with HF is an important aim, and one which is now achievable through the use of primary prevention ICDs, which provide highly effective treatment for life-threatening ventricular arrhythmias. In selected populations of patients with HF and left ventricular dysfunction, randomized trial evidence suggests that the ICD is a well-tolerated, effective, and even cost-effective therapy. However, patients with HF are exposed to competing risks and the prevention of sudden death in HF leads not only to increased survival but also to consequent increases in nonarrhythmic mortality, hospitalization for HF, and death from progressive pump failure. This means that patients with HF should be carefully selected for ICD implantation, with the individual risk of sudden death and HF death being considered as far as possible. Given the difficulties inherent in such individualized risk prediction, it is important to recognize that there is often no correct answer, and each patient must be appropriately counselled and involved in the decision. In order to maximize the benefit afforded by an ICD, all recipients must have optimal medical therapy and be managed by a specialist team with expertise in HF. The evidence suggests that in patients with left ventricular dysfunction, such a complex interdependence exists between arrhythmic sudden death and HF that ICD therapy and optimal management for HF should always be considered together.

References

1. McMurray JJ, Pfeffer MA. Heart failure. *Lancet* 2005;**365**:1877–89.
2. Pfeffer MA, Swedberg K, Granger CB, *et al.* Effects of candesartan on mortality and morbidity in patients with chronic heart failure: the CHARM-Overall programme. *Lancet* 2003;**362**:759–66.
3. Gehi A, Haas D, Fuster V. Primary prophylaxis with the implantable cardioverter-defibrillator: the need for improved risk stratification. *JAMA* 2005;**294**:958–60.
4. Myerburg RJ, Castellanos A. Emerging paradigms of the epidemiology and demographics of sudden cardiac arrest. *Heart Rhythm* 2006;**3**:235–9.
5. Greenberg H, Case RB, Moss AJ, Brown MW, Carroll ER, Andrews ML. Analysis of mortality events in the Multicenter Automatic Defibrillator Implantation Trial (MADIT-II). *J Am Coll Cardiol* 2004;**43**:1459–65.
6. Effect of metoprolol CR/XL in chronic heart failure: Metoprolol CR/XL Randomised Intervention Trial in Congestive Heart Failure (MERIT-HF). *Lancet* 1999;**353**:2001–7.
7. Cleland JG, Massie BM, Packer M. Sudden death in heart failure: vascular or electrical? *Eur J Heart Fail* 1999;**1**:41–5.
8. Engdahl J, Holmberg M, Karlson BW, Luepker R, Herlitz J. The epidemiology of out-of-hospital 'sudden' cardiac arrest. *Resuscitation* 2002;**52**:235–45.
9. Luu M, Stevenson WG, Stevenson LW, Baron K, Walden J. Diverse mechanisms of unexpected cardiac arrest in advanced heart failure. *Circulation* 1989;**80**:1675–80.
10. Leclercq JF, Maisonblanche P, Cauchemez B, Coumel P. Respective role of sympathetic tone and of cardiac pauses in the genesis of 62 cases of ventricular fibrillation recorded during Holter monitoring. *Eur Heart J* 1988;**9**:1276–83.
11. Bayes DL, Coumel P, Leclercq JF. Ambulatory sudden cardiac death: mechanisms of production of fatal arrhythmia on the basis of data from 157 cases. *Am Heart J* 1989;**117**:151–9.
12. Uretsky BF, Thygesen K, Armstrong PW, *et al.* Acute coronary findings at autopsy in heart failure patients with sudden death: results from the assessment of treatment with lisinopril and survival (ATLAS) trial. *Circulation* 2000;**102**:611–16.
13. Bardy GH, Lee KL, Mark DB, *et al.* Amiodarone or an implantable cardioverter-defibrillator for congestive heart failure. *N Engl J Med* 2005;**352**:225–37.
14. Bailey JJ, Berson AS, Handelsman H, Hodges M. Utility of current risk stratification tests for predicting major arrhythmic events after myocardial infarction. *J Am Coll Cardiol* 2001;**38**:1902–11.
15. Huikuri HV, Castellanos A, Myerburg RJ. Sudden death due to cardiac arrhythmias. *N Engl J Med* 2001;**345**:1473–82.
16. Kendall MJ, Lynch KP, Hjalmarson A, Kjekshus J. Beta-blockers and sudden cardiac death. *Ann Intern Med* 1995;**123**:358–67.
17. Domanski MJ, Exner DV, Borkowf CB, Geller NL, Rosenberg Y, Pfeffer MA. Effect of angiotensin converting enzyme inhibition on sudden cardiac death in patients following acute myocardial infarction. A meta-analysis of randomized clinical trials. *J Am Coll Cardiol* 1999;**33**:598–604.
18. Pitt B, Zannad F, Remme WJ, *et al.* The effect of spironolactone on morbidity and mortality in patients with severe heart failure. Randomized Aldactone Evaluation Study Investigators. *N Engl J Med* 1999;**341**:709–17.
19. Waldo AL, Camm AJ, deRuyter H, *et al.* Effect of D-sotalol on mortality in patients with left ventricular dysfunction after recent and remote myocardial infarction. The SWORD Investigators. Survival With Oral D-Sotalol. *Lancet* 1996;**348**:7–12.
20. Echt DS, Liebson PR, Mitchell LB, *et al.* Mortality and morbidity in patients receiving encainide, flecainide, or placebo. The Cardiac Arrhythmia Suppression Trial. *N Engl J Med* 1991;**324**:781–8.
21. Mirowski M, Mower MM, Langer A, Heilman MS, Schreibman J. A chronically implanted system for automatic defibrillation in active conscious dogs. Experimental model for treatment of sudden death from ventricular fibrillation. *Circulation* 1978;**58**:90–4.
22. Mirowski M, Reid PR, Mower MM, *et al.* Termination of malignant ventricular arrhythmias with an implanted automatic defibrillator in human beings. *N Engl J Med* 1980;**303**:322.
23. Mirowski M, Mower MM, Reid PR. The automatic implantable defibrillator. *Am Heart J* 1980;**100**:1089–92.
24. Haffajee C, Martin D, Bhandari A, *et al.* A multicenter, randomized trial comparing an active can implantable defibrillator with a passive can system. Jewel Active Can Investigators. *Pacing Clin Electrophysiol* 1997;**20**:215–19.
25. Kouakam C, Kacet S, Hazard JR, *et al.* Performance of a dual-chamber implantable defibrillator algorithm for discrimination of ventricular from supraventricular tachycardia. *Europace* 2004;**6**:32–42.
26. Daubert JP, Zareba W, Cannom DS, *et al.* Inappropriate implantable cardioverter-defibrillator shocks in MADIT II: frequency, mechanisms, predictors, and survival impact. *J Am Coll Cardiol* 2008;**51**:1357–65.
27. Friedman PA, McClelland RL, Bamlet WR, *et al.* Dual-chamber versus single-chamber detection enhancements for implantable defibrillator rhythm diagnosis: the detect supraventricular tachycardia study. *Circulation* 2006;**113**:2871–9.
28. Cleland JG, Daubert JC, Erdmann E, *et al.* The effect of cardiac resynchronization on morbidity and mortality in heart failure. *N Engl J Med* 2005;**352**:1539–49.
29. Wathen MS, Sweeney MO, DeGroot PJ, *et al.* Shock reduction using antitachycardia pacing for spontaneous rapid ventricular tachycardia in patients with coronary artery disease. *Circulation* 2001;**104**:796–801.
30. Gold MR, Higgins S, Klein R, *et al.* Efficacy and temporal stability of reduced safety margins for ventricular defibrillation: primary results from the Low Energy Safety Study (LESS). *Circulation* 2002;**105**:2043–8.
31. Blatt JA, Poole JE, Johnson GW, *et al.* No benefit from defibrillation threshold testing in the SCD-HeFT (Sudden Cardiac Death in Heart Failure Trial). *J Am Coll Cardiol* 2008;**52**:551–6.
32. Ellenbogen KA, Levine JH, Berger RD, *et al.* Are implantable cardioverter defibrillator shocks a surrogate for sudden cardiac death in patients with nonischemic cardiomyopathy? *Circulation* 2006;**113**:776–82.
33. Alter P, Waldhans S, Plachta E, Moosdorf R, Grimm W. Complications of implantable cardioverter defibrillator therapy in 440 consecutive patients. *Pacing Clin Electrophysiol* 2005;**28**:926–32.
34. Al Khatib SM, Greiner MA, Peterson ED, Hernandez AF, Schulman KA, Curtis LH. Patient and implanting physician factors associated with mortality and complications following implantable cardioverter-defibrillator implantation, 2002–2005. *Circ Arrhythm Electrophysiol* 2008;**1**:240–9.
35. Saksena S. Defibrillation thresholds and perioperative mortality associated with endocardial and epicardial defibrillation lead systems. The PCD investigators and participating institutions. *Pacing Clin Electrophysiol* 1993;**16**:202–7.
36. Mitchell LB, Pineda EA, Titus JL, Bartosch PM, Benditt DG. Sudden death in patients with implantable cardioverter defibrillators: the importance of post-shock electromechanical dissociation. *J Am Coll Cardiol* 2002;**39**:1323–8.
37. Wilson CM, Allen JD, Bridges JB, Adgey AA. Death and damage caused by multiple direct current shocks: studies in an animal model. *Eur Heart J* 1988;**9**:1257–65.
38. Goldenberg I, Moss AJ, Hall WJ, *et al.*, for the Multicenter Automatic Defibrillator Implantation Trial (MADIT) II Investigators. Causes and Consequences of Heart Failure After Prophylactic Implantation of a Defibrillator in the Multicenter Automatic Defibrillator Implantation Trial II. *Circulation* 2006;**113**:2810–17.
39. Hurst TM, Hinrichs M, Breidenbach C, Katz N, Waldecker B. Detection of myocardial injury during transvenous implantation of automatic cardioverter-defibrillators. *J Am Coll Cardiol* 1999;**34**:402–8.

40. Sweeney MO, Wathen MS, Volosin K, *et al.* Appropriate and inappropriate ventricular therapies, quality of life, and mortality among primary and secondary prevention implantable cardioverter defibrillator patients: results from the Pacing Fast VT REduces Shock ThErapies (PainFREE Rx II) trial. *Circulation* 2005;**111**: 2898–905.
41. Ahmad M, Bloomstein L, Roelke M, Bernstein AD, Parsonnet V. Patients' attitudes toward implanted defibrillator shocks. *Pacing Clin Electrophysiol* 2000;**23**:934–8.
42. Hasdemir C, Shah N, Rao AP, *et al.* Analysis of troponin I levels after spontaneous implantable cardioverter defibrillator shocks. *J Cardiovasc Electrophysiol* 2002;**13**:144–50.
43. Poole JE, Johnson GW, Hellkamp AS, *et al.* Prognostic importance of defibrillator shocks in patients with heart failure. *N Engl J Med* 2008;**359**:1009–17.
44. Maisel WH, Stevenson LW. Atrial fibrillation in heart failure: epidemiology, pathophysiology, and rationale for therapy. *Am J Cardiol* 2003;**91**:2–8.
45. Pacifico A, Hohnloser SH, Williams JH, *et al.* Prevention of implantable-defibrillator shocks by treatment with sotalol. d,l-Sotalol Implantable Cardioverter-Defibrillator Study Group. *N Engl J Med* 1999;**340**:1855–62.
46. Burke JL, Hallas CN, Clark-Carter D, White D, Connelly D. The psychosocial impact of the implantable cardioverter defibrillator: a meta-analytic review. *Br J Health Psychol* 2003;**8**:165–78.
47. Mark DB, Anstrom KJ, Sun JL, *et al.* Quality of life with defibrillator therapy or amiodarone in heart failure. *N Engl J Med* 2008;**359**:999–1008.
48. http://www.dft.gov.uk/dvla/medical/ataglance.aspx.
49. Epstein AE, Baessler CA, Curtis AB, *et al.* Public safety issues in patients with implantable defibrillators: a scientific statement from the American Heart Association and the Heart Rhythm Society. *Circulation* 2007;**115**:1170–6.
50. Vijgen J, Botto G, Camm J, *et al.* Consensus statement of the European Heart Rhythm Association: updated recommendations for driving by patients with implantable cardioverter defibrillators. *Europace* 2009;**11**:1097–1107.
51. McIvor ME, Reddinger J, Floden E, Sheppard RC. Study of Pacemaker and Implantable Cardioverter Defibrillator Triggering by Electronic Article Surveillance Devices (SPICED TEAS). *Pacing Clin Electrophysiol* 1998;**21**:1847–61.
52. Cobb LA. Resuscitation from out-of-hospital ventricular fibrillation: 4 years follow-up. *Circulation* 1975;**52**:III223–35.
53. A comparison of antiarrhythmic-drug therapy with implantable defibrillators in patients resuscitated from near-fatal ventricular arrhythmias. The Antiarrhythmics versus Implantable Defibrillators (AVID) Investigators. *N Engl J Med* 1997;**337**:1576–83.
54. Connolly SJ, Gent M, Roberts RS, *et al.* Canadian implantable defibrillator study (CIDS): a randomized trial of the implantable cardioverter defibrillator against amiodarone. *Circulation* 2000;**101**:1297–302.
55. Kuck KH, Cappato R, Siebels J, Ruppel R. Randomized comparison of antiarrhythmic drug therapy with implantable defibrillators in patients resuscitated from cardiac arrest : the Cardiac Arrest Study Hamburg (CASH). *Circulation* 2000;**102**:748–54.
56. Connolly SJ, Hallstrom AP, Cappato R, *et al.* Meta-analysis of the implantable cardioverter defibrillator secondary prevention trials. AVID, CASH and CIDS studies. Antiarrhythmics vs Implantable Defibrillator study. Cardiac Arrest Study Hamburg . Canadian Implantable Defibrillator Study. *Eur Heart J* 2000;**21**:2071–8.
57. Domanski MJ, Epstein A, Hallstrom A, Saksena S, Zipes DP. Survival of antiarrhythmic or implantable cardioverter defibrillator treated patients with varying degrees of left ventricular dysfunction who survived malignant ventricular arrhythmias. *J Cardiovasc Electrophysiol* 2002;**13**:580–3.
58. ACC/AHA/HRS 2008 Guidelines for Device-Based Therapy of Cardiac Rhythm Abnormalities: a report of the American College of Cardiology/American Heart Association Task Force on Practice Guidelines. *Circulation* 2008;**117**:e350–408.
59. Wyse DG, Friedman PL, Brodsky MA, *et al.* Life-threatening ventricular arrhythmias due to transient or correctable causes: high risk for death in follow-up. *J Am Coll Cardiol* 2001;**38**:1718–24.
60. Moss AJ, Hall WJ, Cannom DS, *et al.* Improved survival with an implanted defibrillator in patients with coronary disease at high risk for ventricular arrhythmia. Multicenter Automatic Defibrillator Implantation Trial Investigators. *N Engl J Med* 1996;**335**:1933–40.
61. Buxton AE, Lee KL, DiCarlo L, *et al.* Electrophysiologic testing to identify patients with coronary artery disease who are at risk for sudden death. Multicenter Unsustained Tachycardia Trial Investigators. *N Engl J Med* 2000;**342**:1937–45.
62. Moss AJ, Zareba W, Hall WJ, *et al.* Prophylactic implantation of a defibrillator in patients with myocardial infarction and reduced ejection fraction. *N Engl J Med* 2002;**346**:877–83.
63. Hohnloser SH, Kuck KH, Dorian P, *et al.* Prophylactic use of an implantable cardioverter-defibrillator after acute myocardial infarction. *N Engl J Med* 2004;**351**:2481–8.
64. Steinbeck G, Andresen D, Senges J, Hoffmann E, Seidl K, Brachmann J, IRIS Investigators as Joint Study of the German University Hospitals and German Society of Leading Cardiological Hospital Physicians (ALKK). Immediate Risk-Stratification Improves Survival (IRIS): study protocol. *Europace* 2004;**6**:392–9.
65. Steinbeck G, Andresen D, Seidl K, *et al.*, the IRIS, Investigators. Defibrillator Implantation Early after Myocardial Infarction. *N Engl J Med* 2009;**361**:1427–36.
66. Kadish A, Dyer A, Daubert JP, *et al.*, the Defibrillators in Non-Ischemic Cardiomyopathy Treatment Evaluation (DEFINITE) Investigators. Prophylactic defibrillator implantation in patients with nonischemic dilated cardiomyopathy. *N Engl J Med* 2004;**350**:2151–8.
67. Packer DL, Bernstein R, Wood F, *et al.* Impact of amiodarone versus implantable cardioverter defibrillator therapy on the mode of death in congestive heart failure patients in the SCDHeFT trial. *Heart Rhythm* 2005;**2**:S38–9.
68. Bardy GH, Lee KL, Boehmer JP, *et al.* The progression of congestive heart failure over the course of the sudden cardiac death in heart failure trial (SCD-HeFT). *Heart Rhythm* 2005;**2**:S39.
69. Priori SG, Aliot E, Blomstrom-Lundqvist C, *et al.*Task Force on Sudden Cardiac Death of the European Society of Cardiology. *Eur Heart J* 2001;**22**:1374–450.
70. Update of the guidelines on sudden cardiac death of the European Society of Cardiology. *Eur Heart J* 2003;**24**:13–15.
71. ESC Guidelines for the diagnosis and treatment of acute and chronic heart failure 2008: the Task Force for the Diagnosis and Treatment of Acute and Chronic Heart Failure 2008 of the European Society of Cardiology. *Eur Heart J* 2008;**29**:2388–442.
72. http://www.nice.org.uk/nicemedia/pdf/TA095guidance.pdf.
73. http://www.sign.ac.uk/pdf/sign94.pdf.
74. Hlatky MA, Mark DB. The high cost of implantable defibrillators. *Eur Heart J* 2007;**28**:388–91.
75. Camm J, Klein H, Nisam S. The cost of implantable defibrillators: perceptions and reality. *Eur Heart J* 2007;**28**:392–7.
76. Mark DB, Nelson CL, Anstrom KJ, *et al.* Cost-effectiveness of defibrillator therapy or amiodarone in chronic stable heart failure: results from the Sudden Cardiac Death in Heart Failure Trial (SCD-HeFT). *Circulation* 2006;**114**:135–42.
77. Sanders GD, Hlatky MA, Owens DK. Cost-effectiveness of implantable cardioverter-defibrillators. *N Engl J Med* 2005;**353**:1471–80.
78. Buxton M, Caine N, Chase D, *et al.* A review of the evidence on the effects and costs of implantable cardioverter defibrillator (ICD) therapy in different patient groups, and modelling of cost-effectiveness

and cost-utility for these groups in a UK context. *Health Technol Assess* 2006;**10**:iii–iv, ix–xi, 1–164.

79. Mark DB, Hlatky MA. Medical economics and the assessment of value in cardiovascular medicine: Part I. *Circulation* 2002;**106**:516–20.
80. Zareba W, Piotrowicz K, McNitt S, Moss AJ. Implantable cardioverter-defibrillator efficacy in patients with heart failure and left ventricular dysfunction (from the MADIT II population). *Am J Cardiol* 2005;**95**:1487–91.
81. Yap YG, Duong T, Bland JM, *et al.* Optimising the dichotomy limit for left ventricular ejection fraction in selecting patients for defibrillator therapy after myocardial infarction. *Heart* 2007;**93**:832–6.
82. Wilkoff BL, Cook JR, Epstein AE, *et al.* Dual Chamber and VVI Implantable Defibrillator Trial Investigators. Dual-chamber pacing or ventricular backup pacing in patients with an implantable defibrillator: the Dual Chamber and VVI Implantable Defibrillator (DAVID) Trial. *JAMA* 2002;**288**:3115–23.
83. Gardiwal A, Yu H, Oswald H, *et al.* Right ventricular pacing is an independent predictor for ventricular tachycardia/ventricular fibrillation occurrence and heart failure events in patients with an implantable cardioverter-defibrillator. *Europace* 2008;**10**:358–63.
84. Steinberg JS, Fischer A, Wang P, *et al.*, MADIT II Invetigators. The clinical implications of cumulative right ventricular pacing in the multicenter automatic defibrillator trial II. *J Cardiovasc Electrophysiol* 2005;**16**:359–65.
85. Proclemer A, Ghidina M, Gregori D, *et al.* Impact of the main implantable cardioverter-defibrillator trials in clinical practice: data from the Italian ICD Registry for the years 2005–07. *Europace* 2009;**11**:465–75.
86. Hallstrom AP, Greene HL, Wilkoff BL, Zipes DP, Schron E, Ledingham RB. Relationship between rehospitalization and future death in patients treated for potentially lethal arrhythmia. *J Cardiovasc Electrophysiol* 2001;**12**:990–5.
87. Bristow MR, Saxon LA, Boehmer J, *et al.* Cardiac-resynchronization therapy with or without an implantable defibrillator in advanced chronic heart failure. *N Engl J Med* 2004;**350**:2140–50.
88. Cleland JG, Daubert JC, Erdmann E, *et al.* Longer-term effects of cardiac resynchronization therapy on mortality in heart failure [the CArdiac REsynchronization-Heart Failure (CARE-HF) trial extension phase]. *Eur Heart J* 2006;**27**:1928–32.
89. Moss AJ, Hall WJ, Cannom DS, *et al.* Cardiac-resynchronization therapy for the prevention of heart-failure events. *N Engl J Med* 2009;**361**:1329–38.
90. Linde C, Abraham WT, Gold MR, St John Sutton M, Ghio S, Daubert C. Randomized trial of cardiac resynchronization in mildly symptomatic heart failure patients and in asymptomatic patients with left ventricular dysfunction and previous heart failure symptoms. *J Am Coll Cardiol* 2008;**52**:1834–43.
91. Yao G, Freemantle N, Calvert MJ, Bryan S, Daubert JC, Cleland JG. The long-term cost-effectiveness of cardiac resynchronization therapy with or without an implantable cardioverter-defibrillator. *Eur Heart J* 2007;**28**:42–51.
92. http://www.mcpcil.org.uk/liverpool-care-pathway/pdfs/LCP%20HOSPITAL%20VERSION%2011%20(printable%20version).pdf.
93. Berger JT. The ethics of deactivating implanted cardioverter defibrillators. *Ann Intern Med* 2005;**142**:631–4.
94. Anderson KP. Risk assessment for defibrillator therapy: Il Trittico. *J Am Coll Cardiol* 2007;**50**:1158–60.
95. Stevenson LW, Desai AS. Selecting patients for discussion of the ICD as primary prevention for sudden death in heart failure. *J Card Fail* 2006;**12**:407–12.
96. Levy WC, Mozaffarian D, Linker DT, *et al.* The Seattle Heart Failure Model: prediction of survival in heart failure. *Circulation* 2006;**113**:1424–33.
97. Lee DS, Tu JV, Austin PC, *et al.* Effect of cardiac and noncardiac conditions on survival after defibrillator implantation. *J Am Coll Cardiol* 2007;**49**:2408–15.
98. Bardy GH, Smith WM, Hood MA, *et al.* An entirely subcutaneous implantable cardioverter-defibrillator. *New Engl J Med* 2010;**363**(1):36–44.
99. ACC/AHA/ESC 2006 guidelines for management of patients with ventricular arrhythmias and the prevention of sudden cardiac death: a report of the American College of Cardiology/American Heart Association Task Force and the European Society of Cardiology Committee for Practice Guidelines developed in collaboration with the European Heart Rhythm Association and the Heart Rhythm Society. *Europace* 2006;**8**:746–837.

48

Cardiac resynchronization therapy

Badrinathan Chandrasekaran and Peter J. Cowburn

Introduction

In the last decade, the use of cardiac resynchronization therapy (CRT), also known as biventricular pacing (BVP), has emerged as a new therapeutic option for selected patients with heart failure (HF) and ongoing symptoms despite optimal medical therapy who also have a prolonged QRS interval. CRT, by retiming the failing heart, improves symptoms, reduces hospitalization, and prolongs survival in patients with left ventricular dysfunction and a broad QRS complex.[1–4] CRT improves electromechanical dyssynchrony and maximizes the efficiency of the cardiac contraction sequence, leading to an acute haemodynamic benefit and, over time, a reduction in left ventricular volumes and an improvement in left ventricular ejection fraction (LVEF). A prolonged QRS width (>120 ms) is a marker of benefit from CRT, with approximately 70% of such patients having symptomatic improvement following CRT. Cardiac resynchronization therapy can be delivered on its own as a pacemaker (CRT-P) or in addition to an internal cardiac defibrillator, where it is referred to as CRT-D. Advances in device technology and telecommunications now enable remote monitoring of surrogate markers of HF, offering the ability to predict subclinical deterioration, and thereby potentially preventing HF hospitalization.

Cardiac dyssynchrony

In patients with systolic HF, there is progressive deterioration of left ventricular function with time, known as adverse left ventricular remodelling. Some patients also develop an uncoordinated regional contraction-relaxation pattern, known as dyssynchrony.

Dyssynchrony can be predominantly mechanical or electrical, but more often it is a combination of both. It is associated with changes on the surface ECG including: prolongation of the QRS complex (>120 ms) in 25–50%, left bundle branch block (LBBB) in 15–27%, and first-degree AV block (PR interval >200 ms) in 35%.[5] Dyssynchrony can be between atria and ventricles (atrioventricular, AV), between right and left ventricles (interventricular), between different walls of the left ventricle (intraventricular), or any combination of the three.

The efficiency of the cardiac cycle is dependent on the appropriate timing of AV contraction to achieve maximal filling and ejection. Within the left ventricle, the consequence of dyssynchronous cardiac contraction is regional variation in the timing of contraction of different myocardial segments. There is also a redistribution of myocardial blood flow and regional changes at a molecular level in the expression of stress kinase proteins and proteins involved in calcium handling.[6,7] In turn, there is a reduction in left ventricular filling, and contraction of parts of the left ventricle after closure of the aortic valve, known as postsystolic contraction. In addition, there is an increase in functional mitral regurgitation. AV dyssynchrony exacerbates the process further and leads to a further reduction in left ventricular filling and presystolic mitral regurgitation (MR).

History of pacing in heart failure

Dual-chamber endocardial pacing with a short AV delay (100 ms) was reported to improve LVEF, NYHA class, and exercise duration in studies of small numbers of patients with endstage dilated cardiomyopathy in the early 1990s.[8,9] The benefit occurred predominantly in patients with a long PR interval. The mechanism of benefit appeared to be that a reduction in AV delay led to improved diastolic filling and a reduction in diastolic mitral regurgitation.[9,10] However, these promising results were not confirmed in other studies[11,12] and, indeed, more recently, the DAVID study[13] showed that chronic right ventricular pacing was detrimental for patients with left ventricular systolic dysfunction (LVSD), presumably because of the dyssynchrony created by right ventricular apical pacing.

The haemodynamic effects of temporary pacing with right, left, and simultaneous ventricular activation were described in the 1970s.[14] However, it was only in 1994 that Cazeau and colleagues in France successfully implanted what would now be recognized as a cardiac resynchronization pacemaker in a patient with NHYA class IV HF who had first-degree AV block and LBBB.[15] All four chambers were paced, using a coronary sinus lead to pace the left atrium and an epicardial lead to pace the left ventricular free wall. The patient made a remarkable recovery and this led to further observational studies of biventricular pacing using transvenous leads to pace the left ventricle via cardiac veins. It also stimulated a plethora of research studies looking at the acute haemodynamic effects of atrio-biventricular pacing or CRT.

Acute haemodynamic effects of CRT

Leclercq *et al.*[16] studied the acute haemodynamic effects of biventricular pacing (BVP) in patients with endstage HF and QRS prolongation. Cardiac index (CI) was significantly increased by BVP in comparison with AAI or right ventricular DDD pacing. Pulmonary capillary wedge pressure (PCWP) decreased significantly during BVP compared to AAI pacing. The authors noted that 12/18 patients 'responded' to CRT (which they defined as an increase of 10% or more in CI and a reduction in PCWP of 10% or more), whereas 6 patients were 'nonresponders'.

Kass *et al.*[17] demonstrated that DDD left ventricular free wall pacing raised dP/dt_{max} and pulse pressure compared with sinus rhythm. left ventricular pacing had a greater effect on dP/dt_{max} than BVP. The optimal AV delay averaged 125 ms, and AV delay had less influence on left ventricular function than pacing site. Pacing efficacy was not associated with QRS narrowing. Auricchio *et al.*[18] described similar hemodynamic changes with increased pulse pressure and dP/dt_{max} at patient-specific optimal AV delay in patients with QRS in excess of 150 ms: however, patients with narrower QRS showed predominantly deleterious effects on left ventricular systolic function. Importantly, the acute haemodynamic changes with CRT happen while at the same time modestly lowering myocardial oxygen consumption. By contrast, inotropic agents, such as dobutamine, increase myocardial oxygen demand in achieving similar haemodynamic changes.[19] Given the adverse outcome with inotropic agents in HF, the finding that CRT reduces myocardial oxygen demand offered great hope for the long-term benefits of CRT.

An additional acute benefit from CRT is a reduction in MR. There are a number of mechanisms for functional mitral regurgitation (FMR) in patients with HF, including mitral valve annular dilation, alterations in left ventricular geometry, and left ventricular dyssynchrony.[20] Functional mitral regurgitation is reduced acutely following CRT due to an increase in left ventricular dP/dt_{max} and an increase in transmitral pressure gradient and consequent improvement in closure of the mitral valve leaflets during left ventricular systole.[21] In patients with markedly prolonged AV interval, there may be presystolic MR which can be reduced by improved AV timing. Over time, there may be further reduction in FMR with left atrial and left ventricular remodelling.

Dyssynchrony between papillary muscle contractions also plays a role in the mechanism of mitral regurgitation in patients with HF and QRS prolongation. Mechanical activation strain mapping demonstrate a marked reduction in interpapillary muscle time delay with CRT.[22] Left ventricular dyssynchrony involving the posterior papillary muscle may lead to an immediate reduction in mitral regurgitation with CRT, whereas left ventricular dyssynchrony in the lateral wall may lead to a late response to CRT.[23]

Figure 48.1 demonstrates an acute rise in arterial blood pressure and a fall in pulmonary artery pressure following onset of CRT. Figure 48.2 demonstrates a dramatic reduction in PCWP with onset of CRT in the same patient, with a reduction in the v wave corresponding to mitral regurgitation.

Outcome studies of CRT

There are now 13 randomized controlled trials of CRT with a total of over 6000 patients (Table 48.1).[1–4,24–33] The initial studies required surgical placement of the left ventricular lead.[25,26] However, subsequent developments have made catheter techniques to implant the left ventricular lead transvenously via the coronary sinus the method of choice for delivering CRT. The trials of CRT include a mixture of patients receiving CRT-P and CRT-D.

The early studies demonstrated an improvement in symptoms, exercise capacity, and quality of life measures comparable to, and in some cases better than, those obtained in pharmacological

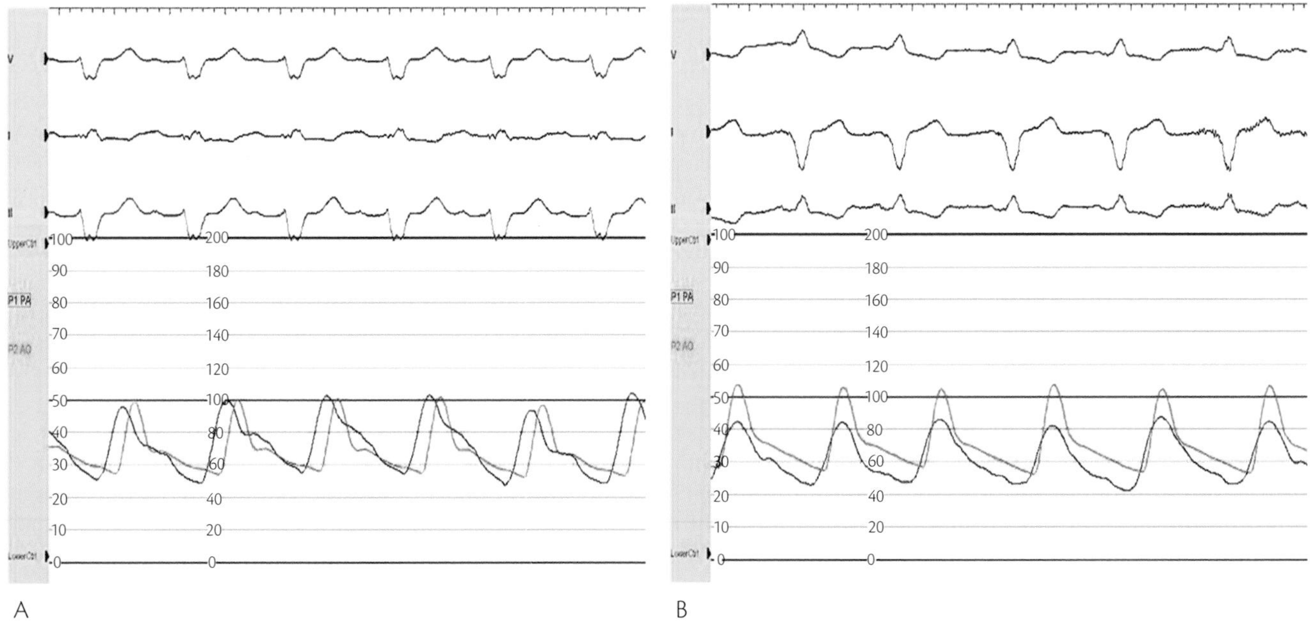

Fig. 48.1 (A) A patient with first-degree heart block and LBBB. Simultaneous aortic and pulmonary artery pressures are shown. There is clear interventricular mechanical delay, with the pulmonary arterial trace preceding the aortic trace. (B) The same patient following commencement of CRT. The PR interval has normalized and the QRS morphology has changed. Aortic pressure has increased and pulmonary artery pressure has fallen. Note the marked reduction in interventricular mechanical delay.

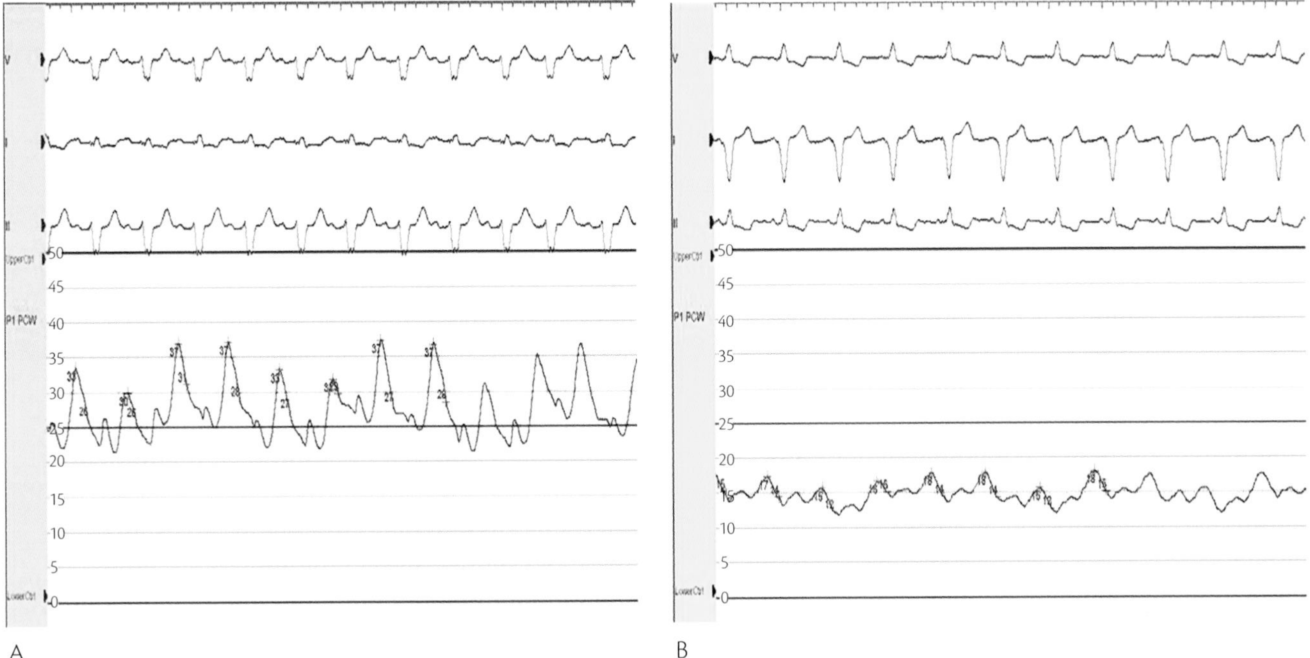

Fig. 48.2 (A) A recording of the pulmonary artery capillary wedge pressure (PCWP) in the same patient as shown in Fig. 48.1. The mean PCWP is elevated in excess of 25 mmHg with a large V wave secondary to mitral regurgitation. (B) The mean PCWP has fallen to 15 mmHg following commencement of CRT. Note how the V wave is much less marked.

studies.[1,2,25–27] The size of the benefit was a 0.5–0.8 point reduction in NYHA class, a 20% increase in six-minute walk distance, and a 10–15% increase in $Vo_{2\ max}$ capacity. Quality of life, assessed predominantly by the Minnesota Living with HF Questionnaire, also improved with CRT. The early studies were disadvantaged by short follow-up times of 3–6 months and they were not powered to assess HF morbidity and mortality.

The much larger COMPANION study compared CRT-D and CRT-P with medical therapy over a 12-month period.[4] It showed that CRT with or without a defibrillator reduced hospital-free survival (CRT-P 19% reduction, CRT-D 20%) and hospitalization for HF (CRT-P 34% reduction, CRT-D 40%) significantly compared with medical therapy alone. The secondary endpoint of all-cause mortality was only significantly reduced by CRT-D (36% reduction, $p < 0.003$), but the study was not suitably powered to assess the effect of CRT-P alone, which itself showed a strong trend towards reducing mortality (24% reduction, $p = 0.059$).

The CARE-HF study[3] was the largest study comparing CRT-P with medical therapy over a mean follow-up of 29.4 months . Both groups were very well treated for a HF study, with 72% on β-blockers and 95% on angiotensin converting enzyme (ACE) inhibitors or angiotensin receptor blockers (ARBs). However, on top of optimal medical therapy, there was a 37% reduction in the primary endpoint of mortality and hospitalization for a major cardiovascular event with CRT-P. All-cause mortality was also reduced by 36% and hospitalization for unplanned HF was reduced by 52% (Fig. 48.3). There was also a significant reduction in sudden arrhythmic death with CRT alone in the extended follow-up of the CARE-HF study,[30] which, taken together with results of the COMPANION study, suggests that there may be only a marginal additional survival benefit of CRT-D compared to CRT-P in patients with advanced HF.

Long-term effects of CRT

Remodelling

A number of randomized studies has demonstrated that CRT leads to a reduction in left ventricular internal dimensions and volumes, and an increase in LVEF compared to medical therapy. Although the majority of the remodelling occurs between 3 and 9 months after CRT, there is ongoing remodelling up to 18 months.[34] Remodelling is less in those with ischaemic heart disease (IHD) and to a lesser extent in those with no mechanical dyssynchrony or right ventricular dysfunction at baseline.[34] A decrease in left ventricular end-systolic volumes (LVESV) of more than 10% following CRT was associated with a lower mortality in one observational study.[35]

At a molecular level, there is a reduction in interstitial fibrosis, the proinflammatory cytokine TNFα, and a reduction in cellular apoptosis.[36] Improvement in left ventricular function following CRT is also associated with favourable changes in genes that regulate the contractile apparatus and pathological hypertrophy.[37] However, left ventricular remodelling only occurs in 50–66% of individuals following CRT and clinical improvement is not confined solely to those patients that exhibit favourable remodelling.[38]

Cardiac energy metabolism and perfusion

Functional studies using positron emission tomography (PET) have demonstrated that CRT increases stroke volume without increasing metabolic demand.[39] Following CRT, there is a more homogeneous pattern of regional myocardial oxygen and glucose metabolism with an increase in global myocardial perfusion reserve.[40,41] These effects of CRT are maintained for at least 13 months, resulting in a return of regional myocardial perfusion pattern similar to that of patients with mild HF and no LBBB.[42]

Table 48.1 The randomized CRT trials

RCT	Authors, country	N	Age (years)	NHYA class	QRS (ms) entry criteria	Mean QRS (ms)	LVEF (%)	LVED (mm)	Follow-up (months)	Primary endpoint	Main result
MUSTIC-SR[1]	Cazeau *et al.* Europe 2001	58	63	III	>150	176	<35	>60	3	6MWT	Positive effect of CRT
MUSTIC-AF[24,a]	Leclerq *et al.* Europe 2002	43	63	III	>200	209	<35	>60	3	6MWT	No significant effect
MIRACLE[2]	Abraham *et al.* USA 2002	453	64	III. IV	>130	167	<35	>55	6	6MWT, QoL, NYHA class	Positive effect of CRT
PATH-CHF[26,c]	Aurrichio *et al.* Germany 2002	41	60	III, IV	>130	175	<35	NA	6	6MWT, peak Vo_2	Positive effect of CRT
PATH-CHF II[25,c]	Aurrichio *et al.* Germany 2003	86	60	≥II	>120	155	<35	NA	3	6MWT, peak Vo_2	No difference in primary endpoint
MIRACLE-ICD[27]	Young *et al.* USA 2003	369	63	III–IV	>130	165	<35	>55	6	6MWT, QoL, NYHA class	Positive effect of CRT
CONTAK-CD[28]	Higgins *et al.* USA 2003	445	66	II–IV	>120	160	<35	NA	6	HF progression	No significant effect of CRT
COMPANION[4]	Bristow *et al.* USA 2004	1520	67	III, IV	>120	160[b]	<35	NA	12	All-cause mortality and hospitalization	12% reduction in primary endpoint
MIRACLE-ICD II[29]	Abraham *et al.* USA 2004	186	60	II	>130	164	<35	>55	6	Peak Vo_2	No significant effect of CRT
CARE-HF[3]	Cleland *et al.* Europe 2005	814	67	III, IV	>120	160[b]	<35	>30/ height	29.4	All-cause mortality and hospitalization	37% reduction in primary endpoint
CARE-HF extension[30]	Cleland *et al.* Europe 2006	813	67	III, IV	>120	160[b]	<35	>30/ height	36.4	All-cause mortality and hospitalization	55% reduction in primary endpoint
HOBIPACE[31,a,c]	Kindermann *et al.* Germany 2006	30	70	NA	NA	174	<35	>60	3	LVEF, LVESV, peak Vo_2	Positive effect of CRT
REVERSE[32]	Linde *et al.* Europe and North America 2008	610	62	I–II	>120	154	<40	>55	12	HF clinical composite response (% worsened)	No difference with CRT
MADIT-CRT[33]	Moss *et al.* Europe and USA 2009	1820	65	I–II	>130	N/A	<30	N/A	28.8	All-cause mortality or nonfatal HF event	44% reduction in primary endpoint

6MWT, six-minute walk test; AF, atrial fibrillation; CARE-HF, CArdiac REsynchronization-Heart Failure; COMPANION, Comparison of Medical Therapy Pacing and Defibrillation Therapy in Heart Failure; HF, heart failure; HOPIPACE, Homburg Biventricular Pacing Evaluation; ICD, implantable cardioverter-defibrillator; LVEDD, left ventricular end-diastolic dimension; LVEF, left ventricular ejection fraction; MADIT-CRT, Multicenter Automated Defibrillator Implantation Trial with Cardiac Resynchronization Therapy; MIRACLE, Multicentre InSync Randomized CLinical Evaluation; MUSTIC, MUltisite STimulation In Cardiomyopathies; N/A, not available; NYHA, New York Heart Association; PATH-CHF, PAcing THerapies in Congestive Heart Failure; QoL, quality of life; REVERSE, REsynchronization reVErsus Remodeling in Systolic left vEntricular dysfunction; SR, sinus rhythm.

[a]Inclusion criteria included indication for right ventricular pacing, therefore comparison of right ventricular pacing vs biventricular pacing.

[b]Median.

[c]Included patients with epicardial left ventricular lead placement.

Cardiac cycle changes

CRT alters cardiac timing so that the proportion of each cardiac cycle spent as isovolumic contraction or relaxation is reduced. The Tei index (the sum of isovolumic contraction and relaxation times divided by the total ejection time) is increased in patients with HF and is reduced with successful CRT.[43,44]

Natriuretic peptides

CRT has potentially beneficial effects on the natriuretic peptides, atrial natriuretic peptide (ANP) and B-type natriuretic peptide (BNP). CRT results in a greater decrease in BNP than medical therapy alone at 3 months, with further reductions at 18 months, correlating with the improvement in left ventricular function.[45] A high BNP at 1 month following CRT is associated with a worse prognosis, and reduction of BNP at 3 months is a strong predictor of an improvement in exercise capacity, LVEF, and MR.[46,47] ANP fell in a subgroup of patients with renal impairment taking part in the MIRACLE study (GFR 30–60 mL/min per 1.73 m^2). In the same group, glomerular filtratration rate increased following CRT. However, noradrenaline, plasma renin activity, aldosterone, and big endothelin were unchanged.[48]

Autonomic nervous system

CRT has a sustained sympathoinibitory effect as measured directly by muscle sympathetic nerve activity (MSNA).[49] Plasma noradrenaline is, however, unchanged.[48–50] In a separate study, MSNA increased by 25% in patients described as 'responders', whereas MSNA was unchanged in 'nonresponders', when CRT was temporarily turned off (to either intrinsic rhythm or right ventricular pacing if pacing dependent).[51] CRT improved heart rate variability

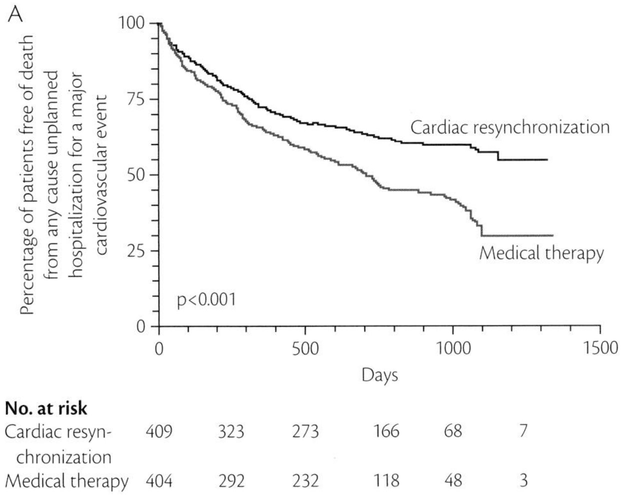

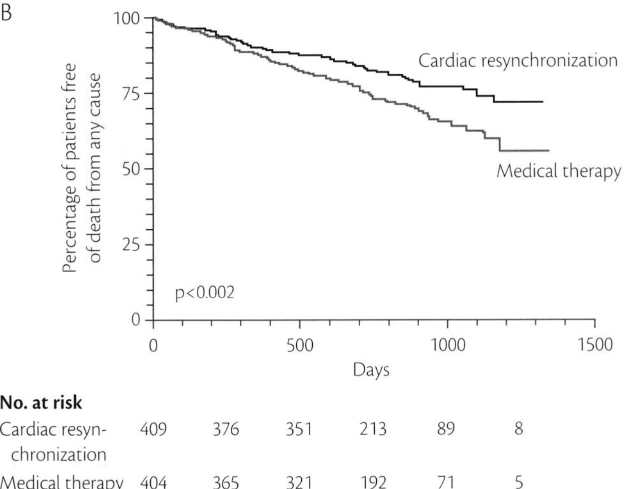

Fig. 48.3 CARE-HF study: Kaplan–Meier estimates of time to primary endpoint (A) and the principle secondary outcome (B). The primary outcome was death from any cause or unplanned hospitalization for a major cardiovascular event. The principle secondary outcome was death from any cause.

(HRV), a sign of improved autonomic function, in patients with symptomatic HF randomized to CRT-ON in the pilot phase of the MIRACLE study.[50]

CRT acutely improves baroreflex sensitivity (BRS).[52] In patients in whom the LVESV had decreased by 15% or more by the 6-month follow-up BRS increased by 30%, whereas in the nonresponders there was no change. Similarly, HRV increased by 30% in the responders.[52] Together, these findings suggest that improvement in autonomic function occurs following CRT and may be part of its beneficial effect.

There is emerging evidence that central sleep apnoea (CSA), which is prevalent in HF patients, may be improved by atrial overdrive pacing and CRT.[53] The exact mechanism is unclear, but may involve stabilization of fluctuating parasympathetic tone.

Patient selection

The current selection criteria for CRT are based on the results of the randomized controlled trials, all of which had similar inclusion criteria. Patients recruited had severe LVSD and symptoms refractory to maximally tolerated medical therapy, and, in particular, had a prolonged QRS width. The European Society of Cardiology (ESC) guidelines for CRT are as follows:

> CRT-P is recommended to reduce morbidity and mortality in patients in NYHA Class III/IV who are symptomatic despite optimal medical therapy, and who have a reduced LVEF (≤35%) and QRS prolongation (QRS width ≥120 ms). CRT-D is recommended for the same indications, where there is expectation of survival with good functional status for > 1 year.[54]

The updated AHA guidelines are similar, [55] but the UK national Institute for Health and Clinical Excellence (NICE) guidelines are a little different:

> CRT-P is recommended for patients currently experiencing, or who have recently experienced, Class III/IV symptoms, and who are in sinus rhythm with either QRS duration ≥150 ms or with QRS of 120–149 ms and mechanical dyssynchrony confirmed by echo. Patients require an LVEF ≤35% and to be on optimal pharmacological therapy. CRT-D is recommended for patients fulfilling the above criteria and separate NICE criteria for an ICD.[56]

The NICE guidelines allow for patients in NYHA class I–II HF to undergo CRT, provided that they have recently had decompensated HF.

Although guidelines tell us which patients can be considered for therapy, the randomized trials give some further insight into clinical characteristics which may affect the likelihood of 'responding' to CRT.

QRS duration

Prolongation of QRS interval is the most widely used criterion for selection for CRT. A QRS width of 120 ms or more was the entry requirement for the majority of the randomized controlled trials, but the QRS width of the patients actually enrolled in the in all the studies was considerably higher (see Table 48.1); the mean QRS duration in patients receiving CRT was 167 ms in MIRACLE[2] and the median QRS was 160 ms in COMPANION and CARE-HF.[3,4] There is evidence to suggest that patients with QRS width greater than 150 ms are more likely to benefit from CRT compared to those with QRS width 120–149 ms,[4,33] a fact which is reflected in the NICE guidelines, which require additional evidence of mechanical dyssynchrony in patients with QRS width 120–149 ms. Patients with right bundle branch block (RBBB) and nonspecific intraventricular delay are also less likely to benefit from CRT than those with LBBB.

The finding that not all patients 'respond' to CRT has led to investigators studying other more detailed methods of identifying dyssynchrony, with two main purposes: first, to try to identify which patients with a broad QRS are less likely to 'respond' to CRT, and thus avoid subjecting them to a complex procedure; and secondly, to see if current guidelines are excluding a subset of patients with a narrow QRS and echocardiographic evidence of dyssynchrony, who may also benefit from CRT.

Dyssynchrony measurements and implications

There is a plethora of different transthoracic echocardiography (TTE) methods for quantifying dyssynchrony, predominantly derived from nonrandomized single-centre studies.[57] The definition of response was not consistent. There is no universally acknowledged 'gold standard' for assessing dyssynchrony and there are large numbers of different echo variables describing radial, longitudinal, and global indices of dyssynchrony.

The PROSPECT study was intended to determine the best echocardiographic predictor of response to CRT.[58] Twelve echocardiographic variables purporting to measure mechanical dyssynchrony, based on both conventional and tissue Doppler-based methods, were measured. Centres underwent training in acquisition methods, with blinded analysis occurring in three core laboratories. Indicators of a positive CRT response were improved clinical composite score (seen in 69% of 426 patients) and at least 15% reduction in LVESV at 6 months (seen in 56% of patients with available data).

The ability of echocardiographic predictors to predict clinical or LVESV response was poor, with very high levels of inter- and intraobserver variability, and highly variable sensitivity and specificity. For all variables, the area under the ROC curve for positive clinical or volumetric response was 0.62 or less.

The PROSPECT trial has caused major controversy. The two sides of the argument are eloquently presented in a detailed review article by Hawkins and colleagues and rebutted in a commentary by Sanderson in the same journal.[57,59] Hawkins *et al.*[57] comment that, rather than identifying the best method of identifying dyssynchrony, the study exposed critical limitations in the 12 echocardiographic measures of dyssynchrony studied and questioned the validity of previous single-centre experiences. They call for clinicians to select patients for CRT solely on the basis of QRS duration, on which the landmark trials are based. Sanderson[59] agrees that this approach is currently to be recommended, but highlights the need to improve our selection criteria to reduce the number of patients who do worse with CRT. Sanderson raises a number of potential flaws with PROSPECT: '. . . [it] was a nonrandomized study, which assessed too many echocardiographic parameters, was funded by a device company and had centre selection based on implantation volumes rather than echocardiography track record'. He summed up PROSPECT to be 'effectively a study of laboratory error rather than a test of a hypothesis'.

Box 48.1 CARE-HF criteria for dyssynchrony on transthoracic echo

Patients with 120 ms < QRS width <150 ms required two out of the following:

1 Aortic pre-ejection time (APET) >140 ms
2 Interventricular delay (IVD) >40 ms
3 Evidence of delayed activation of posterolateral wall, i.e. time to maximal posterolateral wall thickening (M-mode) or systolic velocity (tissue Doppler) greater than time to onset of E-wave (mitral inflow).

The CARE-HF study was the only large randomized study to include echo measures of dyssynchrony prior to enrolment, but only for around 10% of patients who had a QRS width of 120–149 ms (Box 48.1). Simple dyssynchrony measurements were made in most patients, and the probability of not experiencing the primary endpoint (death or unplanned cardiovascular hospitalization) was higher in patients with an interventricular mechanical delay in excess of 49 ms at baseline (where >40 ms is abnormal). However, patients without dyssynchrony at baseline were still less likely to experience the primary outcome if they received CRT.[60] Measurement of interventricular delay is demonstrated in Fig. 48.5.

Other imaging methods used to quantify dyssynchrony are radionuclide ventriculography and cardiac magnetic resonance (CMR) scanning.[61,62] These offer better spatial resolution, but they are inferior to TTE in temporal resolution, which is vital when assessing timing of cardiac events.

Narrow QRS

At present, CRT is only recommended for patients with a prolonged QRS complex. However, up to one-third of patients with advanced HF and a normal QRS width have evidence of mechanical dyssynchrony,[63] raising the possibility that CRT could benefit some

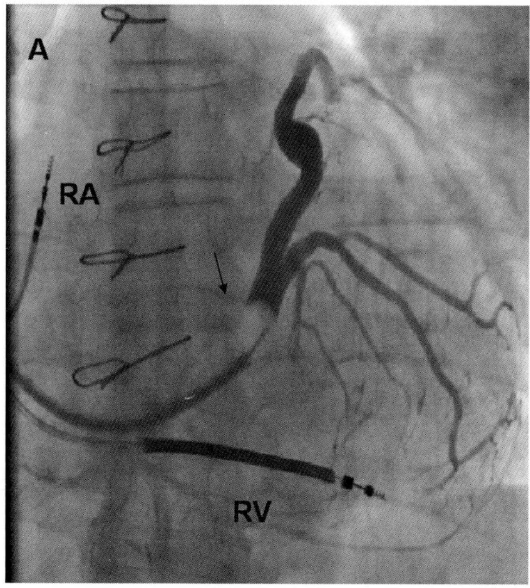

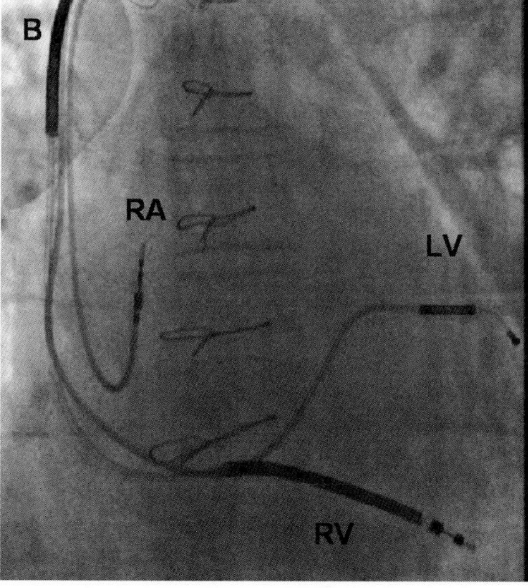

Fig. 48.4 (A) AP projection of coronary sinus venogram using balloon occlusion catheter (arrow) demonstrating a lateral vein. (B) Final positions of right atrial (RA) lead, right ventricular (RV) dual-coil defibrillator lead and left ventricular (LV) lead.

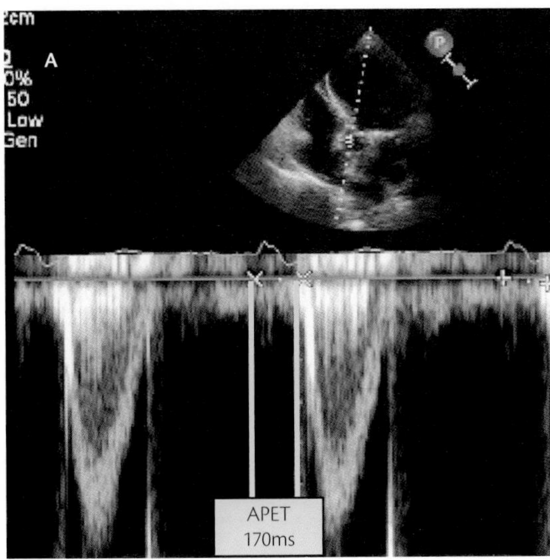

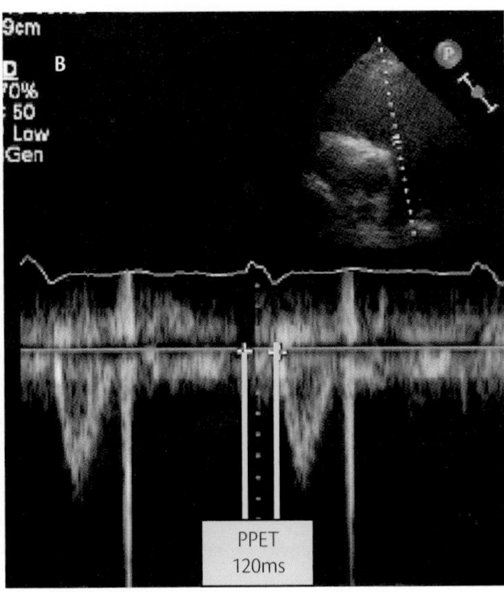

Fig. 48.5 Panel A: Aortic pre-ejection time (APET) =170 ms. Panel B: Pulmonary pre-ejection time (PPET) = 120 ms. The interventricular ventricular delay is 50 ms.

patients with a relatively narrow QRS. The data available for CRT in patients with QRS duration less than 120 ms is limited. A number of small, nonrandomized studies have shown that patients with echo criteria for dyssynchrony and a narrow QRS achieve a similar level of improvement in symptoms and functional capacity to patients with a broad QRS, but with less clear evidence of ventricular remodelling. It should, however, be remembered that NYHA class and six-minute walk times improved in the placebo arm of the MIRACLE trial.

The only randomized study published so far in the narrow QRS patient group was RethinQ.[64] In this study 172 patients with a standard indication for ICD therapy and QRS less than 130 ms underwent CRT-D implantation and were randomized to CRT-on or off. Follow-up was for 6 months; the primary endpoint was increased peak oxygen consumption at 6 months. There was no significant difference in peak oxygen consumption, quality of life, or six-minute walk times with CRT at 6 months. NYHA class improved with CRT, and in the subgroup with QRS 120 ms or more, there was a significant increase in peak oxygen consumption.

Although the results of the RethinQ study were not very encouraging, there have been some interesting haemodynamic studies which have raised the possibility that CRT may have a role in some narrow-QRS patients. Turner *et al.*[65] studied 20 patients with advanced HF and a QRS 120 ms or less. Patients with a wedge pressure greater than 15 mmHg responded to temporary left ventricular pacing with increased cardiac output and decreased wedge pressure. The improvement was seen in association with an increase in QRS duration, providing further evidence that changes in QRS duration do not correlate well with haemodynamic benefits from pacing. The likely mechanism for the improvement was thought to be due to reduced external constraint from both the pericardium and diastolic ventricular interaction across the interventricular septum secondary to raised right ventricular diastolic pressure. More recently, Williams *et al.*[66] studied 30 patients with class III/IV HF, QRS less than 120 ms and no evidence of dyssynchrony on conventional criteria. Cardiac output increased, absolute left ventricular stroke work increased and dP/dt_{max} increased. External constraint was present in 15 patients and was completely abolished by both biventricular and left ventricular pacing. The patients involved in the study have been randomized to a CRT-on or -off trial and the results are awaited with interest. For the present, patients with QRS less than 120 ms should only receive CRT in a research setting.

NYHA class

CRT is proven to be effective in patients with NYHA class III/IV symptoms, yet the vast majority of patients in the clinical trials have been in class III HF.[2–4,27] In the COMPANION study, 217 class IV patients took part; CRT-P and CRT-D improved the time to all-cause mortality and hospitalizations, with a trend for improved mortality.[67] Although CRT-D reduced sudden death, there was no difference between CRT-P and CRT-D when it came to all-cause mortality. COMPANION was, however, a study of ambulatory patients who had not been hospitalized for HF in the last 30 days. CRT has not been proven to be of benefit in acutely decompensated HF in a randomized trial.

There have been a number of case series describing the effects of CRT in inotrope-dependent patients. Cowburn *et al.*[68] described 10 consecutive cases who had been in hospital for a mean of 30 days prior to CRT and who had received inotropic support for a mean of 11 days prior to CRT. The mean QRS was 205 ms. All patients were weaned from inotropic support after a mean of 2 days and all patients were successfully discharge from hospital. Renal function improved, diuretic requirements were reduced, and hyponatraemia was corrected. Seven patients were alive at 1 year. These promising results have been reproduced by others, but it is clear that some of these patients do very badly and that publication bias is likely to lead to reporting of successful series only. A randomized trial is required before CRT becomes standard therapy in this setting.

CRT in mild heart failure

MIRACLE ICD II studied patients in NYHA class II and an indication for an ICD.[29] Patients receiving CRT had a mean QRS duration of 165 ms, yet showed no significant improvement in peak Vo_2, six-minute walk distance, or quality of life. Patients did, however, show evidence of left ventricular remodelling with CRT. Given the fairly high procedural complication rate, it was hard to justify CRT in class II HF on the basis of these results. However, distinguishing a class II from a class III patient is not easy. CARE-HF was a study of class III/IV HF, but when patients were asked to self-assess their NYHA class, 21.5% classed themselves as either class I or II at baseline. There was no statistical interaction between the severity of symptoms and the benefits of CRT on morbidity and mortality.[69]

Two further studies of CRT in milder HF have recently been published. REVERSE studied 610 patients with NYHA class I/II HF with a QRS 120 ms or more and LVEF 40% or less. All patients received CRT devices (predominantly CRT-D) and were then randomly assigned to CRT-ON or OFF for 12 months. Patients receiving CRT showed improved LVESV index and had delayed time to first HF hospitalization.[32] REVERSE was a European/North American Study. The European cohort of 262 patients was followed for 2 years.[70] European patients were less likely to have IHD, a history of hypertension or peripheral vascular disease; they had longer six-minute walk times, lower BMI, and were less likely to receive CRT-D than the US cohort. In this population CRT improved clinical outcomes and led to reverse remodelling. The time to first HF hospitalization or death was delayed by CRT.

MADIT-CRT was the largest study to date to assess the effect of CRT in mild HF.[33] 1820 patients with an ICD indication were randomized to CRT-D or ICD alone in a 3:2 ratio. There was a 34% reduction in the primary endpoint (all-cause death or a nonfatal HF event) with CRT over a mean follow-up of 2.4 years. The superiority of CRT was driven by a 41% reduction in HF events with no difference in mortality. The improved outcome with CRT was found in the subgroup of patients with QRS duration of 150 ms or more, a finding which was also evident in REVERSE.

Taken together, MADIT-CRT and REVERSE support the use of CRT in mildly symptomatic patients when the QRS is 150 ms or more, especially if there has been a prior episode of decompensated HF. Although a mortality benefit has not been shown in these studies, it may be that there is a mortality benefit over a longer follow-up.

CRT in atrial fibrillation

There is almost no data from randomized trials to support the use of CRT in patients with atrial fibrillation (AF). The MUSTIC-AF study recruited 59 patients with chronic AF and a slow ventricular rate requiring pacing.[24] Patients received a biventricular pacemaker and were randomized to 3 months right ventricular pacing or 3 months CRT, crossing over to the alternative therapy for a further 3 months. Only 37 patients completed the crossover phase, and there was no significant difference in exercise capacity between the two treatment phases. The PAVE Study compared chronic biventricular pacing to right ventricular pacing in 184 patients undergoing ablation of the AV node for management of AF with a rapid ventricular response.[71] This was not a study of patients with HF; the mean LVEF was 46%. 6 months post ablation, patients receiving CRT had improved six-minute walk time and had a higher LVEF. The beneficial effect of CRT appeared to be greater in patients with LVEF 45% or less or with NYHA class II/III symptoms.

Part of the problem with AF is that the benefit of CRT is seen when 100% ventricular pacing is achieved. Patients with AF have no capacity to improve AV dyssynchrony, and poor rate control may mean that 100% pacing is hard to achieve unless either a high pacing rate is used or drugs that may be detrimental (amiodarone or rate-limiting calcium antagonists) are used to decrease the intrinsic ventricular rate. A meta-analysis of cohort studies suggested that patients in AF may improve after CRT but with less functional benefit.[72] There are case series suggesting that AV node ablation and CRT improves long-term outcome compared to CRT alone,[73] but others report a similar benefit without need for AV node ablation.[74]

There is a clear need for a large randomized outcome trial in patients with AF, but such a trial may never be carried out, particularly because patients in AF are eligible for CRT according to ESC guidelines and AHA/ACC guidelines (class IIa indication). If the decision is made to proceed with CRT, it is important to be aware that some patients spontaneously revert to sinus rhythm following CRT and some are cardioverted to sinus rhythm at the time of defibrillation threshold testing (for patients receiving CRT-D). It is therefore appropriate to implant an right atrial lead in patients with recent onset AF or in patients where the duration of AF is unknown. If rate control is not adequately achieved by standard medical therapy (β-blockade and digoxin), then AV node ablation should be considered.

CRT in patients with an indication for pacing

The DAVID study suggested that chronic right ventricular apical pacing is associated with an increase in the incidence of HF in patients with LVSD.[13] Therefore every effort must be made to reduce the need for right ventricular apical pacing in patients with HF. Newer pacing algorithms allow patients with sinus node disease to be programmed to atrial pacing, with the back-up of dual-chamber pacing should it become necessary. In patients with LVSD and high degree AV block, CRT improves left ventricular function, quality of life, and exercise capacity compared to right ventricular pacing alone.[31]

Indeed, a recent study has demonstrated that CRT may have advantages over right ventricular apical pacing in patients with normal left ventricular function.[75] Over 1 year of follow-up, right ventricular apical pacing resulted in adverse ventricular remodelling and a reduction in LVEF; these effects were prevented by CRT.

In patients with pre-existing chronic right ventricular pacing who have LVSD and symptomatic HF, upgrading to a biventricular device has been shown to improve acute haemodynamic variables, and the improvement is maintained in the medium term and associated with improvement in symptoms and reduction in admissions for HF.[76] During longer-term follow-up, patients with CRT upgrade appear to gain a similar mortality and morbidity benefit and similar left ventricular reverse remodelling to patients with native LBBB treated with CRT.[77]

CRT outcome by age and sex

As with most randomized controlled trials of HF, the average age of patients recruited for the CRT trials was relatively young at 64 years (see Table 48.1). In the MIRACLE and MIRACLE ICD trials, 174/839 patients were over 75 years old. CRT led to a similar improvement in NYHA class and LVEF regardless of age.[78] Observational studies suggest the benefits of CRT also extend to octogenarians, so there should be no upper age limit for CRT.[79] The role of a primary prevention ICD is less proven in elderly patients, however, as these patients are more likely to die of other noncardiac conditions.

Women are less commonly recruited to clinical trials and are less well represented in the CRT trials. Although numbers are smaller, the benefit from CRT appears similar in men and women.[3,4,33] However, fewer women than men undergo CRT in both the United

States and Europe, for reasons which are unclear. Approximately 25–27% of CRT implants are in women and a relatively higher percentage of these patients received CRT-P (as opposed to CRT-D) when compared with men.[80,81] Although this may represent a sex bias, a meta-analysis reporting on the outcome of 934 women in 5 ICD trials has suggested that primary prevention ICDs offer no prognostic benefit in women.[82]

Aetiology of heart failure

Patients with both ischaemic and nonischaemic causes of HF benefit from CRT.[2,4,32,33] Patients with nonischaemic causes of HF exhibit greater remodelling after CRT which might be expected, as fibrotic scar in IHD patients is unlikely to respond to CRT yet patients with IHD seem to derive equivalent mortality benefit from CRT.[34] Mitral regurgitation is reduced to a similar degree in patients with IHD and nonischaemic cardiomyopathy.[34]

Congenital heart disease and CRT

The role of CRT in patients with congenital heart disease is complicated by the anatomical and physiological heterogeneity of the population and the lack of any randomized trials. The most frequent indication for CRT in case series is as an upgrade in patients with single-site ventricular pacing and HF. Venous access can be challenging (sometimes through surgically redirected atria) and coronary sinus anatomy is very variable. Surgically placed epicardial leads are sometimes required. Evidence from case studies suggests that some patients benefit from CRT, but the risks of the procedure are higher, lead placement may be suboptimal, and some patients may deteriorate following CRT.[83,84] Careful planning before consideration of CRT is therefore essential.

The CRT procedure

The dominant method of CRT implantation is transvenous, using subclavian, axillary, or cephalic veins to access the venous system. Standard endocardial pacing leads are positioned in the right atrial appendage and right ventricle. When implanting a CRT-D system, a single- or dual-coil defibrillator lead is used instead of a right ventricular pacing lead. A variety of preshaped guide catheters are now available to help intubate the coronary sinus (CS). Contrast is sometimes required to guide cannulation, but its use should be minimized. After the CS is cannulated, a balloon occlusion venogram is obtained (Fig. 48.5) in at least two projections (anteroposterior and left anterior oblique) to demonstrate the coronary venous anatomy. The anatomy of the CS is variable and most operators aim to place the left ventricular lead in an epicardial venous tributary overlying the lateral border of the left ventricle.

Placement of the left ventricular lead is more technically challenging than standard pacing, often demanding guide wires or inner preshaped subselection catheters to access the target vein. The left ventricular lead is usually delivered over the wire; once it is positioned, the guide catheters are split and removed. The left ventricular lead can be bipolar or unipolar and most are not actively fixed in the vein. Bipolar leads offer greater options in programming, but the larger profile of the leads tends to make them unsuitable for smaller veins. For larger veins, there are leads with active fixation mechanisms. Advances in the design of equipment for left ventricular lead placement have improved the success rate of implantation, but failure rates of up to 10% are reported due to unsuitable venous anatomy, inadequate pacing thresholds, and diaphragmatic pacing secondary to phrenic nerve stimulation.

Complications of CRT

The majority of the complications are the placement and dislodgement of the left ventricular lead. In a report of over 2000 patients taking part in the MIRACLE, MIRACLE ICD, and InSyncIII studies, the implant attempt succeeded in 91.6% of patients.[85] Dissection or perforation of the CS occurred in 2.2% of patients. A pericardial effusion or tamponade occurred in 0.4% of cases, with one-half of these patients requiring pericardiocentesis; 7.7% of patients required lead revision (predominantly left ventricular lead) during 6-month follow-up. One per cent of patients developed pocket infection, with two-thirds requiring explantation of the device. Procedure related mortality was 0.3%.[85] Similar complication rates are reported from the major clinical trials.

Patients are at risk of other standard complications from device insertion such as a pneumothorax (1%); advisory notices from device manufactures sometimes require generator changes or lead revisions. Intravenous contrast is required for CS venography and to identify the os of the CS if cannulation is difficult. Contrast nephropathy is a serious complication of the procedure and at-risk patients should be prehydrated.[86] Despite these risks, CRT remains a safe and effective procedure.

Left Ventricular Lead Placement

The positioning of the left ventricular lead is limited by coronary venous anatomy, but there is usually a number of options in most patients. Haemodynamic studies have shown that placement of the left ventricular lead over the area of the left ventricular with the most delayed activation results in the maximal rise in left ventricular dP/dt_{max} and pulse pressure.[87] Using noncontact mapping, areas of slow conduction can be identified; haemodynamic benefit is more marked when the chosen pacing site is outside these areas.[88] In the majority of patients, the area of most delayed contraction occurs at the lateral free wall of the left ventricle, which is targeted using lateral or posterolateral veins. The anterior vein is usually orientated away from the free wall, making it less attractive; however, a lateral branch can be used. The left ventricular lead is typically positioned midway between the base and apex of the heart within the chosen vein.

On the basis of early haemodynamic studies, the lateral or posterolateral veins have been preferentially targeted in the clinical trials. However, these veins are not always the best in an individual patient. Van Campen *et al.*[89] studied 9 different pacing configurations in 48 patients. The site most frequently associated with the maximal increase in cardiac output was the combination of left ventricular pacing from a posterolateral vein with right ventricular apical pacing, but only in 29% of patients. Although anteriorly positioned veins have often been considered suboptimal, the combination of right ventricular apical pacing with an anterolateral vein produced optimal haemodynamic benefit in 19% of patients. Individualization of pacing configuration has the potential to improve response to CRT.

In the COMPANION study, functional outcomes were independent of left ventricular lead position.[90] However, this retrospective study has a number of limitations and it would be wrong to suggest that left ventricular lead position is unimportant on the basis of this one study.

Right ventricular lead placement

The optimal position of the right ventricular lead for CRT is controversial. A recent study showed no difference between right ventricular apical and right ventricular high septal pacing sites in terms of overall improvement in clinical outcome and left ventricular reverse remodelling.[91] However, there did appear to be a benefit of right ventricular high septal position when the left ventricular lead was placed in the posterolateral vein and right ventricular apical position was superior with anterolateral left ventricular lead placement (80% of this latter group had a reduction in BNP of >50% post CRT). The study requires confirmation, but has potentially important clinical implications. The right ventricular lead may benefit from repositioning, dependent on final position of the left ventricular lead (most operators position the right ventricular lead first as there is a risk of ventricular standstill during CS cannulation). It may be that it is separation between right ventricular and left ventricular lead tips which is important in achieving optimal resynchronization.[92]

Optimization of CRT

Alterations in pacemaker programming allow changes in timing between atria and ventricle (AV delay) and between right and left ventricle (VV delay). A long AV delay causes late ventricular contraction; diastolic filling time (DFT) is reduced, causing fusion of the E and A waves of the mitral inflow Doppler. The atrial contribution to filling terminates before depolarization of the ventricle, resulting in wasted diastole and suboptimal preload for ventricular contraction.[93]

The goal of AV optimization is to maximize DFT and to allow complete end-diastolic filling before the onset of left ventricular contraction. AV programming of CRT can eliminate 'diastolic' mitral regurgitation. Invasive haemodynamic testing has shown that optimizing the AV delay at implantation results in an acute improvement in left ventricular systolic performance.[18] The most commonly method for AV delay optimization is the iterative method using MV pulse wave Doppler. DFT is measured from the start of the E wave to the end of the A wave. A long AV delay is programmed and reduced in 20-ms steps until the A wave truncates. The interval is then increased in 10-ms increments. The shortest AV delay without A-wave truncation is selected to maximize DFT.[93] Ritter's method, derived from dual-chamber pacing studies, has limited data in HF and is now rarely used.

AV optimization has a clear physiological basis with evidence of acute haemodynamic benefit and was used as standard practice in the major CRT trials. The evidence base for CRT is thus dependent on AV optimization post procedure, and it should be considered standard clinical practice. However, AV optimization is not routinely undertaken in all institutions partly because there is a lack of robust, stand-alone evidence of its benefits, but more commonly because there is lack of appropriately trained staff to undertake what can be a time-consuming procedure. In one small trial, patients randomized to AV optimization had an improved quality of life at 3 months, although objective measures (six-minute walk time, LVEF, or left ventricular volumes) were unchanged.[94]

Optimization is carried out at rest; however, the haemodynamic benefits of CRT may be more marked during exercise, suggesting that optimization should also be carried out at higher heart rates.[95] Most CRT pacemakers can programme a rate-adaptive AV delay to mimic the physiological shortening of AV delay that occurs with exercise, but the clinical value has not been fully evaluated in CRT where an increase in AV delay may actually be of benefit.[96]

VV optimization is intended to restore synchronous ventricular contraction. Suboptimal left ventricular lead position and regional conduction delays can affect ventricular timing; hence tailored ventricular pacing is potentially valuable. Acute haemodynamic studies have shown a benefit from VV optimization.[18,97] Small studies have shown that echocardiographically optimized sequential biventricular pacing can improve left ventricular function, dyssynchrony, and left ventricular filling compared to simultaneous pacing.[98] However, the one randomized trial of VV optimization, RHYTHM II ICD, showed no additional benefit from optimization of VV delay.[99] VV optimization is not currently recommended in routine clinical practice but may be worth attempting in 'nonresponders'.

Optimization of medical therapy

After CRT, patients often have an increase in systolic blood pressure, allowing further up-titration of ACE inhibitors or ARBs. Diuretic requirements may reduce as a result of improved left ventricular performance.[68] Patients are no longer at risk of a β-blocker-induced bradycardia, potentially allowing some patients to be β-blocked for the first time and allowing further up-titration of dose in other patients. Optimization of medical therapy offers the potential to improve patient outcome further, in addition to the benefit achieved through CRT.

CRT response

The issue of CRT 'response' remains controversial. There is no good definition of a 'responder' or 'nonresponder'. The fact that a patient's symptoms may not have improved, or their left ventricular volumes have not reduced, is used by many to indicate lack of 'response', but such an approach ignores the fact the patient may have had a mortality benefit, or might (without the device) have deteriorated further. For example, in a recent observational study of patients with CRT admitted with acute decompensation of their HF (who might therefore be thought to be 'nonresponders'), when the CRT was switched off, the patients' haemodynamic state deteriorated further.[100] Approximately 70% of patients who undergo CRT feel better. However, there is a large placebo response to CRT as demonstrated by improved six-minute walk times and quality of life in the control group of MIRACLE.

The reasons for a lack of symptomatic response to CRT are multifactorial and include poor patient selection, suboptimal lead placement, device programming issues, arrhythmias, or failure to optimize medical therapy. Prior knowledge of CS anatomy and identification of areas with nonviable myocardium may help plan left ventricular lead placement. Contrast-enhanced MRI can identify transmural scar in the posterolateral wall; these patients have been shown not to respond to CRT according to clinical and echo criteria.[101] Factors which predicted a poor response to CRT in the CARE-HF trial were an ischaemic aetiology, high BNP, and severity of mitral regurgitation; patients with low blood pressure and

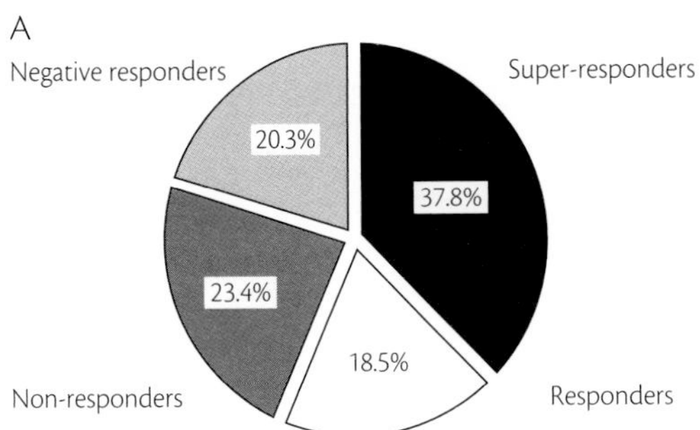

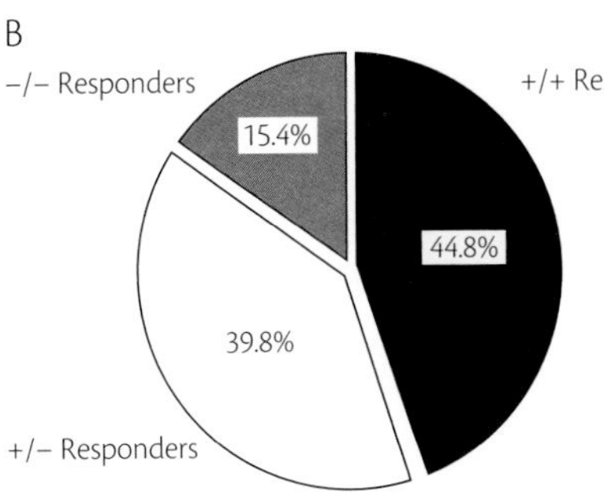

Fig. 48.6 Percentage of responders according to the extent of reduction in LVESV (A) and the combination of clinical response and a reduction in LVESV ≥15% (B).[102]

echocardiographic evidence of interventricular mechanical delay obtained greater benefit from CRT.[60]

Some patients respond spectacularly well to CRT, and some deteriorate. While it is important to identify patients who are most likely to respond, it is perhaps more important to identify patients in whom CRT may actually be harmful. A subanalysis of the PROSPECT study defined super-responders as having a reduction in LVESV of 30% or more, responders a reduction of 15–29%, nonresponders a reduction of 0–14%, and 'negative responders' an increase in LVESV.[102] Super-responders were more frequently female, had nonischaemic HF, a wider QRS complex, and more extensive mechanical dyssynchrony at baseline. The percentage of clinical responders and nonresponders is shown in Fig. 48.6: 15–20% of patients may actually do worse following CRT.

Can we do more to predict which patients may do badly? Acute haemodynamic studies suggest that patients with narrower QRS showed predominantly negative changes.[18] It is clearly impractical to measure dP/dt_{max} invasively on all patients undergoing CRT, but it has been assessed within 24 h of implant noninvasively using echocardiography and has been shown to predict long-term clinical outcome.[103] Another measure of acute haemodynamic benefit is a prompt rise in systolic blood pressure after the onset of CRT; an increase of more than 5 mmHg has recently been shown to predict event-free survival at 2 years.[104] Ideally, we need a method of assessing response at the time of implant so that the operator has the option of testing other lead positions if an inadequate or deleterious response is observed. Measuring systolic blood pressure response using an arterial line is one possibility.

In a study of 75 patients who deteriorated following CRT, a multidisciplinary team following a protocol-driven assessment recommended further management including additional medical therapy, treating underlying arrhythmias, reprogramming the device, and repositioning the left ventricular lead. The most common problem encountered was suboptimal AV timing in 47% of patients; however, 12% of patients had an immediate improvement in haemodynamics when CRT was turned off (the majority of these patients had a narrow QRS).[105]

CRT-P versus CRT-D

The debate as to which patient should receive CRT-P or CRT-D is challenging. CRT-D is approximately four times more expensive that CRT-P and thus cost-effectiveness becomes a major issue.[106] In older patients, CRT-D is less cost-effective than CRT-P. CRT-D should only be considered for patients where there is expectation of survival for more than 1 year with good functional status.

Patients who took part in the clinical trials of CRT and primary prevention ICDs are generally younger than typical patients with HF and have predominantly single-organ disease. Older patients with renal impairment and other comorbidities are less likely to benefit from ICD therapy.[107] COMPANION is the only study to have compared CRT-P with CRT-D, though the results are presented in comparison with medical therapy. CRT-D improved survival compared with medical therapy (36% reduction in mortality), whereas CRT-P nonsignificantly reduced mortality ($p = 0.06$) by 24%. However, although not formally analysed and reported, there was clearly no statistically significant difference between CRT-P and CRT-D in terms of mortality.

Patient perspectives are also highly relevant. A CRT-P device is smaller, has no risk of inappropriate shocks, and is at less risk of device advisories, which have been an ongoing problem with ICDs.[108] An ICD may change the mode of death; in an older patient, a peaceful arrhythmic death, rather than dying in discomfort with refractory HF, may be a patient's preference. Patients often have unrealistic expectations about the life-saving effects of an ICD, due at least in part to inadequate explanation or oversimplification by medical and nursing staff. Realistic advice for a patient receiving an ICD for primary prevention is that for every 100 patients receiving an ICD, over the next 5 years, approximately 30 patients would die anyway, 10–20 patients would have a shock they do not need, 5–15 patients would have other complications from the device, and only 7–8 patients would be saved by the ICD.[109] They should also be aware that some patients choose to have their device inactivated to allow a natural death.

Telemonitoring

Advances in telecommunications and device technology allow the remote monitoring of surrogate markers of HF severity such as patient activity, heart rate variability, and intrathoracic impedance. Such markers may help predict subclinical HF decompensation, allowing medical intervention to ward off hospitalization.[110,111] In order to realize the full potential of telemonitoring, though, device services will need to be reconfigured and more closely integrated with HF clinics. Randomized studies are under way to evaluate the effectiveness of remote monitoring in this setting.

Conclusion

CRT offers an important therapeutic option for patients with advanced HF and a prolonged QRS. Successful CRT depends on appropriate patient selection, successful implantation of the device with optimal left ventricular lead positioning, appropriate device programming, and further optimization of medical therapy. A lack of clinical response should lead to careful reassessment, although it must be appreciated that a lack of clinical response does not mean that the patient will not derive benefit from CRT. Further research is needed to refine the selection criteria for CRT and to optimize left ventricular lead placement at the time of implantation to maximize patient benefit.

References

1. Cazeau S, Leclercq C, Lavergne T, Walker S, Varma C, Linde C et al. Effects of multisite biventricular pacing in patients with heart failure and intraventricular conduction delay. N Engl J Med 2001;**344**:873-880.
2. Abraham WT, Fisher WG, Smith AL, DeLurgio DB, Leon AR, Loh E et al. Cardiac resynchronization in chronic heart failure. N Engl J Med 2002;**346:**1845-1853.
3. Cleland JG, Daubert JC, Erdmann E, Freemantle N, Gras D, Kappenberger L et al. The effect of cardiac resynchronization on morbidity and mortality in heart failure. N Engl J Med 2005;352: 1539-1549.
4. Bristow MR, Saxon LA, Boehmer J, Krueger S, Kass DA, De Marco T et al. Cardiac-resynchronization therapy with or without an implantable defibrillator in advanced chronic heart failure. N Engl J Med 2004;350:2140-2150.
5. Hawkins NM, Petrie MC, MacDonald MR, Hogg KJ, McMurray JJ. Selecting patients for cardiac resynchronization therapy: electrical or mechanical dyssynchrony? Eur Heart J 2006;27:1270-1281.
6. Vernooy K, Verbeek XA, Peschar M, Crijns HJ, Arts T, Cornelussen RN et al. Left bundle branch block induces ventricular remodelling and functional septal hypoperfusion. Eur Heart J 2005;26:91-98.
7. Spragg DD, Leclercq C, Loghmani M, Faris OP, Tunin RS, DiSilvestre D et al. Regional alterations in protein expression in the dyssynchronous failing heart. Circulation 2003;108:929-932.
8. Hochleitner M, Hortnagl H, Ng CK, Hortnagl H, Gschnitzer F, Zechmann W. Usefulness of physiologic dual-chamber pacing in drug-resistant idiopathic dilated cardiomyopathy. Am J Cardiol 1990;66:198-202.
9. Brecker SJ, Xiao HB, Sparrow J, Gibson DG. Effects of dual-chamber pacing with short atrioventricular delay in dilated cardiomyopathy. Lancet 1992;340:1308-1312.
10. Nishimura RA, Hayes DL, Holmes DR, Jr., Tajik AJ. Mechanism of hemodynamic improvement by dual-chamber pacing for severe left ventricular dysfunction: an acute Doppler and catheterization hemodynamic study. J Am Coll Cardiol 1995;25:281-288.
11. Linde C, Gadler F, Edner M, Nordlander R, Rosenqvist M, Ryden L. Results of atrioventricular synchronous pacing with optimized delay in patients with severe congestive heart failure. Am J Cardiol 1995;75:919-923.
12. Gold MR, Feliciano Z, Gottlieb SS, Fisher ML. Dual-chamber pacing with a short atrioventricular delay in congestive heart failure: a randomized study. J Am Coll Cardiol 1995;26:967-973.
13. Wilkoff BL, Cook JR, Epstein AE, Greene HL, Hallstrom AP, Hsia H et al. Dual-chamber pacing or ventricular backup pacing in patients with an implantable defibrillator: the Dual Chamber and VVI Implantable Defibrillator (DAVID) Trial. JAMA 2002;288:3115-3123.
14. Gibson DG, Chamberlain DA, Coltart DJ, Mercer J. Effect of changes in ventricular activation on cardiac haemodynamics in man. Comparison of right ventricular, left ventricular, and simultaneous pacing of both ventricles. Br Heart J 1971;33:397-400.
15. Cazeau S, Ritter P, Bakdach S, Lazarus A, Limousin M, Henao L et al. Four chamber pacing in dilated cardiomyopathy. Pacing Clin Electrophysiol 1994;17(11 Pt 2):1974-1979.
16. Leclercq C, Cazeau S, Le Breton H, Ritter P, Mabo P, Gras D et al. Acute hemodynamic effects of biventricular DDD pacing in patients with end-stage heart failure. J Am Coll Cardiol 1998;32:1825-1831.
17. Kass DA, Chen CH, Curry C, Talbot M, Berger R, Fetics B et al. Improved left ventricular mechanics from acute VDD pacing in patients with dilated cardiomyopathy and ventricular conduction delay. Circulation 1999;99:1567-1573.
18. Auricchio A, Stellbrink C, Block M, Sack S, Vogt J, Bakker P et al. Effect of pacing chamber and atrioventricular delay on acute systolic function of paced patients with congestive heart failure. The Pacing Therapies for Congestive Heart Failure Study Group. The Guidant Congestive Heart Failure Research Group. Circulation 1999;99: 2993-3001.
19. Nelson GS, Berger RD, Fetics BJ, Talbot M, Spinelli JC, Hare JM et al. Left ventricular or biventricular pacing improves cardiac function at diminished energy cost in patients with dilated cardiomyopathy and left bundle-branch block. Circulation 2000;102:3053-3059.
20. Agricola E, Oppizzi M, Galderisi M, Pisani M, Meris A, Pappone C et al. Role of regional mechanical dyssynchrony as a determinant of functional mitral regurgitation in patients with left ventricular systolic dysfunction. Heart 2006;92:1390-1395.
21. Breithardt OA, Sinha AM, Schwammenthal E, Bidaoui N, Markus KU, Franke A et al. Acute effects of cardiac resynchronization therapy on functional mitral regurgitation in advanced systolic heart failure. J Am Coll Cardiol 2003;41:765-770.
22. Kanzaki H, Bazaz R, Schwartzman D, Dohi K, Sade LE, Gorcsan J, III. A mechanism for immediate reduction in mitral regurgitation after cardiac resynchronization therapy: insights from mechanical activation strain mapping. J Am Coll Cardiol 2004;44:1619-1625.
23. Ypenburg C, Lancellotti P, Tops LF, Boersma E, Bleeker GB, Holman ER et al. Mechanism of improvement in mitral regurgitation after cardiac resynchronization therapy. Eur Heart J 2008;29:757-765.
24. Leclercq C, Walker S, Linde C, Clementy J, Marshall AJ, Ritter P et al. Comparative effects of permanent biventricular and right-univentricular pacing in heart failure patients with chronic atrial fibrillation. Eur Heart J 2002;23:1780-1787.
25. Auricchio A, Stellbrink C, Butter C, Sack S, Vogt J, Misier AR et al. Clinical efficacy of cardiac resynchronization therapy using left ventricular pacing in heart failure patients stratified by severity of ventricular conduction delay. J Am Coll Cardiol 2003;42:2109-2116.
26. Auricchio A, Stellbrink C, Sack S, Block M, Vogt J, Bakker P et al. Long-term clinical effect of hemodynamically optimized cardiac resynchronization therapy in patients with heart failure and ventricular conduction delay. J Am Coll Cardiol 2002;39:2026-2033.
27. Young JB, Abraham WT, Smith AL, Leon AR, Lieberman R, Wilkoff B et al. Combined cardiac resynchronization and implantable cardioversion defibrillation in advanced chronic heart failure: the MIRACLE ICD Trial. JAMA 2003;289:2685-2694.
28. Higgins SL, Hummel JD, Niazi IK, Giudici MC, Worley SJ, Saxon LA et al. Cardiac resynchronization therapy for the treatment of heart failure in patients with intraventricular conduction delay and malignant ventricular tachyarrhythmias. J Am Coll Cardiol 2003;42:1454-1459.
29. Abraham WT, Young JB, Leon AR, Adler S, Bank AJ, Hall SA et al. Effects of cardiac resynchronization on disease progression in patients with left ventricular systolic dysfunction, an indication for an implantable cardioverter-defibrillator, and mildly symptomatic chronic heart failure. Circulation 2004;110:2864-2868.
30. Cleland JG, Daubert JC, Erdmann E, Freemantle N, Gras D, Kappenberger L et al. Longer-term effects of cardiac resynchronization therapy on mortality in heart failure [the CArdiac REsynchronization-Heart Failure (CARE-HF) trial extension phase]. Eur Heart J 2006;27:1928-1932.
31. Kindermann M, Hennen B, Jung J, Geisel J, Bohm M, Frohlig G. Biventricular versus conventional right ventricular stimulation for patients with standard pacing indication and left ventricular dysfunction: the Homburg Biventricular Pacing Evaluation (HOBIPACE). J Am Coll Cardiol 2006;47:1927-1937.
32. Linde C, Abraham WT, Gold MR, John Sutton M, Ghio S, Daubert C. Randomized Trial of Cardiac Resynchronization in Mildly Symptomatic Heart Failure Patients and in Asymptomatic Patients

With Left Ventricular Dysfunction and Previous Heart Failure Symptoms. J Am Coll Cardiol 2008;52:1834-1843.

33. Moss AJ, Hall WJ, Cannom DS, Klein H, Brown MW, Daubert JP et al. Cardiac-resynchronization therapy for the prevention of heart-failure events. N Engl J Med 2009;361:1329-1338.
34. Ghio S, Freemantle N, Scelsi L, Serio A, Magrini G, Pasotti M et al. Long-term left ventricular reverse remodelling with cardiac resynchronization therapy: results from the CARE-HF trial. Eur J Heart Fail 2009;11:480-488.
35. Yu CM, Bleeker GB, Fung JW, Schalij MJ, Zhang Q, van der Wall EE et al. Left ventricular reverse remodeling but not clinical improvement predicts long-term survival after cardiac resynchronization therapy. Circulation 2005;112:1580-1586.
36. D'Ascia C, Cittadini A, Monti MG, Riccio G, Sacca L. Effects of biventricular pacing on interstitial remodelling, tumor necrosis factor-alpha expression, and apoptotic death in failing human myocardium. Eur Heart J 2006;27:201-206.
37. Vanderheyden M, Mullens W, Delrue L, Goethals M, De Bruyne B, Wijns W et al. Myocardial gene expression in heart failure patients treated with cardiac resynchronization therapy responders versus nonresponders. J Am Coll Cardiol 2008;51:129-136.
38. Mangiavacchi M, Gasparini M, Faletra F, Klersy C, Morenghi E, Galimberti P et al. Clinical predictors of marked improvement in left ventricular performance after cardiac resynchronization therapy in patients with chronic heart failure. Am Heart J 2006;151:477.
39. Ukkonen H, Beanlands RS, Burwash IG, de Kemp RA, Nahmias C, Fallen E et al. Effect of cardiac resynchronization on myocardial efficiency and regional oxidative metabolism. Circulation 2003;107: 28-31.
40. Nowak B, Sinha AM, Schaefer WM, Koch KC, Kaiser HJ, Hanrath P et al. Cardiac resynchronization therapy homogenizes myocardial glucose metabolism and perfusion in dilated cardiomyopathy and left bundle branch block. J Am Coll Cardiol 2003;41:1523-1528.
41. Knaapen P, van Campen LM, de Cock CC, Gotte MJ, Visser CA, Lammertsma AA et al. Effects of cardiac resynchronization therapy on myocardial perfusion reserve. Circulation 2004;110:646-651.
42. Lindner O, Sorensen J, Vogt J, Fricke E, Baller D, Horstkotte D et al. Cardiac efficiency and oxygen consumption measured with 11C-acetate PET after long-term cardiac resynchronization therapy. J Nucl Med 2006;47:378-383.
43. Duncan AM, Lim E, Clague J, Gibson DG, Henein MY. Comparison of segmental and global markers of dyssynchrony in predicting clinical response to cardiac resynchronization. Eur Heart J 2006;27:2426-2432.
44. St John Sutton MG, Plappert T, Abraham WT, Smith AL, DeLurgio DB, Leon AR et al. Effect of cardiac resynchronization therapy on left ventricular size and function in chronic heart failure. Circulation 2003;107:1985-1990.
45. Fruhwald FM, Fahrleitner-Pammer A, Berger R, Leyva F, Freemantle N, Erdmann E et al. Early and sustained effects of cardiac resynchronization therapy on N-terminal pro-B-type natriuretic peptide in patients with moderate to severe heart failure and cardiac dyssynchrony. Eur Heart J 2007;28:1592-1597.
46. Pitzalis MV, Iacoviello M, Di Serio F, Romito R, Guida P, De Tommasi E et al. Prognostic value of brain natriuretic peptide in the management of patients receiving cardiac resynchronization therapy. Eur J Heart Fail 2006;8:509-514.
47. Kubanek M, Malek I, Bytesnik J, Fridl P, Riedlbauchova L, Karasova L et al. Decrease in plasma B-type natriuretic peptide early after initiation of cardiac resynchronization therapy predicts clinical improvement at 12 months. Eur J Heart Fail 2006;8:832-840.
48. Boerrigter G, Costello-Boerrigter LC, Abraham WT, Sutton MG, Heublein DM, Kruger KM et al. Cardiac resynchronization therapy improves renal function in human heart failure with reduced glomerular filtration rate. J Card Fail 2008;14:539-546.
49. Grassi G, Vincenti A, Brambilla R, Trevano FQ, Dell'Oro R, Ciro A et al. Sustained sympathoinhibitory effects of cardiac resynchronization therapy in severe heart failure. Hypertension 2004;44:727-731.
50. Adamson PB, Kleckner KJ, VanHout WL, Srinivasan S, Abraham WT. Cardiac resynchronization therapy improves heart rate variability in patients with symptomatic heart failure. Circulation 2003;108:266-269.
51. Najem B, Unger P, Preumont N, Jansens JL, Houssiere A, Pathak A et al. Sympathetic control after cardiac resynchronization therapy: responders versus nonresponders. Am J Physiol Heart Circ Physiol 2006;291:H2647-H2652.
52. Gademan MG, van Bommel RJ, Borleffs CJ, Man S, Haest JC, Schalij MJ et al. Biventricular pacing-induced acute response in baroreflex sensitivity has predictive value for midterm response to cardiac resynchronization therapy. Am J Physiol Heart Circ Physiol 2009;297:H233-H237.
53. Luthje L, Renner B, Kessels R, Vollmann D, Raupach T, Gerritse B et al. Cardiac resynchronization therapy and atrial overdrive pacing for the treatment of central sleep apnoea. Eur J Heart Fail 2009;11:273-280.
54. Dickstein K, Cohen-Solal A, Filippatos G, McMurray JJ, Ponikowski P, Poole-Wilson PA et al. ESC Guidelines for the diagnosis and treatment of acute and chronic heart failure 2008: the Task Force for the Diagnosis and Treatment of Acute and Chronic Heart Failure 2008 of the European Society of Cardiology. Developed in collaboration with the Heart Failure Association of the ESC (HFA) and endorsed by the European Society of Intensive Care Medicine (ESICM). Eur Heart J 2008;29:2388-2442.
55. Epstein AE, DiMarco JP, Ellenbogen KA, Estes NA, III, Freedman RA, Gettes LS et al. ACC/AHA/HRS 2008 Guidelines for Device-Based Therapy of Cardiac Rhythm Abnormalities: a report of the American College of Cardiology/American Heart Association Task Force on Practice Guidelines (Writing Committee to Revise the ACC/AHA/NASPE 2002 Guideline Update for Implantation of Cardiac Pacemakers and Antiarrhythmia Devices): developed in collaboration with the American Association for Thoracic Surgery and Society of Thoracic Surgeons. Circulation 2008;117:e350-e408.
56. Barnett D, Phillips S, Longson C. Cardiac resynchronisation therapy for the treatment of heart failure: NICE technology appraisal guidance. Heart 2007;93:1134-1135.
57. Hawkins NM, Petrie MC, Burgess MI, McMurray JJ. Selecting patients for cardiac resynchronization therapy: the fallacy of echocardiographic dyssynchrony. J Am Coll Cardiol 2009;53:1944-1959.
58. Chung ES, Leon AR, Tavazzi L, Sun JP, Nihoyannopoulos P, Merlino J et al. Results of the Predictors of Response to CRT (PROSPECT) trial. Circulation 2008;117:2608-2616.
59. Sanderson JE. Echocardiography for cardiac resynchronization therapy selection: fatally flawed or misjudged? J Am Coll Cardiol 2009;53:1960-1964.
60. Richardson M, Freemantle N, Calvert MJ, Cleland JG, Tavazzi L. Predictors and treatment response with cardiac resynchronization therapy in patients with heart failure characterized by dyssynchrony: a pre-defined analysis from the CARE-HF trial. Eur Heart J 2007;28:1827-1834.
61. Toussaint JF, Lavergne T, Kerrou K, Froissart M, Ollitrault J, Darondel JM et al. Basal asynchrony and resynchronization with biventricular pacing predict long-term improvement of LV function in heart failure patients. Pacing Clin Electrophysiol 2003;26:1815-1823.
62. Westenberg JJ, Lamb HJ, van der Geest RJ, Bleeker GB, Holman ER, Schalij MJ et al. Assessment of left ventricular dyssynchrony in patients with conduction delay and idiopathic dilated cardiomyopathy: head-to-head comparison between tissue doppler imaging and velocity-encoded magnetic resonance imaging. J Am Coll Cardiol 2006;47:2042-2048.
63. Bleeker GB, Schalij MJ, Molhoek SG, Holman ER, Verwey HF, Steendijk P et al. Frequency of left ventricular dyssynchrony in patients with heart failure and a narrow QRS complex. Am J Cardiol 2005;95:140-142.
64. Beshai JF, Grimm RA, Nagueh SF, Baker JH, Beau SL, Greenberg SM et al. Cardiac-resynchronization therapy in heart failure with narrow QRS complexes. N Engl J Med 2007;357:2461-2471.
65. Turner MS, Bleasdale RA, Mumford CE, Frenneaux MP, Morris-Thurgood JA. Left ventricular pacing improves haemodynamic variables in patients with heart failure with a normal QRS duration. Heart 2004;90:502-505.

66. Williams LK, Ellery S, Patel K, Leyva F, Bleasdale RA, Phan TT et al. Short-term hemodynamic effects of cardiac resynchronization therapy in patients with heart failure, a narrow QRS duration, and no dyssynchrony. Circulation 2009;120:1687-1694.
67. Lindenfeld J, Feldman AM, Saxon L, Boehmer J, Carson P, Ghali JK et al. Effects of cardiac resynchronization therapy with or without a defibrillator on survival and hospitalizations in patients with New York Heart Association class IV heart failure. Circulation 2007;115:204-212.
68. Cowburn PJ, Patel H, Jolliffe RE, Wald RW, Parker JD. Cardiac resynchronization therapy: an option for inotrope-supported patients with end-stage heart failure? Eur J Heart Fail 2005;7:215-217.
69. Cleland JG, Freemantle N, Daubert JC, Toff WD, Leisch F, Tavazzi L. Long-term effect of cardiac resynchronisation in patients reporting mild symptoms of heart failure: a report from the CARE-HF study. Heart 2008;94:278-283.
70. Daubert C, Gold MR, Abraham WT, Ghio S, Hassager C, Goode G et al. Prevention of disease progression by cardiac resynchronization therapy in patients with asymptomatic or mildly symptomatic left ventricular dysfunction: insights from the European cohort of the REVERSE (Resynchronization Reverses Remodeling in Systolic Left Ventricular Dysfunction) trial. J Am Coll Cardiol 2009;54:1837-1846.
71. Doshi RN, Daoud EG, Fellows C, Turk K, Duran A, Hamdan MH et al. Left ventricular-based cardiac stimulation post AV nodal ablation evaluation (the PAVE study). J Cardiovasc Electrophysiol 2005;16:1160-1165.
72. Upadhyay GA, Choudhry NK, Auricchio A, Ruskin J, Singh JP. Cardiac resynchronization in patients with atrial fibrillation: a meta-analysis of prospective cohort studies. J Am Coll Cardiol 2008;52:1239-1246.
73. Gasparini M, Auricchio A, Metra M, Regoli F, Fantoni C, Lamp B et al. Long-term survival in patients undergoing cardiac resynchronization therapy: the importance of performing atrio-ventricular junction ablation in patients with permanent atrial fibrillation. Eur Heart J 2008;29:1644-1652.
74. Khadjooi K, Foley PW, Chalil S, Anthony J, Smith RE, Frenneaux MP et al. Long-term effects of cardiac resynchronisation therapy in patients with atrial fibrillation. Heart 2008;94:879-883.
75. Yu CM, Chan JY, Zhang Q, Omar R, Yip GW, Hussin A et al. Biventricular pacing in patients with bradycardia and normal ejection fraction. N Engl J Med 2009;361:2123-2134.
76. Shimano M, Tsuji Y, Yoshida Y, Inden Y, Tsuboi N, Itoh T et al. Acute and chronic effects of cardiac resynchronization in patients developing heart failure with long-term pacemaker therapy for acquired complete atrioventricular block. Europace 2007;9:869-74.
77. Foley PW, Muhyaldeen SA, Chalil S, Smith RE, Sanderson JE, Leyva F. Long-term effects of upgrading from right ventricular pacing to cardiac resynchronization therapy in patients with heart failure. Europace 2009;11:495-501.
78. Kron J, Aranda JM, Jr., Miles WM, Burkart TA, Woo GW, Saxonhouse SJ et al. Benefit of cardiac resynchronization in elderly patients: results from the Multicenter InSync Randomized Clinical Evaluation (MIRACLE) and Multicenter InSync ICD Randomized Clinical Evaluation (MIRACLE-ICD) trials. J Interv Card Electrophysiol 2009;25:91-96.
79. Foley PW, Chalil S, Khadjooi K, Smith RE, Frenneaux MP, Leyva F. Long-term effects of cardiac resynchronization therapy in octogenarians: a comparative study with a younger population. Europace 2008;10:1302-1307.
80. Alaeddini J, Wood MA, Amin MS, Ellenbogen KA. Gender disparity in the use of cardiac resynchronization therapy in the United States. Pacing Clin Electrophysiol 2008;31:468-472.
81. Dickstein K, Bogale N, Priori S, Auricchio A, Cleland JG, Gitt A et al. The European cardiac resynchronization therapy survey. Eur Heart J 2009;30:2450-2460.
82. Ghanbari H, Dalloul G, Hasan R, Daccarett M, Saba S, David S et al. Effectiveness of implantable cardioverter-defibrillators for the primary prevention of sudden cardiac death in women with advanced heart failure: a meta-analysis of randomized controlled trials. Arch Intern Med 2009;169:1500-1506.
83. Janousek J, Tomek V, Chaloupecky VA, Reich O, Gebauer RA, Kautzner J et al. Cardiac resynchronization therapy: a novel adjunct to the treatment and prevention of systemic right ventricular failure. i2004;44:1927-1931.
84. Kiesewetter C, Michael K, Morgan J, Veldtman GR. Left ventricular dysfunction after cardiac resynchronization therapy in congenital heart disease patients with a failing systemic right ventricle. Pacing Clin Electrophysiol 2008;31:159-162.
85. Leon AR, Abraham WT, Curtis AB, Daubert JP, Fisher WG, Gurley J et al. Safety of transvenous cardiac resynchronization system implantation in patients with chronic heart failure: combined results of over 2,000 patients from a multicenter study program. J Am Coll Cardiol 2005;46:2348-2356.
86. Cowburn PJ, Patel H, Pipes RR, Parker JD. Contrast nephropathy post cardiac resynchronization therapy: an under-recognized complication with important morbidity. Eur J Heart Fail 2005;7:899-903.
87. Butter C, Auricchio A, Stellbrink C, Fleck E, Ding J, Yu Y et al. Effect of resynchronization therapy stimulation site on the systolic function of heart failure patients. Circulation 2001;104:3026-3029.
88. Lambiase PD, Rinaldi A, Hauck J, Mobb M, Elliott D, Mohammad S et al. Non-contact left ventricular endocardial mapping in cardiac resynchronisation therapy. Heart 2004;90:44-51.
89. van Campen CM, Visser FC, de Cock CC, Vos HS, Kamp O, Visser CA. Comparison of the haemodynamics of different pacing sites in patients undergoing resynchronisation treatment: need for individualisation of lead localisation. Heart 2006;92:1795-1800.
90. Saxon LA, Olshansky B, Volosin K, Steinberg JS, Lee BK, Tomassoni G et al. Influence of left ventricular lead location on outcomes in the COMPANION study. J Cardiovasc Electrophysiol 2009;20:764-768.
91. Haghjoo M, Bonakdar HR, Jorat MV, Fazelifar AF, Alizadeh A, Ojaghi-Haghjghi Z et al. Effect of right ventricular lead location on response to cardiac resynchronization therapy in patients with end-stage heart failure. Europace 2009;11:356-363.
92. Buck S, Maass AH, Nieuwland W, Anthonio RL, Van Veldhuisen DJ, Van Gelder IC. Impact of interventricular lead distance and the decrease in septal-to-lateral delay on response to cardiac resynchronization therapy. Europace 2008;10:1313-1319.
93. Stanton T, Hawkins NM, Hogg KJ, Goodfield NE, Petrie MC, McMurray JJ. How should we optimize cardiac resynchronization therapy? Eur Heart J 2008;29:2458-2472.
94. Sawhney NS, Waggoner AD, Garhwal S, Chawla MK, Osborn J, Faddis MN. Randomized prospective trial of atrioventricular delay programming for cardiac resynchronization therapy. Heart Rhythm 2004;1:562-567.
95. Whinnett ZI, Davies JE, Willson K, Manisty CH, Chow AW, Foale RA et al. Haemodynamic effects of changes in atrioventricular and interventricular delay in cardiac resynchronisation therapy show a consistent pattern: analysis of shape, magnitude and relative importance of atrioventricular and interventricular delay. Heart 2006;92:1628-1634.
96. Scharf C, Li P, Muntwyler J, Chugh A, Oral H, Pelosi F et al. Rate-dependent AV delay optimization in cardiac resynchronization therapy. Pacing Clin Electrophysiol.2005;28:279-284.
97. Kurzidim K, Reinke H, Sperzel J, Schneider HJ, Danilovic D, Siemon G et al. Invasive optimization of cardiac resynchronization therapy: role of sequential biventricular and left ventricular pacing. Pacing Clin Electrophysiol 2005;28:754-761.
98. Sogaard P, Egeblad H, Pedersen AK, Kim WY, Kristensen BO, Hansen PS et al. Sequential versus simultaneous biventricular resynchronization for severe heart failure: evaluation by tissue Doppler imaging. Circulation 2002;106:2078-2084.
99. Boriani G, Biffi M, Muller CP, Seidl KH, Grove R, Vogt J et al. A prospective randomized evaluation of VV delay optimization in CRT-D recipients: echocardiographic observations from the RHYTHM II ICD study. Pacing Clin Electrophysiol 2009;32 **Suppl 1**:S120-S125.

100. Mullens W, Verga T, Grimm RA, Starling RC, Wilkoff BL, Tang WH. Persistent hemodynamic benefits of cardiac resynchronization therapy with disease progression in advanced heart failure. J Am Coll Cardiol 2009;53:600-607.
101. Bleeker GB, Kaandorp TA, Lamb HJ, Boersma E, Steendijk P, de Roos A et al. Effect of posterolateral scar tissue on clinical and echocardiographic improvement after cardiac resynchronization therapy. Circulation 2006;113:969-976.
102. van Bommel RJ, Bax JJ, Abraham WT, Chung ES, Pires LA, Tavazzi L et al. Characteristics of heart failure patients associated with good and poor response to cardiac resynchronization therapy: a PROSPECT (Predictors of Response to CRT) sub-analysis. Eur Heart J 2009;30:2470-2477.
103. Tournoux FB, Alabiad C, Fan D, Chen AA, Chaput M, Heist EK et al. Echocardiographic measures of acute haemodynamic response after cardiac resynchronization therapy predict long-term clinical outcome. Eur Heart J 2007;28:1143-1148.
104. Tanaka Y, Tada H, Yamashita E, Sato C, Irie T, Hori Y et al. Change in blood pressure just after initiation of cardiac resynchronization therapy predicts long-term clinical outcome in patients with advanced heart failure. Circ J 2009;73:288-294.
105. Mullens W, Grimm RA, Verga T, Dresing T, Starling RC, Wilkoff BL et al. Insights from a cardiac resynchronization optimization clinic as part of a heart failure disease management program. J Am Coll Cardiol 2009;53:765-773.
106. Yao G, Freemantle N, Calvert MJ, Bryan S, Daubert JC, Cleland JG. The long-term cost-effectiveness of cardiac resynchronization therapy with or without an implantable cardioverter-defibrillator. Eur Heart J 2007;28:42-51.
107. Goldenberg I, Vyas AK, Hall WJ, Moss AJ, Wang H, He H et al. Risk stratification for primary implantation of a cardioverter-defibrillator in patients with ischemic left ventricular dysfunction. J Am Coll Cardiol 2008;51:288-296.
108. Maisel WH. Pacemaker and ICD generator reliability: meta-analysis of device registries. JAMA 2006;295:1929-1934.
109. Stevenson LW, Desai AS. Selecting patients for discussion of the ICD as primary prevention for sudden death in heart failure. J Card Fail 2006;12:407-412.
110. Adamson PB, Smith AL, Abraham WT, Kleckner KJ, Stadler RW, Shih A et al. Continuous autonomic assessment in patients with symptomatic heart failure: prognostic value of heart rate variability measured by an implanted cardiac resynchronization device. Circulation 2004;110:2389-2394.
111. Yu CM, Wang L, Chau E, Chan RH, Kong SL, Tang MO et al. Intrathoracic impedance monitoring in patients with heart failure: correlation with fluid status and feasibility of early warning preceding hospitalization. Circulation 2005;112:841-848.

PART XV

Surgical therapy for heart failure

49

Heart transplantation

Nicholas R. Banner, Andre R. Simon, and Margaret M. Burke

Clinical organ transplantation began in the mid-20th century, initially with renal transplants. Surgical techniques for heart transplantation began to be developed during the same period particularly by Cass and Brock in the United Kingdom, and Lower and Shumway in the United States.[1–3] The drugs then available for prophylaxis against rejection were limited to corticosteroids and azathioprine.[4] The first human heart transplant was performed in 1967;[5] the story of the pioneers in this field has been told elsewhere.[6]

The initial results of clinical heart transplantation were disappointing because of relatively ineffective pharmacological immunosuppression, lack of effective monitoring for acute rejection, and lack of therapeutic options for complications including infection and cardiac allograft vasculopathy.[7] The results of organ transplantation improved dramatically following the introduction of ciclosporin as an immunosuppressive agent, first for kidney transplantation and subsequently for the heart and other organs.[8,9]

A number of techniques have been used for heart transplantation. In most cases the recipient's diseased heart is replaced by the donor heart which is inserted in the normal anatomical (orthotopic) position; the anastomoses between donor and recipient great arteries are made end to end. There are, however, several techniques for making the venous or atrial anastomoses. The initial method used by Cass, Brock, Lower, and Shumway was to anastomose the donor atria to the remaining rostral portions of the recipient's atria by creating two atrial anastomoses. The choice of this technique reflected the limitations of surgical materials at that time. Although a 'biatrial' orthotopic transplant performed in that way requires only four vascular anastomoses, the atrial anastomoses are long and can occasionally be subject to technical problems including the creation of a defect between the composite left and right atria; furthermore, there are many points where bleeding can potentially occur. The physiology of the resulting composite atria is abnormal with increased atrial size and wall tension and the technique is associated with an increased incidence of functional tricuspid regurgitation, atrial arrhythmia, and a risk of sinus node injury at the time of implantation).[3] Since the sinus node of the recipient heart remains, two P-waves (donor and recipient) may be visible on the surface ECG.[10]

Subsequently a technique for 'total' orthotopic heart transplantation with separate anastomoses for the superior and inferior vena cavae (SVC and IVC) and the left and right pairs of pulmonary veins was introduced by Yacoub and colleagues, followed by Dreyfus.[11–13] This technique produces the most physiological function of left and right atria but requires a total of six anastomoses, prolongs the surgery, and increases the risk of technical complications. Subsequently a hybrid 'bicaval' technique was introduced by Sievers and colleagues, followed by Sarsam and the Wythenshawe group, whereby a composite left atrial chamber is created as in the 'biatrial' technique, while the right atrium is left intact and separate SVC and IVC anastomoses are fashioned as in the 'total' technique.[14,15] Although this technique increases the complexity of the operation and the overall surgical time, it does not cause an important increase in the ischaemia time for the allograft.[3] There has never been an adequately powered surgical trial to compare these various techniques, but a meta-analysis of the studies available indicates that there are functional advantages from this 'bicaval' technique with improved postoperative haemodynamics (less tricuspid regurgitation, lower right atrial pressure, increased chance of sinus rhythm, and reduced need for pacing).[3] Analysis of the UNOS database indicates that this technique has gradually become the most prevalent in clinical practice and is associated with a low incidence of pacemaker insertion and shortened length of hospital stay while failing to show any improvement in patient survival.[16]

Another form of heart transplantation has been used clinically: the heterotopic heart transplant. In this operation the donor heart is implanted in the right side of the chest and anastomosed to work in parallel with the recipient's own heart. Depending on the pattern of right-sided anastomoses, the heterotopic heart can either function as a left ventricular assist with the donor and recipient left ventricles working in parallel, or a biventricular assist with both left and right ventricles working in parallel. The development of heterotopic transplantation occurred in an era where recipient heart function was probably less impaired than in the current era and when immunosuppression and monitoring for rejection were less effective than they are today. In these circumstances, the recipient's own heart could provide valuable 'back-up' function during episodes of cardiac rejection. With improved prophylaxis and treatment of rejection, this advantage has become significantly less important. The limitations of heterotopic transplantation include more complex surgery and follow-up (e.g. echocardiography and endomyocardial biopsy) coupled with the propensity for late complications from the native heart (e.g. arrhythmia, angina, and systemic embolization). Heterotopic transplantation is associated with lower survival rates and has been used infrequently in recent years.[17]

Heart transplantation was introduced as a treatment for heart failure (HF) at a time when the other therapeutic options were very limited (diuretics and digoxin). In subsequent decades considerable progress has been made in the therapy of chronic HF based principally on the paradigm of neurohormonal antagonism (ACE inhibitors, β-blockers, aldosterone antagonists, and angiotensin receptor blockers) coupled with the use of implantable defibrillators to prevent sudden arrhythmic death and, for selected patients, cardiac resynchronization therapy.[18] In the same time period, immunosuppression and management after heart transplantation have also improved. Heart transplantation has never been tested against medical therapy in a randomized clinical trial. However, the very low medium-term mortality rates after heart transplantation, compared with medical therapy for HF, coupled with the results of studies using statistical modelling, indicate that heart transplantation can provide a long-term benefit for many patients with advanced HF.[19] Far less progress has been made with the medical management of acute HF, and many of the therapies used provide marginal or only temporary benefit to such patients.[20] An increasing proportion of heart transplant operations are being performed on an urgent basis in patients with decompensated HF who have become inotrope dependent.[21] In this group, provided candidates are selected appropriately, heart transplantation is highly efficacious and provides an early survival benefit.[19] However, the scarcity of donor hearts that are suitable for transplantation has prolonged waiting times significantly. This development, coupled with advances in technology, has led to an increased use of ventricular assist devices to maintain patients before heart transplantation ('bridge to transplantation')[22] and now as an alternative therapy for patients who are ineligible for transplantation.[23]

Recipient selection

The International Society for Heart and Lung Transplantation has published guidelines for the care of patients prior to transplantation and case selection.[18,24,25]

For patients with chronic stable HF the decision about transplantation should be made after optimizing medical therapy including the maximum possible use of neurohormonal antagonists and electrical device therapy.[26] The aetiology of the HF should be determined and any alternative treatments (such as high-risk myocardial revascularization when there is evidence of substantial myocardial viability and hibernation) should be considered.[27] Ambulatory HF patients who are on optimal medical therapy can be risk-stratified using the cardiopulmonary exercise test as well as scoring systems such as the HF survival score.[28,29]

Patients with refractory decompensated HF who have become truly inotrope dependent have a dismal prognosis with ongoing medical therapy, and should be considered as candidates for urgent transplantation or mechanical circulatory support.[20]

In all potential candidates, the presence of comorbidity, risk factors, and contraindications to transplantation should be determined. Contraindications may be absolute (e.g. an active malignancy that limits the patient's prognosis and would be exacerbated by pharmacological immunosuppression) or relative (e.g. renal or other organ dysfunction). Many of the risk factors for heart transplantation, such as renal dysfunction and pulmonary hypertension, are usually complications of the HF and directly related to its severity and duration. The dilemma of whether to attempt to transplant such patients has been reduced by the availability of mechanical circulatory support as an alternative strategy to improve the patient's health and make them a more suitable heart transplant candidate in the future.[22]

Treatment of concomitant medical conditions such as cholelithiasis and peptic ulcer disease can reduce the risks at the time of transplant surgery. Preoperative vaccination can be used to reduce the risk of some post-transplant infections, e.g. influenza, pneumococcal pneumonia, chickenpox, and hepatitis B.

Pulmonary hypertension secondary to left HF is an important problem because of the risk of donor right ventricular failure after the transplant procedure. Its prevalence is increasing because of improved survival in chronic HF patients with medical therapy. Right heart catheterization should be used to distinguish passive from reactive pulmonary hypertension with a truly increased resistance to blood flow within the pulmonary circulation. In the case of reactive pulmonary hypertension, the traditional approach has been to use pharmacological testing to assess its reversibility;[24,30,31] however, the reproducibility and predictive value of such tests is moderate at best. In the most recent era, patients with severe pulmonary hypertension have been rendered more suitable for heart transplantation by bridging them with a mechanical left ventricular assist device (LVAD).[32] Device support provides a long-term reduction in left atrial pressure leading to a favourable remodelling in the pulmonary circulation and a regression of reactive pulmonary hypertension.

Mechanical circulatory support prior to transplantation

In the current era, many patients are referred at a very advanced stage of their disease with secondary organ dysfunction, particularly renal failure, chronic congestive hepatopathy, and pulmonary hypertension. In principle, mechanical circulatory support can improve the haemodynamic state of patients with refractory decompensated HF and so make them suitable for transplantation, but this increases the risk of surgery significantly and so referral should be made at an earlier stage whenever possible.

Since HF is a progressive condition, the scarcity of hearts suitable for transplantation and the consequent increase in waiting times has led to many patients deteriorating during the waiting period. Although some can be stabilized with intravenous support until a suitable heart becomes available under an urgent allocation scheme, others need mechanical circulatory support.

Although inotropes may help to produce a short-term improvement in the patient's haemodynamic state and organ function, their efficacy is often limited by the severity of the patient's myocardial dysfunction. In addition, the longer-term use of inotropes has been shown to have a detrimental effect on outcome and so, for the patient who is suitable for surgical therapy, their role should be a temporary one before early transplantation or the implantation of a mechanical circulatory support device.[33]

Historically, the intra-aortic balloon pump has had an important role in maintaining patients prior to transplantation. However, the degree of circulatory support provided is limited and, with increased waiting times, this form of treatment has become increasingly impractical. Therefore, like inotropic therapy, its use is limited to short-term stabilization of the patient and providing an opportunity for more definitive therapy.[34]

Mechanical circulatory support with a LVAD has now become a standard therapy to stabilize and then maintain patients until transplantation becomes possible.[22] Circulatory support can allow physiological recovery of other organ systems, and with modern implantable devices the patient can be rehabilitated and achieve an improved functional status prior to transplant. However, the advantages of this strategy have to be weighed against the increased complexity of the subsequent transplant surgery.

The technology has evolved considerably over the last few decades, with devices progressing from large, external, pneumatically driven, pulsatile pumps to smaller, implantable, electrically driven devices.[35] Currently, the most commonly used devices are the Thoratec HeartMate II (a second-generation device) and the HeartWare HVAD (a third-generation device). These can both provide full left ventricular support and can achieve high systemic flows. Because of their small size, they are easier to implant than first-generation pulsatile devices and are associated with a reduced risk of surgical complications. Their chief limitation is that they provide univentricular support and that this may be inadequate for patients with decompensated HF and very poor right ventricular function. Such patients may also require the use of a right ventricular assist device.[36] An alternative would be to use a total artificial heart that can provide biventricular support and total cardiac replacement.[37] However, this necessitates extensive surgery and the patient becomes totally dependent on the device; the midterm results are far from encouraging (which is problematic when the transplant waiting time is long, as in the United Kingdom).

Patients with implantable second- or third-generation devices can be fully rehabilitated and discharged from hospital. Once they have rehabilitated and achieved a satisfactory nutritional status and organ function, they should be reassessed and listed for transplantation. Time-dependent complications which occur in patients supported with a LVAD include device-related infection, bleeding (particularly gastrointestinal and cerebral), and thromboembolic events.[23] The incidence of device malfunction is much less than it used to be, but accidents causing trauma to the external driveline and operator error are being seen more frequently with long-term support. For all these reasons, it is important that patients who are potentially eligible for transplantation should be listed as soon as possible. Unfortunately some patients develop problems that make it more difficult to transplant them after device implantation (typically HLA sensitization) or that become contraindications to transplantation (e.g. a stroke with substantial neurological deficit).

Surgical planning

Transplantation is a complex process, and detailed plans should be made at the time of listing. Patients who have undergone previous cardiac surgery, particularly, those who have received a LVAD, should undergo CT scanning coupled with a review of the previous surgical records to establish the necessary approach. Preparation of the femoral vessels can facilitate urgent cardiopulmonary bypass if needed during surgical opening of patients already on mechanical support. The exact position of the VAD outflow graft should be known to avoid the risk of catastrophic haemorrhage during opening. Some recipients have particular tissue requirements and a modified operative technique may be needed for those with adult congenital heart disease (ACHD), particularly if there is an abnormal atrial situs.[12,38] Excellent coordination is required to minimize the organ ischaemia time during transplantation. Patients with VADs are sometimes planned to undergo anaesthesia prior to the explant of the donor heart by the retrieval team so as to allow surgery to commence immediately thereafter; this can increase the time for opening and mobilization of the VAD and recipient heart while the donor heart is in transit. The risk of this approach is minimal for patients who are stable on circulatory support.

Donor selection and management

The function of the donor heart may be affected by pre-existing cardiovascular disease in the donor (the majority of donors currently available in the United Kingdom have died from spontaneous intracranial haemorrhage), the management that the donor receives in the intensive care unit, and the impact of myocardial ischaemia during cold storage and transport to the implanting centre.[39]

Brainstem death produces a transient massive increase in sympathetic activity during the period of brainstem ischaemia that often leads to severe hypertension (Cushing's reflex) and catecholamine-mediated injury to the myocardium. Following this there is a progressive loss of homeostatic function including sympathetic tone, neurohormonal regulation, and temperature control. All this contributes to diminished myocardial function and cardiovascular instability. Inadequacies in donor management during this period can exacerbate the situation, e.g. insufficient or excessive volume resuscitation or the excessive use of inotropes and vasopressor agents. Active management of the donor from the time of the diagnosis of brainstem death by either an outreach team from the transplant centre or a separately constituted organ procurement organization helps to increase the yield of usable hearts.[40]

Assessment of the donor heart is based on clinical examination, ECG, and echocardiography coupled with haemodynamic studies using a pulmonary artery flotation catheter (PAFC) and, finally, by direct surgical inspection at the time of organ retrieval coupled with direct haemodynamic measurements. Coronary angiography can be useful for the evaluation of coronary artery disease in older donors but is often not logistically possible in community hospitals.

The ECG can be used to rapidly screen for major abnormalities such as Q waves indicating prior myocardial infarction or signs of left ventricular hypertrophy. Repolarization changes are common after brain death and do not in themselves preclude organ donation. Transthoracic or transoesophageal echocardiography can be used to screen for structural lesions, including valvular heart disease, and to assess ventricular function.[41] Ventricular performance is influenced by the loading conditions (systemic vascular resistance is often low after brainstem death and filling pressures are frequently abnormal). All these factors can be assessed using a PAFC and the results used to direct subsequent therapy. It has been found that left ventricular dysfunction is often reversible after a period of donor resuscitation, so donor hearts should not be declined on the basis of a single echocardiogram showing a low ejection fraction.[41,42]

The Crystal City Conference recommended a four-stage approach to donor assessment and management.[40] In the first phase the patient's volume status and any anaemia should be corrected together with any hypoxaemia or acidosis. Inotropes should be adjusted according to the haemodynamic measurements and whenever possible weaned while maintaining a mean arterial pressure of more than 60 mmHg. Care should be taken to avoid hypothermia. In the second stage an echo should be performed to exclude structural abnormalities and significant left ventricular hypertrophy. If left ventricular function appears adequate (LVEF >45%) organ retrieval may proceed at this stage. In the third phase, if the ejection fraction is inadequate, a hormonal resuscitation package of tri-iodothyronine, arginine vasopressin, and methylprednisolone should be administered together with insulin to control the patient's blood glucose. In this circumstance, a PAFC should be placed to determine the donor's haemodynamic status and assess the suitability of the heart following a period of resuscitation. The evidence for this approach is largely observational and there have been few clinical trials of donor management. This limitation was emphasized by a recent study which found no benefit from hormonal resuscitation as advocated in the Crystal City guidelines.[43] Much of the benefit from the systematic approach to donor management probably lies in the use of objective data, attention to detail, and assessment of serial changes in cardiac function. The final assessment and decision about the donor heart suitability for transplantation is made at the time of retrieval by the surgeon. Transoesophageal echocardiography at this stage can provide a final assessment of ventricular function and the presence or absence of any ventricular hypertrophy. The surgeon should also palpate the coronary arteries. In view of the subjective nature of this assessment process, the experience of the retrieving surgeon is of critical importance.

Donor–recipient matching

The system for donor organ allocation varies between countries. Organs can either be allocated using a 'patient orientated' system where priority is given to patients according to their clinical status within a geographical zone, or a 'centre orientated' system where organs are allocated to individual transplant centres who then use them according to priority. The current system in the United Kingdom is hybrid, where patients can be registered on the national urgent heart allocation scheme provided they meet specific criteria, and there is centre-based allocation of hearts not required for the urgent scheme. Donor–recipient matching requires ABO blood group compatibility, size matching, and a negative virtual or actual HLA cross match in those with preformed antibodies.[44]

Organ retrieval and myocardial protection

The donor operation is usually performed as part of a multiorgan retrieval procedure. At the start of the retrieval, blood flow into the right ventricle is restricted by ligation of the superior caval vein. The inferior caval vein is then opened and the donor heart is vented, to prevent distension, either through an incision into the left atrial appendage or into the left atrium between the inferior pulmonary veins. At this point, the ascending aorta is cross-clamped and cold cardioplegia solution is administered via the aortic root to achieve hypothermic diastolic arrest. A number of solutions are in clinical use and the ideal composition of the cardioplegia and storage solution has not been established.[45,46] The heart is then quickly excised with adequate lengths of aorta, pulmonary artery, venae cavae, and the left atrium intact. Cold storage at 4–8°C is used to transport the heart to the transplant centre. Although most hearts tolerate ischaemia at this temperature for several hours, postoperative cardiac dysfunction and the risk of primary graft failure remain significant problems.[47] The risk associated with the use of hearts from older donors is increased when the organ ischaemia time is prolonged and so care should be taken to minimize the ischaemia time when using a marginal organ donor.[48,49]

Alternative methods for protecting the myocardium have been explored. There has been particular interest in the possibility of transporting hearts in a warm perfused state using an organ care system. Preliminary results have been reported, but a definitive clinical trial has not yet been performed.

Recipient operation (bicaval technique)

A routine orthotopic heart transplant in a patient with nonischaemic dilated cardiomyopathy and no previous cardiac surgery is a routine procedure that has historically been used for training of future surgeons. At the other end of the spectrum, transplants in patients who have undergone multiple previous operations, have abnormal anatomy because of ACHD, or who have had a prior VAD, can be technically challenging. In such cases the donor and recipient surgery needs to be carefully coordinated to allow adequate time for dissection of the recipient heart and haemostasis prior to the arrival of the donor heart, thereby minimizing the organ ischaemia time.

The operation is performed using full cardiopulmonary bypass and most surgeons use a modest degree of hypothermia. Recipient cardiectomy is performed by division of the atria adjacent to the atrioventricular groove and division of the great arteries just distal to the sinotubular junction. This allows the recipient heart to yield homograft valves for other patients. In the bicaval technique, the recipient right atrium is then resected by separating it from the SVC and IVC and from the remnant of the recipient left atrium. The left atrium is then trimmed leaving the posterior wall and surrounding tissue as a bridge between the recipient's four pulmonary veins.[3]

The donor heart is inspected for any damage that may have been sustained during the retrieval process and for the presence of a persistent foramen ovale which, if present, should be closed to eliminate the risk of right-to-left shunting if right ventricular dysfunction should complicate the postoperative course. The donor left atrium is trimmed to remove the pulmonary venous ostia and the posterior wall that lies between them creating a defect that can be anastomosed to the corresponding tissue in the recipient (Figure 49.1). The left atrial anastomosis is performed first and requires particular attention because it will be relatively inaccessible at the end of the procedure. The donor and recipient pulmonary arteries are then trimmed to an appropriate length to avoid kinking or torsion as they are anastomosed end to end. The donor and recipient aortas are then similarly trimmed and anastomosed. At this point, the aortic cross-clamp may be released to re-establish coronary perfusion and minimize the total ischaemia time. The rest of the operation is then performed in a decompressed heart under supportive cardiopulmonary bypass. Suction is used to clear the myocardial venous return to the coronary sinus and right atrium. When the total anticipated ischaemia time is short, some surgeons prefer to complete the SVC and IVC anastomoses before releasing the aortic cross-clamp.

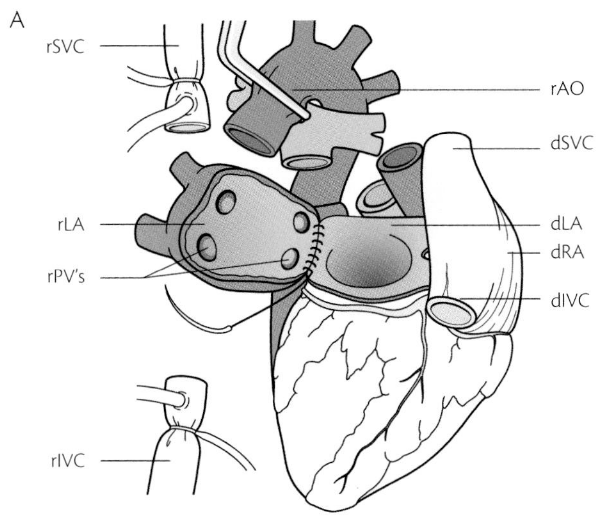

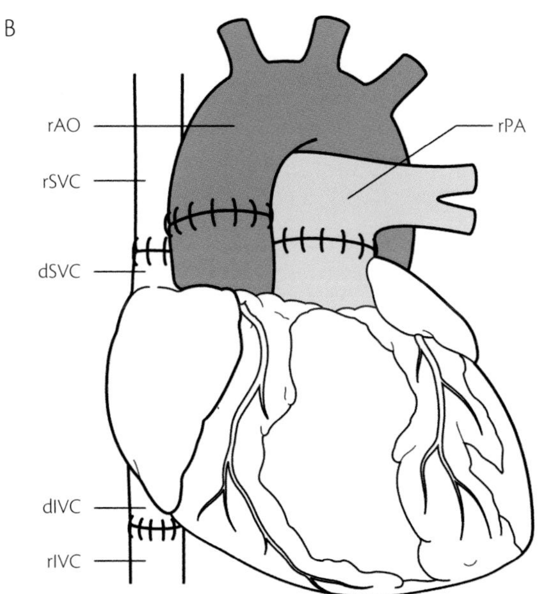

Fig. 49.1 Orthotopic heart transplantation using the bicaval technique. See text for details. AO, aorta; d, donor; IVC, inferior vena cava; LA, left atrium, PA, pulmonary artery; PVs, pulmonary veins; r, recipient; RA, right atrium; SVC superior vena cava.

During the implant procedure, prior to the release of the aortic cross-clamp, many surgeons use repeated infusions of (usually blood-based) cardioplegia to protect the donor heart. Topical cooling with cold saline is also used to protect the myocardium while avoiding slush that may cause freezing injury.

The postischaemic heart is normally kept on supportive cardiopulmonary bypass for a period of up to an hour, keeping the heart 'empty' to minimize myocardial work but maintaining coronary and systemic organ perfusion. The majority of hearts spontaneously return to sinus rhythm following release of the aortic cross-clamp and restoration of coronary perfusion. However, some require internal cardioversion from ventricular fibrillation. Transient atrioventricular block is common but usually resolves within the first few hours. Initial sinus node dysfunction is also common and ultimately requires the implantation of a permanent pacemaker in less than 5% of recipients.

Bleeding can be a particular concern in patients undergoing redo surgery or transplantation following bridging with an LVAD. Provided the patient remains haemodynamically stable, as much dissection as possible should be done before the institution of cardiopulmonary bypass. Early reversal of anticoagulation and the monitoring of haemostatic function with a thromboelastogram can be of assistance in the management of such patients. Platelet transfusion may be required, especially in those who have been receiving dual antiplatelet drug therapy, but the use of blood products appears to be associated with a higher risk of right HF. Care must be taken to avoid technical complications with the anastomoses; the most likely problems are kinking or torsion at the pulmonary anastomosis which can contribute to postoperative right ventricular dysfunction or stenosis at either the SVC of IVC anastomosis. Careful inspection and checking to exclude any significant pressure gradients is important at the end of the procedure. If bleeding should occur from the left atrial anastomosis the patient should be put back onto cardiopulmonary bypass to avoid haemodynamic instability while the suture line is explored, because the postischaemic transplanted heart is particularly vulnerable to any further haemodynamic insult.

Thorough de-airing is essential at the end of the procedure. The use of ice-cold saline for cooling during the procedure reduces the dead space and many surgeons flood the operative field with carbon dioxide to reduce air accumulation. A thorough de-airing drill must be used including the use of mechanical ventilation while restarting circulation through the lungs and venting, either through the left atrium or the left ventricular apex with the patient in a head-down position. Continuous suction from the ascending aorta should be used to protect the coronary and cerebral circulation. A transoesophageal echocardiogram provides additional information about the effectiveness of the de-airing process.

The immediate post-bypass period is of critical importance. It is often at this stage that problems related to donor right ventricular failure become apparent. Pulmonary vascular resistance should be managed with inhaled and systemic vasodilator therapy. Inhaled nitric oxide may be used prophylactically in patients with a known elevation of pulmonary vascular resistance and should be initiated early where there is any sign of right ventricular distension or dysfunction. Once the patient has been separated from cardiopulmonary bypass, a PAFC should be inserted to allow continuous monitoring of cardiac output and pulmonary artery pressures. Some surgeons also use a left atrial line to allow direct monitoring of left-sided filling pressures.[35] Sinus bradycardia and sinus arrest are common at this stage and surgical pacing wires must be placed on the atrium and ventricle. Failure to achieve satisfactory haemodynamics with adequate cardiac output and acceptable filling pressures, without the use of excessive inotropic support, should prompt a complete diagnostic reassessment to exclude technical problems. If necessary, short-term support with temporary ventricular assist devices or venoarterial extracorporeal membrane oxygenation (ECMO) should be considered to reduce myocardial work and maintain coronary perfusion whilst also providing adequate systemic perfusion to avoid a slide into multisystem organ failure.[50,51]

Postoperative care

When the transplanted heart is performing well the patient can be returned to the intensive care unit with only low doses of inotropes being administered. Some centres support the heart rate pharmacologically with an infusion of isoproterenol (isoprenaline), whereas others prefer to use atrial pacing. In the early period, the postischaemic ventricles often have reduced compliance producing a limitation in stroke volume. Therefore, the best cardiac output can usually be achieved at relatively fast heart rate (typically 90–110 beats/min). The overall management plan is similar to that used for patients after coronary bypass surgery, although there are the additional concerns of pharmacological immunosuppression and prophylaxis against infections.

The complications that may occur in the early postoperative period are summarized in Box 49.1 and their differential diagnosis and management have been reviewed in detail elsewhere.[35] Prompt intervention is required to resolve haemodynamic problems and avoid additional injury to the postischaemic cardiac allograft from coronary hypoperfusion, unnecessary right ventricular distension (as a result of volume overload), or the excessive use of inotropes. Such events can exacerbate cardiac dysfunction and trigger a spiral of haemodynamic decline.

For the uncomplicated cardiac transplant, extubation is usually possible following the weaning of nitrous oxide on day 1 or 2, inotropes are slowly weaned during the first postoperative week, and mediastinal and pericardial drains are removed once drainage has ceased, typically on the third or fourth postoperative day. Atrial pacing is usually weaned once inotropic support has stopped, with care to ensure that there is an adequate underlying sinus rate. Minor secondary surgical procedures may be required at this stage, such as the removal of a pacemaker generator or defibrillator that had been used to support the native heart before transplantation, together with any remnant leads. However, this should be done at the time of the transplant whenever possible. The relatively large first-generation pulsatile LVADs (e.g. the HeartMate I) were often disconnected from the recipient heart at the time of transplantation but left *in situ* for several days until the patient had became haemodynamically stable and any coagulopathy had resolved. However, the smaller second- and third-generation devices are removed during the operation.

Box 49.1 Postoperative cardiac and circulatory problems that may occur after orthotopic heart transplantation

- Haemorrhage
  - Surgical
  - Coagulopathic
- Other hypovolaemia
- Pericardial effusion
  - Potential space after resection of enlarged native heart
  - Inflammatory response after surgery
  - Bleeding into pericardial space
  - Complication of rejection (uncommon)
  - Drug complication (sirolimus)
  - Rarely infection (mediastinitis)
- Cardiac tamponade
- Acute right ventricular failure
  - Recipient pulmonary hypertension
  - Primary graft failure
- Acute biventricular failure
  - Primary graft failure
  - Hyperacute rejection
  - Accelerated acute rejection
- Technical anastomotic complications
  - Pulmonary artery (stenosis, torsion)
  - Superior caval vein (stenosis)
  - Inferior caval vein (stenosis)
- Systemic inflammatory response
  - Pre-existing infection (e.g. VAD complication)
  - Prolonged cardiopulmonary bypass
  - As a complication of primary graft failure
  - Pseudosepsis (milrinone accumulation in renal failure)
- Brady- and tachyarrhythmia
  - Sinus node dysfunction
  - Atrioventricular block
  - Atrial arrhythmia, especially atrial flutter
- Acute renal injury
- Hypoalbuminaemia from postoperative catabolism with oedema and effusions

Allograft rejection

Rejection is clinically categorized according to its temporal occurrence (hyperacute, acute, and chronic) and by the underlying mechanism (cellular, antibody-mediated, and mixed). In the nonsensitized patient, cellular rejection is the most common form of acute rejection. The immunological response is initiated and driven by the helper T cell and most of the immunosuppressive drugs in current use act at various stages in the T cell activation cascade (Fig. 49.2).

Antibody-mediated rejection may cause several clinical syndromes. Sensitized patients with preformed donor-specific HLA antibody may be subject to hyperacute rejection which develops in the first few minutes to hours after the operation, and this can be aggressive or even catastrophic in nature. It can be avoided by performing a direct or virtual crossmatch prior to transplantation and avoiding donor–recipient pairs where there is donor-specific antibody in the recipient.[44] ABO-incompatible transplantation can also cause hyperacute rejection in adult patients and should be avoided. Patients with low levels of anti-donor HLA antibody may escape hyperacute rejection but then suffer early accelerated acute rejection in the first few days and weeks after the transplant due to an anamnestic antibody response. Some other patients develop *de novo* HLA donor-specific antibody months or years after the transplant. Many of these cases remain asymptomatic, although the presence of donor-specific antibodies is a risk factor for late allograft failure.[52,53] In other cases, however, acute antibody-mediated rejection with allograft dysfunction may occur.[54]

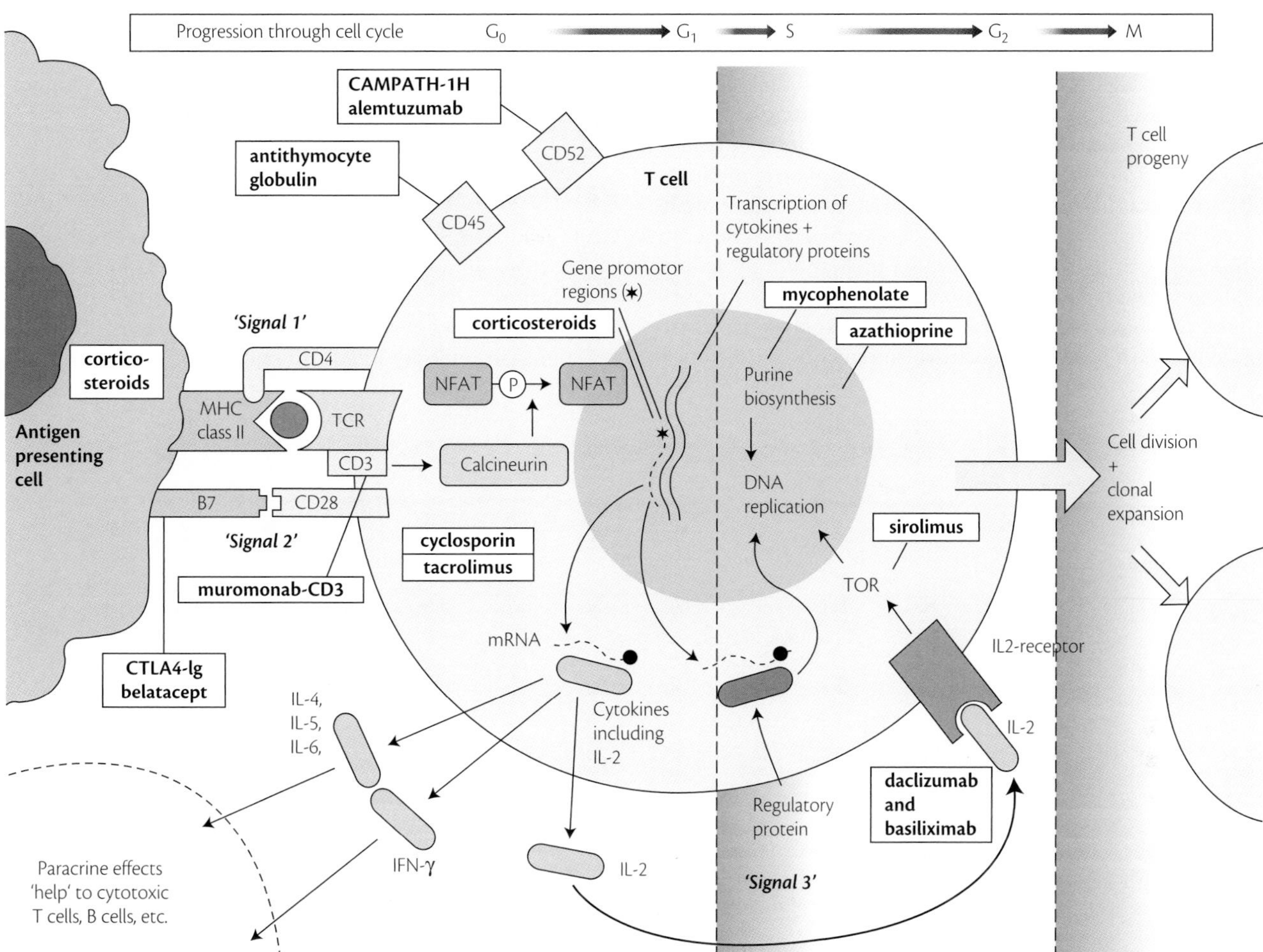

Fig. 49.2 Steps in the T-cell activation cascade: a simplified model of the events which occur during the T-cell activation. The early, calcium-dependent, phase of activation begins when the receptor of a CD4+ helper T-cell (TCR) binds to a complementary MHC class II molecule with an associated peptide in its antigen-presentation grove, '*Signal 1*'. Full activation also requires a second signal ('*Signal 2*') which is caused by binding between complementary adhesion molecules on the surface of the antigen-presenting cell and the T-cell. Signal transduction from the TCR occurs via the CD3 complex. Subsequent intracellular signalling involves the inositol triphosphate/diacylglycerol pathway and mobilization of intracellular calcium. This leads to activation of the protein phosphatase calcineurin. Calcineurin dephosphorylates the nuclear factor of activated T-cells (NFAT), allowing its active moiety to translocate to the nucleus and so bind to the promoter regions of various genes encoding cytokines such as interleukin-2 (IL-2), regulatory proteins and the IL-2 receptor. The pattern of cytokine expression depends on the nature of the T-cell (Th1 or Th2) and can lead to either recruitment of cytotoxic CD8+ T-cells and other effector cells or the provision of help to B-cells for antibody production. The expression of IL-2 leads to autocrine stimulation for the T-cell. Binding of IL-2 to its receptor initiates a second sequence of intracellular signals involving the mammalian target of rapamycin (TOR), which leads to DNA synthesis and replication and which culminates in cell division. The sites of action of various immunosuppressive agents are shown. Polyclonal antithymocyte globulin is shown as binding to the common leucocyte antigen (CD45) although, in reality, it contains antibodies which bind to may different T-cell antigens. CAMPATH-1H (alemtuzumab), a humanized monoclonal against CD52; CTLA4-Ig, the genetically engineered fusion protein between extra cellular domain of CTLA4 (CD152) and the Fc portion of human immunoglobulin that acts as a competitive antagonist for CD28; IFN, interferon; IL, interleukin; MHC, major histocompatibility complex; NFAT, nuclear factor of activated T-cells; TCR, T-cell receptor; TOR; target of rapamycin.

Modified from Banner NR, Lyster H. Pharmacological immunosuppression. In: Banner NR, Polak JM, Yacoub M (eds.) *Lung transplantation*. Cambridge, Cambridge University Press 2003.

Chronic allograft dysfunction may develop many years after the transplant and is principally associated with cardiac allograft vasculopathy, although restrictive cardiomyopathy and, less commonly, dilated cardiomyopathy may also occur. Cardiac allograft vasculopathy is a multifactorial problem in part related to vascular injury caused by previous acute rejection episodes and to chronic injury caused by the presence of donor-specific HLA antibodies as well as to the risk factors for conventional coronary atherosclerosis (e.g. dyslipidaemia, diabetes, hypertension, and smoking).

The gold standard method for diagnosing acute cardiac rejection is the endomyocardial biopsy, first introduced by Philip Caves in 1973.[55,56] Traditionally biopsies have been performed routinely during the first few years after heart transplantation, with the aim of diagnosing rejection at an early stage before cardiac allograft dysfunction has become established.[7] Additional biopsies are performed when there is clinical or other evidence of allograft dysfunction. However, with the current more effective immunosuppression regimens, the yield from routine surveillance biopsies has fallen considerably, diminishing the value of this procedure.[57] Nevertheless, most transplant centres continue to use biopsies in the early phase after transplantation when the risk of rejection is highest and while the immunosuppression is weaned down to the chronic maintenance level. Serious complications of endomyocardial biopsy are rare but include cardiac tamponade, coronary septal branch to right ventricular fistulae, tricuspid regurgitation, myocardial infarction, and infection as well as the complications of vascular access. These risks and the high cost of the procedure have led to a search for alternative, less invasive diagnostic methods. Tests based on cardiac function, particularly echo-Doppler methods, have lacked sufficient sensitivity or specificity.[58,59] Recently attention has been focused on molecular biology and proteomic methods to screen for acute rejection. The AlloMap® is a proprietary method for evaluating the profile of gene expression in circulating white cells. It generates a score which can be used to estimate the likelihood of acute rejection at any stage. Recently it has been demonstrated that the AlloMap® can be used as a screening test to safely reduce the number of routine endomyocardial biopsies that are required beyond 6 months after transplantation.[60]

Pathology of rejection

Acute cellular rejection (ACR) is characterized by an interstitial and perivascular infiltration of T-lymphocytes, also infiltrating vascular endothelium ('lymphocytic intimitis') (Fig. 49.3). Plasma cells, macrophages, and eosinophils may be seen in higher grades of rejection. The intensity and distribution of the infiltrate determines

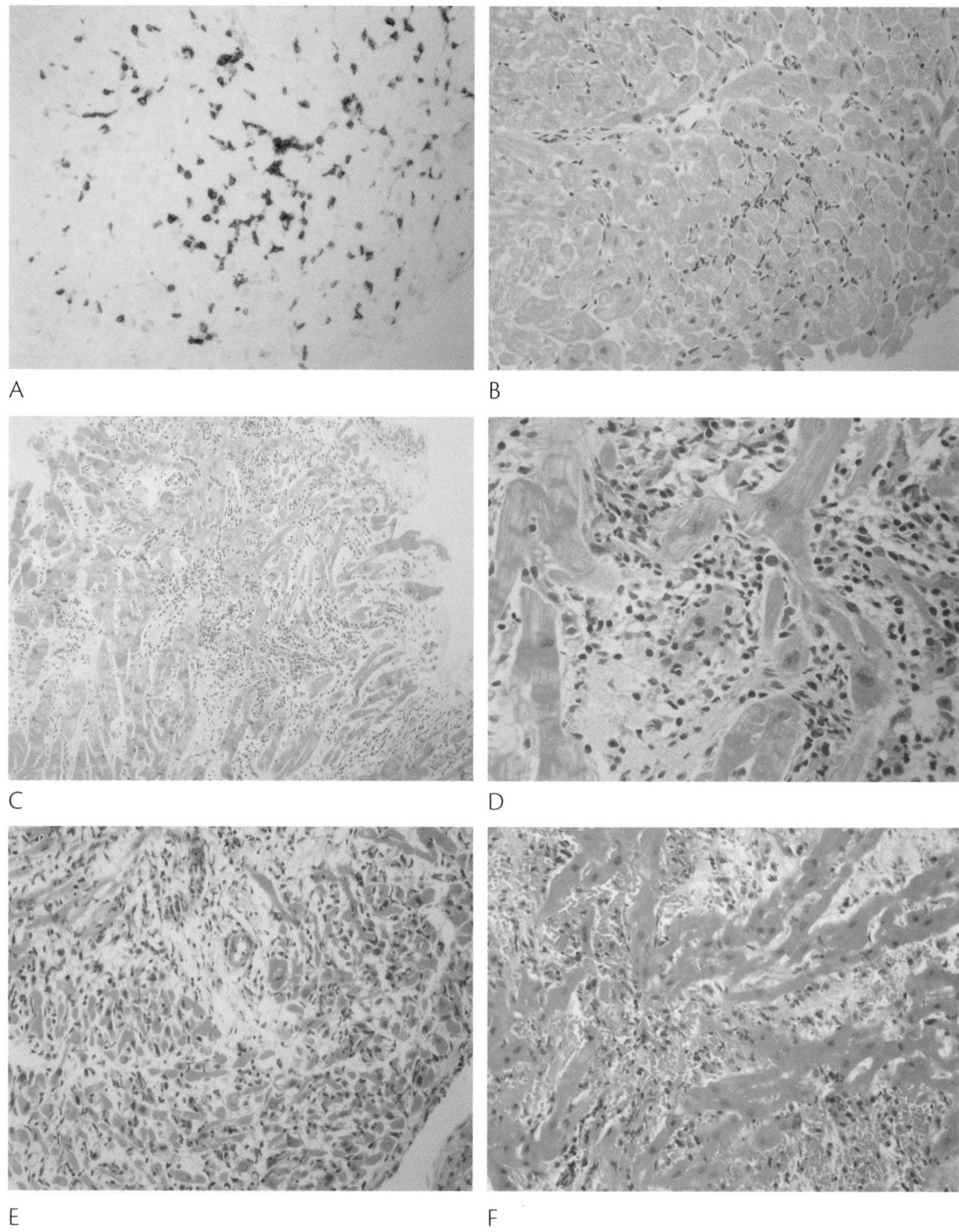

Fig. 49.3 Acute cellular rejection (ACR). (A) ACR is mediated by CD3-positive T-lymphocytes (×100). (B) Mild ACR (ISHLT grade 1R) with a localized perivascular and interstitial lymphocytic infiltrate (×100). (C) Moderate ACR (grade 2R; ×100), with a dense infiltrate of lymphocytes causing some disruption of myocardial architecture and (D) occasional foci of myocytolysis (×400). In severe ACR (grade 3R) a diffuse infiltrate of lymphoid cells (E) with many foci of myocytolysis may dominate the histological picture (×200) or (F) there may be interstitial oedema, haemorrhage, and a mixed inflammatory cell infiltrate with necrotizing vasculitis (×200).

Table 49.1 The 2005 revision of the Working Formulation for classification of acute cellular rejection of the heart

Grade	Category	Description
Grade 0	No rejection	–
Grade 1R	Mild ACR	Multifocal interstitial and/or perivascular mononuclear infiltrates of lymphocytes, some macrophages and occasional eosinophils ± one focus of myocytolysis
Grade 2R	Moderate ACR	Two or more foci of mononuclear cell infiltrates expanding interstitium and with two or more foci of myocyte damage
Grade 3R	Severe ACR	Diffuse mononuclear cell infiltrates expanding interstitium ± oedema ± haemorrhage ± neutrophils ± widespread myocyte necrosis ± vasculitis

ACR, acute cellular rejection; R, revised: this avoids confusion with the grades used in the 1990 Working Formulation.

the grade of ACR in the revised ISHLT grading system, which is graded as mild (1R), moderate (2R), and severe (3R) (Table 49.1).[61] Changes of severe ACR may overlap with those of antibody-mediated rejection. Myocyte damage (myocytolysis) may occur but is inconspicuous relative to the inflammatory infiltrate. It may be present as an occasional focus in mild ACR but is more frequent in moderate and severe ACR.

The diagnosis of antibody-mediated rejection (AMR) is less well standardized (Fig. 49.4).[61] In 2003 a consensus conference on AMR in organ transplants, sponsored by the National Institute of Health, recommended a multidisciplinary approach to diagnosis of AMR based on the results of histology, immunohistology, serology, and graft function studies.[62] They suggested four putative stages of AMR—latent, silent, subclinical, and clinical (Table 49.2). However, this approach has not gained universal acceptance and more research is need to standardize methods and interpretation of results.

Immunosuppression

Many centres use a form of induction therapy with an anti-T-cell antibody to provide additional immunosuppression during the early perioperative period. Agents that have been used for this purpose include monomurab-CD3 (OKT3), antithymocyte globulin (ATG), and the monoclonal antibodies to the IL-2 receptor (basiliximab and daclizumab).[63] Alemtuzumab (CAMPATH-1H) is a humanized antibody against CD52 that can profoundly deplete lymphocytes and which has been used in clinical kidney transplantation; however, there is limited data in heart transplantation and there has been concern about potential cardiac toxicity.[64,65]

The potential benefits of induction therapy include more reliable immunosuppression in the early postoperative period, lower rates of acute rejection, possible host hyporesponsiveness to alloantigen, and, most importantly, renal protection by allowing the delayed introduction of ciclosporin or tacrolimus. Some post-hoc analyses of clinical trials conducted for other purposes suggest that induction therapy may be beneficial.[66,67] However, there is a concern for the potential adverse effects of nonspecific over-immunosuppression including an increased risk of infection or malignancy.[68] Only one large-scale multicentre clinical trial of induction therapy has been conducted in heart transplantation; this compared daclizumab with a placebo control. The daclizumab group had a lower incidence of the composite endpoint of moderate or severe cellular rejection, haemodynamically significant allograft dysfunction, redo transplantation, death, or loss to follow-up within 6 months. However, overall mortality was not different and infection related deaths were more common in a subgroup of the daclizumab patients who also received cytolytic therapy.[69] Based on the evidence currently available, the decision about whether to use induction therapy remains a matter of physician preference and, in some centres, is influenced by the risk profile of the recipient.

The calcineurin inhibitors (CNIs) ciclosporin and tacrolimus are the cornerstones of current immunosuppression regimens. Traditionally these drugs have been used in combination with an antiproliferative agent and corticosteroids.[70] The introduction of the CNI can be delayed by using induction therapy and this strategy may reduce the incidence of perioperative acute renal injury. Mycophenolate has been shown to provide more effective prophylaxis against acute rejection compared with azathioprine, [71] and tacrolimus is somewhat more effective than ciclosporin. [72,73]Therefore most centres currently consider the combination of tacrolimus, mycophenolate, and corticosteroids to be the most effective form of maintenance immunosuppression at least for the first 6–12 months after transplantation.

The target of rapamycin (TOR) inhibitors, sirolimus and everolimus, are another important group of immunosuppressive agents. These drugs provide a prophylaxis against acute rejection that

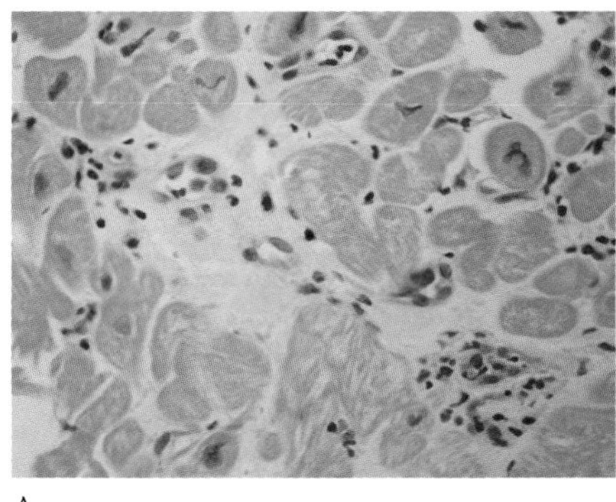
A

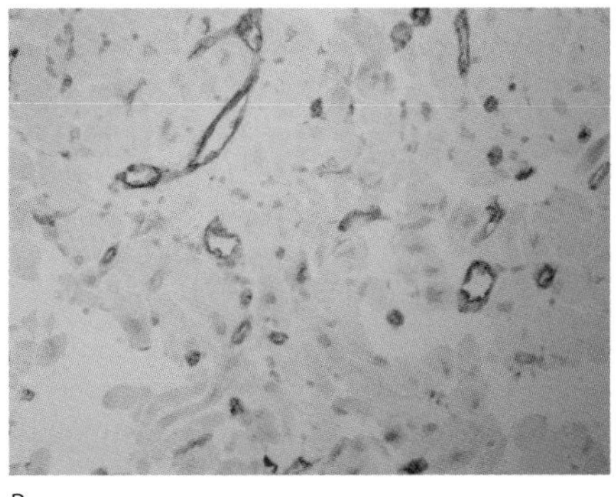
B

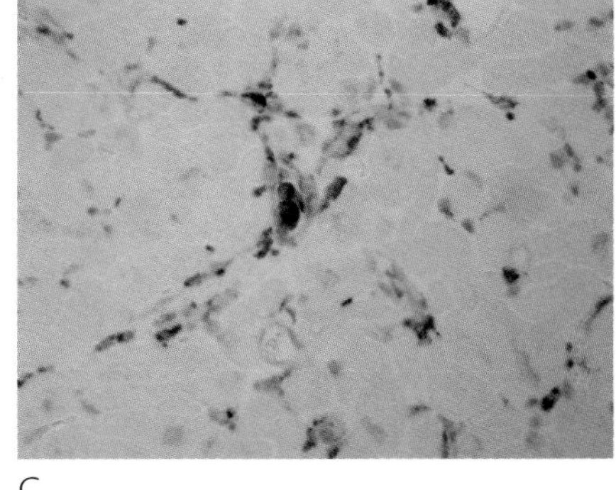
C

Fig. 49.4 Antibody-mediated rejection. (A) Capillary endothelial prominence, intraluminal mononuclear cells and a sparse interstitial mononuclear cell infiltrate (×200). (B) Strong capillary staining for C4d (×200). (C) CD68 staining shows interstitial and intravascular macrophage accumulation (×200).

Table 49.2 Putative stages proposed for evolution of antibody-mediated rejection in solid organ allografts

I	Latent AMR	Detectable circulating antibody to HLA or non-HLA antigens on donor endothelial cells
II	Silent AMR	Detectable circulating antibody to HLA or non-HLA antigens on donor endothelial cells C4d deposition on graft capillary endothelium
III	Subclinical AMR	Detectable circulating antibody to HLA or non-HLA antigens on donor endothelial cells C4d deposition on graft capillary endothelium Histological features of AMR
IV	Clinical AMR	Detectable circulating antibody to HLA or non-HLA antigens on donor endothelial cells C4d deposition on graft capillary endothelium Histological features of AMR Graft dysfunction

AMR, antibody-mediated rejection; HLA, human leucocyte antigen.

is similar to mycophenolate.[74,75] However, the adoption of these drugs as primary immunosuppressive agents after heart transplantation has been limited due to adverse effects, particularly impaired wound healing and increased incidence of postoperative pericardial effusions and of bacterial and fungal infections. They have a number of other dermatological and gastrointestinal side effects; rarely, sirolimus can trigger a severe form of pneumonitis (Fig. 49.5). The TOR inhibitors potentiate CNI nephrotoxicity; however, a recent study suggested this effect can be ameliorated by setting lower target levels for ciclosporin therapy when combined with everolimus.[76]

The TOR inhibitors have a low inherent nephrotoxicity although their use can increase proteinuria. They have antiproliferative properties and have been shown to be effective in primary prophylaxis against cardiac allograft vasculopathy and also in slowing the progression of vasculopathy.[74,75,77] These drugs have also been used in non-CNI maintenance immunosuppression regimens to ameliorate chronic nephrotoxicity.[78,79]

Ciclosporin, tacrolimus, and sirolimus are all metabolized through the cytochrome P450 3A4 pathway and therefore cause, and are subject to, interaction with other drugs metabolized through that pathway.[80] There are genetic polymorphisms in the P450 system and there is a wide variation between individual dose requirements for these drugs. Consequently, the administration of all three agents is adjusted to control the drug level in the blood (therapeutic drug monitoring).

Adjunctive therapy with statins has been found to improve survival and reduce the risk of serious rejection and cardiac allograft vasculopathy (CAV) after heart transplantation.[81,82] Routine prophylaxis against cytomegalovirus and *Pneumocystis jirovecii* has reduced the incidence of these opportunistic infections.[83,84]

Treatment of acute rejection

ACR normally responds to treatment with high-dose intravenous and oral corticosteroids. It is important to ensure that the patient is receiving adequate maintenance immunosuppression and that they are complying with therapy. Repeated or late episodes of acute rejection are often an indication to modify the maintenance regimen. Mild cellular rejection (ISHLT grade 1R) with no evidence of allograft dysfunction usually does not warrant treatment. Episodes of steroid-resistant rejection and those associated with haemodynamic compromise are treated more aggressively with combination of corticosteroids and either antithymocyte globulin or muromonab CD3.[70] The treatment of acute AMR involves antibody removal by either plasmapheresis or immunoadsorption coupled with treatment with high-dose polyspecific immunoglobulin, the B-cell antibody rituximab, or cyclophosphamide. The treatment of AMR is less standardized than for cellular rejection, the therapeutic response more variable, and the long-term outcome more uncertain.[85]

Survival and long-term outcome

The ISHLT Heart Transplant Registry demonstrates that despite the increasing complexity of heart transplant recipients, results have improved progressively. For the most recent cohort transplanted in 2002–2007 the actuarial survival at 1 year is 85%, at 3 years 79%, and at 5 years 73%. For those transplanted between 1992 and 2001, the 10-year actuarial survival is 50%.[63] In contrast to medical therapy, survival is independent of the severity of the HF.[19] Early survival rates tend to be lower in Europe, and this is probably related to the risk profile of the cardiac donors that are available.[21] There is heterogeneity of outcomes between diagnostic groups, with patients with nonischaemic dilated cardiomyopathy having the best overall outcome whilst patients with ACHD have a higher perioperative risk.[21,38] However, if the early postoperative risk is factored out, ACHD patients do at least as well in the long term as the other diagnostic groups. The overall outcome of retransplantation is significantly worse than for *de novo* transplants. However, it appears that the outcome for both ACHD and retransplant cases has improved in the most recent era and this probably reflects both better case selection and perioperative management.[63] Survival after transplantation is also somewhat reduced in patients who have been bridged to transplant with a LVAD as opposed to those undergoing elective transplant and those undergoing heart transplantation following inotropic support. However, this difference is less for patients who have been bridged with the current smaller continuous-flow devices than patients who had received pulsatile support. Functional rehabilitation is excellent, with 93% of patients reporting no limitation in activities at 1 year. However, return-to-work data are less encouraging, with 50% of patients not having returned to work or normal activities at 1 year after transplantation.[63] Quality of life is improved after transplantation.[86]

Heart transplant recipients are at risk of a number of long-term complications. Although the incidence of acute rejection falls dramatically beyond the first few months after transplantation, episodes of late rejection do occur. These are sometimes unexplained but are often related to periods of under-immunosuppression either because of reductions in maintenance immunosuppression because of drug toxicity or because of poor adherence to the drug regimen by the patient.[87] Late rejection episodes are often more difficult to treat because clinical surveillance is less frequent and patients often present when the rejection is well established. Perhaps because of late presentation and association with under-immunosuppression, such episodes are often associated with the *de novo* formulation of anti-donor HLA antibodies, which complicates treatment.

Coronary arterial disease in the transplanted heart (CAV) used to be the leading cause of late death and is still an important cause of mortality (Fig. 49.6). Its aetiology is multifactorial, as outlined above.[88]

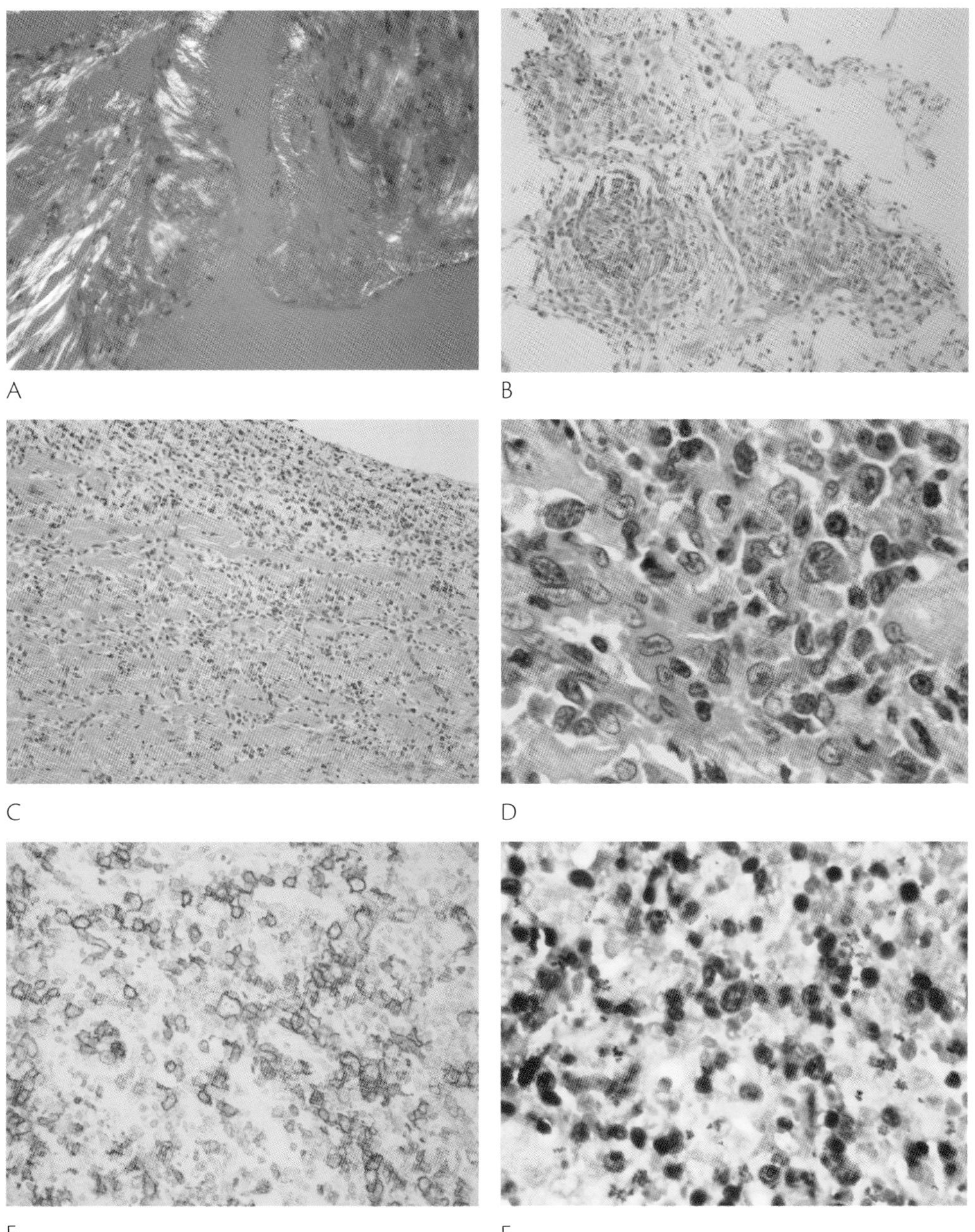

Fig. 49.5 Other complications. (A) Biopsy recurrence of cardiac amyloid 60 months after heart and kidney transplantation for ApoAI Arg60 (variant apolipoprotein AI) amyloidosis (Congo Red ×200 viewed with polarized light). (B) Sirolimus pulmonary toxicity: there is patchy intra-alveolar macrophage-rich exudation in this transbronchial lung biopsy from a heart transplant recipient receiving sirolimus (×200). (C), (D) In EBV-related post-transplant lymphoproliferative disorder in the cardiac allograft cardiac muscle and endocardium are infiltrated by pleomorphic lymphocytes (c ×100, d ×400). (E) The immunophenotype is confirmed as B-cell with immunostaining for CD20. (F) An association with EBV is confirmed by *in situ* hybridization for EBV-encoded RNA (EBERs) which marks the nuclei of the tumour cells (×200; figure kindly provided by Dr Alero Thomas, London School of Hygiene and Tropical Medicine).

Angiographically the disease is often diffuse, affecting both proximal and branch vessels. Its incidence has been reduced as a result of improved prophylaxis against acute rejection and adjunctive therapy with statins.[81,89] For patients who do develop disease, percutaneous coronary intervention with standard or drug-eluting stents can be used to treat focal lesions. However, since the disease is often diffuse and since it has a predilection to affect the secondary and tertiary coronary branches, such intervention often only palliative.[90] Adjunctive therapy with a TOR inhibitor coupled with intensive management of all modifiable coronary risk factors helps to reduce the progression of the disease.[91] Retransplantation may be used in carefully selected cases.[92]

Hypertension is common in orthotopic heart transplant patients and appears to be partly related to the effects of cardiac denervation.[93] CNI inhibitors are also associated with hypertension, which is more of a problem with ciclosporin than with tacrolimus.[94] Treatment can follow conventional lines, although caution is required when using ACE inhibitors in those with significant renal impairment because this and CNIs can both contribute to hyperkalaemia. Some calcium antagonists, notably diltiazem, can also

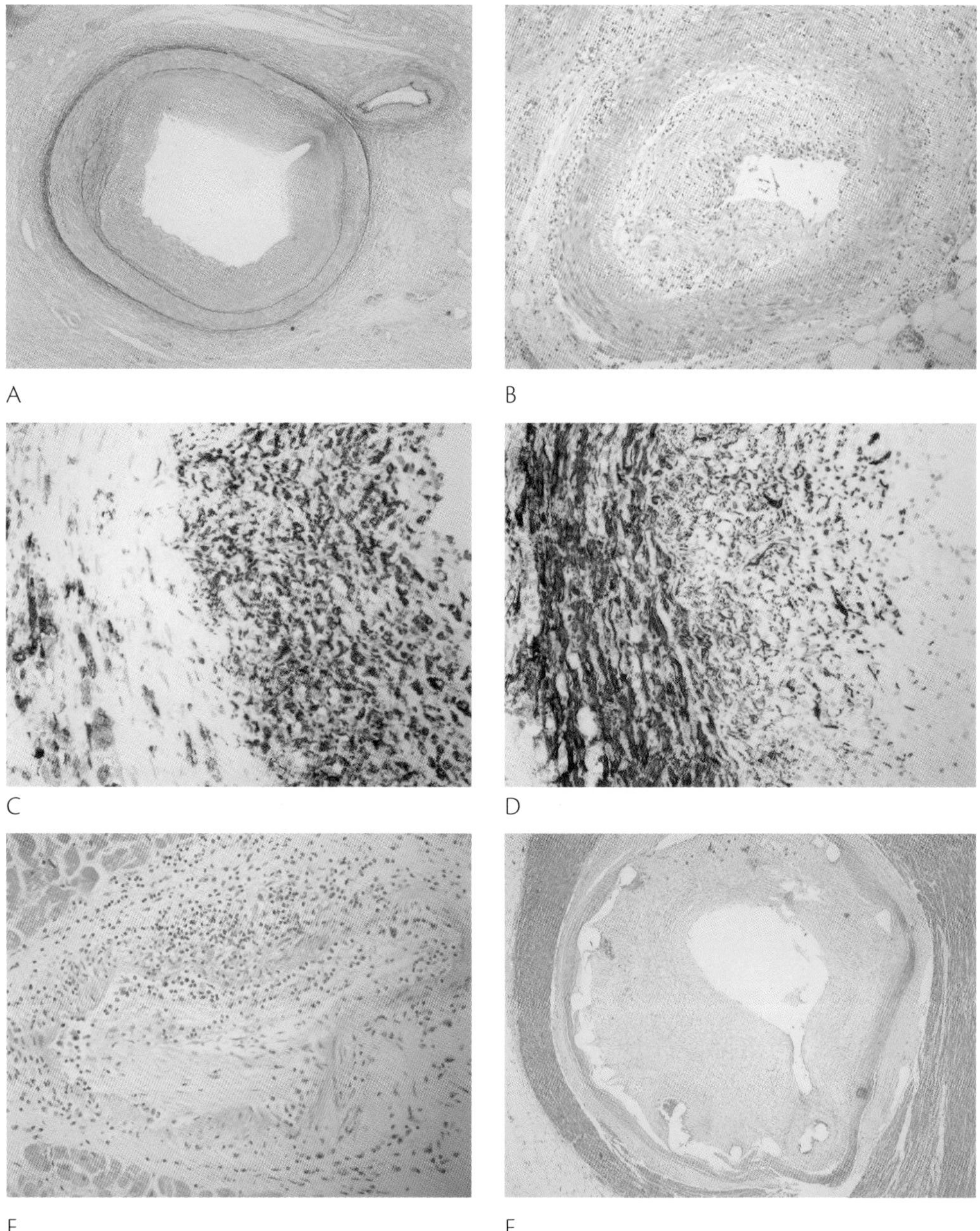

Fig. 49.6 Cardiac allograft vasculopathy (CAV). (A) Typical CAV with circumferential thickening of the intima and good preservation of the internal elastic lamina. A small perforating branch of coronary artery (top right of frame) is normal (Verhoeff's elastic–Van Giesen preparation, ×25). (B) Active cardiac allograft vasculopathy (CAV) with intimal proliferation due to lymphocytic intimitis (×25), (C) numerous macrophages inside media and in adventitia (CD68 ×200), and (D) florid myofibroblastic proliferation (smooth muscle actin ×200). (E) Small-vessel intimitis in an intramyocardial artery (×100). (F) Stented coronary artery with diffuse CAV without plaques but with intimal proliferation causing critical stenosis and sudden death despite insertion some weeks previously of a stent represented by spaces distributed circumferentially just inside the media (×25).

interact with ciclosporin metabolism requiring therapeutic drug monitoring and dose adjustments.

Dyslipidaemia is common in heart transplant patients. This is partly related to their underlying disease and also to the effects of immunosuppressive agents including ciclosporin, tacrolimus, sirolimus, and corticosteroids. Statin therapy is universal after heart transplantation, as described above; however, dose escalation and drug switching may be required in patients with refractory dyslipidaemia. In this circumstance, care is needed when treating patients with ciclosporin because serious drug interactions can occur between some of the statins and there is a risk of rhabdomyolysis and renal failure.[95] In difficult cases it is safer to switch the patient to tacrolimus so as to allow conventional doses of statin therapy to be used.

Chronic kidney disease is common after all forms of organ transplantation.[96] It is related to therapy with CNI inhibitors; however, a number of other factors contribute to this problem including preoperative renal dysfunction related to HF, acute kidney injury, pretransplant diabetes, and recipient age.[97] The severity of renal dysfunction varies considerably between patients but the incidence increases with time and some degree of renal dysfunction is almost universal 10 years after transplantation. Management to prevent progression involves tight control of hypertension and the option of switching the patient to a non-CNI immunosuppression regimen.[79] However, the safety of this approach early after heart transplantation has not been established and renal function rarely returns to normal after late conversion.[79]

The incidence of malignancy is increased in heart transplant recipients mainly due to pharmacological immunosuppression.[98] The most common tumours are nonmelanoma skin cancer and post-transplant lymphoproliferative disease (PTLD). Skin tumours are related to age and cumulative sun exposure occurring, mainly in fair-skinned patients.[99] PTLD usually presents as a non-Hodgkin's lymphoma and the risk is related to Epstein–Barr virus exposure, the intensity of immunosuppression, and use of induction therapy (see Fig. 49.5).[68,100–102] The incidence of many other cancers is also increased after transplantation, but to a lesser extent.[103,104]

Recurrence of the original cardiac disease in the allograft may occur. There is an overlap between the risk factors for convention coronary atherosclerosis and CAV. Some inflammatory and infiltrative diseases may recur after transplantation, e.g. giant cell myocarditis and amyloidosis (see Fig. 49.5).

Conclusion

Heart transplantation remains the gold standard treatment for selected patients with advanced HF. Unlike medical therapy, outcome is independent of the severity of the HF syndrome. However, transplantation is limited by the scarcity of suitable donor hearts. This has led to increasing waiting times and a reliance on mechanical circulatory support to 'bridge' patients to transplantation. The long-term outcome of transplantation is superior to those currently achieved by medical therapy or by long-term mechanical circulatory support. Heart transplant recipients are subject to a number of long-term complications including an increased risk of malignancy, CAV, and chronic kidney disease. Nevertheless most achieve a good level of rehabilitation and an improved quality of life.

References

1. Cass MH, Brock R. Heart excision and replacement. *Guys Hosp Rep* 1959;**108**:285–90.
2. Lower RR, Shumway NE. Studies on orthotopic homotransplantation of the canine heart. *Surg Forum* 1960;**11**:18–19.
3. Schnoor M, Schafer T, Luhmann D, Sievers HH. Bicaval versus standard technique in orthotopic heart transplantation: a systematic review and meta-analysis. *J Thorac Cardiovasc Surg* 2007; **134**(5):1322–31.
4. Banner NR, Lyster H. Pharmacological Immunosuppression. In: Banner NR, Polak JM, Yacoub MH (eds) *Lung transplantation*, pp. 205–42. Cambridge University Press, Cambridge, 2003.
5. Barnard CN. The operation. A human cardiac transplant: an interim report of a successful operation performed at Groote Schuur Hospital, Cape Town. *S Afr Med J* 1967;**41**(48):1271–4.
6. McRae D. *Every second counts: the race to transplant the first human heart.* Putnam, New York, 2006.
7. Hunt SA. Taking heart—cardiac transplantation past, present, and future. *N Engl J Med* 2006;**355**(3):231–5.
8. Calne RY, Rolles K, White DJ, *et al.* Cyclosporin A initially as the only immunosuppressant in 34 recipients of cadaveric organs: 32 kidneys, 2 pancreases, and 2 livers. *Lancet* 1979;**ii**(8151):1033–6.
9. Banner NR, Yacoub MH. Cyclosporine in thoracic organ transplantation. *Transplant Proc* 2004;**36**(2 Suppl):302–8S.
10. Banner NR, Yacoub MH. Physiology of the orthotopic cardiac transplant recipient. *Semin Thorac Cardiovasc Surg* 1990;**2**(3):259–70.
11. Banner NR, Khaghani A, Fitzgerald M, *et al.* The expanding role of cardiac transplantaion. In: Unger F (ed.) *Assisted circulation*, pp. 448–67. Springer-Verlag, Berlin, 1989.
12. Yacoub M, Mankad P, Ledingham S. Donor procurement and surgical techniques for cardiac transplantation. *Semin Thorac Cardiovasc Surg* 1990;**2**(2):153–61.
13. Dreyfus G, Jebara V, Mihaileanu S, Carpentier AF. Total orthotopic heart transplantation: an alternative to the standard technique. *Ann Thorac Surg* 1991;**52**(5):1181–4.
14. Sievers HH, Weyand M, Kraatz EG, Bernhard A. An alternative technique for orthotopic cardiac transplantation, with preservation of the normal anatomy of the right atrium. *Thorac Cardiovasc Surg* 1991;**39**(2):70–2.
15. Sarsam MA, Campbell CS, Yonan NA, Deiraniya AK, Rahman AN. An alternative surgical technique in orthotopic cardiac transplantation. *J Card Surg* 1993;**8**(3):344–9.
16. Weiss ES, Nwakanma LU, Russell SB, Conte JV, Shah AS. Outcomes in bicaval versus biatrial techniques in heart transplantation: an analysis of the UNOS database. *J Heart Lung Transplant* 2008;**27**(2):178–83.
17. Bleasdale RA, Banner NR, Anyanwu AC, Mitchell AG, Khaghani A, Yacoub MH. Determinants of outcome after heterotopic heart transplantation. *J Heart Lung Transplant* 2002;**21**(8):867–73.
18. Jessup M, Banner N, Brozena S, *et al.* Optimal pharmacologic and non-pharmacologic management of cardiac transplant candidates: approaches to be considered prior to transplant evaluation: International Society for Heart and Lung Transplantation guidelines for the care of cardiac transplant candidates—2006. *J Heart Lung Transplant* 2006;**25**(9):1003–23.
19. Banner NR, Rogers CA, Bonser RS. Effect of heart transplantation on survival in ambulatory and decompensated heart failure. *Transplantation* 2008;**86**(11):1515–22.
20. Stevenson LW, Miller LW, Desvigne-Nickens P, *et al.* Left ventricular assist device as destination for patients undergoing intravenous inotropic therapy: a subset analysis from REMATCH (Randomized Evaluation of Mechanical Assistance in Treatment of Chronic Heart Failure). *Circulation* 2004;**110**(8):975–81.
21. Thekkudan J, Rogers CA, Thomas HL, van der Meulen JH, Bonser RS, Banner NR. Trends in adult heart transplantation: a national survey from the United Kingdom Cardiothoracic Transplant Audit 1995–2007. *Eur J Cardiothorac Surg* 2010;**37**(1):80–6.
22. Miller LW, Pagani FD, Russell SD, *et al.* Use of a continuous-flow device in patients awaiting heart transplantation. *N Engl J Med* 2007;**357**(9):885–96.
23. Slaughter MS, Rogers JG, Milano CA, *et al.* Advanced heart failure treated with continuous-flow left ventricular assist device. *N Engl J Med* 2009;**361**(23):2241–51.
24. Mehra MR, Kobashigawa J, Starling R, *et al.* Listing criteria for heart transplantation: International Society for Heart and Lung Transplantation guidelines for the care of cardiac transplant candidates—2006. *J Heart Lung Transplant* 2006;**25**(9):1024–42.
25. Gronda E, Bourge RC, Costanzo MR, *et al.* Heart rhythm considerations in heart transplant candidates and considerations for ventricular assist devices: International Society for Heart and Lung Transplantation guidelines for the care of cardiac transplant candidates—2006. *J Heart Lung Transplant* 2006;**25**(9):1043–56.
26. Jessup M, Abraham WT, Casey DE, *et al.* 2009 focused update: ACCF/AHA Guidelines for the Diagnosis and Management of Heart Failure in Adults: a report of the American College of Cardiology Foundation/American Heart Association Task Force on Practice Guidelines: developed in collaboration with the International Society for Heart and Lung Transplantation. *Circulation* 2009;**119**(14):1977–2016.

27. Thekkudan J, Dronavalli VB, Bonser RS. Myocardial revascularization for heart failure. In: Banner NR, Jessup M (eds) *Advanced heart failure*, pp. 525–40. Elsevier, Philadelphia, 2009.
28. Mancini DM, Eisen H, Kussmaul W, Mull R, Edmunds LH Jr, Wilson JR. Value of peak exercise oxygen consumption for optimal timing of cardiac transplantation in ambulatory patients with heart failure. *Circulation* 1991;**83**(3):778–86.
29. Aaronson KD, Schwartz JS, Chen TM, Wong KL, Goin JE, Mancini DM. Development and prospective validation of a clinical index to predict survival in ambulatory patients referred for cardiac transplant evaluation. *Circulation* 1997;**95**(12):2660–7.
30. Kirklin JK, Naftel DC, Kirklin JW, Blackstone EH, White-Williams C, Bourge RC. Pulmonary vascular resistance and the risk of heart transplantation. *J Heart Transplant* 1988;**7**(5):331–6.
31. Chen JM, Levin HR, Michler RE, Prusmack CJ, Rose EA, Aaronson KD. Reevaluating the significance of pulmonary hypertension before cardiac transplantation: determination of optimal thresholds and quantification of the effect of reversibility on perioperative mortality. *J Thorac Cardiovasc Surg* 1997;**114**(4):627–34.
32. Adamson RM, Dembitsky WP, Jaski BE, *et al.* Left ventricular assist device support of medically unresponsive pulmonary hypertension and aortic insufficiency. *Asaio J* 1997;**43**(4):365–9.
33. Lyster H, Banner NR. Intravenous inotropic agents. In: Banner NR, Jessup M (eds) *Advanced heart failure*, pp. 307–24. Elsevier, Philadelphia, 2009
34. Lindsay AC, Khaghani A, Dalby MCD. Intraaotic balloon and other counterpulsation techniques. In: Banner NR, Jessup M (eds) *Advanced heart failure*, pp. 557–68. Elsevier, Philadelphia, 2009.
35. Banner NR, Hamour I, Lyster H, Burke M, Boscoe MJ, Dreyfus G. Postoperative care of the heart transplant patient. In: O'Donnell JM, Nacul FE (eds) *Surgical intensive care medicine*, 2nd edition, pp. 599–619. Springer, New York, 2010.
36. Dang NC, Topkara VK, Mercando M, *et al.* Right heart failure after left ventricular assist device implantation in patients with chronic congestive heart failure. *J Heart Lung Transplant* 2006;**25**(1):1–6.
37. Copeland JG, Smith RG, Arabia FA, *et al.* Cardiac replacement with a total artificial heart as a bridge to transplantation. *N Engl J Med* 2004;**351**(9):859–67.
38. Patel ND, Weiss ES, Allen JG, *et al.* Heart transplantation for adults with congenital heart disease: analysis of the United network for organ sharing database. *Ann Thorac Surg* 2009;**88**(3):814–21; discussion 21–2.
39. Smith M. Management of the multiple organ donor. *Surgery* 1998;**16**:180–3.
40. Zaroff JG, Rosengard BR, Armstrong WF, *et al.* Consensus conference report: maximizing use of organs recovered from the cadaver donor: cardiac recommendations, March 28–29, 2001, Crystal City, Va. *Circulation* 2002;**106**(7):836–41.
41. Venkateswaran RV, Bonser RS, Steeds RP. The echocardiographic assessment of donor heart function prior to cardiac transplantation. *Eur J Echocardiogr* 2005;**6**(4):260–3.
42. Zaroff JG, Babcock WD, Shiboski SC, Solinger LL, Rosengard BR. Temporal changes in left ventricular systolic function in heart donors: results of serial echocardiography. *J Heart Lung Transplant* 2003;**22**(4):383–8.
43. Venkateswaran RV, Steeds RP, Quinn DW, *et al.* The haemodynamic effects of adjunctive hormone therapy in potential heart donors: a prospective randomized double-blind factorially designed controlled trial. *Eur Heart J* 2009;**30**(14):1771–80.
44. Stehlik J, Islam N, Hurst D, *et al.* Utility of virtual crossmatch in sensitized patients awaiting heart transplantation. *J Heart Lung Transplant* 2009;**28**(11):1129–34.
45. Havel M, Owen AN, Simon P. Basic principles of cardioplegic management in donor heart preservation. *Clin Ther* 1991;**13**(2):289–303.
46. Jahania MS, Sanchez JA, Narayan P, Lasley RD, Mentzer RM Jr. Heart preservation for transplantation: principles and strategies. *Ann Thorac Surg* 1999;**68**(5):1983–7.
47. Banner NR, Thomas HL, Curnow E, Hussey JC, Rogers CA, Bonser RS. The importance of cold and warm cardiac ischemia for survival after heart transplantation. *Transplantation* 2008;**86**(4):542–7.
48. Russo MJ, Chen JM, Sorabella RA, *et al.* The effect of ischemic time on survival after heart transplantation varies by donor age: an analysis of the United Network for Organ Sharing database. *J Thorac Cardiovasc Surg* 2007;**133**(2):554–9.
49. Patel J, Kobashigawa JA. Cardiac transplantation: the alternate list and expansion of the donor pool. *Curr Opin Cardiol* 2004;**19**(2):162–5.
50. Marasco SF, Lukas G, McDonald M, McMillan J, Ihle B. Review of ECMO (extra corporeal membrane oxygenation) support in critically ill adult patients. *Heart Lung Circ* 2008;**17**(Suppl 4):S41–7.
51. Chou NK, Chi NH, Ko WJ, *et al.* Extracorporeal membrane oxygenation for perioperative cardiac allograft failure. *Asaio J* 2006;**52**(1):100–3.
52. Terasaki PI. Humoral theory of transplantation. *Am J Transplant* 2003;**3**(6):665–73.
53. Terasaki PI, Cai J. Human leukocyte antigen antibodies and chronic rejection: from association to causation. *Transplantation* 2008;**86**(3):377–83.
54. Lones MA, Czer LS, Trento A, Harasty D, Miller JM, Fishbein MC. Clinical-pathologic features of humoral rejection in cardiac allografts: a study in 81 consecutive patients. *J Heart Lung Transplant* 1995;**14**(1 Pt 1):151–62.
55. Caves PK, Billingham ME, Schulz WP, Dong E, Jr., Shumway NE. Transvenous biopsy from canine orthotopic heart allografts. *Am Heart J* 1973 Apr;**85**(4):525–30.
56. Caves PK, Stinson EB, Billingham ME, Shumway NE. Serial transvenous biopsy of the transplanted human heart. Improved management of acute rejection episodes. *Lancet* 1974;**1**(7862):821–6.
57. Hamour IM, Burke MM, Bell AD, Panicker MG, Banerjee R, Banner NR. Limited utility of endomyocardial biopsy in the first year after heart transplantation. *Transplantation* 2008;**85**(7):969–74.
58. Valantine HA, Fowler MB, Hunt SA, *et al.* Changes in Doppler echocardiographic indexes of left ventricular function as potential markers of acute cardiac rejection. *Circulation* 1987;**76**(5 Pt 2):V86–92.
59. Desruennes M, Corcos T, Cabrol A, *et al.* Doppler echocardiography for the diagnosis of acute cardiac allograft rejection. *J Am Coll Cardiol* 1988;**12**(1):63–70.
60. Pham MX, Teuteberg JJ, Kfoury AG, *et al.* Gene-expression profiling for rejection surveillance after cardiac transplantation. *N Engl J Med* 2010;**362**(20):1890–900.
61. Stewart S, Winters GL, Fishbein MC, *et al.* Revision of the 1990 working formulation for the standardization of nomenclature in the diagnosis of heart rejection. *J Heart Lung Transplant* 2005;**24**(11):1710–20.
62. Takemoto SK, Zeevi A, Feng S, *et al.* National conference to assess antibody-mediated rejection in solid organ transplantation. *Am J Transplant* 2004;**4**(7):1033–41.
63. Taylor DO, Stehlik J, Edwards LB, *et al.* Registry of the International Society for Heart and Lung Transplantation: Twenty-sixth Official Adult Heart Transplant Report-2009. *J Heart Lung Transplant* 2009;**28**(10):1007–22.

64. Woodside KJ, Lick SD. Alemtuzumab (Campath 1H) as successful salvage therapy for recurrent steroid-resistant heart transplant rejection. *J Heart Lung Transplant* 2007;**26**(7):750–2.
65. Watson CJ, Bradley JA, Friend PJ, *et al.* Alemtuzumab (CAMPATH 1H) induction therapy in cadaveric kidney transplantation—efficacy and safety at five years. *Am J Transplant* 2005;**5**(6):1347–53.
66. Eisen HJ, Hobbs RE, Davis SF, *et al.* Safety, tolerability and efficacy of cyclosporine microemulsion in heart transplant recipients: a randomized, multicenter, double-blind comparison with the oil based formulation of cyclosporine—results at six months after transplantation. *Transplantation* 1999;**68**(5):663–71.
67. Reichart B, Meiser B, Vigano M, *et al.* European Multicenter Tacrolimus (FK506) Heart Pilot Study: one-year results—European Tacrolimus Multicenter Heart Study Group. *J Heart Lung Transplant* 1998;**17**(8):775–81.
68. Opelz G, Dohler B. Lymphomas after solid organ transplantation: a collaborative transplant study report. *Am J Transplant* 2004;**4**(2):222–30.
69. Hershberger RE, Starling RC, Eisen HJ, *et al.* Daclizumab to prevent rejection after cardiac transplantation. *N Engl J Med* 2005;**352**(26):2705–13.
70. Hunt SA, Haddad F. The changing face of heart transplantation. *J Am Coll Cardiol* 2008;**52**(8):587–98.
71. Kobashigawa J, Miller L, Renlund D, *et al.* A randomized active-controlled trial of mycophenolate mofetil in heart transplant recipients. Mycophenolate Mofetil Investigators. *Transplantation* 1998;**66**(4):507–15.
72. Kobashigawa JA, Miller LW, Russell SD, *et al.* Tacrolimus with mycophenolate mofetil (MMF) or sirolimus vs. cyclosporine with MMF in cardiac transplant patients: 1-year report. *Am J Transplant* 2006;**6**(6):1377–86.
73. Grimm M, Rinaldi M, Yonan NA, *et al.* Superior prevention of acute rejection by tacrolimus vs. cyclosporine in heart transplant recipients—a large European trial. *Am J Transplant* 2006;**6**(6):1387–97.
74. Eisen HJ, Tuzcu EM, Dorent R, *et al.* Everolimus for the prevention of allograft rejection and vasculopathy in cardiac-transplant recipients. *N Engl J Med* 2003;**349**(9):847–58.
75. Keogh A, Richardson M, Ruygrok P, *et al.* Sirolimus in de novo heart transplant recipients reduces acute rejection and prevents coronary artery disease at 2 years: a randomized clinical trial. *Circulation* 2004;**110**(17):2694–700.
76. Lehmkuhl HB, Arizon J, Vigano M, *et al.* Everolimus with reduced cyclosporine versus MMF with standard cyclosporine in de novo heart transplant recipients. *Transplantation* 2009;**88**(1):115–22.
77. Mancini D, Pinney S, Burkhoff D, *et al.* Use of rapamycin slows progression of cardiac transplantation vasculopathy. *Circulation* 2003;**108**(1):48–53.
78. Groetzner J, Kaczmarek I, Schulz U, *et al.* Mycophenolate and sirolimus as calcineurin inhibitor-free immunosuppression improves renal function better than calcineurin inhibitor-reduction in late cardiac transplant recipients with chronic renal failure. *Transplantation* 2009;**87**(5):726–33.
79. Lyster H, Leaver N, Hamour I, Palmer A, Banner NR. Transfer from ciclosporin to mycophenolate-sirolimus immunosuppression for chronic renal disease after heart transplantation: safety and efficacy of two regimens. *Nephrol Dial Transplant* 2009;**24**(12):3872–5.
80. Banner NR, Lyster H, Yacoub MH. Clinical immunosuppression using the calcineurin-inhibitors ciclosporin and tacrolimus. In: Pinna LA, Cohen P(eds) *Inhibitors of protein kinases and protein phophatases, handbook of experimental pharmacology,* pp. 321–59. Springer-Verlag, Berlin, 2005.
81. Kobashigawa JA, Moriguchi JD, Laks H, *et al.* Ten-year follow-up of a randomized trial of pravastatin in heart transplant patients. *J Heart Lung Transplant* 2005;**24**(11):1736–40.
82. Wenke K, Meiser B, Thiery J, *et al.* Simvastatin initiated early after heart transplantation: 8-year prospective experience. *Circulation* 200;**107**(1):93–7.
83. Paya C, Humar A, Dominguez E, *et al.* Efficacy and safety of valganciclovir vs. oral ganciclovir for prevention of cytomegalovirus disease in solid organ transplant recipients. *Am J Transplant* 2004;**4**(4):611–20.
84. Fishman JA. Prevention of infection caused by *Pneumocystis carinii* in transplant recipients. *Clin Infect Dis* 2001;**33**(8):1397–405.
85. Singh N, Pirsch J, Samaniego M. Antibody-mediated rejection: treatment alternatives and outcomes. *Transplant Rev (Orlando)* 2009;**23**(1):34–46.
86. Grady KL, Jalowiec A, White-Williams C. Improvement in quality of life in patients with heart failure who undergo transplantation. *J Heart Lung Transplant* 1996;**15**(8):749–57.
87. Butler JA, Peveler RC, Roderick P, Smith PW, Horne R, Mason JC. Modifiable risk factors for non-adherence to immunosuppressants in renal transplant recipients: a cross-sectional study. *Nephrol Dial Transplant* 2004;**19**(12):3144–9.
88. Rahmani M, Cruz RP, Granville DJ, McManus BM. Allograft vasculopathy versus atherosclerosis. *Circ Res* 2006;**99**(8):801–15.
89. Edelman ER, Danenberg HD. Rapamycin for cardiac transplant rejection and vasculopathy: one stone, two birds? *Circulation* 2003;**108**(1):6–8.
90. Lee MS, Tarantini G, Xhaxho J, *et al.* Sirolimus- versus paclitaxel-eluting stents for the treatment of cardiac allograft vasculopathy. *JACC Cardiovasc Interv* 2010;**3**(4):378–82.
91. Raichlin E, Bae JH, Khalpey Z, *et al.* Conversion to sirolimus as primary immunosuppression attenuates the progression of allograft vasculopathy after cardiac transplantation. *Circulation* 2007;**116**(23):2726–33.
92. Tjang YS, Tenderich G, Hornik L, Korfer R. Cardiac retransplantation in adults: an evidence-based systematic review. *Thorac Cardiovasc Surg* 2008;**56**(6):323–7.
93. Taegtmeyer AB, Crook AM, Barton PJ, Banner NR. Reduced incidence of hypertension after heterotopic cardiac transplantation compared with orthotopic cardiac transplantation: evidence that excision of the native heart contributes to post-transplant hypertension. *J Am Coll Cardiol* 2004;**44**(6):1254–60.
94. Taylor DO, Barr ML, Radovancevic B, *et al.* A randomized, multicenter comparison of tacrolimus and cyclosporine immunosuppressive regimens in cardiac transplantation: decreased hyperlipidemia and hypertension with tacrolimus. *J Heart Lung Transplant* 1999;**18**(4):336–45.
95. Ballantyne CM. Statins after cardiac transplantation: which statin, what dose, and how low should we go? *J Heart Lung Transplant* 2000;**19**(6):515–17.
96. Ojo AO, Held PJ, Port FK, *et al.* Chronic renal failure after transplantation of a nonrenal organ. *N Engl J Med* 2003;**349**(10):931–40.
97. Hamour IM, Omar F, Lyster HS, Palmer A, Banner NR. Chronic kidney disease after heart transplantation. *Nephrol Dial Transplant* 2009;**24**(5):1655–62.
98. Ippoliti G, Rinaldi M, Pellegrini C, Vigano M. Incidence of cancer after immunosuppressive treatment for heart transplantation. *Crit Rev Oncol Hematol* 2005;**56**(1):101–13.
99. Lindelof B, Sigurgeirsson B, Gabel H, Stern RS. Incidence of skin cancer in 5356 patients following organ transplantation. *Br J Dermatol* 2000;**143**(3):513–19.
100. Wasson S, Zafar MN, Best J, Reddy HK. Post-transplantation lymphoproliferative disorder in heart and kidney transplant patients: a single-center experience. *J Cardiovasc Pharmacol Ther* 2006;**11**(1):77–83.

101. Swinnen LJ, Costanzo-Nordin MR, Fisher SG, *et al.* Increased incidence of lymphoproliferative disorder after immunosuppression with the monoclonal antibody OKT3 in cardiac-transplant recipients. *N Engl J Med* 1990;**323**(25):1723–8.

102. Opelz G, Daniel V, Naujokat C, Dohler B. Epidemiology of pretransplant EBV and CMV serostatus in relation to posttransplant non-Hodgkin lymphoma. *Transplantation* 2009;**88**(8):962–7.

103. Penn I. Tumors after renal and cardiac transplantation. *Hematol Oncol Clin North Am* 1993;**7**(2):431–45.

104. Crespo-Leiro MG, Alonso-Pulpon L, Vazquez de Prada JA, *et al.* Malignancy after heart transplantation: incidence, prognosis and risk factors. *Am J Transplant* 2008;**8**(5):1031–9.

50

Revascularization and remodelling surgery

John R. Pepper

Introduction

There is a wide spectrum of clinical presentations of coronary heart disease ranging from mild asymptomatic single-vessel disease, through multivessel disease with mild or moderate left ventricular dysfunction, to severe endstage ischaemic cardiomyopathy. As the severity of left ventricular disease increases, so does the potential benefit of surgical intervention to the patient's outcome. Unfortunately the clarity of the specific indications for coronary artery bypass grafting decreases. For example, in a patient with multivessel coronary artery disease and moderate left ventricular dysfunction, the indications for coronary artery bypass grafting (CABG) are clear and well-defined by multiple large-scale prospective and retrospective studies. In contrast, for a patient with severe ischaemic cardiomyopathy and potentially graftable coronary arteries who is being evaluated for a variety of treatment options including medical treatment, resynchronization therapy, percutaneous coronary intervention, coronary bypass grafting, valvular reconstruction, ventricular remodelling, mechanical assistance, and transplantation, the exact role of CABG is not so clear.

Nevertheless, there is persuasive experimental and clinical evidence that revascularization and perfusion of ischaemic or injured myocardium enhances cardiomyocyte integrity and contractility, thereby augmenting ventricular function. Thus the drive to revascularize is strong. In this high-risk population, the challenge is to identify those patients who will derive the most long-term benefit while incurring the least perioperative risk.

Pathophysiology

The pathophysiology of advanced heart failure (HF) has been extensively reviewed.[1,2] The common pathology in all cases of systolic HF is that of impaired myocyte contractility, activation of the renin–angiotensin–aldosterone and sympathoadrenal systems, leading subsequently to ventricular remodelling: myocyte hypertrophy, fibroblast proliferation, and fibrosis, and eventually to dilatation and increased sphericity of the ventricle. Specific pathological processes are present in ischaemic HF which are relevant to surgical treatment.

Ischaemic HF is brought about by two mechanisms: (1) impaired contractility of poorly perfused regions of myocardium supplied by stenotic coronary arteries, and (2) noncontractile or poorly contractile regions of scarred myocardium following myocardial infarction (MI). Impaired contractility of poorly perfused myocardium due to coronary artery disease was first described by Rahimtoola[3] who coined the term 'hibernating myocardium'. It was suggested that this occurred as a result of cardiomyocytes down-regulating their function and metabolism in the presence of hypoxia, as a means of surviving. More recently, it has been suggested that hibernating myocardium may be a result of repeated episodes of ischaemia causing myocardial stunning.[4] Such ischaemic, hibernating myocardium has been shown to improve its function upon revascularization.

Dilatation of the ventricle

Ventricular dilatation occurs in all cases of HF. The ventricle dilates in an attempt to maintain stroke volume in the setting of decreased myocardial contractility. In the case of ischaemic HF, expansion of the infarct area in the early days of recovery following a moderate-to large-sized MI may be responsible for the initial stages of ventricular dilatation. In the longer term, adverse ventricular remodelling is responsible for continued ventricular dilatation.

Following MI, loss of contractile function in the infarct-related region of the ventricle increases wall stress in the remote myocardium. Myocytes in regions immediately adjacent to the infarct area also become dysfunctional with decreased contractility. Eccentric hypertrophy of myocytes occurs with extra intracellular sarcomeres (contractile proteins) laid down in series.[5] This is thought to be the main mechanism of ventricular dilatation. Slippage of myocytes also occurs and contributes further to ventricular dilatation. This may be due to activation of matrix metalloproteinases (MMPs) which dissolve the intermyofibrillar collagen struts in the extracellular matrix. MMP activation may also be responsible for thinning of the infarcted segment.[5] The result is that the ventricular chamber diameter and volume increases and the ventricle assumes a more spherical shape.[5]

The increase in ventricular chamber diameter results in a raised tension or stress at the ventricular wall to support any given intraventricular pressure. This occurs in accordance with Laplace's law which states that $T = P \times R/2h$ (where T is circumferential ventricular wall stress, P is intraventricular pressure, R is radius of curvature, and h is wall thickness). The increase in ventricular wall stress has several adverse effects: (1) oxygen consumption is increased as the increased wall stress results in the ventricle facing an increased workload at the beginning of systole, (2) subendocardial perfusion is compromised, and (3) myocyte systolic shortening is impaired.[6]

The increase in ventricular diameter further compromises ventricular function. First, the increased ventricular size means that the ventricle operates on a flat portion of the Frank–Starling curve.[5] Secondly, the more spherical shape of the dilated ventricle alters the orientation of myofibrils. Normally most myofibrils lie obliquely to the axis of the heart, such that a 15% shortening during systole achieves a 60% ejection fraction. In the dilated, spherical ventricle, Ingel and colleagues[7] have shown that most of the myofibrils lie in a transverse direction to the axis of the heart and a 15% shortening during systole only achieves an ejection fraction of 30%. The problem is further compounded in areas of infarcted myocardium where nonfunctional myocytes and scar tissue exist. Such areas of akinesia or dyskinesia further compromise the efficiency of ventricular systole.

The increased ventricular wall stress is a potent stimulus for further myocyte hypertrophy. The elongation of myocytes by eccentric hypertrophy is out of proportion to an increase in its thickness by concentric hypertrophy so that ventricular wall stress continues to be significantly raised. Progressive adverse ventricular remodelling occurs as long as ventricular wall stress is raised, leading eventually to endstage HF.[5]

Revascularization of hibernating myocardium

The aim of myocardial revascularization, whether by CABG or percutaneous coronary intervention (PCI), is: (1) to correct myocardial ischaemia and hence prevent further adverse ventricular remodelling and MIs, and (2) to improve myocardial contractility in regions of ischaemic hibernating myocardium that have been shown to be viable.

The determination of hibernating myocardium and viability can be made by stress echocardiography or by various nuclear imaging techniques such as PET, SPECT, or thallium or by cardiovascular magnetic resonance imaging (CMR) with gadolinium enhancement.[8] It has been reported that the improvement in left ventricular function after CABG is related to the number of viable segments present; at least eight viable segments should be present to ensure an absolute improvement in ejection fraction of at least 5%.[9] The early randomized trials of CABG versus medical treatment excluded patients with HF symptoms (NYHA class >II) and those with severe impairment of left ventricular function (ejection fraction <35% in the CASS study and <50% in the ECSS study).[10] Subgroup analysis of 160 trial patients who had an ejection fraction of less than 50% and three-vessel coronary artery disease or proximal left main stem or proximal left anterior descending artery stenosis showed that the 10-year survival in those who had CABG was better compared to those who were treated with medication (79% vs 61%, $p = 0.01$). The survival advantage for CABG was present regardless of the severity of impairment of left ventricular function.

This survival advantage with CABG in patients with impaired left ventricular function has been consistently reported in the other early randomized trials.[11,12] No trial included patients with left ventricular ejection fraction (LVEF) less than 35%, but registry data from CASS[13] and the Duke University Cardiovascular Database[14] indicated that coronary bypass surgery carried a distinct survival advantage in patients with the worst ventricular function, most extensive coronary artery disease, and most severe angina. It should be emphasized that most of these patients presented with angina and not HF. Only 4% of the trial patients had HF symptoms and only 7.2% had an ejection fraction less than 40%. In addition, advances in the medical treatment of advanced HF in the last decade have improved survival significantly. The results of these early randomized studies may therefore not be applicable at the present day in a patient with advanced ischaemic HF, i.e. a patient with NYHA class III and IV HF symptoms and an ejection fraction less than 30%.

Several more recent nonrandomized studies have reported that CABG in patients with advanced ischaemic HF can be performed with an acceptable risk (operative mortality of 1.7–5.3%) and improves ejection fraction by up to 40% above the baseline value. The reported 5-year survival is 60–75%.[15–19] The larger studies are summarized in Table 50.1. Unfortunately, complete data is not reported for many of these studies and the patient population is not uniform across the studies. Hibernation studies were performed preoperatively in some studies[17,18] but not in others.[16] In addition, only 23–43% of patients had HF symptoms preoperatively. Accurate reporting of ventricular function, HF symptoms, and NYHA functional class at late follow-up is absent from most studies. This is important, as many of the benefits noted in the studies may not be sustained at late follow-up. Recurrence of HF symptoms is reported in 53% of patients at 5 years by Luciani.[17] However, only 48% of patients in this study had hibernation studies preoperatively. More favourable results are reported by Lorusso's group[18] which performed hibernation studies in all patients (18% recurrence of HF symptoms at 4 years, 40% at 8 years). Interestingly, the same study reports that left ventricular function, although improving significantly immediately postoperatively (ejection fraction 40 ± 2% compared to 28 ± 9%, $p < 0.01$), subsequently fell at late follow-up and was only marginally better compared to preoperatively (ejection fraction 30 ± 9% compared with 28 ± 9%). This decline in left ventricular function at late follow-up is also reflected in the NYHA functional class (35% in NYHA class III and IV at 8 years compared to 24% immediately postoperatively).

There is some evidence that recurrence of HF symptoms after CABG for ischaemic HF may be related to the severity of ventricular dilatation. Yamaguchi *et al.*[20] reported a recurrence of HF following CABG in 69% of patients when the left ventricular end-systolic volume index (LVESVI) was greater than 100 mL/m^2, compared to only 15% when the LVESVI was less than 100 mL/m^2 ($p < 0.01$). Five-year survival was also worse when LVESVI was greater than 100 mL/m^2 (53.5% vs 85%; $p < 0.01$). Similarly, Louie *et al.*[21] reported a failure of CABG in 27% of patients with

Table 50.1 Results of CABG in ischaemic cardiomyopathy (studies with more than 100 patients)

Study	n	Baseline			Follow-up					Outcome			
		NYHA	EF (%)	LV size	NYHA	EF (%)	LV size	EF change (%)	LV size reduction	Hospital mortality (%)	Event free survival (%)	Actuarial survival (%)	Period (years)
Athanasuleas 2001 (RESTORE Study)	439	N/A	29	LVESVI 109 mL/m^2	N/A	39	LVESVI 69 mL/m^2	10	LVESVI 40 mL/m^2 (37% of baseline)	6.6	85	89.2	1.5
Di Donato 2001	245	N/A	35	LVESVI 112 mL/m^2	N/A	48	LVESVI 46 mL/m^2	13	LVESVI 66 mL/m^2 (59% of baseline)	8.1	98	89.9	1
											95.8	87.7	2
											82.1	74	3
Mickleborough 2004	285	III & IV (83%)	24	LVESVI 97 mL/m^2	III & IV (34%)	34	LVESVI 65 mL/m^2	10	LVESVI 32 mL/m^2 (33% of baseline)	2.8	N/A	92	1
												82	5
												62	10
O'Neill 2006	220	III & IV (66%)	22	LVESVI 120 mL/m^2	III & IV (15%)	32	LVESVI 77 mL/m^2	10	LVESVI 43 mL/m^2 (36% of baseline)	1	N/A	92	1
												90	3
												80	5
Menicanti 2007	488	2.7	33	LVESV 145ml	1.6	40	LVESV 40ml	7	LVESV 105ml (72% of baseline)	4.9	N/A	63	10
Jones 2009 (STICH Trial)	501	III & IV (48%)	28	LVESVI 83 mL/m^2	III & IV (15%)	N/A	LVESVI 67 mL/m^2	N/A	LVESVI 16 mL/m^2 (19% of baseline)	5.2	42	72	4

EF, ejection fraction; LV, left ventricular; NYHA, New York Heart Association class.

ischaemic cardiomyopathy undergoing CABG for HF symptoms, all of whom had a left ventricle that was significantly more dilated compared with those in whom CABG was successful (left ventricular end-diastolic diameter of 81 mm vs 68 mm). In these patients, it may be necessary to perform some form of ventricular restoration surgery in addition to CABG.

Diabetes mellitus in patients with coronary artery disease is associated with a poor outcome. Evidence from the SAVE trial[22] showed that diabetic patients were more prone to HF after MI. But those with diabetes exhibited less left ventricular cavity dilation than control patients without diabetes.[23] In a prospective study of 129 patients (31 diabetic, 98 nondiabetic), Rizello and colleagues[24] assessed myocardial viability before and after myocardial revascularization. LVEF increased in 44% of diabetic and in 40% of nondiabetic patients. LVEF only improved in patients with viable myocardium. Indeed, viability was the only predictor of both early (30 days) and late (5 years) survival.

There has been a widespread reluctance among HF physicians to refer patients with HF for higher-risk coronary surgery, not only because of the lack of a high level of evidence but because of the difficulty in predicting outcome in an individual patient. A recent prospective study from Japan by Mizuno and coworkers[25] studied 31 diabetic and 33 nondiabetic patients with ischaemic cardiomyopathy before and after surgical revascularization. At 6 months after revascularization, subepicardial perfusion was markedly improved in both populations. In contrast, subendocardial perfusion markedly improved only in the nondiabetic patients and was little changed in the diabetic patients. Improvement in left ventricular function was greater in nondiabetics and persistent HF was found more often in the diabetic patients. Diabetes appears to be an important clinical modifier of the remodelling process. This is one of the first studies to demonstrate the intramural heterogeneity of recovery of myocardial perfusion and its relation to persistent HF after surgical revascularization.

Nonrandomized studies have reported that CABG in patients with advanced ischaemic HF can be performed with an acceptable risk and that it improves ejection fraction and NYHA functional class. There is concern that these improvements may not be sustained in the long term and many of these patients have a recurrence of HF symptoms with deterioration in ventricular function within 5 years. Patient selection is crucial and those with severely dilated ventricles may do less well with CABG alone. Of interest, is not only the influence of CABG on long-term survival in patients with advanced ischaemic HF, but also its impact on functional capacity, quality of life, heart function, and whether any benefits are sustained in the long term. Other factors in patient selection may also be important such as the presence of good target coronary vessels for revascularization, complete revascularization, absence of right HF, or raised pulmonary artery pressures.[17,26] In cases where the left ventricle is significantly dilated, e.g. above a LVESVI of 100 mL/m^2, some sort of ventricular restoration surgery may be necessary in addition to myocardial revascularization.

Ventricular restoration

The aim of ventricular restoration is to restore the size, shape, and geometry of the dilated left ventricle towards normal. Restoration of ventricular size reverses many of the pathophysiological processes described earlier by decreasing ventricular wall stress.[27] This in turn enhances myocardial perfusion, decreases oxygen consumption, and enables improved contractility of myocytes. Restoration of ventricular shape and geometry towards a more elliptical structure also leads to greater efficiency of ventricular systole as previously described. Ventricular restoration is achieved by resection of myocardium and reconstructing the remaining ventricle into a more elliptical shape. Several different techniques for ventricular restoration can be used depending on the underlying cause of the cardiomyopathy.

As Buckberg[28] has pointed out, there are certain specific questions that need to be asked before surgical remodelling occurs:

- How much asynergy exists?
- Is there sufficient compensatory muscle to resume function?
- What is the ventricular volume?

Ischaemic cardiomyopathy

Ventricular restoration in ischaemic cardiomyopathy, also referred to as ventricular restoration surgery (VRS), is most commonly performed using the Dor procedure.[29] The modified linear closure technique described by Mickleborough[30] is also sometimes used. The Dor procedure was initially described for the resection of left ventricular aneurysms and was later modified for use in ischaemic cardiomyopathy. Both techniques involve resection of the akinetic or dyskinetic anterior free wall of the left ventricle (Fig. 50.1). Typically, these patients have had an anterior MI with scarring and akinesia or dyskinesia of the left ventricle anterior free wall which may extend on to the septum. This segment of nonfunctional

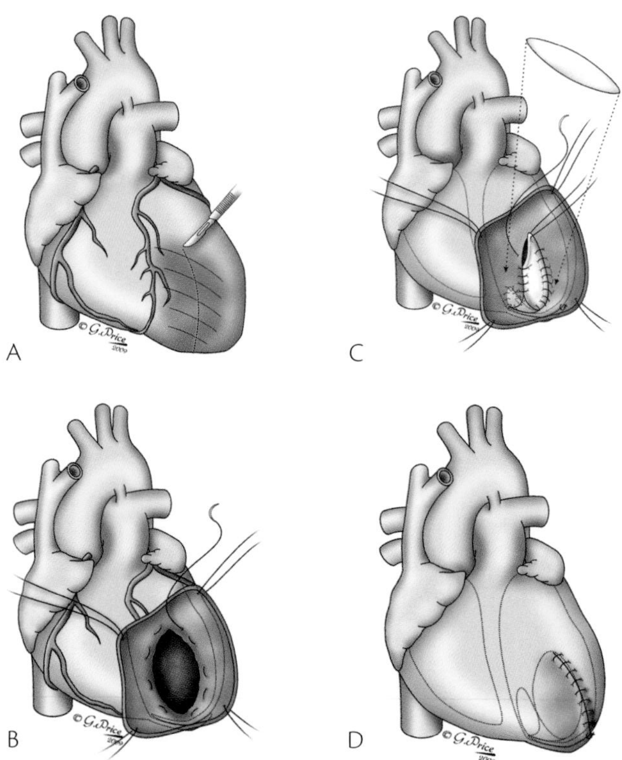

Fig. 50.1 Dor procedure: (A) incision in anterior wall of left ventricle; (B) encircling endoventricular suture to reduce left ventricular volume; (C) placement of oval patch; (D) closure of left ventricle over the patch.

myocardium is resected. In order to reshape the ventricle an endoventricular suture is placed to reduce the size of the defect. This judgement, which will determine the final stroke volume of the left ventricle, can be guided by the use of a balloon of known volume. In the Dor procedure, an oval Dacron patch is then placed which excludes the infarcted part of the septum from the rest of the ventricle. The size of the patch is tailored to the required size of the ventricle, and the shape of the patch is tailored such that it helps restore the geometry of the left ventricle towards a more elliptical configuration (Fig. 50.1b, c). VRS adds about 20 minutes to the duration of an operation for CABG and has not been found to increase the operative risk.[31] CABG is always performed at the same time. The aim is to (1) recruit hibernating myocardium and hence enhance myocardial contractility; (2) resect nonfunctional akinetic or dyskinetic myocardium and hence improve the efficiency of ventricular contraction; and (3) restore the left ventricle to its normal size, shape, and geometry with the benefits discussed previously. In a nonrandomized study involving 814 patients, Dor[32] reported an increase in LVEF from 22% to 38%, and an increase in cardiac index from 1.7 to 2.5 L/min/m^2 following surgery. The operative mortality was 6.6%. Survival at 10 years was 80% in those with an ejection fraction of 30–40% preoperatively and 60% in those with an ejection fraction less than 30%.

Numerous nonrandomized studies have been reported.[33–36] The three larger studies with more than 200 patients each are summarized in Table 50.2. These studies report a hospital mortality of 2.8%-8.1%, an absolute improvement in ejection fraction of 10–13% above baseline (or a relative improvement of up to 40% above baseline), and an improvement in NYHA functional class. The benefits of VRS appear to be sustained. In the RESTORE trial Athanasuleas and coworkers[33] examined how VRS affected early and late survival in postanterior infarction CHF patients. The investigators applied VRS to 1198 postinfarction patients between 1998 and 2008. Anteroseptal, apical, and anterolateral left ventricular scarred segments were identified and excluded by an intracardiac patch. Concomitant procedures included CABG in 95% of patients, mitral valve repair in 22%, and mitral valve replacement in 1%. Overall 30-day mortality after SVR was 5.3% (8.7% with mitral repair vs 4.0% without repair, $p < 0.001$). Perioperative mechanical support was uncommon (<9%). Global systolic function improved postoperatively. Ejection fraction increased from 29.6% ± 11.0% preoperatively to 39.55 ± 12.3% postoperatively ($p < 0.001$). The LVESVI decreased from 80.4 ± 51.4 preoperatively to 56.6 ± 34.3 mL/min postoperatively ($p < 0.001$). Overall 5-year survival was 68.6% ± 2.8%. Logistic regression analysis identified LVEF of <30%, LVESVI of at least 80 mL/min^2, advanced NYHA functional class, and age of at least 75 years as risk factors for death. In this study, 85% of patients were free of congestive HF symptoms at 18 months. Five-year freedom from hospital readmission for CHF was 78%. Similarly, Di Donato[34] reported an event-free survival of 82.1% at 3 years. Actuarial survival was 89.2% at 18 months in the RESTORE study and 74% at 3 years in Di Donato's study.

The results of these nonrandomized studies are encouraging. They suggest that VRS in these very sick patients can be performed with acceptable hospital mortality, and improves ejection fraction and functional capacity. The early results of up to 3 years suggest that the improvement in congestive HF symptoms is sustained. The 3-year actuarial survival also appears impressive considering the patient population. Clearly, patient selection is important. The ideal patient may be one who has had an anterior MI with akinesia or dyskinesia of the left ventricle anterior free wall, dilatation of the

Table 50.2 Results of ventricular restoration surgery in ischaemic cardiomyopathy (studies with more than 100 patients)

Study	n	Baseline		Follow-up			Hospital mortality (%)	Event-free survival (%)	Actuarial survival (%)	Period (years)
		NYHA	EF (%)	NYHA	EF (%)	EF change (%)				
Anderson, 1997	203	III or IV (92%)	34	III & IV (34%)			6.0		87	1
									59	5
									38	7
Trachiotis, 1998	156		<25				3.8		90	1
									64	5
									49	7
									24	10
	588		25–34				3.4		91	1
									75	5
									58	7
									42	10
Luciani, 2000	167	III & IV (24%)	28		38	10	1.7	78	94	1
								47	75	5
								42		7
Lorusso, 2001	120	III & IV (43%)	28	III & IV (24%)	30	2	1.6		80	1
								60	60	8

EF, ejection fraction; NYHA, New York Heart Association class.

left ventricle, good target coronary vessels which can be grafted, and viable hibernating myocardium. The results of VRS may not be as good in patients who have pathology outside the left ventricle such as right ventricular failure or raised pulmonary artery pressures.

The need for a randomized trial has been widely recognized and the design much discussed.[37] The Hypothesis 2 substudy of the Surgical Treatment for Ischemic Heart Failure (STICH) has recently been reported by Jones *et al.*[38] This substudy compared CABG alone with the combined procedure of CABG with surgical ventricular reconstruction. Eligible patients were required to have coronary artery disease amenable to CABG, a LVEF of 35% or less, and a dominant anterior region of myocardial akinesia or dyskinesia that was amenable to surgical ventricular reconstruction. All patients received standard medical and device treatment for HF. In total, 1000 patients were recruited from 96 medical centres in 23 countries. The patients in the two study groups were closely matched for demographic characteristics, comorbidity, the proportion who were on HF drugs, CCS angina class, NYHA class, coronary anatomy, and the extent of anterior myocardial akinesia or dyskinesia. Both groups of patients were equally successful in improving the postoperative CC angina and NYHA class. There was similar improvement in the six-minute walk test and similar reductions in symptoms. As one would expect, there was a greater reduction in the end-systolic volume index with the combined procedure (16 mL/m^2 of body surface area), as compared with CABG alone (5 mL/m^2). Unfortunately these data were obtained from only 373 patients at baseline and at 4 months.

The primary outcome of the trial was a composite of death from any cause or hospitalization for cardiac causes. There was no difference in the occurrence of the primary outcome between the CABG group (59%) and the combined procedure group (58%). The 30-day surgical rates of death for CABG alone (5%) and for the combined procedure (6%) were similar and low overall, and no difference in the rate of death from any cause was observed in a mean follow-up period of 48 months.

On the basis of this trial, Eisen[39] stated in an editorial that the routine use of surgical ventricular reconstruction in addition to CABG cannot be justified. There may be specific subgroups of patients who might benefit from the combined procedure, but such an effect is not apparent so far in the results of the STICH trial and may be difficult to detect, given the heterogeneity of the study population.

There were several major problems with the conduct of this trial.[40] Myocardial viability was assessed in only 20% of the patients, so it is not clear whether the study was examining the treatment of scar tissue or hibernating myocardium. The conduct of the surgery also raises questions: 501 SVR procedures were performed in 127 sites over 5 years, an average of 0.7 SVR operations per site per year. Were steps taken to assure the eligibility of the surgeons and effectiveness of the units? The ESVI was reduced by only 19% in STICH, which compares unfavourably with a 36% reduction in the RESTORE study. In 41% of patients undergoing the Dor procedure in STICH a Dacron patch was not used, whereas in the RESTORE studies all patients received a patch. This raises the question of whether operative procedures were inadequate in a large proportion of the patients randomized to the Dor procedure. Despite the caution of Eisen,[39] it will be important to examine the subgroups in detail to identify those patients who may benefit from the Dor procedure.

Myocardial protection

Effective protection in these operations can be challenging but is essential to prevent the vulnerable left ventricular endocardium from undergoing subendocardial necrosis. A review of protection during the Dor procedure in the 1198-patient RESTORE study[41] showed a fairly even distribution between cold blood cardioplegia and continuous perfusion in the beating heart on cardiopulmonary bypass. The beating heart method was used more frequently in older patients and those with the lowest ejection fractions, larger left ventricular volumes, and more advanced HF. There was a tendency, which did not achieve statistical significance, towards a higher 5-year survival in this subset.

The safety of the beating heart method was shown in acute studies. Preferential subendocardial blood flow occurred during perfusion in chronically dilated hearts, whereas cardioplegia caused diminished subendocardial perfusion. Higher perfusion pressures are required during blood cardioplegia or beating heart methods because of the vascular remodelling which occurs in the coronary bed of failing versus normal hearts.

Flexibility is a critical factor in planning protection strategies in failing hearts.

Ventricular restraint devices

New treatments such as the Acorn CoCap and Paracor cardiac support device (CSD) have been evaluated with respect to their usefulness in limiting adverse ventricular remodelling. Dynamic cardiomyoplasty was the precursor of passive prosthetic ventricular support. Unfortunately the results from animal and clinical studies were inconsistent and limited, despite frequently observed clinical benefit. In a canine model of chronic dilated cardiomyopathy, Patel and colleagues[42] suggested that the haemodynamic benefit of cardiomyoplasty was due to the passive effect of the skeletal muscle wrap around the heart. The relief of wall stress produced by girdling of the conditioned muscle wrap was shown to stabilize the remodelling process of HF, preventing progressive deterioration of systolic and diastolic function. These studies led to the development of a device that would relieve wall stress, similar to the skeletal muscle wrap.

The device that has been studied most extensively is the CorCap CSD (Acorn Cardiovascular Inc., St. Paul, Minnesota, USA) It is a multifilament polyester mesh implant which is placed around both ventricles to decrease diastolic wall stress without resultant constriction (Fig. 50.2). Mann and colleagues[43] assessed the safety and efficacy of the CSD in 300 patients with HF. Of the 300 patients enrolled, 193 were randomized to mitral surgery alone or mitral surgery plus CSD. The 107 patients who did not need mitral surgery were randomized to medical treatment or medical treatment plus CSD. The primary endpoint was a composite based on changes in clinical status, the need for major cardiac procedures for worsening HF, and a change in NYHA class. All patients had an LVEF of less than 35%, a LVEDD of 60 mm or greater, and a six-minute walk test of less than 450 m. The proportional odds ratio for the primary endpoint favoured treatment with the CSD (1.73; 95% CI 1.07–2.79; $p = 0.024$). When compared with the baseline, LVEF increased significantly at 12 months ($p = 0.0009$) in the CSD-treated group compared with controls ($p = 0.65$), but the changes in LVEF between groups were not significant ($p = 0.45$). Therefore the CorCap CSD may have a role in preventing adverse

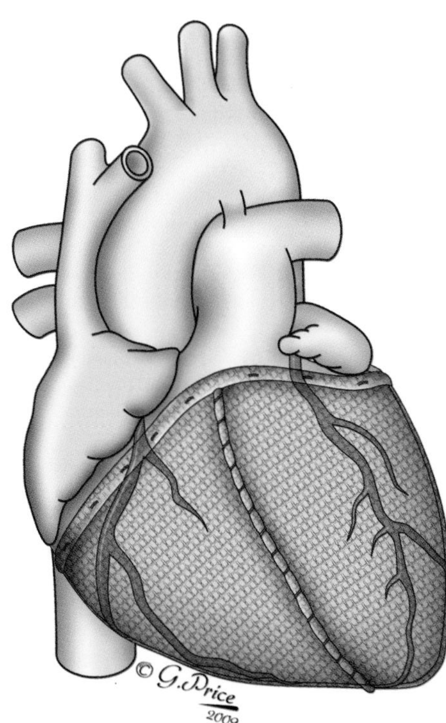

Fig. 50.2 Acorn restratint device: the left and right ventricles are enclosed in a polyester mesh.

remodelling after MI. It requires an operation for its insertion but this could be through a small anterior thoracotomy.

A more recent development, the Paracor device, is currently being assessed in clinical trials in Europe and the United States. This is an elastic nitinol mesh that is designed to mechanically reinforce the heart to retard or hopefully halt the remodelling process. It can be deployed in a minimally invasive fashion. Klodell and coworkers have reported their early results.[44] Fifty patients in NYHA class II or III underwent the procedure, which was well tolerated. At 6 months there was a significant improvement in the six-minute walk (+65.7 m, $p = 0.002$) and Minnesota Living with Heart Failure scores (−15.7, $p = 0.002$). Long-term functional results are not yet available.

Conclusion

Recent advances in medical treatment have greatly improved symptom control and survival in HF, but morbidity and mortality continue to remain significant especially in the advanced stages of HF. This may be because medical treatment alone neither corrects the cause, nor reverses all of the pathophysiological changes that occur in advanced HF, especially those related to ventricular dilatation and alteration in the geometry of the ventricle. It is likely that significant numbers of patients with advanced HF, especially that due to ischaemic heart disease, will benefit from surgery. A combination of surgical treatments may be necessary depending on the pathological changes present.

Clinical studies on revascularization of ischaemic, hibernating myocardium are promising but more randomized studies are needed to confirm its long-term efficacy. Similarly, large non randomized studies have shown that VRS combined with CABG in ischaemic cardiomyopathy improves cardiac function and functional capacity and may improve survival. The results of the STICH trial were disappointing, but the design of the trial has been heavily criticized.

Advanced HF is a complex disease leading to many different pathologies and the ideal treatment for each patient may need to be tailored individually. Some patients may need a combination of different treatments. The armamentarium is enlarging and the future appears promising for these very sick patients.

References

1. Beltrami CA, Finato N, Rocco M, *et al.* The cellular basis of dilated cardiomyopathy in humans. *J Mol Cell Cardiol* 1995;**27**:291–305.
2. Nadal-Ginard B, Kajstura J, Leri A, *et al.* Myocyte death, growth and regeneration in cardiac hypertrophy and failure. *Circ Res* 2003;**92**:139–50.
3. Rahimtoola SH. The hibernating myocardium. *Am Heart J* 1989;**95**:204–9.
4. Wijns W, Vatner SF, Camici PG. Hibernating myocardium. *N Engl J Med* 1998;**339**:173–81.
5. Baig MK, Mahon, McKenna WJ, *et al.* The pathophysiology of advanced heart failure. *Am Heart J* 1998;**135**: S216–30.
6. Bogaert J, Bosmans H, Maes A, Suetens P, Marchal G, Rademakers FE. Remote myocardial dysfunction after acute anterior myocardial infarction: impact of left ventricular shape on regional function: a magnetic resonance myocardial tagging study. *J Am Coll Cardiol* 2000;**35**:1525–34.
7. Ingel NB Jr. Myocardial fibre architecture and left ventricular function. *Technol Health Care* 1997;**5**:45–52.
8. Chareonthaitawee P, Gersh BJ, Arooz PA, Gibbons RJ. Revascularisation in severe left ventricular dysfunction: the role of viability testing. *J Am Coll Cardiol* 2005;**46**:567–74.
9. Pagano D, Townend JN, Littler WA, Horton R, Camici PG, Bonser RS. Coronary artery bypass surgery as treatment for ischemic heart failure: the predictive value of viability assessment with quantitative positron emission tomography for symptomatic and functional outcome. *J Thorac Cardiovasc Surg* 1998;**115**:791–9.
10. Yusuf S. Effect of coronary artery bypass grafting on survival: overview of 10-year results from randomised trials by the Coronary Artery Bypass Graft Trialist Collaboration. *Lancet* 1994;**344**:563–70.
11. Rahimtoola SH. A perspective on the three large multicenter randomised clinical trials of coronary artery bypass surgery for chronic stable angina. *Circulation* 1985;**73**(Suppl V):123–35.
12. Passamani E, Davis KB, Gillespie MJ, *et al.* A randomised trial of coronary artery bypass surgery: survival of patients with low ejection fraction. *N Engl J Med* 1985;**312**:1665–71.
13. Alderman EL, Fisher LD, Litwin P, *et al.* Results of coronary artery surgery in patients with poor left ventricular function (CASS). *Circulation* 1983;**68**:785–95.
14. Bounous EP, Mark DB, Pollock BG, *et al.* Surgical survival benefits for coronary disease patients with left ventricular dysfunction. *Circulation* 1988;**78**(Suppl III):1151–7.
15. Tolis GA, Korkolis DP, Kopf GS, Elefteriades JA. Revascularisation alone (without mitral valve repair) suffices in patients with advanced ischemic cardiomyopathy and mild to moderate mitral regurgitation. *Ann Thorac Surg* 2002;**74**:1476–81.
16. Trachiotis GD, Weintraub WS, Johnston TS, Jones EL, Guyton RA, Craver JM. Coronary artery bypass grafting in patients with advanced left ventricular dysfunction. *Ann Thorac Surg* 1998;**66**:1632–9.
17. Luciani GB, Montalbano G, Casali G, Mazzucco A. Predicting long-term functional results after myocardial revascularisation in ischaemic cardiomyopathy. *J Thorac Cardiovasc Surg* 2000;**120**:478–89.
18. Lorusso R, La Canna G, Ceconi C, *et al.* Long-term results of coronary artery bypass grafting procedure in the presence of left ventricular dysfunction and hibernating myocardium. *Eur J Cardiothorac Surg* 2001;**20**:937–48.

19. Elefteriades J, Edwards R. Coronary bypass in left heart failure. *Semin Thorac Cardiovasc Surg* 2002;**14**:125–32.
20. Yamaguchi A, Ino T, Adachi H, *et al.* Left ventricular volume predicts postoperative course in patients with ischaemic cardiomyopathy. *Ann Thorac Surg* 1997;**65**:434–8.
21. Louie HW, Laks H, Milgalter E, Drinkwater D, Hamilton M, Brunken R, Stevenson L. Ischaemic cardiomyopathy. Criteria for coronary revascularisation and cardiac transplantation. *Circulation* 1991;**94**(suppl III):290–5.
22. Pfeffer MA, Braunwald E, Moye LA, Basta L, Brown EJ Jr, Cuddy TE. Effect of captopril on mortality and morbidity in patients with left ventricular dysfunction after myocardial infarction: results of the survival and ventricular enlargement trial. The SAVE Investigators. *N Engl J Med* 1992;**327**:669–77.
23. Solomon SD, St John SM, Lamas GA, *et al.* Ventricular remodelling does not accompany the development of heart failure in diabetic patients after myocardial infarction. *Circulation* 2002;**106**:1251–5.
24. Rizello V, Poldermans D, Biagini E, *et al.* Benefits of coronary revascularisation in diabetic and non-diabetic patients with ischaemic cardiomyopathy: role of myocardial viability. *Eur J Heart Fail* 2006;**8**:314–20.
25. Mizuno R, Fujimoto S, Saito Y, Nakamura S. Depressed recovery of subendocardial perfusion in persistent heart failure after complete revascularisation in diabetic patients with hibernating myocardium. *Heart* 2009;**95**:830–4.
26. Jones EL, Weintraub WS. The importance of completeness of revascularisation during long-term follow up after coronary artery operations. *J Thorac Cardiovasc Surg* 1996;**112**:227–37.
27. Schenk S, McCarthy PM, Starling RC, *et al.* Neurohormonal response to left ventricular reconstruction surgery in ischaemic cardiomyopathy. *J Thorac Cardiovasc Surg* 2004;**128**:38–43.
28. Buckberg GD. Congestive heart failure: treat the disease, not the symptom return to normalcy. *J Thorac Cardiovasc Surg* 2001;**121**(4):628–37.
29. Dor V, Kreitmann P, Jourdan J. Interest of 'physiological' closure (circumferential plasty on contractive areas) of left ventricle after resection and endocardiectomy for aneurysm or akinetic zone comparison with classical technique about a series of 209 left ventricular resections. *J Cardiovasc Surg* 1985;**26**:73.
30. Mickleborough LL, Carson S, Ivanov J. Repair of dyskinetic or akinetic left ventricular aneurysm: results obtained with a modified linear closure. *J Thorac Cardiovasc Surg* 2001;**121**:675–82.
31. Maxey TS, Reece TB, Ellman PL, *et al.* Coronary artery bypass with ventricular restoration is superior to coronary artery bypass alone in patients with ischemic cardiomyopathy. *J Thorac Cardiovasc Surg* 2004;**127**:428–34.
32. Dor V, Di Donato, Sabatier M, Montiglio F, Civaia F;RESTORE Group. Left ventricular reconstruction by endoventricular circular patch plasty repair: a 17 year experience. *Semin Thorac Cardiovasc Surg* 2001;**13**:435–47.
33. Athanasuleas CL, Stanley AW Jr, Buckberg GD, Dor V, DiDonato M, Blackstone EH. Surgical anterior ventricular endocardial restoration (SAVER) in the dilated remodelled ventricle after anterior myocardial infarction. RESTORE group. Reconstructive Endoventricular Surgery, returning Torsion Original Radius Elliptical Shape to LV. *J Am Coll Cardiol* 2001;**37**(5):1210–13.
34. Di Donato M, Toso A, Maioli M, Sabatier M, Stanley AWH, Dor V, RESTORE Group. Intermediate survival and predictors of death after ventricular restoration. *Semin Thorac Cardiovasc Surg* 2001;**13**(4):468–475.
35. Mickleborough LL, Merchant N, Ivanov J, Rao V, Carson S. Left ventricular reconstruction: early and late results. *J Thorac Cardiovasc Surg* 2004;**128**(1):27–37.
36. Suma H, Isomura T, Horii T, Hisatomi K. Left ventriculoplasty for ischemic cardiomyopathy. *Eur J Cardiothorac Surg* 2001;**20**:319–23.
37. Velazquez EJ, Lee KL, O'Connor CM, *et al.* Rationale and design of the Surgical Treatment for Ischemic Heart Failure (STICH) Trial. *J Thorac Cardiovasc Surg* 2007;**134**:1540–7.
38. Jones RH, Velazquez EJ, Michler RE, *et al.*, for the STICH Hypothesis 2 Investigators. *N Engl J Med* 2009;**360**:1705–17.
39. Eisen HJ. Surgical ventricular reconstruction for heart failure. *N Engl J Med* 2009;**360**:1781–4.
40. Buckberg GD. Questions and answers about the STICH trial: a different perspective. *J Thorac Cardiovasc Surg* 2005;**130**:245–9.
41. Athanasuleas C, Siles W, Buckberg G, and the RESTORE Group. Myocardial protection during surgical ventricular restoration. *Eur J Cardiothorac Surg* 2006;**295**: S231–7.
42. Patel HJ, Polidori DJ, Pilla JJ, *et al.* Stabilisation of chronic remodelling by asynchronous cardiomyoplasty in dilated cardiomyopathy: effects of a conditioned muscle wrap. *Circulation* 1997;**96**:3665–71.
43. Mann DL, Acker MA, Jessup M. Acorn Trial Principal Investigators and Study Coordinators. Clinical evaluation of the CorCap cardiac support device in patients with dilated cardiomyopathy. *Ann Thorac Surg* 2007;**84**:1226–35.
44. Klodell CT, Aranda JM, McGiffin DC, *et al.* Worldwide surgical experience with the Paracor HeartNet cardiac restraint device. *J Thorac Cardiovasc Surg* 2008;**135**:188–95.

51

Ventricular assist devices, including intra-aortic balloon pumps

Emma J. Birks and Mark S. Slaughter

Heart failure (HF) is a major problem associated with high morbidity and mortality, and the prognosis from heart failure is worse than that for myocardial infarction or carcinoma of the bowel, breast, or prostate.[1] Medical therapy with ACE inhibitors, β-blockers, angiotensin 2 inhibitors, and aldosterone antagonists, together with resynchronization therapy, has improved the survival of many with HF, but there remain a large group of patients who, despite optimal medical therapy, are in NYHA class III/IV HF with a very poor prognosis. Unfortunately the numbers of useable donor hearts available to perform heart transplantation for these patients has significantly decreased over recent years and the number is totally inadequate for the population who require heart transplantation.

Left ventricular assist devices (LVADs) are rapidly evolving and are being increasingly used to treat patients with advanced HF. They are very efficient artificial hearts that assist the circulation and they are being inserted into an increasing number of patients with advanced HF. The LVAD technology itself is also evolving very quickly. They were initially inserted as a bridge to transplantation in patients with advanced HF with deteriorating clinical status who were unable to wait any longer for heart transplantation. They were mostly inserted into patients who, despite inotropic ± intra-aortic balloon pump (IABP) support, had deteriorating NYHA class IV HF and usually also end-organ dysfunction. Not only are LVADs life saving in these deteriorating patients who might otherwise die before a donor heart becomes available, but they also improve secondary organ function prior to transplantation, reduce pulmonary hypertension, and allow for improvement of nutritional status. The decrease in donors means that an increasing number of patients have been requiring support with a LVAD for survival when their clinical status deteriorates.

There is also now compelling evidence that with LVAD unloading, recovery of the patient's myocardial function can occur, this can be sufficient to allow device removal and avoid the need for transplantation (together with immunosuppression and its associated complications) and leave the patient with an excellent quality of life. This means that the precious resource of a donor organ can be used for another needy individual. This indication, known as 'bridge to recovery' is a newer and expanding indication.

The future use of these devices, however, particularly as survival continues to increase, is their much wider use as destination therapy. This means the insertion of the device lifelong as an alternative to transplantation. The current generation of devices are much more durable than their predecessors and have a lower complication rate, hence patients can be maintained on them for much longer with lower morbidity and destination therapy has now become a very realistic option for these patients to expand rather than replace the pool of patients that can be treated.

Early referral of the deteriorating patient and insertion of the LVAD before the onset of severe end-organ dysfunction is extremely important. Factors affecting early survival and reversal of organ dysfunction include chronicity of disease, intrinsic end-organ functional reserve, comorbid conditions, and age. Early intervention improves outcome enormously—the stress of surgery superimposed on a fragile patient with advanced disease contributes to poor outcomes in the short and the long term.

Intra-aortic balloon pumps

The IABP is the most commonly used cardiac assist device. The major physiological effects of the IABP are reduction of left ventricular afterload and an increase in aortic root coronary perfusion pressure. Cardiac output increases because of improved myocardial contractility brought about by increased coronary blood flow and reduced afterload and preload. Several variables are known to affect the physiological performance of the IABP in clinical practice, including location, timing, cardiac rhythm, and blood pressure. The position of the balloon should be just downstream of the left subclavian artery, and the balloon should fit the aorta so that during inflation it nearly occludes the vessel. For adults balloon volumes of 30–40 mL significantly improve both left ventricular unloading and diastolic coronary perfusion pressure over smaller volumes. Inflation should be timed to coincide with closure of the aortic valve, which, for clinical purposes, is the dicrotic notch of the aortic blood pressure trace. Deflation should occur as late as possible to maintain the duration of the augmented diastolic blood pressure but before the aortic valve opens and the ventricle ejects. For practical purposes, deflation is timed to occur with the onset of the electrocardiographic R wave. Optimal performance requires a regular heart rate with an easily identified R wave or a good arterial pulse tracing with a discrete aortic dicrotic notch. Balloon pumps trigger from the R wave or from the arterial pressure tracing. During tachycardia the IABP should be timed to inflate every other beat. Every effort should be made to establish a regular rhythm so that the IABP can be timed properly.

The IABP is usually inserted into the common femoral artery either by the percutaneous technique or by surgical cut-down. The balloon should be positioned so that when it is inflated it does not occlude the left subclavian artery. Intravenous heparin is given while the patient is on the IABP. When removing a percutaneously inserted IABP pressure should be applied to the puncture site for at least 30 min to obtain haemostasis. Complications from the use of the IABP include leg ischaemia, infection at the insertion site, bleeding, and rarely balloon rupture, thrombosis within the balloon, sepsis, false aneurysm, lymph fistula, and femoral neuropathy.

A meta-analysis of controlled trials of IABP counterpulsation versus percutaneous LVADs for the treatment of cardiogenic shock recently showed[2] that after device implantation, percutaneous LVAD patients had a higher cardiac index and mean arterial pressure and lower pulmonary capillary wedge pressure (PCWP) than IABP patients. However, a similar 30-day mortality was observed using percutaneous LVAD compared to IABP and no significant difference was observed in the incidence of leg ischaemia. Bleeding was more significantly observed in the patients receiving percutaneous LVAD. Hence although percutaneous LVAD provides superior haemodynamic support in patients with cardiogenic shock compared to IABP, the use of these more powerful devices did not improve early survival, suggesting these results do not yet support percutaneous LVAD as a first-choice approach in the medical management of cardiogenic shock.

Ventricular assist devices

The devices used have evolved over the years and are still rapidly evolving. They can broadly be divided into first-, second-, and third-generation devices according to their principle of operation.

First-generation devices

The first-generation devices are pulsatile positive displacement pumps, the main ones being the Heartmate I, Thoratec PVAD, and Novacor. The Heartmate I, which has been inserted in over 5000 patients, is made of titanium with a polyurethane diaphragm and has a pusher-plate actuator; it can be powered pneumatically or electrically. A cannula is placed in the apex of the left ventricle and blood flows through a Dacron conduit, in which there is a porcine valve, to the pump and returns into a Dacron outflow graft through another porcine valve and returns to the ascending aorta (Fig. 51.1). The Heartmate I is unique because its blood pumping surface consists of titanium microspheres and a fibrillar textured inner surface that promotes the formation of a 'pseudointima' that seems to resist thrombogenesis. This means that the only anticoagulant with this pump needed is aspirin. Power is supplied by two external batteries (approximately the size of videocamera batteries) and an external controller that weighs less than 300 g, via a driveline that passes through the skin. The pumping can be performed in either a fixed-rate mode or an automatic mode in which stroke volume is maintained at 97% full and the rate is varied in response to preload. This device can pump up to 10 L/min. The Heartmate I has undergone several design improvements and evolved from the pneumatic to the vented electric (VE) to the XVE. The current XVE has had several design improvements compared to the earlier version—a strengthened percutaneous lead to reduce kinking and occlusion and improve fatigue resistance, a bend relief for the outflow graft to prevent kinking and repositioning to prevent the diaphragm 'buckling,' a major cause of diaphragm rupture. The valves have also been modified to prevent commissural dehiscence and incompetence, which previously limited the lifespan of the pump.

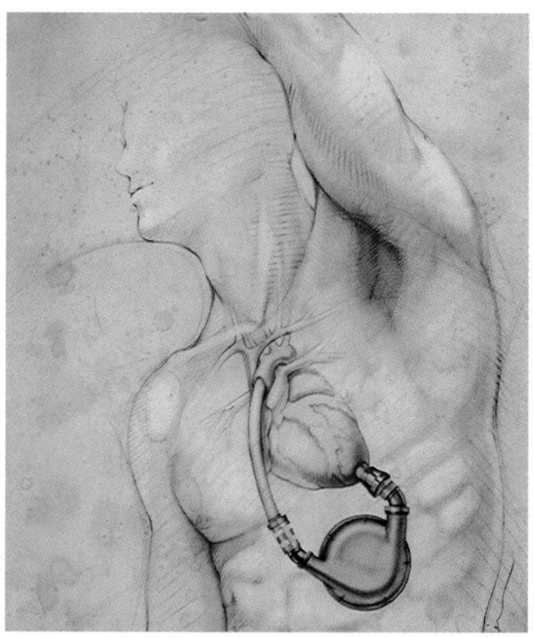

Fig. 51.1 The Heartmate I pulsatile left ventricular assist device drains blood from the failing left ventricle through the inlet cannula to the pump and back to the aorta.

The Thoratec paracorporeal ventricular assist device (PVAD) has been inserted in over 3000 patients; it has a 65-mL stroke volume pumping chamber and two mechanical valves. It has the advantage that it can be used as an LVAD or RVAD, or two together as a BIVAD. Alternating positive and negative air pressure by a console or portable pneumatic driver produces a beat rate of 40–110 beats/min and a flow rate of 1.3–7.2 L/min. The PVAD is positioned outside the body (paracorporeal) on the anterior abdominal wall with cannulas crossing into the chest wall. Warfarin (INR 2.5–3.5) and aspirin anticoagulation is required for this pump. There is also now an implantable version of this pump, the

IVAD. The Novacor LVAD was implanted in over 1600 patients for durations of up to 6.1 years but has now been discontinued.

The pulsatile volume-displacement devices provide excellent haemodynamic support and improve survival but have constraints, particularly the need for extensive surgical dissection, the presence of a large-diameter lead (which is more prone to infection), an audible pump, the need for medium–large body habitus, and quite limited long-term durability. Hence, although many of the original publications are about patients receiving these devices, they are being used less now.

Second-generation devices

The second-generation axial flow pump devices are being inreasingly used now. These are continuous-flow rotary pumps that have only one moving part, the rotor, unlike the the first-generation devices (and hence are more durable). They are also smaller (principally through elimination of the blood sac or reservoir necessary for a pulsatile system), quieter, and tend to have a less traumatic surgical implantation. They have smaller drivelines and hence tend to have lower rates of driveline infection.

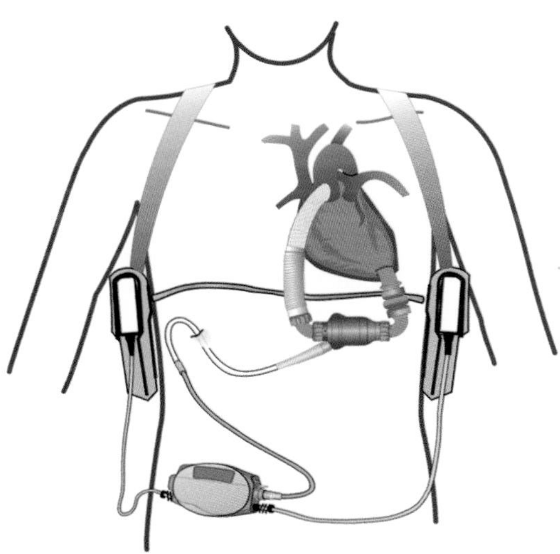

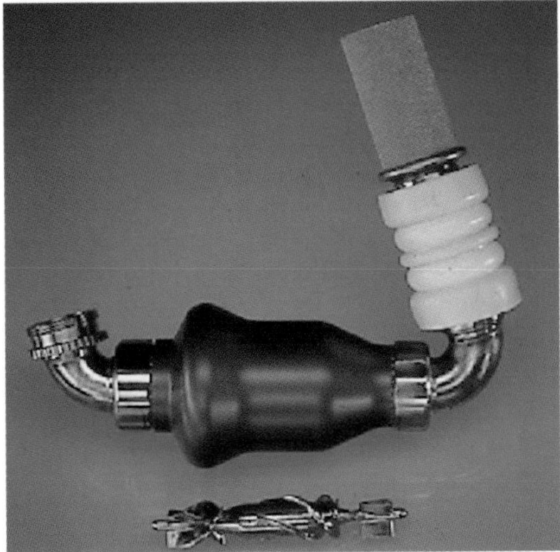

Fig. 51.2 The Heartmate II axial flow left ventricular assist device.

The Heartmate II device is a continuous-flow axial blood pump (Fig. 51.2) with an internal rotor with helical blades that curve around a central shaft. As the blood flows around the pump rotor, the spinning action of the rotor, with its three curving blades, introduces a radial or tangential velocity to the blood flow and imparts kinetic energy to the blood, which then flows past the outlet stator vanes. The twisted shape of the outlet stator vanes converts the radial velocity of the blood flow to an axial direction. The pump weighs 350 g and measures approximately 7.0 cm in length and 4.0 cm at its largest diameter. It can generate up to 10 L/min of flow at a pressure of 100 mmHg. The axial-flow design and absence of blood sac eliminates the need for venting (currently required for the first generation of implantable pumps) thus reducing the size of the percutaneous drive lead and also eliminating the need for internal one-way valves. Again blood drains through the inflow cannula in the apex of the LV to the pump and returns back to the ascending aorta (Fig. 51.2).

The Jarvik 2000 is an axial-flow continuous-flow pump which has an intraventricular position with the whole pump sitting within the left ventricular cavity (Fig. 51.3). The pump weighs 85 g, measures 2.4 cm in diameter and is 5.5 cm long. The single moving component is the impeller located in the centre of the titanium housing. A brushless direct-current motor, contained within the housing, creates the electromagnetic force necessary to rotate the impeller. Blood flow is directed through the outlet graft by stator blades located near the pump outlet and it returns to either the ascending or descending aorta. The pump can generate up to 7 L/min maximum. Pump implantation with the outlet graft in the descending aorta can result in stasis and clot formation in the aortic root, hence an intermittent low-speed controller can be used which drops the pump speed for 9 s every minute to allow the aortic valve to open. Furthermore, many units anastomose the graft to the ascending and not the descending aorta, resulting in few static complications in patients implanted in this way.[3] Because this pump has no pocket, serious pump infections are rare.

The Berlin Heart Incor is also an axial-flow pump. As blood passes into the Incor it first passes the inducer, which guides the laminar flow on to the actual impeller, which is suspended by a magnetic bearing and floats free of contact with other parts. The impeller operates between speeds of 5000 and 10 000 rotations/min. The stationary diffuser behind the rotor has specially aligned blades which reduce the rotational effect of the blood flow and adds additional pressure to assist the transport of blood in the outflow cannula to the aorta.

The MicroMed-De-Bakey VAD is another axial-flow rotary pump. It has an elbow-shaped inflow cannula that inserts into the apex of the left ventricle, a pump housing unit that houses the impeller (which is actuated by an electromagnet), a Dacron outflow conduit graft and an ultrasonic flow probe that encircles the outflow graft and provides direct, online measurements of pump flow.

Third-generation devices

Heartware and Duraheart are magnetic levitation third-generation pumps that are now being tested in clinical use. Heartware (Fig. 51.4) is a centrifugal pump that has only one moving part, the

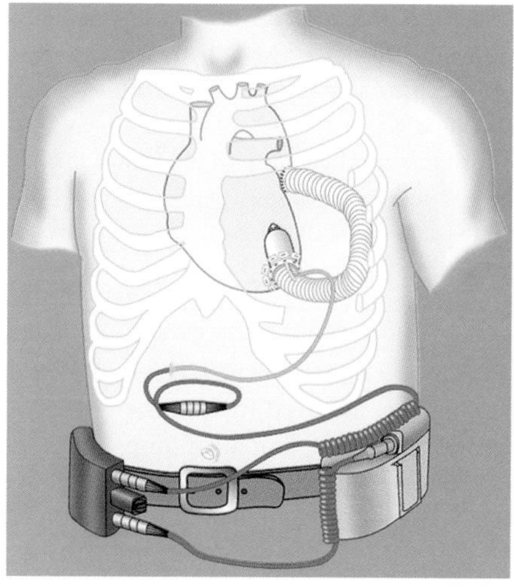

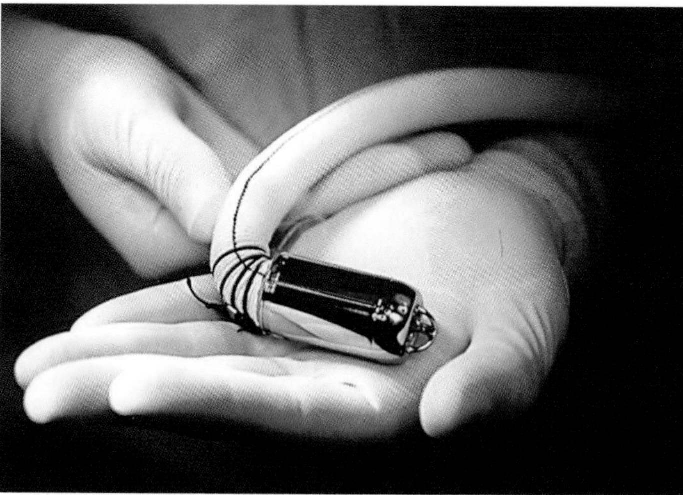

Fig. 51.3 The Jarvik 2000 left ventricular assist device. Note the intraventricular position of the device.

impeller, and no mechanical bearings. The impeller spins at rates between 2000 and 3000 rotations/min to generate up to 10 L/min of blood flow. The total size is equivalent to 50 mL, making it implantable in the pericardial space, directly adjacent to the heart. The impeller is suspended within the pump housing through a combination of passive magnets and a hydrodynamic thrust bearing. This hydrodynamic suspension is achieved by a gentle incline on the upper surfaces of the impeller blades. When the impeller spins, blood flows across these inclined surfaces, creating a 'cushion' between the impeller and the pump housing. At no point is there contact between the impeller and the housing chamber. Device reliability is enhanced through the use of dual motor stators with independent drive circuitry, allowing a seamless transition between dual- and single-stator mode if required. The inflow cannula is integrated with the device itself, ensuring proximity between the heart and the pumping mechanism and hence facilitating ease of implant and ensuring optimal blood flow characteristics. The impeller has a wide blade to help minimize risk of pump-induced haemolysis or thrombus.

Because Heartware has no bearings and runs at a lower rotation rate it is likely to have a very long durability; it is also much smaller than previous devices and easier to implant surgically. HeartWare remains under investigation, and although it has been awarded the CE trademark, its use in the United States has not yet been approved by the Food and Drug Administration (FDA). The Duarheart also incorporates a centrifugal-flow rotary pump with an active magnetically levitated impeller featuring three position sensors and magnetic coils that optimize blood flow, while minimizing device wear and tear. It is also undergoing US bridge to transplant trials. Although these third-generation devices are only just starting to be used, they are anticipated to last for 5–10 years. Smaller versions of the third-generation devices are currently in development and undergoing animal testing.

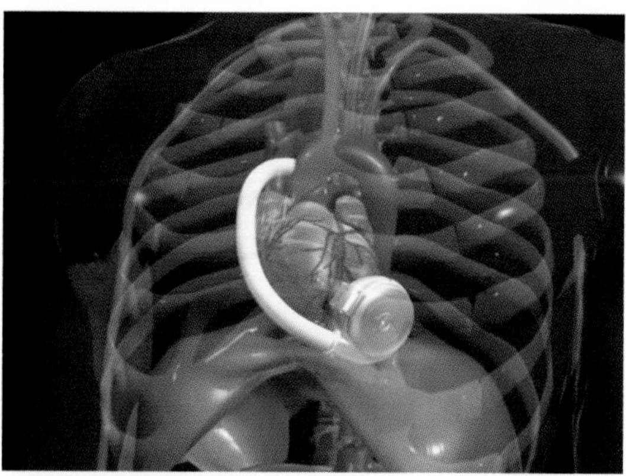

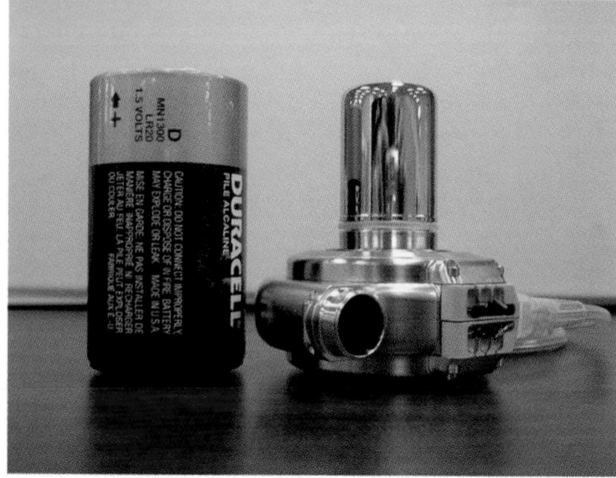

Fig. 51.4 The Heartware magnetic levitation left ventricular assist device.

Clinical role of ventricular assist devices

LVADs are being increasingly inserted into patients with advanced HF. Initially this was mainly as a bridge to transplant, but now it is also as a bridge to recovery and increasingly is likely to be as destination therapy.

Bridge to transplantation

For patients with advanced medical urgency status 1A (United Network for Organ Sharing classification) the death rate in 1999 was 58% compared to 20% for medical urgency status 1B and 13% for regular urgency status 2.[4] Hence LVAD- and inotrope-supported patients stand to gain most from transplantation. LVAD insertion for bridge to transplantation is usually considered either because of cardiogenic shock and deteriorating clinical status (when it is felt the patient will not survive long enough to receive a donor organ) or if the patient develops secondary organ dysfunction such that transplantation becomes contraindicated. Support from the device allows renal function, nutritional status, and pulmonary vascular resistance to improve for subsequent transplantation which usually takes several weeks or months. Transplantation should only be considered once these improvements have occurred.

In the multicentre evaluation of the Heartmate VE LVAD as a bridge to transplantation 71% of 280 patients survived to transplantation or device removal,[5] and in the Cleveland Clinic experience of 277 LVADs 69% survived to transplantation.[6] From 60% to 75% survival to transplantation has been reported in other early series.[7,8] However, these data are all from the first-generation pumps which are associated with higher mortality.

Data are now becoming available from the second-generation pumps, which would be expected to have a better outcome because of their smaller size, easier surgical implantation, and lower complication rates. Miller *et al.*[9] published a prospective multicentre study of 133 NYHA class IV patients on a transplant waiting list who underwent implantation of a Heartmate II device as a bridge to transplantation. All were on inotropic support (except 11% who were intolerant because of arrythmias) and 41% were also IABP-dependent. After 180 days, 100 (75%) patients had reached the principal outcome of transplantation, recovery, or survival on ongoing support with eligibility for transplantation. Patients on Heartmate II support had improvement in NYHA class, six-minute walk time, functional status, and quality of life. An additional 5 (4%) were alive and ongoing but not yet eligible for transplantation and another 3 (2%) were alive but had had a device replacement, i.e. overall survival was 81% at 6 months. Interestingly, 4 patients removed themselves from the transplant waiting list as they preferred to continue mechanical support. The overall survival of patients who underwent transplantation, recovered their cardiac function, or continued to receive mechanical circulatory support while remaining a candidate for transplantation was estimated to be 70% at 1 year.[9] These 133 patients, enrolled from March 2005 to May 2006, represented the primary cohort. Enrolment continued after this, and Pagani *et al.*[10] published the results of 281 of 469 patients enrolled by April 2008 who had completed study endpoints or had at least 18 months of follow-up with ongoing device support. Of these, 79% had either received a transplant, been explanted due to myocardial recovery, or remained alive on a VAD at 18 months. Of the 55.8% (n = 157) who received a transplant, post-transplant survival was 96% at 30 days and 86% at 1 year. During the study period 78% of patients were discharged from the hospital with a VAD, after a median postsurgery stay of 25 days.

Data are beginning to emerge for the third-generation devices. Thirty-five patients who received the Duraheart had an actuarial survival of 78% at 2 years and 86% of 1-month survivors were discharged home.[11] Fifty patients have received the Heartware device in Europe and Australia with a 96% 30-day and 86% 1-year survival[12] compared to a predicted survival in the same 50 patients if treated with medical therapy of 93% at 30 days and 57% at 1 year.

An analysis[13] of 48 982 patients on the transplant waiting list in the United States between 1990 and 2005 (era 1, 1990–4; era 2, 1995–9; era 3, 2000–5) showed that between eras 1 and 3 (i.e. between 1990 and 2005) the 1-year survival on the heart transplant waiting list has improved from 49.5% to 69% for status 1 patients, i.e. those who require continuous inotropic or mechanical circulatory support (IABP, LVAD, ECMO, total artificial heart) or ventilation, have a life expectancy <7 days without transplantation, or are considered a justifiable exceptional case. For status 2 candidates (those who meet the general criteria for heart transplantation but do not meet status 1 criteria) the 1-year survival improved from 81.8% to 89.4% over the same period. For status 2 candidates, demographics, aetiology, and markers of severe HF did not substantially change throughout the period, indicating that improved outcomes most likely represent improvements in HF therapy. In the current era of medical therapy, the 1-year survival of status 2 candidates without transplantation (81.4%) is approaching the outcome of heart transplantation,[14] although it should be remembered that 40% of status 2 candidates listed in the early 2000s worsened and required upgrading to status 1.[15] In the most recent era (2000–5) the majority of patients listed as UNOS status I candidates were hospitalized at the time of listing (82%), including 56% in the intensive care unit (ICU). The majority (71%) required continuous inotropic infusions or balloon pump support (12%) or were on mechanical circulatory support (23%). In comparison, in era 1 (1990–5), although 87% were hospitalized, only 20% were in the ICU, 14.6% required inotropes, 3.4% required balloon pump support, and 8.4% were on mechanical circulatory support. Despite the improvements in survival of transplant candidates, the survival of status 1 patients continues to depend on urgent cardiac replacement therapy: 52.4% of those listed between 2000 and 2005 died within 6 months without heart transplantation. Although the use of mechanical circulatory support has increased and the presence of mechanical circulatory support on the day of listing as a bridge to heart transplantation had increased from 8.4% in era 1 to 22.8% in era 3, given the high 6-month mortality in this group without heart transplantation, it is likely that mechanical circulatory support is still being very underused in this population.

Bridge to recovery

A small number of patients supported with a LVAD have shown significant improvement in their myocardial function [16] and there is now compelling evidence that prolonged near-complete unloading of the left ventricle with the use of an LVAD is associated with structural reverse remodelling that can be accompanied by functional improvement.[17] This can be sufficient in some cases to allow explantation of the device.[16–20] Although the exact proportion of patients in which this is possible is unknown it has been reported to be only 5–24% in previous series.[18–21] At Harefield we evolved a strategy which combines mechanical unloading using LVAD support with specific pharmacological interventions firstly to maximize the incidence of recovery in patients with dilated cardiomyopathy and secondly to improve durability of recovery following explantation.[17,22–24] Briefly, the pharmacological interventions of the first phase of the therapy are designed to act on component parts of the myocardium with the aim of reversing the pathological hypertrophy, remodelling, and normalizing cellular metabolic function. The underlying cardiac function is regularly tested throughout the process while the pump is off. When maximal reverse remodelling has been achieved, as judged by echocardiographic measurements of left ventricular dimensions with the pump switched off (under full heparinization), clenbuterol is given as the second phase. This drug has been shown to induce physiological hypertrophy in several experimental models, including those with pressure overload hypertrophy.[25,26] Using this strategy it has been possible to promote recovery and allow removal of the pump in 73% of a prospective series of patients[17] with chronic HF due to dilated cardiomyopathy receiving the Heartmate I device. Furthermore, these patients remain well 9 years later, suggesting this recovery is durable, and they have a good quality of life.[27] Subsequently the same protocol was applied to a prospective series of patients receiving the Heartmate II continuous-flow pump and 60% recovered sufficiently for the pump to be removed. Hence LVADs can be used as a platform for myocardial recovery. In these patients we have also observed reversal of many molecular changes seen at the time of LVAD implantation.[28–32] Recovery of patients on an LVAD provides an ideal and so far unique opportunity to study the molecular mechanisms that occur during reverse remodelling as the patient recovers. Myocardial samples, obtained at the time of device insertion and removal, along with serum samples, provide an ideal opportunity to explore the myocardial and circulating factors involved in recovery of human HF.

Destination therapy

The future use of these devices, particularly as survival increases, is likely to lie in their wider use as destination therapy and this is already happening in the United States. Successful experience in the bridge-to-transplant patients, particularly among those who had prolonged periods of support, justified evaluating these devices as long-term or destination therapy for chronic HF. The first-generation pulsatile devices had many moving parts, making them susceptible to device failure, but the axial and magnetic levitation devices have less and are much more durable, making destination therapy now a very viable alternative.

The first randomized trial (REMATCH—The Randomized Evaluation of Mechanical Assistance for the Treatment of Congestive Heart Failure[33]) randomized 129 patients with end-stage failure at 20 experienced cardiac transplant centres to receive either optimal medical therapy (OMM) or a Heartmate I LVAD as permanent therapy. Patients were in NYHA class IV for at least 60 of 90 days despite maximal medical therapy and they were ineligible for cardiac transplantation. The median age was 69 years. One-year survival in the LVAD group was 52% compared to 25% in the OMM group, and 2-year survival was 23% compared to 8% in the OMM group. Overall, all-cause mortality was reduced by 48%. Interestingly, 1-year survival for patients under 60 years of age was 74%. Both NYHA class and quality of life were better at follow-up in the LVAD group. The survival benefit was particularly significant for those on inotropes (survival benefit $p = 0.0014$ for LVAD compared to OMM[34]). There was a significant improvement in survival for LVAD patients enrolled during the second half of the trial (1 January 2000–July 2001) compared with the first half (May 1998–31 December 1999),[35] reflecting improvements in patient management and device modifications even throughout this period of the trial. The 1-year survival in the second half of the trial patients was 59% vs 44% in the first half ($p = 0.029$) and the 2-year survival 38% vs 21%. The Minnesota Living with Heart Failure scores also improved significantly over the course of the trial.[35] Terminal HF caused the majority of deaths in the medical therapy group, whereas the most common cause of deaths in the device group were sepsis (41% of deaths) and failure of the device (17% of deaths).[33] The adverse event rate was also significantly lower as the trial progressed and the rates per patient-year of sepsis, renal failure, and infection were significantly lower for those enrolled during the second half of the trial.[35] A further study of patients implanted with the first-generation Heartmate I device at four high-volume centres following REMATCH from January 2003 to December 2004 showed improved 90% and 61% 30-day and 1-year survival respectively.[36] The death rates due to sepsis and device failure were respectively 8.3 times and 2.2 times lower than in REMATCH. Overall patients were 2.1 times less likely to experience an adverse event and there were reductions of 66%, 63%, 89%, and 92% in neurologic dysfunction, sepsis, site infection, and for combined and suspected device failure respectively.

The INTrEPID trial was a prospective nonrandomized clinical trial comparing outcome with the Novocor first-generation pulsatile pump with medical therapy. Again the LVAD-treated patients had superior survival rates at 6 months (46% vs 22%) and 12 months (27% vs 11%). Patients experienced no improvement in NYHA functional class with medical therapy, whereas 85% of the LVAD patients had either no symptoms or minimal HF symptoms. Quality of life measures improved in the LVAD group.[37]

Introduction of axial-flow and centrifugal designs have improved LVAD survival further and reduced complications. Results of a trial randomizing the Heartmate II continuous-flow pump against the pulsatile Heartmate I device with a 2:1 randomization have recently been published.[38] 134 patients received the HMII and 66 received the HMI between March 2005 and May 2007. The median age was 64 years, nearly 80% were on intravenous inotropes at the time of randomization, and 22% and 23% respectively were on IABP support. The median duration of support was 1.7 years for the continuous-flow device and 0.6 years for the pulsatile pump, with 86% and 76% respectively being discharged home on the device after a median length of stay of 27 and 28 days.[38] The percentage of time spent out of hospital on the device was significantly longer on the HMII compared to the HMI patients. One- and 2-year survival was 68% and 58% respectively with the continuous-flow device and 55% and 24% respectively for the pulsatile device.[38] Early and sustained improvements in functional capacity were seen in each group and the quality of life improved in both groups. There were significant reductions in the rates of major adverse events among patients with a continuous-flow device including device-related infection (0.9 vs 0.48 events/patient year), non-device-related infection (1.33 vs 0.76 events/patient year or local infection and 1.11 vs 0.39 for sepsis), right HF, respiratory failure, renal failure (0.34 vs 0.1 events/patient year) and cardiac arrhythmia.[38] Twenty of the 59 patients with the Heartmate I device required pump replacement with 21 pump replacements and the rate was 0.51 events/patient year versus 0.06 events/patient year for the continuous-flow pump arm ($p < 0.001$). There was a 38% relative reduction in the rate of rehospitalization in patients with a continuous compared to a pulsatile device.[38]

The results of the REMATCH trial led to FDA approval of the Heartmate VE for destination therapy in the United States in November 2002, and in January 2009 the FDA approved the Heartmate II for its use as destination therapy.

Bridge to decision

Despite the improvements in the field of mechanical circulatory support observed in the last few years, the group of patients who present with severe HF in an extremely critical condition or 'moribund' state are still a difficult group of patients to deal with, usually because of the presence of endstage organ failure and/or uncertain neurological status in a ventilated patient. The outcome remains poor in these very critically ill patients. The Levitronix short-term VAD (Fig. 51.5) can be used as a 'bridge to decision' in these extremely sick patients who have contraindications to the implantation of a long-term VAD or urgent transplantation at the time of presentation, if these contraindications are considered acute and potentially reversible, prior to deciding if a more expensive device or transplant should be used. Using short-term, low-cost devices such as the Centrimag in this setting is very effective in stabilizing the haemodynamic state, improving the end-organ function, extubating the patient to allow assessment of their neurological status, and providing an opportunity to assess further their clinical condition.[39] Short-term, low-cost devices that can be inserted with minimal surgical invasiveness in such sick patients, often with coagulopathy, provide immediate haemodynamic stability and recovery for further assessment of these patients either for bridge to transplantation, bridge to recovery, or a long-term device. They can then be upgraded to a longer-term device when the patients are in a much better condition—usually extubated, with normalized renal and liver function and with sepsis under control. Alternatively, some patients can be bridged straight to transplantation[40] from the Levitronix device or straight to recovery, especially if they have a disease in which their myocardial function has the potential to recover in a short time, e.g. myocarditis or post MI.

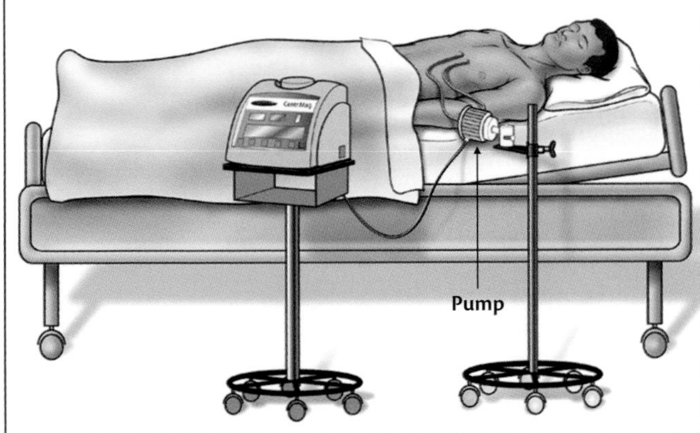

Fig. 51.5 The Levitronix Centrimag short-term device. Cannulation is from the left atrium to the aorta and the pump sits outside the body.

Complications of ventricular assist devices

LVADs are not without complications: perioperative haemorrhage, right HF, abdominal and cerebral bleeding, infection, thromboembolism, haemolysis, and device failure can be a problem. Earlier insertion of the LVAD before the development of multiorgan failure improves survival and lessens the risk of these complications. With evolving LVAD technology some of these complications are now improving.

Early complications following device insertion include right ventricular failure and perioperative haemorrhage—although this remains common, it is much less of a problem with the newer continuous-flow pumps, which involve a less traumatic surgical implantation than the bulkier pulsatile pumps. Often the underlying disease has a biventricular component and when the LVAD supports the left side of the heart and a normal cardiac output is returned to the right side, the right side can fail more and sometimes additional RVAD support is needed. Most commonly this can be removed again after a short period. Abdominal complications caused by the device were common with the bulkier pulsatile devices, in particular the Heartmate I device which is inserted into the abdomen, and can lead to gastrointestinal obstruction, fistula, and adhesions in some cases. These abdominal complications are rare with the axial flow pumps and with the devices that are not implanted into the abdomen. However, with continuous-flow pumps bleeding can occur from arteriovenous malformations of the intestine that are found incidentally in normal adults,[41] and this bleeding is worsened by the anticoagulation these patients require.

Later complications include infection, thromboembolism, cerebral bleeding, haemolysis, and device failure. Infection can occur in the pump, in the pump pocket, and around the driveline. The smaller surface area of foreign material of the axial flow pumps, the minimal movement of the device inside the body, and the smaller driveline compared to the pulsatile pumps results in lower infection rates with the axial-flow pump devices. (0.37 vs 3.49 driveline infections per patient-year for the Heartmate II vs Heartmate I devices in the recently published trial[9]). However, driveline infection remains a significant problem late after device implantation. The future direction is to operate LVADs through a transcutaneous energy transfer system to avoid the need for an external driveline. In terms of thromboembolism, pump thrombosis is a complication that can occur causing obstruction of the pump; it usually manifests as an increased power consumption of the pump, which is seen as an increased wattage. Although it can be successfully treated with tyrofiban/tPA, it is associated with a high mortality and can require a pump change. Although most thromboembolism is avoided by the anticoagulation these patients require, thromboembolic stroke can still be a problem. As these patients are anticoagulated, bleeding complications such as intracerebral haemorrhage can occur. This is becoming a significant problem late after device implantation and it is important to

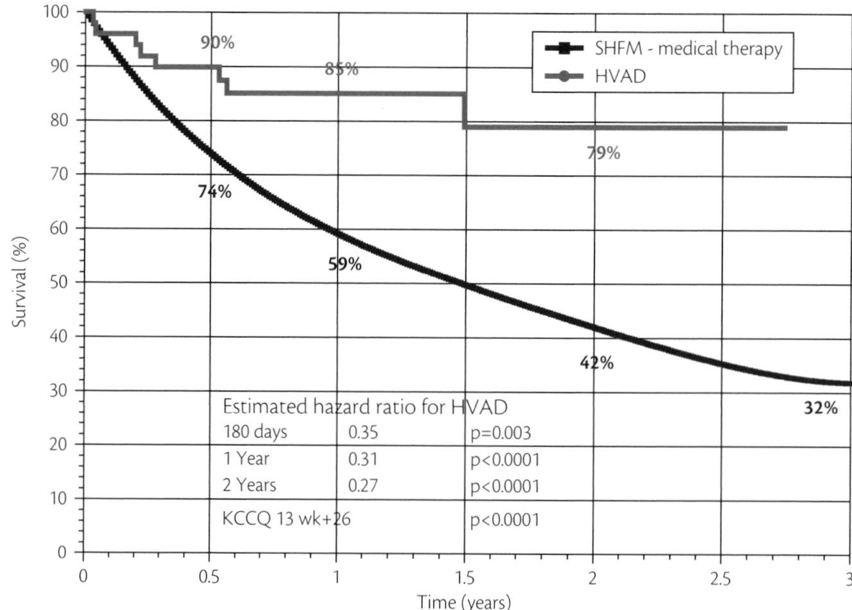

Fig. 51.6 Survival in patients in the European trial following treatment with Heartware (red line) compared to their predicted survival with medical therapy (blue line).[12]

control the patients blood pressure well to reduce the risk of an intracerebral bleed. In the randomized trial of continuous versus pulsatile flow pumps the leading cause of death in each group was from cerebral haemorrhage.[38]

Device failure is another serious problem that can occur, particularly late after device insertion. There can be failure of the external components (which can usually be replaced), or of the internal components (which can be life threatening). Device failure is more common with the first-generation pulsatile pumps as they have more moving parts and also have valves which can degenerate leading to valvular regurgitation. However, they do have a hand pump back-up system (manually operated by the patient or their carer, both of whom are trained in this procedure). Consequently device failure can be associated with low morbidity and mortality[42] if appropriately managed. The second-generation axial-flow pumps have only one moving part, the rotor. They are threfore more durable and have a lower rate of device failure. The third-generation magnetic levitation pumps have no bearings to wear out and are expected to be much more durable. The possibility of changing the device in device failure should be considered. Patients on LVADs are now discharged home into the community while on the devices. They and their carers are trained about the device, including what to do in the event of device failure. Haemolysis is an unusual problem and is only usually significant enough to result in clinical compromise when it is due to thrombus in the pump.

Conclusions, the future, and evolving role

LVADs are now being inserted into an increasing number of patients with advanced HF. As the devices and patient management improve the complications lessen and patient survival improves, justifying the earlier referral of patients for VAD implantation. Earlier referral of patients significantly reduces the risks of these complications and improves survival and long-term outcome further, and the vicious circle of treating these patients with such a poor prognosis can be broken. Sustained reversal of severe HF (myocardial recovery) can be achieved with LVAD therapy, particularly when combined with pharmacological therapy. This can allow explantation of the device in a high proportion of patients with nonischaemic cardiomyopathy, avoiding the need for transplantation, immunosuppression, and its associated complications, leaving the patient with a good quality of life and allowing the precious resource of a donor organ to be used for another needy individual. VADs can hence be used as a platform to induce myocardial recovery and may well be combined with other novel therapies such as stem cells in the future.

These devices are rapidly evolving, which—together with better patient management and selection—is resulting in improved survival and a lower rate of complications and is also likely to lead to lower cost. The role of VADs as an alternative to transplantation, i.e. destination therapy, is increasing rapidly in patients with advanced HF. It appears that as device design, patient selection and management, and the promptness of referral continues to improve, the outcome for many patients with advanced HF will improve further.

References

1. Stewart S, MacIntyre K, Hole DJ, Capewell S, McMurray JJ. More 'malignant' than cancer? Five-year survival following a first admission for heart failure. *Eur J Heart Fail* 2001;**3**(3): 315–22.
2. Cheng JM, Den Uil CA, Hoeks SE, *et al.* Percutaneous left ventricular assist devices vs. Intra-aortic balloon pump counterpulsation for treatment of cardiogenic shock: a meta-analysis of controlled trials. *Eur Heart J* 2009;**30**(17):2102–8.
3. Haj-Yahia S, Birks EJ, Rogers P, *et al.* Midterm experience with the Jarvik 2000 axial flow left ventricular assist device. *J Thorac Cardiovasc Surg* 2007;**134**(1):199–203.
4. Deng MC. Cardiac transplantation. *Heart* 2002;**87**:177–84.

5. Frazier OH, Rose EA, Oz MC, *et al.* Multicenter clinical evaluation of the Heartmate vented electric left ventricular assist sytem in patients awaiting heart transplantation. *J Thorac Cardiovasc Surg* 2001;**122**:1186–95.
6. Navia JL, McCarthy PM, Hoercher KJ, *et al.* Do left ventricular assist device (LVAD) bridge-to-transplantation outcomes predict the results of permanent LVAD implantation? *Ann Thorac Surg* 2002;**74**(6):2051–62.
7. El-Banayosy A, Arusoglu L, Kizner L, *et al.* Predictors of survival in patients bridged to transplantation with the Thoratec VAD device: a single-centre retrospective study on more than 100 patients. *J Heart Lung Transplant* 2000;**19**:964–8.
8. Sun BC, Catanese KA, Spanier TB, *et al.* 100 long-term implantable left ventricular assist devices: the Columbia Presbyterian interim experience. *Ann Thorac Surg* 1999;**68**(2):688–94.
9. Miller LW, Pagani FD, Russell SD, *et al.*; HeartMate II Clinical Investigators. Use of a continuous-flow device in patients awaiting heart transplantation. *N Engl J Med* 2007;**357**(9):885–96.
10. Pagani F, Miller LW, Russell SD, *et al.* Extended mechanical circulatory support with a continuous-flow rotary left ventricular assist device. *J Am Coll Cardiol* 2009;**54**:312–21.
11. Nojiri C, Fey O, Jaschke F, *et al.* Long-term circulatory support with the Duraheart Maglev centrifugal left ventricular assist system for advanced heart failure patients eligible to transplantation:European Experiences. *J Heart Lung Transplant* 2008;**27**(2S):S245.
12. Levy W, Wieselthaler GM, O'Driscoll G, *et al.* Application of the Seattle Heart Failure Model to the Heartware third generation LVAD. Presented at the American Heart Association Sessions, Orlando, 2009.
13. Lietz K, Miller LW. Improved survival of patients with end-stage heart failure listed for heart transplantation. *J Am Coll Cardiol* 2007;**50**(13):1282–90.
14. Taylor DO, Edwards LB, Boucek MM, *et al.* Registry of the International Society for Heart and Lung Transplantation: twenty-fourth official adult heart transplant report 2007. J Heart Lung Transplant 2007;**26**(8):769–81.
15. Mokadam NA, Ewald GA, Damiano RJ, Moazami N. Deterioration and mortality among patients with United Network for Organ Sharing status 2 heart disease: caution must be exercised in diverting organs. *J Thorac Cardiovasc Surg* 2006;**131**:926–6.
16. Frazier OH, Benedict CR, Radovacevic B, *et al.* Improved Left ventricular function after chronic ventricular unloading. *Ann Thorac Surg* 1996;**62**:675–82.
17. Birks EJ, Tansley PD, Hardy J, *et al.* Left ventricular assist device and drug therapy for the reversal of heart failure. *N Engl J Med* 2006;**355**(18):1873–84.
18. Dandel M, Weng Y, Siniawski H, Potapov E, Lehmkuhl HB, Hetzer R. Long-term results in patients with idiopathic dilated cardiomyopathy after weaning from left ventricular assist devices. *Circulation* 2005;**112**(9 Suppl):I37–45.
19. Simon MA, Kormos RL, Murali S, *et al.* Myocardial recovery using ventricular assist devices: prevalence, clinical characteristics, and outcomes. *Circulation* 2005;**112**(9 Suppl):I32–6.
20. Farrar DJ, Holman WR, McBride LR, *et al.* Long-term follow-up of Thoratec ventricular assist device bridge-to-recovery patients successfully removed from support after recovery of ventricular function. *J Heart Lung Transplant* 2002;**21**(5): 516–21.
21. Mancini DM, Beniaminovitz A, Levin H, *et al.* Low incidence of myocardial recovery after left ventricular assist device implantation in patients with chronic heart failure. *Circulation* 1998;**98**:2383–9.
22. Yacoub MH. A novel strategy to maximise the efficacy of LVADs as a bridge to recovery. *Eur Heart J* 2001;**22**:534–40.
23. Yacoub MH, Birks EJ, Tansley P, Henein MY, Bowles CT. Bridge to recovery:The Harefield Approach. *J Congestive Heart Fail Circ Support* 2001;**2**(1):27–30.
24. Yacoub MH, Tansley P, Birks EJ, Bowles CT, Banner NR, Khaghani A. A novel combination therapy to reverse end-stage heart failure. *Transplantation Proc* 2001;**33**:2762–4.
25. Wong K, Boheler K, Bishop J, *et al.* Pharmacological modulation pressure overload cardiac hypertrophy changes in ventricular function, extracellular matrix and gene expression. *Circulation* 1997;**96**:2239–46.
26. Wong K, Boheler KR, Bishop J, *et al.* Clenbuterol induces cardiac hypertrophy with normal functional, morphological and molecular features. *Cardiovasc Res* 1998 Jan;**37**(1):115–22.
27. George RS, Yacoub MH, Bowles CT, *et al.* Quality of life following LVAD removal for myocardial recovery. *J Heart Lung Transplant* 2008;**27**:165–72.
28. Birks EJ, Hall JL, Barton PJ, *et al.* Gene profiling changes in cytoskeletal proteins during clinical recovery after left ventricular-assist device support. *Circulation* 2005;**112**(9 Suppl): I57–64.
29. Hall JL, Birks EJ, Grindle S, *et al.* Molecular signature of recovery following combination left ventricular assist device (LVAD) support and pharmacologic therapy. *Eur Heart J* 2007;**28**(5): 613–27.
30. Latif N, Yacoub MH, George R, Barton PJ, Birks EJ. Changes in sarcomeric and non-sarcomeric cytoskeletal proteins and focal adhesion molecules during clinical myocardial recovery after left ventricular assist device support. *J Heart Lung Transplant* 2007;**26**(3):230–5.
31. Cullen ME, Yuen AH, Felkin LE, *et al.* Myocardial expression of the arginine:glycine amidinotransferase gene is elevated in heart failure and normalized following recovery: potential implications for local creatine synthesis. *Circulation* 2006;**114**:16–20.
32. Terracciano CMN, Harding SE, Tansley PT, Birks EJ, Barton PJR, Yacoub MH. Changes in sarcolemmal Ca entry and sarcoplasmic reticulum Ca content in ventricular myocytes from patients with end-stage heart failure following myocardial recovery after combined pharmacological and ventricular assist device therapy. *Eur Heart J* 2003;**24**:1329–39.
33. Rose EA, Gelijins AC, Moskowitz AJ, *et al.* Long-term use of a left ventricular assist device for end-stage heart failure. *New Engl J Med* 2001;**345**(20):1435–43.
34. Stevenson LW, Miller LW, Desvigne-Nickens P, *et al.* Left ventricular assist device as destination for patients undergoing intravenous inotropic therapy. A subset analysis from REMATCH (Randomized Evaluation of Mechanical Assistance for the Treatment of Congestive Heart Failure). *Circulation* 2004;**110**:975–81.
35. Park SJ, Tector A, Piccioni W, *et al.* Left ventricular assist devices as destination therapy: a new look at survival. *J Thorac Cardiovasc Surg* 2005;**129**(1):9–17.
36. Long JW, Kfoury AG, Slaughter MS, *et al.* Long term destination therapy with the Heartmate XVE left ventricular assist device: improved outcome since the REMATCH study. *Congest Heart Fail* 2005;**11**(3):133–8.
37. Rogers JG, Butler J, Lansman SL, *et al.*; INTrEPID Investigators. Chronic mechanical circulatory support for inotrope-dependent heart failure patients who are not transplant candidates: results of the INTrEPID Trial. *J Am Coll Cardiol*;**50**(8):741–7.
38. Slaughter MS, Rogers JG, Milano CA, *et al.*; HeartMate II Investigators. Advanced heart failure treated with continuous-flow left ventricular assist device. *N Engl J Med* 2009;**361**(23):2241–51.
39. De Robertis F, Rogers P, Amrani M, *et al.* Bridge to decision using the Levitronix CentriMag short-term ventricular assist device. *J Heart Lung Transplant* 2008;**27**(5):474–8.

40. Haj-Yahia S, Birks EJ, Amrani M, *et al.* Bridging patients after salvage from bridge to decision directly to transplant by means of prolonged support with the CentriMag short-term centrifugal pump. *J Thorac Cardiovasc Surg* 2009;**138**(1):227–30.
41. Letsou GV, Shah N, Gregoric ID, Myers TJ, Delgado R, Frazier OH, Gastrointestinal bleeding from arteriovenous malformations in patients supported by the Jarvik 2000 axial-flow left ventricular assist device. *J Heart Lung Transplant* 2005;**24**(1):105–9.
42. Birks EJ, Tansley PD, Yacoub MH, *et al.* Incidence and clinical management of life-threatening Left ventricular assist device (LVAD) failure. *J Heart Lung Transplant* 2004;**23**(8):964–9.

52

Mitral valve surgery in heart failure

Andrew Murday

Introduction

Functional, or secondary, mitral regurgitation (MR) develops as part of the process of remodelling which in turn occurs as a result of left ventricular failure. Although this complication can result whatever the primary pathology causing the left ventricular failure, the pathophysiological process varies to a certain extent depending on the aetiology. There is some confusion in the literature with respect to ischaemic MR, with some authors calling all ischaemic MR functional. For the sake of clarity, this chapter deals with functional MR resulting from left ventricular failure which for the sake of argument I will define as a left ventricular ejection fraction (LVEF) of less than 35%.

Functional MR is a common consequence of left ventricular systolic dysfunction (LVSD) and it has an important bearing on both symptoms and outcome in patients suffering from heart failure (HF). In a study of 2057 patients with symptomatic HF and with a LVEF of less than 40% but without structural valve disease, 56.2% had some degree of MR and in 29.8% of these it was moderate or severe. Furthermore, the presence of moderate or severe MR was associated with a significantly higher mortality at 1, 3, and 5 years (Fig. 52.1). In a multivariate analysis, MR of any degree was an independent predictor of death.[1]

The success of mitral valve surgery, and in particular the flourishing of mitral valve repair techniques, along with the ever-increasing burden of patients with HF, has led to the adaptation of repair techniques, originally developed to correct structural abnormalities of the mitral valve, to attempt to halt or even reverse the remodelling process.

As much as 40 years ago it was appreciated that an adequate mitral valve repair might have advantages over valve replacement so long as 'such repair would hold up over a long period of time'.[2] During that era of cardiac surgery most patients coming to valve surgery had either congenital abnormalities or, more commonly, rheumatic heart disease. Subsequently, through the 1970s Carpentier and his colleagues in Paris were developing more complex techniques to repair mitral valves with degenerative as well as rheumatic pathology.[3]

The first published series of patients undergoing repair for functional MR in 1995[4] heralded a rapid expansion in the number of patients with a combination of left ventricular failure and MR being put forward for surgery. Subsequently, in the absence of appropriate randomized clinical trials it has become less clear which patients should undergo this procedure and even what procedure should be offered.

The surgical literature, although replete with studies of mitral valve surgery for structural abnormalities, is not so well furnished with respect to correction of functional regurgitation. Much of this subjective literature is also devalued by primitive assessment of the degree of MR. From the earliest years of open heart surgery onwards there have been nonrandomized comparisons of mitral repair versus replacement[5] and although there are several ongoing randomized trials there are no trials yet published which measure the effect of mitral valve surgery in HF. Thus, as is so often the case in heart surgery, we must fall back on evidence based on cohort studies and, to some extent, inadequately tested conjecture.

The reader should also bear in mind that mitral valve surgery is only one weapon in the surgeon's armamentarium against HF and that it can be employed in combination with other procedures such as revascularization, ventricular remodelling, and mechanical ventricular assist.[6]

Pathophysiology

The three principle components of left ventricular remodelling which contribute to the development of MR are annular dilatation, papillary muscle displacement, and discoordination of ventricular contraction resulting from dyssynchrony. One effect of the latter two processes is to cause tethering of the mitral leaflets. Once MR has developed, the consequent increase in volume loading of the ventricle leads to an increase in ventricular cavity volumes, greater transmural tension, and yet more ventricular dilatation.

Carpentier's original pathophysiological classification of MR consisted of three types (figure) according to leaflet motion: normal (type I), increased (type II), or restricted (type III) (Fig. 52.2).[7] This classification was designed to help in the decision-making process

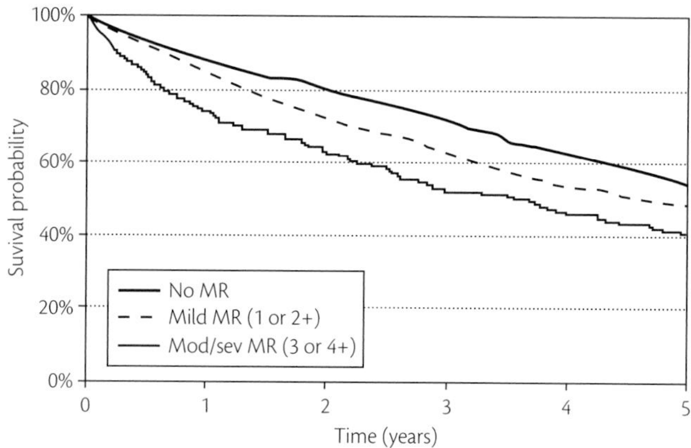

Fig. 52.1 Unadjusted Kaplan–Meier survival estimates are shown. Patients with moderate or severe (Mod/sev) mitral regurgitation (MR) are represented by the light line, those with mild MR by the dashed line, and those with no MR by the dark line.
From Trichon BH, Felker M, Shaw LK, Cabell CH, O'Connor CM. Relation of frequency and severity of mitral regurgitation to survival among patients with left ventricular systolic dysfunction and heart failure. *Am J Cardiol* 2003;**91**:538–43.

before and during valve repair. Thus, type I MR can be resolved by an annuloplasty of some kind, type II by elimination of prolapse, and type III by relieving whatever is causing the restrictive motion. In both dilated and ischaemic cardiomyopathy, the posterior leaflet can be restricted by an outward, paradoxical motion of the left ventricular wall at the base of a papillary muscle. This has come to be known as type IIIb leaflet motion. In many patients more than one mechanism may be at work at the same time.

To some extent the mechanism of MR is dependent on the underlying pathology. Functional regurgitation is either type I, as a result of annular dilatation, or type IIIb, as a result of abnormal ventricular wall motion leading to leaflet tethering. In idiopathic dilated cardiomyopathy, the process can be considered to be passive although there can still be both annular dilatation and leaflet tethering as result of ventricular dilatation. In ischaemia there is the possibility of an active component to leaflet tethering with the potential for reversing this by revascularization. There is no direct evidence for this and experimental models of ischaemia of the papillary muscles, in the absence of ventricular dilatation, failed to produce MR.[8]

It might seem logical that the presence of MR is associated with a reduction in left ventricular afterload. Indeed, it is not uncommon to hear the view that restoration of mitral competence in the presence of left ventricular dysfunction might result in worsening HF because the mitral valve is no longer acting as a safety valve for the ventricle. In fact, there is evidence that the opposite is more likely to be the case. Physiological studies, albeit in patients with chronic MR resulting from structural valve abnormalities, have demonstrated that there is an increase in mean, peak, and end-systolic stress[9] when compared to controls without MR, all three being measures of afterload. Furthermore, the increase in afterload is greater in the presence of reduced ventricular function. At face value this would suggest that restoration of mitral competence, providing that it can be achieved safely, is always going to be to the patient's advantage. There is also evidence that once functional MR is corrected there is an arrest and reversal of remodelling. This has been demonstrated in the ACORN trial in which elimination of MR with repair or replacement, in patients with a LVEF of less than 35%, was associated with progressive reduction in left ventricular end-diastolic volume and left ventricular end-systolic volume and an increase in LVEF compared with the preoperative baseline up to 24 months after surgery.[10]

Preservation of left ventricular function in the face of mitral valve surgery is particularly important when dealing with a ventricle whose function is impaired in the first place. Nonrandomized studies suggested, from an early stage in the evolution of mitral valve repair techniques, that repair was associated with better preservation of left ventricular function than replacement and that this was linked to lower operative mortality and morbidity.

There is evidence that the advantage which repair holds over replacement is the result of the preservation of the subvalvar apparatus and the consequent maintenance of left ventricular geometry. Nearly 50 years ago Dr C. Walton Lillehei, one of the greatest of the founding fathers of modern cardiac surgery, published experimental and clinical studies which demonstrated that mitral valve replacement with preservation of the subvalvar apparatus significantly reduced the ill-effects of mitral valve replacement on left ventricular function.[11] More recent publications have born this out to the extent that mitral valve replacement with preservation of the subvalvar apparatus may be just as good as mitral valve repair with respect to ventricular function and geometry.[12,13] There is one small randomized controlled trial of mitral valve replacement comparing preservation of posterior leaflet attachments with preservation of all chordal structures,[14] the findings of which support the contention that mitral valve replacement with preservation of all chordal attachments is as efficacious as valve repair in preserving left ventricular function.

Surgical options

There are only two fundamental questions in surgery: 'what to do?' and 'when to do it?' With respect to functional MR, the first can be simply expressed as 'repair or replace?'

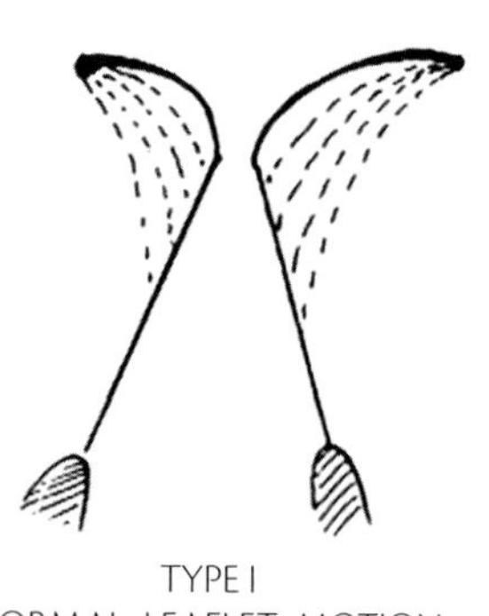

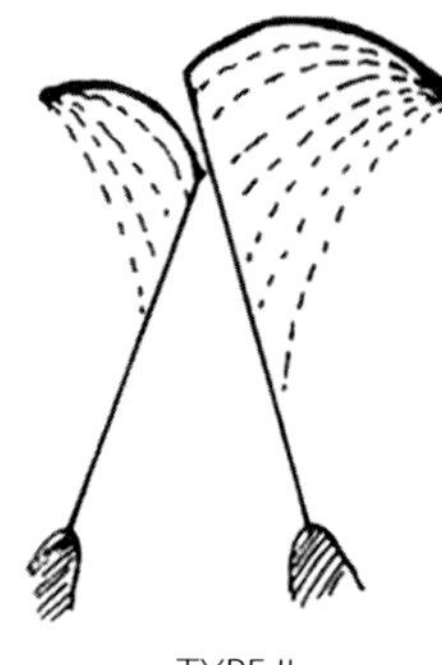

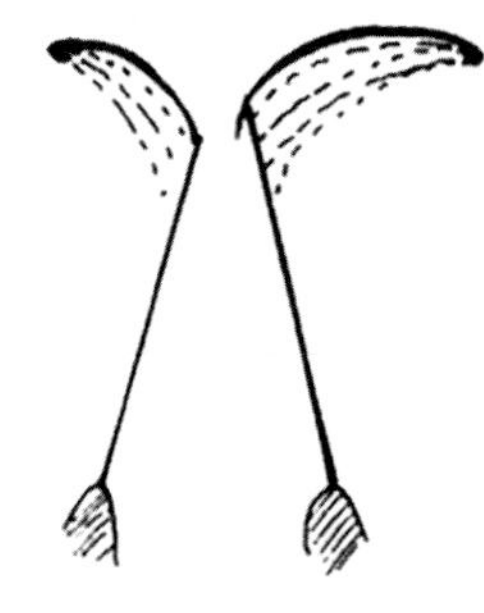

Fig. 52.2 The Carpentier classification of the pathophysiology of mitral regurgitation.
From Carpentier A. Cardiac valve surgery—the 'French correction'. *J Thorac Cardiovasc Surg* 1983;**86**:323–37.

Before the advent of valve prostheses there was a profusion of techniques described for repair of MR. Most of them were varying forms of suture annuloplasty.[15–18] Reed and his colleagues brought a greater application of pathophysiological and haemodynamic principles to the subject.[19] They had become aware that annular dilatation predominantly affected the posterior part of the annulus, that part to which the posterior leaflet is attached. Their suture repair technique left the unaffected anterior annulus unaltered but reduced the posterior annulus to a measured length corresponding to a reduced but adequate mitral valve orifice area. In due course these same principles governed the development of the rigid and semirigid annuloplasty rings developed by Carpentier and others.

The initial generation of valve prostheses at the start of the 1960s brought with them a host of new complications, so that for many surgeons valve repair was maintained while they awaited the development of 'safe' prostheses. When that happened, through the 1970s and 1980s, the torch of valve repair was kept alight by a group of vocal advocates. They subsequently provided evidence that convinced the rest of the surgical community that repair was safer than replacement both initially and in the long term after surgery, so that repair became the gold standard.[20] Unfortunately, throughout these changing times, there were no randomized controlled trials to confirm or refute the evidence of cohort studies and, as we shall see, it is still unclear whether repair or replacement is the most appropriate procedure for functional MR.[21]

The principal repair technique used to correct both type I and type IIIb components in functional MR is that of reduction annuloplasty. The surgical technique consists of sizing for an annuloplasty ring in the same way as in a patient with structural valve disease. When carrying out a repair in the face of functional MR, an annuloplasty two sizes smaller than the obturator or sizer is chosen. The prosthesis is then sutured in place in the usual way. This was first reported by Bolling and colleagues in a series of 16 patients, 12 with idiopathic dilated cardiomyopathy and 4 with irreversible ischaemic cardiomyopathy and all with a LVEF of less than 25% assessed by left ventricular angiography or radionuclide ventriculography. The early results in terms of symptomatology and left ventricular reverse remodelling were remarkably good.[4] There were no operative deaths and 1-year actuarial survival was 75%. The patients showed marked symptomatic improvement and an improvement in left ventricular function. Subsequent authors have mirrored these findings.[22,23]

However, in larger and later studies the benefits were not so clear cut. In a cohort of 126 patients, including both ischaemic and dilated cardiomyopathy, undergoing reduction mitral annuloplasty the 30-day mortality was 4.8%. Furthermore, surgery in this group of patients did not confer a survival advantage compared with a matched group who did not undergo surgery and in whom confounding clinical variables were controlled by propensity scoring. This finding held true whatever the aetiology of the HF.[24]

One of the trade-offs between repair and replacement rests on the incidence of recurrence of regurgitation after repair. After valve replacement the incidence of regurgitation should approach zero. Since the life expectancy of patients with severe left ventricular function is relatively poor no matter what, they are unlikely to suffer the consequences of bioprosthetic valve degeneration so that the hazards of mechanical valve replacement can be avoided.[25] Valve repairs for structural valve disease are robust and reoperation rates for subsequent failure are low. The situation after reduction mitral annuloplasty for functional MR is not so clear. Certainly high rates of recurrent regurgitation have been found in patients with an ischaemic aetiology following annuloplasty,[26] with moderate or severe regurgitation present in 57% of patients at an average follow-up of 28 months after surgery despite satisfactory initial echocardiographic outcomes. Providing the initial annuloplasty is sufficiently restrictive and the prosthetic ring does not dehisce, the recurrence must be due to a type IIIb mechanism.

This is borne out in a study of a subgroup of 117 patients from the ACORN trial, all with idiopathic dilated cardiomyopathy. Of these patients 25 had at least moderate MR within 6 months of surgery.[27] Those patients with recurrent MR failed to show the improvement in left ventricular dimensions and function compared with the patients with competent mitral valves following surgery. Preoperative anterior leaflet tethering strongly correlated with recurrence of MR after surgical repair. After annuloplasty the posterior leaflet is fixed and passive and in effect is maximally restricted, so that it is the type IIIb motion of the anterior leaflet which becomes the predominant lesion in these patients. When that lesion exists prior to surgery then it comes to prominence postoperatively. There is little doubt that further developments in valve repair will be required to overcome this difficulty.

There exist a whole range of different designs of annuloplasty prostheses, including complete and incomplete rings of all degress of flexibility. While there is echocardiographic evidence that flexible rings result in better ventricular function following repair for structural valve disease,[28] there is no good evidence that this is reflected in clinical outcome.[29] Indeed, there is limited evidence that, at least in ischaemic aetiology, a complete rigid ring gives the best results for functional MR.[30]

As to when to operate, there really is no evidence on which to base surgical practice. At present it would seem reasonable to exhaust all other therapies before advising any patient to go forward to what is a relatively high-risk procedure with a limited outcome. We need to see the results of the ongoing randomized clinical trials in the hope that these will provide some clues as to which patients might benefit most from correction of functional regurgitation.

Summary

Functional MR occurs commonly as part of the remodelling process resulting from left ventricular failure. Surgical correction of the regurgitation either by repair or replacement can be effective, although there are no randomized clinical trial results to substantiate this claim, and little evidence to guide timing of mitral surgery for functional regurgitation. Reduction annuloplasty is the most favoured means of surgical correction, although mitral valve replacement with preservation of all the subvalvular structure should not be discounted, especially if restrictive motion of the anterior mitral leaflet is present preoperatively.

References

1. Trichon BH, Felker M, Shaw LK, Cabell CH, O'Connor CM. Relation of frequency and severity of mitral regurgitation to survival among patients with left ventricular systolic dysfunction and heart failure. *Am J Cardiol* 2003;**91**:538 –43.
2. Reed GE. Repair of mitral regurgitation. *Am J Cardiol* 1973;**31**:494–6.
3. Carpentier A, Chavaud S, Fabiani JN, *et al.* Reconstructive surgery of mitral valve incompetence: ten-year appraisal. *J Thorac Cardiovasc Surg* 1980;**79**:338–48.

4. Bolling SF, Deeb M, Brunsting LA, Bach DS. Early outcome of mitral valve reconstruction in patients with end-stage cardiomyopathy. *J Thorac Cardiovasc Surg* 1995;**109**:676–83.
5. Kerth WJ, Sharma G, Hill JD, Gerbode F. A comparison of the late results of replacement and of reconstructive procedures for acquired mitral valve disease. *J Thorac Cardiovasc Surg* 1971;**61**:14–22.
6. A Pitsis, N Aikaterini, V Bougioukas, *et al.* Elective bridging to recovery after repair: the surgical approach to ventricular reverse remodeling. *Artif Organs* 2008;**32**:730–4.
7. Carpentier A. Cardiac valve surgery—the 'French correction'. *J Thorac Cardiovasc Surg* 1983;**86**:323–37.
8. Otsuji Y, Handschumacher MD, Liel-Cohen N, *et al.* Mechanism of ischemic mitral regurgitation with segmental left ventricular dysfunction: three-dimensional echocardiographic studies in models of acute and chronic progressive regurgitation. *J Am Coll Cardiol* 2001;**37**:641–8.
9. Corin WJ, Monrad ES, Murakami T, Nonogi H, Hess OM, Krayenbuehl HPL. The relationship of afterload to ejection performance in chronic mitral regurgitation. *Circulation* 1987;**76**:59–67.
10. Acker MA, Bolling S, Shemin R, *et al.* Mitral valve surgery in heart failure: insights from the Acorn clinical trial. *J Thorac Cardiovasc Surg* 2009;**132**:568–77.
11. Lillhei CW, Levy MJ, Bonnabeau RC. Mitral valve replacement with preservation of papillary muscles and chordae tendineae. *J Thorac Cardiovasc Surg* 1964;**47**:532–43.
12. David TE, Uden DE, Strauss HD. The importance of the mitral apparatus in left ventricular function after correction of mitral regurgitation. *Circulation* 1983;**68**(suppl II):II76–82.
13. Rozich JD, Carabello BA, Usher BW, Kratz JM, Bell AE, Zile MR. Mitral valve replacement with and without chordal preservation in patients with chronic mitral regurgitation: mechanisms for difference in postoperative ejection performance. *Circulation* 1992;**86**:1718–26.
14. Yun KL, Sintek CF, Miller DG, *et al.* Randomized trial comparing partial versus complete chordal-sparing mitral valve replacement: effects on left ventricular volume and function. *J Thorac Cardiovasc Surg* 2002;**123**:707–14.
15. Davila JC, Glover RP. Circumferential suture of the mitral valve for the correction of regurgitation. *Am J Cardiol* 1958;**2**:267.
16. Kay JH, Egerton WS, Zubiate P. The surgical treatment of mitral insufficiency and combined mitral stenosis and insufficiency with use of the heart-lung machine. *Surgery* 1961;**50**:67.
17. Wooler GH, Nixon PGF, Grimshaw VA, Watson DA. Experiences with the repair of the mitral valve in mitral incompetence. *Thorax* 1962;**17**:49.
18. Anderson AM, Cobb LA, Bruce RA, Merendino KA. Evaluation of mitral annuloplasty for mitral regurgitation. *Circulation* 1962;**26**:26.
19. Reed GE, Tice DA, Clauss RH. Asymmetric exaggerated mitral annuloplasty: repair of mitral insufficiency with haemodynamic predictability. *J Thorac Cardiovasc Surg* 1965;**49**:753–61.
20. Enriquez-Sarano M, Schaff HV, Frye RL. Mitral regurgitation: what causes the leakage is fundamental to the outcome of valve repair. *Circulation* 2003;**108**:253–6.
21. Magne J, Girerd N, Senechal M, *et al.* Mitral repair versus replacement for ischaemic mitral regurgitation. *Circulation* 2009; **120**(suppl 1):S104–11.
22. Rothenbergurger M, Rukosujew A, Hammel D, *et al.* Mitral valve surgery in patients with poor ventricular function. *Thorac Cardiovasc Surg* 2002;**50**:351–4.
23. Gummert JF, Rahmel A, Bucerius J *et al.* Mitral valve repair in patients with end-stage cardiomyopathy: who benefits? *Eur J Cardiothorac Surg* 2003;**X**:1017–22.
24. Wu AH, Aaronson KD, Bolling SF, Pagani FD, Welch K, Koelling TM. Impact of mitral annuloplasty on mortality risk in patients with mitral regurgitation and left ventricular dysfunction. *J Am Coll Cardiol* 2005;**45**:381–7.
25. Miller DG. Ischemic mitral regurgitation redux—to repair or to replace. *J Thorac Cardiovasc Surg* 2001;**122**:1059–62.
26. Serri K, Bouchard D, Demers P, *et al.* Is a good perioperative echocardiographic result predictive of durability in ischaemic mitral valve repair? *J Thorac Cardiovasc Surg* 2006;**131**:565–73.
27. Lee AP-W, Acker M, Kubo, *et al.* Mechanisms of recurrent functional mitral regurgitation after mitral valve repair in nonischemic dilated cardiomyopathy. *Circulation* 2009;**119**:1606–14.
28. David TE, Komeda M, Pollick C, Burns RJ. Mitral valve annuloplasty: the effect of the type on left ventricular function. *Ann Thorac Surg* 1989;**47**:524–7.
29. Chee T, Haston R, Togo A, Raja SG. Is a flexible mitral annuloplasty ring superior to a semi-rigid or rigid ring in terms of improvement in symptoms and survival. *Interact Cardiovasc Thorac Surg* 2008;**7**:477–84.
30. Onorati F, Rubino AS, Marturano D, *et al.* Mid-term echocardiographic results with different rings following restrictive mitral annuloplasty for schaemic cardiomyopathy. *Eur J Cardiothorac Surg* 2009;**36**:250–60.

PART XVI

Ventilatory strategies in heart failure

53

Ventilatory strategies in acute heart failure

Mhamed Mebazaa and Alexandre Mebazaa

Ventilatory support and positive end-expiratory pressure (PEEP) are pivotal treatments of cardiogenic pulmonary oedema. As recently recommended, it should be introduced within minutes of admission at hospital for acute heart failure (HF) and ideally at home in case of prehospital management. Ventilatory support is one of the few tools that have been proven to change short-term outcome in acute HF.

Effect of PEEP on pulmonary dysfunction

The primary cause of hypoxaemia in cardiogenic pulmonary oedema is the intrapulmonary shunt related to the filling of alveolar by oedema fluid. PEEP will keep the alveoli open during inspiration and expiration. PEEP will augment functional residual capacity (FRC) thereby decreasing intrapulmonary shunting. As a consequence, arterial oxygen content will rise, leading to a greater oxygen transport. Furthermore, the increase in airway and alveolar pressure toward positive values tends by itself to reduce pulmonary oedema.

Pulmonary oedema also worsens the work of breathing. Indeed, oedema fluid reduces pulmonary compliance and engorgement of blood vessels—by reducing the caliber of the peripheral airways—increases airway resistance. This may lead to hypercapnia and impaired consciousness might occur as the consequence of respiratory exhaustion. Ventilatory support and PEEP can allow the alveoli and bronchi to stay open and ultimately improve pulmonary compliance by reducing lung water. Those effects of PEEP will improve oxygenation, reduce congestion of the small airways, and reduce hypercapnia.

Effects of PEEP on cardiac dysfunction

PEEP and ventilator support will have two beneficial effects on the heart: (1) decreasing left ventricular preload by reducing venous return and (2) reducing left ventricular afterload.

Heart–lung interactions during mechanical ventilation have been extensively described. By increasing intrathoracic pressure, PEEP reduces right ventricular preload. Thus, when the heart is congestive, PEEP will reduce the venous return to the right and ultimately the left ventricles. Indeed, PEEP also increases the right ventricular afterload leading to a reduction of left ventricular preload.

PEEP and ventilator support have also direct beneficial effects of left ventricular function. PEEP reduces transmural pressure of both the left ventricle and the initial 'intrathoracic' portion of the aorta. Those effects will lead to reduced left ventricular afterload, improved myocardial oxygen consumption, and a better left ventricular contraction. The latter may lead to improved cardiac index.

Levels of PEEP in acute HF

In most cases of acute HF, pulmonary congestion is the main clinical sign and left ventricular function is often maintained. Accordingly, only moderate levels of PEEP (5–10 cmH_2O) are needed to improve Pa_{O_2} by increasing alveolar recruitment, thereby increasing FRC and reducing intrapulmonary shunt. In few patients with signs of congestion and reduced cardiac output, PEEP might improve cardiac index. By contrast, in patients with low pulmonary capillary wedge pressure (PCWP), PEEP may reduce cardiac index.

Noninvasive ventilation is the optimal tool in acute heart failure

Noninvasive ventilation (NIV) is a modality of ventilatory support without endotracheal intubation and sedation. It is usually delivered through a face mask but sometimes through a helmet. NIV is now recognized as a very simple and efficient treatment of acute pulmonary oedema due to acute HF. NIV has a rapid and tremendous effect on severe pulmonary oedema and is associated with a low cost-effectiveness ratio. NIV improves dyspnoea, oxygenation, and hypercapnia. Many NIV techniques require less than 1 h training and can be used by every physician or nurse in charge of patients suffering from acute HF and pulmonary oedema.

Two NIV techniques are particularly effective in cases of cardiogenic pulmonary oedema: noninvasive pressure support ventilation (NIPSV) and continuous positive airway pressure (CPAP). NIPSV provides (1) pressure support during the inspiratory phase and (2) PEEP. Of note, NIPSV is similar to bilevel positive airway pressure (BiPAP). Pressure support actively helps the patient during the inspiration. It requires the use of a mechanical ventilator with energy, air, and oxygen inputs. Thus during NIPSV, the patient makes a very small effort that triggers the inspiratory flow. CPAP is less sophisticated (no ventilator is required) and the most widely used NIV technique. Unlike NIPSV, in CPAP there is no active help in the inspiratory phase of respiration (no pressure support) and breathing is entirely spontaneous. CPAP requires a device that provides a high air/oxygen flow into the face mask. A flow higher than the patient's maximum instantaneous inspiratory flow allows maintenance of a constant positive pressure.

CPAP and NIPSV are both indicated as soon as possible after admission for cardiogenic pulmonary oedema. Three recent meta-analyses showed that early application of NIV in patients with acute cardiogenic pulmonary oedema reduces both the need for intubation and short-term mortality; however, in a large randomized controlled trial, NIV improved clinical parameters but not mortality. NIV should not be used in patients who cannot cooperate or if there is an immediate need of endotracheal intubation as a result of progressive life-threatening hypoxia.

A PEEP of 5–7.5 cmH_2O should be applied first and titrated to clinical response up to 10 cmH_2O; Fio_2 delivery should be at least 0.40. Usually NIV is applied 30 min/h until the patient's dyspnoea and oxygen saturation remain improved without NIV.

The two potential adverse effects of NIV are worsening of severe right ventricular failure and pneumothorax.

Mechanical ventilation is rarely indicated in acute heart failure

Sometimes, intubation and invasive mechanical ventilation are needed in case of respiratory exhaustion, haemodynamic instability, cardiogenic shock, impaired consciousness, and/or severe cardiac arrhythmias. Some of the ventilator parameters should be carefully chosen.

- Volume assist-control ventilation is a frequently used mode in which the ventilator delivers the same tidal volume (V_T) during each inspiration, whether it be patient-triggered or machine initiated. Following tracheal intubation, patients should be (at least transiently) ventilated under 100% O_2 ($Fio_2 = 1$) until arterial blood gases are tested (c.30 min later). The value of Pao_2 after Fio_2 increases to 1 will be helpful in assessing the severity of gas exchange abnormalities (including shunt), guiding therapy (addition of PEEP), and evaluating the response to therapy. Pao_2 should be kept between 80 and 100 mmHg.
- In order to avoid worsening pulmonary function, V_T should be less than 6 mL/kg and, most importantly, end-inspiratory plateau pressure (which best approximates end-inspiratory lung volume at the bedside) should be kept below 30 cmH_2O.
- Moderate levels of PEEP (3–5 cmH_2O) should be applied initially and adjusted according to haemodynamic tolerance (blood pressure and cardiac index should be maintained), effect on oxygenation, and plateau pressure. Higher levels of PEEP (15–18 cmH_2O) should no longer be used.
- Respiratory rate should be set between 15 and 20 breaths/min and adjusted according to $Paco_2$. The ratio of inspiratory to expiratory time (I:E) should be usually set at 1/1.

Box 53.1 Algorithm in case of worsening hypoxaemia during mechanical ventilation

1. Increase Fio_2 to 100%.
2. Check expired flow meter and tubing.
3. In case of unilateral murmurs, chest radiograph is needed:
   - Suspected elective intubation: deflate the cuff of the endotracheal tube and pull the tube slightly, ideally using fibroscopy, in order to leave 3–4 cm between the tip of the tube and the carina.
   - Suspected pneumothorax: consider chest tube insertion if needed.
   - Suspected atelectasis: perform endotracheal suctioning, check humidification device.

Under mechanical ventilation, arterial oxygenation, and hypercapnia should be improved within the first hour. In case oxygenation worsens, Box 53.1 provides an algorithm that should be followed to detect any complication relating to mechanical ventilation.

When the patient's condition is improved (e.g. if the patient is awake with Fio_2 <40–50%), discontinuation of mechanical ventilation should be considered as soon possible to minimize related complications. However, patients must also satisfy a number of criteria before extubation is contemplated. The classical criteria for extubation are absence of uncontrolled ongoing infection (temperature ≤38°C), haemodynamic stability without vasopressors or moderate levels of dopamine or dobutamine, no sedation or sedative infusion, adequate cough, and adequate neurological status.

When patients meet these described criteria, enteral feeding should be stopped within 6 h preceding the weaning trial. A 30-min T-piece trial helps evaluate a patient's ability to sustain spontaneous breathing. The patient is disconnected from the ventilator, and left to breathe spontaneously through an endotracheal tube with oxygen added laterally through an adaptor at the upper extremity of the tube (hence the term T-piece or T-tube). The first successful T-piece trial should be followed by extubation.

Conclusion

It is recommended to apply NIV, essentially CPAP, as early as possible in patients suffering from acute cardiogenic pulmonary oedema. CPAP should be applied 30 min/h until dyspnoea and oxygenation is improved. NIV improves both lung and heart functions.

References

1. Peter JV, Moran JL, Phillips-Hughes J, *et al.* Effect of non-invasive positive pressure ventilation (NIPPV) on mortality in patients with acute cardiogenic pulmonary oedema: a meta-analysis. *Lancet* 2006;**367**:1155–63.

2. Masip J, Roque M, Sanchez B, *et al.* Noninvasive ventilation in acute cardiogenic pulmonary edema: systematic review and meta-analysis. *JAMA* 2005;**294**:3124–3130.
3. Dickstein K, Cohen-Solal A, Filippatos G, *et al.*; ESC Guidelines for the diagnosis and treatment of acute and chronic heart failure 2008: the Task Force for the Diagnosis and Treatment of Acute and Chronic Heart Failure 2008 of the European Society of Cardiology. Developed in collaboration with the Heart Failure Association of the ESC (HFA) and endorsed by the European Society of Intensive Care Medicine (ESICM). *Eur Heart J* 2008;**29**:2388–44.

PART XVII

Disease management

54

Multidisciplinary heart failure management programmes

Ali Vazir and Suzanna Hardman

Introduction

In the early 21st century, heart failure (HF) guidelines and other consensus documents recommend a multidisciplinary approach to the management of people with this diagnosis.[1–8] This trend towards, and aspiration to, the involvement of a range of health care professionals in the care of a particularly vulnerable patient group does not appear controversial. It seems intuitive that this would deliver best care, and is an approach welcomed by patient groups. But how robust is the evidence for this approach, and which components of these multidisciplinary services confer benefit and in what health care contexts? To what extent are they then applicable to other populations and health care environments? The literature is extensive, diverse, and complex, which explains the repeated meta-analyses undertaken, and both published and planned Cochrane reviews.

In this chapter we explore the background to, and evidence for, different models of multidisciplinary working, and conclude by arguing for a more consistent implementation of care for those with HF.

HF management programmes tend to focus on the care of patients who have been admitted to hospital; this group has a high readmission rate and subsequent mortality, so there is much to be gained by improving care. Worryingly, 60% or more of HF patients continue to present in advanced HF, as acute admissions. This failure to make an early robust diagnosis and implement best care in the community is then frequently confounded by a failure to optimize management in the hospital setting.[8] This is not intended to underestimate the difficulty, or time involved, in making a robust diagnosis in patients who are often, though not invariably, elderly, and who frequently suffer from a range of other conditions or comorbidities. These problems are further confounded by the lack of access to natriuretic peptide testing and echocardiography, both in primary care and in acute hospital settings. Following stabilization, the introduction of drugs—angiotensin-converting enzyme (ACE) inhibitors, β-blockers, and aldosterone antagonists—that prolong life and reduce hospital readmissions can be time consuming, and the optimization of these drugs more so. Too many patients leave hospital without an adequate diagnosis or even the introduction of basic life-enhancing medication,[8,9] and optimization of the medical therapy is unusual. Hence the inevitable cycle of inadequate treatment and early readmissions, with psychological and physical deterioration and high mortality, is established. Yet the length of hospital stay in the United Kingdom is long relative to Europe and the United States, suggesting that care is not well organized. These failures are confounded by other factors including insufficient discharge planning or poor follow-up. In this context poor patient self-care behaviour, including increased risk of non-compliance with medication and lifestyle change, or lack of symptom recognition,[10,11] should be no surprise. The management of patients with HF can be further complicated by behavioural, psychosocial, and financial considerations. Collectively these factors may contribute to 50% of HF exacerbations[3] and over one-third of hospital readmissions. HF is one of the commonest causes of either admission or readmission to hospital in adults over 65,[4] with about 2% of the NHS budget spent on HF-related care in the United Kingdom, though in absolute terms the United Kingdom spends less per patient on HF care than France, Germany, or the United States (see Fig. 54.1)[12] where outcomes are often better. Irrespective of these differentials, HF care is regarded as expensive across Europe, the United States, and Australia, with a high proportion of the costs attributable to hospitalization.[5]

Inadequately diagnosed and managed, a diagnosis of HF continues to carry an unacceptably high mortality.[8,13] For these reasons, in recent years there has been a growing interest in the development of more effective strategies for the care of patients with HF, including the use of HF management programmes. These programmes are designed to improve outcomes through a multidisciplinary approach with structured follow-up including patient education, outpatient optimization of medical treatment, psychosocial support, and better access to care when needed. The multidisciplinary teams may include any of a wide number of health care professionals, though inclusion of a HF nurse is usual, and in some HF management programmes may be the only intervention. The content and structure of HF management programmes vary from one

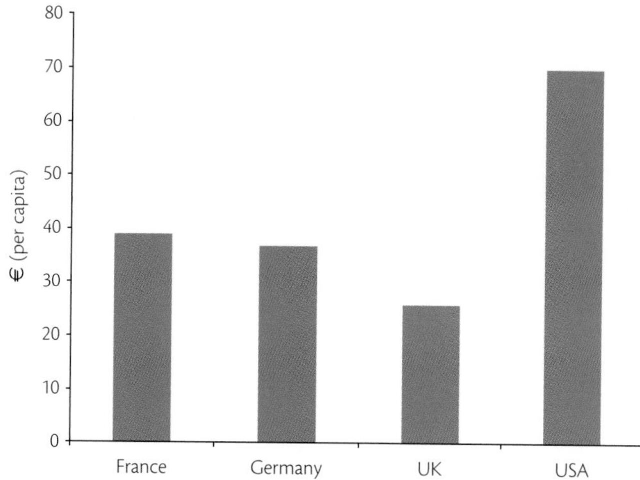

Fig. 54.1 Absolute expenditure for heart failure in France, Germany, the United Kingdom, and the United States.

Data adapted from Bundkirchen A, Schwinger RHG. Epidemiology and economic burden of chronic heart failure. *Eur Heart J Suppl* 2004;**6**(D):D57–60.

health care setting to another, but they appear to be most effective where tailored to meet local needs and available infrastructure.[14] With a few important exceptions,[15–18] inpatient care is not formally optimized (and rarely described) before recruitment, and the focus of interventions tends to be on subsequent outpatient care with an emphasis on reducing readmissions. Whilst this is an important consideration, an opportunity to reduce early (inpatient) and subsequent mortality and further reduce the readmission rate is often lost. These differences may explain the wide range of mortalities for the total cohorts reported from different studies (see Table 54.1), where similarly high-risk patients have been the focus of a range of interventions. Support for this thesis comes from the demonstration that one of the predictors of long-term outcome for patients who have been admitted to hospital with HF, from the 2009 National HF audit for England and Wales, is the number of (HF) drugs a patient is taking at the time of discharge (see Fig. 54.2) and better outcome for those whose management includes cardiologists and care within specialist wards.[8]

Attempts to understand and to interpret the diverse range of studies relating to HF programmes for patients who have been admitted to hospital, should recognize the considerable impact the quality of inpatient care for HF patients will have on immediate and long-term outcomes, and the extent to which any subsequent intervention confers benefit. Papers often provide little detail of this, but where standard inpatient HF care is minimal it will likely serve to exaggerate the benefits of the intervention under scrutiny. In contrast, good standard inpatient clinical care may make it more difficult for any intervention to demonstrate additional benefit (though should be reflected in mortality outcomes for the overall cohort). Similarly, in the literature there is often a dearth of information describing the standard availability of, and access to, HF and other services across the wider health communities. Yet this context may also exert important differential influences on the short- and longer-term patient outcomes, and the ability to demonstrate benefits of any intervention. A further complexity that impacts on an individual's response to a diagnosis of HF, including any advice, is the illness beliefs of that person—a complexity we should recognize but which is for the most part beyond the scope of this chapter.[19,20]

Evidence base for multidisciplinary heart failure management programmes

One of the first published reports of multidisciplinary HF management programmes was a pilot study performed in the early 1990s by Rich and colleagues, exploring the feasibility of a multidisciplinary HF management programme in elderly patients.[21] The subsequent study was a randomized controlled trial in 282 patients, powered to show a reduction in survival at 90 days without readmission. The randomized intervention—nurse-led education with review of medication by a geriatric cardiologist and intensive follow-up at home—did not achieve significance for the primary endpoint, but a range of secondary endpoints relating to readmissions were significant in favour of the intervention, and this appeared both to be cost-effective and to improve quality of life when compared with usual care. Other studies of home-based interventions and other multidisciplinary interventions followed, with numerous publications involving many thousands of patients, but only a relatively small proportion of these were randomized controlled trials, rarely blinded, and some more statistically robust than others.[22]

Stewart's work from Adelaide, Australia, examined the impact of a nurse-led intervention, with access to multidisciplinary input, on patients with recurrent hospitalization for HF.[23] The home visit was undertaken within 2 weeks of leaving hospital and included a thorough clinical assessment, review of medications, and identification of factors likely to provoke readmission. This resulted in a high level of additional input from others including GPs, cardiologists, pharmacists, and a range of social support. This was followed by telephone calls at 3 and 6 months. No detail is given of inpatient care, but reference to short admissions and the relatively high overall subsequent mortality might suggest no formal programme of inpatient optimization. The intervention significantly reduced the combined primary endpoint of the frequency of unplanned readmissions plus all-cause out-of-hospital deaths at 6 months, but there was no impact on out-of-hospital deaths or all-cause mortality at 6 months. The unplanned readmission rates were similar for the two groups, but overall unplanned bed usage was significantly less in the intervention group. Following a hospital admission the background level of care from a range of professionals was high, and services much more accessible than in the United Kingdom and some other European countries. Thus, typical follow-up for the patients receiving usual care included both a cardiology outpatient appointment and an appointment with their primary care physician within 14 days, and subsequent regular review by both. The study thus raised a number of interesting questions as to its reproducibility in other, less well-resourced, health care systems. An interesting finding was a trend towards increased elective bed usage in the intervention group, with most of this due to surgical intervention that had earlier been delayed when the patients were unstable. If we assume this contributed to the well-being of these patients, the finding illustrates the hazards of employing reduced bed usage as a surrogate for good care for patients with HF. Stewart had earlier reported a very similar study[24] where the intervention had also conferred benefit on their rather unusual combined primary endpoint of frequency of unplanned readmissions plus

Table 54.1 A range of heart failure studies illustrating wide variation in mortality in usual care

Study	Sample size	Age	Summary findings	Usual care mortality
Home-based intervention				
Rich and colleagues (US, 1995)	282	79	Nurse-led education, social service consultation, review of medications and planning for early discharge, as a multidisciplinary intervention, did not significantly modify the combined primary endpoint of 'survival for 90 days without readmissions' when compared with the control group (p = 0.09), though the trend was in favour of the intervention	12.1% at 3 months
Jaarsma and colleagues (Netherlands, 1999)	179	73	RCT to assess the effect of education and support by a nurse on self-care and resource utilization in patients with HF. The increase in self-caring behaviour observed in all patients was significantly greater in the intervention group than in the control group, beyond 1 month. No significant effects were found on the use of health care resources	17% at 9 months
Cline and colleagues (Sweden, 1998)	190	76	Prospective randomized trial to assess the impact of nurse-led education and nurse follow-up clinics on time to hospitalization, days in hospital and health care costs. Of these outcome measures the intervention only had a significant effect on time to hospitalization (p < 0.05), though elsewhere a trend in favour of the intervention was noted	28% at 12 months
Stewart and colleagues (Australia, 1998)	97	75	RCT to assess the effect of a home-based intervention involving a pharmacist, nurse, and others as needed, on the combined endpoint of 'frequency of re-admissions and out of hospital deaths'. This intervention resulted in a significantly reduced event rate at 6 months (p = 0.03)	25% at 6 months
Blue and colleagues (UK, 2001)	165	75	Nurse-led education beginning in hospital with high-intensity subsequent support and protocol led up-titration of medicines. A RCT with a combined primary endpoint of 'time to all-cause death or rehospitalization because of worsening HF'. A significant difference in this event rate was found in favour of the intervention (p < 0.05) at 12 months	31% at 12 months
Krumholz and colleagues (US, 2002)	88	74	RCT designed to demonstrate a reduction in the primary combined end point of 'readmission or death at 12 months', where the randomized intervention was a nurse-led education initiative with phone calls to identify deterioration, but not to modify treatment per se. This intervention conferred significant benefit in terms of this combined endpoint and appeared cost-effective	29.5 % at 12 months
Telemonitoring-based intervention				
Goldberg and colleagues (US, 2003)	280	59	RCT, in a relatively young cohort, of daily monitoring of weight and symptoms using a technology-based approach, to assess impact upon rehospitalization rates at 180 days. There was no significant impact on the primary endpoint but the intervention conferred mortality benefit in the population studied	19% at 6 months
Cleland and colleagues (European, 2005)	426	68	RCT of telemonitoring versus telephone support, compared with usual care. The primary endpoint was a combined endpoint of 'days dead or hospitalized at 12 months', with no significant difference between the groups. However notable differences in mortality are reported	48% at 12 months
Dar and colleagues (UK, 2009)	182	70	RCT of usual care versus telemonitoring. There was no significant difference in the primary endpoint of 'days alive and out of hospital at 6 months'	5.4% at 6 months
Clinic-based intervention				
McDonald and colleagues (Ireland, 2002)	98	71	RCT, following inpatient optimization of treatment and predischarge clinical stability for all. The subsequent randomized intervention of nurse-led HF clinics for patient and family conferred significant benefit in terms of the primary combined endpoint of 'mortality or HF readmission' (p = 0.04), in the context of an overall low mortality rate	6.4% at 3 months
Doughty and colleagues (New Zealand, 2002)	197	73	Cluster RCT to assess the effect of an integrated HF management programme (involving educationof patients and their families with follow-up shared between primary and secondary care) on the primary combined endpoint of 'death or hospital readmission'. There was no significant impact of the intervention on the combined event rate when compared with usual care	24.7% at 12 months
Kasper and colleagues (US, 2002)	200	62	RCT of a multidisciplinary input involving a personal treatment plan, devised by a HF cardiologist and nurse implemented, supported by frequent phone calls and GP support for other conditions. There was no significant effect of the intervention on the primary combined endpoint of 'all-cause mortality and HF readmissions', but as with other studies benefit in terms of secondary outcomes	13.2% at 6 months
Stromberg and colleagues (Sweden, 2003)	106	78	Patients admitted to hospital with HF were randomized to either nurse-led HF clinics or usual care. The primary endpoint was all-cause mortality or all-cause hospital admissions at 12 months and the event (death or readmission) rate was significantly reduced (p < 0. 03)	24% at 3 months, and 37% at 12 months
Jaarsma and colleagues (Netherlands, 2008)	1023	71	Multicentre RCT of moderate vs high-intensity nurse-led disease management compared with usual care (involving cardiology follow-up). Neither the moderate intensity nor the high-intensity intervention reduced the primary endpoint of 'time to death or rehospitalization because of HF'	29% at 18 months

HF, heart failure; RCT, randomized controlled trial.

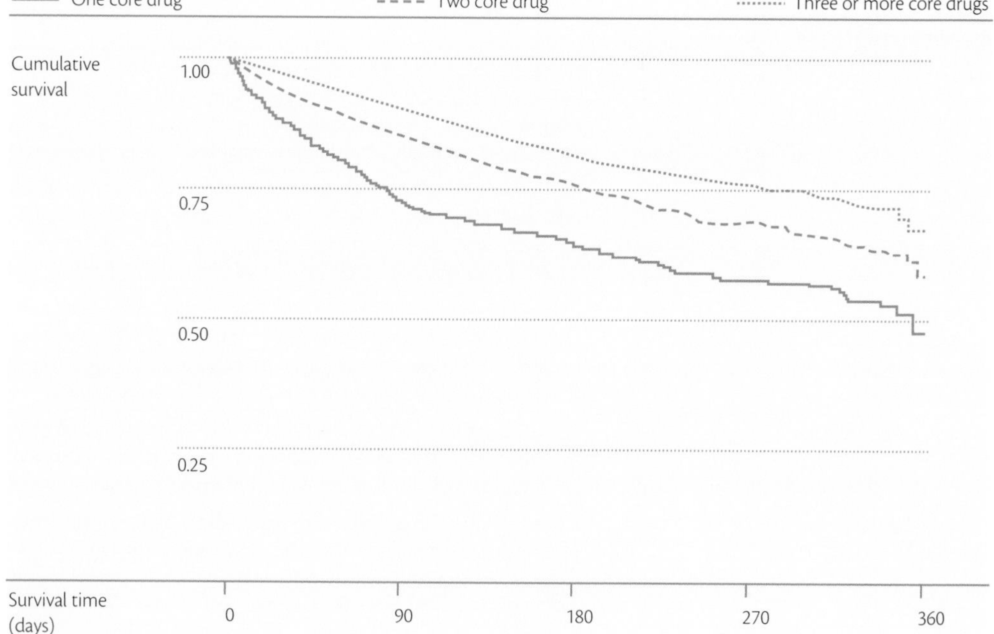

Fig. 54.2 Cumulative survival of heart failure patients over the course of a year. Patients on only one core drug have a worse prognosis compared to heart failure patients on two, whereas those taking three, or more core drugs for heart failure have the best survival.

all-cause out-of-hospital deaths at 6 months.[23,25] The combining of these study cohorts and long-term follow-up suggest that the early intervention, delivered in the context of a well-resourced and well-supported health care community, continued to deliver considerable late benefit to the patients including reduced mortality (Fig. 54.3), lower readmission rates, and related cumulative bed day usage, while being highly cost-effective.[26] In discussing these late benefits the authors make an important point, which may be key to an effective multidisciplinary grouping: as the improved outcomes are observed by those involved in the ongoing care of the patients, good practice is reinforced and perpetuated over time.

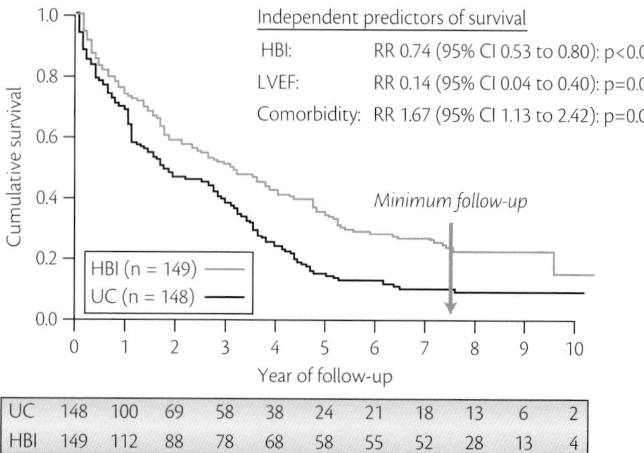

UC	148	100	69	58	38	24	21	18	13	6	2
HBI	149	112	88	78	68	58	55	52	28	13	4

Fig. 54.3 All-cause mortality, and the impact of a home-based intervention (HBI), on mortality in a group of patients hospitalized for heart failure and then randomized to either usual care or HBI with all patients followed up for a minimum of 7.5 years.
From Inglis SC, Pearson S, Treen S, Gallasch T, Horowitz JD, Stewart S. Extending the horizon in chronic heart failure: effects of multidisciplinary, home-based intervention relative to usual care. *Circulation* 2006;**114**(23):2466–73, with permission.

From Scotland came further evidence of the effectiveness of nurse-led interventions, supported by the local HF cardiologists, in reducing HF readmissions.[25] These patients were not required to receive any predetermined standard of inpatient care, but following recruitment (from the cohort undergoing echocardiography, in whom echocardiography confirmed that the HF failure was due to left ventricular systolic dysfunction, LVSD) were randomized either to intervention or to standard care under the admitting physician and subsequently their GP. Those randomized to intervention received input from the HF nurse during that admission and then a home visit within 48 h and subsequent intensive input with visits at 1, 3, and 6 weeks and then at 3, 6, 9 and 12 months. The nurses additionally made 10 phone calls at prespecified time-points and encouraged further contact from the patient and their carers. The nurse input combined education with encouraging the patient's awareness of symptoms, and psychological support. The HF nurses also aimed to up-titrate drugs, using written protocols. The primary endpoint was a combined endpoint of all-cause mortality or hospital admission for HF at 12 months, for which a significant difference was reported in favour of those receiving the intervention; though, had the very different inpatient mortalities (during the index admission) not been included, statistical significance would not have been reached.[22] At 12 months HF readmissions and related bed usage were both significantly reduced, but there was no impact on all-cause admissions, all-cause hospital bed usage, or all-cause mortality, which was of the order of 30% for the total cohort, and similar to that of Stewart *et al.*[24]

McDonald's group, from Ireland, report a rather different approach, initially as a pilot and subsequently as a randomized controlled trial.[16] In this study all patients with HF received inpatient optimization of care, including echocardiography, and medical therapy (then defined for those with impaired systolic function as diuretics, digoxin, and ACE inhibitors at maximally tolerated doses). They were required to satisfy predefined clinical and stability criteria before discharge. Those randomized to the active intervention received three or more consultations with a nurse specialist and dietician while inpatients, and subsequently were telephoned within 3 days of leaving hospital and weekly thereafter. Both these telephone calls and the HF clinic appointments at 2, 6, and 12 weeks allowed for clinical reassessment and reinforcement of the educational messages. In clinic appointments, intravenous infusions of diuretics could be administered when necessary. In contrast, following optimization of inpatient care, including pre-discharge clinical stability, the control group were referred back to their primary physician for any ongoing care. The study achieved statistical significance for the primary combined endpoint of death or HF readmission at 12 weeks, with the intervention conferring benefit. Although this paper is not without its own statistical quirks,[22] arguably its greatest interest lies in the very low mortality at 3 months (7.1%) for the entire cohort, which it can be argued reflects the strategy of inpatient optimization of care.

In this context the mortality rates we reported from a randomized controlled trial of a low-intensity, nurse-led, self-management intervention, in patients who were hospitalized for HF due to LVSD and recruited when stable following a routine strategy of cardiology-led inpatient optimization of care, are of interest.[17,18] It is of note that the patients in this cohort were elderly and high risk, with multiple comorbidities, and referred from primary care populations noted to have a year-on-year excess cardiovascular mortality, when compared with the United Kingdom, London, and similar Primary Care Trusts.

This study was designed to explore the possibility that a low-intensity, nurse-led, self-management intervention using a problem-solving strategy would reduce HF readmissions. Following recruitment, those randomized to the intervention were visited by a nurse twice while in hospital and then again at home within 10 days of leaving hospital. Thereafter the nurse phoned the patients once, but was available by phone should the patient initiate further telephone contact.

In all other respects there was no difference in the HF care between the two randomized cohorts which included a hospital-wide, protocol-driven, shared-care strategy involving cardiologists and the admitting physicians, aimed at early diagnosis and subsequent inpatient optimization of ACE inhibitors, diuretics including aldosterone receptor antagonists, and, for some, initiation of β-blockade. Patients were allowed home when they were clinically and biochemically stable without treatment changes for 48 h. Thereafter all patients had early and continued cardiology review. The broader context was that when the study was designed and undertaken there were no HF nurses employed either by the hospital or by the local community, and there were no GPs with a special interest in HF. Provisional results, reported elsewhere, demonstrated no difference in the readmission rates at either 3 or 12 months between the two randomized groups. The all-cause mortality for the total cohort was relatively low at both 3 months[17] (and similar to MacDonald's study), and again at 12 months (17.6%). We would suggest this reflects the early inpatient optimization of care for all.[18]

Interestingly, using post-hoc subset analyses, we demonstrated a differential response between those admitted with a pre-existing diagnosis and those admitted with a new diagnosis (incident HF). In the latter group the randomized intervention conferred benefit in terms of reduced HF readmissions and bed usage at 12 months (see Fig. 54.4), and importantly there was no mortality penalty, but rather a trend towards improved mortality.[18]

Thus far we have explored in some detail just a few publications from an extensive literature. Elsewhere papers argue for the benefits of nurse-led HF clinics,[27] strategies around patient education,[28,29] the use of nurses and or pharmacists to effect the up-titration of drugs using agreed protocols and treatment algorithms [30] as hospital outpatient led initiatives,[16,27,31–33] or community-based approaches including programmes where home visits are key.[23–26,29,34] Many of the studies use phone calls to reinforce care and provide increased access to additional care. The phone calls can provide reassurance and allow patients the opportunity to discuss symptoms, treatment, and side effects where contact with a programme has already been established.[16,18,24,25,32,35] Phone calls may be less well received where there has been no prior contact, or where the patients are elderly or have some degree of mental impairment. The literature may be especially vulnerable to publication bias here, in favour of studies with positive outcomes. Patients who are elderly, immobile, or less mentally alert may derive particular benefit from home visits, but this can be a much more costly intervention than clinic-led care. Increasingly in some health care systems this community care is being devolved to other health care professionals who may have little or no specific training in the area of HF.

Remote monitoring is undoubtedly an emerging model for delivering components of HF care, either to a large group of individuals who may not have access to traditional programmes, or as an adjunct to other programmes of HF care. The subject is dealt with in detail elsewhere, but involves daily monitoring of symptoms and signs measured by patients, family, or caregivers at home, so allowing patients to remain under close supervision[36] in their own home. A range of equipment may be installed in the home allowing variables such as blood pressure, heart rate, oxygen saturation,

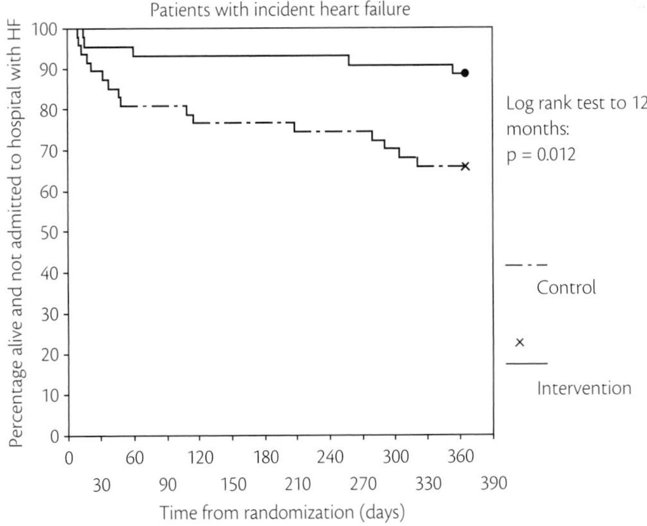

Fig. 54.4 The impact of a low-intensity self-management intervention on event-free survival for patients admitted to hospital with incident heart failure (due to left ventricular systolic dysfunction). Results based on post-hoc subset analysis of a randomized controlled blinded trial.

From Zaphiriou A, Mulligan K, Hargrave P, *et al.* Improved outcomes following hospitalisation in patients with a new diagnosis of heart failure: Results from a randomised controlled trial of a novel, nurse-led self-management intervention *Heart* 2006;**92**: A119–A120.

weight, symptoms, and medication compliance to be recorded and transmitted. This then allows a designated health care worker to remotely advise on changes in care. The success of remote monitoring is highly dependent on patient education and the ease with which the equipment can be used, both by those setting it up and by those endeavouring to use it. Central to its effectiveness is patient, and or carer, education, which is usually time consuming, and more difficult in those with cognitive impairment. Currently there appears to be no consensus regarding which variables are most helpful to monitor. New equipment, additional monitoring parameters, and increasingly sophisticated technologies are under development.[36] Nonetheless, themes discussed earlier re-emerge from the telemonitoring literature, namely that the extent of the benefit appears greatest where baseline care is less well developed. This may explain in part the differences in outcomes between the Trans-European Network Initiative (TENS-HMS)[13] and those of the Home-HF study.[37] 'Usual care' from the Trans-European Network Initiative reported the highest 12-month mortality of 48%, but it was also high both in those receiving home telemonitoring, at 29%, and in those receiving nurse telephone support, at 27%. In contrast, in the Home-HF study, *6 month* mortality rates were 9.8% for the intervention group and 5.4% in the usual care group, though the study had not been powered to demonstrate a mortality difference. The message from this may be simple and appears to be supported by details of those patients studied: namely, that baseline HF care for the patients being recruited from three hospitals in north-west London was probably better than that received by their counterparts recruited from hospitals in the United Kingdom, Germany and the Netherlands. The home telemonitoring from TENS-HMS did not reduce readmissions, but the mean duration of stay was shorter by 6 days for those randomized to home telemonitoring, whereas Home-HF reported no reduction in days alive and out of hospital but avoided readmissions via the emergency department and was cost neutral.

The HF literature exploring the impact of various interventions ranges from tiny studies to large, well-devised randomized controlled trials with an accompanying range of outcomes, so the extensive literature also includes systematic reviews and meta-analyses.[22,38,39] All recognize the heterogeneity of the included studies (even in the absence of descriptors of standard care) and so exclude and group the studies in a range of different ways.[22,38,39] McAllister and Holland both endeavoured to report on whether multidisciplinary strategies improve outcomes for HF patients, with the main emphasis on mortality and readmissions. McAllister's group concluded that where follow-up included a specialized multidisciplinary team both HF admissions and mortality were improved, whereas interventions designed to enhance self-care and telephone follow-up or telemonitoring reduced admissions but had no impact on mortality. In contrast, Holland's group found that it was the postdischarge interventions which combined education with self-management strategies that reduced mortality alongside readmissions. As ever, the answer lies in the detail, much of which goes unpublished in the interest of brevity.[38,39]

So, can the limitations of meta-analyses and structured reviews be overcome by larger studies? The Coordinating study evaluating Outcomes of Advising and Counselling in Heart Failure (COACH),[32] aimed at examining the effect of education and an intense support programme by HF nurses on top of frequent visits with a cardiologist, is of considerable interest in this context, and poses some fundamental questions which challenge earlier accepted conclusions relating to HF care. As so often, there is no detail surrounding the quality or norm for inpatient care or whether inpatient optimization is usual. Of note is a reduction from NYHA class III or IV on admission to NHYA class II/III for the vast majority by discharge, though curiously no patients were rendered asymptomatic despite high levels of prescribing of ACE inhibitors/angiotension receptor blockers (83%), diuretics (95%), and β-blockers (66%). These figures of course do not tell us anything about dose levels or timing of up-titration. All patients saw a cardiologist on at least four occasions and additionally as dictated clinically. On this background of usual care there was a three-way randomization to a control group, a basic support group (where there was a nurse-led programme of structured education and outpatient visits, but no home-based intervention), or an intensive nurse-led support programme where contacts with the nurse were monthly over the 18-month study period, and included two home visits and some multidisciplinary input from a physiotherapist, dietitian, and social worker. This multicentre study recruited and randomized more than 1000 patients from across the Netherlands with a mean age 71 ± 11 years, of whom 38% were women, and then followed them up over an 18-month period. Although there was no significant difference in the primary endpoint of time to death or rehospitalization and the number of days lost to death or hospitalization, the all-cause mortality for the entire cohort (with no significant differences between the groups) was relatively low at around 21–22% at 12 months. The COACH authors conclude that the patients in the control group were already well managed, making it more difficult to improve the outcome with the added intervention. We concur with that conclusion, noting that the mortality rate at 12 months is substantially lower than that of many published studies,[23–25] but in keeping with our own.[18] The authors further note that hospital admissions may be beneficial (where care is carefully and appropriately targeted at the patients needs), rather than deleterious, noting that in the intervention groups a nonsignificant trend to reduction in mortality was accompanied by more frequent, shorter hospital admissions.

Box 54.1 Patient priorities for heart failure service

- Access to quick and accurate diagnosis without delays in the pathway
- Good links between the services, organizations, and professions
- Having a point of contact and someone to coordinate care requirements
- Easy access to specialist advice and medication
- Access to specialist services such as rehabilitation and counselling
- Regular follow-up and ability to seek advice at short notice
- Information
- Honesty about prognosis

Source: Health Care Commission survey 2007.

Table 54.2 The multidisciplinary heart failure team. These components of the team are not intended to be either comprehensive or exclusive but rather a suggested model for those establishing or improving existing services

Key members of HF team (suggested minimum)	Other expertise/services periodically required for HF patients	Comments
Consultant cardiologist with an interest in HF (service lead)	Rehabilitation	Ideally in some form for all, but to date few benefit
GP	Electrophysiology/ device implantation/ revascularization	Need to have established access for those who require this when indicated
HF nurse specialist	Imaging	Timely high-quality echocardiography for all. Other imaging will be needed to establish aetiology, prognosis, and intervention in some
	Social services	
	Palliative care/end of life planning	These teams may serve to up-skill the core HF team and selectively provide input to individual patients
	Input from health care professionals with other expertise e.g. renal, diabetes, respiratory, haematology, care of the elderly, renal, diabetes, surgeons, psychologists, and others	The challenge for the future is to deliver high-quality care with a balance between general and specialist care for those with more than one long-term condition
	Pharmacists	Can be a key component of delivering multidisciplinary care, and a valuable and as yet underused resource for inpatients

GP, general practitioner; HF, heart failure.

So what might we conclude? A critical reading of the literature and recognition of its limitations should not in any way discourage, but rather support, the establishment of effective and responsive multidisciplinary teams for the care of people with known or suspected HF. Encouragingly, these aims are consistent with the patients' priorities that emerged from the Health Care Commission within England (see Box 54.1).

To date the emphasis of these groupings has been community based but a number of studies and emerging audit data argue powerfully, in addition, for an improvement in hospital care where best outcomes can be achieved when patients are proactively identified, and ongoing care, including early echocardiography, is led by a (HF) cardiologist, and ideally within a specialist ward where a range of health care professionals will be involved to ensure rapid stabilization and inpatient optimization of treatment. As the patient recovers opportunities for education arise and should be embraced—and this is the ideal time for first contacts with those who will be involved in their care when they leave hospital. This often involves a HF nurse specialist who may subsequently see the patients in clinics or their own homes, but might equally be a number of others. Discharge planning should include plans for primary care and cardiology review, rehabilitation, β-blocker up-titration and ongoing opportunities for individuals to understand their condition. It is important that the patient knows whom to contact and how to do so in the early days following a hospital admission when they may be most vulnerable. For individual

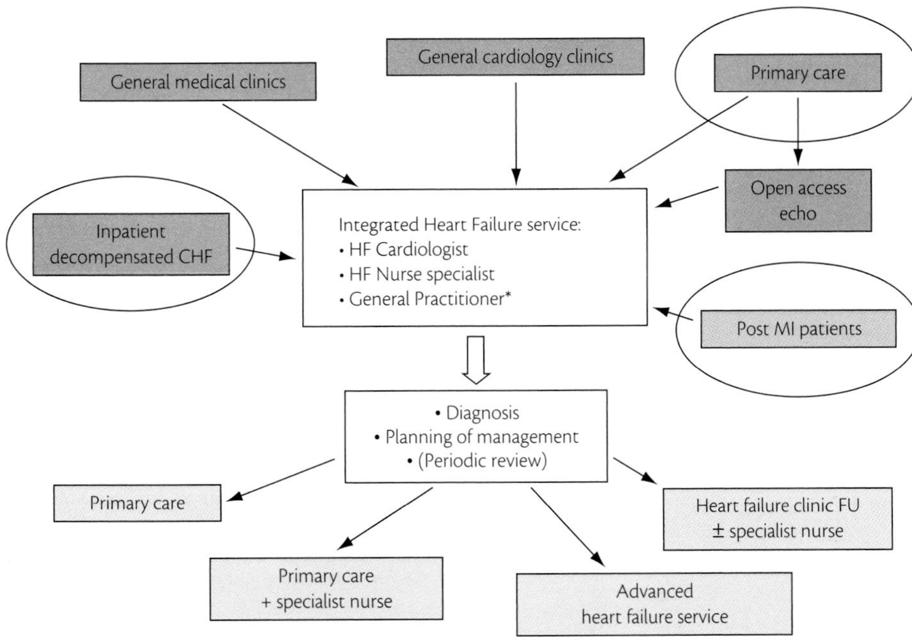

Fig. 54.5 Model of an integrated heart failure service. Like Table 54.3, this emphasizes the need for multidisciplinary working across the different health care domains.
Adapted from McDonagh TA. Lessons from the management of chronic heart failure. *Heart* 2005;**91**(Suppl 2):ii24–7, with permission.

patients, input from others may make the difference between ongoing improvement and an early, unplanned readmission. The nature of this input may be diverse—certain needs will be identified before the patient goes home but others may only become apparent in the days after leaving hospital and this argues for an early home assessment which, wherever possible, should be inclusive of spouse or carer.

And so we see the emerging need for an established multidisciplinary team, ideally led by the HF cardiologist who has been involved with the care of the patient during the index admission, working closely with the GP and HF nurse specialist, but with access to many others. The skill in building this team is to establish mechanisms of support, mutual trust, and learning so that the patient's changing needs may be met in a timely fashion and delivered in a cost-effective manner across the different health care communities. Table 54.2 summarizes important components of a multidisciplinary HF team. This team will include people who may never directly meet many of the patients but their expertise can be drawn upon. It is essential that when discussions occur that they include a clinician who knows the patient well.

Thus, rather than an overriding obsession with length of stay the HF community needs to focus on the quality of care during an index HF admission and thereafter within the patient's community, recognizing that for some timely and planned readmissions may be part of a health care strategy that delivers a much lower mortality rate than we have seen hitherto, and an improved quality of life. Timely access to a range of expertise through a multidisciplinary team is essential for the patient, with the HF cardiologist, a HF nurse specialist, and the GP ideally at the centre of this care delivery (Fig. 54.5). This will allow specialist input when necessary alongside the input of the generalist, which is also critical given the wide range of comorbidities that confound and complicate the problems of this patient group. Over time, continuity of care and (wherever practicable) self-management will reduce the intensity of support needed by some and allow individual patients to re-establish their sense of normality.

References

1. Hunt SA, Abraham WT, Chin MH, *et al.* 2009 focused update incorporated into the ACC/AHA 2005 Guidelines for the Diagnosis and Management of Heart Failure in Adults: a report of the American College of Cardiology Foundation/American Heart Association Task Force on Practice Guidelines: developed in collaboration with the International Society for Heart and Lung Transplantation. *Circulation* 2009;**119**(14):e391–479.
2. McDonagh TA. Lessons from the management of chronic heart failure. *Heart* 2005;**91**(Suppl 2):ii24–7.
3. National Institute for Clinical Excellence. *NICE clinical guidance: Management of chronic heart failure in adults in primary and secondary care.* NICE, 2003.
4. Scottish Intercollegiate Guidelines Network. *Management of chronic heart failure: a national clinical guideline.* SIGN, Edinburgh, 2007.
5. Dickstein K, Cohen-Solal A, Filippatos G, *et al.* ESC guidelines for the diagnosis and treatment of acute and chronic heart failure 2008: the Task Force for the diagnosis and treatment of acute and chronic heart failure 2008 of the European Society of Cardiology. Developed in collaboration with the Heart Failure Association of the ESC (HFA) and endorsed by the European Society of Intensive Care Medicine (ESICM). *Eur J Heart Fail* 2008;**10**(10):933–89.
6. The NHS Information Centre for Health and Social Care. *National Heart Failure Second Audit Report for the audit period between July 2007 and March 2008.* National Clinical Audit Support Programme, http://www.ic.nhs.uk, 2008.
7. National Institute for Clinical Excellence. *NICE clinical guidance: Management of chronic heart failure in adults in primary and secondary care (partial update).* NICE, 2010.
8. NHS Information Centre for Health and Social Care. *National Heart Failure Third Audit Report for the audit period between April 2008 and March 2009.* National Clinical Audit Support Programme, http://www.ic.nhs.uk; 2009.
9. Cleland JG, Swedberg K, Cohen-Solal A, *et al.* The Euro Heart Failure Survey of the EUROHEART survey programme. A survey on the quality of care among patients with heart failure in Europe. The Study Group on Diagnosis of the Working Group on Heart Failure of the European Society of Cardiology. The Medicines Evaluation Group Centre for Health Economics University of York. *Eur J Heart Fail* 2000;**2**(2):123–32.
10. Evangelista LS, Dracup K. A closer look at compliance research in heart failure patients in the last decade. *Prog Cardiovasc Nurs* 2000;**15**(3):97–103.
11. van der Wal MH, Jaarsma T, van Veldhuisen DJ. Non-compliance in patients with heart failure; how can we manage it? *Eur J Heart Fail* 2005;**7**(1):5–17.
12. Bundkirchen A, Schwinger RHG. Epidemiology and economic burden of chronic heart failure. *Eur Heart J Suppl* 2004;**6**(D):D57–60.
13. Cleland JG, Louis AA, Rigby AS, Janssens U, Balk AH. Noninvasive home telemonitoring for patients with heart failure at high risk of recurrent admission and death: the Trans-European Network-Home-Care Management System (TEN-HMS) study. *J Am Coll Cardiol* 2005;**45**(10):1654–64.
14. Yu DS, Thompson DR, Lee DT. Disease management programmes for older people with heart failure: crucial characteristics which improve post-discharge outcomes. *Eur Heart J* 2006;**27**(5):596–612.
15. McDonald K, Ledwidge M, Cahill J, *et al.* Elimination of early rehospitalization in a randomized, controlled trial of multidisciplinary care in a high-risk, elderly heart failure population: the potential contributions of specialist care, clinical stability and optimal angiotensin-converting enzyme inhibitor dose at discharge. *Eur J Heart Fail* 2001;**3**(2):209–15.
16. McDonald K, Ledwidge M, Cahill J, *et al.* Heart failure management: multidisciplinary care has intrinsic benefit above the optimization of medical care. *J Card Fail* 2002;**8**(3):142–8.
17. Zaphiriou A, Mulligan K, Cowie MR, Newman S, Hardman SM. Should we assume that low-intensity interventions benefit patients admitted to hospital with heart failure in all health care systems? *Circulation* 2005;**112**(17):2794.
18. Zaphiriou A, Mulligan K, Hagrave P, *et al.* Improved outcomes following hospitalisation in patients with a new diagnosis of heart failure: Results from a randomised controlled trial of a novel, nurse-led self-management intervention. *Heart* 2006;**92**:A119–120.
19. Mulligan K, Zaphiriou A, Hargrave P, *et al.* Quality of life in heart failure is related to mood and illness beliefs rather than left ventricular dysfunction. *Eur Heart J* 2005;**26**:601.
20. Mulligan K, Zaphiriou A, Hargrave P, *et al.* A self-management intervention in heart failure: differential impact on newly diagnosed patients. *Psychol Health* 2006;**21**:109.
21. Rich MW, Beckham V, Wittenberg C, Leven CL, Freedland KE, Carney RM. A multidisciplinary intervention to prevent the readmission of elderly patients with congestive heart failure. *N Engl J Med* 1995;**333**(18):1190–5.
22. Taylor S, Bestall J, Cotter S, *et al.* Clinical service organisation for heart failure. *Cochrane Database Syst Rev* 2005;(2):CD002752.

23. Stewart S, Marley JE, Horowitz JD. Effects of a multidisciplinary, home-based intervention on unplanned readmissions and survival among patients with chronic congestive heart failure: a randomised controlled study. *Lancet* 1999;**354**(9184):1077–83.
24. Stewart S, Pearson S, Horowitz JD. Effects of a home-based intervention among patients with congestive heart failure discharged from acute hospital care. *Arch Intern Med* 1998;**158**(10):1067–72.
25. Blue L, Lang E, McMurray JJ, *et al.* Randomised controlled trial of specialist nurse intervention in heart failure. *BMJ* 2001;**323**(7315):715–18.
26. Inglis SC, Pearson S, Treen S, Gallasch T, Horowitz JD, Stewart S. Extending the horizon in chronic heart failure: effects of multidisciplinary, home-based intervention relative to usual care. *Circulation* 2006;**114**(23):2466–73.
27. Stromberg A, Martensson J, Fridlund B, Levin LA, Karlsson JE, Dahlstrom U. Nurse-led heart failure clinics improve survival and self-care behaviour in patients with heart failure: results from a prospective, randomised trial. *Eur Heart J* 2003;**24**(11):1014–23.
28. Koelling TM, Johnson ML, Cody RJ, Aaronson KD. Discharge education improves clinical outcomes in patients with chronic heart failure. *Circulation* 2005;**111**(2):179–85.
29. Krumholz HM, Amatruda J, Smith GL, *et al.* Randomized trial of an education and support intervention to prevent readmission of patients with heart failure. *J Am Coll Cardiol* 2002;**39**(1):83–9.
30. Blue L, McMurray J. How much responsibility should heart failure nurses take? *Eur J Heart Fail* 2005;**7**(3):351–61.
31. Doughty RN, Wright SP, Pearl A, *et al.*Randomized, controlled trial of integrated heart failure management: The Auckland Heart Failure Management Study. *Eur Heart J* 2002;**23**(2):139–46.
32. Jaarsma T, van der Wal MH, Lesman-Leegte I, *et al.* Effect of moderate or intensive disease management program on outcome in patients with heart failure: Coordinating Study Evaluating Outcomes of Advising and Counseling in Heart Failure (COACH). *Arch Intern Med* 2008;**168**(3):316–24.
33. Kasper EK, Gerstenblith G, Hefter G, *et al.* A randomized trial of the efficacy of multidisciplinary care in heart failure outpatients at high risk of hospital readmission. *J Am Coll Cardiol* 2002;**39**(3):471–80.
34. Cline CM, Israelsson BY, Willenheimer RB, Broms K, Erhardt LR. Cost effective management programme for heart failure reduces hospitalisation. *Heart* 1998;**80**(5):442–6.
35. Riegel B, Carlson B, Kopp Z, LePetri B, Glaser D, Unger A. Effect of a standardized nurse case-management telephone intervention on resource use in patients with chronic heart failure. *Arch Intern Med* 2002;**162**(6):705–12.
36. Clark RA, Inglis SC, McAlister FA, Cleland JG, Stewart S. Telemonitoring or structured telephone support programmes for patients with chronic heart failure: systematic review and meta-analysis. *BMJ* 2007;**334**(7600):942.
37. Dar O, Riley J, Chapman C, *et al.* A randomized trial of home telemonitoring in a typical elderly heart failure population in North West London: results of the Home-HF study. *Eur J Heart Fail* 2009;**11**(3):319–25.
38. Holland R, Battersby J, Harvey I, Lenaghan E, Smith J, Hay L. Systematic review of multidisciplinary interventions in heart failure. *Heart* 2005;**91**(7):899–906.
39. McAlister FA, Lawson FM, Teo KK, Armstrong PW. A systematic review of randomized trials of disease management programs in heart failure. *Am J Med* 2001;**110**(5):378–84.

55

End of life

Miriam Johnson

The clinical course of heart failure (HF) has been transformed by the development of therapies (medication, devices, and surgery) targeted at the pathophysiological mechanisms underlying its perpetuation and progression. Over the last decade, the prognosis has improved and it is likely that the 1-year survival figures often quoted[1] are now less bleak. However, given that HF is a progressive disease, patients who have not suffered a sudden cardiac death from arrhythmia ultimately enter an end stage which may be prolonged, and carries a significant daily symptom burden, affecting both themselves and their caregivers. With increasing use of implantable defibrillators, more patients may eventually live to experience such endstage disease. In addition, comorbidities, often smoking related, are common. Comorbidities add to the symptom load, affect optimum cardiac management, and may be the final cause of death.

End-of-life care is not always delivered well, particularly in secondary care settings where the emphasis may still be on life-prolonging interventions. The dying phase may not be recognized or acknowledged.[2,3] Despite Hinton's observations 50 years ago[4] that patients with HF and renal failure often died in distress, those with nonmalignant disease still have unequal access to services skilled in end-of-life care; more than 95% of patients seen by hospice services in the United Kingdom have cancer. In the United Kingdom, the Department of Health has declared end-of-life care to be a national priority.[5] To this end, a national End of Life Strategy is to be implemented throughout the National Health Service,[6] and tools such as the Liverpool Care of the Dying Pathway (LCP)[7] and the Gold Standards Framework (GSF)[8] have been recommended. Such a central drive is welcome, but several challenges remain in the care of the patient dying from HF; the main one being the difficulties clinicians, patients, and their carers may have in recognizing the end stage of the illness.

Recognition of endstage heart failure

> It appears to me a most excellent thing for the physician to cultivate Prognosis; for by foreseeing and foretelling . . . thus a man will be the more esteemed to be a good physician, for he will be the better able to treat those aright who can be saved, having long anticipated everything; and by seeing and announcing beforehand those who will live and those who will die. . . . Hippocrates.[9]

Hippocrates recognized the importance of prognostication and it remains a vital part of clinical management. Prognostication helps to frame the potential benefits and burdens of medical intervention, not only in terms of the individual patient's best interests, but also with regard to the best use of health care resources. He stated strongly that physicians should 'refuse to treat those who are overmastered by their diseases, realizing that in such cases medicine is powerless'. However, perhaps because of increasing therapeutic possibilities, it is tempting for the clinician to focus on any hope of prolonging a patient's life and to give less attention to the skill of prognostication. The recent greater emphasis on patient choice with regard to place of care and place of death, coupled with recent publications presenting the voice of patients and caregivers, show that many patients and their caregivers have a poor understanding of what HF is, its treatment, and likely clinical course.[10–14] Patients with HF therefore have less access to supportive and palliative services, despite a well-documented high psychological morbidity, and less chance to be involved in planning the last stage of their lives, than do patients with cancer.

Trajectories

Performance status is a useful prognostic sign. One of the main difficulties in recognizing the dying phase of patients with HF is that the trajectory of their performance status is one of gradual decline interspersed by periods of decompensation followed by recovery to a level almost equal to their predecompensation state.[15] Performance will deteriorate more quickly in the last few months of the patient's life, but still follow the pattern of dips and recovery; there may even be an initial indication of recovery from the final episode of deterioration that leads to death. Thus, patients, their caregivers, and clinicians may have been through the cycle of anxiety induced by decompensation followed by relief at restoration several times and it can be difficult to recognize the one decompensation from which there will be no recovery.

In contrast, the disease trajectory of a patient with lung cancer is said to be more predictable, with a rapid decline to death over the last 1–2 months of life.[15] However, in practice, patients with cancer can also follow a declining trajectory interspersed with acute events followed by recovery. Individual patients with HF have an even more chaotic trajectory than typically shown,[16] and their experience is often characterized by daily fluctuations in how they feel. In addition, many patients have concurrent chronic lung disease and chronic kidney disease which further complicates the clinical situation.

However, despite the difficulties, there are clinical features that make it possible to see the background deterioration in overall stage of HF. It is important to assess this background context when making management decisions about individual patients in order to allow relevant discussions with the patient and their caregivers about the aims and likely success of various treatment options.

Markers of worsening heart failure

It is important to recognize signs of worsening HF that should trigger sensitive conversations with the patient about the stage of their illness and to allow them and their carers to work out together realistic hopes and goals in light of their decline. Awareness of a patient's wishes, such as the wish to be able to die at home and not be readmitted to hospital, is important. Even if the patient dies suddenly at home, the caregiver will be aware of the patient's wishes and an inappropriate use of an emergency ambulance and futile attempt at cardiopulmonary resuscitation (CPR) can be avoided. For those who die of progressive HF, recognition of this stage allows access to support (social services and financial), symptom control, and advanced planning and coordination of care (including out of hours care) in order to allow the patient to be cared for in the place of their choosing. Most patients, given the choice, express a wish to die at home, but currently nearly two-thirds will die in hospital.[17]

There are many clinical scoring systems for HF that attempt to aid prognostication. They range from the simple New York Heart Association (NYHA) classification to more complex scores including age, aetiology of HF, QRS duration, and biochemical markers such as brain natriuretic peptide, serum creatinine, and serum sodium.[18–24] More simple systems have been suggested using NHYA status, age, and comorbidities.[25] However, in practice, looking at a patient's course in the context of what has been happening over the past 3–6 months is usually adequate. The patient with worsening and persistent hypotension, sufficient to render intolerance of cardiac drugs; persistent hyponatraemia and deteriorating renal function; increasing doses of diuretics; repeated hospital admissions with episodes of decompensation (especially those without an apparent precipitating factor); loss of body mass; and worsening fatigue all indicate an irreversible decline in health status.

Communication

Patients with HF often have inadequate understanding of their disease, the stage of their disease, and the aims of treatment, and thus have little say in their care at the end of life.[10,11,13,26,27] Barnes *et al.*[28] found that few patients with HF had had any discussion regarding prognosis with any health care professional. Sensitive communication to explore what a patient already understands and what they are able to take in is important, both to redress this balance and to ensure informed consent for treatment. There are understandable concerns from clinicians about removing hope, and, indeed, entering such discussions is often difficult for clinician, patient, and carer. However, evidence from the fields of oncology and renal medicine shows that, although these conversations are hard, on balance they are welcomed by patients and their carers.[29–31] Interestingly, many participants in Rogers's study willingly discussed death and dying with the researcher.[13] Moving a patient's goals from the hopelessly unrealistic to the hopefully achievable may maintain hope, and build trust with their clinician—the majority valuing honesty if delivered with concern. However, an individual approach taking cultural aspects into account is important. For example, a study exploring the views of elderly patients with HF, who attached less importance to the concept of individual autonomy, showed that many would not want an explicit acknowledgement of the imminence of death.[32] Conversely, patients may wish to discuss issues related to death and dying but their family members may feel unable to cope with such a conversation.[33] In addition, a few patients may be dealing with their illness using denial, again underlining why a blanket approach is inappropriate, and time taken assessing the level of information the patient is able to cope with is important. However, complete denial is unusual, and it is possible to facilitate a discussion, preferably including their caregivers, to establish what their wishes would be 'if the illness got seriously worse' given that they 'aren't as well as they were'.[34]

One particular area of communication that can cause anxiety to clinician, patient, and caregiver is that of CPR decisions. There is a considerable amount of confused thinking about this subject among clinicians and patients.[35] The current British Medical Association advice is clear: clinicians are under no obligation to offer a futile intervention.[36] Although discussion abounds as to what is medically futile or not,[37–40] in the patient dying from end-stage HF an attempt at CPR is highly unlikely to have any clinically meaningful successful outcome.[35] The clinician is therefore not under obligation to offer such an intervention. However, it may be appropriate to discuss the decision with the patient, in the context of a general conversation about the current seriousness of the illness. Most are able to understand that only treatments which have a reasonable chance of benefiting the patient should be employed, rather than those that will not (such as cardiac surgery, further cardiac medication or insertion of devices, and an attempt at CPR). It is therefore part of a more wide-reaching discussion about what can be offered to the patient rather than a bald 'taking away' of an option. However, these discussions should be assessed on an individual basis and there is no requirement specifically to talk about CPR if it is considered futile by the medical team and it is likely that a discussion is likely to cause unnecessary distress to the patient.[36]

If the patient is happy for the clinician to discuss their care with the family, it is often useful to mention specifically that 'natural death' will be allowed; some family members are worried that there will be an inappropriate attempt at CPR and are relieved there will not, while others have an unrealistic expectation of what an attempted CPR could achieve and would be distressed if an attempt is not made at the time of death. It may be that family members are more concerned that a futile intervention will be attempted inappropriately.[33] The discussion is particularly important for the patient who wishes to die at home, and clarity with the whole family can often prevent an inappropriate and distressing call to the emergency services. Any conversation should be held with great sensitivity, exploring patient and family expectations of CPR, being aware that wildly overoptimistic views may be held, either as a result of a previously successful CPR much earlier on in the illness, or as a result of media portrayals. Any decision and conversation about CPR should be documented in the patient's medical case records and communicated to other staff. Finally, patients and caregivers may change their opinions about both place of care and CPR, and these decisions should be looked at as an ongoing process.[35,41]

Care of the dying

The process of recognizing dying follows the principle of assessing a patient's current presentation within the context of their individual illness trajectory as discussed above. A tool which provides both a framework for decision -making and prompts for care is the Liverpool Care Pathway for the Dying (LCP),[7] which although developed initially for the hospital setting, has now been adapted for use in communities, hospices and nursing homes. The decision as to whether the patient is dying is outlined in Table 55.1. Clinicians can be concerned about the inherent uncertainty that can still be present even a few days before death, and worry about missing the occasional patient who may yet recover. It should be reassuring to them that there is provision within the LCP documentation to give a trial of therapy, as long as there are: clear therapeutic targets to justify continued use; the decision is clearly noted within the 'variance' documentation; and reviewed at least daily. This then allows clinical discretion, but minimizes the risk of ambivalent and inappropriate prescribing in a dying patient simply because clinicians have not allowed themselves to recognize that the patient is likely to be dying. The benefits of starting a patient on the LCP include specific prompts for caregivers: to assess patient and caregiver understanding and spiritual needs; to advise on practical needs such as where a relative can stay, or get a wash and a drink; to pay regular attention to symptom control with appropriate and safe advanced prescribing of medication; and to discontinue futile interventions (2-hourly turns, futile drug medication, blood tests, active CPR status). The decisions and arrangements should be by the usual clinical team caring for the patient, and not entrusted to an out-of-hours, often very junior, doctor. The systematic documentation and prompts of care also mean that continuity of care is less disrupted by staff changeovers or bank/locum staff.

Table 55.1 Decision-making tool for the Liverpool Care Pathway

The multiprofessional team agree the patient is dying . . .	Current clinical presentation taken in the context of the individual's trajectory (previous admissions with decompensation, not tolerating cardiac drugs, persistent hypotension, persistent hyponatraemia, renal dysfunction, etc.)
. . . and all potentially reversible clinical issues have been considered and an attempt at reversal deemed futile	E.g. inotrope treatment, attempt at CPR (including ICD), further intervention such as LVAD, transplantation, valve replacement surgery, pacing
The patient has at least two of the following four: Bedbound Only able to take sips of water Unable to manage oral medication Decreased conscious level	These more categorical issues are of course only relevant in the context of the two points above. The national audit for the care of the dying indicate that where these criteria are met, the average length of time spent on the LCP is 48 h

CPR, cardiopulmonary resuscitation; ICD, implantable cardioverter device; LCP, Liverpool Care Plan; LVAD, left ventricular assist device.

The skills required in caring for the dying HF patient are largely the same as those for the cancer patient. Although the LCP documentation was originally devised for cancer patients, it has proved directly transferable to HF patients with the addition of a reminder to check whether an implantable cardioverter-defibrillator (ICD), if present, has been reprogrammed to pacemaker mode only. A national audit of the use of the LCP confirmed that it can be used effectively for patients dying of HF.[42,43] The five symptoms commonly encountered in the dying patient remain the same: pain; nausea/vomiting; agitation/distress; breathlessness; excess secretions. The general principles of symptom control should be followed: assessment of the cause of the symptom (e.g. urinary retention or hypoxia may be a cause of agitation); reverse what can be reversed (catheterize the bladder, give oxygen); and palliate what cannot be reversed (e.g. sedation for agitation if no apparent underlying reversible cause or persistent despite attempt at reversal). Care of skin, mouth, bowels, and bladder likewise remain generic skills which should be provided for any patient dying irrespective of disease and will not be discussed here.

However, there are a few issues pertinent to patients with HF that need to be borne in mind.

Use of strong opioids

Patients may require strong opioids for ischaemic pain, breathlessness or severe Cheyne–Stokes respiration (rarely this may be so extreme that the patient may rouse in distress on restarting breathing after a prolonged apnoeic spell). The evidence base for the use of opioids in breathlessness comes from work primarily in chronic lung disease and cancer, although there are some small, underpowered studies in patients with HF.[44–47] Some patients appear to respond better than others, although predicting which patients might benefit is difficult;[48] a therapeutic trial in the breathless individual with HF is therefore appropriate. Strong opioids are poor sedatives because, although they may cause drowsiness, they may also cause agitation if the dose is not carefully titrated against pain or breathlessness. They should thus not be used simply for sedation. Clinicians may forget that a parenteral dose of morphine is equivalent to approximately 2–3 times that dose if given orally; 10 mg parenteral morphine is equivalent to 30 mg oral morphine. The implication is that for a patient who is not already taking strong opioids ('opioid naive'), an initial small dose of 2.5–5 mg diamorphine or morphine should be given intravenously or subcutaneously, and the effect monitored. Diamorphine is highly water soluble and thus often used in the United Kingdom for parenteral administration in palliative care.

If repeated doses are needed, then a continuous subcutaneous infusion (CSCI) of diamorphine, the dose based on the previous 24-h opioid requirement, or an empirical starting dose of 5–10 mg/24 h, may save the patient repeated injections, and the trauma of unsuccessful attempts to find venous access. If the patient is established on oral opioids but can now no longer manage them, the opioids should be converted to a CSCI, remembering that the 24-h oral morphine dose is equivalent to approximately one-third of the dose when given parenterally—for example, a patient who has been on 30 mg/day oral morphine would be converted to 10 mg diamorphine (or morphine)/24 h by CSCI. The response should always be carefully monitored and the dose adjusted according to effect.

If there is poor renal function, morphine or diamorphine and metabolites can accumulate, leading to agitation, confusion and hallucinations, and ultimately respiratory depression. The dose should be reduced, the dosing interval increased, and continuous infusion avoided. If there is advanced kidney disease (eGFR <30 mL/min), morphine and diamorphine should be avoided altogether and fentanyl or alfentanil for injection used instead.[49] Unless the patient is already established on a fentanyl transdermal patch, this formulation is not recommended in the dying patient as the dose–response delay is too cumbersome to manage appropriately if the patches are started in the last 48 h or so of life. Recently published LCP–renal failure guidelines endorsed by the Department of Health, the Renal Association, and the British Renal Society, advocate an initial immediate dose of 25 µg of fentanyl in the opioid naive patient, followed by a CSCI of 100–250 µg/24 h if the patient has required three or more doses in a 24-h period.[49]

Oedema

Pulmonary oedema does not seem to occur frequently in the dying patient, presumably because of minimal oral fluid intake at that stage. However, it can still occur and be distressing for all concerned. In this situation furosemide can be given by CSCI, which is particularly useful when intravenous access is difficult or impossible in a dying patient with little peripheral circulation. The infusion must be sited in an area where there is no peripheral oedema: even in the most oedematous patient, there is usually an area on the upper chest wall that is free of fluid. Diuresis and natriuresis has been demonstrated using this route of administration in a placebo-controlled trial in normal volunteers[50] and in a case series of patients with decompensated HF.[51] However, subcutaneous furosemide remains something of an unknown: for example, the oral/subcutaneous dose equivalent is not clear, and an empirical approach is needed with daily review. If effective, the subcutaneous route of administration may prevent a hospital admission close to the end of life as it is simple to administer a CSCI in the patient's home.

There is some evidence that a continuous 24-h intravenous infusion generates a more effective diuresis than repeated boluses to the same total dose.[52,53] It must be remembered, however, that in practice, at this stage, higher doses of loop diuretic may be needed because of diuretic resistance due to renal dysfunction and renal tubule cell hypertrophy. In conjunction with poor peripheral perfusion, furosemide may thus result in limited benefit.

Peripheral oedema is a more common problem than pulmonary oedema: it causes discomfort and increases the risk of complicating pressure sores and cellulitis. Again, parenteral diuretics may help, but the oedema can prove very resistant. Excellent nursing care with attention to pressure-relieving aids and good skin care is mandatory. Itch may also be a problem in patients with endstage HF, and the use of aqueous cream with menthol may help both the skin and the itch.

Breathlessness

Even in the absence of pulmonary oedema, breathlessness may be distressing in the patient dying from HF and is closely associated with anxiety. Opioids and the flow of cool air may be helpful.[54] A small dose (e.g. 2.5–5 mg diamorphine) of opioid should be given and the response assessed. If there is benefit, a CSCI should be started.

Although there is little evidence that oxygen therapy will benefit the patient's breathlessness, a trial of oxygen therapy[55,56] may be worth while unless the patient is unconscious and completely settled. However, correction of hypoxia is more likely to help any remaining cognition rather than help breathlessness; oxygen therapy may be no more effective than a fan causing a draught of cold air across the face for relieving breathlessness *per se*.[54,57–59] If there is no benefit from oxygen, it should be stopped.

When the patient is in the dying phase, breathlessness may require sedation with benzodiazepines. Earlier on in the disease, the use of benzodiazepines should be restricted (because of the risk of falls and memory impairment) to intermittent use for panic, or even avoided by using an anxiolytic antidepressant such as mirtazepine. If the patient is semiconscious but restless due to breathlessness-induced agitation, the effect of a subcutaneous dose of a quick-acting benzodiazepine such as midazolam 2.5–5 mg should be assessed. If it is effective, but the patient requires repeat doses, then a CSCI with an initial midazolam dose of 10 mg/24 h should be started and titrated according to effect. If the patient is still conscious, then the level of sedation and level of relief from distress can be negotiated with them: some patients would rather have some distress but still be awake enough to converse with their family, some wish for 'time out' with the short-term sedation-induced sleep afforded by bolus doses, and still others would rather be asleep continually and unaware of their distress. In the latter case, it is good practice to discuss the situation with the palliative care team. In a patient who is dying over 48–72 h, such deep sedation does not hasten death, but makes the patient comfortable while they die.[60] However, if a patient is not in the dying phase, then deep sedation is not an appropriate approach for the management of breathlessness. A clear assessment and distinction must be made, and if there is any doubt, a second opinion should be sought. At all stages it is vital to maintain clear communication with the patient's family, as sedation is an area of practice which is easily misunderstood.

Nausea and excess respiratory secretions ('death rattle')

Patients with HF have several reasons to be nauseated, including gut oedema and liver congestion. In the dying patient, drug-related nausea (e.g. from spironolactone and digoxin) is less of an issue as the patient is often unable to take oral medication. Theoretically, the antiemetic cyclizine should be avoided in HF,[61] but in the dying patient, if it is the only antiemetic available, it should not be withheld because of potential cardiac adverse effects.

The 'death rattle' can be a problem even if there is no pulmonary oedema. The noise of excess respiratory secretions can be distressing for attendant family and staff, although the patient may not be disturbed by it at this stage.[62–64] Changing patient position may be sufficient to reduce the noise, and occasionally suction can be helpful if the secretions are severe and the patient is so deeply unconscious that the gag reflex is absent. The traditionally accepted drug treatment option is anticholinergic medication such as hyoscine butylbromide, hyoscine hydrobromide, or glycopyrrhonium. However, the effectiveness of anticholinergics has recently been questioned, although robust clinical trials are difficult in the dying.[65,66] They are an option if the situation appears to be distressing the patient and other avenues have failed to help. However, there should be careful review of effectiveness to prevent the continued administration of an unhelpful drug. Anticholinergic drugs could adversely affect cardiac function, but they should not be withheld from a dying patient if a therapeutic trial appeared to show benefit. Of the three options, hyoscine butylbromide and glycopyrrhonium have fewer central effects and reduce the risk of anticholinergic-induced agitation.

Pacemakers and implantable defibrillators

A patient with a pacemaker may request that it be turned off. Although ethically this is accepted as part of withdrawing treatment, it is important to assess fully what is behind the patient's request.[67] It may be because they believe that they will not be able to die if it is still functioning, or that it will greatly prolong the dying process. Simple reassurance that it is quite possible to die with a pacemaker functioning may be all that is required. It is also important to counsel the patient and family that the effect of turning the pacemaker to its lowest setting is difficult to predict. If the patient has become totally pacemaker dependent, then death may indeed be hastened or even immediate. However, if the patient is not dependent, little may happen at all, or the symptoms that were present at pacemaker insertion may return just at a time of life where comfort is mandatory.

The issue of reprogramming an ICD to pacemaker mode only is different, but again comes under the ethical heading of withdrawal of treatment.[68,69] Discharge of an ICD in a patient who is dying is highly unlikely to prolong life, for the same reasons as an attempt at CPR is futile. Even patients who are not imminently dying, but who have endstage HF with an ejection fraction of less than 30%, are unlikely to have significant survival benefit from an ICD.[70–72] However, there is a risk that the dying patient may receive repeated shocks while fully conscious, unless the mode of death is asystole.[73,74] It is therefore important that conversations regarding the likely benefits or otherwise of an active ICD should be started as early as possible in patients with severe HF so that there is time while the patient is well enough to attend the pacemaker clinic to have the device reprogrammed. However, this often does not happen, either because there is little warning of deterioration, because there is staff reticence to broach the subject, or the patient is reluctant to enter discussion. Local systems should therefore be in place for technicians to reprogramme devices in hospital, hospice, or the patient's home if that is their preferred place of care and they are too unwell to travel to the clinic. In the hospital and hospice setting, magnets big enough to inactivate ICD discharge can be available to use in an emergency but should not be relied upon as the main solution.

Frank and open discussion with the family, carers, and the patient is an important priority should be meticulously documented. Many people have the misperception that 'turning off' an ICD is synonymous with 'turning off' the patient. As is the case with decisions about CPR, decisions about ICDs should be seen as potentially changing over the months prior to death.[41]

Coordination of care

One of the main potential problems in caring for the dying is fragmentation of care. HF patients may see clinicians from primary, secondary, tertiary, and voluntary sector care. It is not unusual for a patient to be under the care of a different consultant on each hospital admission and a patient may never be reviewed by a cardiologist. There is a risk that each admission deals only with the immediate problem and does not look at the overall situation. Clinic appointments may also only deal with any immediate problem, as there are great time constraints in most clinics. The patient may be seen by a succession of different doctors with varying levels of experience. As a result, the risk is that no overall plan is made with the patient and that there is little helpful communication with the primary care physician. Patients often do not know who they should call if they should run into problems and can 'fall between the stools' of the different areas of the health service.

The NHS Cancer Plan of 2000 recognized this as a problem in oncology and introduced the concept of a 'keyworker'.[75] The keyworker has helped the patient's care to be coordinated throughout their illness and has made information and planning consistent. An additional role is to aid communication, particularly between primary and secondary care. The keyworker may be a nurse specialist, doctor, or district nurse depending on the stage of the illness. The keyworker works closely in conjunction with the multidisciplinary team (MDT) which meets to discuss the management of each patient at diagnosis. Many cardiology units are developing the MDT model, with the MDT including cardiologists, HF nurse specialists (HFNSs), and cardiac surgeons. In practice, many HFNSs act as keyworkers. Where they have a remit across primary and secondary care, there are significant benefits in end of life planning.[34]

The MDT approach has also been applied in primary care in order to coordinate end-of-life care for patients, initially with cancer, but more recently extended to all patients irrespective of diagnosis. Growing from the realization that most inappropriate admissions to hospital at the end of life were out of hours and triggered by poor symptom control and/or caregiver exhaustion, the GSF[8] has been developed and is now recommended by the UK Department of Health. The GSF provides a prompt for the primary care MDT to ensure there is a designated keyworker, that there is coordination with out-of-hours services, that preferred place of care is known, that financial assistance has been applied for, and that an overall plan of care has been made. Patients are discussed at the GSF meeting if the clinician 'would not be surprised if the patient died in the next year', in addition to other markers (see Box 55.1). In practice, primary care clinicians may feel more nervous of recognizing that their HF patients are at end stage compared to cancer patients about whom they may feel more confident, and this is an area where it is helpful for secondary care clinicians to communicate clearly to their colleagues in primary care when the patient is reaching the end stage of their disease.

Supporting a patient's wish to die in their preferred place is a challenge for those caring for HF patients, but not impossible. Dying at home may be possible if the patient has a family or caregiver who concurs with their wish but is less likely if they do not.[76] Support for patients wishing to die at home may come from social service carers, and be helped by coordination with other services such hospice-at-home, where available, Marie Curie nurses, and out-of-hours palliative care support phone lines, which exist in

Box 55.1 Suggested patient clinical features for inclusion in GSF meetings

Cancer

- Any patient whose cancer is metastatic or inoperable
- Patient thought to be in the last year of life by the care team—the 'surprise' question

Heart failure (at least two criteria should be met)

- CHF NYHA stage III or IV—CHF symptoms at rest
- Patient thought to be in the last year of life by the care team—the 'surprise' question
- Repeated hospital admissions with symptoms of HF
- Difficult physical or psychological symptoms despite optimal tolerated therapy

General indicators:

- Weight loss—more than 10% weight loss over 6 months
- General physical decline
- Serum albumin <25 g/L
- Reduced performance status/Karnofsky score <50%
- Dependence in most activities of daily living

many areas of the United Kingdom. (Although Marie Curie is a cancer charity, there has been a recent agreement for the nurses to help support patients dying from any illness.) Other patients may wish to die in their local hospice. The UK hospice service is still patchy, but there is a growing recognition and willingness to accept patients with any diagnosis, not just cancer.[77] Knowledge of local services is important for the primary care and cardiology teams so that the best possible option for the patient can be organized.

Summary and conclusions

The most important and potentially the most difficult aspect of end-of-life care for patients with HF is the recognition that they are now dying. Taking the patient's current clinical presentation within the context of their individual disease trajectory is vitally important and requires careful assessment. Coordination of care and communication of management plans between clinical teams, ideally using a keyworker such as the HFNS, may help prevent revolving-door admissions during the last few months of life, and prevent an inappropriate emergency admission around the time of death. Advance planning tools, such as GSF, do exist in primary care, and discussion about the stage of the disease and the possible aims of treatment should be a feature of the growing cardiology MDTs.

Sensitive communication tailored to the individual patient and their family about their understanding and wishes should allow appropriate planning of services and care for the patient who prefers to die at home or in a hospice.

Prompts of care for the dying patient, such as the LCP, are relevant for HF patients and contain useful decision-making suggestions to help the team recognize that the patient is dying.

Excellent extended team working and communication skills should result in a patient dying in the place of their choice, with their symptoms well controlled and their family well supported. That the NHS Darzi Report[5] has raised end-of-life care to a national UK priority is appropriate. Hinton's observations that 'discomfort was not necessarily greatest in those dying from cancer; patients dying from HF, or renal failure, or both, had most physical distress. . .'[4] should be addressed at last.

References

1. Cowie MR, Wood DA, Coats AJ, *et al.* Survival of patients with a new diagnosis of heart failure: a population based study. *Heart* 2000;**83**:505–10.
2. Mills M, Davies HT, Macrae WA. Care of dying patients in hospital. *BMJ* 1994;**309**(6954):583–6.
3. Rogers A, Karlsen S, Addington-Hall JM. Dying for care: the experiences of terminally ill cancer patients in hospital in an inner city health district. *Palliat Med* 2000;**14**(1):53–4.
4. Hinton JM. The physical and mental distress of the dying. *Q J Med* 1963;**32**:1–21.
5. Darzi A. *High quality care for all: NHS Next Stage Review final report.* Department of Health, London, 2008.
6. Department of Health. *End of Life Care Strategy—promoting high quality care for all adults at the end of life.* Department of Health, London, 2008.
7. Ellershaw J, Murphy D, Bloger M, Agar R. *The Liverpool Care Pathway for the dying patient (LCP).* Marie Curie Palliative Care Institute, Liverpool, 2007; Available from: http://www.endoflifecareforadults.nhs.uk/eolc/files/F2091-LCP_pathway_for_dying_patient_Sep2007.pdf.
8. Thomas K. *The Gold Standards Framework: a programme for community palliative care.* Department of Health 2009; Available from: http://www.goldstandardsframework.nhs.uk/.
9. Hippocrates. *Book of Prognostics* (Adams F, transl). Dodo Press, Gloucester, 2009.
10. Boyd KJ, Murray SA, Kendall M, Worth A, Frederick BT, Clausen H. Living with advanced heart failure: a prospective, community based study of patients and their carers. *Eur J Heart Fail* 2004;**6**(5):585–91.
11. Buetow SA, Coster GD. Do general practice patients with heart failure understand its nature and seriousness, and want improved information? *Patient Educ Couns* 2001;**45**(3):181–5.
12. Murray SA, Boyd K, Kendall M, Worth A, Benton TF, Clausen H. Dying of lung cancer or cardiac failure: prospective qualitative interview study of patients and their carers in the community. *BMJ* 2002;**325**(7370):929.
13. Rogers AE, Addington-Hall JM, *et al.* Knowledge and communication difficulties for patients with chronic heart failure: qualitative study. *BMJ* 2000;**321**(7261):605–7.
14. Exley C, Field D, Jones L, Stokes T. Palliative care in the community for cancer and end-stage cardiorespiratory disease: the views of patients, lay-carers and health care professionals. *Palliat Med* 2005;**19**(1):76–83.
15. Murray SA, Kendall M, Boyd K, Sheikh A. Illness trajectories and palliative care. *BMJ* 2005;**330**(7498):1007–11.
16. Gott M, Barnes S, Parker C, *et al.* Dying trajectories in heart failure. *Palliat Med* 2007;**21**(2):95–9.
17. ONS. *Mortality Statistics: General. DH1 No. 36*, 2003 [Web Page]. ONS, 2009. Available from: http://www.statistics.gov.uk/downloads/theme_health/Dh1_36_2003/DH1_2003.pdf.
18. Mancini DM, Eisen H, Kussmaul W, Mull R, Edmunds LH Jr, Wilson JR. Value of peak exercise oxygen consumption for optimal timing of cardiac transplantation in ambulatory patients with heart failure. *Circulation* 1991;**83**(3):778–86.
19. Metra M, Nodari S, Parrinello G, *et al.* The role of plasma biomarkers in acute heart failure. Serial changes and independent prognostic value of NT-proBNP and cardiac troponin-T. *Eur J Heart Fail* 2007;**9**(8):776–86.

20. Metra M, Nodari S, Parrinello G, *et al.* Worsening renal function in patients hospitalised for acute heart failure: clinical implications and prognostic significance. *Eur J Heart Fail* 2008;**10**(2):188–95.
21. Rothenburger M, Wichter T, Schmid C, *et al.* Aminoterminal pro type B natriuretic peptide as a predictive and prognostic marker in patients with chronic heart failure. *J Heart Lung Transplant* 2004;**23**(10):1189–97.
22. Koelling TM, Joseph S, Aaronson KD. Heart failure survival score continues to predict clinical outcomes in patients with heart failure receiving beta-blockers. *J Heart Lung Transplant* 2004;**23**(12):1414–22.
23. Lee DS, Austin PC, Rouleau JL, Liu PP, Naimark D, Tu JV. Predicting mortality among patients hospitalized for heart failure: derivation and validation of a clinical model. *JAMA* 2003 Nov 19;**290**(19):2581–7.
24. Levy WC, Mozaffarian D, Linker DT, *et al.* The Seattle Heart Failure Model: prediction of survival in heart failure. *Circulation* 2006;**113**(11):1424–33.
25. Barnes S, Gott M, Payne S, *et al.* Predicting mortality among a general practice-based sample of older people with heart failure. *Chronic Illn* 2008;**4**(1):5–12.
26. Murray SA, Kendall M, Grant E, Boyd K, Barclay S, Sheikh A. Patterns of social, psychological, and spiritual decline toward the end of life in lung cancer and heart failure. *J Pain Symptom Manage* 2007;**34**(4):393–402.
27. Rogers A, Addington-Hall JM, McCoy AS, *et al.* A qualitative study of chronic heart failure patients' understanding of their symptoms and drug therapy. *Eur J Heart Fail* 2002;**4**(3):283–7.
28. Barnes S, Gott M, Payne S, *et al.* Communication in heart failure: perspectives from older people and primary care professionals. *Health Soc Care Community* 2006;**14**(6):482–90.
29. Davison SN, Simpson C. Hope and advance care planning in patients with end stage renal disease: qualitative interview study. *BMJ* 2006;**333**(7574):886.
30. Fallowfield LJ, Jenkins VA, Beveridge HA. Truth may hurt but deceit hurts more: communication in palliative care. *Palliat Med* 2002;**16**(4):297–303.
31. Michel DM, Moss AH. Communicating prognosis in the dialysis consent process: a patient-centered, guideline-supported approach. *Adv Chronic Kidney Dis* 2005 Apr;**12**(2):196–201.
32. Gott M, Small N, Barnes S, Payne S, Seamark D. Older people's views of a good death in heart failure: implications for palliative care provision. *Soc Sci Med* 2008;**67**(7):1113–21.
33. Small N, Barnes S, Gott M, *et al.* Dying, death and bereavement: a qualitative study of the views of carers of people with heart failure in the UK. *BMC Palliat Care* 2009;**8**:6.
34. Johnson MJ, Parsons S, Raw J, Williams A, Daley A. Achieving preferred place of death—is it possible for patients with chronic heart failure? *Br J Cardiol* 2009;**16**:194–6.
35. Agard A, Hermeren G, Herlitz J. Should cardiopulmonary resuscitation be performed on patients with heart failure? The role of the patient in the decision-making process. *J Intern Med* 2000 Oct;**248**(4):279–86.
36. *Decisions relating to cardiopulmonary resuscitation: A joint statement from the British Medical Association, the Resuscitation Council (UK) and the Royal College of Nursing.* British Medical Association, London, 2007.
37. Schneiderman LJ, Jecker NS, Jonsen AR. Medical futility: its meaning and ethical implications. *Ann Intern Med* 1990 Jun 15;**112**(12):949–54.
38. Schneiderman LJ, Jecker NS, Jonsen AR. Medical futility: response to critiques. *Ann Intern Med* 1996;**125**(8):669–74.
39. Swanson JW, McCrary SV. Medical futility decisions and physicians' legal defensiveness: the impact of anticipated conflict on thresholds for end-of-life treatment. *Soc Sci Med* 1996 Jan;**42**(1):125–32.
40. Vayrynen T, Kuisma M, Maatta T, Boyd J. Medical futility in asystolic out-of-hospital cardiac arrest. *Acta Anaesthesiol Scand* 2008;**52**(1):81–7.
41. Withell B. Patient consent and implantable cardioverter defibrillators: some palliative care implications. *Int J Palliat Nurs* 2006;**12**(10):470–5.
42. Marie Curie Cancer Care Institute, Royal College of Physicians (RCP) Clinical Effectiveness and Evaluations Unit (CEEu). *National Care of The Dying Audit—Hospitals (NCDAH). Generic Report 2006/2007.* Department of Health End of Life Programme 2007. Available from: http://www.liv.ac.uk/mcpcil/liverpool-care-pathway/pdfs/NCDAHGENERICREPORTFINAL-Auglockedpdf.pdf.
43. LCP Central Team UK MCPCIL. *Can the LCP be used for all patients in the last hours/days of life irrespective of their diagnosis?* Liverpool Care Pathway for the Dying Patient Briefing Paper, MCPCIL, 2009. Available from: http://www.liv.ac.uk/mcpcil/liverpool-care-pathway/pdfs/lcp-briefing-paper-specific-diagnostic-groups-may09.pdf.
44. Abernethy AP, Currow DC, Frith P, Fazekas BS, McHugh A, Bui C. Randomised, double blind, placebo controlled crossover trial of sustained release morphine for the management of refractory dyspnoea. *BMJ* 2003;**327**(7414):523–8.
45. Currow DC, Ward AM, Abernethy AP. Advances in the pharmacological management of breathlessness. *Curr Opin Support Palliat Care* 2009;**3**(2):103–6.
46. Jennings L. Systematic review of the use of opioid drugs in the palliative treatment of dyspnoea. *Palliat Med* 1999;**13**(4):354.
47. Johnson MJ, McDonagh TA, Harkness A, McKay SE, Dargie HJ. Morphine for the relief of breathlessness in patients with chronic heart failure—a pilot study. *Eur J Heart Fail* 2002;**4**(6):753–6.
48. Currow DC, Plummer J, Frith P, Abernethy AP. Can we predict which patients with refractory dyspnea will respond to opioids?. *J Palliat Med* 2007;**10**(5):1031–6.
49. DH Renal NSF Team, Marie Curie Palliative Care Institute. *Guidelines for LCP drug prescribing in advanced chronic kidney disease (estimated GFR rate <30mls/min).* MCPCIL, 2008. Available from: http://www.renal.org/pages/media/Guidelines/National%20LCP%20Renal%20Symptom%20Control%20Guidelines%20(05.06.08)%20(printable%20pdf).pdf.
50. Verma AK, da Silva JH, Kuhl DR. Diuretic effects of subcutaneous furosemide in human volunteers: a randomized pilot study. *Ann Pharmacother* 2004;**38**(4):544–9.
51. Goenaga MA, Millet M, Sanchez E, Garde C, Carrera JA, Arzellus E. Subcutaneous furosemide. *Ann Pharmacother* 2004;**38**(10):1751.
52. Dormans TP, van Meyel JJ, Gerlag PG, Tan Y, Russel FG, Smits P. Diuretic efficacy of high dose furosemide in severe heart failure: bolus injection versus continuous infusion. *J Am Coll Cardiol* 1996;**28**(2):376–82.
53. Lahav M, Regev A, Ra'anani P, Theodor E. Intermittent administration of furosemide vs continuous infusion preceded by a loading dose for congestive heart failure. *Chest* 1992;**102**:725–31.
54. Schwartzstein RM, Lahive K, Pope A, Weinberger SE, Weiss JW. Cold facial stimulation reduces breathlessness induced in normal subjects. *Am Rev Respir Dis* 1987;**136**(1):58–61.
55. Currow DC, Fazekas B, Abernethy AP. Oxygen use-patients define symptomatic benefit discerningly. *J Pain Symptom Manage* 2007;**34**(2):113–4.
56. Booth S, Wade R, Johnson M, Kite S, Swannick M, Anderson H. The use of oxygen in the palliation of breathlessness. A report of the expert working group of the Scientific Committee of the Association of Palliative Medicine. *Respir Med* 2004;**98**(1):66–77.
57. Currow DC, Agar M, Smith J, Abernethy AP. Does palliative home oxygen improve dyspnoea? A consecutive cohort study. *Palliat Med* 2009;**23**(4):309–16.
58. Booth S, Wade R. Oxygen or air for palliation of breathlessness in advanced cancer. *J Roy Soc Med* 2003;**96**(5):215–18.
59. Uronis HE, Abernethy AP. Oxygen for relief of dyspnea: what is the evidence? *Curr Opin Support Palliat Care* 2008;**2**(2):89–94.
60. de GA, Dean M. Palliative sedation therapy in the last weeks of life: a literature review and recommendations for standards. *J Palliat Med* 2007;**10**(1):67–85.

61. Tan LB, Bryant S, Murray RG. Detrimental haemodynamic effects of cyclizine in heart failure. *Lancet* 1988;**i**(8585):560–1.
62. Wee B, Coleman P, Hillier R, Holgate S. Death rattle: its impact on staff and volunteers in palliative care. *Palliat Med* 2008;**22**(2):173–6.
63. Wee BL, Coleman PG, Hillier R, Holgate SH. The sound of death rattle II: how do relatives interpret the sound?. *Palliat Med* 2006;**20**(3):177–81.
64. Wee BL, Coleman PG, Hillier R, Holgate SH. The sound of death rattle I: are relatives distressed by hearing this sound? *Palliat Med* 2006;**20**(3):171–5.
65. Bennett M, Lucas V, Brennan M, Hughes A, O'Donnell V, Wee B. Using anti-muscarinic drugs in the management of death rattle: evidence-based guidelines for palliative care. *Palliat Med* 2002;**16**(5):369–74.
66. Wee B, Hillier R. Interventions for noisy breathing in patients near to death. *Cochrane Database Syst Rev* 2008;(**1**):CD005177.
67. Mueller PS, Hook CC, Hayes DL. Ethical analysis of withdrawal of pacemaker or implantable cardioverter-defibrillator support at the end of life. *Mayo Clin Proc* 2003;**78**(8):959–63.
68. Berger JT. The ethics of deactivating implanted cardioverter defibrillators. *Ann Intern Med* 2005 Apr 19;**142**(8):631–4.
69. Berger JT, Gorski M, Cohen T. Advance health planning and treatment preferences among recipients of implantable cardioverter defibrillators: an exploratory study. *J Clin Ethics* 2006;**17**(1):72–8.
70. Ermis C, Lurie KG, Zhu AX, *et al.* Biventricular implantable cardioverter defibrillators improve survival compared with biventricular pacing alone in patients with severe left ventricular dysfunction. *J Cardiovasc Electrophysiol* 2004;**15**(8):862–6.
71. Setoguchi S, Nohria A, Rassen JA, Stevenson LW, Schneeweiss S. Maximum potential benefit of implantable defibrillators in preventing sudden death after hospital admission because of heart failure. *CMAJ* 2009;**180**(6):611–6.
72. Marijon E, Trinquart L, Otmani A, *et al.* Competing risk analysis of cause-specific mortality in patients with an implantable cardioverter-defibrillator: The EVADEF cohort study. *Am Heart J* 2009;**157**(2):391–7.
73. Nambisan V, Chao D. Dying and defibrillation: a shocking experience. *Palliat Med* 2004;**18**(5):482–3.
74. Goldstein NE, Lampert R, Bradley E, Lynn J, Krumholz HM. Management of implantable cardioverter defibrillators in end-of-life care. *Ann Intern Med* 2004;**141**(11):835–8.
75. Department of Health. *The NHS cancer plan: a plan for investment, a plan for reform.* Department of Health, London, 2000.
76. Agar M, Currow DC, Shelby-James TM, Plummer J, Sanderson C, Abernethy AP. Preference for place of care and place of death in palliative care: are these different questions?. *Palliat Med* 2008;**22**(7):787–95.
77. Gibbs LM, Khatri AK, Gibbs JS. Survey of specialist palliative care and heart failure: September 2004. *Palliat Med* 2006;**20**(6):603–9.

56

Monitoring

Jillian P. Riley and Martin R. Cowie

Introduction

Heart failure (HF) is a chronic condition with the risk of episodic deterioration ('decompensation'). Aims of therapy include stabilization of the syndrome, improvement in the prognosis and quality of life, and the avoidance of hospitalization. Early detection of deterioration is a key component of HF management programmes, with the goal of adjusting therapy to restabilize the syndrome rapidly and to avoid the need for emergency hospitalization.

HF management programmes were developed to help ensure patients received appropriate multiprofessional input to their treatment, education, and monitoring. They were designed to help fill the gap that often existed between discharge from hospital and the traditional outpatient clinic review. Many patients decompensated during this high-risk period, resulting in readmission to hospital. However, despite such programmes becoming more widespread, perhaps as many as 30% of patients are still readmitted within 12 months of hospital discharge,[1] with some of the admissions preventable with better monitoring.

This chapter discusses the key elements of monitoring of patients with HF, including what and who should be monitored, the frequency of monitoring, and the different methods of monitoring.

Monitoring is a key component of disease management

Professional guidelines suggest that all patients recently hospitalized with HF (and other 'high-risk' patients) should enter a HF management programme.[2,3] Only around 20% of such patients in England do so at the present time.[4] Many of the key components of such a programme relate to monitoring (Box 56.1). Meta-analysis suggests that the various types of disease management programmes are similarly effective in terms of reducing mortality and rehospitalizations.[5]

Monitoring can take many forms: supported self-monitoring, clinic attendance, home visits, or remote monitoring. Most modern programmes combine several different approaches, tailoring the care to the needs of the patient and family, and taking account of the local resources and expertise available in both primary and secondary care. Such a tailored approach, matching the model of care to the severity of the condition, is in keeping with current health care policy in the developed world: most attention is focused on those with more complex needs ('case management'), built on a platform of good disease management in general and with increasingly expert patients who are supported to self-care (Fig. 56.1).[6]

Elderly patients, or those with multiple co-morbidities, will have more complex healthcare needs that place them at higher risk of hospitalization. They benefit from more intensive case management.

A recent randomized study from the Netherlands confirms the value of a more tailored approach, reporting that more intensive management for all patients is not necessarily better than a less intensive approach.[7]

Models of monitoring

Traditional periodic monitoring

Historically, patients with HF were not taught to self-monitor but were reviewed periodically by a doctor working in either primary or secondary care. Even in the high-risk period after hospital discharge it was traditional to arrange hospital clinic review some weeks after discharge. At that visit the doctor would assess the patient and determine if changes to treatment were required. In the United Kingdom, with very few physicians with a special interest in the condition, many patients would be discharged back to primary care review alone. Such patients might perhaps be reviewed in other clinics, due to comorbidities such as diabetes, where the HF syndrome might or might not be reassessed. It is little surprise that this model of monitoring was associated with poor outcomes, including a high rate of emergency rehospitalizations. Such a model is now considered outdated and substandard.

Self-monitoring

There is much that the patient and their family can do to monitor how well the HF syndrome is controlled. Professional monitoring

Box 56.1 Recommended components of heart failure management programmes

- Multidisciplinary approach frequently led by HF nurses in collaboration with physicians and other related services
- First contact during hospitalization, early follow-up after discharge through clinic and home-based visits, telephone support and remote monitoring
- Target high-risk, symptomatic patients
- Increased access to healthcare (telephone, remote monitoring, and follow-up)
- Facilitate access during episodes of decompensation
- Optimized medical management
- Access to advanced treatment options
- Adequate patient education with special emphasis on adherence and self-care management
- Patient involvement in symptom monitoring and flexible diuretic use
- Psychosocial support to patients and family and/or caregiver

Source: European Society of Cardiology Guidelines 2008.[3]

is likely to be supplemental to this self-monitoring. Self-monitoring should facilitate self-management, where a patient adjusts their therapy depending on the control of the HF syndrome. Typically this would involve a patient adjusting the dose of diuretic depending on changes in their weight.

Where they wish, patients and their families should be helped to become involved in monitoring their HF. They will need advice on how to monitor symptoms of HF easily and on the significance of any changes in symptoms, weight, or other measurements such as blood pressure or pulse. Simple management strategies and information on when and where to seek professional help can then help the patient self-manage.

Patients experience a variety of symptoms, which complicates their ability to recognize the importance of symptoms and to identify their cause as HF-related.[8–10] Older age, depression, and cognitive dysfunction may decrease self-care ability.

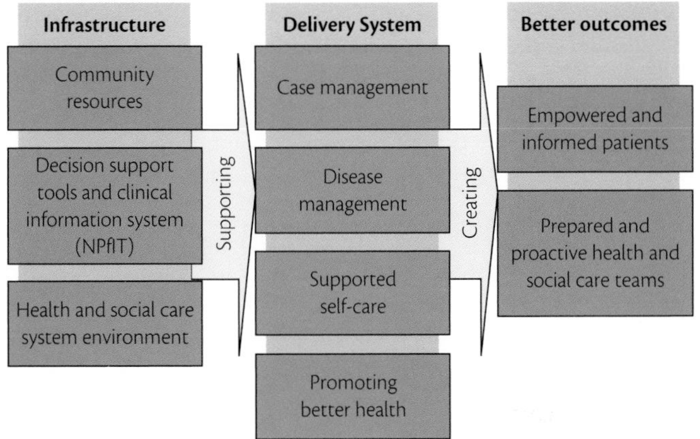

Fig. 56.1 The NHS and Social Care long-term conditions model, proposed by the UK Department of Health.[6]

To be effective, self-monitoring requires the local HF service to be easily accessible to the patient and their family/carer. Although most HF services provide a telephone advice line (at least during working hours Monday through Friday), a proportion of patients will be reluctant to use this for fear of interrupting the professional and uncertainty regarding the significance of their symptoms. Telemonitoring can be useful in this situation and patients may develop expertise through the timely feedback provided by the monitored data and from the health professional contact triggered by abnormal results.

Remote monitoring

Heart failure typically affects elderly people, and their limited mobility and lack of social support may make hospital clinic attendance problematic. Home visits can bridge the gap, but are costly in terms of travel time for the health professional, limiting the case load that a specialist nurse can take on. Telehealth ('healthcare at a distance') has the potential to widen access to high-quality care and to provide this care closer to home than the traditional, usually hospital-based, model can. Telemonitoring—the remote monitoring of patients using information technology—has developed rapidly in the past decade.

There are several types of remote monitoring, from simple to complex:

- Telephone support from a health care professional: the patient monitors their symptoms and weight and reports these during a structured telephone call from a health care professional.
- Patient-initiated electronic monitoring with transfer of physiological data and symptom record from the patient in their home to the health care professional, using a telephone or broadband connection.
- Implanted device monitoring, where a defibrillator or cardiac resynchronization device, or an implanted haemodynamic monitor, can transmit data wirelessly to a near-patient unit that is connected to a telephone or broadband connection. These systems are described in more detail later in this chapter.

What should be monitored?

The UK National Institute for Health and Clinical Excellence (NICE) has made recommendations for monitoring of HF (Box 56.2).[2] These recommendations are based on consensus on what constitutes good clinical practice, rather than on specific randomized controlled trials. The ideal variable to monitor would be simple and convenient to measure, reproducible, sensitive to changes in the control of HF, specific for this condition, and would change rapidly enough to give an early warning of decompensation. No such variable has been identified. In practice, several measurements are relied on to detect decompensation. The patient's history, signs, and symptoms, supplemented where possible with physiological data, are combined with skilled clinical interpretation.

Symptom monitoring

The typical signs and symptoms of clinical deterioration of chronic HF are increasing fluid retention, breathlessness, and effort intolerance, but can include less specific symptoms such as fatigue, cough, and poorer cognition. In many, but not all, patients and

Box 56.2 Recommendations for the monitoring of patients with CHF[2]

All patients with CHF require monitoring. This monitoring should include:*

- a clinical assessment of functional capacity, fluid status, cardiac rhythm (minimum of examining the pulse), cognitive status, and nutritional status
- a review of medication, including need for changes and possible side effects
- serum urea, electrolytes, and creatinine

More detailed monitoring will be required if the patient has significant comorbidity, or has deteriorated since the previous review.

The frequency of the monitoring should depend on the clinical status and stability of the patient. The monitoring interval should be short (days to 2 weeks) if the clinical condition or medication has changed, but is required at least 6-monthly for stable patients with proven HF.

Patients who wish to be involved in their monitoring of their condition should be provided with sufficient education and support from their health care professional to do this, with clear guidelines as to what to do in the event of deterioration.

*This is a minimum. Patients with comorbidities or coprescribed medications will require further monitoring. Monitoring serum potassium is particularly important if a patient is taking digoxin or spironolactone. Source: NICE.[2]

episodes, deterioration is gradual and it should be possible to detect such deterioration if the patient or HF team is monitoring the clinical condition. Many patients are aware of symptoms for several weeks but only seek professional help when they became intolerable.[11]

In some patients, and in some episodes, the deterioration may be abrupt and thus could not be detected earlier by closer monitoring. Such deterioration might occur as a result of sudden changes in cardiac rhythm (such as the onset of atrial fibrillation) or incidental infection (particularly chest or urinary tract infection).

Some telemonitoring systems ask patients questions about a range of symptoms which can be useful in identifying deterioration (particularly if combined with daily weight monitoring). From our experience in the Home-HF study,[12] patients often find it difficult to say if any specific symptom is better or worse than the day before. Changes are often subtle and noticed at different time points during the day, making it difficult to decide if they relate to a change in the overall condition or to differing activities.

The New York Heart Association (NYHA) classification of HF[13] provides some structure to symptom monitoring by health care professionals by grading the severity of HF according to a broad classification of functional limitation. It is relatively easy to score but its value is limited by poor sensitivity to small change and poor reproducibility among clinicians.[14] There is also limited agreement between patients and their clinicians.[15]

Patients tend to measure change in their symptoms by the effect on their activities of daily living rather than more abstract concepts: they may notice a change in their ability to go out shopping, tidy the garden, or walk to their friend's house, and so behavioural questioning may be more effective at monitoring change in symptoms.

The six-minute walk test is a more reliable tool to monitor changes in functional capacity,[16] but is rarely done in routine practice. However, it is of less value where functional capacity is limited by comorbidity, such as osteoarthritis.

Body weight

An early sign of worsening HF in many patients is increasing fluid retention, and in theory daily monitoring of weight using accurate scales should be useful in identifying decompensation early. Such an approach is standard practice in HF management programmes, and is recommended in professional guidelines.[2,3,17]

There is some evidence that the speed of weight gain is more sensitive and specific for HF decompensation than absolute weight change, with an increase of more than 2 kg over a period of 72 h being clinically significant.[3] For more effective monitoring, the weight increase should be the weight above 'dry' weight; that is, the steady weight achieved following any change in diuretic therapy and where there are no signs of fluid overload. To allow for normal weight change, 'dry' weight should be recalculated periodically (every 1–2 months). This is particularly important after discharge from hospital, when patients generally feel better and start to eat more and therefore may put on muscle or fat rather than merely fluid weight.

The significance of an increase in body weight of 2 kg depends upon patient size, and such a weight increase in a patient weighing only 40 kg is likely to be more significant than in someone of 120 kg. Attempts have been made to correct for patient size, with different patients being given different guidelines for identifying possible increasing fluid retention.

Despite the widespread use of weight monitoring, its accuracy is limited. In an attempt to establish the sensitivity and specificity of weight gain in correctly identifying clinical deterioration, Lewin and colleagues[18] recruited patients with established HF, predominately (70%) left ventricular systolic dysfunction (LVSD), and compared the patients' daily weight diary against clinical examination. They concluded that a weight gain of more than 2 kg over 48–72 h demonstrated good specificity (97%) but poor sensitivity (9%) for predicting clinical deterioration. A weight increase of more than 2% above dry weight had a similar specificity (94%) with only marginal improvement in sensitivity (17%). Although such weight increase is highly specific for decompensation, these results suggest that the lack of such a change cannot be taken to exclude decompensation. Attention must therefore also be directed at assessment of symptoms or other physiological measurements that may reflect overall HF status. Patients who are able to self-care should also be aware that while weight monitoring is useful, they should seek help if they notice an increase in symptoms regardless of any weight change.

Data from a home telemonitoring study in patients with left ventricular ejection fraction (LVEF) less than 40% also showed that relying only on weight monitoring is unlikely to be of great value in detecting decompensation, even when using more complex calculations of weight change. Weight gain started around 14 days prior to a hospital admission with worsening HF, but substantial weight gain was seen in only around 20% of patients.[19] Continuous weight monitoring demonstrated that weight gain starts much earlier than expected, may be considerably less than that suggested in guidelines, and that patients may present with worsening HF without any weight increase.

It may be that the cause of decompensation influences the number of days over which weight gain occurs. For example, weight gain resulting from worsening left ventricular function or nonadherence to angiotensin converting enzyme (ACE) inhibitors or β-blockers may be more insidious, whereas infection, arrhythmias, or noncompliance with diuretic medication may cause a more rapid increase in volume and may even precipitate HF decompensation before any change in weight is noticed.

For weight monitoring to be reliable it requires consistency in its monitoring; patients should be encouraged to weigh themselves at the same time each morning, wearing similar clothing. Although these suggestions appear straightforward, patients are likely to monitor their weight at a time they find convenient and in clothing that may differ in weight from one day to the next. This does not necessarily imply inadequate knowledge or understanding of weight monitoring, but reflects the everyday reality of living with HF and the attempt to integrate self-monitoring into their daily lives. In some cases, although monitoring is done very carefully, instructions on when to inform the HF team about changes are not followed, often because the patient or family do not feel the weight change is important or they do not wish to 'bother' the professionals.

Another limitation of relying on weight monitoring alone to determine fluid status is that patients with advanced HF may develop cachexia and a stable weight over time may mask volume overload combined with reducing muscle and fat mass.

Despite the above limitations, daily weight measurement is easy to monitor and is considered the cornerstone of daily monitoring in most HF management programmes. As argued above, it is best combined with monitoring of other variables, including symptoms.

Peripheral oedema/swollen ankles

In many patients, increasing fluid retention may be most marked in the legs. Monitoring of ankle swelling is a routine component of clinical monitoring for HF deterioration. However, perhaps as much as 5 L of excess fluid is present before oedema is noticed by most patients. Patients frequently find it difficult to identify when their ankles are more swollen than usual and may only notice change when it is so severe that they no longer can wear their normal shoes.

In the patient with venous insufficiency, it may be difficult to distinguish dependent oedema resulting from HF from the normal state. Often the oedema is asymmetrical, particularly if the patient has had venous harvesting for bypass surgery, and patients often concentrate on the better leg, denying that fluid is building up.

In some patients, particularly those with failure of the right ventricle or tricuspid regurgitation, accumulation of fluid may be more marked in the abdomen than in the legs. Patients may notice an increase in girth, with their clothes or belt becoming tighter, or increased pulsation in their neck as the venous pressure increases. In our experience, it is rare for patients to identify decompensation early through these signs.

Blood pressure

Detection of significant hypotension (including postural hypotension) is important in the clinical review of a patient. It may point towards intravascular fluid depletion due to excessively high diuretic usage, or a low cardiac output, or sepsis, or inappropriately high dosage of neurohormonal antagonists. For some patients, the control of hypertension is also critical to the control of the HF syndrome. Many patients monitor their own blood pressure at home, and it can be easily monitored remotely.

Arrhythmia

Arrhythmia is common in patients with HF. Ventricular arrhythmia may be life-threatening and atrial arrhythmia (such as atrial fibrillation) may cause symptom deterioration. Both complicate management decisions. Heart rate monitoring (supplemented by rhythm monitoring if possible and appropriate) may help identify problems that requires further investigation.

Single-lead ECG monitoring has been added to external telemonitoring equipment. However, it increases the complexity of monitoring and to date there is no evidence of additional benefit.[20,21] Heart rate monitoring alone is easier and may be sufficient in many cases. Where devices such as cardiac resynchronization therapy (CRT) or a dual-chamber implantable cardioverter-defibrillator (ICD) are implanted, device interrogation can provide potentially continuous information (but more often daily or less frequently) on both heart rate and rhythm.

Blood tests

Renal function is often impaired in patients with HF, and deterioration is associated with a poor prognosis. Intercurrent illness (such as infection) can have a profound effect on renal function, as can the introduction and up-titration of therapies such as ACE inhibitors, angiotensin receptor blockers, β-blockers or aldosterone antagonists. Regular monitoring of serum biochemistry (in particular serum potassium, urea, and creatinine) is important and structured follow-up can ensure this is not missed. Biochemistry should be checked within 2 weeks of the introduction or up-titration of new medication and otherwise at a minimum of 6-monthly intervals. Intercurrent illness should trigger a check of HF status, including renal function. The introduction of drugs such as nonsteroidal anti-inflammatory drugs (NSAIDs), either prescribed or obtained over the counter, can markedly impair renal function in patients with HF.

Other blood tests may be required as part of routine monitoring: anaemia is increasingly common as HF advances, as is diabetes, so a check on the full blood count and plasma glucose should be made periodically. Thyroid and liver function may be deranged by amiodarone. Urate is often high in patients with HF on diuretic therapy, and repeated attacks of acute gout may occur if allopurinol is not used.

Plasma natriuretic peptide serial monitoring

Several randomized trials have assessed whether the serial measurement of plasma B-type natriuretic peptide (BNP) or NT-proBNP might aid the management of patients with HF. Early studies suggested the clinical outcome was better if a target BNP or NT-proBNP was used to titrate diuretics and ACE inhibitors, but a more recent and larger randomized trial found little evidence of benefit, except in a post-hoc subgroup of those aged less than 75 years.[22] The 2010 partial update to the NICE guidance on the management of HF suggests that serial measurement of plasma BNP should be considered for certain patients being followed up in specialist practice, particularly if they have been recently hospitalized or there have been problems in up-titrating their drug therapy.[23]

The degree to which plasma natriuretic peptides fall during a hospitalization for HF is a good indicator of the subsequent risk of readmission, and might be used to target closer follow-up for some patients when the plasma level fails to fall during admission.[24] Near-patient testing of plasma BNP is advancing rapidly, and it is likely that a home-based test will be available in the near future. Near-patient testing of electrolytes and creatinine is unlikely to become available in the near future.

Monitoring adherence to medication

Monitoring adherence to medication is problematic but it is estimated that between 20% and 50% of patients mismanage their medication.[25,26] Patients with HF are likely to have multiple comorbidities, cognitive decline, social isolation, and depression, all of which adversely affect their ability to adhere to medication regimes.

Patients may choose not to comply with medication from concern about side effects, or they may simply forget; they may be unable to refill the drug prescription, or be unsure how to take the medication or of its value. In some countries, there may be economic constraints. Nonadherence with medication has been implicated in possibly as many as 30% of hospital admissions with HF.[27] Electronic monitoring of medication adherence is possible and may provide insights into particular issues. Some telemonitoring systems also provide reminders to patients regarding their medication.

Nutrition

Weight loss is a poor prognostic factor in HF. There is a variety of contributors to weight loss including inadequate dietary intake, loss of appetite, and malabsorption of nutrients.

The simplest method of monitoring nutritional status is through recording the body weight and the European Society of Cardiology (ESC) guidance states that a decrease of more than 6% of total body weight within 6 months is suggestive of cachexia.[3] Monitoring of appetite and interest in eating can easily become part of regular monitoring and may identify potential malnutrition.

Monitoring for increased anxiety, depression and cognitive dysfunction

As many as 40% of patients with HF may become moderately depressed or anxious.[28,29] Depression is an independent risk factor for mortality,[30] increases symptom reporting,[29] decreases quality of life, and (alongside anxiety) can decrease self-care ability.

Cognitive decline through age, depression, or chronic illness is also a potential influence on patient outcome and is likely to make self-care more difficult. There are scoring tools to quantify decline in cognitive function, but they may have limited value in elderly people or in routine clinical practice.

Physiological monitoring through implanted devices

Some of the newer models of implantable CRT devices include features with the potential to monitor and identify preclinical signs of worsening HF remotely. For example, intrathoracic impedance can be measured between the right ventricular lead and the generator of a pacing device. Accumulating intrathoracic fluid decreases the impedance. Evidence for the value of intrathoracic impedance monitoring in detection of worsening HF is emerging, although it is unlikely to be sensitive enough on its own to aid decision-making.[31–33] False-positive results may trigger an increase in health care utilization.

Other devices include sensors capable of monitoring circulatory pressures (including right ventricular, pulmonary artery and left atrial pressures), heart rate variability,[34,35] and mean daily physical activity with movement detectors.[35] The feasibility of using trends in these variables to assist early intervention and prevent overt clinical deterioration has been established, but results of larger studies are awaited to determine their exact role.[36] Currently the strongest evidence exists for monitoring pulmonary artery pressure, which is discussed further below.

In the future, it is likely that data from devices will be combined with traditional indicators such as vital signs, weight change, and symptoms to indicate clinical status and detect worsening HF more reliably. Patients with advanced HF are most likely to benefit.

The evidence for benefit of remote monitoring

Telephone monitoring

The DIAL trial[37] enrolled 1518 stable outpatients in Argentina, and used a centralized call centre together with protocol-driven phone calls focusing on symptom monitoring, adjustment of medication, and patient education. All phone calls were nurse-initiated: initially at 2-weekly intervals, after which the frequency was based on the clinical condition. The study population was relatively young with a mean age of 65 years and 80% had LVSD. There was a statistically significant 20% reduction in the number of patients who died or were admitted to hospital with HF, largely attributable to the reduction in the number of patients admitted with worsening HF. Mortality was unaffected. Importantly, patients were generally on evidence-based medication at randomization but more patients in the control arm stopped taking their medication or reported non-adherence with other lifestyle advice, demonstrating the benefit of regular monitoring on adherence with treatment of proven benefit.

Other studies of telephone monitoring in different health care settings provide further evidence of benefit and when combined in a meta-analysis indicate a significant reduction in HF-related hospital admission, a trend towards a reduction in mortality, but no effect on all-cause admission.[38] The limitations of such models are that the phone calls are primarily initiated by the professional at preset times (usually protocol-driven) and they are thus unable to detect more rapid changes in the condition.

Telemonitoring

Telemonitoring uses patient-initiated remote electronic monitoring and involves the transmission of information from the patient (usually in their home) to the health professional (Fig. 56.2). In most cases, data are transmitted using a domestic telephone line; manufacturers are developing equipment with wireless transmission. Telemonitoring enables frequent (usually daily) assessment of clinical variables by a health professional, early identification of clinical deterioration, and early patient management (either remotely or through early recall to clinic for review). There is no consensus as to which variables provide the most useful data. There is a balance between accurate patient assessment and overburdening the patient.

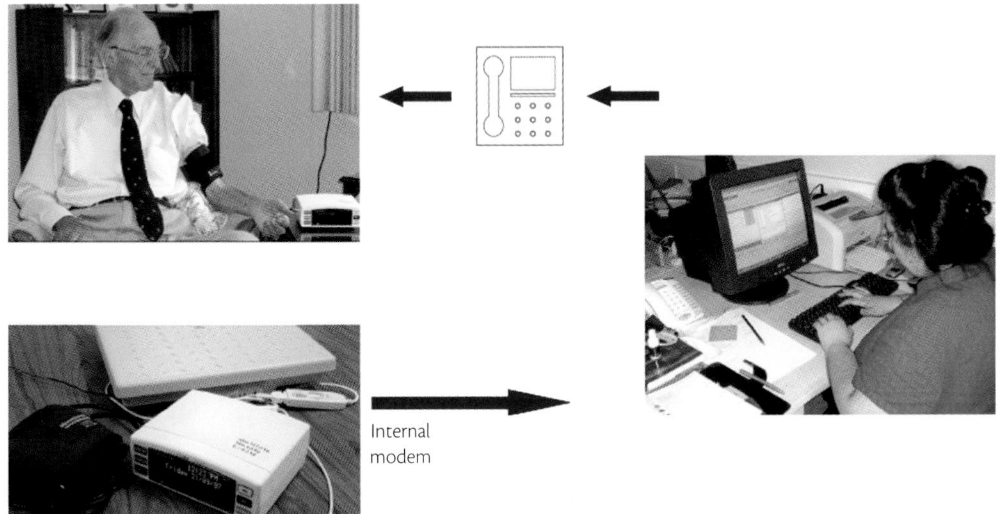

Fig. 56.2 The telemonitoring cycle: data collected from the patient is transmitted to the health care professional, who views the data and its trends, and may telephone the patient to make a fuller assessment of his/her condition before giving advice or arranging clinical review.
From Riley J, Cowie MR. Telemonitoring in heart failure. *Heart* 2009;**95**:1964–8, with permission from BMJ Publishing Group Ltd.

The Trans-European Network-Home-Care Management System (TEN-HMS) study randomized 426 patients (mean age 67 years) with LVSD (LVEF <40%) in NYHA class II–IV to home telemonitoring, nurse telephone support, or usual care. This multicentre study recruited patients from 16 centres and 3 European countries. There was no statistically significant effect on HF-related hospitalization or average length of stay for such admissions. Although it was not a primary outcome, there was a statistically significant reduction in mortality in the telemonitoring group compared to usual care. A greater number of patients in the telemonitored group was ultimately on optimal drug therapy than in the usual care group.[21]

We have reported the results of a randomized trial of home telemonitoring (Home-HF)in a typical elderly HF population (mean age 71, 45% >75 years), which included those with either preserved or impaired left ventricular systolic function. We compared 6 months of daily telemonitoring with specialist HF care in 182 patients discharged from three district hospitals in west London, United Kingdom. We found no difference in the primary outcome of all-cause hospitalization, but did find a significant decrease in the proportion of hospitalizations for HF that were as an emergency (usual care 81% vs telemonitoring 36%, p = 0.01). We also found a reduction in the number of emergency department attendances and secondary care clinic visits with telemonitoring.[12]

A recent meta-analysis including around 800 patients suggested that telemonitoring was associated with a 38% reduction in risk of all-cause mortality with no effect on all-cause hospitalization.[39] The reduction in mortality may not be seen in a more elderly population, but the technology can enable specialist services to care for more patients, with an improvement in patient experience. Home-based technology is generally easy to use, and studies consistently report very high levels of usage (>80%). Systems are likely to be adopted widely in European health care practice, and will lead to a major change in the way HF clinicians interact with patients.[40]

Remote monitoring of implantable devices

Rapid advances in health care technology have led to the possibility of remotely monitoring a large number of physiological variables using implanted therapeutic devices, such as CRT or ICD. Using either a bedside monitoring device or a portable 'interrogator' placed over the device, the patient can be remotely monitored, with the data being transferred to a central station. If patients feel unwell or have concerns about their heart or device function, they can trigger a download from the device to the health professional. Using a web-based system, the professional can monitor device performance and a number of physiological variables.

Such remote monitoring reduces rather than eliminates all face-to-face contact, and an annual face-to-face clinic visit is recommended for clinical examination.[41] A recent audit of 97 patients at our centre demonstrated a 70% reduction in face-to-face pacing clinic visits with the introduction of remote monitoring. In 84% of the remote scheduled pacing checks, no further action was required.[42] There are early indicators that remote monitoring of implantable devices considerably increases the number of patients who can be safely cared for by one practitioner and extends the reach of effective monitoring programmes. Good communication between the electrophysiology department, pacing technologist, and HF team is essential.

How often data should be examined is unclear, as is the value of individual physiological variables monitored (discussed earlier in chapter). Large clinical trials are under way to test the clinical value of such monitoring in terms of patient outcome and health care expenditure.[36]

Currently, the strongest evidence exists for monitoring pulmonary artery pressure. A randomized controlled study of the addition of data from an implanted haemodynamic monitor to usual clinical review reported a statistically nonsignificant 21% reduction in HF hospitalizations or urgent care visits requiring intravenous therapy in the 134 patients with advanced HF in the active arm, compared with 140 randomized to the control arm.[43] An algorithm indirectly estimated pulmonary artery pressure from measured right ventricular pressure in this device. Directly measured pulmonary artery pressure appears to be more useful, with recent data (as yet unpublished) from the CHAMPION study reporting a 30% reduction in HF hospitalization over 6 months in patients with an implantable pulmonary artery pressure monitoring device in NYHA class III.

Frequency of monitoring

It is often not possible, or indeed necessary, to follow all patients with the same level of intensity. The period of greatest vulnerability remains the period immediately following hospital discharge. Only a minority of patients are readmitted, but it is best to schedule a review soon after hospital discharge and preferably within 10 days. A major difficulty in establishing the frequency of subsequent follow-up is the substantial difference in the intensity of interventions in the studies demonstrating benefit from management programmes, with follow-up varying from a single home visit[44] to weekly home visits for older or unstable patients.[45] The positive outcomes of the early studies were largely derived from trials in patients with LVSD where 'usual' care was very poor. The generalizability to current patients, particularly where 'usual' care has improved, is unclear.

The COACH study (Coordinating study evaluating Outcome of Advising and Counselling), a multicentre study of over 1000 patients in the Netherlands, was designed to establish the optimal frequency of professional monitoring in a more general HF population.[7] Patients were randomized to one of three groups: (1) outpatient cardiologist clinic visit within 2 months of discharge and 6-monthly thereafter; (2) the addition of nine outpatient nurse visits; or (3) a total of four visits to the cardiologist, and twenty contacts with the nurse (with the greatest intensity within the first month of hospital discharge), and multidisciplinary team contact for lifestyle advice. Patients were followed up for a period of 18 months. The study reported no difference in the risk of death or HF-related hospital admission between the groups. There was also no difference in the total number of days lost to death or all-cause hospitalization. Importantly, there was a substantial increase in contact with the secondary care HF team in all groups and this was frequently triggered by an increase in symptoms. The study has been interpreted as providing evidence that HF programmes need to be adaptive to patient need, pointing to the need for an open access follow-up service, with varying levels of support.

Who should be monitored more frequently?

A 6-monthly clinical review, including a check of symptom control, cardiac rhythm, medication, and blood chemistry may be sufficient when the patient's condition is stable. An annual review by a cardiologist may also be useful. Patients with advanced HF, those undergoing therapy changes, and those with a history of frequent decompensation will benefit from more frequent monitoring. Patients who have multiple comorbidities or renal failure, are elderly, or are on multiple medications may also benefit from more frequent monitoring, but this must be done carefully to prevent confusion from too many visits and too many changes to medication.

Patients with implanted devices such as CRT, ICD, or combined CRT-D will require technical checks on the devices.[41] Patients with long-term ventricular assist devices will have follow-up organized by the implanting centre, as will patients after heart transplantation.

Where should monitoring take place?

Current UK government policy promotes health care that is easily accessible and adaptive to patient need, with a focus on the delivery of care in the community.[6] A secondary care specialist is usually involved with the initial introduction of medication, but optimization can be safely carried out in primary care. This process is best guided by a management plan, shared between primary and secondary care. Once the patient is on optimized medication, the GP and community HF nurse can continue to monitor the majority of patients with only an annual review by a consultant cardiologist (either in secondary care or a satellite community clinic). Patients with more complex needs, such as elderly people or those with comorbidities, may benefit from care delivery by a case manager or care coordinator (often a community matron). Based in primary care, the care coordinator is well placed to liaise regularly with the multidisciplinary community health care team and social care services to ensure the right services are offered at the right time.

Who should be involved in monitoring?

Cardiologists and specialist nurses have played a central role in HF management in most studies and are key members of the HF team in clinical practice. Not all patients need to be seen at all time points by a secondary care specialist. Where primary care services are well-developed, the GP and community nurse should be involved in the routine monitoring of the stable patient. Monitoring must be incorporated into the activities of the multidisciplinary team,[46] with timely (and accurate) communication between primary, secondary, and tertiary care being vital. Where monitoring also involves technical checks on implanted devices, communication must also be good between those responsible for the technology and the HF multidisciplinary team.

Health care professional education

Education and training underpin effective monitoring. Subspecialist HF training is now recognized in the United Kingdom but there are differences in medical specialist training across Europe: HF is not recognized as a subspecialty in all countries. The European Heart Failure Curriculum for Nurses has attempted to provide some standardization, but HF education is usually local and country specific. In the United Kingdom, nurses and some allied professionals (such as pharmacists) obtain further qualifications to expand their role to include the prescription of medications and so manage their own patient caseload.[47] Training in remote monitoring is essential, as it requires decision-making in response to different cues than is usual in traditional face-to-face clinical contacts. There is the risk that more data leads to more frequent, but not necessarily effective, changes in the management plan and increased health care utilization. Remote monitoring cannot replace more traditional care, but should be integrated into a multiprofessional disease management programme, enabling more patients to access high-quality care.

Conclusions

Monitoring of patients with HF happens in a variety of settings: primary, secondary, and tertiary care. The level of complexity varies from patient to patient, and varies during the course of an individual's illness. Final decisions will be needed on when to stop monitoring for the active control of HF and move towards monitoring for symptom relief and end-of-life care (see Chapter 55). Organizations need to develop systems that are adaptive and individualized; both adding and removing components as needs change.

The management of HF is complex and patient expectations for care are increasing. A variety of new monitoring systems is becoming available. Many enable remote monitoring, which increases patient convenience and improves the experience of care. The systems also increase the amount of data that can be monitored and may complicate decision-making. The evidence base for telemonitoring is increasing, but better guidance is needed to help identify patients most likely to benefit from intensive monitoring and to manage the increased data effectively. Although the health care professional is important, the patient and their family are central to the success of monitoring.

References

1. Jhund P, MacIntyre K, Simpson CR, *et al.* Long-term trends in first hospitalisation for heart failure and subsequent survival between 1986 and 2003. A population study of 5.1 million people. *Circulation* 2009;**119**:515–23.
2. National Institute of Clinical Excellence. *National clinical guideline for management of chronic heart failure in primary and secondary care*, 2003. Available at: http://www.nice.org.uk/nicemedia/pdf/Full_HF_Guideline.pdf (accessed 12 June 2010).
3. Dickstein K, Cohen-Solal A, Filippatos G, *et al.* European Society of Cardiology Guidelines for the diagnosis and treatment of chronic heart failure. *Eur Heart J* 2008;**29**:2388–442.
4. Nicol ED, Fittall B, Roughton M, Cleland JGF, Dargie H, Cowie MR. NHS heart failure survey: a survey of acute heart failure admissions in England:Wales and Northern Ireland. *Heart* 2008;**94**:172–7.
5. Roccaforte R, Demers C, Baldassarre F, *et al.* Effectiveness of comprehensive disease management programmes in improving clinical outcomes in heart failure patients. A meta-analysis. *Eur J Heart Fail* 2005;**7**:1133–44.
6. Department of Health. *Supporting people with long term conditions: An NHS and Social Care model to support local innovation and integration*, 2005. Available at: http://www.dh.gov.uk/en/Publicationsandstatistics/Publications/PublicationsPolicyAndGuidance/DH_4100252 (accessed 22 January 2010).
7. Jaarsma T: van der Wal M, Lesman-Leegte I *et al.* Effect of moderate or intensive disease management program on outcome in patients with heart failure. *Arch Intern Med* 2008;**168**(3):316–24.
8. Rogers A, Addington-Hall J, Abery A, *et al.* Knowledge and communication difficulties for patients with chronic heart failure. *BMJ* 2000;**321**:605–7.
9. Horowtiz CR, Rein SB, Leventhal H. A story of maladies, misconceptions and mishaps: Effective management of heart failure. *Soc Sci Med* 2004;**58**:631–43.
10. Clark AM, Freydberg CN, McAlister FA, Tsuyuki RT, Armstrong PW, Strain LA. Patient and informal caregivers' knowledge of heart failure: necessary but insufficient for effective self-care. *Eur J Heart Fail* 2009;**11**:617–21.
11. Schiff GD, Fung S, Speroff T, McNutt RA. Decompensated heart failure: symptoms, patterns of onset and contributing factors. *Am J Med* 2003;**114**:625–30.
12. Dar O, Riley J, Chapman C, *et al.* A randomized trial of home telemonitoring in a typical elderly heart failure population in North West London: results of the Home-HF study. *Eur J Heart Fail* 2009;**11**:319–25.
13. The Criteria Committee of the New York Heart Association. *Nomenclature and criteria for diagnosis of diseases of the heart and great vessels*, 9th edition. Little, Brown, Boston, 1994.
14. Raphael C, Briscoe C, Davies J *et al.* Limitations of the New York Heart Association functional classification system and self-reported walking distances in chronic heart failure. *Heart* 2007;**93**:476–82.
15. Goode KM, Nabb S, Cleland JGF, Clark AL. A comparison of patient and physician-rated New York Heart Association Class in a community-based heart failure clinic. *Journal of Cardiac Failure* 2008;**14**:379–87.
16. Rostagno C, Olivo G, Comeglio M, *et al.* Prognostic values of 6-minute walk corridor test in patients with mild to moderate heart failure: comparison with other methods of functional evaluation. *Eur J Heart Fail* 2003;**5**:247–52.
17. American Heart Association. ACC/AHA 2005 Guideline Update for the Diagnosis and Management of Chronic Heart Failure in the Adult. *Circulation* 2005;**112**:154–235.
18. Lewin J, Ledwidge M, O'Loughlin C, McNally C, McDonald K. Clinical deterioration in established heart failure: What is the value of BNP and weight gain in aiding diagnosis. *Eur J Heart Fail* 2005;**7**:953–7.
19. Zhang J, Goode KM, Cuddihy PE, Cleland JFG. Predicting hospitalisation due to worsening heart failure using daily weight measurement: analysis of the Trans-European Network-Home-Care Management System (TEN-HMS) study. *Eur J Heart Fail* 2009;**11**:420–7.
20. Capomolla S, Pinna G, La Rovere M, *et al.* Heart failure case disease management program: a pilot study of home telemonitoring versus usual care. *Eur Heart J* 2004;**6**(F1):F91–8.
21. Cleland JGF, Louis AA, Rigby AS, Janssens U, Balk AHMM. Noninvasive home telemonitoring for patients with heart failure at high risk of recurrent admission and death. *J Am Coll Cardiol* 2005;**45**(10):1654–64.
22. Pfisterer M, Buser P, Rickli H, *et al.* BNP-guided vs symptom-guided heart failure therapy. The trial of intensified vs standard medical therapy in elderly patients with congestive heart failure (TIME-CHF) randomized trial. *JAMA* 2009;**301**:383–92.
23. National Institute for Clinical Excellence. *Guidance on the management of chronic heart failure in the adult in primary or secondary care—partial update.* NICE, 2010.
24. Bettencourt P, Azevedo A, Pimenta J, *et al.* N-terminal-pro-brain natriuretic peptide predicts outcome after hospital discharge in heart failure patients. *Circulation* 2004;**110**:2168–74.
25. Haynes RB, McDonald HP, Garg AX, Monatgue P. Interventions for helping patients to follow prescriptions for medications. *Cochrane Database of Systematic Reviews,* 2002. Available at: http://www.thecochranelibrary.com (accessed 12 June 2010).
26. Kripalani S, Yao X, Haynes B. Interventions to enhance medication adherence in chronic medical conditions: a systematic review. *Arch Intern Med* 2007;**167**:540–9.
27. Nieminen MS, Brutsaert D, Dickstein K, *et al.* EuroHeart failure survey II (EHFS I): a survey on hospitalised acute heart failure patients; description of population. *Eur Heart J* 2006;**27**:2725–36.
28. Guck TP, Elsasser GN, Kavan MG, *et al.* Depression and congestive heart failure. *Congestive Heart Failure* 2003;**9**:163–9.
29. Ramasamy R, Hildebrandt T, O'Hea E, *et al.* Psychological and social factors that correlate with dyspnea in heart failure. *Psychosomatics* 2006;**47**:430–4.
30. Jiang W, Hasselblad V, Krishnan RR, *et al.* Patients with CHF and depression have greater risk of mortality and morbidity than patients without depression. *J Am Coll Cardiol* 2002;**39**:919–21.
31. Yu CM, Wang L, Chau E, *et al.* Intrathoracic impedance monitoring in patients with heart failure: correlation with fluid status and feasibility of early warning preceding hospitalization. *Circulation* 2005;**112**:841–8.
32. Vollman D, Nagele H, Schauerte P, *et al.* Clinical utility of intrathoracic impedance monitoring to alert patients with an implanted device of deteriorating chronic heart failure. *Eur Heart J* 2007;**28**:1835–40.
33. Cowie MR, Conraads V, Tavazzi L, Yu CM, on behalf of the SENSE-HF Investigators. Rationale and design of a prospective trial to assess the sensitivity and positive predictive value of implantable intrathoracic impedance monitoring in the prediction of heart failure hospitalizations: the SENSE-HF Study. *J Card Fail* 2009;**15**:394–400.

34. Adamson PB, Smith AL, Abraham WT, *et al.* Continuous autonomic assessment in patients with symptomatic heart failure. *Circulation* 2004;**110**:2389–94.
35. Braunschweig F, Mortensen PT, Gras D, *et al.* Monitoring of physical activity and heart rate variability in patients with chronic heart failure using cardiac resynchronisation devices. *Am J Cardiol* 2005;**95**:1104–7.
36. Braunschweig F, Ford I, Conraads V, *et al.* Can monitoring of intrathoracic impedance reduce morbidity and mortality in patients with chronic heart failure? Rationale and design of the Diagnostic Outcome Trial in Heart Failure (DOT-HF). *Eur J Heart Fail* 2008;**10**:907–16.
37. GESICA investigators. Randomised trial of telephone intervention in chronic heart failure: DIAL trial. *BMJ* 2005;**331**:425–427.
38. McAlister FA, Stewart S, Ferrua S, McMurray J. Multidisciplinary strategies for the management of heart failure patients at high risk for admission. A systematic review of randomized trials. *J Am Coll Cardiol* 2004;**44**(4):810–19.
39. Clark R, Inglis S, McAlister F. Telemonitoring or structured telephone support programmes for patients with chronic heart failure: systematic review and meta-analysis. *BMJ* 2007;**334**:942–51.
40. Riley J, Cowie MR. Telemonitoring in heart failure. *Heart* 2009;**95**:1964–8.
41. Wilkoff BL, Auricchio A, Brigada J, *et al.* HRS/EHRA Expert consensus on the monitoring of cardiovascular implantable devices (CIEDI): description of techniques, indications, personnel, frequency and ethical considerations. *Europace* 2008;**10**:707–25.
42. Trembath L, Azucena C, Stain N, Cowie MR. Remote monitoring for CRT-D leads to substantial reduction in the need for 'routine' visits to a pacing clinic. *Eur J Heart Fail Suppl* 2009;**8**(2):112.
43. Bourge RC, Abraham WT, Adamson PB, *et al.* On behalf of the COMPASS-HF Study Group. Randomized controlled trial of an implantable continuous hemodynamic monitor in patients with advanced heart failure. *J Am Coll Cardiol* 2008;**51**:1073–9.
44. Stewart S, Pearson S, Horowitz JD. Effects of a home-based intervention among patients with congestive heart failure discharged from acute hospital care. *Arch Intern Med* 1998;**158**:1067–72.
45. Blue L, Lang E, McMurray J, *et al.* Randomised controlled trial of specialist nurse intervention in heart failure. *BMJ* 2001;**323**:715–18.
46. Swedberg K, Cleland J, Cowie MR, *et al.* Successful treatment of heart failure with devices requires collaboration. *Eur J Heart Fail* 2008;**10**:1229–35.
47. Department of Health. *The non-medical prescribing programme*, 2009. Available at: http://www.dh.gov.uk/en/Healthcare/Medicinespharmacyandindustry/Prescriptions/TheNon-MedicalPrescribingProgramme/index.htm (accessed 22 January 2010).

PART XVIII

Future therapies

57

The future

Andrew L. Clark, Henry J. Dargie, Roy S. Gardner, and Theresa A. McDonagh

Heart failure (HF) continues to challenge professionals in all areas of health care, yet remains one of the most rewarding medical conditions to treat. Enormous advances in pharmacological care have led to a doubling in life expectancy for patients with chronic HF; a renewed emphasis on the central haemodynamic abnormalities of HF has led to the widespread uptake of cardiac resynchronization therapy (CRT); and changes in the delivery of health care together with improved monitoring of patients have greatly increased the likelihood of patients receiving the care they need.

No textbook of cardiology is complete without a *tour d'horizon* considering possible new developments over the next 5–10 years: HF therapy has progressed dramatically in the last 30 years, and will continue to do so over the next 30.

Acute heart failure

The bulk of the research to date in HF has been on chronic HF, and only recently has there been a new emphasis on acute HF. The interest is driven in large part by pharmaceutical developments—new drugs need to find their niche. One difficulty with dealing with acute HF and acute HF trials has been the classification and definition of acute HF syndromes: it is important that the defining process is tightened up.

Novel vasodilator drugs being studied in acute HF include cinaciguat and relaxin.[1,2] Some new drugs share more than one mode of action: chimeric natriuretic peptides such as CD-NP have both venodilatory and natriuretic effects.[3,4] Similarly, some novel positive inotropic agents being tested in clinical trials have other properties. Isataroxime is a Na^+,K^+-ATPase inhibitor which increases SERCA2a activity and is both inotropic and lusitropic.[5] Urocortins also exhibit powerful inotropic and lusitropic effects.[6] There are novel myocardial protection agents in development. Adenosine regulators such as acadesine have anti-ischaemic effects and ameleriorate glucose uptake and free fatty acid oxidation, thereby increasing ATP synthesis.[7] We will see many clinical trials of these novel agents reporting in the next few years.

Therapy for acute HF will become much more evidence-based: the traditional treatments will be subjected to clinical trials, and newer agents being developed and reaching market will have their roles defined. Making sure the right drugs are tested in appropriate populations may be a challenge. For example, the vaptans need to be tested in HF patients with hyponatraemia, endothelin antagonists in HF patients with pulmonary hypertension, and tumour necrosis factor (TNF) antagonists in HF patients with a raised TNF.

Pharmacological developments

The neurohormonal explanation for the pathophysiology of chronic HF and its progression led to the modern treatment regime of angiotensin converting enzyme (ACE) inhibition, β-blockade, and aldosterone antagonism. However, a limit does seem to have been reached: essentially neutral results of trials testing the addition of further neurohormonal antagonists, such as endothelin antagonists (bosentan) and combined ACE/neutral endopeptidase inhibitors (omapatrilat), suggest that any further interference with neurohormones may cause trouble.

Controversies still remain as to which is the better 'triple therapy': should patients on ACE inhibitor plus β-blocker be offered either an angiotensin receptor antagonist or an aldosterone antagonist? The question is unlikely to be answered directly, but there will be new data on aldosterone antagonists, particularly eplerenone, in the next few years.

Other developments in the neurohormonal field include the combination of the angiotensin receptor blocker (ARB) valsartan and a neutral endopeptidase (NEP) inhibitor in a single molecule. The NEP inhibitor increases the concentrations of natriuretic peptides in the circulation by preventing their breakdown. Clinical trials are under way.

Moving away from the neurohormonal field, other agents attracting interest include myosin ATPase activators. These drugs potentially improve myocardial contractility by accelerating the productive phosphate-release step of the crossbridge cycle.[8] They prolong stroke volume, improving the energy efficiency of the contractile apparatus rather than by increasing dP/dt (and hence increasing myocardial oxygen demand) as conventional inotropes do. Clinical studies are at an early stage.

Metabolic therapy

Some lines of evidence suggest that the failing heart is starved of energy.[9,10] For example, a major change in advancing HF is depletion of phosphocreatine.[11] Such changes lead to the suggestion that therapy directed at cardiac metabolism may have a role. One possible target is to modulate the substrates used for energy production. Fatty acids are the dominant fuel for myocytes (at least in some circumstances) and whereas, weight for weight, oxidation of fatty acids produces more ATP than oxidation of glucose, it takes more oxygen per mole of ATP produced to oxidize lipid.

Perhexiline and etomoxir both inhibit carnitine palmitoyltransferases (CPT) 1, the enzyme responsible for transporting fatty acids into mitochondria. Trimetazidine inhibits fatty acid oxidation. The use of such agents results in a shift towards predominant glucose metabolism, and small-scale clinical studies have suggested that they may have a role in HF therapy.[12–14] Other metabolic approaches include modifying insulin and glucose metabolism with metformin.

Metabolic manipulation is at an early stage of development and larger-scale clinical trials with hard endpoints are now needed.

Individualizing treatment

An important part of HF management will be the individualizing of treatment. The present practice of trying to give all treatments to all patients may not last. Clear examples of the trend include treating only those with iron deficiency with intravenous iron, and only those with left bundle branch block with a CRT device.

If knowledge of the human genome is to make an impact in 'ordinary' medicine, then it will be in trying to select the appropriate therapies for the right patients. Genome-wide association studies of, for example, genetic loci associated with hypertension,[15] hold the promise that individually targeted medication regimes will eventually be possible. However, the most promising single genetic polymorphism area widely researched so far has perhaps been the insertion/deletion polymorphism in the gene coding for angiotensin converting enzyme and its relation to the risk of ischaemic heart disease: conflicting results have not led to any advance in therapy.[16]

It is unlikely that the answer will be so simple as to depend on a single polymorphism in a single gene: individual enzymes and gene products function only in relation to other enzymes and gene products. A particular polymorphism might have different effects in different environments. Chains of potentially polymorphic enzymes lead to the production of the different active neurohormones, as well as to potentially polymorphic receptors and then polymorphisms in downstream signalling pathway enzymes; in addition, there are polymorphisms in the enzymes responsible for breaking down the neurohormones.[17]

Nevertheless, despite these complications, it is possible that an individual patient presenting with HF in the future might be genotyped rapidly, and specific therapy targeted to that person's individual genetic make-up will be used.[18] Perhaps the first area where an individualized approach might be practicable is in those cases of familial cardiomyopathy with a single-gene defect underlying HF.

Implantable devices

The biggest changes with implantable devices will be in patient selection. As with pharmacological therapy, the selection of patients for device therapy is very broad brush at present; for patients receiving a CRT device, only about two-thirds experience a sustained symptomatic benefit, and for patients with an implantable cardioverter-defibrillator (ICD), only a small proportion ever receives an appropriate shock.

Studies already under way will expand and refine the selection criteria for CRT, and address whether (and which) patients in atrial fibrillation or with narrow QRS complexes might benefit. There will be important refinements in technique, allowing careful selection of which potential lead position creates the greatest benefit, and allowing easier positioning of the left ventricular lead in that position.

For ICDs, the indications are likely to narrow markedly as new methods will make the assessment of which patients are at greatest risk of ventricular tachyarrhythmia more precise. The technology will continue to improve: new pacemakers are being developed with a total volume of only 1 cm^3, and miniaturization of defibrillators will follow. The burden of an ICD for the patients will thereby decrease, and perhaps incidentally save money for pressed health care systems.

Other developments include the possibility of using devices as neural stimulators: for example, a stimulator positioned in the neck can be used to produce vagal simulation to the heart, thereby redressing the sympathovagal imbalance of chronic HF (see Fig. 57.1).[19,20]

Monitoring

Ever more sophisticated monitoring of patients is becoming possible (see Chapter 56). As more and more patients have devices implanted, the remote and, importantly, automatic, monitoring of patients will become widespread. On-board 'add-ons' already in

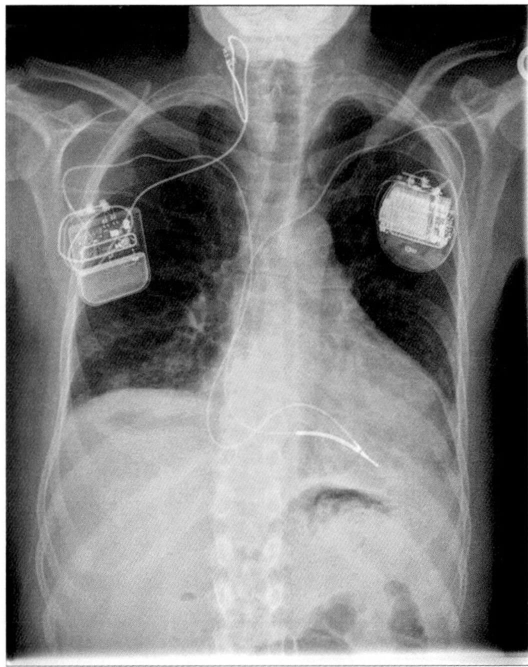

Fig. 57.1 Chest radiograph of patient with a defibrillator implanted on the left and a vagal stimulator on the right. The device on the right-hand side of the patient uses an intracardiac lead for detection and a cuff wrapped around the vagus nerve in the neck to deliver appropriately timed vagal stimulation.

use can now measure variables such as activity level and intrathoracic impedance, and newer devices capable of monitoring mixed venous oxygen saturation and even left atrial pressure are being developed. Remote programming of the devices is also possible.

Simplification of telemonitoring equipment is also moving apace. Home telemonitoring can be burdensome, and newer devices simply attached to the skin as patches can detect changes in cutaneous impedance, heart rate, and rhythm and transmit information to the centre using wireless technology via a mobile phone.

Mechanical help

CRT improves the mechanical function of the heart without the cost of positive inotropic drug therapy (see Chapter 48). Its success has refocused attention on the underlying mechanics of HF, rather than the secondary effects of neurohormonal activation. Advances in left ventricular assist device (LVAD) therapy make long-term survival with a device implanted as 'destination therapy' a present reality,[21] and the technology will continue to advance. Currently, the source of greatest morbidity with LVADs is drive-line infection, and efforts are being made to have fully implantable systems with internal batteries (see Chapter 51).

Inevitably, devices that can be implanted percutaneously are already being assessed,[22] and will become more reliable, and easier to insert. Their widespread use might not only tide patients over an initial episode of cardiogenic shock, but become in turn destination therapy for some patients.

If such devices actually become sufficiently reliable and cheap, it holds out the possibility that the HF syndrome might even become a thing of the past.

Stem cell therapy

The possibility of using pluripotent stem cells to replace damaged organs is very appealing, and has been suggested for a range of conditions including chronic HF. Initial reports were extremely enthusiastic: small, noncontrolled, nonrandomized studies from enthusiasts were reported as showing improvements in many clinical variables. Some patients have heard enough to come to clinic and demand stem cell therapy, convinced that some dramatic intervention may be possible.

There are many potential hurdles to an effective stem cell therapy: which stem cells to use, how to deliver them, and the timing of delivery (Box 57.1). Other remaining problems include that of persuading implanted cardiomyocytes to remain in the heart, and persuading those that do remain to continue to function. In some situations, fewer than 1% of transplanted cells survive.[26]

Clinical trial results have not provided compelling evidence for the use of stem cells as yet. The most promising overall concept appears to be the use of intracoronary injections of mesenchymal stem cells in patients with HF due to coronary artery disease. A meta-analysis of 18 randomized and nonrandomized trials including 999 patients found that stem cell treatment improved left ventricular ejection fraction by 3.7%, with small decreases in scar size and left ventricular volume. Whether such a small benefit translates into a clinical benefit is not at all clear.

A final possibility for cell therapy is the possibility of persuading surviving differentiated cardiac myocytes to divide and replace damaged cells. There is some evidence that cardiac cells can divide,[27] and recruiting the patient's native cells is obviously attractive. One possible source of appropriate cells is cardiac progenitor cells isolated from endomyocardial biopsies. A trial, CADUCEUS,[28] is under way to assess whether the cells help in clinical practice.

For the moment, despite much promise, stem cell therapy for chronic HF is a rather distant dream. Testing of new strategies should surely only take place with in the context of carefully controlled clinical trials to avoid the overdramatizing of results that subsequently prove illusory.

Box 57.1 Important considerations in stem cell therapy

Source of stem cells

- Embryonic stem cells are perhaps the purest form of stem cell, and will form lineages leading to cardiovascular cells.[23] Difficulties with their use include lack of availability, the possibility of teratoma formation and immunological tolerance, including graft versus host disease.
- Mesenchymal stem cells can be derived from many tissues, including bone marrow. They can be induced to differentiate into cardiac myocytes, but more easily mature into osteoblasts and chondrocytes. A major problem with their use has been their tendency to heterotopic calcification.[24]
- Myoblasts derived from skeletal muscle have been tried clinically: however, they differentiate into mature skeletal muscle cells and fail to couple with adjoining cardiac myocytes. Their use has been associated with an increased risk of arrhythmia.[25]
- Bone marrow-derived stem cells can be transformed into cardiac myocytes. Their use clinically has been associated with a very small increase in left ventricular ejection fraction.
- Stem cells induced from a patient's somatic cells can be induced to form myocyte lineages, but fears about teratoma or neoplasm development persist, as for embryonic stem cells.

Route of stem cell delivery

- Delivery directly into damaged myocardium by injection, perhaps at the time of coronary artery surgery, has been tried.
- Intracoronary delivery is the other major technique tried so far.

Timing of stem cell delivery

- Should the stem cells be transplanted immediately peri-infarct, or at a time when healing (and potentially scar formation) has taken place? The best option is not yet clear.

Prevention

Writing from the perspective of physicians in the developed world, it is all too easy to think of chronic HF as a problem controllable with medication, and the major challenge being delivery of care. For much of the world's population, access to health care is a major challenge, and the high-technology world of Westernized medicine is not practical. However, it is in the developing nations that HF is increasing in incidence and prevalence. The greatest intervention that can be made to help potential patients with HF is to prevent their getting HF in the first place.

As with other great health care advances in the past (such as the control of infectious disease with improvements in sanitation and the development of vaccination), the greatest impact is in the arena of public health. As ischaemic heart disease will continue to be the commonest cause of HF, tobacco control is perhaps the single most important measure to prevent HF.[29] Other measures, such as the widespread availability of a 'polypill' treating other risk factors for heart disease (antihypertensives, a statin, aspirin)[30] may have something to offer, but the long struggle to be free of tobacco remains perhaps the biggest single challenge for HF.[31,32]

References

1. Lapp H, Mitrovic V, Franz N, *et al.* Cinaciguat (BAY 58–2667) improves cardiopulmonary hemodynamics in patients with acute decompensated heart failure. *Circulation* 2009;**119**:2781–8.
2. Teerlink JR, Metra M, Felker GM, *et al.* Relaxin for the treatment of patients with acute heart failure (Pre-RELAX-AHF): a multicentre, randomised, placebo-controlled, parallel-group, dose-finding phase IIb study. *Lancet* 2009;**373**:1429–39.
3. Lisy O, Huntley BK, McCormick DJ, Kurlansky PA, Burnett JC Jr. Design, synthesis, and actions of a novel chimeric natriuretic peptide: CD-NP. *J Am Coll Cardiol* 2008;**52**:60–8.
4. Lee CY, Chen HH, Lisy O, *et al.* Pharmacodynamics of a novel designer natriuretic peptide, CD-NP, in a first-in-human clinical trial in healthy subjects. *J Clin Pharmacol* 2009;**49**:668–73.
5. Gheorghiade M, Blair JE, Filippatos GS, *et al.* Hemodynamic, echocardiographic, and neurohormonal effects of istaroxime, a novel intravenous inotropic and lusitropic agent: a randomized controlled trial in patients hospitalized with heart failure. *J Am Coll Cardiol* 2008;**51**:2276–85.
6. Davidson SM, Rybka AE, Townsend PA. The powerful cardioprotective effects of urocortin and the corticotropin releasing hormone (CRH) family. *Biochem Pharmacol* 2009;**77**:141–50.
7. Engler RL. Harnessing nature's own cardiac defense mechanism with acadesine, an adenosine regulating agent: importance of the endothelium. *J Card Surg* 1994;**9**(3 Suppl):482–92.
8. Bragadeesh TK, Mathur G, Clark AL, Cleland JG. Novel cardiac myosin activators for acute heart failure. *Expert Opin Investig Drugs* 2007;**16**:1541–8.
9. Wollenberger A. On the energy-rich phosphate supply of the failing heart. *Am J Physiol* 1947;**150**:733–6.
10. Ingwall JS, Weiss RG. Is the failing heart energy starved? On using chemical energy to support cardiac function. *Circ Res* 2004;**95**:135–45.
11. Ten Hove M, Chan S, Lygate C, *et al.* Mechanisms of creatine depletion in chronically failing rat heart. *J Mol Cell Cardiol* 2005;**38**:309–13.
12. Vitale C, Wajngaten M, Sposato B, Gebara O, Rossini P, Fini M, Volterrani M, Rosano GM. Trimetazidine improves left ventricular function and quality of life in elderly patients with coronary artery disease. *Eur Heart J* 2004;**25**:1814–21.
13. Lee L, Campbell R, Scheuermann-Freestone M, *et al.* Metabolic modulation with perhexiline in chronic heart failure: a randomized, controlled trial of short-term use of a novel treatment. *Circulation* 2005;**112**:3280–8.
14. Schmidt-Schweda S, Holubarsch C. First clinical trial with etomoxir in patients with chronic congestive heart failure. *Clin Sci* 2000;**99**:27–35.
15. Ehret GB. Genome-wide association studies: contribution of genomics to understanding blood pressure and essential hypertension. *Curr Hypertens Rep* 2010;**12**:17–25.
16. Rudnicki M, Mayer G. Significance of genetic polymorphisms of the renin-angiotensin-aldosterone system in cardiovascular and renal disease. *Pharmacogenomics* 2009;**10**:463–76.
17. Ingelman-Sundberg M, Sim SC, Gomez A, Rodriguez-Antona C. Influence of cytochrome P450 polymorphisms on drug therapies: pharmacogenetic, pharmacoepigenetic and clinical aspects. *Pharmacol Ther* 2007;**116**:496–526.
18. de Boer RA, van der Harst P, van Veldhuisen DJ, van den Berg MP. Pharmacogenetics in heart failure: promises and challenges. *Expert Opin Pharmacother* 2009;**10**:1713–25.
19. Schwartz PJ, De Ferrari GM, Sanzo A, *et al.* Long term vagal stimulation in patients with advanced heart failure. First experience in man. *Eur J Heart Fail* 2008;**10**:884–91.
20. De Ferrari GM, Sanzo A, Schwartz PJ. Chronic vagal stimulation in patients with congestive heart failure. *Conf Proc IEEE Eng Med Biol Soc* 2009:2037–9.
21. Richmond C. Obituary. Peter Houghton. *Guardian*, London, 18 December 2007.
22. Cheng JM, den Uil CA, Hoeks SE, *et al.* Percutaneous left ventricular assist devices vs. intra-aortic balloon pump counterpulsation for treatment of cardiogenic shock: a meta-analysis of controlled trials. *Eur Heart J* 2009;**30**:2102–8.
23. Kehat I, Kenyagin-Karsenti D, Snir M, *et al.* Human embryonic stem cells can differentiate into myocytes with structural and functional properties of cardiomyocytes. *J Clin Invest* 2001;**108**:407–14.
24. Yoon YS, Park JS, Tkebuchava T, Luedeman C, Losordo DW. Unexpected severe calcification after transplantation of bone marrow cells in acute myocardial infarction. *Circulation* 2004;**109**:3154–7.
25. Menasche P, Alfieri O, Janssens S, *et al.* The Myoblast Autologous Grafting in Ischemic Cardiomyopathy (MAGIC) trial: first randomized placebo-controlled study of myoblast transplantation. *Circulation* 2008;**117**:1189–2000.
26. Pagani FD, DerSimonian H, Zawadzka A, *et al.* Autologous skeletal myoblasts transplanted into ischemia-damaged myocardium in humans: histological analysis of cell survival and differentiation. *J Am Coll Cardiol* 2003;**41**:879–88.
27. Bergmann O, Bhardwaj RD, Bernard S, *et al.* Evidence for cardiomyocyte renewal in humans. *Science* 2009;**324**:98–102.
28. Marbán E. Cardiosphere-derived autologous stem cells to reverse ventricular dysfunction (CADUCEUS), 2009. ClinicalTrials.gov identifier: NCT00893360.
29. Teo KK, Ounpuu S, Hawken S, *et al.*; INTERHEART Study Investigators. Tobacco use and risk of myocardial infarction in 52 countries in the INTERHEART study: a case-control study. *Lancet* 2006;**368**:647–58.
30. Yusuf S, Pais P, Afzal R, *et al.* Effects of a polypill (Polycap) on risk factors in middle-aged individuals without cardiovascular disease (TIPS): a phase II, double-blind, randomised trial. *Lancet* 2009;**373**:1341–51.
31. Baleta A. Africa's struggle to be smoke free. *Lancet* 2010;**375**:107–8.
32. Cheng MH. WHO's Western Pacific region agrees tobacco-control plan. *Lancet* 2009;**374**:1227–8.

Index

Locators in italics indicate tables; locators in bold indicate figures.